AF829037

Pediatric Musculoskeletal Infections

Mohan V. Belthur • Ashish S. Ranade
Martin J. Herman
James A. Fernandes
Editors

Pediatric Musculoskeletal Infections

Principles & Practice

Springer

Editors
Mohan V. Belthur
Department of Child Health &
Orthopedics, University of Arizona
College of Medicine, Phoenix, AZ, USA

Department of Orthopedics, Phoenix
Children's Hospital, Phoenix, AZ, USA

Martin J. Herman
Drexel University College of Medicine
Philadelphia, PA, USA

Orthopedic Surgery
St. Christopher's Hospital for Children
Philadelphia, PA, USA

Ashish S. Ranade
Blooming Buds Centre for Pediatric
Orthopedics
Deenanath Mangeshkar Hospital
Pune, Maharashtra, India

James A. Fernandes
Orthopedics
Sheffield Children's
NHS Foundation Trust
Sheffield, UK

ISBN 978-3-030-95793-3 ISBN 978-3-030-95794-0 (eBook)
https://doi.org/10.1007/978-3-030-95794-0

© Springer Nature Switzerland AG 2022
This work is subject to copyright. All rights are reserved by the Publisher, whether the whole or part of the material is concerned, specifically the rights of translation, reprinting, reuse of illustrations, recitation, broadcasting, reproduction on microfilms or in any other physical way, and transmission or information storage and retrieval, electronic adaptation, computer software, or by similar or dissimilar methodology now known or hereafter developed.
The use of general descriptive names, registered names, trademarks, service marks, etc. in this publication does not imply, even in the absence of a specific statement, that such names are exempt from the relevant protective laws and regulations and therefore free for general use.
The publisher, the authors and the editors are safe to assume that the advice and information in this book are believed to be true and accurate at the date of publication. Neither the publisher nor the authors or the editors give a warranty, expressed or implied, with respect to the material contained herein or for any errors or omissions that may have been made. The publisher remains neutral with regard to jurisdictional claims in published maps and institutional affiliations.

This Springer imprint is published by the registered company Springer Nature Switzerland AG
The registered company address is: Gewerbestrasse 11, 6330 Cham, Switzerland

This book is dedicated to the resiliency of all children the world over with bone and joint infections and their parents in their journey. We hope that it will help clinicians and health professionals to reduce mortality, morbidity following pediatric musculoskeletal infections and improve the quality of life of children with musculoskeletal infections.

We would also like to dedicate this book to our families for their unwavering support, gift of time, patience, and sacrifice through this journey.

Foreword

I have been involved with teaching, examining, and setting up institutions to manage children's orthopaedics on a global level for more than 30 years. Infection of the musculoskeletal system remains a massive part of this work. A part that we hoped in the optimism of last century would diminish with time, but sadly has not. Indeed, it continues to comprise some 10–20% of cases in children's orthopaedic clinics globally and shows no sign of diminishing, indeed appears to be increasing. In my own experience in sub-Saharan Africa in the late 1990s with the increase in HIV prevalence, the non-HIV bacterial fungal and other musculoskeletal infections increased exponentially.

Children in low-income countries are often malnourished and anaemic; therefore, they are particularly susceptible to infections in all anatomical systems. De novo infective conditions of the musculoskeletal system if diagnosed early, with appropriate culture and sensitivity, can be treated relatively simply with antibiotics. If diagnosed late, then the treatment is more invasive and often needs surgery, firstly to help clear the infection by removing all the destroyed tissue. Then, at a later stage, more complex surgery is required to reconstruct the part, be it the bone or joint in limb or spine that has been destroyed by the infection.

Improvements in antibiotics and delivery of these antibiotics have resulted in the establishment of evidence-based techniques that give good results and can reduce or even abolish the gap between eradication of the infection and reconstruction of the part.

These trends in management demonstrate the importance of the combination of disciplines in diagnosis and treatment in children's musculoskeletal infections. It is crucial that experts in imaging, microbiology, pharmacology, surgery, and rehabilitation combine in an interdisciplinary approach to the problem.

In high-income countries, with good Internet service, it is possible within a few hours for clinicians to find advice on management of their complex infective cases. This book brings all that advice together in one place, with instructive case reports, snippets of wisdom, and practical learning that are not always reproduced in academic papers. In low-income settings, where Internet is limited, this book becomes even more valuable as all the information is there on the treating clinician's desk.

I have reviewed all the sections of this book. The editors have engaged experts from all around the world and bring together a combination of wisdom and experience that is unsurpassed in children's orthopaedic infection. The book can be read as a source of advice for difficult cases as needed or as an instructional manual for trainees and learners at all levels.

The editors and chapter authors are to be congratulated, firstly, for their work for putting together a book that is unsurpassed in its scholarship in this area of children's orthopaedics, and, secondly, because this book will save lives and limbs, and improve outcomes for many children in many countries.

Chris Lavy OBE, MD, MCh, FCS, FRCS
Professor of Orthopedic and Tropical Surgery,
University of Oxford, Oxford, UK
Honorary Professor, London School of Hygiene
and Tropical Medicine, London, UK
Consultant Orthopedic and Spine Surgeon,
Nuffield Department of Orthopedics,
Rheumatology and Musculoskeletal Sciences,
Oxford, UK

Foreword

The renowned editors and international authors have created a masterpiece that provides the reader with a comprehensive and practical guide to better understanding pediatric musculoskeletal infections and related conditions. Musculoskeletal infections (MSKI) in children are a major public health problem that brings many disciplines together – primary care, nursing, medical specialists, surgical specialists, research, public health, and public policy. By creating one comprehensive reference for the variety of conditions related to pediatric MSKI, this book will improve the lives of many children globally. I am most impressed with the quality, diversity, and expertise of the many authors that the editors brought together for this historic first edition. Since musculoskeletal infections are so common in children, this book will be useful to medical students, residents, fellows, and pediatric healthcare professionals.

Before the arrival of antibiotics, mortality from MSKI was estimated to be about 40%. Currently, sepsis-related global case fatality remains at 25% and is disproportionately higher in low- and middle-income countries (LMIC), where critical care is resource dependent and subject to health disparities. As a result, approximately 85% of sepsis cases and related deaths globally occur in LMIC, especially sub-Saharan Africa and South-East Asia. Children under 5 years in particular experience this health disparity, as seen in mortality statistics. Although overall case fatality is improving, survivors of septic shock have significantly less long-term health-related quality of life. There is also a correlation of severity of the infection and poor functional outcome.

Musculoskeletal infections remain a challenge for several reasons: lack of education in the population and healthcare providers, limited access, and associated trauma often confusing the clinical presentation. Globally, acute hematogenous osteomyelitis (AHO) is the most common MSKI in approximately two thirds of patients, with children under 5 years the most susceptible. Dr. Antonio Loro (Chap. 10) put this condition in perspective globally, stating that early osteomyelitis is one of the worst treated diseases in primary care. Chronic osteomyelitis is likewise a major problem in the developing world and is exacerbated by insufficient medical care and poor access to food supply and hygiene, especially in rural areas. It is also one of the most common reasons for surgery for children in LMIC. Besides AHO, tuberculosis is the next most common infection, with 10% affecting the MSK system and one half of these involving the spine. Surgical care has been shown to be cost effective in LMIC, and this book provides the information to safely provide this care.

The book is divided into 5 sections and 39 chapters. The first section on general principles is especially useful. The authors of Chap. 3 describe the musculoskeletal tissue injury that occurs with infections and the complex regulated pathway described as the acute phase response (APR). The purpose of the APR is initially for survival and later for tissue repair. However, the severity of the initial infection and the resulting tissue response also increase the child's risk for adverse outcomes such as ARDS, thrombosis, multiorgan dysfunction, and even death. The authors describe this as a double-edged sword; while a well-coordinated APR is necessary for fighting the infection, an excessive APR leads to adverse outcomes. Markers of the APR response such as CRP, platelet count, and the neutrophil to lymphocyte ratio can be accurate predictors of the severity of the APR and possible adverse outcomes. Chapter 4 on imaging describes MRI as the standard for evaluating MSKI, although a challenge to access in LMIC. MRI and FAST-sequence MRI can effectively differentiate pyomyositis, osteomyelitis, and septic arthritis. Chapter 5 discusses the mimics of infection including chronic non-infectious osteitis (CNO), which was formerly termed chronic recurrent multifocal osteomyelitis (CRMO), Langerhans cell histiocytosis, and more rare conditions such as scurvy. Chapter 6 describes Staphylococcus as the most important organism for MSKI, representing 65% of these culture positive infections in the USA, with 37.4% being MRSA. Staphylococcus aureus is so effective because it hijacks parts of the APR such as coagulation and fibrinolysis, thus evading the host immune response. Because of institutional and geographic variability in these percentages, prediction rules cannot be generalized.

The remainder of the book is thoughtfully divided into sections of acute, chronic, region specific, and uncommon infections. Since the book is multi-authored, each chapter can stand and be read on its own. Many pearls of wisdom are to be found in these pages. Among those I found useful are:

- When disseminated disease is suspected, avoid 'satisfaction of search'. Look beyond the most painful joint.
- Eradication of bone infections may require more than one surgery, particularly in the management of multi-focal disease, or when bone-soft tissue reconstruction is required. Explain this to the parents before the first surgery.
- The severity of the infection determines the severity of sequela
- Infections that are more severe and lead to adverse outcomes typically involve infection of multiple tissues or systemic infections involving multiple body parts.
- MRI should be ordered in a thoughtful, interdisciplinary fashion. This can help avoid excessive use.
- When ordering radiographs, remember the principles of ALARA- As low as reasonably achievable.
- New molecular techniques to distinguish MRSA from MSSA allow the transition from vancomycin to a more appropriate and safer bactericidal drug using a semisynthetic penicillin or a first-generation cephalosporin.

This may reduce the risk of acute kidney injury which is common among children in the ICU who are treated with vancomycin.
- Tuberculosis should be considered in endemic areas or in confusing cases and cultures obtained.
- Subacute osteomyelitis, which was previously termed "Brodie abscess", does not always need surgery. Since it occurs near the physis, it is important to follow these patients until maturity for growth arrest.
- Importance of the health of the periosteum, physis, cartilage and surrounding tissues for recovery and long-term prognosis
- The Masquelet technique for bone gap management following osteomyelitis (Chap. 27) is especially useful in developing countries where bone loss from chronic osteomyelitis is so common.

Although this is only the first edition, one can readily see that this already is an important reference for the treatment of musculoskeletal infections in children. Progress will continue to be made in the clinical care of children, in research, and in health policy and equity. New conditions and treatments will be described, so there will be future editions of this book. I hope you enjoy reading this first edition as much as I have and will use it frequently in your care of these children.

Richard Schwend, MD, FAAP
Rex Diveley Endowed Professor of Orthopedics Research
UMKC KUMC, Director Research
Interim Chair Department of Orthopedics and Musculoskeletal Sciences
Children's Mercy Hospital
Kansas City, MO, USA

Preface

Background Pediatric musculoskeletal infections are common globally and represent about 1–2% of all pediatric hospital admissions in the developed world and about 10–20% of admissions in the developing countries. If untreated or treated inappropriately or inadequately, pediatric bone and joint infections can cause significant mortality and morbidity resulting in a huge functional and economic burden to the family and the community at large. This represents a significant public health problem. The last decade has witnessed a lot of advances in this field with respect to early diagnosis, management, and prevention/treatment of complications.

Why this book? To the best of our knowledge, there is no comprehensive, easily accessible textbook on this topic to guide clinicians in early diagnosis and comprehensive management of pediatric musculoskeletal infections.

Structure The book is organized into five sections:

1. General Principles
2. Acute Musculoskeletal Infections
3. Chronic Musculoskeletal Infections & Sequelae of Musculoskeletal Infections
4. Anatomic Region-Specific Considerations in Musculoskeletal Infections
5. Uncommon Musculoskeletal Infections

Illustrative case examples will aid the reader in simplifying the treatment algorithm for the specific infection. The call-out boxes will help in determining the appropriate treatment and avoiding pitfalls. Efforts have been made to cite the most relevant scientific literature to help evidence-based decision-making. We understand that in certain scenarios, the literature support is not available. We are fortunate to have authors from many countries and from a wide range of specialties contribute to this book. Each author group has outlined the treatment principles and discussed their treatment approach. Each author group provides a global perspective on treating specific musculoskeletal infections to address the unique challenges faced by physicians and healthcare personnel all over the world. We hope this knowledge will benefit children with musculoskeletal infections worldwide by reducing mortality and morbidity, and improving their quality of life.

Phoenix, AZ, USA — Mohan V. Belthur
Pune, Maharashtra, India — Ashish S. Ranade
Philadelphia, PA, USA — Martin J. Herman
Sheffield, UK — James A. Fernandes

Acknowledgments

We are grateful to:

1. Rashmi Oka, creator of the drawings, for her perseverance, hard work, and dedication to do her best, picture by picture.

2. Kathy Zeblisky (librarian @ Phoenix Children's Hospital) for her time and efforts spent researching the literature.

Contents

Part I General Principles

1 **Epidemiology of Musculoskeletal Infections** 3
Gauri A. Oka, Ashish S. Ranade, and Mohan V. Belthur

2 **The Microbiology of Musculoskeletal Infections and Antibiotic Therapies** 17
Jesus Vallejo, Anish P. Sanghrajka, and J. Chase McNeil

3 **Pathology of Musculoskeletal Infections** 35
Stephanie N. Moore-Lotridge and Jonathan G. Schoenecker

4 **Imaging Modalities to Diagnose Musculoskeletal Infections** . . . 51
Caroline M. Blakey, Penny Broadley, Binu T. Kurian, and James A. Fernandes

5 **Infection Mimics: Differential Diagnoses of Musculoskeletal Infections** 69
Yushane Celestine Shih and Mihir M. Thacker

6 **MRSA and Virulent MSSA Infections** 95
Stephanie N. Moore-Lotridge, Monique R. Bennett, Cullen P. Moran, Jonathan G. Schoenecker, and Isaac P. Thomsen

7 **Systemic Effects of Musculoskeletal Infections and ICU Management** 109
Rudolph Wong, Michael Lintner Rivera, Vishal Gunnala, Shilpa Kalane, and David Tellez

8 **Local Antibiotic Drug Delivery Systems for Musculoskeletal Infections** 133
Jessica Burns, Martin McNally, and Janet Conway

9 **Evidence-Based Management of Pediatric Musculoskeletal Infections** 151
Scott B. Rosenfeld, Kishore Mulpuri, and Lawson A. Copley

10 **Paediatric Musculoskeletal Infections: A LMIC Perspective** . . . 165
Loro Antonio, Horn Anria, Franceschi Fulvio, and Mohan V. Belthur

Part II Acute Musculoskeletal Infections

11 Acute Hematogenous Osteomyelitis 191
Scott B. Rosenfeld and Lawson A. Copley

12 Septic Arthritis 203
Sreeharsha V. Nandyala, Martin J. Herman, and Mininder S. Kocher

13 Pyomyositis 221
Ashish S. Ranade, Nirmal Raj Gopinathan, Neeraj Vij, and Mohan V. Belthur

14 Musculoskeletal Infections in the Neonate 235
Atul R. Bhaskar and Ashok N. Johari

15 Subacute Osteomyelitis 253
Hitesh Shah and Benjamin Joseph

16 Surgical Site Infections in Pediatric Orthopedic Surgery 263
Aditya Thandoni and Martin J. Herman

17 Surgical Site Infection in Spine Surgery 281
Anthony A. Catanzano Jr and Vidyadhar V. Upasani

18 Infections Related to External Fixators 301
James Widnall and Selvadurai Nayagam

Part III Chronic Musculoskeletal Infections and Their Sequelae

19 Chronic Hematogenous Osteomyelitis 321
Deepika Pinto and Alaric Aroojis

20 Chronic Post-traumatic Osteomyelitis 339
Ian Singleton, Premal Naik, Levent Eralp, and Mohan V. Belthur

21 Chronic Recurrent Multifocal Osteomyelitis (Chronic Non-infective Osteitis) 371
Grainne M. Murray, Ethan S. Sen, and Athimalaipet V. Ramanan

22 Pathological Fractures with Osteomyelitis 383
Manoj Padman, Scott B. Rosenfeld, and Mohan V. Belthur

23 Post Infective Deformities: Strategies for Limb Reconstruction 411
Mohan V. Belthur, Melissa Esparza, James A. Fernandes, and Milind M. Chaudhary

24 **Sequelae of Septic Arthritis of the Hip and Late Reconstruction** 495
In-Ho Choi and Hyung-Chul Cho

25 **Post Infective Bone Gap Management of the Upper Extremity** 511
Milind M. Chaudhary, Ashish S. Ranade, and James A. Fernandes

26 **Post Infective Bone Gap Management of the Lower Extremity** 543
Timothy Nunn, Sandeep Patwardhan, and Gamal Ahmed Hosny

27 **Post Infective Bone Gap Management: Induced Membrane Technique** 561
Richard Gouron

Part IV Region Specific Musculoskeletal Infections

28 **Epiphyseal Osteomyelitis** 577
Maulin M. Shah, Anil Agarwal, and Prateek Rastogi

29 **Pediatric Hand Infections** 587
Casey M. Codd, Scott H. Kozin, and Joshua M. Abzug

30 **Pediatric Foot Infections** 601
Laurence Wicks, Vrisha Madhuri, and Richard Gardner

31 **Tuberculosis of the Axial Skeleton** 629
Arjun Dhawale, K. Venugopal Menon, and Anil K. Jain

32 **Tuberculosis of the Appendicular Skeleton** 659
Chang Ho Shin and Won Joon Yoo

33 **Non-tuberculous Infections of the Spine** 675
Kelly Gillock, Archana Malik, and Martin J. Herman

Part V Uncommon Musculoskeletal Infections

34 **Musculoskeletal Infections in Immunocompromised Children** 693
Sara Louise Dorman, John P. Cashman, and William James Harrison

35 **Fungal Infections** 713
Mandar Agashe, Binoti Sheth, and Mohan V. Belthur

36 **Necrotising Fasciitis** 743
Arne Schröder and Christina Oetzmann von Sochaczewski

37 Gas Gangrene 761
Parmanand Gupta and Hitesh Shah

38 Meningococcal Infections 773
Sam Weston-Simons, Mohan V. Belthur,
and James A. Fernandes

39 Brucellosis, Hydatid Disease, and Viral Osteomyelitis 795
Nirmal Raj Gopinathan, Jagdish Menon,
and James A. Fernandes

Index 809

Editors and Contributors

About the Editors

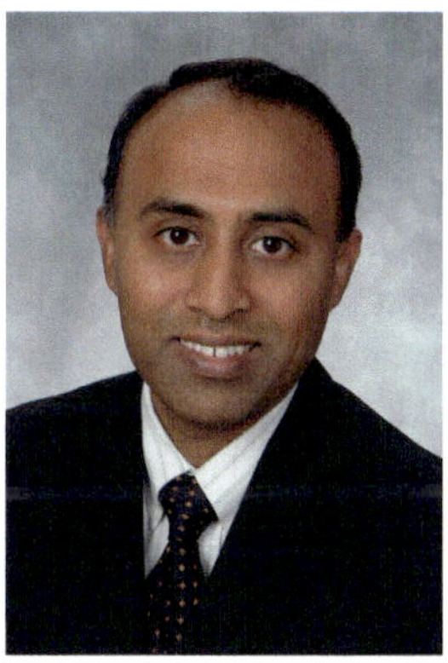

Mohan V. Belthur MD, MS, FRCS (Tr & Orth), FRCSC, Associate Professor, Department of Orthopaedics, The University of Arizona College of Medicine & Phoenix Children's Hospital, Phoenix, AZ, USA.

Dr. Belthur is committed to providing the best orthopedic care and service to his patients, by being compassionate, competent, and conscientious. He strives relentlessly to improve the quality of life of children, adolescents, and young adults with musculoskeletal problems by engaging, empathizing, educating, enlisting their help, and empowering them and their families. He is involved in clinical research projects that are impactful and make a difference to the lives of disabled children. He is passionate about teaching and mentoring learners from all walks of the health profession. He is interested in global health and works with non- profit organizations to reduce the burden of childhood musculoskeletal disorders in low- and middle-income countries.

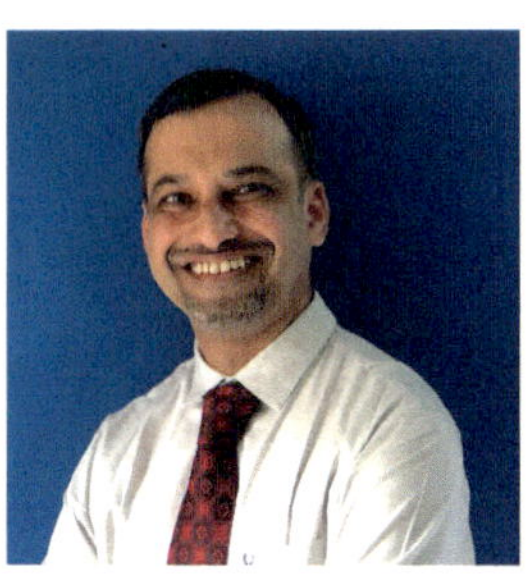

Ashish S. Ranade MBBS, MS Orth, FRCS (Glasg), Consultant Orthopedic Surgeon, Blooming Buds Centre for Pediatric Orthopaedics, Deenanath Mangeshkar Hospital & Research Centre, Pune, India

Dr. Ranade is a pediatric orthopedic surgeon who is trained in the UK, the USA, and India. He believes in giving the best treatment by putting patients and their families first. While practicing in India for more than a decade, he has seen musculoskeletal infections and their complications in diverse forms. The desire to give the best possible outcome to every child with such complex problems sparked his interest in musculoskeletal infections. He hopes that this book will help tremendously all those who treat musculoskeletal infections in children. In addition to a busy clinical practice, he is very much involved in teaching, writing, and doing clinical research. He strives to keep his knowledge up to date and loves to learn new things.

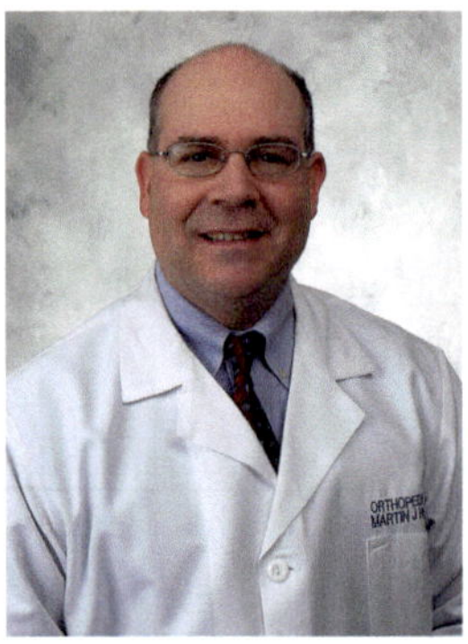

Martin J. Herman MD, Professor of Orthopedic surgery, Drexel University College of Medicine, Chief of Orthopedic Surgery, St. Christopher's Hospital for Children, Philadelphia, PA, USA

Dr. Herman has been practicing pediatric orthopedic surgery, teaching and mentoring trainees, and writing about pediatric orthopedic conditions for over 25 years. The diagnosis and treatment of musculoskeletal infections have evolved in many important ways. This textbook is the first of its kind that is solely dedicated to these complex and potentially catastrophic diseases. It is our hope that these pages will serve as a guide for those dedicated to the care of children with these varied conditions and who are committed to improving outcomes.

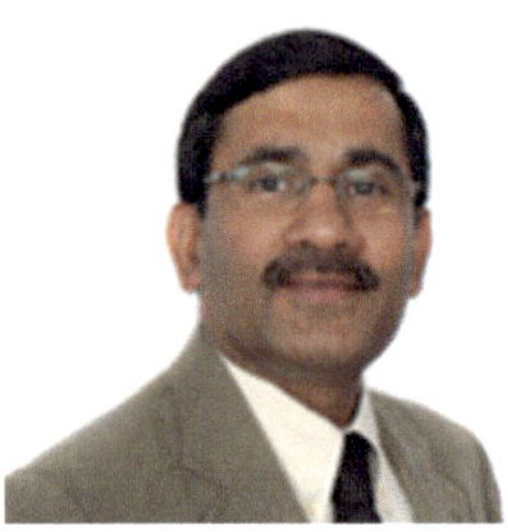

James A. Fernandes MS Orth, FRCS (Glas), FRCS Tr & Orth(Eng), Consultant Orthopedic Surgeon, Sheffield Children's NHS Foundation, Western Bank, Sheffield, UK

Mr. Fernandes trained in India and the UK, practicing in his specialist area of pediatric orthopedics since 1990. He has been a part of the center of excellence in Sheffield since 2000 in pediatric limb reconstruction and general pediatric orthopedics; training, mentoring, and teaching many a fellow over the years; and treating children of the UK and from Europe. His interests in musculoskeletal infections stem from his background in India, where the burden is high; therefore, his primary aim is to support those who treat especially the sequela of these infections.

Contributors

Joshua M. Abzug Department of Orthopaedics, University of Maryland School of Medicine, Baltimore, MD, USA

Anil Agarwal Department of Paediatric Orthopaedics, Chacha Nehru Bal Chikitsalaya, Delhi, India

Mandar Agashe Agashe's Paediatric SuperSpeciality Clinic, Mumbai, India

Childrens' Hip Preservation Services, (CHiPS), SRCC Childrens' Hospital, Mumbai, India

BJ Wadia Hospital for Children, Mumbai, India

Horn Anria Division of Orthopaedic Surgery, University of Cape Town, South Africa, Cape Town, South Africa

Red Cross War Memorial Children's Hospital, Cape Town, South Africa

Loro Antonio Department of Orthopedic Surgery, CoRSU Rehabilitation Hospital, Kisubi, Uganda

Alaric Aroojis Department of Paediatric Orthopaedics, Bai Jerbai Wadia Hospital for Children, Mumbai, India

Mohan V. Belthur Department of Child Health & Orthopedics, University of Arizona College of Medicine, Phoenix, AZ, USA

Department of Orthopedics, Phoenix Children's Hospital, Phoenix, AZ, USA

Monique R. Bennett Vanderbilt University Medical Center, Department of Pediatrics, Division of Infectious Diseases, and the Vanderbilt Institute for Infection, Immunology, and Inflammation, Nashville, TN, USA

Atul R. Bhaskar RN Cooper Hospital - HBT Medical College, Bombay Hospital Institute of Medical Sciences, Mumbai, Maharashtra, India

Caroline M. Blakey Department of Paediatric Orthopaedics, Trauma and Spinal Surgery, Sheffield Children's NHS Foundation Trust, Sheffield, UK

Penny Broadley Department of Paediatric Radiology, Sheffield Children's NHS Foundation Trust, Sheffield, UK

Jessica Burns Department of Child Health, The University of Arizona College of Medicine – Phoenix, Phoenix, AZ, USA

Phoenix Children's Hospital, Phoenix, AZ, USA

John P. Cashman Sheffield Childrens Hospital, Sheffield, UK

Anthony A. Catanzano Jr Rady Children's Hospital, San Diego, San Diego, CA, USA

Milind M. Chaudhary International Deformity & Lengthening Institute, Akola, Maharashtra, India

Hyung-Chul Cho Department of Orthopedic Surgery, Chung-Ang University Hospital, Seoul, South Korea

In-Ho Choi Department of Orthopedic Surgery, Chung-Ang University Hospital, Seoul, South Korea

Department of Orthopedic Surgery, Seoul National University Hospital, Seoul, South Korea

Division of Pediatric Orthopaedics, Seoul National University Children's Hospital, Seoul, Republic of Korea

Casey M. Codd Department of Orthopaedics, University of Maryland School of Medicine, Baltimore, MD, USA

Janet Conway International Center for Limb Lengthening, Rubin Institute for Advanced Orthopaedics, Sinai Hospital of Baltimore, Baltimore, MD, USA

Lawson A. Copley Department of Orthopaedic Surgery, Texas Scottish Rite Hospital for Children and Children's Health System of Texas, University of Texas Southwestern, Dallas, TX, USA

Arjun Dhawale Department of Orthopaedics, Bai Jerbai Wadia Hospital for Children, Mumbai, India

Department of Orthopaedics, Sir H.N. Reliance Foundation Hospital, Mumbai, India

Sara Louise Dorman Sheffield Childrens Hospital, Sheffield, UK

Levent Eralp Istanbul Medical School, University of Istanbul, Istanbul, Turkey

Melissa Esparza Department of Child Health & Orthopedics, University of Arizona College of Medicine, Phoenix, AZ, USA

Department of Orthopedics, Phoenix Children's Hospital, Phoenix, AZ, USA

James A. Fernandes Sheffield Children's Hospital NHS Foundation Trust, University of Sheffield, Sheffield, UK

Franceschi Fulvio Consultant Paediatric Orthopaedic Surgeon, Trento, Italy

Richard Gardner CURE International, Grand Rapids, MI, USA

Kelly Gillock Drexel University College of Medicine in Philadelphia, Philadelphia, PA, USA

Nirmal Raj Gopinathan Division of Paediatric Orthopaedics, Department of Orthopaedic Surgery, Post Graduate Institute of Medical Education and Research, Chandigarh, India

Richard Gouron Department of Pediatric Orthopedic Surgery, Amiens University Medical Center and Jules Verne University of Picardie, Amiens, France

Service d'Orthopédie Pédiatrique, CHU Amiens, Groupe Hospitalier Sud, Amiens, France

Vishal Gunnala Department of Critical Care, Phoenix Children's Hospital, Phoenix, AZ, USA

Department of Child Health, University of Arizona College of Medicine, Phoenix, AZ, USA

Parmanand Gupta Government Medical College and Hospital, Chandigarh, India

William James Harrison Countess of Chester Hospital NHS Foundation Trust, Chester, UK

Martin J. Herman Drexel University College of Medicine, Philadelphia, PA, USA

Orthopedic Surgery, St. Christopher's Hospital for Children, Philadelphia, PA, USA

Gamal Ahmed Hosny Benha University, Kalyubia, Egypt

Anil K. Jain Department of Orthopaedics, University College of Medical Sciences, New Delhi, India

Ashok N. Johari Children's Orthopaedic Centre, Mahim, Mumbai, India

Benjamin Joseph Kasturba Medical College, Manipal Academy of Higher Education, Manipal, Karnataka, India

Shilpa Kalane Deenanath Mangeshkar Hospital, Pune, India

Mininder S. Kocher Department of Orthopaedic Surgery, Boston Children's Hospital, Harvard Medical School, Boston, MA, USA

Scott H. Kozin Department of Orthopedics, Shriners Hospital, Philadelphia, PA, USA

Binu T. Kurian Department of Trauma and Orthopaedic Surgery, St. John's Medical College Hospital, Bangalore, India

Vrisha Madhuri Paediatric Orthopaedic Department, Ida Scudder Chair for Clinical Research, Adjunct Scientist, Centre for Stem Cell Research, Christian Medical College and Hospital, Vellore, Tamil Nadu, India

Archana Malik St. Christopher's Hospital for Children, Department of Radiology, Philadelphia, PA, USA

Martin McNally Oxford Bone Infection Unit, Oxford University Hospitals, Oxford, UK

J. Chase McNeil Department of Pediatrics, Section of Infectious Diseases, Baylor College of Medicine, Houston, TX, USA

Jagdish Menon Department of Orthopaedic Surgery, Jawaharlal Institute of Postgraduate Medical Education and Research, Pondicherry, India

Stephanie N. Moore-Lotridge Vanderbilt University Medical Center, Department of Orthopaedics, Nashville, TN, USA

Cullen P. Moran Vanderbilt University School of Medicine, Nashville, TN, USA

Kishore Mulpuri Department of Orthopaedic Surgery, BC Children's Hospital, University of British Columbia, Vancouver, BC, Canada

Grainne M. Murray Department of Paediatric Rheumatology, University Hospitals Bristol NHS Foundation Trust, Bristol, UK

Premal Naik NHL Municipal Medical College, Rainbow Super-speciality Hospital & Children's Orthopaedic Centre, Ahmedabad, Gujarat, India

Sreeharsha V. Nandyala Boston Children's Hospital, Harvard Medical School, Boston, MA, USA

Selvadurai Nayagam Alder Hey Children's Hospital, Liverpool, UK

Royal Liverpool University and Broadgreen University Hospitals, Liverpool, UK

Timothy Nunn CURE Ethiopia Children's Hospital, Addis Ababa, Ethiopia

Gauri A. Oka Department of Community Medicine, Bharati Vidyapeeth Deemed to be University Medical College, Bharati Hospital and Research Centre, Pune, Maharashtra, India

Manoj Padman Centre for Paediatric Orthopaedics & Disabilities, Paediatric Orthopaedics, Rainbow Children's Hospital, Fortis Memorial Research Institute, Delhi NCR, New Delhi, India

Sandeep Patwardhan Sancheti Institute for Orthopaedics and Rehabilitation, Pune, India

Deepika Pinto Department of Paediatric Orthopaedics, Bai Jerbai Wadia Hospital for Children, Mumbai, India

Athimalaipet V. Ramanan Department of Paediatric Rheumatology, University Hospitals Bristol NHS Foundation Trust, Bristol, UK

Translational Health Sciences, Bristol Medical School, University of Bristol, Bristol, UK

Ashish S. Ranade Blooming Buds Centre for Pediatric Orthopaedics, Deenanath Mangeshkar Hospital, Pune, Maharashtra, India

Prateek Rastogi Department of Paediatric Orthopaedics, Chacha Nehru Bal Chikitsalaya, Delhi, India

Michael Lintner Rivera, MD Department of Critical Care, Phoenix Children's Hospital, Phoenix, AZ, USA

Department of Child Health, University of Arizona College of Medicine, Phoenix, AZ, USA

Scott B. Rosenfeld Department of Orthopaedic Surgery, Texas Children's Hospital, Baylor College of Medicine, Houston, TX, USA

Anish P. Sanghrajka Department of Trauma and Orthopaedics, Norfolk & Norwich University Hospitals, Norfolk, UK

Jonathan G. Schoenecker Vanderbilt University Medical Center, Department of Orthopaedics, Nashville, TN, USA

Department of Pediatrics, Department of Pathology Microbiology and Immunology, and Vanderbilt Center for Bone Biology, Nashville, TN, USA

Vanderbilt University, Department of Pharmacology, Nashville, TN, USA

Arne Schröder Department of Paediatrics, Municipal Hospital Dortmund, Dortmund, Germany

Ethan S. Sen Department of Paediatric Rheumatology, Great North Children's Hospital, Newcastle upon Tyne, UK

Faculty of Medical Sciences, Newcastle University, Newcastle upon Tyne, UK

Hitesh Shah Kasturba Medical College, Manipal Academy of Higher Education, Manipal, Karnataka, India

Maulin M. Shah Orthokids Clinic, Ahmedabad, Gujarat, India

Binoti Sheth Department of Orthopaedics, LTMGH and LTM Medical College, Mumbai, India

Yushane Celestine Shih Nemours Children's Hospital, Delaware, Department of Orthopedic Surgery, Wilmington, DE, USA

Chang Ho Shin Division of Pediatric Orthopaedics, Seoul National University Children's Hospital, Seoul, Republic of Korea

Department of Orthopaedic Surgery, Seoul National University College of Medicine, Seoul, Republic of Korea

Ian Singleton University of Arizona College of Medicine – Phoenix, Phoenix, AZ, USA

Christina Oetzmann von Sochaczewski Division of Paediatric Surgery, Department of Surgery, University Medical Centre Bonn, Bonn, Germany

David Tellez Department of Critical Care, Phoenix Children's Hospital, Phoenix, AZ, USA

Department of Child Health, University of Arizona College of Medicine, Phoenix, AZ, USA

Mihir M. Thacker Nemours Children's Hospital, Delaware, Department of Orthopedic Surgery, Wilmington, DE, USA

Aditya Thandoni Drexel University College of Medicine, Philadelphia, PA, USA

Isaac P. Thomsen Vanderbilt University Medical Center, Department of Pediatrics, Division of Infectious Diseases, and the Vanderbilt Institute for Infection, Immunology, and Inflammation, Nashville, TN, USA

Vidyadhar V. Upasani Rady Children's Hospital, San Diego, San Diego, CA, USA

Jesus Vallejo Department of Pediatrics, Section of Infectious Diseases, Baylor College of Medicine, Houston, TX, USA

K. Venugopal Menon Department of Orthopaedics, Bharati Vidyapeeth University, Pune, India

Neeraj Vij University of Arizona College of Medicine – Phoenix, Phoenix, AZ, USA

Sam Weston-Simons Evelina London Children's Hospital, Guy's and St Thomas' NHS Foundation Trust, London, UK

Laurence Wicks CURE International, Grand Rapids, MI, USA

James Widnall Alder Hey Children's Hospital, Liverpool, UK

Rudolph Wong Department of Critical Care, Phoenix Children's Hospital, Phoenix, AZ, USA

Department of Child Health, University of Arizona College of Medicine, Phoenix, AZ, USA

Won Joon Yoo Division of Pediatric Orthopaedics, Seoul National University Children's Hospital, Seoul, Republic of Korea

Department of Orthopaedic Surgery, Seoul National University College of Medicine, Seoul, Republic of Korea

Part I

General Principles

Epidemiology of Musculoskeletal Infections

1

Gauri A. Oka, Ashish S. Ranade, and Mohan V. Belthur

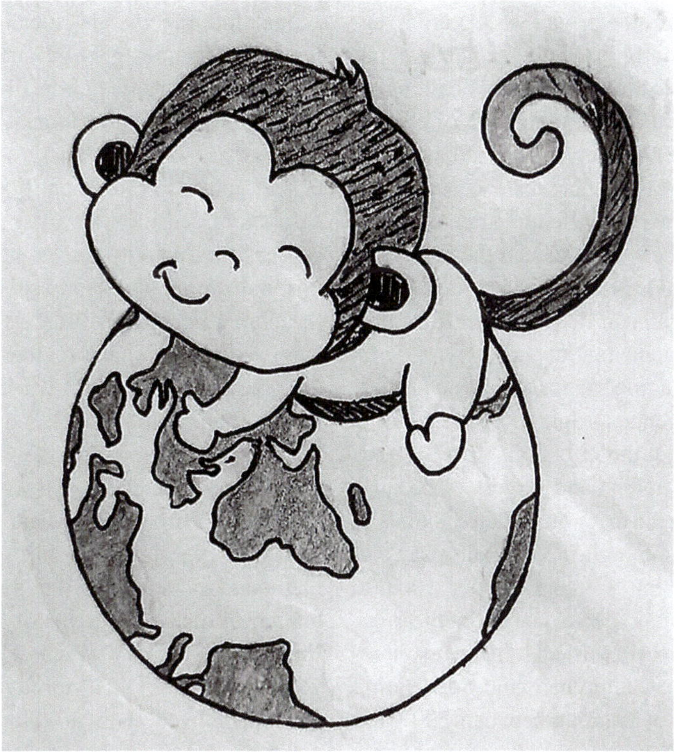

G. A. Oka (✉)
Department of Community Medicine, Bharati Vidyapeeth Deemed to be University Medical College, Bharati Hospital and Research Centre, Pune, Maharashtra, India
e-mail: gauri.oka@bharatividyapeeth.edu

A. S. Ranade
Blooming Buds Centre for Pediatric Orthopaedics, Deenanath Mangeshkar Hospital, Pune, Maharashtra, India
e-mail: ranadea2@gmail.com

M. V. Belthur
Department of Child Health & Orthopedics, University of Arizona College of Medicine, Phoenix, AZ, USA

Department of Orthopedics, Phoenix Children's Hospital, Phoenix, AZ, USA
e-mail: mbelthur@phoenixchildrens.com

© Springer Nature Switzerland AG 2022

M. V. Belthur et al. (eds.), *Pediatric Musculoskeletal Infections*,
https://doi.org/10.1007/978-3-030-95794-0_1

Introduction Epidemiology is defined as the study of the distribution and determinants of health and disease and the application of this science to the control of diseases. Of the three main tenets of epidemiology, the first is the measurement of disease frequency in different populations or population subgroups. The second is to understand how the disease or health-related event is distributed in the population by time, place, and person characteristics. The third tenet is to test etiological hypotheses and identify the determinants (causes or risk factors) of the disease to formulate prevention and control strategies.

Musculoskeletal infections (MSKI) are a significant cause of morbidity in the pediatric population [1]. Often, the diagnosis can be challenging and is usually based on a combination of clinical and radiological evaluation, as well as laboratory investigations. Delayed diagnosis can lead to disastrous consequences affecting not only the patients but also their families and the society in which they live. Understanding the epidemiology of MSKI in children can help better inform prevention and management strategies.

Musculoskeletal infections in children primarily have a hematogenous origin. Some cases have been reported where the infections were secondary to penetrating trauma and surgery or because of contiguous spread from an affected site. The incidence of MSKI in high-income European settings ranges between 1.4 and 25 per 100,000 people [2–5]. There is sparse data about the prevalence and incidence of MSKI from resource-limited settings. A Cambodian study presenting retrospective data of patients between 2007 and 2011 reported an incidence of 13.8/100,000 hospital patients [6], while Ugandan data from 2018 reports a MSKI prevalence of 10.5% in hospital and outreach pediatric patients [7].

This chapter discusses the global burden of MSKI in children, as well as the epidemiological aspects of the following musculoskeletal infections:

1. Osteomyelitis
2. Septic arthritis
3. Pyomyositis
4. Spine infections
5. Tuberculosis
6. Hand infections
7. Foot infections
8. Surgical site infections
9. Fungal infections

Global Burden of MSKI in Children

Burden of disease refers to the socioeconomic impact of poor health. Diseases impact not only the health and well-being of a nation but also development, affecting education and knowledge acquisition, income and social status, productivity and economic growth, and other direct and indirect components of human development such as gender equality and human rights [1, 8–14].

Beyond mortality statistics, different methods can be considered to quantify the burden of disease expressed in terms of socioeconomic costs such as productivity losses, care and treatment, hospitalization, and handicap. To better describe the global burden of disease (GBD) across diseases, risk factors, and regions and to overcome the specific problems of each country, the World Health Organization (WHO) developed standard methodology to measure the GBD including the disability adjusted life year (DALY), years lived with a disability (YLD), years of life lost (YLL), and life expectancy at birth. The most used method is the approach that measures the global burden of disease in terms of disability adjusted life years (DALYs) which is a combination of years of life lost (YLL) through premature death and years lived with disability (YLD). It is a combination of both mortality and morbidity caused by a disease condition and is applied to populations rather than to individuals [1–3]. Bickler et al. recommend that the burden of surgical conditions should be expressed as DALYs, that unmet surgical need be expressed as potential DALYs avertable, and that DALYs averted be used as a measure of the impact of surgical care [15].

The GBD uses validated, standardized methods across databases to estimate the GBD for each condition. This allows us to identify diseases with the most burden and differentiate those that cause death versus those that result in poor health. The response (timing and allocation of resources) to a disease condition depends on its socioeconomic impact. This method based on economic and ethical fairness principles has been used by the WHO and different countries to compare disease effects within and between populations and to understand changes over time, for health situation assessment, priority setting, and policy-making, and allows cost-effective, equitable allocation of scarce resources (money, material, and manpower) for a variety of health-related conditions [1, 8–12, 15].

The GBD study has estimated that the burden of nontraumatic musculoskeletal conditions was 2.5% of the entire global burden in 2004. This increased to 4.4% in 2010 and to 5.9% in 2016, according to recent estimates [8–12]. Infectious diseases are causing about 15 million deaths annually with more than 80% in Africa. Tuberculosis is the second leading infectious disease, causing about two million deaths every year. Beyond mortality figures, the health impact of several infectious diseases can be measured by severe and permanent disabilities and deformities affecting approximately 1 billion people in the world and causing millions of DALYs.

However, there are no good data for the common pediatric conditions, especially globally, and estimating GBD for the pediatric musculoskeletal conditions has been difficult [1, 15]. Recent studies have shown that the most common pediatric orthopedic conditions causing musculoskeletal impairment (MSI) are infection, trauma, clubfoot, limb deformity, DDH, and neuromuscular conditions [1]. These conditions not only contribute to GBD but also cause significant MSI into adult life. The burden of MSI in children <16 years has been estimated to be around 2.6% of the population [1]. They have a long period of time of YLD for the individual and DALYs for the population. These conditions can be treated appropriately with a combination of prevention, early diagnosis, and combined nonoperative (medical, orthosis/prosthesis, and rehabilitation) and surgical management, which is more effective when provided early rather than later in the disease natural history. Because of the long YLD and the large proportion of children in a population, these pediatric musculoskeletal conditions can contribute greatly to the GBD, now and later [8–12, 16–20].

Osteomyelitis In LMICs, untreated acute septic arthritis and osteomyelitis remain a common cause of chronic osteomyelitis and late sequelae. Osteomyelitis continues to be a worldwide problem because of inappropriate and inadequate treatment mainly due to the lack of availability of antibiotics and lack of access to basic and specialized healthcare. Untreated chronic osteomyelitis leads to poor overall health, disability, social isolation, and restriction from school. There are 12 million children with osteomyelitis in the least developed countries [1]. In New Zealand, the prevalence of osteomyelitis is around 1 in 4000 population with Maori and Pacific Islander dominance [21]. In Uganda, 10% of all outpatient visits were for osteomyelitis, and 80% of cases were in patients younger than age 20 years [22]. Osteomyelitis accounts for 15% of all pediatric inpatient days, 7.8% of all pediatric surgical admissions, and about 3.5% of all surgical procedures. In 32% of these operations, the patients were children aged between 10 and 14 years. The tibia was the bone most frequently involved (31%), and sequestrectomy was the most frequent surgical procedure (60%) [22]. To decrease this burden in LMICs, improved diagnosis and more timely treatment of acute osteomyelitis are needed. Osteomyelitis disproportionately affects the young and is a clinical and surgical burden, best treated early rather than late. Unfortunately, there are no published DALY or YLD data for pediatric osteomyelitis or septic arthritis [21–25].

In HICs, the prevalence of osteomyelitis is about 3–13 per 100,000 population. The CORTICES group reported that at large, academic pediatric tertiary care centers, pediatric orthopedic services consult on an average of 3000 "rule-out" MSKI cases annually. These patients account for nearly one in ten orthopedic consultations, and one in three of these are culture positive. Extrapolation estimates that 45,000 children are evaluated annually for MSKI, and 15,000 cases have culture-positive disease. There is large regional variation in the burden of MSKI across the United States [26, 27].

In HICs, musculoskeletal conditions accounted for 13.5% of hospital visits and 5.4% of hospital charges in the pediatric population. Musculoskeletal infections as a primary diagnosis accounted for 1.8% of all hospital discharges for musculoskeletal-related conditions and 0.1% of all hospital discharges in children and adolescents. When the primary diagnosis was a musculoskeletal infection, the hospital charges averaged $46,000 with a mean of 6.3 days in the hospital. Total hospital charges for primary diagnoses of musculoskeletal infections in 2012 were $419 million [10].

Septic arthritis The reported incidence of bacterial arthritis in children ranges from 1 to 37 cases per 100,000, depending upon the study population. The estimated incidence in the United States is between 3 and 4 per 100,000 children <20 years, based on hospital discharge data. The estimated incidence in LMICs is higher and is around 20–30 per 100,000 population [28].

Tuberculosis (TB) Tuberculosis is a major global public health problem, with latent TB affecting about 2 billion people. Globally there were 10.4 million incident cases of TB in 2016, 331,00 multidrug-resistant cases, and 19,800 extensively drug-resistant cases. Tuberculosis is the second leading infectious disease, causing about two million deaths every year. The incidence of TB is about 2–3 per 100,000 in the United States and 25 per 100,000 in the EU [29]. Overall, musculoskeletal involvement is seen in less than 10% of all cases of TB, and half of these affect the axial skeleton. The proportion of children with TB is smaller; however, TB of the spine remains a serious cause of paralysis worldwide. Incident cases of TB and musculoskeletal TB contribute to DALYs for the population. A systematic analysis for the Global Burden of Disease study 2010 showed that tuberculosis was an important cause of YLD in sub-Saharan Africa [4–6].

Surgical site infections (SSI) The prevalence of pediatric orthopedic surgical site infections is about 2.5–4%. Musculoskeletal SSI are devastating adverse events that may become life-threatening conditions. They create an additional burden on total healthcare expenditures and can lead to functional impairment, long-lasting disability, or even permanent handicap, with the inevitable social and economic burdens [30, 31].

Cost-effective analysis (CEA) Using the per capita income, the World Bank has introduced four levels of income, namely, high income, higher middle income, lower middle income, and lower income [32]. Murray et al. [33] utilized the DALY to develop CEA as an analytical tool that correlates the effectiveness of a health intervention to its costs, in terms of dollar per DALY averted. Recent data for CEA show that surgical care is cost-effective in low- and middle-income countries (LMICs) compared with the much higher surgical care costs in the United States and other high-income countries (HICs). As a response to these data and much persistence from surgical leadership, the WHO has recently promoted essential surgical services through their Emergency and Essential Surgical Care Project (EESC) and Global Initiative [34, 35].

Summary Because of a long YLD and the large proportion of children in a population, pediatric musculoskeletal infections can contribute greatly to the GBD, now and later, especially in LMIC countries. Pediatric MSKI should be part of future GBD studies. DALYs should be determined so that policy-makers can allocate appropriate resources for these conditions that may affect children and families for generations. Prevention and appropriate treatment of pediatric MSKI should become WHO essential surgical services. Recommendations from the Global Initiative for Children's Surgery (GICS) for optimizing children's surgical care include establishing standards and integrating them into national surgical plans for each level of care, a children's hospital for each country, establishment and support of regional

Table 1.1 Incidence of some MSKI in children

MSKI	HIC	LMIC	Comment
AHO [26, 36–38]	3–13 per 100,000	80–100 per 100,000	
SA [28, 39, 40]	3–5 per 100,000	20–30 per 100,000	
Pyomyositis [41–43]	Unknown	10–20 per 100,000	1–4% of hospital admissions
TB [29]	3–25 per 100,000	136 per 100,000	About 10% involve MSK system

training hubs for all children's surgical specialties, and establishing regional research support centers. Table 1.1 depicts the incidences of some MSKI in children.

Epidemiology of Specific Infections

Osteomyelitis

Osteomyelitis is classified as acute if the duration of the illness is less than 2 weeks, subacute if the duration of the illness is between 2 weeks to 3 months, and chronic, if for longer durations [44].

Incidence The incidence of pediatric osteomyelitis in developed countries ranges from 1 to 13/100,000 [36, 37, 45–47] and up to 80–100/100,000 in developing countries [36, 38]. Acute hematogenous osteomyelitis (AHO) is the most common form of osteomyelitis constituting two-thirds of all MSKI [46, 48]. There has been no evidence to show a racial predilection [49].

Mortality The mortality in acute hematogenous OM has dropped sharply from the pre-antibiotic era to the current times. Data from a few studies report that there is no mortality with acute hematogenous osteomyelitis. However, the exact mortality data is lacking.

Morbidity Osteomyelitis is associated with bacteremia and prolonged duration of hospitalization with long-term sequelae and limb-threatening complications [50]. Osteomyelitis can lead to secondary septic arthritis.

Affected sites According to Stevenson et al., the long bones, namely, the tibia (up to 70%), femur (almost 40%) and the humerus, are the most frequently affected bones in children [37, 46, 51, 52]. Among other bones, the calcaneum is the commonest (10%) [53]. The femur (26.9%) only slightly overtakes the tibia (26%) according to the systematic review by Dartnell et al. These are followed by the pelvis (9.2%), humerus (8.1%), foot (7.7%), and forearm (4.8%) [36].

Causative microorganisms The most common microorganisms causing acute hematogenous osteomyelitis in children are *Staphylococcus aureus* [(methicillin-sensitive *Staphylococcus aureus* (MSSA) and methicillin-resistant *Staphylococcal aureus* (MRSA)] and *Streptococcus* species. Other common microorganisms are *Enterobacter*, *Kingella kingae*, *Haemophilus influenzae* in an unimmunized child, *Neisseria gonorrhoeae*, and *Candida* [53]. Atypically, superinfection with group A *Streptococcus* or varicella can be found in immunocompromised patients; *Pseudomonas aeruginosa* and *Salmonella* can complicate puncture wounds in the foot and sickle cell disease, respectively. Methicillin-resistant *Staphylococcus aureus* is found in more than 70% of pediatric osteomyelitis in some regions, followed by other staphylococcal and streptococcal species. Pneumococcus and Panton-Valentine leukocidin-producing *Staphylococcus aureus* are responsible for more severe and complicated osteomyelitis [36, 54].

Seasonal variations Seasonal variation has been reported for pediatric acute hematogenous osteomyelitis with peak occurrence in the summer season [55].

Patient Factors

Age and sex Children younger than 5 years of age are most prone to develop acute hematogenous osteomyelitis [53, 56]. Children from low-income regions are more likely to have higher hospitalization rates [4]. Boys are more likely affected than girls (1.9:1) [6]. Male-to-female ratios were 1.6–1.8 (between 2006 and 2012) in the United States based on the Kids' Inpatient Database [4].

Risk factors Sickle cell disease is a risk factor due to its effect on the microvasculature leading to infarction of the bone [36]. Children with respiratory distress syndrome, an umbilical artery catheter, and conditions associated with heightened susceptibility to infection (e.g., prematurity, low birth weight, and small size for age) are more vulnerable [39].

Septic Arthritis

Septic arthritis is an infection of the synovium and structures within the joint. It is a potentially fatal disease that can cause permanent joint destruction and death [39, 57].

Incidence An annual incidence of 1 in 100,000 has been reported from developed countries (data from the United States) [40], while a higher incidence of 1/20,000 to 1/5000 has been reported from Africa [39, 58]. A serial cross-sectional study in the United States found a decrease in the annual hospitalization rates of 4.23, 3.64, and 3.28 per 100,000 children in 2006, 2009, and 2012, respectively. Septic arthritis along with osteomyelitis has been seen in 10.6–13% of hospitalizations for septic arthritis [5].

Morbidity The distinctive anatomy, namely, the presence of vessels between the metaphysis and epiphysis and presence of intracapsular metaphyses, predisposes a bone infection to result in secondary septic arthritis. Without prompt and effective treatment, this could result in long-term disability due to functional joint impairment or limb asymmetry because of destruction of the articular cartilage and the epiphyseal growth plate.

Affected joints The most frequently affected joints are the hip and the knee. The ankle, elbow, shoulder, sacroiliac, and metatarsophalangeal joints are less-commonly affected. Monoarticular presentation is most common [59].

Causative microorganisms *Staphylococcus aureus* is the most common causative organism with MRSA, MSSA with PVL-positive *Staphylococcus* causing the most serious infections. Other pathogens are *Streptococcus* species, *Enterobacter*, *Kingella kingae*, and *Haemophilus influenzae* type b (found to be decreasing due to vaccination in developed countries) [57]. *Salmonella* species have been commonly found in Malawian, Kenyan, and Zambian infants with sickle cell disease [40, 59].

Patient Factors

Age and sex Infants and toddlers are the most frequently affected with a predilection for male children.

Risk factors Risk factors include respiratory distress syndrome, an umbilical artery catheter, prematurity, low birth weight, and sickle cell disease [39]. Rosenfeld found adjacent infections in 59% of septic arthritis cases in the form of osteomyelitis, subperiosteal abscess, or intramuscular abscess [60]. Septic arthritis caused by *H. influenzae* has been shown to coexist with osteomyelitis in 22% of cases [59].

Socioeconomic/cultural influences Hospitalization rates for septic arthritis were found to be higher in children from low- or very low-income areas with the highest rates seen among Black children, followed by children of Asian and Hispanic origin [5].

Pyomyositis

Pyomyositis is a bacterial intramuscular infection beginning with an early stage of muscular inflammation, leading subsequently to formation of single or multiple abscesses, symptomatically mimicking osteomyelitis and septic arthritis. Pyomyositis may be primary (hematogenous spread) or secondary and may complicate contiguous bone and joint infection [2, 61].

Incidence Pyomyositis is endemic to tropical countries and constitutes 1–4% of all surgical admissions [41–43]. The incidence is much lower in the United States and other temperate regions but is increasing. An increasing linear trend was noted by Maravelas et al. [42].

Mortality There is limited information on mortality due to pyomyositis, with the reported rates varying between 0% and 10% from countries like the United States, Brazil, sub-Saharan Africa, and India [42, 43].

Morbidity Tropical pyomyositis was found to contribute to 1% of all hospital admissions in South America, while in various countries of Africa, the number was much higher at 4–27% [43].

Affected sites Muscle involvement is usually single but can be multifocal. Common sites include the obturator internus, iliopsoas, and quadriceps femoris muscles. Gluteus medius and minimus, adductor longus, piriformis, external oblique, internal oblique, and transverse abdominis are also affected more frequently compared to other sites.

Causative microorganisms The most common causative organisms are *Staphylococcus aureus* (both MSSA and MRSA) (90% in tropical areas, 75% in temperate zones) and group A *Streptococcus* (1–5%), while the less common bacterial causes include group B, C, and G *Streptococcus*, pneumococcus, *Haemophilus* species, and Gram-negative bacilli. Community-acquired PVL-producing MRSA largely accounts for infections in the temperate regions [62].

Seasonal variations Cases are found throughout the year but have been found to peak during May to July [63, 64], persisting through October [61].

Patient Factors

Age and sex Age range is between 1 week and 15 years, peaking between 2 and 5 years with a 2:1 to 3:1 male preponderance [43, 65]. Maravelas et al. report that almost one quarter (24%) of the patients are younger than 20 years, with greater incidence in children between 5 and years of age [42].

Risk factors Preceding muscular injuries, severe exercise, lacerations, insect bites, malnutrition, leukemia, lymphoma, steroid use, underlying infections such as pulmonary tuberculosis, malaria, urinary tract infection, and HIV are the known risk factors. Pyomyositis has been reported in healthy pediatric populations in the tropics, while associated immunocompromised status is frequently found in the temperate regions [41, 64].

Socioeconomic/cultural influences According to data published from Texas, USA, in 2006, about 65% of children with pyomyositis over a 6-year period were Blacks and Hispanics [61].

Spine Infections

Based on etiology, spinal infections can be divided into pyogenic or nonspecific, granulomatous or specific (such as tuberculosis, brucellosis, fungal), and parasitic [66]. Pediatric spondylodiscitis encompasses vertebral osteomyelitis, spondylitis, and infectious discitis. The infection can spread to the spinal cord causing catastrophic neurologic complications.

Incidence Pediatric nontuberculous spondylodiscitis, unlike that in adults, is rare. Overall, the incidence corresponds to 2–4% of infectious bone diseases [67]. Vertebral osteomyelitis accounts for 1–2% of all children with osteomyelitis [68]. Primary pyogenic spinal infections are uncommon with a very low incidence between one and two per year per 32,500 pediatric hospital evaluations or one in 250,000 among the pediatric population [69].

Mortality Currently, the mortality is lower than 5% due to advances in diagnosis and management [66].

Morbidity Nontuberculous spondylodiscitis can be benign in the older child but, in infants, can lead to serious spinal deformities and segmental instabilities due to extensive bony destruction, severe kyphosis, and irreversible neurologic complications if the infection spreads into the spinal canal or epidural space [70].

Affected sites Discitis occurs almost exclusively in the lumbar region, while vertebral osteomyelitis affects the lumbosacral, thoracolumbar, and cervical regions.

Causative microorganisms *Staphylococcus aureus* is the most common microorganism (30–80%) responsible for spinal infections followed by *Kingella kingae* [71]. Coagulase-negative staphylococci, several *Streptococcus* species, and *Escherichia coli* are other causative pathogens [69–71].

Patient Factors

Age and sex Spondylodiscitis is generally seen in younger children less than 5 years of age who present with no or low-grade fever [68, 69]. Vertebral osteomyelitis typically occurs in older children (peaking around adolescence) who present with fever and back pain in the lumbar, thoracic, or cervical regions. A significant male preponderance is seen [69]. The infantile form has profoundly serious manifestations. Children between 6 months and 4 years of age constitute 60% of childhood spondylodiscitis cases [69].

Tuberculosis

Tuberculosis affects a huge population of the world. It is a major cause of skeletal infection in many LMIC countries. The majority of the cases are diagnosed in the WHO regions of Southeast Asia (44% of the total cases) followed by Africa (25% cases) and the Western Pacific (18%). The cases diagnosed in other parts of the globe are as follows: the Eastern Mediterranean region (8.2%), the Americas (2.9%), and Europe (2.5%). Globally, an estimated 10.0 million (range, 8.9–11.0 million) people were diagnosed with TB in 2019. Of this group, children (age <15 years) constitute 12% of cases, i.e., approximately one million children are affected with TB. This number has been decreasing very slowly in the last few years [29]. Of all the cases with tuberculosis, less than 10% (approximately 5–6%) of cases are bone and joint tuberculosis [72], which approximately amounts to 50–60,000 new cases of bone and joint tuberculosis diagnosed every year.

Tuberculosis of the axial skeleton (vertebral column) is the most common form of skeletal tuberculosis. Spine involvement constitutes approximately 50% of all cases of skeletal tuberculosis. The most commonly affected areas in the spine are the thoracic spine or the thoracolumbar junction. Other areas that are affected include the hip, knee, foot, elbow, wrist, and shoulder. The hip and the knee constitute the majority of extraspinal tuberculosis sites [72–74]. In a minority of cases, tuberculosis may present as tuberculous dactylitis, or cold abscess. In the foot, the common areas of involvement are the calcaneus and the talus [75]. Multifocal involvement accounts for in 5–10% of all osteoarticular cases [76].

In children, an uncommon but peculiar presentation of tuberculosis is primary epiphyseal osteomyelitis. The most common site of involvement is the distal femoral epiphysis [77–79].

Multidrug-resistant (MDR) tuberculosis remains a challenge. Globally in 2019, 3.3% of new TB cases and 17.7% of previously treated cases had MDR/rifampicin-resistant tuberculosis. Worldwide in 2019, close to half a million people developed rifampicin-resistant TB (RR-TB), of which 78% had multidrug-resistant TB (MDR-TB). There is limited information on the exact burden of MDR TB in extraspinal tuberculosis in children. In a study from South Africa, 10.5% of children with extraspinal TB (TB involving hip, knee, foot) were found to be multidrug resistant [80]. Despite TB being a notifiable disease in several countries, there is a lack of epidemiological information about musculoskeletal tuberculosis in children. Going forward, registries or study groups are necessary to provide reliable data on bone and joint tuberculosis in children.

Hand Infections

Hand infections can be classified into septic arthritis, osteomyelitis, and flexor tenosynovitis; superficial spreading infections, such as cellulitis and necrotizing fasciitis; and closed space infections with collections of purulence [81].

Incidence Hand infections have been reported following 4–40% of various types of injuries in children [81].

Morbidity Due to varied presentations of children with hand infections, the chances of delayed diagnoses are high. As a result, a superficial infection could spread and progress to osteomyelitis and/or septic arthritis and result in significant morbidity or even amputation.

Affected sites The distal phalanges are the most common sites (38%), followed by the proximal phalanges and any of the metacarpals (in case of osteomyelitis) [82].

Causative microorganisms *Staphylococcus aureus* is the most commonly implicated microorganism. MRSA accounts for up to 65% of *Staphylococcus aureus* infections [82]. *Kingella kingae* has been reported to cause flexor tenosynovitis. In rare cases, *Streptococcus* species and coccidiomycosis may cause osteomyelitis. Bite wounds from both animals and humans can lead to Gram-negative anaerobic infections from organisms such as *Eikenella*, *Pasteurella*, and *Bacteroides*. Atypical infections are caused by various species of mycobacterium (*tuberculosis*, *marinum*) and fungi (sporotrichosis, coccidioidomycosis, cryptococcosis) [81].

Patient Factors

Risk factors Injuries, animal and human bites, and nosocomial infections are the most common causes of hand infections in children. Behaviors such as finger or thumb-sucking or biting predispose a child to develop these infections. Hematogenous spread is seen in osteomyelitis of the hand. Septic arthritis, though rare, is most commonly found in the fingertips. Immunosuppression may be a contributing factor to the development of infections in a child's hand.

Foot Infections

Incidence The calcaneus is the most common site of infection in the foot. Calcaneal osteomyelitis rates have been reported to be between 3% and 10% of all cases of pediatric osteomyelitis, with hematogenous origin reported in 43–63% of all pediatric calcaneal osteomyelitis cases [83].

Morbidity Complications of calcaneal osteomyelitis include chronic infection, growth arrest, leg length discrepancy, and spontaneous arthrodesis of the surrounding joints [84].

Affected sites Aside from the calcaneus, the talus, cuboid, and navicular bones are other sites of foot osteomyelitis.

Causative microorganisms *Staphylococcus aureus* is most commonly responsible in immunocompetent children, while *Salmonella* species are known to cause infections in immunocompromised children [85]. Pseudomonas infections are associated with thorn prick injuries or nail puncture wounds through the sole of a shoe.

Patient Factors

Age, sex There is no consistent age of occurrence for acute osteomyelitis of the calcaneus. Studies report age ranges of less than 2 years to 9 years, with an average age of about 7.6 years [84] and a male preponderance.

Risk factors Direct trauma due to penetrating injuries and hematogenous spread are important risk factors. Often, a delay in presentation, and hence, a delay in diagnosis and treatment, is seen due to atypical presentation. A history of prior injury or illness may not be present in a large proportion of cases.

Surgical Site Infections

The rate of infection after elective pediatric orthopedic surgery is less than 5% [86]. In a study from the United Kingdom involving elective non-spinal procedures, the infection rate was 4%. The most common organism was *Staphylococcus aureus*, and there were no infections with MRSA [30]. Most postoperative infections are caused by contamination of the surgical site with naturally occurring skin flora organisms, with *Staphylococcus aureus* and *Staphylococcus epidermidis* predominant. Infection after pediatric spine surgery forms an important group as the treatment may be prolonged and may involve readmission and surgical pediatric musculoskeletal infection (MSKI), epidemiology of, intervention. The infection rate after idiopathic scoliosis surgery is 1% [87, 88]. The infection rate is much higher in neuromuscular scoliosis; the reported rate is 12–14%, with 60% of patients having Gram-negative sepsis [89, 90].

The Kirschner wire is the most commonly used implant in pediatric orthopedic surgery. Very few studies have described Pediatric musculoskeletal infection (MSKI), epidemiology of, infections following the use of k wires. The reported rate is between 1% and 2% [91, 92]. The risk of serious infectious complications from the smooth wire in pediatric patients is low. The most common pathogen is MSSA followed by *Pseudomonas aeruginosa*.

Fungal Infections

A fungus is a member of the group of eukaryotic organisms that includes microorganisms such as yeasts and molds, as well as the more familiar mushrooms. They have a worldwide distribution, and about 120,000 species have been described, with over 300 that can be pathogenic to humans.

Fungi are silent killers, causing the death of over two million people every year, making fungal disease one of the top global causes of death, even ahead of TB and malaria. Globally, over 300 million people of all ages are estimated to suffer from a serious fungal infection every year. Vulnerable people from countries in the global south are disproportionately affected, and those afflicted with fungal disease live with difficult challenges secondary to morbidity, the inability to work, and the social stigma associated with the disease. Limited data on the number of patients diagnosed and poor measurement of disease morbidity means that the true scale of the problem is unknown [93, 94].

Although invasive fungal infections contribute substantially to human morbidity and mortality and their impact on human health is steadily growing, fungal musculoskeletal infections are still considered an uncommon disease. There has been a worldwide increase in the burden of invasive fungal musculoskeletal infections in children in recent times, due to the growing number of patients at risk. Travel and immigration have affected the geographic localization of several important fungal infections, which may be seen in nonendemic areas. The most common fungi causing musculoskeletal infections in children are *Candida*, *Aspergillus*, dimorphic fungi like *Blastomyces*, *Coccidioides*, *Histoplasma*, and *Cryptococcus*. Less common pathogens include *Sporothrix*, non-aspergillus filamentous fungi (hyaline *Hyphomycetes*, *Mucormycetes*, dematiaceous fungi), and eumycetes. There is a wide variation in the geographic distribution of musculoskeletal infection due to various types of fungal species.

Box 1.1 Key Learning Points

- Acute hematogenous osteomyelitis is the most common MSKI.
- Children <5 years are commonly affected.
- The tibia is the most commonly affected bone in osteomyelitis.
- The hip and knee are the commonly affected joints in septic arthritis.
- *Staphylococcus aureus* is the commonest pathogen.

References

1. Schwend RM. The burden of pediatric musculoskeletal diseases worldwide. Orthop Clin North Am. 2020;51:207–17.
2. Saavedra-Lozano J, Falup-Pecurariu O, Faust SN, et al. Bone and joint infections. Pediatr Infect Dis J. 2017;36:788–99.
3. Paakkonen M, Peltola H. Management of a child with suspected acute septic arthritis. Arch Dis Child. 2012;97:287–92.
4. Okubo Y, Nochioka K, Testa M. Nationwide survey of pediatric acute osteomyelitis in the USA. J Pediatr Orthop Part B. 2017;26:501–6.
5. Okubo Y, Nochioka K, Marcia T. Nationwide survey of pediatric septic arthritis in the United States. J Orthop. 2017;14:342–6.
6. Stoesser N, Pocock J, Moore CE, et al. The epidemiology of pediatric bone and joint infections in Cambodia, 2007-11. J Trop Pediatr. 2013;59:36–42.
7. Alves K, Penny N, Kobusingye O, Olupot R, Katz JN, Sabatini CS. Pediatric musculoskeletal disease in Kumi District, Uganda: a cross-sectional survey. Int Orthop. 2018;42:1967–73.
8. Murray C. Quantifying the burden of disease: the technical basis for disability-adjusted life years. Bull World Health Organ. 1994;72:429–45.
9. Murray C, Lopez AD. The global burden of disease: a comprehensive assessment of mortality and disability from diseases, injuries, and risk factors in 1990 and projected to 2020: Summary, 1996.
10. Murray C, Acharya A. Understanding DALYs. J Health Econ. 1997;16:703–30.
11. Vos T, Alemu Abajobir A, Hassen Abate K, et al. Global, regional, and national incidence, prevalence, and years lived with disability for 328 diseases and injuries for 195 countries, 1990-2016: a systematic analysis for the Global Burden of Disease Study 2016. Lancet. 2017;390:1211–59.
12. Joshipura M, Mock C, Gosselin RA. Global burden of musculoskeletal conditions. In: Gosselin R, Spiegel D, Foltz M, editors. Global orthopedics. New York, Cham: Springer; 2014. p. 9–11.
13. Poultsides L, Liaropoulos L, Malizos K. The socioeconomic impact of musculoskeletal infections. J Bone Jt Surg Am. 2010;92:e13.
14. Malizos KN. Global forum: the burden of bone and joint infections: a growing demand for more resources. J Bone Jt Surg Am. 2017;99-A:e20. (1–7).
15. Bickler S, Ozgediz D, Gosselin R, et al. Key concepts for estimating the burden of surgical conditions and the unmet need for surgical care. World J Surg. 2010;34:374–80.
16. Rosenfeld SB, Schroeder K, Watkins-Castillo SI. The economic burden of musculoskeletal disease in children and adolescents in the United States. J Pediatr Orthop. 2018;38:e230–6.
17. Atijosan O, Simms V, Kuper H, Rischewski D, Lavy C. The orthopaedic needs of children in Rwanda: results from a national survey and orthopaedic service implications. J Pediatr Orthop. 2009;29:948–51.
18. Matheson JI, Atijosan O, Kuper H, Rischewski D, Simms V, Lavy C. Musculoskeletal impairment of traumatic etiology in Rwanda: prevalence, causes, and service implications. World J Surg. 2011;35:2635–42.
19. Alves K, Penny N, Kobusingye O, Olupot R, Katz JN, Sabatini C. Paediatric musculoskeletal disease in Kumi District, Uganda: a cross-sectional survey. Int Orthop. 2018;42:1967–73.
20. Qudsi RA, Roberts HJ, Bhashyam AR, et al. A self-reported needs assessment survey of pediatric orthopaedic education in Haiti. J Surg Educ. 2018;75:140–6.
21. Street M, Puna R, Huang M, Crawford H. Pediatric acute hematogenous osteomyelitis. J Pediatr Orthop. 2015;35:634–9.
22. Stanley CM, Rutherford GW, Morshed S, Coughlin RR, Beyeza T. Estimating the healthcare burden of osteomyelitis in Uganda. Trans R Soc Trop Med Hyg. 2010;104:139–42.
23. Munshi B, MacFater W, Hill AG, McCaig EH. Paediatric osteomyelitis in Fiji. World J Surg. 2018;42:4118–22.
24. Bickler SW, Sanno-Duanda B. Epidemiology of paediatric surgical admissions to a government referral hospital in the Gambia. Bull World Health Organ. 2000;78:1330–6.
25. Jones HW, Beckles VLL, Akinola B, Stevenson AJ, Harrison WJ. Chronic haematogenous osteomyelitis in children. An unsolved problem. J Bone Joint Surg Br. 2011;93-B:1005–10.
26. Schoenecker J, The Children's Orthopaedic Trauma and Infection Consortium for Evidence Based Study (CORTICES) Group. Defining the volume of consultations for musculoskeletal infection encountered by pediatric orthopaedic services in the United States. PLoS One. 2020;15:e0234055.
27. Koehler R, Baldwin KD, Copley LA, et al. The epidemiology and regional burden of musculoskeletal infection in pediatric orthopaedics. Pediatrics. 2018; https://doi.org/10.1016/j.solener.2019.02.027.
28. The World Health Organization. The world health report 2003 – shaping the future. Geneva: World Health Organization; 2003.
29. World Health Organization. Global tuberculosis report 2020: executive summary. Geneva: World Health Organization; 2020.
30. Jones S, Shepherd J, Robinson K, Khandekar SA. Surgical site infection following elective non-spinal paediatric orthopaedic surgery: a prospective review. J Pediatr Orthop Part B. 2019;28:89–93.
31. de Chagas MQL, Costa AMM, Mendes PHB, Gomes SC. Analysis of surgical site infections in pediatric

patients after orthopedic surgery. Rev Paul Pediatr. 2017;35:18–24.
32. Serajuddin U, Hamadeh N. New World Bank country classifications by income level: 2020–2021. 2020. https://blogs.worldbank.org/opendata/new-world-bank-country-classifications-income-level-2020-2021. Accessed 10 Feb 2021.
33. Murray C, Kreuser J, Whang W. Cost-effectiveness analysis and policy choices: investing in health systems. Bull World Health Organ. 1994;72:663–74.
34. Spiegel DA, Abdullah F, Price RR, Gosselin RA, Bickler SW. World Health Organization global initiative for emergency and essential surgical care: 2011 and beyond. World J Surg. 2013;37:1462–9.
35. Goodman LF, St-Louis E, Yousef Y, et al. The global initiative for children's surgery: optimal resources for improving care. Eur J Pediatr Surg. 2018;28:51–9.
36. Dartnell J, Ramachandran M, Katchburian M. Haematogenous acute and subacute paediatric osteomyelitis. J Bone Jt Surg – Ser B. 2012;94 B:584–95.
37. Iliadis AD, Ramachandran M. Paediatric bone and joint infection. EFORT Open Rev. 2017;2:7–12.
38. Jaramillo D, Dormans JP, Delgado J, Laor T, St Geme JW III. Hematogenous osteomyelitis in infants and children: imaging of a changing disease. Radiology. 2017;283:629–43.
39. Gigante A, Coppa V, Marinelli M, Giampaolini N, Falcioni D, Specchia N. Acute osteomyelitis and septic arthritis in children: a systematic review of systematic reviews. Eur Rev Med Pharmacol Sci. 2019;23:145–58.
40. Kang S-N, Sanghera T, Mangwani J, Paterson JMH, Ramachandran M. The management of septic arthritis in children. Systematic review of the english language literature. J Bone Jt Surg [Br]. 2009;91B:1127–33.
41. Comegna L, Guidone PI, Prezioso G, et al. Pyomyositis is not only a tropical pathology: a case series. J Med Case Rep. 2016; https://doi.org/10.1186/s13256-016-1158-2.
42. Maravelas R, Melgar TA, Vos D, Lima N, Sadarangani S. Pyomyositis in the United States 2002–2014. J Infect. 2020;80:497–503.
43. Shittu A, Deinhardt-Emmer S, Vas Nunes J, Niemann S, Grobusch MP, Schaumburg F. Tropical pyomyositis: an update. Trop Med Int Heal. 2020;25:660–5.
44. Peltola H, Paäkkonen M. Acute osteomyelitis in children. N Engl J Med. 2014;370:352–60.
45. Riise ØR, Kirkhus E, Handeland KS, et al. Childhood osteomyelitis-incidence and differentiation from other acute onset musculoskeletal features in a population-based study. BMC Pediatr. 2008;8:45.
46. Cohen E, Lifshitz K, Fruchtman Y, Eidelman M, Leibovitz E. Current data on acute haematogenous osteomyelitis in children in Southern Israel: epidemiology, microbiology, clinics and therapeutic consequences. Int Orthop. 2016;40:1987–94.
47. Blyth M, Kincaid R, Craigen M, Bennet G. The changing epidemiology of acute and subacute haematogenous osteomyelitis in children. J Bone Jt Surg [Br]. 2001;83-B:99–102.
48. Pääkkönen M, Peltola H. Bone and joint infections. Pediatr Clin N Am. 2013;60:425–36.
49. Frank G, Mahoney HM, Eppes SC. Musculoskeletal infections in children. Pediatr Clin N Am. 2005;52:1083–106.
50. Cooper AM, Shope AJ, Javid M, Ali P, Chinoy MA, Parvizi J. Musculoskeletal infection in pediatrics. J Bone Jt Surg Am. 2019;101-A:e133. (1–7).
51. Yeo A, Ramachandran M. Acute haematogenous osteomyelitis in children. BMJ. 2014;348:g66.
52. Stevenson AJ, Jones HW, Chokotho LC, Beckles VLL, Harrison WJ. The Beit CURE classification of childhood chronic haematogenous osteomyelitis – a guide to treatment. J Orthop Surg Res. 2015;10:1–10.
53. Agarwal A, Aggarwal AN. Bone and joint infections in children: acute hematogenous osteomyelitis. Indian J Pediatr. 2016;83:817–24.
54. Thakolkaran N, Shetty A. Acute hematogenous osteomyelitis in children. Ochsner J. 2019;19:116–22.
55. Lindsay EA, Tareen N, Jo C-H, Copley LA. Seasonal variation and weather changes related to the occurrence and severity of acute hematogenous osteomyelitis in children. J Pediatric Infect Dis Soc. 2018;7:e16–23.
56. Calvo C, Núñez E, Camacho M, et al. Epidemiology and management of acute, uncomplicated septic arthritis and osteomyelitis spanish multicenter study. Pediatr Infect Dis J. 2016;35:1288–93.
57. García-Arias M, Balsa A, Mola EM. Septic arthritis. Best Pract Res Clin Rheumatol. 2011;25:407–21.
58. Rutz E, Spoerri M. Septic arthritis of the paediatric hip – a review of current diagnostic approaches and therapeutic concepts. Acta Orthop Belg. 2013;79:123–34.
59. Agarwal A, Aggarwal AN. Bone and joint infections in children: septic arthritis. Indian J Pediatr. 2016;83:825–33.
60. Rosenfeld S, Bernstein DT, Daram S, Dawson J, Zhang W. Predicting the presence of adjacent infections in septic arthritis in children. J Pediatr Orthop. 2016;36:70–4.
61. Pannaraj PS, Hulten KG, Gonzalez BE, Mason EO, Kaplan SL. Infective pyomyositis and myositis in children in the era of community-acquired, methicillin-resistant Staphylococcus aureus infection. Clin Infect Dis. 2006;43:953–60.
62. Chattopadhyay B, Mukhopadhyay M, Chatterjee A, Biswas PKA, Chatterjee N, Debnath NB. Tropical pyomyositis. N Am J Med Sci. 2013;5:600–3.
63. Borgesálvaro HD, Faragher B, Lalloo DG. Pyomyositis in the upper Negro river basin, Brazilian Amazonia. Trans R Soc Trop Med Hyg. 2012;106:532–7.
64. Verma S, Singhi SC, Marwaha RK, Singhi P, Singh S, Singh M. Tropical pyomyositis in children: 10 years experience of a tertiary care hospital in Northern India. J Trop Pediatr. 2013;59:243–5.

65. Taksande A, Vilhekar K, Gupta S. Primary pyomyositis in a child. Int J Infect Dis. 2009;13:149–51.
66. Principi N, Esposito S. Infectious discitis and spondylodiscitis in children. Int J Mol Sci. 2016; https://doi.org/10.3390/ijms17040539.
67. De Moraes Barros M, Fucs P, Meves R, Yamada HH. Spinal infections in children: a review. Int Orthop. 2012;36:387–95.
68. Fernandez M, Carrol CL, Baker CJ. Discitis and vertebral osteomyelitis in children: an 18-year review. Pediatrics. 2000;105:1299–304.
69. Dayer R, Alzahrani MM, Saran N, et al. Spinal infections in children: a multicentre retrospective study. Bone Jt J. 2018;100B:542–8.
70. Garron E, Viehweger E, Launay F, Guillaume JM, Jouve JL, Bollini G. Nontuberculous spondylodiscitis in children. J Pediatr Orthop. 2002;22:321–8.
71. Gouliouris T, Aliyu SH, Brown NM. Spondylodiscitis: update on diagnosis and management. J Antimicrob Chemother. 2010;65:iii11–24.
72. Leonard MK, Blumberg HM. Musculoskeletal tuberculosis. Microbiol Spectr. 2017; https://doi.org/10.1128/microbiolspec.TNMI7-0046-2017.
73. Tuli S. Tuberculosis of the skeletal system: bones, joints, spine and bursal sheaths. 5th ed. New Delhi: Jaypee Brothers Medical Publishers (P) Ltd.; 2016.
74. Held MF, Hoppe S, Laubscher M, et al. Epidemiology of musculoskeletal tuberculosis in an area with high disease prevalence. Asian Spine J. 2017;11:405–11.
75. Agarwal A, Qureshi NA, Khan SA, Kumar P, Samaiya S. Tuberculosis of the foot and ankle in children. J Orthop Surg. 2011;19:213–7.
76. Agarwal A. Paediatric osteoarticular tuberculosis: a review. J Clin Orthop Trauma. 2020;11:202–7.
77. Shah MM, Gupta G, Makadia AS, Rabbi Q. Primary Epiphyseal Osteomyelitis (PEO) in 18 children: a rare entity with atypical features. J Pediatr Orthop. 2020;40:361–6.
78. Yoo WJ, Choi IH, Yun Y-H, et al. Primary epiphyseal osteomyelitis caused by mycobacterium species in otherwise healthy toddlers. J Bone Jt Surg Am. 2014;96:e145.
79. Agarwal A, Gupta N, Mishra M, Agrawal N, Kumar D. Primary epiphyseal and metaepiphyseal tubercular osteomyelitis in children: a series of 8 cases. Acta Orthop Belg. 2016;82:797–805.
80. Firth GB, Lescheid J, Camacho M, et al. Extraspinal osteoarticular multidrug-resistant tuberculosis in children: a case series. South African Med J. 2017;107:983–6.
81. Kroonen L. Pediatric hand infections. In: Pediatr. up. extrem. San Diego: Springer Science Business Media; 2014. p. 1–25.
82. Flevas DA, Syngouna S, Fandridis E, Tsiodras S, Mavrogenis AF. Infections of the hand: an overview. EFORT Open Rev. 2019;4:183–93.
83. Mooney ML, Haidet K, Liu J, Ebraheim NA. Hematogenous calcaneal osteomyelitis in children: a systematic review of the literature. Foot Ankle Spec. 2017;20:63–8.
84. Leigh W, Crawford H, Street M, Huang M, Manners S, Puna R. Pediatric calcaneal osteomyelitis. J Pediatr Orthop. 2010;30:888–92.
85. Abdulla M, Khaled YS, Kapoor H. Salmonella osteomyelitis of the calcaneum bone in an immunocompetent child. J Pediatr Orthop Part B. 2014;23:270–3.
86. Khoshbin A, So JP, Aleem IS, Stephens D, Matlow AG, Wright JG. Antibiotic prophylaxis to prevent surgical site infections in children: a prospective cohort study. Ann Surg. 2015;262:397–402.
87. Newton PO, Bastrom TP, Yaszay B. Patient-specific risk adjustment improves comparison of infection rates following posterior fusion for adolescent idiopathic scoliosis. J Bone Jt Surg Am. 2017;99:1846–50.
88. Du JY, Poe-Kochert C, Thompson GH, Son-Hing JP, Hardesty CK, Mistovich RJ. Risk factors for early infection in pediatric spinal deformity surgery: a multivariate analysis. Spine Deform. 2019;7:410–6.
89. Janjua MB, Toll B, Ghandi S, et al. Risk factors for wound infections after deformity correction surgery in neuromuscular scoliosis. Pediatr Neurosurg. 2019;54:108–15.
90. Minkara AA, Matsumoto H, Glotzbecker M, et al. A multicenter study of the epidemiology of deep surgical site infections in children with nonidiopathic early-onset scoliosis including associated pathogens. Spine Deform. 2019;7:647–51.
91. Tosti R, Foroohar A, Pizzutillo PD, Herman MJ. Kirschner wire infections in pediatric orthopaedic surgery. J Pediatr Orthop. 2015;35:69–73.
92. Varik K, Kirsimägi U, Värimäe E, Eller M, Lõivukene R, Kübarsepp V. Incidence and risk factors of surgical wound infection in children: a prospective study. Scand J Surg. 2010;99:162–6.
93. Gamaletsou MN, Walsh TJ, Sipsas NV. Epidemiology of fungal osteomyelitis. Curr Fungal Infect Rep. 2014;8:262–70.
94. Fungal Disease Frequency – Gaffi | Gaffi - Global Action Fund for Fungal Infections. https://www.gaffi.org/why/fungal-disease-frequency/. Accessed 9 Feb 2021.

The Microbiology of Musculoskeletal Infections and Antibiotic Therapies

2

Jesus Vallejo, Anish P. Sanghrajka, and J. Chase McNeil

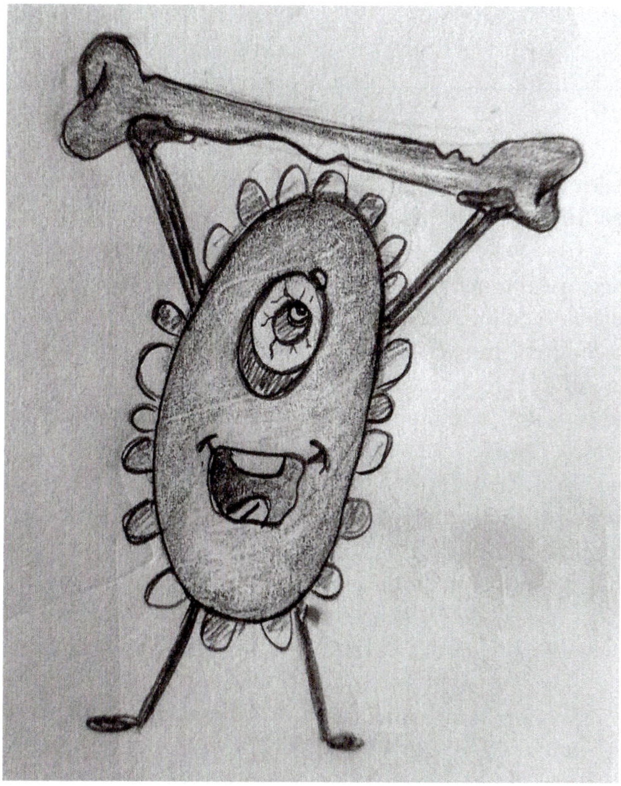

J. Vallejo · J. C. McNeil (✉)
Department of Pediatrics, Division of Infectious Diseases, Baylor College of Medicine, Houston, TX, USA
e-mail: jvallejo@bcm.edu; jm140109@bcm.edu

A. P. Sanghrajka
Department of Trauma and Orthopaedics, Norfolk & Norwich University Hospitals, Norfolk, UK

© Springer Nature Switzerland AG 2022
M. V. Belthur et al. (eds.), *Pediatric Musculoskeletal Infections*,
https://doi.org/10.1007/978-3-030-95794-0_2

Introduction

Antimicrobial therapy is a critical component in the management of childhood osteoarticular infections. Given the nature of infectious diseases, knowledge of the likely causative organisms is essential in the selection of empiric therapy. The microbiology of osteoarticular infections in children varies tremendously with pathogenesis, epidemiology, and clinical presentation. In addition, questions often arise as to the optimal duration and route of therapy. In this chapter, we will review relevant literature regarding the microbial etiologies and antimicrobial management of osteoarticular infections in children.

Microbiology

Acute Osteoarticular Infections (Osteomyelitis and Septic Arthritis)

Staphylococcus aureus is the most common cause of hematogenous acute osteoarticular infections (AOIs) in children. In a 2012 meta-analysis, Dartnell et al. [1] reported that *S. aureus* was identified in ~66% of culture-positive osteomyelitis cases. McNeil et al. [2] reported that *S. aureus* was the most common pathogen (62.8%) causing acute osteomyelitis at Texas Children's Hospital (TCH) in Houston, Texas. *S. aureus* also is the most common cause of acute septic arthritis. In a study by Branson et al., *S. aureus* accounted for 47.7% of all septic arthritis cases [3].

The prevalence of community-associated methicillin-resistant *S. aureus* (CA-MRSA) varies by geographic location and has changed in the United States over the past 20 years [4, 5]. Between 2001 and 2004, CA-MRSA caused 62.9% of *S. aureus* AOIs at TCH [6]. These investigators noted that AOIs caused by *S. aureus* strains carrying the genes encoding Panton-Valentine leukocidin (PVL), an exotoxin which promotes lysis of leukocytes, were associated with more severe local disease and a greater systemic inflammatory response compared with AOI caused by PVL negative strains. More recent studies have demonstrated a substantial decline in CA-MRSA [4, 5]. McNeil et al. have reported that between 2011 and 2017, MRSA caused only 27.6% of staphylococcal acute hematogenous osteoarticular infections in children [7]. This study also found that *agr* group III *S. aureus* strains were associated with increased risk of orthopedic sequelae. In contrast, carriage of PVL or methicillin resistance was not a predictor of long-term orthopedic complications.

In contrast to the United States, CA-MRSA-associated AOI has a significantly lower prevalence in Europe (2.5% Spain, 8.5% France) and is rare in the United Kingdom [8]. In a randomized controlled trial of 131 culture-positive acute osteomyelitis in Finish children, no cases of MRSA infection occurred [9].

Streptococcus pyogenes (Group A *Streptococcus*, GAS) may cause AOIs in older infants and children. In two different studies, it has accounted for 6.8–8% of acute osteomyelitis cases [1, 2]. Similarly, in a recent study, GAS was the second most common cause (8.9%) of septic arthritis [3].

Streptococcus pneumoniae AOIs are well-described but relatively uncommon, accounting for <1% of osteomyelitis [2, 10]. In a 16-year review, Olarte et al. reported that AOIs accounted for only 3% of all invasive pneumococcal disease [11]. Septic arthritis (56.7%) was the most common AOI reported in this series, and patients were more likely to be less than 3 years of age.

Streptococcus agalactiae (Group B *Streptococcus*, GBS) is a well-described cause of AOIs in infants younger than 3 months of age [12, 13]. AOI is, however, a relatively rare manifestation of GBS disease. In one study, AOIs accounted for only 4% of GBS late-onset invasive disease [14].

Kingella kingae is a significant cause of osteomyelitis and septic arthritis in children under the age of 4 years [15]. This organism is often difficult to isolate in culture but identification may be aided with the use of molecular diagnostics. Since the introduction of nucleic acid amplification tests in Switzerland, *K. kingae* now accounts for 51% of confirmed AOIs in children 6–48 months of age [16]. In contrast, other pyogenic bacteria accounted for <5% of OAI in this age group.

Nontyphoidal *Salmonella* species (NTS) may cause AOIs in children with major sickle cell hemoglobinopathies and rarely in otherwise healthy children with exposure to reptiles or a history of preceding gastrointestinal symptoms [17, 18]. Kaplan et al. recently reported that in an area with endemic CA-MRSA, NTS remain the most common cause (61%) of AOIs in children with sickle cell hemoglobinopathies [19].

Brodie's Abscess

Brodie's abscess is a subacute form of hematogenous osteomyelitis that is characterized by intraosseous abscess formation. A paucity of systemic symptoms along with the absence of a clear history of trauma make the diagnosis challenging. In two recent studies (including a systematic review), *S. aureus* was the most common (60–67%) pathogen reported to be isolated from Brodie's abscesses [20, 21]. Other less common pathogens identified from a Brodie's abscess include *Salmonella* spp., *K. kingae*, and *Pseudomonas* spp. [20]. It is important to note that in up to 33% of such cases, a pathogen is not identified [21].

Penetrating Trauma/Direct Inoculation Osteomyelitis

Non-hematogenous osteomyelitis can occur as a result of contiguous spread of infection to bones and/or joints from adjacent soft tissues or via direct inoculation into the bone as a result of trauma, surgery (e.g., hardware placement, sternotomy, etc.), or a poorly healing decubitus ulcer.

In pediatric AOIs following penetrating trauma or direct inoculation, the most commonly isolated organisms include *S. aureus*, *Enterobacter* spp., and fungi [22]. Polymicrobial infections also are common (38.2%) in trauma-related AOI. In soil-contaminated wounds, less commonly implicated pathogens include *Enterococcus* species, anaerobes, and nontuberculous mycobacteria [23]. *Pseudomonas aeruginosa* is a common cause of puncture wound osteomyelitis, especially when a history of a puncture wound through a shoe is present [24]. In small case series, the presence of retained foreign bodies, particularly organic material (such as twigs, grass, etc.), has been strongly associated with either fungal or mycobacterial osteomyelitis [22, 25, 26]. Importantly, however, skin flora such as *S. aureus* and streptococci also have been frequently implicated in cases of puncture wound osteomyelitis.

Discitis and Vertebral Osteomyelitis

The etiology of discitis is controversial. It has been proposed that discitis in children represents low-grade infection and is on one end of the spectrum of vertebral osteomyelitis. When disk biopsy is performed, the yield for a pathogen ranges from 0 to 62.6%, with *S. aureus* being the most common isolate [27–29]. In one series from France, *K. kingae* was identified as the cause of discitis in 27% of cases [29]. This study, however, did not provide data on the source of the culture (i.e., blood vs. tissue culture).

S. aureus is isolated in most cases of vertebral osteomyelitis [27, 30]. However, in a review of the literature, Correa et al. reported that *Salmonella* spp. caused 12% of cases of childhood vertebral osteomyelitis [30]. Vertebral osteomyelitis can also be an atypical presentation of *Bartonella henselae* infection. Tuberculosis and brucellosis should also be considered if symptoms and radiographs suggest chronic infection (discussed in Chaps. 16, 17, and 30).

Chronic Osteomyelitis (CO)

CO develops as a complication of primary acute hematogenous osteomyelitis in less than 5% of cases. In these cases, *S. aureus* is the most common pathogen isolated [31, 32]. CO may also develop more commonly as a complication of non-hematogenous osteomyelitis (e.g., from a contiguous focus of infection or post-traumatic osteomyelitis). In a recent pediatric study, the most commonly isolated organism in cases of CO from a contiguous focus of infection was *Pseudomonas* spp. [32]. Dubey et al. reported that CO from a contiguous focus of infection was polymicrobial in 33% of cases (including skin flora and gram-negative bacilli) [33]. Polymicrobial infections are also common in CO that develops as a complication of hardware-associated and trauma-associated infections.

Fungal Osteomyelitis

Fungi can cause osteomyelitis via (1) direct inoculation after surgery or traumatic injuries with open wounds or those contaminated with soil, (2) contiguous extension from a nearby focus of infection, and (3) rarely, hematogenous dissemination. Hematogenous fungal osteomyelitis is most frequently caused by *Candida* spp. and is unusual in healthy children, but it does occur in premature neonates and immunocompromised patients. In one series that included pediatric patients, the most common *Candida* species recovered were *C. albicans* (65%) followed by *C. tropicalis* (16%), *C. glabrata* (8%), and *C. parapsilosis* (7%) [34]. Children with chronic granulomatous disease are at risk of developing fungal osteomyelitis caused by *Aspergillus* spp. infection [35]. *Blastomyces dermatitidis*, *Coccidioides immitis*, *Histoplasma capsulatum*, and *Cryptococcus neoformans* can cause osteomyelitis in endemic regions in both normal and immunosuppressed patients [36].

Microbiology of Infections Associated with Orthopedic Implants

Implant-related infection in children undergoing orthopedic surgery is significantly less of a problem than in the adult population. In a study investigating surgical site infection (SSI) in children undergoing procedures without an orthopedic implant, an SSI rate of 1% was found overall; the SSI rate was 1.8% for those undergoing musculoskeletal surgical procedures [37]. Perhaps as a consequence of this low incidence, most reports of complications for orthopedic surgical interventions in children in the literature do not report rates of infection. In a study of 138 children undergoing hip surgery, only 2 required reoperation for deep infection (1.4%) [38]. Spinal surgery in children carries higher rates of infection than operations on the limbs, with rates of 10% reported in the literature [39]. Consequently, the biggest body of work examining hardware-related infection in children, and the responsible pathogens, is in the context of spinal surgery. Neuromuscular conditions such as cerebral palsy appear to significantly increase the risk of SSI and deep infection (fourfold for proximal femoral osteotomy [40] and up to tenfold for spinal surgery [41]).

Studies show that *S. aureus* is the most common pathogen in these cases, whatever the underlying pathology [40, 41]. Other commonly implicated organisms are the coagulase-negative staphylococci (e.g., *S. epidermidis*), gram-positive anaerobic cocci, *Pseudomonas*, and *Enterobacteriaceae* (the latter two being much more prevalent in non-idiopathic, neuromuscular-type cases). These organisms are also the most commonly implicated in prosthetic joint infection in the adult population. Almost half of implant-related infections are polymicrobial [41].

The causative bacteria species varies with the time elapsed between surgery and presentation of infection. Spinal instrumentation infections have often been characterized as early onset vs. late onset in the literature. Early-onset infections have variably been defined as those occurring from 30 days to 6 months post-surgery [42–46]. Early-onset infections have often been associated with the more virulent organisms such as *S. aureus*, while later infections may be caused by more indolent organisms such as *S. epidermidis*.

Infections associated with orthopedic hardware are typically caused by microorganisms that may exist in biofilms [47], making them very difficult to treat (summarized in Table 2.1). With a sufficiently high microbial density, the high volume of released cell-to-cell signaling molecules

Table 2.1 Features of the biofilm contributing to difficulty eradicating infection

Increased horizontal gene transfer for antibiotic resistance
Bacteria enter dormant "persister" state with metabolic inactivity
Limited antibiotic penetration
Antibiotic binding and degradation within the EPS
Antibiotic concentration gradient resulting in sublethal concentrations increasing antibiotic tolerance
EPS limits polymorphonuclear leukocyte and granulocyte function
Impaired antibody reactions to bacteria within a mature biofilm

activates genes involved in biofilm production. These microorganisms form an organized, complex community within a self-produced extracellular polymeric substance (EPS) comprising polysaccharides, proteins, lipids, and extracellular DNA. The EPS binds these cells to the surface of the implant and to each other, shielding them from the host's immune responses and from antimicrobial agents [48].

The biofilm bacteria communicate through chemical ("quorum sensing") [49] or electrical signals which can modulate gene expression within the bacterial cells allowing diversity and the ability to adapt to a changing environment [48]. The close proximity of cells within biofilms facilitates horizontal gene transfer, allowing them to share virulence and antibiotic resistance genes. While the peripheral bacteria in the biofilm consume nutrients, the bacteria in the central area of the biofilm are left with a relative deprivation of nutritional resource, causing them to enter a dormant metabolically inactive "persister" state [48]. This increases these cells' ability to withstand high concentrations of antibiotic [50], particularly as the activity of many antimicrobials (such as β-lactams) is dependent on active cell replication.

Once established, biofilm-related implant infections can be extremely difficult to identify and also to eradicate. The minimum biofilm eradication concentration (MBEC) is the concentration of an antimicrobial agent required to kill a bacterial biofilm and is generally 100–1000 times greater than its minimum inhibitory concentration (MIC) [51]. Furthermore, the impaired immune response in the presence of foreign material results in a one-million-fold reduction in the bacterial load required for abscess formation [48].

Medical Management

Acute Hematogenous Osteomyelitis (AHO)

Empiric Therapy

Given the predominance of *S. aureus* as a pathogen of acute hematogenous osteoarticular infection, empiric therapy should, in general, be directed toward this agent unless risk factors for other organisms exist. As the pathogens that cause both osteomyelitis and septic arthritis are very similar, the approach to empiric therapy in general is the same for both diseases. The European Society for Pediatric Infectious Diseases (ESPID) recently published guidelines for the management of osteomyelitis and septic arthritis in children [8]. In regions with a low prevalence of methicillin-resistant *S. aureus* (MRSA), therapy with either an antistaphylococcal penicillin (ASP, e.g., nafcillin, flucloxacillin, etc.) or first-generation cephalosporin (1GC, e.g., cefazolin, cephalexin, etc.) is recommended (Tables 2.2 and 2.3, Fig. 2.1). While not specifically endorsed by the ESPID guidelines, ceftriaxone also has in vitro activity against methicillin-susceptible *S. aureus* (MSSA) and may be a reasonable alternative.

Historically, many experts have preferred ASPs over 1GCs; however several studies have shown that use of 1GCs are associated with similar outcomes to ASPs in serious MSSA infections outside the central nervous system (CNS) [52–54]. Additionally, some authors have expressed concerns that excessive production of β-lactamases may occur in the setting of serious deep-seated *S. aureus* infection leading to clinically significant inactivation of 1GCs (the so-called cefazolin inoculum effect) [55]. However, in a recent multicenter observational study of MSSA AHO in children, use of a 1GC relative to alternative therapy was not associated with treatment failure even when the inoculum effect was

Table 2.2 Suggested pathogen-specific agents for AHO

Pathogen	Suggested agents
Methicillin-susceptible *S. aureus*	Nafcillin, flucloxacillin, dicloxacillin Cefazolin, cephalexin Vancomycin Clindamycin Daptomycin Ceftaroline Linezolid Trimethoprim-sulfamethoxazole
Methicillin-resistant *S. aureus*	Vancomycin Clindamycin Daptomycin Ceftaroline Linezolid Trimethoprim-sulfamethoxazole
Group A *Streptococcus*	Penicillin (drug of choice) Ampicillin, amoxicillin Cefazolin, cephalexin Ceftriaxone, oral third-generation cephalosporins Vancomycin Clindamycin Linezolid
Kingella kingae	Cephalosporins Penicillins (if known to be β-lactamase negative) Trimethoprim-sulfamethoxazole
Salmonella spp.	Cephalosporins Ampicillin (if susceptible) Fluoroquinolones
Pneumococcus	Penicillin Ampicillin, amoxicillin Third-generation cephalosporins Fluoroquinolones
Haemophilus influenzae	Ampicillin/amoxicillin (if known to be β-lactamase-negative) Third-generation cephalosporins
Gonococcus	Ceftriaxone/cefotaxime + azithromycin[a]

Note: This table is not intended to be comprehensive in terms of pathogens or antimicrobials. Therapy should always ultimately be guided by antimicrobial susceptibility testing and clinical judgment

[a]Concomitant empiric treatment of *Chlamydia trachomatis* is generally recommended with gonococcal infection

accounted for [56]. Based on available evidence, ASPs and 1GCs appear equally efficacious in the treatment of MSSA AHO and other serious infections outside the CNS.

Overall, the likelihood of osteoarticular infection being caused by MRSA would be expected to be influenced by the prevalence of MRSA in the community as well as individual patient risk factors. The ESPID guidelines recommend providing empiric coverage for MRSA when the proportion of *S. aureus* that are methicillin-resistant exceeds 10–15% locally ([8] Fig. 2.1). Vancomycin is generally regarded as the agent of choice for serious MRSA infections in children [57]. In patients with musculoskeletal infection who are critically ill, some experts recommend a combination of vancomycin with an antistaphylococcal β-lactam pending culture data. Clindamycin may also be considered an alternative for empiric therapy for MRSA in noncritically ill patients and avoids the potential nephrotoxicity of vancomycin. Clindamycin has been demonstrated to be effective in the treatment of serious MRSA infections and well tolerated in children [58, 59]. Rising rates of clindamycin-resistant *S. aureus* in certain regions can make selection of empiric therapy challenging; some centers have reported clindamycin resistance in up to 20% of isolates [60]. Per ESPID guidelines, clindamycin can be considered for empiric therapy of AHO in regions in which the clindamycin resistance rate is <10–15% provided the patient is not critically ill. Interestingly, some investigators have reported that clindamycin resistance may be more common among MSSA than MRSA in certain regions [4]. Linezolid may be considered an alternative agent for coverage of MRSA in areas of relatively high clindamycin resistance. Daptomycin and ceftaroline have also been used successfully to treat staphylococcal AHO although experience is limited with these agents [61–63]. All of these agents also have the advantage of reliably providing coverage for GAS (although penicillin is the drug of choice).

In children <5 years of age, additional coverage for *K. kingae* may be necessary [8], particularly in the regions requiring empiric therapy directed at MRSA. *K. kingae* are universally resistant to vancomycin and frequently clindamycin as well. Importantly, *K. kingae* may rarely produce a β-lactamase [64], although sensitivity

Table 2.3 Potential antimicrobial agents in osteoarticular infections, routes of administration, and adverse events

Class	Examples of Specific Drug	IV/PO	Adverse Events	Comments
Antistaphylococcal penicillins	Nafcillin, oxacillin, flucloxacillin	IV	Neutropenia, transaminase elevation, phlebitis, nephritis	Not active against MRSA, *Kingella*
	Dicloxacillin, flucloxacillin	PO		
First-generation cephalosporins	Cefazolin	IV	Neutropenia, transaminase elevation, nephritis	Not active against MRSA
	Cephalexin	PO		
Glycopeptides	Vancomycin	IV	Nephrotoxicity, cytopenias, infusion reactions, rash	Careful monitoring of renal function is advised
Lincosamides	Clindamycin	IV/PO	Transaminase elevation, antibiotic-associated diarrhea (common), *Clostridium difficile* diarrhea (rare)	High oral bioavailability. Liquid formulation often has a foul taste. Clindamycin resistance among staphylococci is common in some regions
Oxazolidinones	Linezolid	IV/PO	Neutropenia, thrombocytopenia (common), transaminase elevation, peripheral neuropathy (rare), optic neuropathy (rare)	High oral bioavailability. Tyramine-containing foods should be avoided. Close monitoring for adverse events is advised. Costs may limit utilization
Lipopeptide	Daptomycin	IV	Rhabdomyolysis (rare), transaminase elevation	Data are limited in children with osteoarticular infections. In animal models, daptomycin appears to be inactivated by pulmonary surfactant
"Fifth-generation cephalosporins"	Ceftaroline	IV	Cytopenias, rash, abdominal pain	Data are limited in children with osteoarticular infections
Sulfonamides	Trimethoprim-sulfamethoxazole	IV/PO	Cytopenias, rash, nephritis, Stevens-Johnson syndrome (rare)	Data are limited in children with osteoarticular infections
Penicillin/aminopenicillins	Penicillin G, penicillin V potassium, ampicillin, amoxicillin	IV/PO	Cytopenias, rash, nephritis, diarrhea, vomiting, antibiotic-associated diarrhea (more common with high doses of amoxicillin)	Considered the drugs of choice for Group A *Streptococcus* as well as pneumococcus strains that are penicillin susceptible
Third-generation cephalosporins	Ceftriaxone, cefotaxime	IV	Cytopenias, rash, nephritis, transaminase elevation, antibiotic-associated diarrhea	
	Cefdinir, cefixime	PO		

testing cannot be routinely performed by most clinical laboratories. ASPs do not provide reliable coverage for *K. kingae* (oxacillin MIC_{90} = 6 μg/ml); however they are susceptible to cephalosporins (cefazolin MIC_{90} = 0.5 μg/ml and cefuroxime MIC_{90} = 0.19 μg/ml) [64, 65]. As such, special attention to empiric therapy choices is warranted in young children.

Other situations in which to consider broadening empiric therapy beyond that for staphylococci and streptococci include immunocompromised hosts (including asplenic or hemoglobinopathy patients), those with significant animal exposures, antecedent gastrointestinal illness, or the under-immunized [18, 19].

As with any infectious disease, definitive antibiotic choice should be guided by culture and sensitivity data when available.

Duration of Therapy in AHO

Small retrospective studies in the 1970s of osteomyelitis found that a treatment of ≤3 weeks of antibiotics was associated with a higher rate of treatment failure and/or progression to chronic infection compared to patients treated for a longer period of time [66, 67]. While these studies

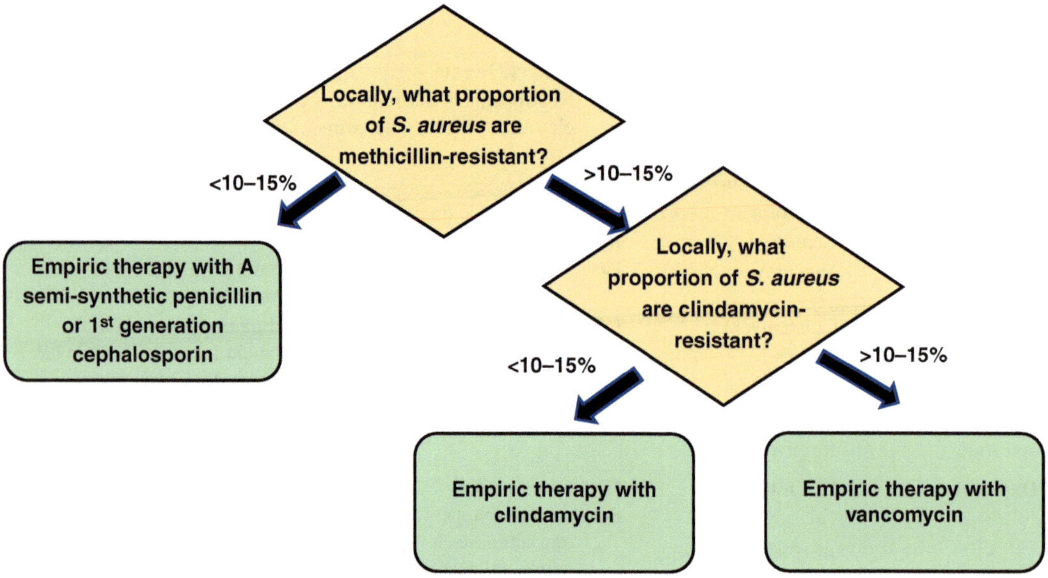

Fig. 2.1 Selection of empiric antistaphylococcal therapy in noncritically ill children with AHO. The suggested algorithm is based in part on ESPID guidelines (Reference [8]) for selection of antistaphylococcal therapy. Clinicians should consider individual patient risk factors for other pathogens and should incorporate this into selection of empiric therapy. This figure should not substitute for sound clinical judgment. Definitive antibiotic choice should be informed by culture and sensitivity data when available

are limited, they have informed the common practice in North America of treating osteomyelitis with approximately 4–6 weeks of therapy [68, 69]. A more recent randomized controlled trial in Finland found similar outcomes between patients treated with 20 days of therapy compared to ≥30 days [9]; these investigators also used serial measurements of C-reactive protein (CRP) to help guide discontinuation of therapy. While this was a well-designed and important study, the study population did not include any cases of disease due to MRSA and relatively few patients required surgical intervention. This is notable as MRSA AHO (particularly that due to the dominant strain in North America, USA300) has often been associated with a more complicated clinical course including prolonged fever, large abscesses, the need for multiple debridements, venous thromboses, and septic pulmonary emboli [6, 70, 71]. Thus, extrapolating the results of this study to populations with a high incidence of MRSA is challenging. The ESPID guidelines recommend 3–4 weeks of antimicrobial therapy but acknowledge that longer therapy may be necessary with select pathogens (e.g., MRSA or *Salmonella* spp.), very young children, and those with extensive disease or with infection of the pelvis or spinal column [8]. By contrast, the common practice in North America is to treat patients for 4–6 weeks of total therapy [2, 69]. Irrespective of the precise duration, the patient's signs/symptoms of infection should be resolved and the inflammatory markers normalized (or nearly so) prior to discontinuation of therapy.

Transition to Oral Therapy

Early transition to oral therapy has become an increasingly accepted practice in the management of pediatric AHO. Zaoutis et al. [72] conducted a large multicenter observational study in which the outcomes of children with AHO who were discharged on oral antibiotics were compared to those who received prolonged intravenous therapy. The authors found no difference in rates of treatment failure between the two study groups. Similarly, a recent clinical trial of adults

Table 2.4 Proposed criteria for transition to oral antibiotics

Consider transition to oral antimicrobials when the following are met:
Finalization of culture and susceptibility testing
If bacteremic, documentation of sterilization of blood cultures
Resolution of fever
Pain manageable with oral analgesics
Improvement in mobility
Down-trending CRP
Able to tolerate oral antibiotics and food

with either acute or chronic osteomyelitis found that the use of oral-stepdown antibiotics was non-inferior to prolonged IV therapy [73]. In addition, outpatient parenteral antimicrobial therapy (OPAT) typically requires the placement of a central venous line (CVC, either in the form of a tunneled line or a peripherally inserted central catheter [PICC]). The use of CVCs in the management of AHO are associated with complications specific to the catheter in 30–42% of patients [74, 75], many of which require emergency room visits and/or hospital admission. Additionally, another multicenter observational study found that children with AHO treated with OPAT via PICC had a >3.5-fold increased risk of adverse events compared to those treated with oral antibiotics [76]. In summation, the potential risks may not justify the theoretical benefits of higher serum drug levels in patients receiving OPAT compared to oral antimicrobials. The ESPID guidelines support transition to oral therapy once clinical improvement has been demonstrated (e.g., afebrile, reduced pain, improved mobility, down-trending C-reactive protein, tolerating oral medications, etc.) [8]. Proposed criteria for transition to oral antibiotics are provided in Table 2.4. Notably, both observational and clinical trial data suggest that the presence of a positive blood culture should not in and of itself justify prolonged parenteral therapy [77, 78]. However, it is generally recommended to have evidence of blood culture sterilization in bacteremic patients prior to transition to oral antibiotics. It is worth noting that certain situations arise in which completing all therapy with parenteral antibiotics may be needed such as in the case of multidrug-resistant pathogens, extensive disease with concomitant thrombophlebitis or septic emboli, or in immunocompromised hosts; however, robust studies do not exist to support these practices.

Potential agents for oral therapy include dicloxacillin, cephalexin, clindamycin, linezolid, or other oral β-lactams with selection based on the sensitivity of the organism isolated. Trimethoprim-sulfamethoxazole (TMP-SMX) is a potential therapeutic option which would provide coverage for both *S. aureus* and *K. kingae* although published data on the use of this agent in AHO are scant [79]. Importantly, GAS exhibits in vitro resistance to TMP-SMX. Regardless of the precise treatment regimen prescribed, careful follow-up is appropriate for all patients with musculoskeletal infections.

Combined Medical and Surgical Management

While most patients with osteomyelitis or pyomyositis can be successfully treated with medical therapy alone, the value of surgical intervention in specific situations with AOI should not be understated. Surgical debridement and/or drainage of purulent collections may provide therapeutic benefit by relieving pressure and hastening clinical resolution, as well as the opportunity for obtaining specimens for culture. A recent single-center observational study of *S. aureus* AHO in children found that early surgical intervention is associated with improved long-term outcomes [7]. Further work is needed to better understand the optimal role of surgical intervention in all cases of AHO. This topic is discussed in greater detail in other chapters in this text.

In principle, for patients for whom surgical intervention is planned, the administration of systemic antimicrobial therapy prior to obtaining cultures may reduce culture yield. The desire to maximize culture yield must be balanced with the potential risks of decompensation in a child with an untreated serious infection. In a single-center series, however, among patients requiring operative intervention for AHO, the yield of deep culture remained >70% with up to 72 hours of antibiotic pretreatment [2]. Moreover, we would strongly recommend prompt antibiotic treatment in children with AOI exhibiting signs/symptoms of sepsis.

Hematogenous Septic Arthritis

Empiric Therapy of Septic Arthritis

As the microbiology of hematogenous septic arthritis is very similar to that of AHO, empiric therapy should include an antistaphylococcal agent with the selection of specific agents as discussed above. For septic arthritis, there are a few notable caveats to remember, however [8]. For septic arthritis in sexually active adolescents, coverage for *Neisseria gonorrhoeae* should be considered particularly in the setting of a pustular skin rash. Gonococcal arthritis should also be included in the differential diagnosis of newborns with known or suspected septic arthritis. In such situations, the addition of a third-generation cephalosporin should be considered. For children ≤5 years old with septic arthritis, *K. kingae* is high in the microbiologic differential diagnosis as is the case with AHO; notably, *K. kingae* more frequently causes isolated septic arthritis than osteomyelitis [80].

Duration of Therapy

Historically, many experts have recommended different durations of antimicrobial therapy for septic arthritis depending on the organism identified. It has been recommended to treat septic arthritis due to streptococci, *H influenzae*, or *K. kingae* for 2–3 weeks, while *S. aureus* and gram-negative bacilli (including *Salmonella*) should be treated for ≥3 weeks [81]. With regard to septic arthritis, the ESPID guidelines recommend 2–3 weeks of effective therapy [8]. However, the guidelines acknowledge that a longer duration of therapy may be needed with complex disease or those with virulent pathogens (e.g., MRSA or *Salmonella* spp.). Notably, the potential for concomitant osteomyelitis, which may prompt an extension in therapy duration, must also be considered. In case series, 22–64% of children with septic arthritis have concomitant osteomyelitis [3, 82]. Some experts have advocated for obtaining radiographs in children with septic arthritis near the end of their course of antibiotic treatment to assess for evidence of osteomyelitis [83], as follow-up radiographs have illustrated abnormalities in up to 42% of patients.

A shorter duration of therapy than that recommended by the ESPID guidelines, however, may be effective in highly select cases. In Finland, Peltola et al. [84] conducted a randomized controlled trial of a short (10 days) vs. long course of therapy (30 days) in children with septic arthritis without osteomyelitis; most patients in this study transitioned to oral antibiotics after 3–4 days of parenteral therapy. The investigators noted no difference in outcome between patients receiving 10- and 30-day duration of antimicrobial therapy. Notably, however, approximately 18% of cases in this study were due to *H. influenzae* type b, and there were no cases of disease due to MRSA making extrapolation of this data to other populations challenging.

Gonococcal arthritis is typically approached differently than other causes of hematogenous septic arthritis. For gonococcal arthritis/arthritis-dermatitis syndrome, the use of ceftriaxone (or cefotaxime) daily for at least 7 days along with a single dose of azithromycin is recommended by the US Centers for Disease Control and Prevention (CDC) guidelines [85]. Such patients should also be screened for other sexually transmitted infections including HIV, syphilis, and *Chlamydia trachomatis*.

Oral Antibiotics for Septic Arthritis

Similar to AHO, most patients with septic arthritis can be transitioned to oral antibiotic therapy once the patient has demonstrated clinical improvement. Studies have shown similar outcomes for children with septic arthritis treated with approximately 7 days of parenteral therapy followed by oral transition compared to those receiving a longer course of IV therapy [86–88]; some investigators have successfully transitioned septic arthritis patients to oral antibiotics after as short as 2 days of parenteral therapy [84]. As with

AHO, definitive oral antibiotics should be selected based on culture and susceptibility data.

Surgical management via arthrotomy or arthrocentesis is critical in the management of septic arthritis and will be discussed in detail in Chap. 8.

Treating Culture Negative AHO and Septic Arthritis

In 24–43% of cases of AHO and septic arthritis, a pathogen is not definitively identified [2, 3, 89]. This situation can create a degree of uncertainty for providers and anxiety for patients/parents. However, a number of studies have shown that therapy can be administered presumptively against staphylococci and streptococci in most situations with high rates of success [90, 91]. Treatment duration and monitoring should in general be similar between culture-negative AOI and culture-positive cases.

Therapy Considerations for Non-hematogenous Osteomyelitis

Direct Inoculation Osteomyelitis

Little high-quality data exist to guide treatment decisions for patients with osteomyelitis arising from direct inoculation or open trauma. Debridement/drainage of infected tissues and removal of foreign bodies are generally regarded as important for treatment success.

While *S. aureus* is the most prominent cause of trauma-related osteomyelitis, gram-negative pathogens (particularly *Enterobacter* spp.) also frequently play a role. Moreover, up to 38% of these infections are polymicrobial in case series [22]. As such, some experts recommend the inclusion of empiric coverage for gram-negative pathogens in addition to staphylococci [22].

With a prolonged incubation period between trauma and presentation with symptoms or with foreign bodies in situ, providers should consider the potential for both fungi and atypical *Mycobacteria*. In such cases, given the diversity of possible organisms, culture and/or molecular microbiology data are essential to guide antimicrobial choices.

No controlled studies exist to inform treatment duration in children with osteomyelitis related to penetrating trauma. In case series, the duration of therapy has ranged from 28 days to several months [22, 33]. In one single center series, the median duration of therapy was 34 days with >85% experiencing no long-term sequelae [22].

Osteomyelitis Arising from a Contiguous Focus

Osteomyelitis in children may also develop as a result of spread from a contiguous focus. Similar to other musculoskeletal infections, staphylococci and streptococci are prominent pathogens; however, gram-negative bacilli (including *Pseudomonas* spp.) and anaerobes are also frequently isolated; these infections are also commonly polymicrobial [32, 92]. No studies exist regarding the optimal antibiotic treatment regimen or duration of therapy in children; even in adult patients, there is a paucity of high-quality data. Studies in adults with osteomyelitis underlying pressure ulcers found no benefit to antibiotic durations beyond 6 weeks, and, in some cases, short durations of therapy along with surgical intervention may be satisfactory [93]. Moreover, in limited studies, duration of therapy has not been clearly associated with likelihood of treatment failure/success [94]. Despite this, practice is variable among both adult and pediatric providers with durations of therapy ranging from 4 weeks to >6 months [32, 33, 95]. Notably, high rates of reinfection/secondary infection have been described with osteomyelitis associated with decubiti [32]. Surgical management, coverage of defects, and/or pressure off-loading are important in promoting healing. Case series of adults with pelvic/sacral osteomyelitis associated with decubiti have described high cure rates with combined medical and surgical approaches along with wound coverage [96]. One adult retrospective study found that combined medical and surgical management was associated with a lower rate of readmission than either medical or surgical intervention alone, although the sample size in this study limited statistical inference [92]. Given the limitations in available data, we would recommend at least 4 weeks of antimicrobials along with surgical management; patients should be regularly reassessed for the persistence of signs/symptoms of infection. Specific empiric antimicrobials should include coverage for gram-positive agents (i.e., staphylococci) as well as gram-negative bacilli and anaerobes when appropriate (including disease involving the feet or sacrum/pelvis). Final antibiotic choices should be guided by the results of culture/susceptibility testing.

Therapy Considerations for Orthopedic Hardware Infections

Treatment of implant-related infections can be broadly divided into three strategies:

- Debridement of all infected tissues with device retention and long-term (e.g., 3 months or more) antimicrobial therapy
- Surgical removal of all infected tissues including the implant, followed by reimplantation (single or two stage)
- Long-term suppressive oral antimicrobial therapy (usually for those in whom surgery is contraindicated)

The primary determinant between replacement of all implants and retention is duration of symptoms, which in turn relates to the formation and maturation of a biofilm. Table 2.5 summarizes one example of treatment strategy based on duration of infection [97].

Table 2.5 Treatment strategies for orthopedic implant infection

	Acute (immature biofilm)	Chronic (mature biofilm)
Perioperative	<4 weeks after surgery	≥4 weeks after surgery
Hematogenous	<3 weeks duration symptoms	≥3 weeks symptom duration
Treatment	Debridement and retention	Removal of prosthesis

Data regarding the management of orthopedic implant infections in children are limited; however, the Infectious Diseases Society of America (IDSA) has published guidelines for the management of prosthetic joint infection (PJI) in adults [98]. These guidelines suggest that debridement and implant retention (DAIR) may be an option when the following criteria are met: (1) duration of symptoms is <3 weeks, (2) < 30 days since the implant was placed, (3) well-fixed prosthesis, (4) absence of a sinus tract, and (5) the organisms are susceptible to oral antibiotics. With longer durations of infection, it is thought that the biofilm will be well-established, necessitating implant removal. Recent literature, however, has reported that DAIR can have reasonable rates of success in cases of infection within up to 90 days of the index procedure [99]. It should be remembered that implant retention is only an option when the implant is stable and there is no significant bone loss or weakness.

Empirical antibiotics should be commenced after samples for culture have been taken (provided the patient is clinically stable) and then followed by specific, targeted antibiotics when culture results become available. Empiric therapy should generally include an agent or combination of agents active against staphylococci and *Pseudomonas*.

The optimal antimicrobial agent in these cases should have bactericidal activity against surface adherent, slow-growing, and biofilm-producing microorganisms. Rifampicin has been demonstrated to fulfil these requirements for both methicillin-sensitive and resistant staphylococcal infections in laboratory and clinical studies (including a randomized controlled trial) [50, 100]. Rifampicin should not be administered as a monotherapy as staphylococci rapidly develop antimicrobial resistance. Quinolones, such as ciprofloxacin, have also been shown to be an effective agent, because of their bioavailability, antimicrobial activity, and tolerability [100].

The duration of antibiotics required in these cases is usually between 6 and 12 weeks in those with implant removal, making oral agents more convenient and avoiding the need for indwelling long-term venous catheters. While specific pediatric data are limited, the IDSA PJI guidelines recommend 3–6 months of oral suppressive antimicrobials (including at least one biofilm active agent) for cases managed with DAIR or one-stage implant exchange [98].

This oral regimen is usually commenced after a 2-week duration of either intravenous flucloxacillin (or nafcillin or cefazolin) or vancomycin, for MSSA and MRSA, respectively, along with oral rifampicin in combination. For streptococcal and *Enterococcus faecalis* infections, a 1-week course of intravenous penicillin G (or ampicillin depending on susceptibility) followed by oral amoxicillin is recommended. As with all musculoskeletal infection, close collaboration between orthopedists and infectious disease specialists is recommended in cases of orthopedic hardware infection.

Treatment Considerations for Pyomyositis, Bacterial Myositis

Data are limited to inform clinicians regarding the optimal management of pyomyositis/bacterial myositis in children. Given that the vast majority of culture-positive cases involve *S. aureus*, empiric therapy can be directed against this pathogen in most patients [101–103]. Notably, within staphylococci, CA-MRSA may more often contribute to pyomyositis than MSSA [103]. In immunocompromised hosts or those with central venous lines, a variety of other organisms including *Enterobacteriaceae* and *Candida* may contribute to pyomyositis, and thus expanded coverage is warranted in these clinical scenarios. Drainage of purulent collections is often needed and has been performed in 38% to >90% cases in reported series [102, 104]. The precise optimal duration of therapy is unclear and has varied in the literature from 2 to 6 weeks and is often guided by clinical examination as well as inflammatory marker trends (erythrocyte sedimentation rate and CRP) [101, 103, 104]. Following drainage and clinical defervescence, most patients can be transitioned to oral antimicrobials. This topic is discussed in more detail in Chap. 9.

Treatment Consideration for Mycobacterial Musculoskeletal Infection

Mycobacteria spp. may rarely contribute to musculoskeletal infections. *M. tuberculosis* (TB) of bones, particularly the spine (Pott's disease) is well-described. In general, treatment of skeletal TB relies on the same antimicrobials as that used to treat pulmonary TB and should ultimately be guided by the susceptibility of the organism. When drug-resistant TB is *not* clinically suspected, initial treatment with a combination of rifampin, isoniazid, pyrazinamide, and ethambutol (RIPE) should be administered for 2 months followed by 7–10 months of isoniazid and rifampin [105]. Supplementation with pyridoxine (vitamin B6) is generally recommended in patients receiving isoniazid. When drug-resistant TB is known or suspected (such as in patients with previous residence in an area endemic for multidrug-resistant [MDR] TB or contact with a source case with MDR-TB), the use of other agents including fluoroquinolones or aminoglycosides is often warranted; consultation with an expert in mycobacterial disease is recommended.

Nontuberculous mycobacteria (NTM) may also contribute to osteoarticular infection either following penetrating trauma or as a manifestation of disseminated disease in an immunocompromised host. Among NTM there is tremendous species- and strain-specific variability in antimicrobial susceptibility, making selection of empiric therapy extremely challenging. As with TB, consultation with an expert is highly advisable. In general NTM infections of bone should be managed with surgical debridement along with at least 3–6 months of active therapy. A thorough treatment of mycobacterial disease of the skeleton is provided in Chaps. 16 and 17.

Treatment Considerations for Fungal Musculoskeletal Infections

A variety of fungi may cause osteomyelitis or other musculoskeletal infections, albeit relatively rarely. *Candida* osteomyelitis may develop in the immunocompromised or those with central venous lines or as a manifestation of disseminated candidiasis (particularly in neonates). Evidence-based guidelines from the IDSA, which are primarily geared toward an adult patient population, recommend 6–12 months of targeted antifungals for osteomyelitis caused by *Candida* spp. [106]. Notably, several case reports/series exist of infants and children being successfully treated with courses of antifungal therapy of 4–6 weeks [107, 108]. While therapy should be chosen based on antifungal susceptibility testing of the *Candida* isolate, potential therapeutic options include amphotericin formulations, triazoles, and echinocandins; side effect profile and individualized patient characteristics (such as the need for CNS or renal penetration or comorbid conditions) should inform antifungal choice.

Blastomyces and *Coccidioides* are endemic mycoses which have a predilection for causing osteoarticular disease; coccidioidomycosis in particular may have a tropism for the spine. IDSA guidelines recommend 1–2 weeks of amphotericin induction therapy followed by at least 1 year of itraconazole therapy for *Blastomyces* infections [109]. For coccidioidomycosis of the skeleton, use of a triazole (i.e., fluconazole) is recommended unless disease is severe. With severe *Coccidioides* of the skeleton, an initial induction period with amphotericin is advised by some experts. Treatment of *Coccidioides* of the skeleton is often continued for many years [110]. A number of dematiaceous fungi have been isolated in cases of osteomyelitis following penetrating trauma (e.g., *Cladosporium*, *Curvularia*, etc.) as well as *Aspergillus* and *Rhizopus* spp.; such cases have received surgical debridement in addition to antifungal regimens lasting from 6 weeks to 9 months or longer [22]. A thorough discussion of fungal musculoskeletal infections and their management is provided in Chap. 27.

Conclusion

Antimicrobial treatment is a critical component of the management of childhood osteoarticular infection, making knowledge of the likely pathogens essential. *S. aureus* is by far the most common causative organism for all forms of musculoskeletal infection (osteomyelitis, septic arthritis, or pyomyositis), with MRSA being a much greater problem in the United States than in Europe. *K. kingae* is now recognized as a significant cause of AOIs, accounting for half of cases in 6–48-month-olds. Based on this knowledge, empiric treatment with either an antistaphylococcal β-lactam, clindamycin or vancomycin is appropriate in the majority of cases of AOI. A cephalosporin may be preferred in children under the age of 5 years as this provides coverage for *K. kingae*. In regions where the proportion of *S. aureus* in the community that is methicillin resistant is over 10–15%, vancomycin or clindamycin should be the treatment of choice.

The evidence supports shorter courses of antibiotics than traditionally given, with 3–4 weeks of total treatment for osteomyelitis and 2–3 weeks for septic arthritis; early transition to oral antimicrobial therapy is considered preferable and has been shown to not compromise clinical outcomes.

AOI is an overarching term for a wide spectrum of disease severity, and so the clinician must be careful not to generalize treatments and regimens without distinguishing the complex cases from the simple ones. The value of experience and expertise with a multidisciplinary approach between the orthopedic surgeon, pediatrician, and microbiologist/infectious disease specialists cannot be overstated in managing these cases.

References

1. Dartnell J, Ramachandran M, Katchburian M. Haematogenous acute and subacute paediatric osteomyelitis: a systematic review of the literature. J Bone Joint Surg Br. 2012;94(5):584–95.
2. McNeil JC, Forbes AR, Vallejo JG, Flores AR, Hulten KG, Mason EO, et al. Role of operative or interventional radiology-guided cultures for osteomyelitis. Pediatrics. 2016;137:e20154616.
3. Branson JN, Vallejo JG, Flores AR, Hulten KG, Mason EO, Kaplan SL, et al. The contemporary microbiology and rates of concomitant osteomy-

elitis in acute septic arthritis. Pediatr Infect Dis J. 2017;36:267–73.
4. Hulten KG, Mason EO, Lamberth LB, Forbes AR, Revell PA, Kaplan SL. Analysis of invasive community-acquired methicillin-susceptible Staphylococcus aureus infections during a period of declining CA-MRSA infections at a large children's hospital. Pediatr Infect Dis J. 2018;37(3):235–41.
5. Sutter DE, Milburn E, Chukwuma U, Dzialowy N, Maranich AM, Hospenthal DR. Changing susceptibility of Staphylococcus aureus in a US pediatric population. Pediatrics. 2016;137(4):e20153099.
6. Bocchini CE, Hulten KG, Mason EO Jr, Gonzalez BE, Hammerman WA, Kaplan SL. Panton-valentine leukocidin genes are associated with enhanced inflammatory response and local disease in acute hematogenous Staphylococcus aureus osteomyelitis in children. Pediatrics. 2006;117(2):433–40.
7. McNeil JC, Vallejo JG, Kok EY, Sommer LM, Hulten KG, Kaplan SL. Clinical and microbiologic variables predictive of Orthopedic complications following S. aureus acute hematogenous osteoarticular infections in children. Clin Infect Dis. 2019;69(11):1955–61.
8. Saavedra-Lozano J, Falup-Pecurariu O, Faust SN, Girschick H, Hartwig N, Kaplan S, et al. Bone and joint infections. Pediatr Infect Dis J. 2017;36(8):788–99.
9. Peltola H, Paakkonen M, Kallio P, Kallio MJ, Osteomyelitis-Septic Arthritis Study Group. Short-versus long-term antimicrobial treatment for acute hematogenous osteomyelitis of childhood: prospective, randomized trial on 131 culture-positive cases. Pediatr Infect Dis J. 2010;29(12):1123–8.
10. Bradley JS, Kaplan SL, Tan TQ, Barson WJ, Arditi M, Schutze GE, et al. Pediatric pneumococcal bone and joint infections. The Pediatric Multicenter Pneumococcal Surveillance Study Group (PMPSSG). Pediatrics. 1998;102(6):1376–82.
11. Olarte L, Romero J, Barson W, Bradley J, Lin PL, Givner L, et al. Osteoarticular infections caused by Streptococcus pneumoniae in children in the post-pneumococcal conjugate vaccine era. Pediatr Infect Dis J. 2017;36(12):1201–4.
12. Edwards MS, Baker CJ, Wagner ML, Taber LH, Barrett FF. An etiologic shift in infantile osteomyelitis: the emergence of the group B streptococcus. J Pediatr. 1978;93(4):578–83.
13. Rubin LG, Shin J, Kaur I, Scheuerman O, Levy I, Long SS. Frequency of multifocal disease and pyogenic arthritis of the hip in infants with osteoarticular infection in three neonatal intensive care units. J Pediatr. 2020;227:157–62.
14. Berardi A, Rossi C, Lugli L, Creti R, Bacchi Reggiani ML, Lanari M, et al. Group B streptococcus late-onset disease: 2003-2010. Pediatrics. 2013;131(2):e361–8.
15. Juchler C, Spyropoulou V, Wagner N, Merlini L, Dhouib A, Manzano S, et al. The contemporary bacteriologic epidemiology of osteoarticular infections in children in Switzerland. J Pediatr. 2018;194(190–6):e1.
16. Samara E, Spyropoulou V, Tabard-Fougere A, Merlini L, Valaikaite R, Dhouib A, et al. Kingella kingae and osteoarticular infections. Pediatrics. 2019;144:6.
17. Chambers JB, Forsythe DA, Bertrand SL, Iwinski HJ, Steflik DE. Retrospective review of osteoarticular infections in a pediatric sickle cell age group. J Pediatr Orthop. 2000;20(5):682–5.
18. Boguniewicz J, Rubiano Landinez A, Kaplan SL, Lamb GS. Comparison of musculoskeletal infections due to nontyphoidal salmonella species and Staphylococcus aureus in immunocompetent children. Pediatr Infect Dis J. 2019;38(10):1020–4.
19. Kaplan J, Ikeda S, McNeil JC, Kaplan SL, Vallejo JG. Microbiology of osteoarticular infections in patients with sickle hemoglobinopathies at Texas Children's Hospital, 2000-2018. Pediatr Infect Dis J. 2019;38(12):1251–3.
20. van der Naald N, Smeeing DPJ, Houwert RM, Hietbrink F, Govaert GAM, van der Velde D. Brodie's abscess: a systematic review of reported cases. J Bone Jt Infect. 2019;4(1):33–9.
21. Foster CE, Taylor M, Schallert EK, Rosenfeld S, King KY. Brodie abscess in children: a 10-year single institution retrospective review. Pediatr Infect Dis J. 2019;38(2):e32–e4.
22. McNeil JC, Vallejo JG, Hulten KG, Kaplan SL. Osteoarticular infections following open or penetrating trauma in children in the post-community-acquired methicillin-resistant Staphylococcus aureus era: the impact of Enterobacter cloacae. Pediatr Infect Dis J. 2018;37(12):1204–10.
23. Gaglani MJ, Friedman J, Hawkins EP, Campbell JR. Infections complicating lawn mower injuries in children. Pediatr Infect Dis J. 1996;15(5):452–5.
24. Jacobs RF, McCarthy RE, Elser JM. Pseudomonas osteochondritis complicating puncture wounds of the foot in children: a 10-year evaluation. J Infect Dis. 1989;160(4):657–61.
25. Kesson AM, Bellemore MC, O'Mara TJ, Ellis DH, Sorrell TC. Scedosporium prolificans osteomyelitis in an immunocompetent child treated with a novel agent, hexadecylphospocholine (miltefosine), in combination with terbinafine and voriconazole: a case report. Clin Infect Dis. 2009;48(9):1257–61.
26. Stripeli F, Pasparakis D, Velegraki A, Lebessi E, Arsenis G, Kafetzis D, et al. Scedosporium apiospermum skeletal infection in an immunocompetent child. Med Mycol. 2009;47(4):441–4.
27. Fernandez M, Carrol CL, Baker CJ. Discitis and vertebral osteomyelitis in children: an 18-year review. Pediatrics. 2000;105(6):1299–304.
28. Afshari FT, Rodrigues D, Bhat M, Solanki GA, Walsh AR, Lo WB. Paediatric spondylodiscitis: a 10-year single institution experience in management and clinical outcomes. Childs Nerv Syst. 2020;36(5):1049–54.
29. Garron E, Viehweger E, Launay F, Guillaume JM, Jouve JL, Bollini G. Nontuberculous spon-

dylodiscitis in children. J Pediatr Orthop. 2002;22(3):321–8.
30. Correa AG, Edwards MS, Baker CJ. Vertebral osteomyelitis in children. Pediatr Infect Dis J. 1993;12(3):228–33.
31. Bar-On E, Weigl DM, Bor N, Becker T, Katz K, Mercado E, et al. Chronic osteomyelitis in children: treatment by intramedullary reaming and antibiotic-impregnated cement rods. J Pediatr Orthop. 2010;30(5):508–13.
32. McNeil JC, Joseph M, Sommer LM, Vallejo JG. The contemporary epidemiology, microbiology and management of chronic osteomyelitis in US children. Pediatr Infect Dis J. 2021;40(6):518–24.
33. Dubey L, Krasinski K, Hernanz-Schulman M. Osteomyelitis secondary to trauma or infected contiguous soft tissue. Pediatr Infect Dis J. 1988;7(1):26–34.
34. Gamaletsou MN, Kontoyiannis DP, Sipsas NV, Moriyama B, Alexander E, Roilides E, et al. Candida osteomyelitis: analysis of 207 pediatric and adult cases (1970-2011). Clin Infect Dis. 2012;55(10):1338–51.
35. Gamaletsou MN, Rammaert B, Bueno MA, Moriyama B, Sipsas NV, Kontoyiannis DP, et al. Aspergillus osteomyelitis: epidemiology, clinical manifestations, management, and outcome. J Infect. 2014;68(5):478–93.
36. Henry MW, Miller AO, Walsh TJ, Brause BD. Fungal musculoskeletal infections. Infect Dis Clin N Am. 2017;31(2):353–68.
37. Ciofi Degli Atti ML, Serino L, Piga S, Tozzi AE, Raponi M. Incidence of surgical site infections in children: active surveillance in an Italian academic children's hospital. Ann Ig. 2017;29(1):46–53.
38. Druschel C, Heck K, Pennekamp PH, Wimmer M, Funk JF, Placzek R. Avoiding drainage after major hip surgery in children is a viable option: results from a retrospective comparative study. Int Orthop. 2016;40(1):129–33.
39. Maesani M, Doit C, Lorrot M, Vitoux C, Hilly J, Michelet D, et al. Surgical site infections in pediatric spine surgery: comparative microbiology of patients with idiopathic and nonidiopathic etiologies of spine deformity. Pediatr Infect Dis J. 2016;35(1):66–70.
40. Kolman SE, Ruzbarsky JJ, Spiegel DA, Baldwin KD. Salvage options in the cerebral palsy hip: a systematic review. J Pediatr Orthop. 2016;36(6):645–50.
41. Mackenzie WG, Matsumoto H, Williams BA, Corona J, Lee C, Cody SR, et al. Surgical site infection following spinal instrumentation for scoliosis: a multicenter analysis of rates, risk factors, and pathogens. J Bone Joint Surg Am. 2013;95(9):800–6, S1–2.
42. Kowalski TJ, Berbari EF, Huddleston PM, Steckelberg JM, Mandrekar JN, Osmon DR. The management and outcome of spinal implant infections: contemporary retrospective cohort study. Clin Infect Dis. 2007;44(7):913–20.
43. Ho C, Skaggs DL, Weiss JM, Tolo VT. Management of infection after instrumented posterior spine fusion in pediatric scoliosis. Spine (Phila Pa 1976). 2007;32(24):2739–44.
44. Hedequist D, Haugen A, Hresko T, Emans J. Failure of attempted implant retention in spinal deformity delayed surgical site infections. Spine (Phila Pa 1976). 2009;34(1):60–4.
45. Khoshbin A, Lysenko M, Law P, Wright JG. Outcomes of infection following pediatric spinal fusion. Can J Surg. 2015;58(2):107–13.
46. Glotzbecker MP, Gomez JA, Miller PE, Troy MJ, Skaggs DL, Vitale MG, et al. Management of spinal implants in acute pediatric surgical site infections: a Multicenter study. Spine Deform. 2016;4(4):277–82.
47. Gristina AG. Biomaterial-centered infection: microbial adhesion versus tissue integration. Science. 1987;237(4822):1588–95.
48. Davidson DJ, Spratt D, Liddle AD. Implant materials and prosthetic joint infection: the battle with the biofilm. EFORT Open Rev. 2019;4(11):633–9.
49. Vuong C, Gerke C, Somerville GA, Fischer ER, Otto M. Quorum-sensing control of biofilm factors in Staphylococcus epidermidis. J Infect Dis. 2003;188(5):706–18.
50. Zimmerli W, Trampuz A, Ochsner PE. Prosthetic-joint infections. N Engl J Med. 2004;351(16):1645–54.
51. Olson ME, Ceri H, Morck DW, Buret AG, Read RR. Biofilm bacteria: formation and comparative susceptibility to antibiotics. Can J Vet Res. 2002;66(2):86–92.
52. Rao SN, Rhodes NJ, Lee BJ, Scheetz MH, Hanson AP, Segreti J, et al. Treatment outcomes with cefazolin versus oxacillin for deep-seated methicillin-susceptible Staphylococcus aureus bloodstream infections. Antimicrob Agents Chemother. 2015;59(9):5232–8.
53. Li J, Echevarria KL, Hughes DW, Cadena JA, Bowling JE, Lewis JS 2nd. Comparison of cefazolin versus oxacillin for treatment of complicated bacteremia caused by methicillin-susceptible Staphylococcus aureus. Antimicrob Agents Chemother. 2014;58(9):5117–24.
54. McDanel JS, Perencevich EN, Diekema DJ, Herwaldt LA, Smith TC, Chrischilles EA, et al. Comparative effectiveness of beta-lactams versus vancomycin for treatment of methicillin-susceptible Staphylococcus aureus bloodstream infections among 122 hospitals. Clin Infect Dis. 2015;61(3):361–7.
55. Miller WR, Seas C, Carvajal LP, Diaz L, Echeverri AM, Ferro C, et al. The cefazolin inoculum effect is associated with increased mortality in methicillin-susceptible Staphylococcus aureus bacteremia. Open forum. Infect Dis. 2018;5(6):ofy123.
56. McNeil JC, Sommer LM, Boyle M, Hogan P, Vallejo JG, Hulten KG, et al. Cefazolin inoculum effect and methicillin-susceptible Staphylococcus aureus osteoarticular infections in children. Antimicrob Agents Chemother. 2020;64(9):e00703–20.
57. American Academy of Pediatrics Committee on Infectious Diseases. Staphylococcal infections. In: Pickering LK, Baker C, Kimberlin DW, Long SS, editors. Red book: 2012 report of the committee

on infectious diseases. 29th ed. Elk Grove Village: American Academy of Pediatrics; 2012. p. 653–68.
58. Martinez-Aguilar G, Avalos-Mishaan A, Hulten K, Hammerman W, Mason EO Jr, Kaplan SL. Community-acquired, methicillin-resistant and methicillin-susceptible Staphylococcus aureus musculoskeletal infections in children. Pediatr Infect Dis J. 2004;23(8):701–6.
59. Kaplan SL, Mason EO Jr, Feigin RD. Clindamycin versus nafcillin or methicillin in the treatment of Staphylococcus aureus osteomyelitis in children. South Med J. 1982;75(2):138–42.
60. Al-Zubeidi D, Burnham CA, Hogan PG, Collins R, Hunstad DA, Fritz SA. Molecular epidemiology of recurrent cutaneous methicillin-resistant infections in children. J Pediatric Infect Dis Soc. 2014;3(3):261–4.
61. Erturan G, Holme H, Smith R, Dodds R, Iyer S. Successful use of daptomycin in Panton-Valentine leucocidin positive Staphylococcus aureus paediatric osteomyelitis. Int J Surg Case Rep. 2012;3(7):238–41.
62. Syriopoulou V, Dailiana Z, Dmitriy N, Utili R, Pathan R, Hamed K. Clinical experience with daptomycin for the treatment of gram-positive infections in children and adolescents. Pediatr Infect Dis J. 2016;35(5):511–6.
63. Williams AW, Newman PM, Ocheltree S, Beaty R, Hassoun A. Ceftaroline fosamil use in 2 pediatric patients with invasive methicillin-resistant Staphylococcus aureus infections. J Pediatr Pharmacol Ther. 2015;20(6):476–80.
64. Yagupsky P. Antibiotic susceptibility of Kingella kingae isolates from children with skeletal system infections. Pediatr Infect Dis J. 2012;31(2):212.
65. Tran Quang V, Bidet P, Birgy A, Caseris M, Basmaci R, Bonacorsi S. Susceptibility testing of Kingella kingae to cefazolin. Clin Microbiol Infect. 2018;24(3):312–3.
66. Dich VQ, Nelson JD, Haltalin KC. Osteomyelitis in infants and children. A review of 163 cases. Am J Dis Child. 1975;129(11):1273–8.
67. Blockey NJ, Watson JT. Acute osteomyelitis in children. J Bone Joint Surg Br. 1970;52(1):77–87.
68. Osteomyelitis KP. In: Cherry JD, Harrison GJ, Kaplan SL, Steinbach WJ, Hotez PJ, editors. Feigin and Cherry's textbook of pediatric infectious diseases, vol. 1. 8th ed. Philadelphia: Elsevier; 2019. p. 516–29.
69. Krogstad P. Hematogenous osteomyelitis in children: management. In: UpToDate Online. [web-based textbook]. Baron EL (ed), UpToDate, Waltham, MA, 2019. Available from: https://www.uptodate.com/contents/hematogenous-osteomyelitis-in-children-management?search=osteomyelitis%20treatment%20children&source=search_result&selectedTitle=1~150&usage_type=default&display_rank=1.
70. Gonzalez BE, Hulten KG, Dishop MK, Lamberth LB, Hammerman WA, Mason EO Jr, et al. Pulmonary manifestations in children with invasive community-acquired Staphylococcus aureus infection. Clin Infect Dis. 2005;41(5):583–90.
71. Hawkshead JJ 3rd, Patel NB, Steele RW, Heinrich SD. Comparative severity of pediatric osteomyelitis attributable to methicillin-resistant versus methicillin-sensitive Staphylococcus aureus. J Pediatr Orthop. 2009;29(1):85–90.
72. Zaoutis T, Localio AR, Leckerman K, Saddlemire S, Bertoch D, Keren R. Prolonged intravenous therapy versus early transition to oral antimicrobial therapy for acute osteomyelitis in children. Pediatrics. 2009;123(2):636–42.
73. Li HK, Rombach I, Zambellas R, Walker AS, McNally MA, Atkins BL, et al. Oral versus intravenous antibiotics for bone and joint infection. N Engl J Med. 2019;380(5):425–36.
74. Ruebner R, Keren R, Coffin S, Chu J, Horn D, Zaoutis TE. Complications of central venous catheters used for the treatment of acute hematogenous osteomyelitis. Pediatrics. 2006;117(4):1210–5.
75. Barrier A, Williams DJ, Connelly M, Creech CB. Frequency of peripherally inserted central catheter complications in children. Pediatr Infect Dis J. 2012;31(5):519–21.
76. Keren R, Shah SS, Srivastava R, Rangel S, Bendel-Stenzel M, Harik N, et al. Comparative effectiveness of intravenous vs oral antibiotics for postdischarge treatment of acute osteomyelitis in children. JAMA Pediatr. 2015;169(2):120–8.
77. McNeil JC, Kaplan SL, Vallejo JG. The influence of the route of antibiotic administration, methicillin-susceptibility, vancomycin duration and serum trough concentration on outcomes of pediatric Staphylococcus aureus bacteremic osteoarticular infection. Pediatr Infect Dis J. 2017;36(6):572–7.
78. Paakkonen M, Kallio PE, Kallio MJ, Peltola H. Does bacteremia associated with bone and joint infections necessitate prolonged parenteral antimicrobial therapy? J Pediatric Infect Dis Soc. 2015;4(2):174–7.
79. Messina AF, Namtu K, Guild M, Dumois JA, Berman DM. Trimethoprim-sulfamethoxazole therapy for children with acute osteomyelitis. Pediatr Infect Dis J. 2011;30(12):1019–21.
80. Dubnov-Raz G, Ephros M, Garty BZ, Schlesinger Y, Maayan-Metzger A, Hasson J, et al. Invasive pediatric Kingella kingae infections: a nationwide collaborative study. Pediatr Infect Dis J. 2010;29(7):639–43.
81. Krogstad P. Septic arthritis. In: Cherry JD, Harrison GJ, Kaplan SL, Steinbach WJ, Hotez PJ, editors. Feigin and Cherry's textbook of pediatric infectious diseases, vol. 1. 7th ed. Philadelphia: Elsevier Saunders; 2014. p. 727–34.
82. Montgomery CO, Siegel E, Blasier RD, Suva LJ. Concurrent septic arthritis and osteomyelitis in children. J Pediatr Orthop. 2013;33(4):464–7.
83. Jackson MA, Burry VF, Olson LC. Pyogenic arthritis associated with adjacent osteomyelitis: identification of the sequela-prone child. Pediatr Infect Dis J. 1992;11(1):9–13.
84. Peltola H, Paakkonen M, Kallio P, Kallio MJ, Osteomyelitis-Septic Arthritis Study Group. Prospective, randomized trial of 10 days versus 30 days of antimicrobial treatment, including a short-

term course of parenteral therapy, for childhood septic arthritis. Clin Infect Dis. 2009;48(9):1201–10.
85. Workowski KA, Bolan GA, Centers for Disease Control and Prevention. Sexually transmitted diseases treatment guidelines, 2015. MMWR Recomm Rep. 2015;64(RR-03):1–137.
86. Ballock RT, Newton PO, Evans SJ, Estabrook M, Farnsworth CL, Bradley JS. A comparison of early versus late conversion from intravenous to oral therapy in the treatment of septic arthritis. J Pediatr Orthop. 2009;29(6):636–42.
87. Jaberi FM, Shahcheraghi GH, Ahadzadeh M. Short-term intravenous antibiotic treatment of acute hematogenous bone and joint infection in children: a prospective randomized trial. J Pediatr Orthop. 2002;22(3):317–20.
88. Newton PO, Ballock RT, Bradley JS. Oral antibiotic therapy of bacterial arthritis. Pediatr Infect Dis J. 1999;18(12):1102–3.
89. Arnold SR, Elias D, Buckingham SC, Thomas ED, Novais E, Arkader A, et al. Changing patterns of acute hematogenous osteomyelitis and septic arthritis: emergence of community-associated methicillin-resistant Staphylococcus aureus. J Pediatr Orthop. 2006;26(6):703–8.
90. Floyed RL, Steele RW. Culture-negative osteomyelitis. Pediatr Infect Dis J. 2003;22(8):731–6.
91. Paakkonen M, Kallio MJ, Kallio PE, Peltola H. Significance of negative cultures in the treatment of acute hematogenous bone and joint infections in children. J Pediatric Infect Dis Soc. 2013;2(2):119–25.
92. Bodavula P, Liang SY, Wu J, VanTassell P, Marschall J. Pressure ulcer-related pelvic osteomyelitis: a neglected disease? Open forum. Infect Dis. 2015;2(3):ofv112.
93. Marriott R, Rubayi S. Successful truncated osteomyelitis treatment for chronic osteomyelitis secondary to pressure ulcers in spinal cord injury patients. Ann Plast Surg. 2008;61(4):425–9.
94. Russell CD, Tsang SJ, Simpson A, Sutherland RK. Outcomes, microbiology and antimicrobial usage in pressure ulcer-related pelvic osteomyelitis: messages for clinical practice. J Bone Jt Infect. 2020;5(2):67–75.
95. Kaka AS, Beekmann SE, Gravely A, Filice GA, Polgreen PM, Johnson JR. Diagnosis and Management of osteomyelitis associated with Stage 4 pressure ulcers: report of a query to the emerging infections network of the Infectious Diseases Society of America. Open forum. Infect Dis. 2019;6(11):ofz406.
96. Dudareva M, Ferguson J, Riley N, Stubbs D, Atkins B, McNally M. Osteomyelitis of the pelvic bones: a multidisciplinary approach to treatment. J Bone Jt Infect. 2017;2(4):184–93.
97. Izakovicova P, Borens O, Trampuz A. Periprosthetic joint infection: current concepts and outlook. EFORT Open Rev. 2019;4(7):482–94.
98. Osmon DR, Berbari EF, Berendt AR, Lew D, Zimmerli W, Steckelberg JM, et al. Diagnosis and management of prosthetic joint infection: clinical practice guidelines by the Infectious Diseases Society of America. Clin Infect Dis. 2013;56(1):e1–e25.
99. Lowik CAM, Parvizi J, Jutte PC, Zijlstra WP, Knobben BAS, Xu C, et al. Debridement, antibiotics, and implant retention is a viable treatment option for early periprosthetic joint infection presenting more than 4 weeks after index arthroplasty. Clin Infect Dis. 2020;71(3):630–6.
100. Zimmerli W, Widmer AF, Blatter M, Frei R, Ochsner PE. Role of rifampin for treatment of orthopedic implant-related staphylococcal infections: a randomized controlled trial. Foreign-Body Infection (FBI) Study Group. JAMA. 1998;279(19):1537–41.
101. Mitsionis GI, Manoudis GN, Lykissas MG, Sionti I, Motsis E, Georgoulis AD, et al. Pyomyositis in children: early diagnosis and treatment. J Pediatr Surg. 2009;44(11):2173–8.
102. Moriarty P, Leung C, Walsh M, Nourse C. Increasing pyomyositis presentations among children in Queensland, Australia. Pediatr Infect Dis J. 2015;34(1):1–4.
103. Pannaraj PS, Hulten KG, Gonzalez BE, Mason EO Jr, Kaplan SL. Infective pyomyositis and myositis in children in the era of community-acquired, methicillin-resistant Staphylococcus aureus infection. Clin Infect Dis. 2006;43(8):953–60.
104. Spiegel DA, Meyer JS, Dormans JP, Flynn JM, Drummond DS. Pyomyositis in children and adolescents: report of 12 cases and review of the literature. J Pediatr Orthop. 1999;19(2):143–50.
105. American Academy of Pediatrics Committee on Infectious Diseases. Tuberculosis. In: Kimberlin DW, Brady MT, Jackson MA, Long SS, editors. RedBook 2018 report of the committee on infectious diseases. 31st ed. Elk Grove Village: American Academy of Pediatrics; 2018. p. 829–53.
106. Pappas PG, Kauffman CA, Andes DR, Clancy CJ, Marr KA, Ostrosky-Zeichner L, et al. Clinical practice guideline for the management of candidiasis: 2016 update by the Infectious Diseases Society of America. Clin Infect Dis. 2016;62(4):e1–50.
107. Harris MC, Pereira GR, Myers MD, Cardin AJ, Razdan B, Pleasure J, et al. Candidal arthritis in infants previously treated for systemic candidiasis during the newborn period: report of three cases. Pediatr Emerg Care. 2000;16(4):249–51.
108. McCullers JA, Flynn PM. Candida tropicalis osteomyelitis: case report and review. Clin Infect Dis. 1998;26(4):1000–1.
109. Chapman SW, Dismukes WE, Proia LA, Bradsher RW, Pappas PG, Threlkeld MG, et al. Clinical practice guidelines for the management of blastomycosis: 2008 update by the Infectious Diseases Society of America. Clin Infect Dis. 2008;46(12):1801–12.
110. Galgiani JN, Ampel NM, Blair JE, Catanzaro A, Geertsma F, Hoover SE, et al. 2016 Infectious Diseases Society of America (IDSA) clinical practice guideline for the treatment of coccidioidomycosis. Clin Infect Dis. 2016;63(6):e112–46.

Pathology of Musculoskeletal Infections

3

Stephanie N. Moore-Lotridge and Jonathan G. Schoenecker

MSKI in Pediatric Patients

Few conditions are as enigmatic or carry higher stakes for a child than MSKI. Pediatricians, pediatric orthopedic surgeons, and infectious disease physicians are frequently called upon to evaluate children with suspected MSKI. For example, the Children's Orthopaedic Trauma and Infection Consortium for Evidence-based Studies (CORTICES) group determined that pediatric MSKI accounts for nearly 1 in 10 orthopedic consultations at academic pediatric tertiary care centers [1]. Under the umbrella of pediatric MSKI, there are numerous diagnoses based on tissue location, such as pyomyositis (muscle), osteomyelitis (bone), cellulitis (skin), or septic arthritis (joint space). Importantly, the severity of the infection can vary relative to the pathogen's virulence and dissemination. For example, MSKI can happen both focally at a single site (Fig. 3.1) or be multifocal throughout multiple tissue types (Fig. 3.2) in addition to being disseminated within the bloodstream.

S. N. Moore-Lotridge
Vanderbilt University Medical Center, Department of Orthopaedics, Nashville, TN, USA
e-mail: stephanie.n.moore@vanderbilt.edu

J. G. Schoenecker (✉)
Vanderbilt University Medical Center, Department of Orthopaedics, Nashville, TN, USA

Department of Pediatrics, Department of Pathology Microbiology and Immunology, and Vanderbilt Center for Bone Biology, Nashville, TN, USA

Vanderbilt University, Department of Pharmacology, Nashville, TN, USA
e-mail: jon.schoenecker@Vanderbilt.Edu

Why Does MSKI Occur in Children?

While bacteria travel through the circulation and the musculoskeletal systems each day, they rarely take hold to cause clinical infection. Though chance will play a role in determining when and where MSKI will occur, it has been established that "trauma" to musculoskeletal tissue is a major predisposing factor [2, 3]. For example, when a traumatic injury occurs in the skeletal muscle, a hematoma can form and serve as a focal nidus for infection [4]. However, many times, MSKIs in children occur spontaneously, without a known predisposing injury. Bacteria, like mesenchymal stem cells or cancers, have a tropism for the microenvironment regenerating tissue [5, 6]; thus, growing bone and muscle during a child's development can mimic regenerative tissue following an injury, predisposing it to a similar relative risk of being targeted by bacteria. Specifically, bacteria express virulence factors with lock and key mechanisms that can directly interact with factors expressed by regenerative or growing muscle and bone [6]. Furthermore, the unique characteristics of the physis, such as robust "tortuous" vascularity [7] and its relative immune-

© Springer Nature Switzerland AG 2022
M. V. Belthur et al. (eds.), *Pediatric Musculoskeletal Infections*,
https://doi.org/10.1007/978-3-030-95794-0_3

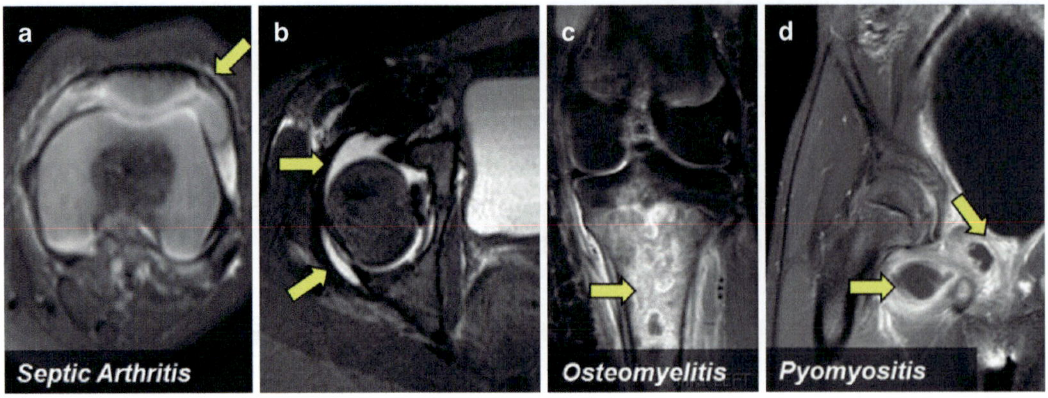

Fig. 3.1 Examples of focal MSKI. Septic arthritis surrounding the (**a**) knee and (**b**) hip indicated by MRI. (**c**) Intraosseous osteomyelitis lesion of the proximal tibia visualized by MRI. (**d**) Pyomyositis lesions within the musculature of the hip visualized by MRI. Yellow arrows indicate the infection site. (*Figure permission: Schoenecker Laboratory*)

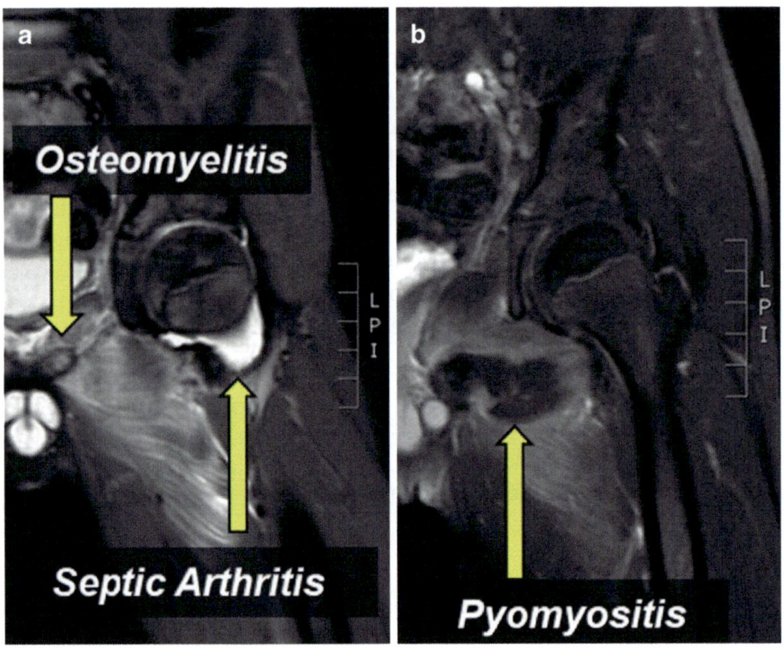

Fig. 3.2 Infection involving multiple tissues surrounding the hip. Most severe cases of musculoskeletal infection of the hip or the knee do not involve an isolated tissue type. In these MRI cuts, there is evidence of both (**a**) osteomyelitis in addition to septic arthritis and (**b**) pyomyositis in the same patient. This is typical of cases of hip and knee infections where pathogens rarely stay isolated to the joint. (*Figure permission: Schoenecker Laboratory*)

privileged nature [8], can likewise predispose these sites to initiation of infection. Together, these molecular factors support the long-standing observation that developing children are susceptible to "spontaneous" infections predominately at or around major joints. For reasons not completely understood, lower extremities are far more susceptible to spontaneous MSKI than upper extremities, with the femur (hip and knee) being the most susceptible [9].

Clinical Presentation

Independent of the musculoskeletal infection type, pediatric patients commonly present with complaints of pain, decreased range of motion, inability/refusal to bear weight, and systemic signs of infection, such as a fever. While deep tissue infections, such as deep pyomyositis and osteomyelitis, may show minimal alteration to the skin, soft tissue infections, such as superficial

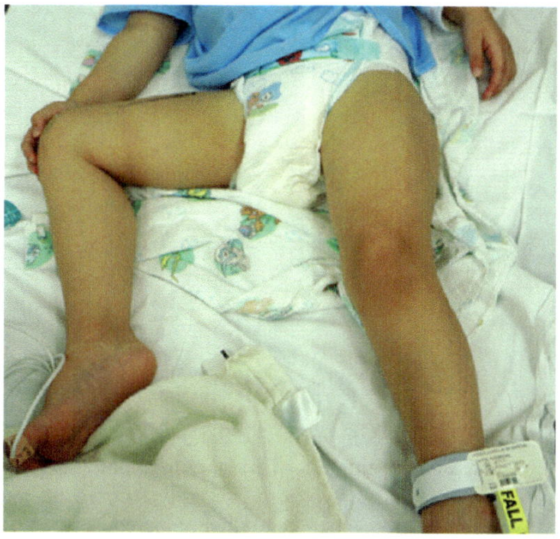

Fig. 3.3 Exam findings of a flexed, externally rotated, and abducted hip are the most concerning as they indicate infection around the hip in children. (*Figure permission: Schoenecker Laboratory*)

pyomyositis, can present with erythema and a swollen appearance. Due to significant swelling associated with musculoskeletal infections, pediatric patients can experience pain, effusion that hinders motion, and subsequent anxiety associated with pain [10]. As such, when the hip is involved, patients most often hold their hips in a flexed, abducted, and externally rotated position (Fig. 3.3). When the knee or elbow is involved, patients will likewise present with an unwillingness to move the joint, adopting a semi-flexed position. As the infection progresses, further tissue damage and swelling can cause increased pressure within the joint capsule, ultimately depriving the joint of its necessary blood supply. For this reason, patients are left in their most comfortable position rather than immobilized in an extended position [11, 12].

Imaging Is Essential when Working Up an MSKI

In current practice, MRI has become the gold standard for accurately determining the anatomical location(s) and tissue types infected in children with suspected MSKI. Given the superior soft tissue resolution, MRI and FAST-sequence MRI can both effectively differentiate pyomyositis, osteomyelitis, and septic arthritis. If the child is young enough to necessitate sedation for a full MRI to be performed, a FAST-sequence MRI can be employed [13]. While cases of isolated MSKI do occur, infections that are more severe and lead to adverse outcomes typically involve infection of multiple tissues (e.g., bone, muscle, and the intra-articular space) or systemic infections involving multiple body parts (e.g., bone and lung) [14–16] (Fig. 3.2). When disseminated disease is suspected, the investigative team must be sure to avoid "satisfaction of search" by not expanding their search for additional infected sites beyond the most painful joint (Fig. 3.4). Thus, MRI can be extremely beneficial when assessing disease severity and directing surgical intervention.

- While cases of isolated MSKI do occur, infections that are more severe and lead to adverse outcomes typically involve infection of multiple tissues or systemic infections involving multiple body parts.
- When disseminated disease is suspected, the investigative team must be sure to avoid "satisfaction of search" and look beyond the most painful joint.

More frequent utilization of MRI during the evaluation of pediatric patients with suspected MSKI has dramatically improved our understanding of MSKI pathology. For example, just one decade ago, pericapsular hip pyomyositis was considered a tropical infection; however, now it is a common diagnosis in temperate climates [17–21]. At one center, by employing routine FAST-sequence MRI, pericapsular hip pyomyositis was found to be twice as common as an isolated septic hip [17]. The distinction of this diagnosis is clinically relevant, as draining an aseptic hip with a sympathetic effusion is not only unnecessary but also may potentially allow dissemination from the pyomyositis into the

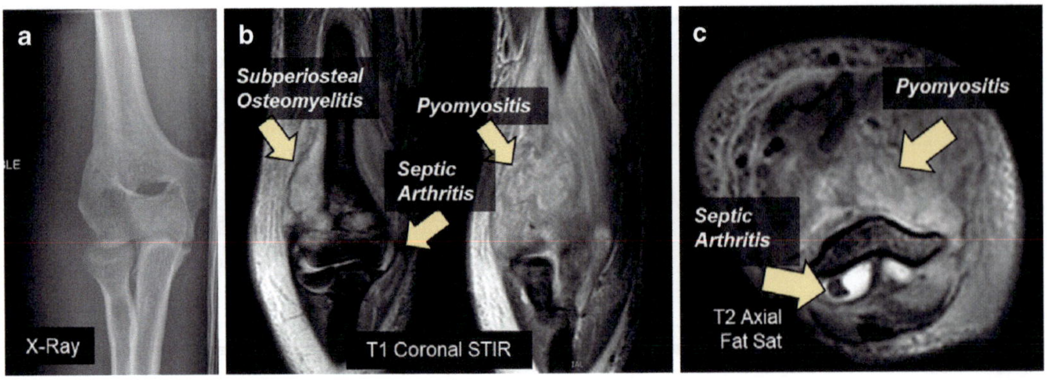

Fig. 3.4 Case example of multifocal infection. A 16-year-old presented with a painful elbow joint. X-ray (**a**) did not reveal diagnostic information, and ultrasound (not shown) was suggestive of a septic joint. An elbow FAST-sequence MRI was performed non-sedated in less than 15 minutes, revealing invaluable diagnostic information for culture and debridement. (**b**) MRI (T1 coronal STIR sequence) and (**c**) axial T2 Fat-Sat illustrated evidence of simultaneous subperiosteal osteomyelitis, septic arthritis, and pyomyositis. Without this information, culture and surgical debridement would have been primarily focused on the intra-articular space and potentially intraosseous, whereas the primary focus of the infection was extra-articular in the muscle and subperiosteal space. (*Figure permission: Schoenecker Laboratory*)

intra-articular space. Furthermore, routine use of FAST-sequence MRI has similarly revealed heterogeneity of infectious pathologies around the knee with synovitis, isolated osteomyelitis, and bursitis occurring at a greater frequency than isolated septic arthritis [22]. Taken together, these studies illustrate that to help direct treatment, a sensitive and multidimensional assessment of muscle and bone is required. Additional information on imaging modalities to diagnose MSKI can be found in Chap. 4.

Musculoskeletal Infections Are a Form of Continuous Injury

Musculoskeletal tissue injury evokes a cascade of carefully regulated pathways that are collectively known as the acute-phase response (APR). The two principal roles of the APR are (1) survival and (2) tissue repair. These objectives are tackled in temporal order, such that during the "survival" phase, damage control is initiated by a coordinated effort between coagulation and the survival inflammatory response to temporarily isolate compartments with a fibrin/platelet seal. Additionally, this sealant promotes the reduction of bleeding as well as the egress of survival inflammatory cells that help reduce the susceptibility to infection. For example, neutrophils, in cooperation with the host's coagulation response, work to trap bacteria in DNA-neutrophil extracellular traps (DNA-NETS) and fibrin webs and release chemotoxins to kill pathogens. Meanwhile, macrophages clear the trapped bacteria [13]. Once survival is ensured, the APR transitions to a reparative inflammatory response that paves the way for revascularization and regeneration of the damaged tissues. In the context of an isolated injury, such as an elbow fracture, the APR is a regulated and coordinated series of events occurring over 6 weeks, allowing for a timely recovery [23, 24] (Fig. 3.5).

Unlike an acute injury, in the context of an MSKI, tissue damage is continual as the infection worsens or spreads. After invading the body, bacterial proliferation and the expression of virulence factors allow pathogens to evade the host containment mechanisms (fibrin/DNA webs) and migrate through tissue planes causing damage to neighboring tissue. Thus, as opposed to single isolated infections, the APR in combinatory infections is more exuberant and correlates with

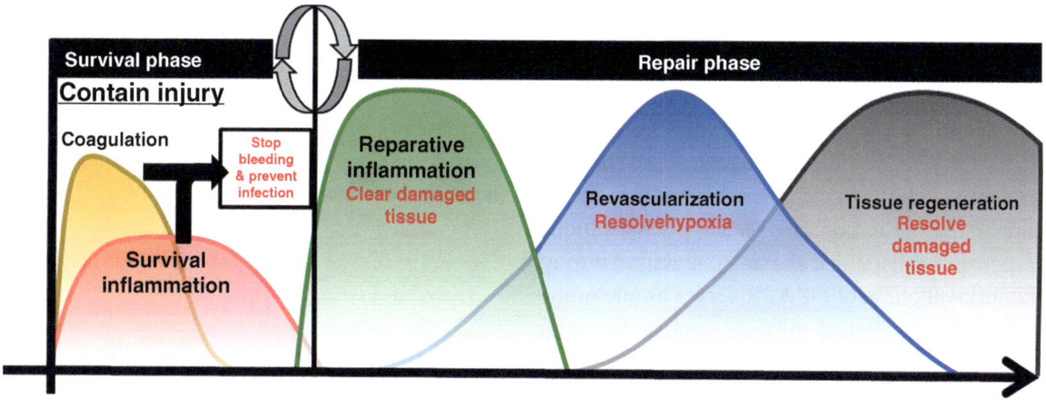

Fig. 3.5 The acute-phase response – the body's response to injury. To ensure survival following an injury, the body must first contain the injury by resolving bleeding and preventing infection. This is accomplished through the coordinated activation of the coagulation cascade (i.e., hemostasis) and the survival inflammatory response. Once bleeding has been stopped and any infectious pathogens are contained, the body can transition to the "reparative phase" where inflammatory components, such as macrophages, can enter the tissue and begin to clear dead cellular debris, bacteria, and damaged tissue. Once cleared, revascularization and tissue regeneration of the damaged tissues can occur to reestablish the pre-injury physiologic state. (*Figure permission: Schoenecker Laboratory*)

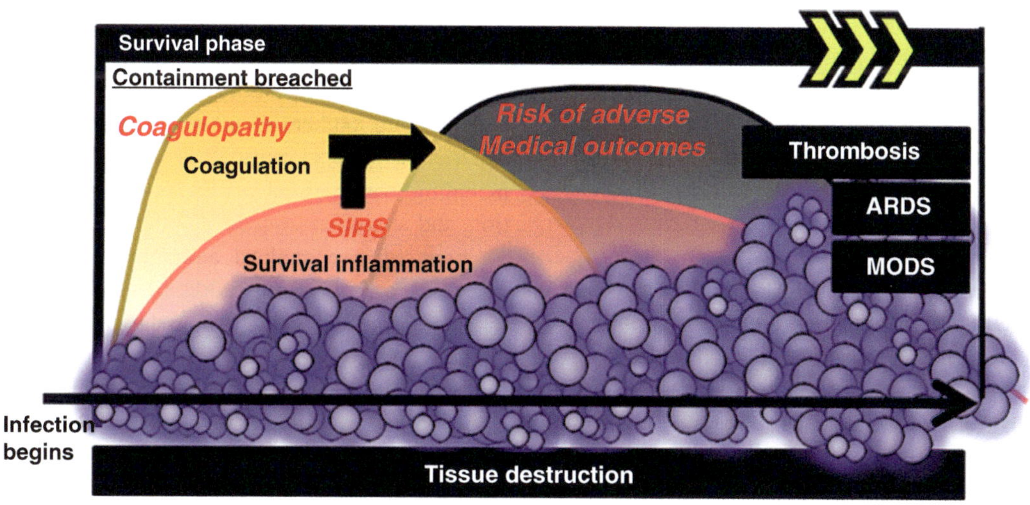

Fig. 3.6 Exuberant acute-phase response during an MSKI. As the infection progresses, the survival phase of the APR will progressively increase in magnitude as it attempts to respond to the growing infection and tissue destruction. The duration and severity of activation of coagulation and survival inflammation proportionally increase the patient's risk for adverse medical outcomes such as thrombosis, acute respiratory distress syndrome (ARDS), multiorgan dysfunction (MODS), and ultimately death. *Figure permission: Schoenecker Laboratory*

the amount of tissue infected and the duration of the infection. Furthermore, in addition to the "volume" of an infection, the bacteria's capacity to hijack many of the acute-phase reactants can further drive an exuberant "survival" APR (Fig. 3.6). As a result, the regulated and coordinated nature of the APR can be lost [6, 23] due to this continuous and invasive nature of MSKI.

Bacterial Hijacking of the APR

The significance of MSKI in APR aberration is in part due to the coevolution over millions of years of bacteria to develop mechanisms to "hijack" and utilize the host APR to their advantage to support dissemination and evade the host immune response. As discussed above, coagulation during the survival phase of the APR serves as one of the initial defense mechanisms against bacterial invasion by immobilizing bacteria with fibrin clots and recruiting leukocytes to the site of infection through integrin expression on fibrin [6]. However, bacteria like *S. aureus* utilize the coagulation system to support abscess formation, thus allowing the bacteria to proliferate with protection from the host immune response [6]. Once a quorum within the abscess is reached, *S. aureus* utilizes plasmin, a critical fibrinolytic enzyme, to break apart the fibrin abscess allowing the bacteria to disseminate [6].

Unsurprisingly, many bacteria have developed virulence factors that manipulate the fibrinolytic system to avoid being trapped by procoagulant factors like fibrin. As plasmin is the critical protease for the fibrinolytic system, *S. pyogenes*, *S. aureus*, *E. coli*, *B. burgdorferi*, *N. meningitidis*, and *P. aeruginosa* all hijack plasmin activity as a means to cleave fibrin clots, laminin basement membranes, and DNA nets to escape containment and disseminate [6]. Together, these virulence factors help to explain why bacteria commonly associated with musculoskeletal infections often disseminate among various anatomical tissue compartments (bone, muscle, joint space, or in circulation). This ongoing evolutionary battle between the host APR and the pathogen's capacity to hijack these mechanisms will continue to evolve. Therefore, awareness and continual reeducation of the interplay between the APR and bacterial infections of the musculoskeletal system will aid in the diagnosis, prognostication of disease severity, and treatment of MSKI henceforth [6, 23, 25].

> The APR activates proportionally to the severity of the infection. *S. aureus* hijacks elements of the host APR, specifically both coagulation and fibrinolysis, to evade the host immune response, allowing the infection to progress and subsequently disseminate.

Morbidity and Mortality Is Relative to a Prolonged or Exuberant APR

When dysregulated, an exuberant survival APR drives inflammation and coagulation to pathologic levels, leading to adverse musculoskeletal and medical outcomes in pediatric patients with MSKI. Adverse medical outcomes can include thrombotic events such as deep vein thrombosis, pulmonary emboli, or septic emboli [23, 26], as well as the need for interventions such as ICU admission or placement on ECMO. Given the essential role for vascularity in developing bone, patients with exuberant survival APRs can also experience adverse musculoskeletal outcomes including avascular necrosis, loss of joint function, and abnormal limb development (Fig. 3.7). To limit adverse medical and musculoskeletal outcomes, rapid identification, diagnosis, and treatment of an MSKI are essential to mitigate an exuberant or prolonged APR. Additional details about adverse medical and musculoskeletal outcomes following MSKI and associated treatment can be found in Chaps. 6 and 22.

Assessing the Severity of a Musculoskeletal Infection

Fortunately, modern medicine has dramatically reduced the mortality from MSKI, which was estimated as high as 40% in the pre-antibiotic era [27, 28]. Although few pediatric patients succumb to MSKI in the United States, MSKI continues to cause significant morbidity in children through

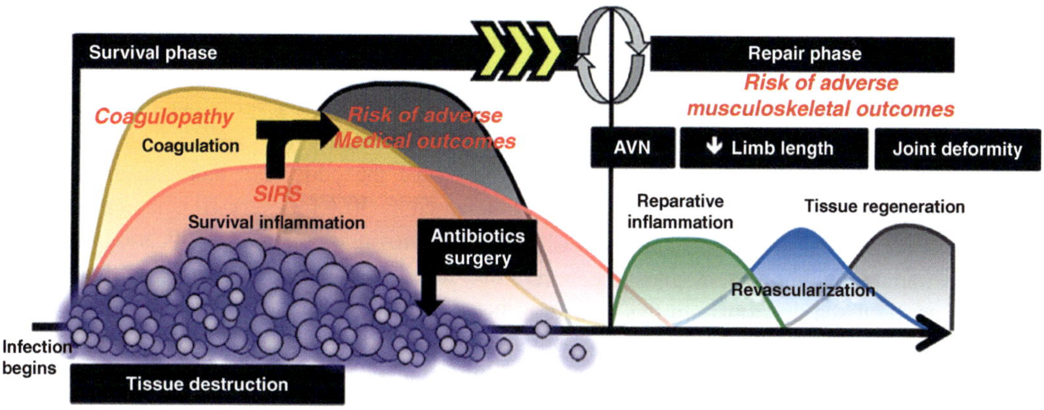

Fig. 3.7 The acute-phase response following treatment for MSKI. Through intervention with surgical debridement and antibiotic administration, the pathogen onslaught can be reduced. This allows the survival phase of the APR to be sufficient to stop bleeding and trap the remaining bacteria. However, as a result of the exuberant survival APR activated in response to infection, patients may still experience adverse musculoskeletal outcomes such as avascular necrosis (AVN), limb length discrepancies, joint deformity, or impaired tissue healing following the resolution of the infection. (*Figure permission: Schoenecker Laboratory*)

adverse medical and musculoskeletal outcomes [14, 22, 26, 29, 30]. The incidence and severity of these adverse medical and musculoskeletal outcomes increase in proportion to the severity of the infection. As noted above, the severity of an infection is a summation of the pathogen's virulence and dissemination, combined with the exuberance of the body's APR to the pathogen.

- MSKI continues to cause significant morbidity in children through adverse medical and musculoskeletal outcomes.
- The incidence and severity of these adverse medical and musculoskeletal outcomes increase in proportion to the severity of the infection.

Identification of the Pathogen Can Aid in Assessing Disease Severity

In cases of presumed MSKI, rapid identification of the causative organisms by culturing allows for earlier narrowing of antibiotic therapy, thus decreasing the overuse of broad-spectrum antibiotics. In addition to directing pharmacologic intervention, knowledge of the causative pathogen can likewise inform the clinical care team about the severity of the infection given that pathogens vary in their expression of virulence factors and capacity to hijack the APR. For example, the two most common bacteria that infect children, *S. pyogenes* and *S. aureus*, produce virulence factors that increase disease severity by allowing the pathogen to rapidly disseminate across tissue planes and into the bloodstream [6]. Alternatively, pathogens such as *Kingella kingae*, which has been rising in incidence as a causative pathogen for septic arthritis in children younger than 2 years of age, express relatively fewer virulence factors and are often associated with a minimal APR [31–34]. For these reasons, knowledge of the causative pathogen not only aids in directing antibiotic therapy but likewise can inform treating physicians about disease severity and risk of adverse outcomes. Please see Chap. 2 for more information on microbiology of MSKI and Chap. 6 for a deeper discussion of *S. aureus* virulence factors.

Classification System for MSKI Severity in Pediatric Patients

Presently, many studies assessing pediatric MSKI divide patient populations relative to their diagnosis base on the tissue type that is infected [13, 35]. An inherent limitation to this practice is that clinical presentation, treatment, and patient prognosis are highly variable within each diagnostic cohort [36], and as discussed previously in this chapter, MSKIs are often not isolated to a single tissue. For these reasons, classification systems based on MSKI severity and degree of dissemination have been developed [14, 29] to stratify patients with suspected MSKI into three categories: inflammation (noninfectious), local infection, and disseminated infection [14] (Table 3.1). Utilizing these criteria, cases of disseminated disease were found to be positively correlated with both prolonged hospital stays and elevated markers of the APR. As such, a subsequent study demonstrates that CRP, pulse rate, and temperature together could accurately predict MSKI severity classification at the time of presentation [29]. Specifically, this model found that the odds of a more severe outcome increased by 30% for every 10 U increase in CRP [29]. Improving upon this classification system, it was noted that pediatric patients with disseminated disease who did or did not experience complications had varying APR profiles [15]; thus, a fourth category (disseminated infection + complication) has been established (Table 3.1). Since this classification system does not rely on anatomic diagnosis or identification of tissue involvement, early identification of disease severity, and therefore patient prognosis, is possible. Future prospective studies are warranted to validate the clinical utility of this classification system and model.

Table 3.1 Classification system for MSKI severity

	Inflammatory(noninfectious)	Local infections	Disseminated infections	Disseminated infection + complication
Definition	All of the following (if available) must be TRUE: Negative blood culture Negative local culture The criteria for "local" or "disseminated infections" are not met	One of the following must be TRUE: Imaging diagnostic for osteomyelitis or pyomyositis in one anatomical site Local culture positive AND/OR fluid/tissue consistent with infection (grossly purulent, cell count >50,000, and/or positive PCR) One positive blood culture The criteria for "disseminated infections" are not met	For two or more anatomic sites, at least one of the following must be TRUE: Imaging diagnostic for osteomyelitis or pyomyositis Local culture positive AND/OR fluid/tissue consistent with infection (grossly purulent, cell count >50,000, and/or positive PCR) Two or more positive blood culture	In addition to meeting the criteria for "disseminated infections," at least one of the following must be TRUE: Thromboembolic disease such as: Deep vein thrombosis Pulmonary embolism Avascular necrosis Multiorgan failure Pleural effusion Pathologic fracture Limb/joint deformity Amputation Sequestration/involucrum Death
Example	Transient synovitis	Isolated distal femoral osteomyelitis with no subperiosteal abscess Isolated septic hip	Distal fibular osteomyelitis with subperiosteal abscess Septic hip with surrounding pyomyositis	Patient with proximal femur osteomyelitis with subperiosteal abscess and adjacent pyomyositis that experiences multiple venous thromboembolisms

Laboratory Measure of the APR to Assess MSKI Severity

Accurately determining the severity of an MSKI is essential to managing patient morbidity and the risk of adverse medical and musculoskeletal outcomes. In addition to identifying the causative pathogen and locating the site(s) of the infection, clinical laboratory draws can be used to assess the exuberance of the infection provoked APR. One such well-validated laboratory measure, C-reactive protein (CRP) is a dynamic acute-phase reactant that becomes elevated in response to inflammation [13]. In current clinical practice, CRP is utilized as both a diagnostic and prognostic tool at the time of consultation for MSKI. In prior studies, CRP has been found to be effective for early diagnosis of an infection within 4–6 hours of symptom onset. Given that CRP levels rapidly elevate in proportion to the amount of tissue inflammation, admission CRP levels have been demonstrated to sensitively predict the severity of an MSKI [14], while assessment of peak CRP levels has been demonstrated to be a strong predictor of adverse vascular outcomes in patients with MSKI, such as venous thromboembolism. Specifically, it was found that for every 20 mg/L increase in peak CRP, the risk of thrombosis increased by 29% [15]. Beyond prognosticating the severity of MSKI and risk of adverse outcomes, serial measures of CRP have been proposed as a means to assess response to treatment. In MSKIs, if a treatment is effective, the CRP and other acute-phase reactants should begin to return to normal levels [23]. If values do not return to baseline or continue to increase within ~48 hours of intervention, this may indi-

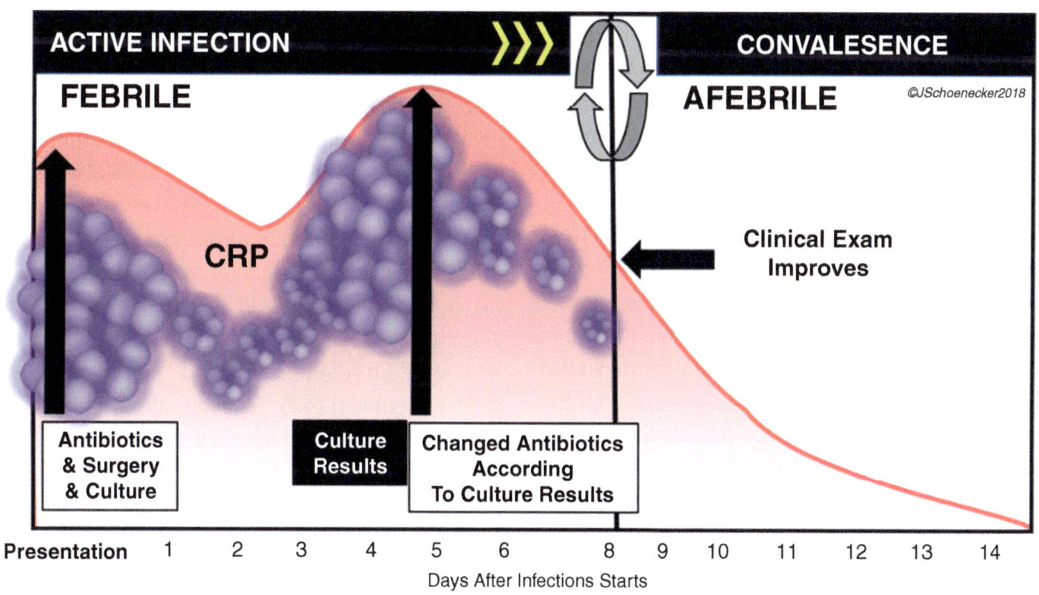

Fig. 3.8 Utility of serial laboratory values of the APR. Trends in CRP can be useful for assessing disease severity and treatment efficacy in pediatric patients with MSKI, as seen in this representative patient data. Early treatment with antibiotics and surgery can reduce the infectious burden, thereby leading to a decrease in CRP over the first 2 days. However, if CRP begins increasing again, this can indicate to the treating physician that further intervention may be necessary. At this time, culture results showed inadequate therapy, and antibiotics were adjusted. After this point, the CRP once again began trending downward and the clinical exam improved. The body then entered the convalescent stage where tissue repair can begin. This case highlights the importance of both culture-directed therapy and the capacity for serial APR measures to assist with patient care. (*Figure permission: Schoenecker Laboratory*)

cate to the medical team that the prior treatment was insufficient and further intervention is likely necessary (Fig. 3.8).

- In addition to identifying the causative pathogen and locating the site(s) of the infection, clinical laboratory draws can be used to assess the exuberance of the infection provoked APR.
- Serial laboratory measures of the APR can aid the medical team in determining if the prior treatment was sufficient or if further intervention is necessary.

Another classically measured plasma APR value is the erythrocyte sedimentation rate (ESR). In the context of injury or infection, ESR has been examined as a surrogate measure for fibrinogen and the ongoing containment of the injury to prevent bleeding and reduce susceptibility to infection (Fig. 3.5). Compared to CRP, ESR is a less sensitive marker for the APR and can also produce misleading data for assessing infections given that confounding conditions, such as pregnancy, obesity, and anemia, all result in an elevated ESR [37, 38]. Furthermore, reflective of fibrinogen's role in containment, ESR is a longer acting and less dynamic acute-phase reactant. Therefore, while ESR may not perform well at admission for predicting the presence of an infection, monitoring ESR may be useful to assess disease severity and risk of adverse medical and musculoskeletal outcomes [39].

Cellular Markers of the Acute-Phase Response

In addition to plasma acute-phase reactants, changes in cellular effectors can also be sensitive indicators of the "survival' APR (Fig. 3.9a). Broadly, white blood cell (WBC) counts are commonly utilized to assess the presence of an infection. However, WBC counts are one of the least sensitive measures for the diagnosis of a pediatric MSKI. In addition to being variable with age, prior studies have demonstrated a wide range in the incidence of elevated WBC counts (25–73%) among osteomyelitis patients. Furthermore, similar WBC values have been reported in pediatric patients with inflammatory (noninfectious) etiologies, local infections, and disseminated infection. This demonstrates that elevated WBC counts alone are not sufficient to confirm the presence or assess the severity of a MSKI [29].

Alternatively, analysis of specific subtypes of leukocytes, such neutrophils, lymphocytes, and their relative proportions, has been found to be more sensitive for assessing the presence or severity of an infection. As opposed to measuring the WBC without a differential, which is "like trying to decide who won an election by just counting how many people voted,[1]" understanding a differential provides invaluable information regarding the infection and can tell you "who is winning the election." Neutrophils are an essential cellular player in innate immunity that activate in response to the APR and bacterial invasion. In addition to directly binding and phagocytosing pathogens, neutrophils also aid in trapping and killing bacteria in the extracellular space by producing neutrophil extracellular traps (NETs), reactive oxygen species, and other cytotoxic molecules [40, 41] (Fig. 3.9b). Given these essential roles, neutrophils are the most abundant leukocyte in circulation, and their levels are tightly regulated [42]. As such, elevation in neutrophil number has long been utilized as a prognostic indicator of infection. However, when evaluating the severity of infection, neutrophil count alone does not perform well [43]. For these reasons, many studies have begun to examine cellular ratios, such as the neutrophil to lymphocyte ratio (NLR), as more sensitive predictors of disease severity and prognosticators of patient outcomes.

While not yet commonly utilized in pediatric MSKI, NLR has been demonstrated in numerous studies to sensitively detect infections and prog-

[1]Dr. Isaac Thomsen – Vanderbilt University Pediatric Infectious Disease

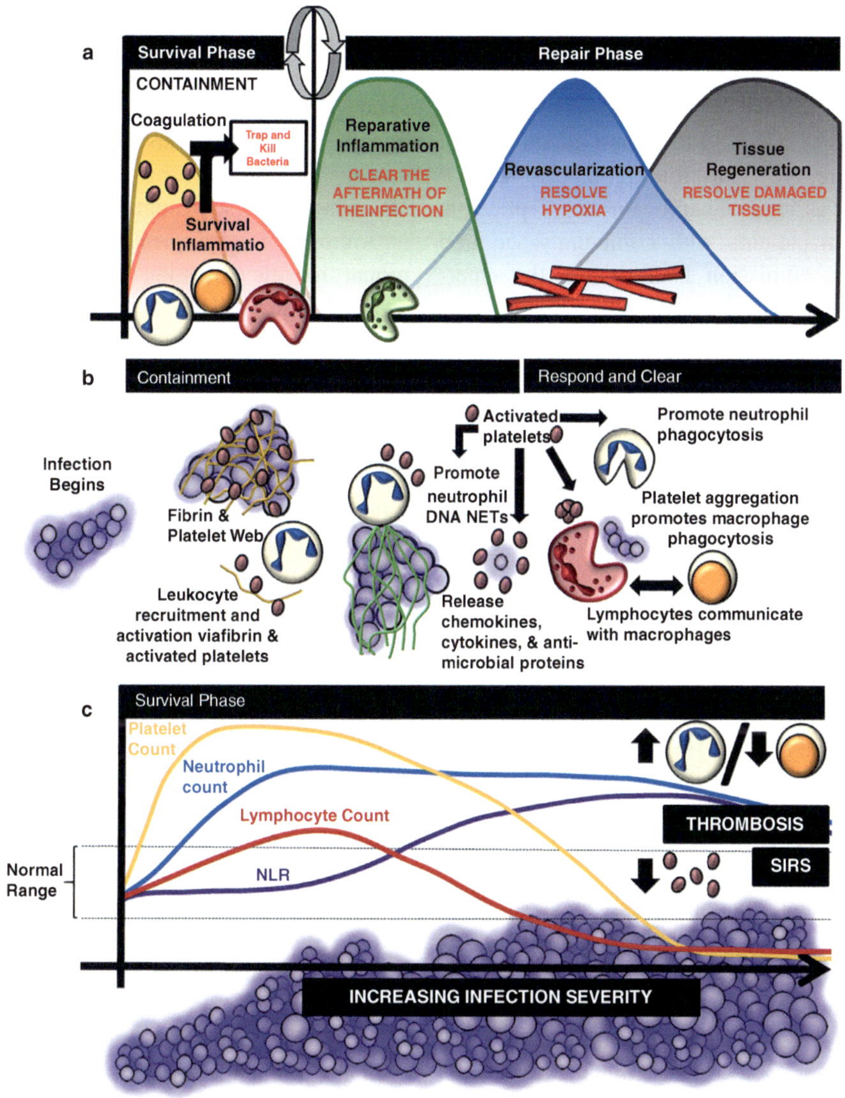

Fig. 3.9 The cellular APR following infection. Always get a differential. (**a**) Following the establishment of an infection and the associated tissue destruction, much like an acute injury, the body must first stop bleeding and contain the infection. This is accomplished through the coordinated activities of the coagulation and survival inflammatory systems during the "survival" phase of the APR. (**b**) Coagulation components, specifically fibrin and platelets, aid in containing the bacteria to the site of infection in addition to serving as a platform for recruitment of leukocytes. Through these interactions, an important second containment mechanism is activated – the production of NETs. As the infection is contained, pro-inflammatory macrophages and neutrophils begin to phagocytose invading pathogens. Through engulfing the pathogens, macrophages can then communicate with lymphocytes as part of the innate immune response. Together, these coordinated activities of the coagulation and survival inflammatory systems are essential to control, contain, and combat an infection. (**c**) As the infection progresses and increases in severity, the cellular components of the APR can become dysregulated. Platelets, which initially increase in number to assist with fighting an infection, can begin to diminish when the infection is exuberant and prolonged, reflecting their consumption, sequestration, or clearance from circulation. Likewise, neutrophils and lymphocytes both elevate in response to infection. As the infection increases in severity and/or prolongs, lymphocytopenia can occur, resulting in a greater NLR. Thus, measures of decreasing platelet count and increasing NLR together have been found in cases of adult infection to associate with poor outcomes such as thrombosis and systemic inflammatory response syndrome (SIRS). While less examined to date, there is ample scientific premise for the use of both platelet count and NLR as a means to assess severity and outcome in patients with pediatric MSKI. (*Figure permission: Schoenecker Laboratory*)

nosticate disease severity and patient outcomes (Fig. 3.9c). For example, in patients hospitalized for fever with an unknown origin, NLR was found to be higher in patients with a bacterial infection than in those with a viral infection [44]. Furthermore, NLR was able to outperform CRP and WBC as an early indicator for septicemia [45–47]. In patients with community-acquired pneumonia, admission NLR within the emergency department was able to predict disease severity and outcomes with a higher prognostic accuracy than CRP, WBC, or either cellular measure alone [48]. Finally, when considering patient outcomes, elevated NLR was an independent marker for mortality in patients with bacteremia [49] and a strong positive predictor for treatment failure and 90-day mortality in adult patients with septic arthritis [50].

Finally, a small but essential cellular marker of the APR are platelets. As the first line of defense against pathogen invasion, platelets are capable of directly interacting with bacteria [51, 52], engulfing bacteria [53], and releasing bactericidal molecules from their granules. Furthermore, platelets can also interface with the innate immune response, leading to the release of a myriad of chemokines, cytokines, and the formation of platelet-lymphocyte aggregates, which together play an essential role in supporting the containment and removal of pathogens by the innate immune response that is critical to survival [54, 55]. As part of these activities, both abnormally high as well as abnormally low platelet counts have been associated with detection of infection and adverse outcomes [56, 57] (Fig. 3.9b and c).

Combatting an Exuberant APR with Surgical Debridement and Antibiotic Administration

As noted above, regulation of the survival APR is critical, such that continuous exuberant activation of the APR can lead to adverse outcomes and account for the majority of morbidity and mortality in pediatric patients with MSKI. Therefore, the APR may be viewed as a "double-edged sword." While a well-coordinated survival APR is essential for combating and eliminating an infection, a prolonged, excessive survival APR can drive adverse outcomes [23]. Together, these concepts present a paradox for surgeons, physicians, and healthcare professionals caring for these patients.

Antibiotics and surgical debridement are paramount for the cessation of continuous injury caused by the MSKI [6, 23] (Fig. 3.8). In collaboration with antibiotic administration that pharmacologically targets the pathogen, surgical debridement of the infected tissue is often required to reduce the infectious burden and mitigate the associated survival APR. Numerous factors should be considered when directing surgical intervention in these patients. For example, any patient who is physiologically unstable secondary to an MSKI should be considered for urgent surgical debridement. This is particularly important in cases of rapidly progressing and destructive musculoskeletal infections, such as necrotizing fasciitis [58]. Beyond these cases, the indications for surgery become less defined. In general, abscesses will not resolve on their own; thus, drainage and debridement are required. Depending on the location and severity of the MSKI, drainage and debridement can be done at the bedside or with a small radiographically guided procedure. However, when the infection lies deeper within tissues behind vital structures, involves multiple tissues, or has formed more complex fluid collections, operative debridement might be necessary to clear the infection [59]. Additional details about antibiotic administration and management of patients with MSKI can be found in Chaps. 2, 34, and 35.

Conclusion

Pediatric MSKIs have diverse pathology with variable clinical presentation, heterogeneity of anatomic location, and a range of possible adverse medical and musculoskeletal outcomes. Given that MSKI is a form of continuous injury, as the infection progresses, an exuberant APR is activated relative to the severity of the disease.

Timely and accurate evaluation of patients with suspected MSKI is essential to direct treatment to limit the possibility of an exuberant APR, thereby reducing the risk of adverse medical and musculoskeletal outcomes.

Box 3.1 Key Learning Points

- Pediatric MSKI can range markedly in severity, influencing the patient's risk for adverse medical and musculoskeletal outcomes.
- The severity of an infection is a summation of the virulence and dissemination of the pathogen, combined with the level to which the body responds to the pathogen (i.e., APR).
- Clinically, diagnostic imaging and serial laboratory values assessing the APR are powerful predictors of MSKI severity.
- Together, these data can aid in directing timely and accurate treatment for MSKI, ultimately aimed at limiting the possibility of an exuberant APR to reduce the risk of adverse outcomes.

References

1. Schoenecker JG, The Children's Orthopaedic Trauma and Infection Consortium for Evidence Based Study (CORTICES) Group. Defining the volume of consultations for musculoskeletal infection encountered by pediatric orthopaedic services in the United States. PLoS One. 2020;15(6):e0234055.
2. Morrissy RT, Haynes DW. Acute hematogenous osteomyelitis: a model with trauma as an etiology. J Pediatr Orthop. 1989;9(4):447–56.
3. Whalen JL, Fitzgerald RH Jr, Morrissy RT. A histological study of acute hematogenous osteomyelitis following physeal injuries in rabbits. J Bone Joint Surg Am. 1988;70(9):1383–92.
4. Stannard JP, Robinson JT, Anderson ER, McGwin G Jr, Volgas DA, Alonso JE. Negative pressure wound therapy to treat hematomas and surgical incisions following high-energy trauma. J Trauma. 2006;60(6):1301–6.
5. Alshryda S, Howard JJ, Huntley JS, Schoenecker JG. The pediatric and adolescent hip: essentials and evidence. Springer Nature Switzerland AG 2019.
6. Rosenfeld S, Bernstein DT, Daram S, Dawson J, Zhang W. Predicting the presence of adjacent infections in septic arthritis in children. J Pediatr Orthop. 2016;36(1):70–4.
7. Hobo T. Zur Pathogenese der akuten haematogenen osteomyelitis. Acta Sch Med Univ Kioto. 1921;4:1–29.
8. Cunningham R, Cockayne A, Humphreys H. Clinical and molecular aspects of the pathogenesis of Staphylococcus aureus bone and joint infections. J Med Microbiol. 1996;44(3):157–64.
9. Yi J, Wood JB, Creech CB, Williams D, Jimenez-Truque N, Yildirim I, et al. Clinical epidemiology and outcomes of pediatric musculoskeletal infections. J Pediatr. 2021;234:236–244.e2.
10. Peltola H, Vahvanen V. A comparative study of osteomyelitis and purulent arthritis with special reference to aetiology and recovery. Infection. 1984;12(2):75–9.
11. Nade S. Acute septic arthritis in infancy and childhood. J Bone Joint Surg Br. 1983;65(3):234–41.
12. Soto-Hall R, Johnson LH, Johnson RA. Variations in the intra-articular pressure of the hip joint in injury and disease. A probable factor in avascular necrosis. J Bone Joint Surg Am. 1964;46:509–16.
13. Moore-Lotridge SN, Gibson BH, Duvernay MT, Martus JE, Thomsen IP, Schoenecker JG. Pediatric musculoskeletal infection. JPOSNA. 2020;2:2.
14. Mignemi ME, Benvenuti MA, An TJ, Martus JE, Mencio GA, Lovejoy SA, et al. A novel classification system based on dissemination of musculoskeletal infection is predictive of hospital outcomes. J Pediatr Orthop. 2018;38(5):279–86.
15. Amaro E, Marvi TK, Posey SL, Benvenuti MA, An TJ, Dale KM, et al. C-reactive protein predicts risk of venous thromboembolism in pediatric musculoskeletal infection. J Pediatr Orthop. 2019;39(1):e62–e7.
16. Copley LA, Barton T, Garcia C, Sun D, Gaviria-Agudelo C, Gheen WT, et al. A proposed scoring system for assessment of severity of illness in pediatric acute hematogenous osteomyelitis using objective clinical and laboratory findings. Pediatr Infect Dis J. 2014;33(1):35–41.
17. Mignemi ME, Menge TJ, Cole HA, Mencio GA, Martus JE, Lovejoy S, et al. Epidemiology, diagnosis, and treatment of pericapsular pyomyositis of the hip in children. J Pediatr Orthop. 2014;34(3):316–25.
18. Comegna L, Guidone PI, Prezioso G, Franchini S, Petrosino MI, Di Filippo P, et al. Pyomyositis is not only a tropical pathology: a case series. J Med Case Rep. 2016;10(1):1–6.
19. Shuler FD, Buchanan GS, Stover C, Johnson B, Modarresi M, Jasko JJ. Pyomyositis mistaken for septic hip arthritis in children: the role of MRI in diagnosis and management. Marshall J Med. 2018;4(2):22.
20. Chotai PN, Hsiao MS, Pathak I, Banh D, Abdou M, Abdelgawad AA. Pediatric pelvic pyomyositis: initial MRI can be misleading. J Pediatr Orthop B. 2016;25(6):520–4.

21. Levitt DL, Byer R, Miller AF. Point-of-care ultrasound to diagnose pyomyositis in a child. Pediatr Emerg Care. 2019;35(1):69–71.
22. Gibian JT, Daryoush JR, Wollenman CC, Johnson SR, Henry A, Koehler RJ, et al. The heterogeneity of pediatric knee infections: a retrospective analysis. J Pediatr Orthop. 2020;40(6):314–21.
23. Benvenuti M, An T, Amaro E, Lovejoy S, Mencio G, Martus J, et al. Double-edged sword: musculoskeletal infection provoked acute phase response in children. Orthop Clin North Am. 2017;48(2):181–97.
24. Oelsner WK, Engstrom SM, Benvenuti MA, An TJ, Jacobson RA, Polkowski GG, et al. Characterizing the acute phase response in healthy patients following Total joint arthroplasty: predictable and consistent. J Arthroplast. 2017;32(1):309–14.
25. Blyth MJ, Kincaid R, Craigen MA, Bennet GC. The changing epidemiology of acute and subacute haematogenous osteomyelitis in children. J Bone Joint Surg Br. 2001;83(1):99–102.
26. Mantadakis E, Plessa E, Vouloumanou EK, Michailidis L, Chatzimichael A, Falagas ME. Deep venous thrombosis in children with musculoskeletal infections: the clinical evidence. Int J Infect Dis. 2012;16(4):e236–e43.
27. Ciampolini J, Harding KG. Pathophysiology of chronic bacterial osteomyelitis. Why do antibiotics fail so often? Postgrad Med J. 2000;76(898):479–83.
28. Song KM, Sloboda JF. Acute hematogenous osteomyelitis in children. J Am Acad Orthop Surg. 2001;9(3):166–75.
29. Benvenuti MA, An TJ, Mignemi ME, Martus JE, Mencio GA, Lovejoy SA, et al. A clinical prediction algorithm to stratify pediatric musculoskeletal infection by severity. J Pediatr Orthop. 2019;39(3):153–7.
30. Alshryda S, Huntley JS, Banaszkiewicz PA. Paediatric orthopaedics: an evidence-based approach to clinical questions. Cham: Springer International Publishing; 2016.
31. Adebiyi EO, Ayoade F. Kingella Kingae. Treasure Island: StatPearls Publishing; 2019.
32. Wong M, Williams N, Cooper C. Systematic review of kingella kingae musculoskeletal infection in children: epidemiology, impact and management strategies. Pediatric Health Med Ther. 2020;11:73–84.
33. Yagupsky P, Erlich Y, Ariela S, Trefler R, Porat N. Outbreak of Kingella kingae skeletal system infections in children in daycare. Pediatr Infect Dis J. 2006;25(6):526–32.
34. Yagupsky P, Porsch E, St Geme JW. *Kingella kingae*: an emerging pathogen in young children. Pediatrics. 2011;127(3):557–65.
35. Fayad LM, Carrino JA, Fishman EK. Musculoskeletal infection: role of CT in the emergency department. Radiographics. 2007;27(6):1723–36.
36. Calhoun JH, Manring MM, Shirtliff M. Osteomyelitis of the long bones. Semin Plast Surg. 2009;23(2):59–72.
37. Bottiger LE, Svedberg CA. Normal erythrocyte sedimentation rate and age. Br Med J. 1967;2(5544):85–7.
38. Sox HC Jr, Liang MH. The erythrocyte sedimentation rate. Guidelines for rational use. Ann Intern Med. 1986;104(4):515–23.
39. Michail M, Jude E, Liaskos C, Karamagiolis S, Makrilakis K, Dimitroulis D, et al. The performance of serum inflammatory markers for the diagnosis and follow-up of patients with osteomyelitis. Int J Low Extrem Wounds. 2013;12(2):94–9.
40. Kobayashi SD, Voyich JM, Burlak C, DeLeo FR. Neutrophils in the innate immune response. Arch Immunol Ther Exp. 2005;53(6):505–17.
41. An TJ, Benvenuti MA, Mignemi ME, Thomsen IP, Schoenecker JG. Pediatric musculoskeletal infection: hijacking the acute-phase response. JBJS Rev. 2016;4(9):e4.
42. Kobayashi SD, Malachowa N, DeLeo FR. Influence of microbes on neutrophil life and death. Front Cell Infect Microbiol. 2017;7:159.
43. de Jager CPC, van Wijk PTL, Mathoera RB, de Jongh-Leuvenink J, van der Poll T, Wever PC. Lymphocytopenia and neutrophil-lymphocyte count ratio predict bacteremia better than conventional infection markers in an emergency care unit. Crit Care. 2010;14(5):R192.
44. Naess A, Mo R, Nilssen SS, Eide GE, Sjursen H. Infections in patients hospitalized for fever as related to duration and other predictors at admittance. Infection. 2014;42(3):485–92.
45. Loonen AJ, de Jager CP, Tosserams J, Kusters R, Hilbink M, Wever PC, et al. Biomarkers and molecular analysis to improve bloodstream infection diagnostics in an emergency care unit. PLoS One. 2014;9(1):e87315.
46. Lowsby R, Gomes C, Jarman I, Lisboa P, Nee PA, Vardhan M, et al. Neutrophil to lymphocyte count ratio as an early indicator of blood stream infection in the emergency department. Emerg Med J. 2015;32(7):531–4.
47. Naess A, Nilssen SS, Mo R, Eide GE, Sjursen H. Role of neutrophil to lymphocyte and monocyte to lymphocyte ratios in the diagnosis of bacterial infection in patients with fever. Infection. 2017;45(3):299–307.
48. de Jager CP, Wever PC, Gemen EF, Kusters R, van Gageldonk-Lafeber AB, van der Poll T, et al. The neutrophil-lymphocyte count ratio in patients with community-acquired pneumonia. PLoS One. 2012;7(10):e46561.
49. Terradas R, Grau S, Blanch J, Riu M, Saballs P, Castells X, et al. Eosinophil count and neutrophil-lymphocyte count ratio as prognostic markers in patients with bacteremia: a retrospective cohort study. PLoS One. 2012;7(8):e42860.
50. PE Schwab, Varady N, Chen A. Novel marker for septic hip and knee arthritis: neutrophil-to-lymphocyte ratio is a strong predictor of treatment failure and postoperative 90-day mortality. Orthopaed Proc. 2019;101-B(Supp_14):63–.
51. Kerrigan SW. The expanding field of platelet-bacterial interconnections. Platelets. 2015;26(4):293–301.

52. Ali RA, Wuescher LM, Dona KR, Worth RG. Platelets mediate host defense against Staphylococcus aureus through direct bactericidal activity and by enhancing macrophage activities. J Immunol. 2017;198(1):344–51.
53. McNicol A, Israels SJ. Beyond hemostasis: the role of platelets in inflammation, malignancy and infection. Cardiovasc Hematol Disord Drug Targets. 2008;8(2):99–117.
54. Klinger MHF, Jelkmann W. Role of blood platelets in infection and inflammation. J Interf Cytokine Res. 2002;22(9):913–22.
55. Kral JB, Schrottmaier WC, Salzmann M, Assinger A. Platelet interaction with innate immune cells. Transfus Med Hemother. 2016;43(2):78–88.
56. Riise ØR, Kirkhus E, Handeland KS, Flatø B, Reiseter T, Cvancarova M, et al. Childhood osteomyelitis-incidence and differentiation from other acute onset musculoskeletal features in a population-based study. BMC Pediatr. 2008;8(1):45.
57. Assinger A, Schrottmaier WC, Salzmann M, Rayes J. Platelets in sepsis: an update on experimental models and clinical data. Front Immunol. 2019;10:1687–.
58. Hysong AA, Posey SL, Blum DM, Benvenuti MA, Benvenuti TA, Johnson SR, et al. Necrotizing fasciitis: pillaging the acute phase response. JBJS. 2020;102(6):526–37.
59. Mignemi M, Copley L, Schoenecker J. Evidence-based treatment for musculoskeletal infection. In: Paediatric orthopaedics. Springer; 2017. p. 403–18.

4 Imaging Modalities to Diagnose Musculoskeletal Infections

Caroline M. Blakey, Penny Broadley, Binu T. Kurian, and James A. Fernandes

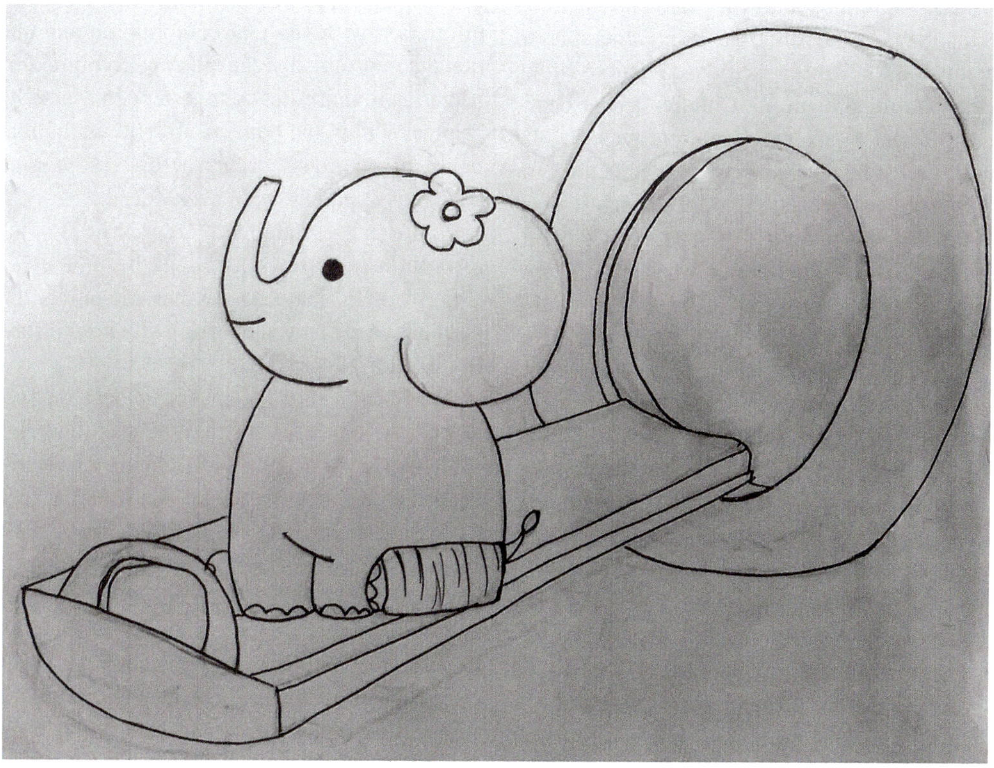

C. M. Blakey (✉)
Department of Paediatric Orthopaedics, Trauma and Spinal Surgery, Sheffield Children's NHS Foundation Trust, Sheffield, UK
e-mail: caroline.blakey1@nhs.net

P. Broadley
Department of Paediatric Radiology, Sheffield Children's NHS Foundation Trust, Sheffield, UK
e-mail: penny.broadley@nhs.net

B. T. Kurian
Department of Trauma and Orthopaedic Surgery, St. John's Medical College Hospital, Bangalore, India
e-mail: binu.k@stjohns.in

J. A. Fernandes
Sheffield Children's Hospital NHS Foundation Trust, University of Sheffield, Sheffield, UK
e-mail: james.fernandes@nhs.net

© Springer Nature Switzerland AG 2022
M. V. Belthur et al. (eds.), *Pediatric Musculoskeletal Infections*,
https://doi.org/10.1007/978-3-030-95794-0_4

Introduction

In children, osteoarticular infection is a condition that continues to evolve. The incidence of paediatric osteomyelitis has increased around the world, with the complexity of disease and virulence of infection also rising [1–3].

Careful history taking in the assessment of a child presenting with possible infection is critical. Symptoms can range from classical joint swelling and reluctance to weight bear, with associated fever, to pyrexia of unknown origin or in an infant isolated pseudoparalysis. The history can be clouded by features such as recent trauma or immunocompromise following varicella infection and antibiotic use. Children are vulnerable to osteomyelitis at highly vascularised regions of the skeleton during growth [2]. Children are susceptible to different organisms at different ages, and the clinician must be aware of risks for infection, for example, in the neonatal period. Examination can be difficult and requires skill and patience, particularly in the child who doesn't want to be examined. Refusal to weight bear can be enough to raise concerns. Serology can be an excellent marker of infection and its severity but does not always correlate and can be normal in the presence of immunocompromise and in younger children.

The consequences of infection, particularly when not managed promptly, can be devastating. Joint destruction, growth disturbance and sepsis are examples. Imaging techniques can lead to prompt, targeted therapy and play a critical role in the work up and monitoring of children with suspected infection. Options for imaging techniques have advanced in line with the complexity of disease, but the approach to imaging must consider the affordability, practicality, necessity and implications to the child. In this chapter we discuss the imaging techniques utilised in the diagnosis of paediatric osteoarticular infection and their potential indications.

Radiography

Conventional radiographs should always be part of initial investigations where there is suspicion of osteoarticular infection. Whilst 90% of X-rays are likely to be normal in the early presentation [4], they are rapid and accessible and remain a very useful investigation, with a relatively low radiation dose. Whilst radiographs cannot exclude acute infection, they may help to identify differential diagnosis such as fracture, oncological process or, in the limping child, conditions such as Perthes' disease or slipped capital femoral epiphysis.

In the presence of acute infection, subtle signs of deep soft tissue swelling may be seen. There may be joint effusion, and periarticular muscle planes may be elevated (Fig. 4.1).

The sensitivity of radiographs for infection increases with the passage of time. Bone changes may be seen, with or without periosteal involvement, but changes can take between 1 and 3 weeks to appear in some cases. Leucocytic infiltration with vascular compression and nutritional compromise of the marrow, combined with bacterial toxicity, leads to osteopenia and lytic changes within the bone. A 30–50% reduction in bone mass must occur before radiographic change is apparent [5, 6] (Fig. 4.2).

Endosteal scalloping, representing focal resorption of cortical bone may become evident (Fig. 4.3). In some aggressive osteomyelitis, a permeative lucency is seen reflecting rapid spread of infection (Fig. 4.4).

Septic arthritis is often not evident on radiographs. A joint effusion may be seen and rarely subluxation and dislocation. There may be signs of periarticular infection. Joint sepsis may occur through direct haematogenous dissemination. Extension from a metaphyseal abscess is often seen in infants since there is direct vascular channels across the physis. In older children perforation of the metaphyseal cortex may contaminate the joint. Increased intraarticular pressure may result in joint subluxation. Subluxation and dislocation can be seen in the infected hip joint (Fig. 4.3). The capsule becomes stretched in the presence of fluid and pus, or the capsule can rupture as infectious material is relieved into the periarticular space [7]. Without early treatment, chondrolytic enzymes rapidly result in cartilage degeneration, with irreversible deformity (Fig. 4.5). There may be tamponade of nutrient blood vessels with signs of avascular necrosis (Fig. 4.6).

Brodie's abscess describes a subacute haematogenous osteomyelitis with intraosseous abscess seen typically in the metaphysis of children with unfused physis [8]. The radiographic appear-

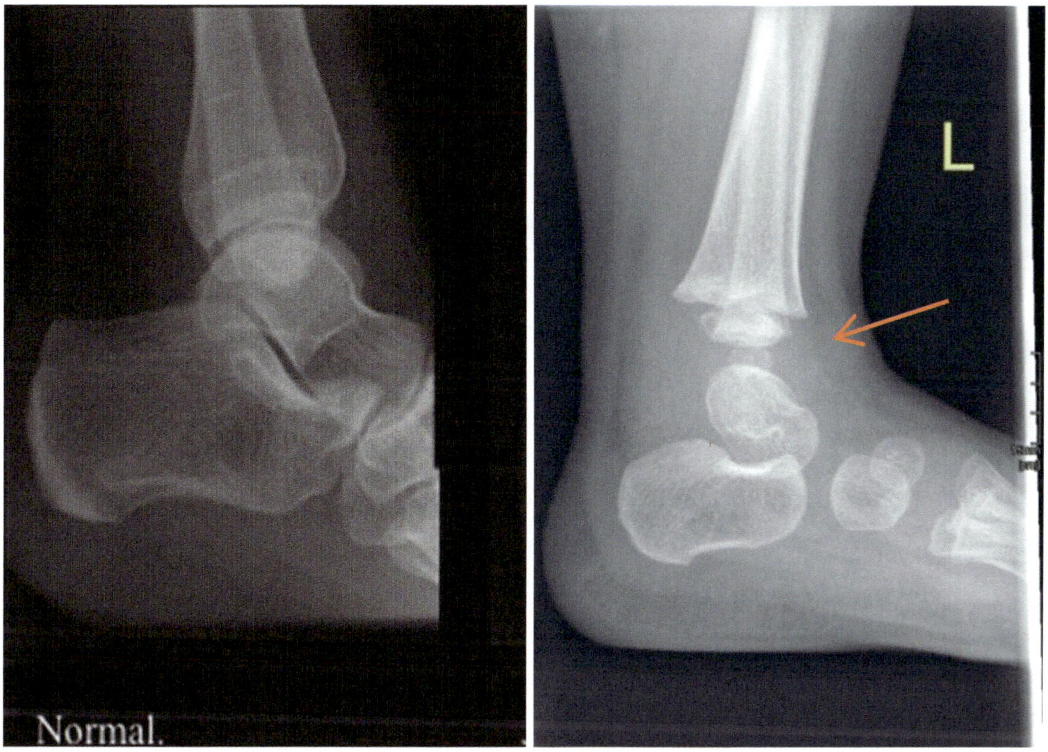

Fig. 4.1 Lateral radiographs of ankle joint demonstrating elevated periarticular muscle/tendon planes and joint effusion (red arrow)

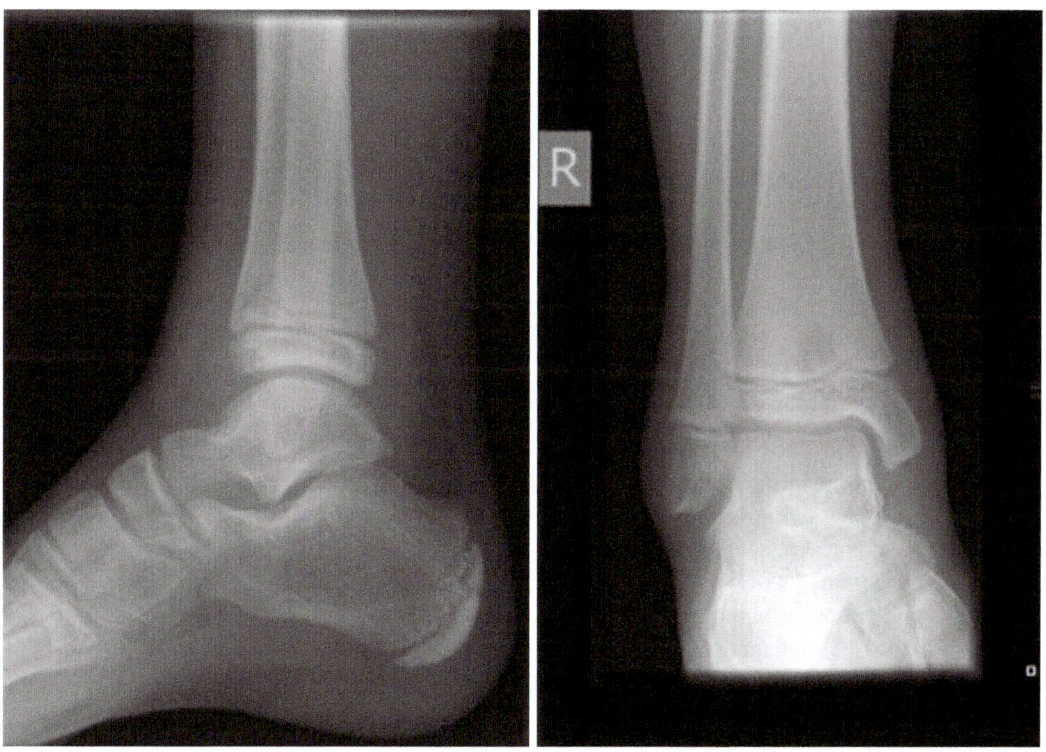

Fig. 4.2 Subtle ill-defined metaphyseal lucency with soft tissue swelling in early osteomyelitis

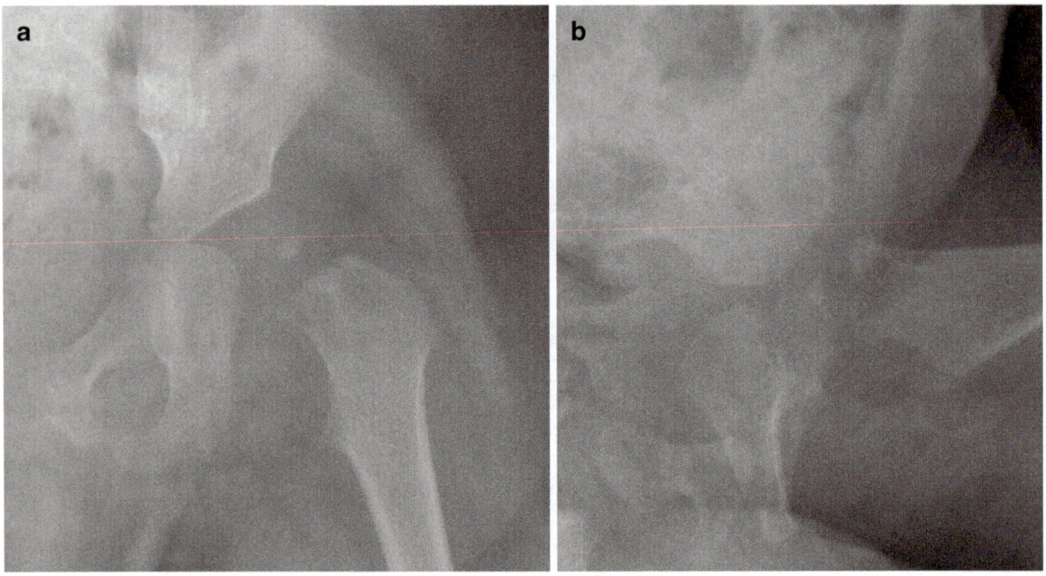

Fig. 4.3 (**a**, **b**) AP and lateral left hip in an infant. Note lateralisation of hip on AP view. There is endosteal scalloping, lucency of the metaphysis extending to the physis

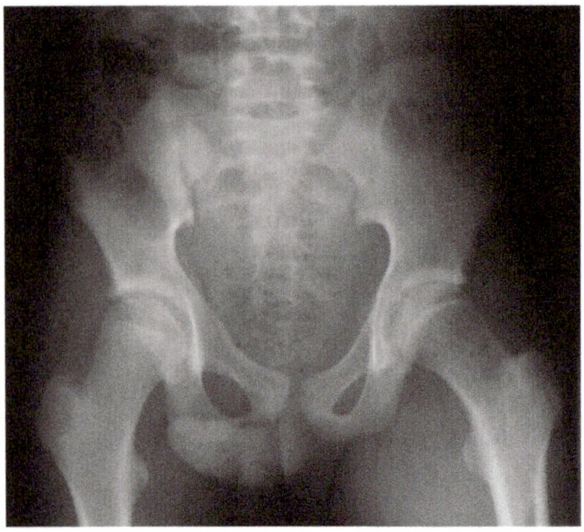

Fig. 4.4 AP pelvis and both hips demonstrating permeative lucency of the left proximal femoral metaphysis

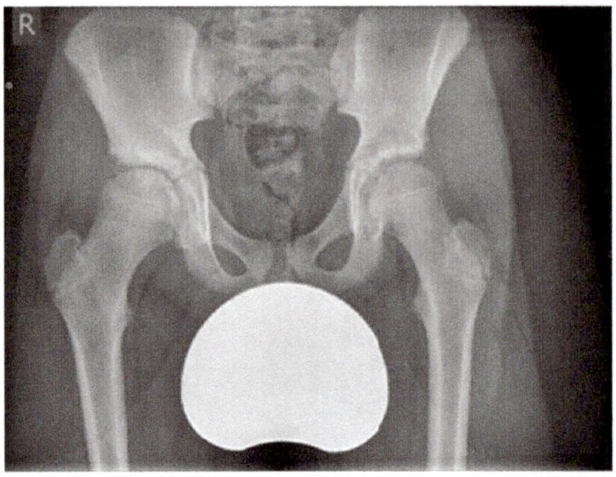

Fig. 4.5 Post-septic sequelae right hip with chondrolysis and loss of joint space. Coxa magna and secondary incongruency

ances are of a well-defined lucency often with a sclerotic rim within the metaphysis but may extend across the physis (Fig. 4.7). An epiphyseal/metaphyseal abscess is more frequent after physeal closure or in younger infants (<18 months) when an interconnecting vascular communication exists across the physis [9]. Inflammatory markers are often normal, and plain radiograph not always typical but classically demonstrates a lytic lesion orientated along the long axis of the bone, with a pathognomonic channel extending towards the growth plate, described as the 'serpentine sign'. The infection is contained within a dense reactive sclerosis, hence little systemic inflammatory response. Sequestrum may be identified within the lucency.

Radiographs can demonstrate the late effects of osteomyelitis (Fig. 4.8). Sequestrum and sclerotic bone are signs of protracted infection. The formation of involucrum, sinus tracts and soft tissue fistulas all points towards chronicity of osteomyelitis. Chronic osteomyelitis can present with cortical sclerosis (Fig. 4.9).

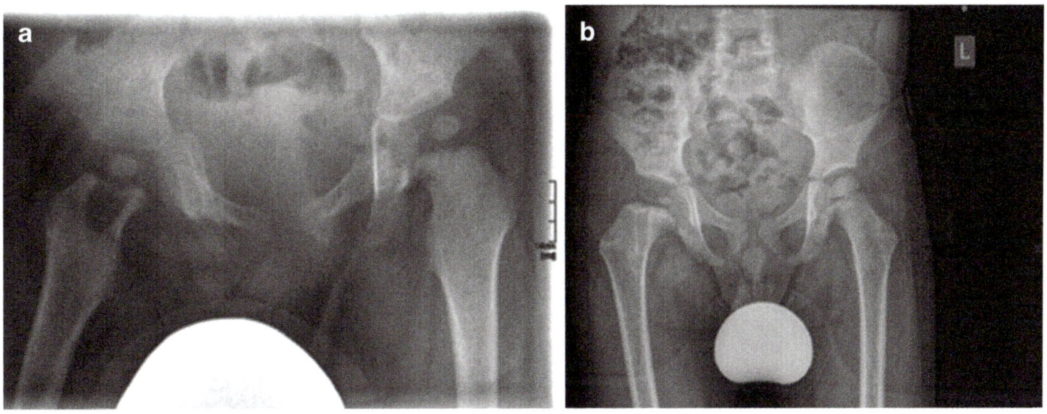

Fig. 4.6 Right hip osteomyelitis with secondary AVN. The child presented at age 6 months (**a**) with follow-up film shown at 3 years of age (**b**)

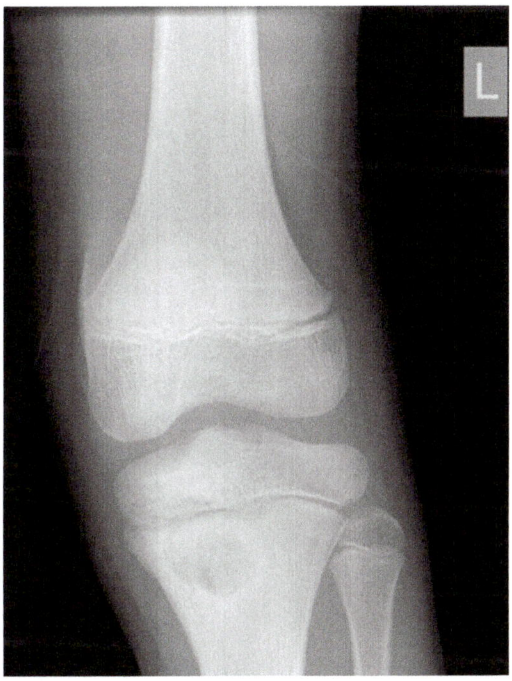

Fig. 4.7 Brodie's abscess of the proximal tibial metaphysis

Ultrasonography

Sonography generates images from sound waves reflected from tissues. It gives excellent resolution of the subcutaneous tissue, muscles and tendons as well as the joint and periosteum and is well tolerated. The unossified structures of the paediatric joint are well seen. There are no contraindications. It avoids radiation and is often quick and easy to access. It can be performed at the bedside and does not require the child to be completely still, avoiding the need for anaesthesia. In deep joints, such as the hip, it can be used to detect effusions difficult to identify clinically. These features, particularly for the timely treatment of suspected joint sepsis, make it a very valuable modality for early diagnosis of infection in children. A high-resolution linear probe can provide excellent images of superficial joints. A more general-purpose curved array probe may be needed for deeper joints in larger patients. The use of colour or power Doppler enables blood flow to be seen and is an important component of the study. Increased vascularity can be seen where there is inflammation and absence of blood flow where there is fluid in a collection. Careful use of the greyscale is required to differentiate the unossified epiphysis from fluid. The comparison of the contralateral limb or adjacent joints is useful in assessing variations in ossification which can be normal. It is operator dependent but highly sensitive, and effusions as low as 1 ml can be detected.

The limitations of ultrasound are that it can be technically difficult in an upset child. Joints can be hard to examine if the joint is flexed and cannot be straightened. It is not possible to examine every aspect of a bone in most areas of the body due to adjacent structures. It is most effective looking at an area of concern and is less useful for screening of a large area as the periosteal changes are subtle. It should be used combined with radiography since the techniques are complementary. Fractures are generally more easily identified on plain film. The exception to this is

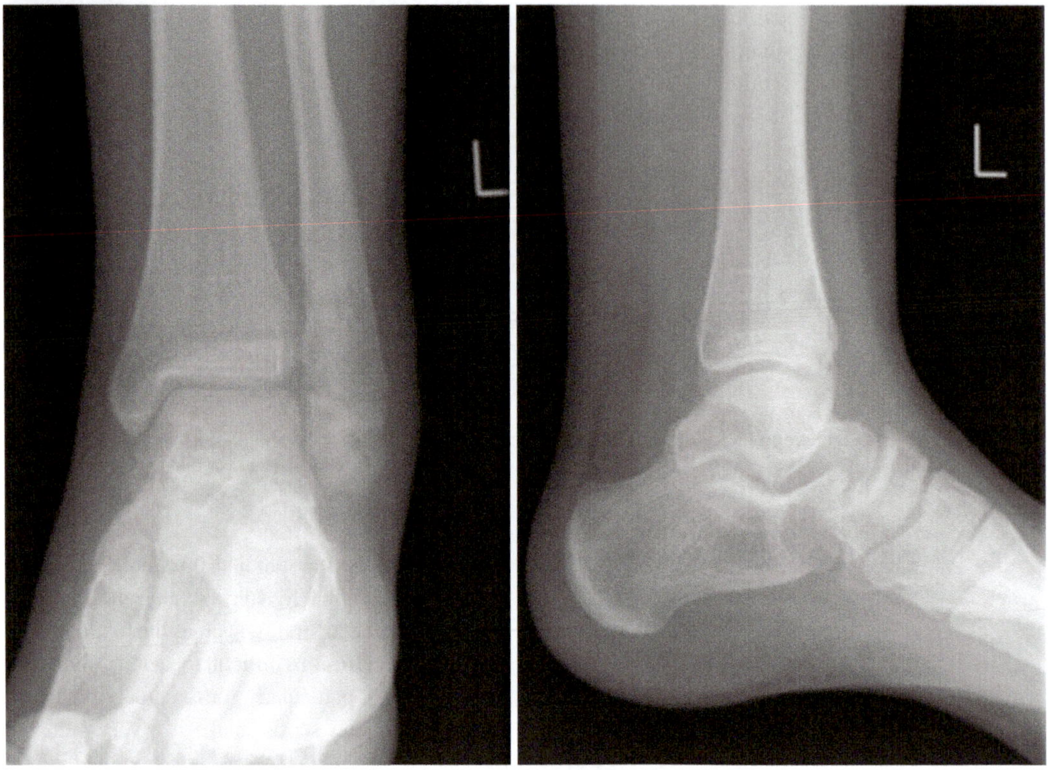

Fig. 4.8 Chronic osteomyelitis of the left distal fibula with sclerosis and medullary cavities. Fibular overgrowth can also be seen

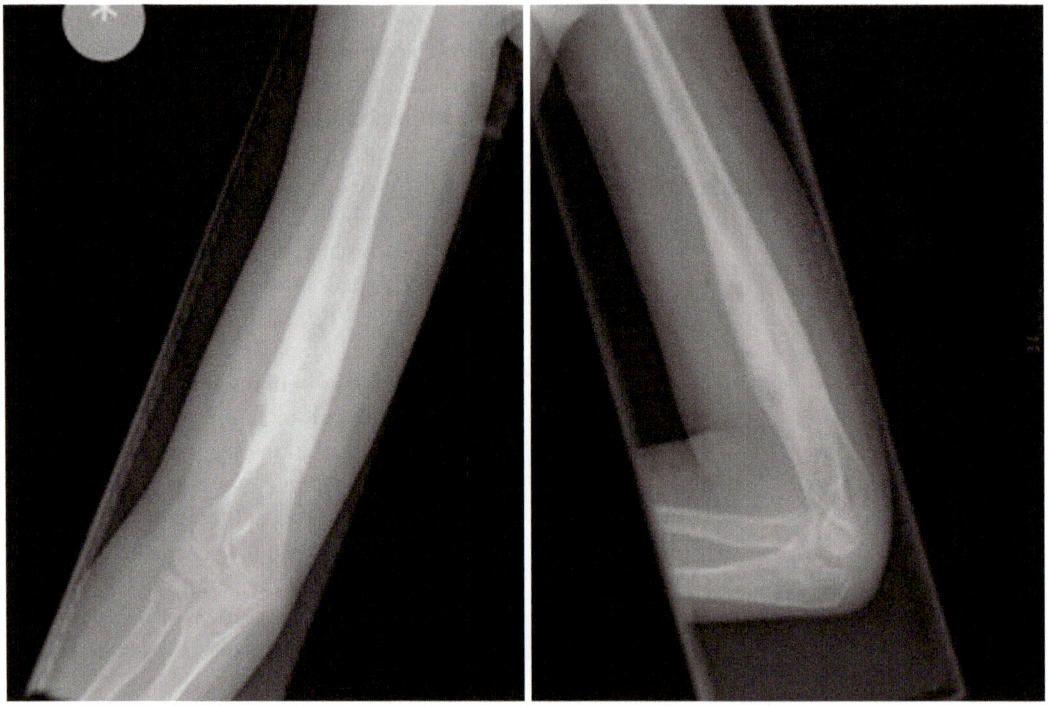

Fig. 4.9 Cortical sclerosis of the left distal humerus in the presence of chronic osteomyelitis

where there is physeal separation of an unossified epiphysis, ultrasound is superior.

The hip is the most common joint to present with septic arthritis in children. Early detection and intervention are imperative to avoid rapid joint destruction. Hip effusion can be visualised on ultrasound as a relatively hypoechoic fluid anterior to the proximal femoral neck and posterior to the iliopsoas muscle. It appears as a hypoechoic stripe, which lifts the anterior joint capsule (Fig. 4.10). In a child, displacement of the anterior capsule more than 5 mm from the anterior cortex of the femoral neck has been used as diagnostic criteria for a hip effusion [10, 11].

The classic presenting criteria of fever, non-weight bearing, erythrocyte sedimentation rate >40 and a peripheral white blood count of >12,000 [12] help predict the likelihood of septic arthritis, but not all children present with these features. This is particularly true in children under the age of 1 and those who have other immunocompromising pathologies. Ultrasound helps to give additional information and build the clinical picture and may also be useful to guide needle aspiration.

The absence of joint fluid can be used to help rule out septic arthritis, but it is more difficult to differentiate between septic and non-septic joint fluid. The echogenicity of the fluid on ultrasound is not specific for infection. Anechoic fluid does not exclude infection, nor does echogenic fluid necessarily correspond to infection, and may be due to proteinaceous fluid from chronic inflammation. The size of an effusion is also non-discriminatory. Increased adjacent soft tissue perfusion may be present on power Doppler but in both inflammatory and infective effusions [10]. Where there is subperiosteal pathology, ultrasound can be helpful in the exclusion of a mass lesion [13, 14].

In addition, the absence of effusion does not eliminate periarticular osteomyelitis or adjacent pyomyositis which both can present with similar symptoms. Ultrasound can however identify periosteal lift and subperiosteal abscess formation, visualised as a band of spindle-shaped subperiosteal fluid, bordered by a line of increased echogenicity representing the elevated periosteum (Fig. 4.11). An abscess can form as the pressure of acute osseous infection is relieved through the cortex into the subperiosteal space. Subperiosteal abscess can be the primary infection with no medullary change, a result of presumed haematogenous seeding to the vascular growing tissue beneath the periosteum. Colour Doppler will demonstrate an avascular periosteal collection with peripheral hyperaemia. These findings precede radiographic changes by several days and help guide treatment where advanced imaging is delayed or not accessible [14].

In chronic osteomyelitis cortical defects and fistula may be seen [10] (Fig. 4.12) (Box 4.1).

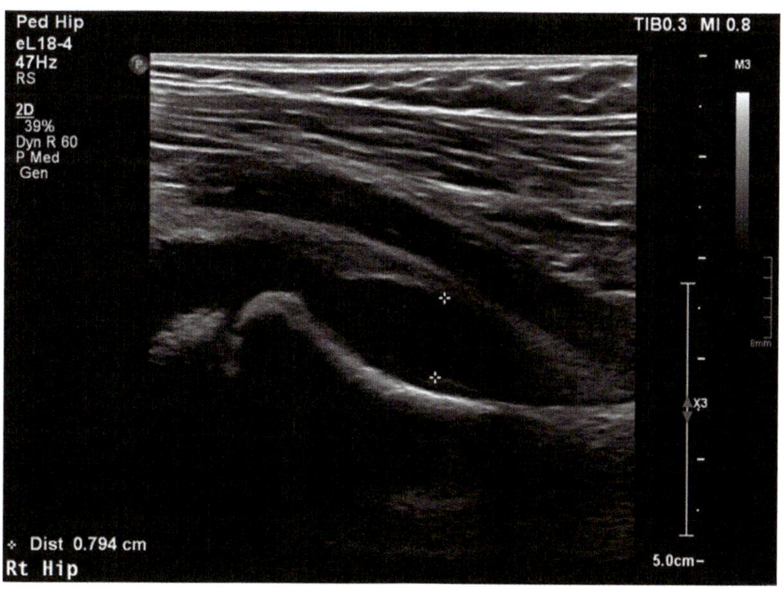

Fig. 4.10 Right hip effusion. The hypoechoic fluid can be seen anterior to the femoral neck

Box 4.1 Advantages and Disadvantages

	Advantages	Disadvantages
X-ray	Quick, affordable, helps exclude alternative diagnosis	Normal in early infection. Low sensitivity and specificity
USS	Excellent resolution of soft tissues and joints. No sedation requirement	User dependent. Not appropriate for large area scanning
CT	Excellent bony resolution for identifying sequestra/involucrum. Short scanning time	Significant radiation dose. Poor resolution of soft tissues
MRI	Gold standard for infection. High sensitivity and specificity. Excellent delineation of soft tissue planes and bony involvement. Large areas can be scanned to localise infection	Sedation/general anaesthesia may be required in younger children. Longer scanning time
Scintigraphy	Simple bone scan highly sensitive. Advancing techniques with indication in complex infection	Scan duration and radiation dose

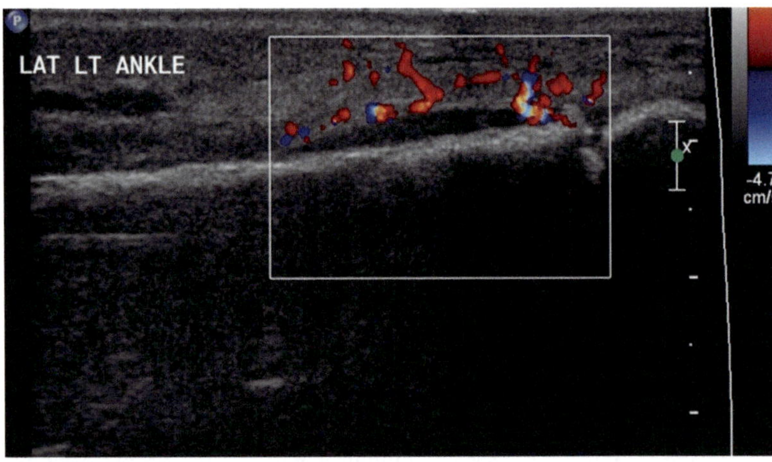

Fig. 4.11 Ultrasound of left distal fibula showing a subperiosteal abscess. There is elevation of periosteum and adjacent hyperaemia on colour Doppler

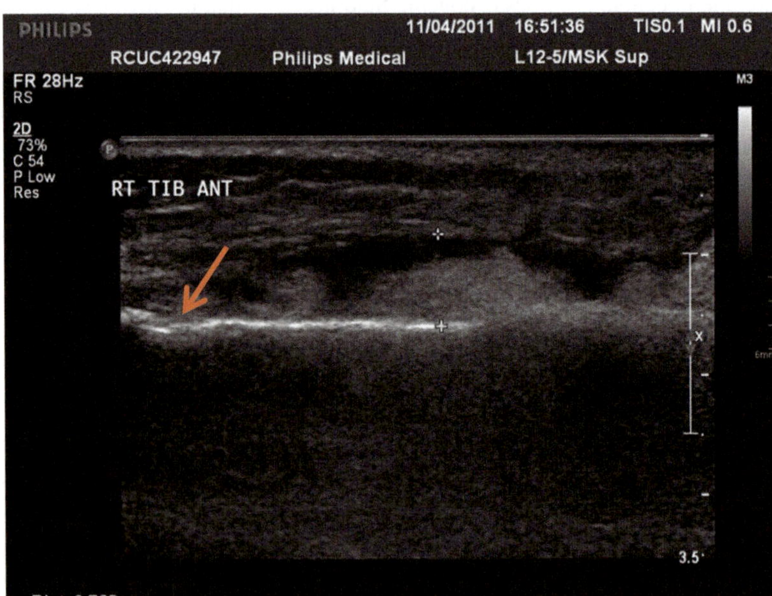

Fig. 4.12 Chronic osteomyelitis with cortical defects (arrow) and a subperiosteal collection

Magnetic Resonance Imaging

Magnetic resonance imaging (MRI) has become the gold standard investigation for diagnosing osteoarticular infection [3, 15]. High-resolution multiplanar images are generated from the radiofrequencies returned from body tissues in the magnet. Large and small field of view images can be performed which will demonstrate bones, unossified cartilage and surrounding soft tissues with a very high sensitivity for pathology identified as oedema. MRI is positive for infection before changes on plain radiograph, and there is no radiation dose (Fig. 4.13).

MRI is considered highly sensitive (84%) and highly specific (60%) for detection of osteomyelitis [16]. Where a joint effusion has been diagnosed, there is frequently osteomyelitis affecting the adjacent bone, especially in young children. MRI can detect unsuspected osteomyelitis of the adjacent bone [17] (Fig. 4.14). MRI allows rapid assessment of the suspected site of infection with high-resolution, multiplanar images and is particularly valuable for areas otherwise difficult to examine or image such as the pelvis [18] (Fig. 4.15). Excellent delineation of the extent of osseous involvement can be achieved, at the same time allowing assessment of surrounding soft tis-

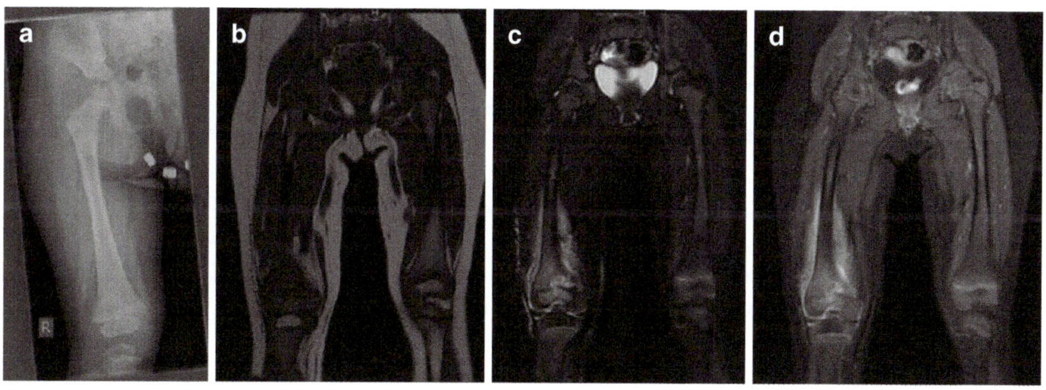

Fig. 4.13 (**a–d**) Osteomyelitis of the right distal femur with only very subtle X-ray changes (**a**). Note low-signal change on T1 imaging (**b**) with high signal on T2 (**c**). Post-contrast imaging demonstrates a small collection (**d**)

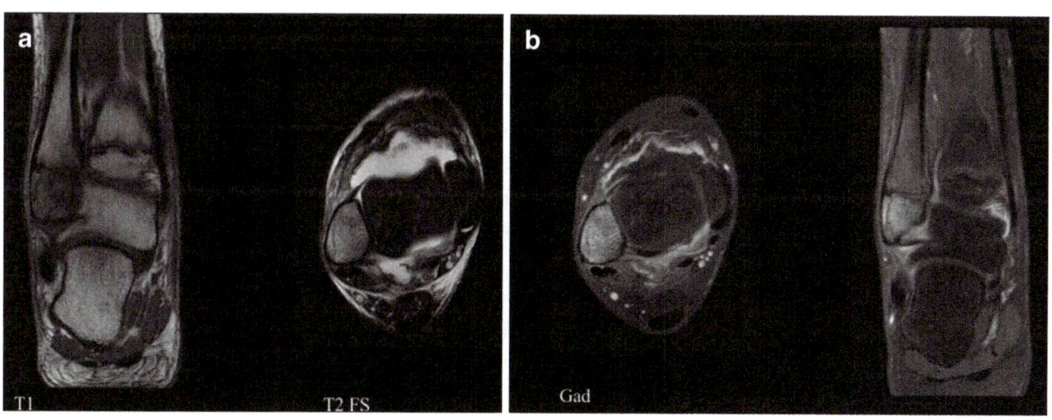

Fig. 4.14 (**a**, **b**) Fibular osteomyelitis with ankle joint effusion. There is low signal on T1 (**a**) and high signal on T2FS (**b**) within the distal fibular metaphysis and epiphysis in keeping with oedema. No soft tissue mass. There is a large joint effusion with high signal on T2FS but no enhancement which may be septic or reactive. These findings together are high likely to be due to infection

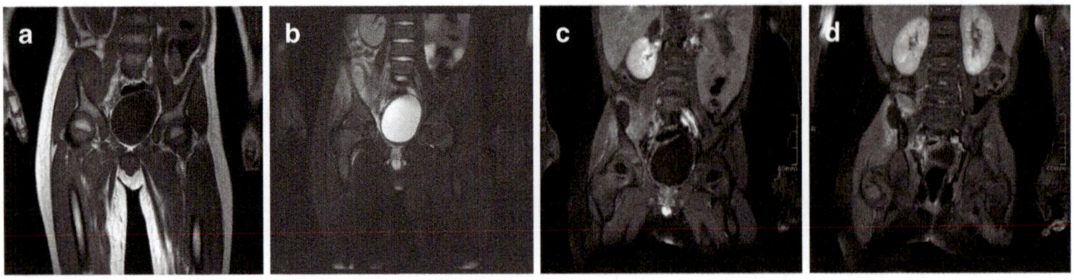

Fig. 4.15 (**a**–**d**) Osteomyelitis of the ileum with adjacent psoas abscess

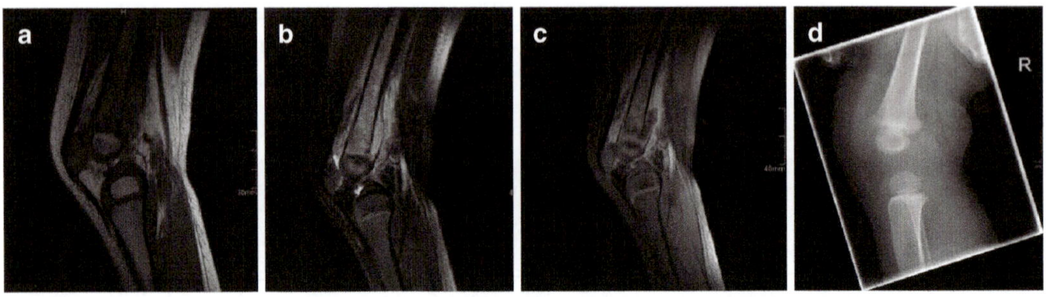

Fig. 4.16 (**a**–**d**) Osteomyelitis of distal femur with dorsal subperiosteal collection: (**a**) T1, (**b**) T2FS, (**c**) post-gadolinium, (**d**) normal X-ray

sues and adjacent joints including the unossified epiphyses. With the absence of ionising radiation, whole body MRI can safely be performed in infants and young children, within a reasonable scan time, to assess multifocal disease or to quickly identify areas of oedema indicating the site of a lesion in a child not using a limb. A large area can be scanned using a water-sensitive sequence such as STIR, before focusing on the limb segment of concern with smaller field of view. Sequences with and without contrast can optimally provide information to aid management. Where the pelvis and lower limbs show no areas of concern, the scan should be extended to include the spine [19].

Findings on MRI will depend on the pulse sequences (T1- or T2-) and the stage of disease. A number of different sequences are used, each providing different and complimenting information. T1 provides excellent anatomical delineation of the bone, joint and surrounding soft tissues and confirms which is low signal on T1. An area of bone infection will have increased fluid content, demonstrated by low-signal-intensity marrow on T1-weighted images compared to adjacent muscle and high signal on T2-weighted imaging within the marrow and surrounding soft tissues. Fat-saturated T2 imaging is used to increase the conspicuity of high-signal lesions. The use of gadolinium increases definition of hyperaemic lesions and allows collections to be differentiated from areas of diffuse inflammation or soft tissue mass [17]. It can be used to differentiate oedema from collections by demonstrating lack of enhancement of fluid collections or joint effusions although this is only useful on the sequences immediately after injection as contrast leaches into fluid with time (Fig. 4.16). Lack of contrast uptake may also be due to vascular compromise (Fig. 4.17).

Fatty marrow has high signal on T1 and T2 which makes low-signal T1 non-fat-containing lesions very conspicuous. The presence of haematopoietic marrow which is intermediate signal on T1 and T2 particularly in infants, but also in the metaphysis of older children, makes differentiation of normal from abnormal marrow more difficult. Gadolinium enhancement is very useful in these circumstances, delineating pathology within red marrow [3]. Imaging of the contralateral leg or

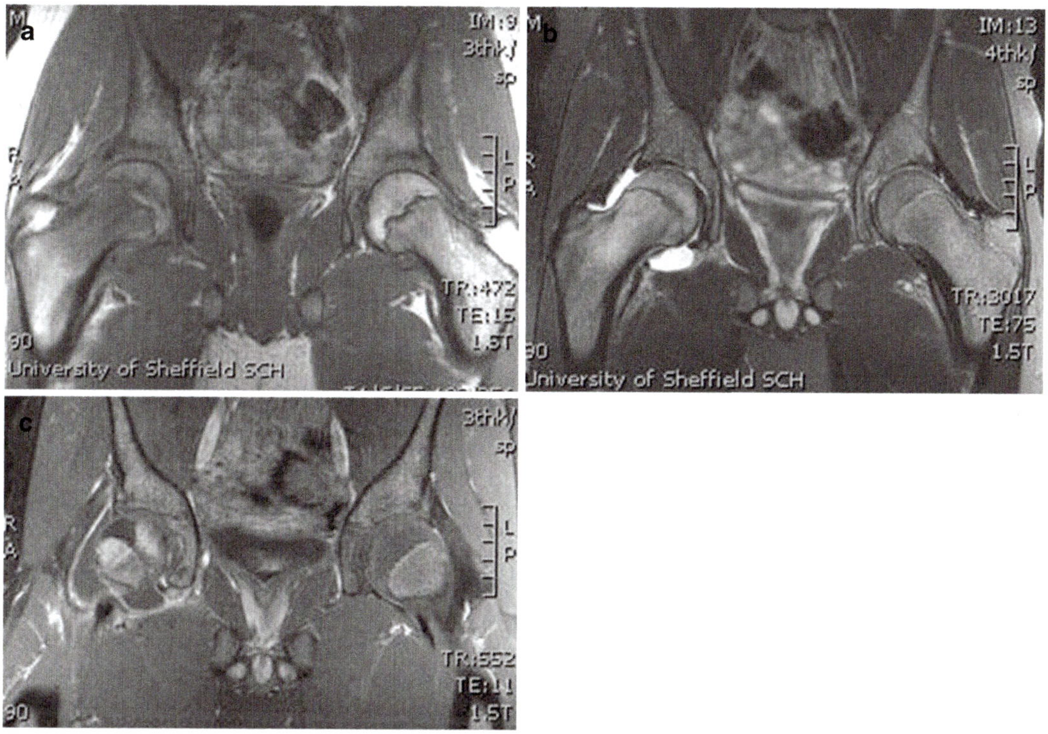

Fig. 4.17 (**a**–**c**) Osteomyelitis of the proximal femur. Femoral neck and head marrow are low signal on T1 (**a**) and high signal on T2 (**b**) in keeping with fluid. There is a large joint effusion which is high signal on T2 (**b**) and does not show enhancement (**c**). The right femur enhances with contrast, but there is some segmental under perfusion of the femoral head (**c**)

whole pelvis can also be very useful in assessing the signal characteristics of the normal marrow in a child in cases of difficulty. However, T1 and T2 fat-saturated imaging and T1FS with enhancement are optimal for assessing infection (Box 4.2).

Box 4.2 Key Sequences for MR Imaging of Acute Infection

A typical MRI examination for acute infection would include the following:

- T1 sequence – defining anatomy and to confirm the presence of fluid/oedema (low signal/black).
- A T2 fluid-sensitive sequence with fat saturation such as T2FS or STIR – very sensitive for water/oedema (high signal/white).
- T1 fat saturation both before and after IV contrast – the contrast is high signal on T1 and is taken up by normal structures. Uptake is increased in areas of hyperaemia and inflammation.

It must be remembered that a high-signal bone lesion on water-sensitive sequences is non-specific. As well as the imaging characteristics, consideration of the clinical picture, distribution and nature of the lesions is imperative, and biopsy maybe required. The differential diagnoses include lymphoma, Ewing's tumour and histiocytosis, stress injury and inflammatory lesions such as osteoid osteoma, as well as CRMO [15]. Previous trauma without secondary infection is less often a diagnostic question. Physeal separation in very young children can be due to infection but also should raise the possibility of inflicted injury in appropriate circumstances. MRI does not differentiate between infected and reactive effusions. Mass lesions will typically enhance with contrast, and this can be helpful in differentiating infection from tumour. Diffusion imaging can also be helpful in characterising lesions [20].

Practical limitations of MRI imaging are that it is contraindicated in cases with some electrical implants and with recent metal work. Most surgical implants are compatible with MRI and this is always checked before scanning. Metal work in the vicinity of the area scanned produces artefact and can make the scan non-diagnostic in the worst-case scenario. Metal artefact reduction software is available on some scanners. The scan sequences can be modified to avoid those particularly affected by metal, but the study quality is negatively affected.

In young children sedation or general anaesthesia may be required, which remains the drawback of MRI. The patient has to remain immobile and tolerate the enclosed space and loud noise of the scanner, which can be difficult depending on the age of the child and expected scan duration. Good analgesia before the scan where appropriate is essential. With the neonate asleep following a feed, a study may be possible with the feed and wrap technique. Patient play specialists can help with distraction techniques for older children to avoid the need for sedation. The ability to view a DVD from the scan table is particularly useful. Long sequences should be avoided where possible. There is a trade-off, however, between image quality and scan time which is made at the time of the scan to optimise the study.

It has been reported that the reoperation rate is 2.8x higher for the management of joint infection without preoperative MRI and patients are likely to undergo longer hospital admissions and total antibiotic duration. If adjacent infections are not recognised, surgical debridement may be inadequate. MRI can be useful in differentiating suppurative arthritis from transient synovitis of the hip, looking for oedema of the adjacent bone exclusively associated with septic arthritis or identifying contralateral (asymptomatic) joint effusion and signal-intensity alterations and enhancement in surrounding soft tissues associated with transient synovitis [21].

The trend towards routine MRI looking for periarticular infection in the presence of clinical septic arthritis may however risk delay to theatre. Some authors have attempted to stratify which patients with clinical signs of septic arthritis are at risk of adjacent bony infection based on age, inflammatory blood markers and delay to presentation [17]. MRI is a powerful but expensive modality, it is not always necessary, and its use should be considered on a case to case basis.

Computed Tomography

Computed tomography (CT) provides very quick images with excellent bone spatial and contrast resolution. Features of infection are similar to those on plain radiographs. Periosteal reaction and medullary and cortical destruction can be seen, and the multiplanar imaging allows assessment of bone without overlap of surrounding structures (Fig. 4.18). Sequestrum appears as a sclerotic lesion with a lucent rim (Fig. 4.19). Although subtle bone changes can be identified on CT, they are not apparent as early as on MRI, and there is much less visualisation of the soft tissues. For this reason, CT is less useful in acute infection. CT also requires a significant radiation dose. However, where MRI is not available or contraindicated, CT can be used to help to characterise a lesion, in conjunction with plain film or bone scan for localisation.

CT is superior to MRI in the detection of intramedullary gas. The speed of scans is an advantage with low requirement for sedation or anaesthesia.

The value of CT in osteoarticular infection is primarily mapping bone change in subacute and chronic osteomyelitis and in aiding preoperative planning for sequestra, involucrum and sinuses. It is also very good for mapping physeal tethers, which may avoid the need for MRI [22]. CT is also a good modality for image-guided biopsy and aspiration of deep structures, particularly in the spine [23].

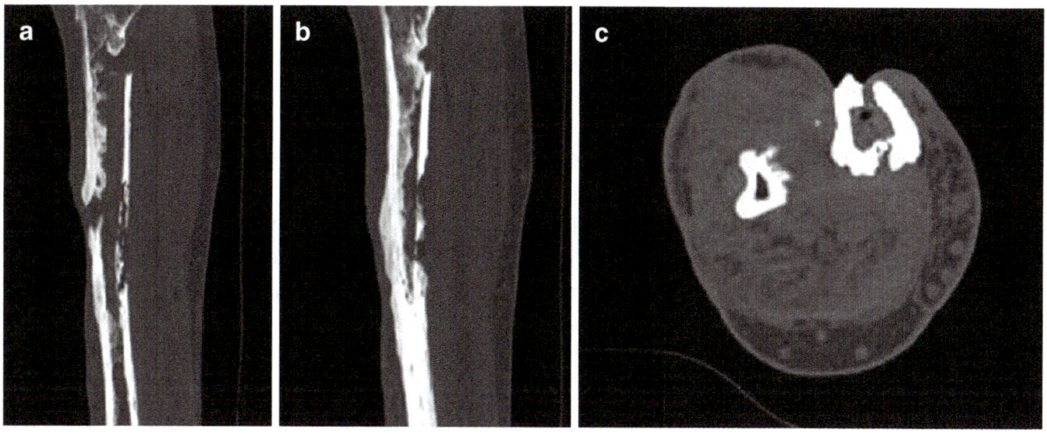

Fig. 4.18 (**a–c**) Chronic osteomyelitis of the right tibia with sequestrum, involucrum and cortical destruction

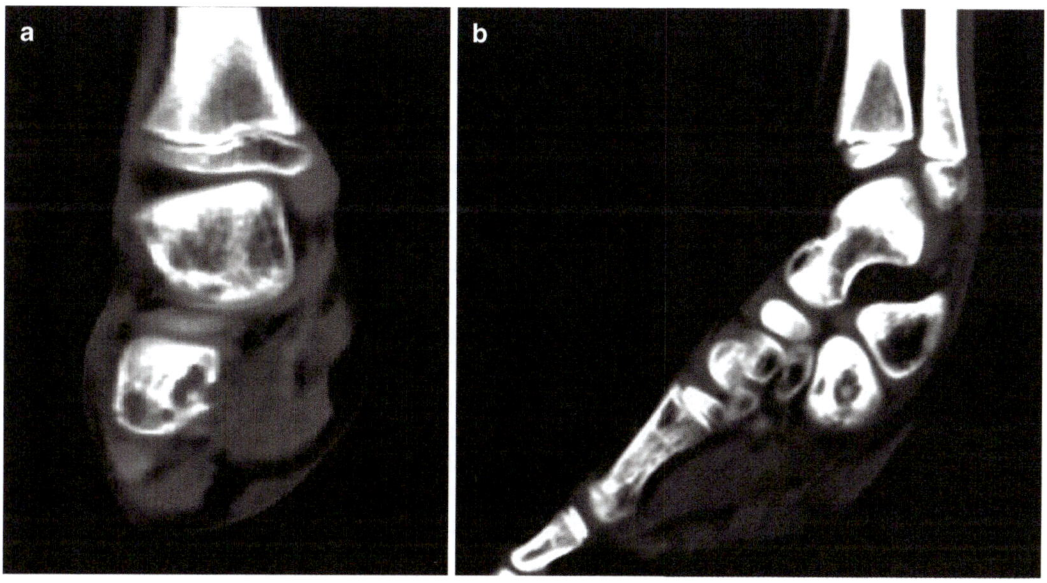

Fig. 4.19 (**a** and **b**) Coronal and sagittal CT. Chronic osteomyelitis cuboid with sequestrum and cortical defect

Even in the presence of chronic osteomyelitis, the sensitivity and specificity of CT are considered to be low (67% and 50%, respectively [16]).

Scintigraphy

Triple-phase bone scan can detect and localise osteomyelitis before it is evident on X-ray, showing increased activity 24–48 hours after the onset of symptoms [24]. Images are produced following an injection of radiotracer, technetium-99m methylene diphosphonate (99mTc-MDP), followed by a series of images indicating areas of increased blood flow. All three phases, blood flow, blood pool and delayed phase (angiographic, tissue and bone phases), will depict increased activity in the presence of osteomyelitis. Sequential images are taken during the injection and following injection for the blood flow and pool phases showing accumulation of isotope in tissues of increased vascularity [25].

The bone phase is performed 4 hours after the injection when the isotope has become incorporated into the bone matrix as calcium-phosphate salts. The areas with increased bone turnover will have increased activity on the scan. This may be areas of inflammation or tumour but also the physis where there is bone growth and bone repair following fracture or surgery. Planar imaging typically takes 25 minutes. The child is required to be very still during each phase of the scan but is a little less enclosed than in an MRI scanner, and it is not noisy. Although it is better tolerated than MRI, very young children are likely to require sedation or anaesthesia.

The bone scan is very sensitive for bone pathology and will generally identify the site or sites of bone infection before it is apparent on X-ray (Fig. 4.20). Sensitivity has been reported as high as 94%, a little lower in neonates [6]. It is however non-specific, showing all areas of high bone turnover, and does not provide any information on soft tissue change. Some infections, particularly staphylococcal, do not always show early on bone scans [26]. There is a significant radiation dose delivering an effective dose of approximately 2.8 mSv for a 1-year-old.

Where MRI is not available or contraindicated, bone scan can be very useful in the investigation of infection particularly in conjunction with ultrasound for soft tissue change and radiographs to delineate bone abnormality.

Where there is metalwork in place, nuclear medicine bone scans have an advantage over CT and MRI in that although there will be a photopenic defect where the metal work is, there is no artefact generated so the bone immediately around the metal work can be seen clearly. If there is increased bone turnover due to surgical healing, this will have increased activity on bone scan.

The localisation of abnormal activity on the planar image can be improved with the use of SPECT which gives cross-sectional images of the bone scan by measuring gamma rays. This is particularly useful in areas of overlapping structures such as the pelvis and spine. SPECT also improves the contrast. Although this takes an additional 25 minutes to perform, it does not require any further radiation dose. The half-life of the radioactive tracer is longer.

Nuclear medicine cameras in conjunction with CT, CT SPECT, enable a CT scan to be done at the same examination and superimposed on the bone scan image. This CT scan can be very low dose to provide localisation information only or diagnostic quality. In the context of infection in children if diagnostic quality CT is used, it can be limited to the exact area of increased activity on the bone scan keeping the dose to a minimum.

Other scintigraphic approaches, such as white cell-labelled imaging, are less frequently used in children. White blood cell-labelled imaging depends largely on neutrophil-driven processes such as bacterial infection. It is very specific and useful in differentiating active infection from metal work, fracture or chronic infection with ongoing healing which may appear similar in other modalities such as MRI [27] (Fig. 4.21).

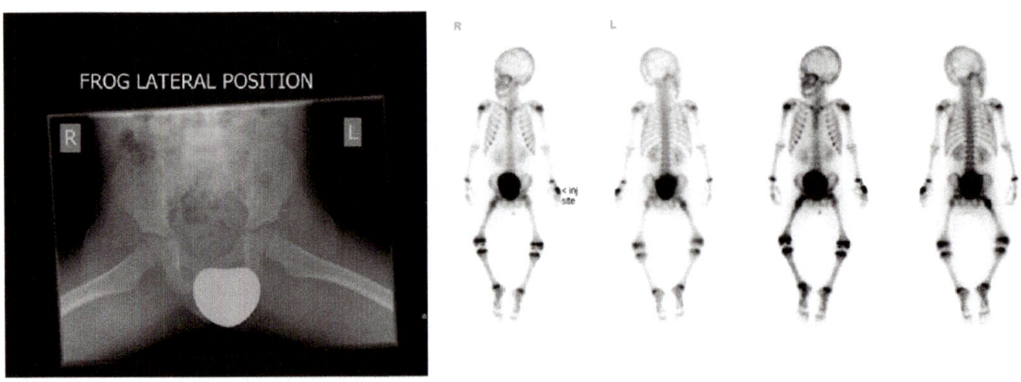

Fig. 4.20 Bone scan showing abnormal uptake within the proximal right femur in the presence of a normal X-ray, highly suspicious of infection. Normal uptake at the physes can be seen

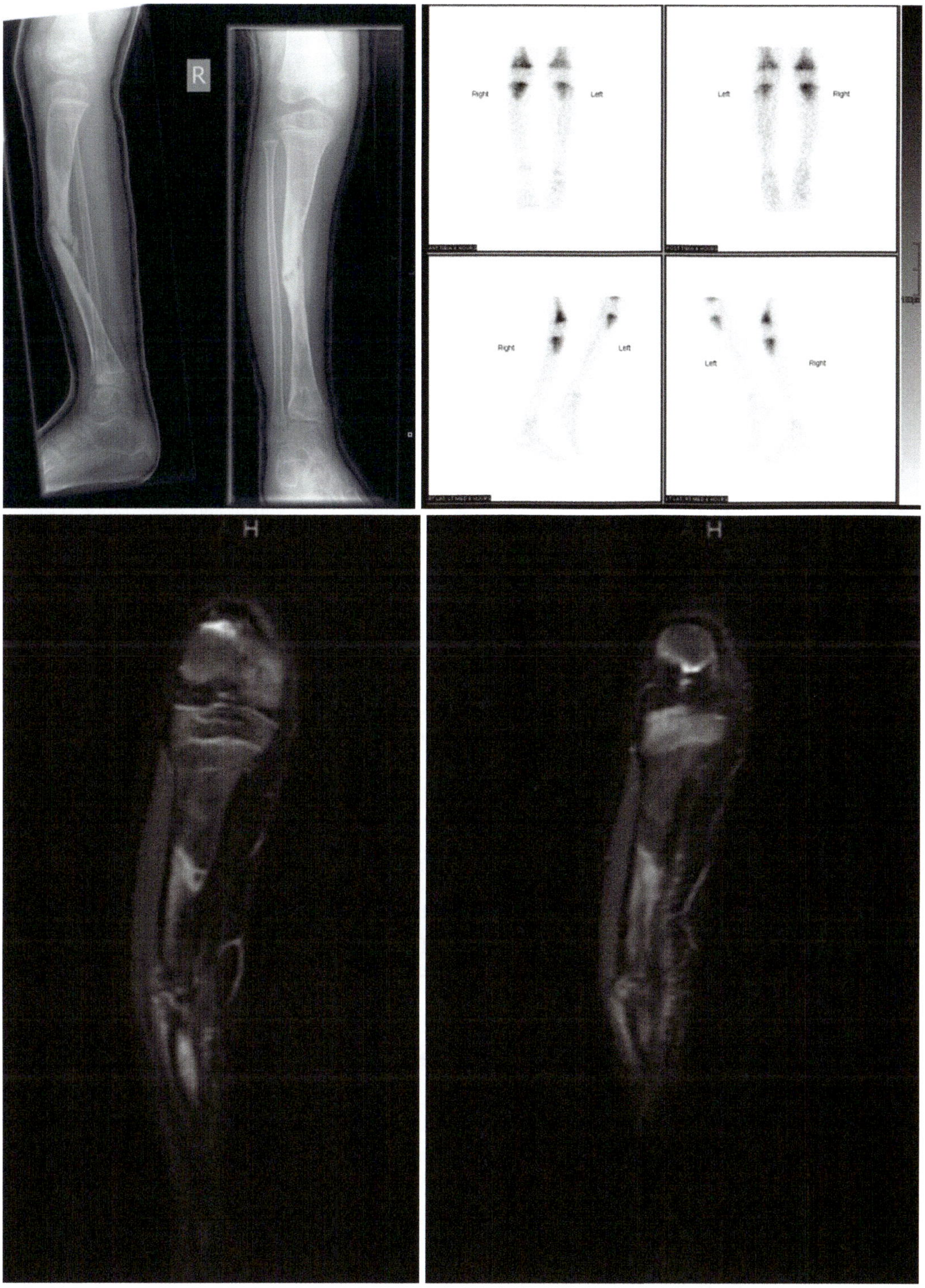

Fig. 4.21 Surgical planning for a case with chronic and refractory osteomyelitis of the right tibia. The radiograph shows sclerosis of the diaphysis with non-union of a pathological fracture. MRI shows oedema in the diaphysis non-specific for ongoing infection or granulation tissue and oedema. The white cell scan shows no activity at the site of concern. Note the uptake within metaphyseal red marrow

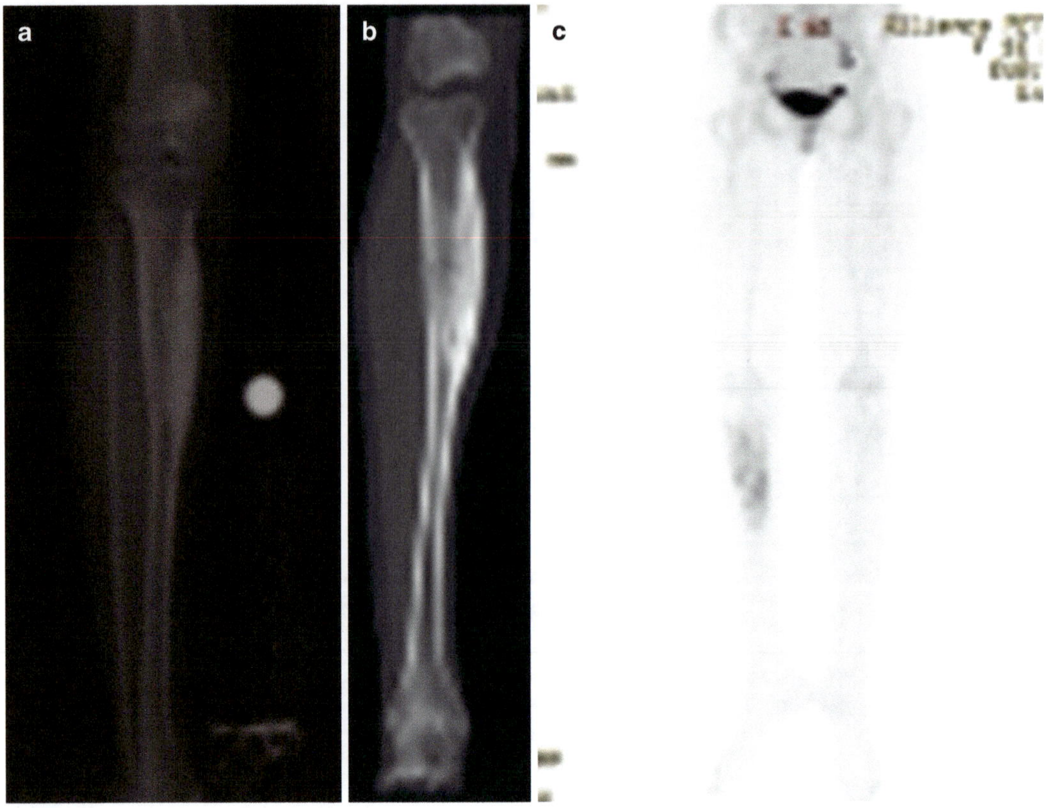

Fig. 4.22 (a–c) X-ray, CT and PET-CT right proximal tibial chronic osteomyelitis

The use of SPECT increases the sensitivity. White cell scans also show high activity at sites of red marrow, and consideration is required using the contralateral limb, current MRI appearances and if needed a further marrow colloid scan to avoid a false-positive scan for infection. It is less useful if the predominant cellular response is not neutrophilic, in TB, for example. The technique requires large volumes of blood be taken prior to the scan, and the scan acquisition time can be an issue for children.

Positron emission tomography (PET-CT) detects areas of high metabolic activity by detecting the decay of the radiotracers as they produce small particles called positrons. They have a narrow window of pickup. PET-CT is very sensitive and high resolution in the context of an unexplained pyrexia. It is however non-specific. There is a significant radiation dose and requires a child to be very still for the duration of the scan. PET-CT may have a role in very complex cases, for example, refractory chronic osteomyelitis in adolescence, but the use of this technology in children is still evolving [28, 29] (Fig. 4.22).

In the future, radiolabelled anti-granulocyte antibodies, antibody fragments and radiolabelled peptides that target bacteria may provide new avenues for imaging bone infection.

References

1. Gafur OA, Copley LAB, Hollmig ST, Browne RH, Thornton LA, Crawford SE. The impact of the current epidemiology of pediatric musculoskeletal infection on evaluation and treatment guidelines. J Pediatr Orthop. 2008;28(7):777–85.
2. Arnold JC, Bradley JS. Osteoarticular infections in children. Infect Dis Clin North Am [Internet]. 2015;29(3):557–74. Available from:. https://doi.org/10.1016/j.idc.2015.05.012.
3. Jaramillo D, Dormans JP, Delgado J, Laor T, St Geme JW. Hematogenous osteomyelitis in infants and children: imaging of a changing disease. Radiology. Radiological Society of North America Inc. 2017;283:629–43.

4. Tumeh SS, Aliabadi P, Weissman BN, McNeil BJ. Disease activity in osteomyelitis: role of radiography. Radiology. 1987;165(3):781–4.
5. Bonakdar-pour A, Gaines V. The radiology of osteomyelitis. Orthop Clin North Am. 1983;14(1):21–37.
6. Treves S, Khettry J, Broker F, Wilkinson R, Watts H. Early scintigraphic detection in children. Pediatrics. 1976;57:173–86.
7. Boeck D. Osteomyelitis and septic arthritis in children. Acta Orthop Belg. 2005;71(5):505–15.
8. van Der N, Smeeing DPJ, Houwert RM, Hietbrink F, Govaert GAM, van Der D. Brodie's abscess: a systematic review of reported cases. J Bone Jt Infect. 2019;4(1):33–9.
9. Trueta J. The three types of acute haematogenous osteomyelitis. A clinical and vascular study. J Bone Jt Surg Br. 1959;41:671–80.
10. Chau CLF, Griffith JF. Musculoskeletal infections: ultrasound appearances. Clin Radiol. 2005;60:149–59.
11. Robben SGF. Ultrasonography of musculoskeletal infections in children. Eur Radiol Suppl. 2004;14(4):65–77.
12. Rule CP, Between D, Arthritis S, Synovitis T. Kocher validation article. 2004.
13. Madej T, Flak-Nurzyńska J, Dutkiewicz E, Ciechomska A, Kowalczyk J, Wieczorek AP. Ultrasound image of malignant bone tumors in children. An analysis of nine patients diagnosed in 2011–2016. J Ultrason [Internet]. 2018;18(73):103–11. Available from: http://jultrason.pl/index.php/issues/volume-18-no-73/ultrasound-image-of-malignant-bone-tumors-in-children-an-analysis-of-nine-patients-diagnosed-in-2011-2016?aid=618.
14. Moraux A, Gitto S, Bianchi S. Ultrasound features of the Normal and pathologic periosteum. J Ultrasound Med. 2019;38(3):775–84.
15. Guillerman RP. Osteomyelitis and beyond. Pediatr Radiol. 2013;43(SUPPL. 1):S193–S203.
16. Termaat MF, Raijmakers PGHM, Scholten HJ, Bakker FC, Patka P, Haarman HJTM. The accuracy of diagnostic imaging for the assessment of chronic osteomyelitis. J Bone Jt Surg. 2005;87(11):2464–71.
17. Monsalve J, Kan JH, Schallert EK, Bisset GS, Zhang W, Rosenfeld SB. Septic arthritis in children: frequency of coexisting unsuspected osteomyelitis and implications on imaging work-up and management. Am J Roentgenol. 2015;204(6):1289–95.
18. Connolly SA, Connolly LP, Drubach LA, Zurakowski D, Jaramillo D. MRI for detection of abscess in acute osteomyelitis of the pelvis in children. Am J Roentgenol. 2007;189(4):867–72.
19. Lindsay AJ, Delgado J, Jaramillo D, Chauvin NA. Extended field of view magnetic resonance imaging for suspected osteomyelitis in very young children: is it useful? Pediatr Radiol. 2019;49(3):379–86.
20. Harish S, Chiavaras MM, Kotnis N, Rebello R. MR imaging of skeletal soft tissue infection: utility of diffusion-weighted imaging in detecting abscess formation. Skelet Radiol. 2011;40(3):285–94.
21. Yang WJ, Im SA, Lim GY, Chun HJ, Jung NY, Sung MS, et al. MR imaging of transient synovitis: differentiation from septic arthritis. Pediatr Radiol. 2006;36:1154–8.
22. Wang DC, Deeney V, Roach JW, Shah AJ. Imaging of physeal bars in children. Pediatr Radiol. Springer Verlag. 2015;45:1403–12.
23. Hoang D, Fisher S, Oz OK, La Fontaine J, Chhabra A. Percutaneous CT guided bone biopsy for suspected osteomyelitis: diagnostic yield and impact on patient's treatment change and recovery. Eur J Radiol. 2019 May;1(114):85–91.
24. Palestro CJ. Radionuclide imaging of osteomyelitis. In: Seminars in nuclear medicine. W.B. Saunders; 2015. p. 32–46.
25. DiPoce J, Jbara ME, Brenner AI. Pediatric osteomyelitis: a scintigraphic case-based review. Radiographics. 2012;32:865–78.
26. Browne LP, Mason EO, Kaplan SL, Cassady CI, Krishnamurthy R, Guillerman RP. Optimal imaging strategy for community-acquired Staphylococcus aureus musculoskeletal infections in children. Pediatr Radiol. 2008;38(8):841–7.
27. Govaert GA, IJpma FF, McNally M, McNally E, Reininga IH, Glaudemans AW. Accuracy of diagnostic imaging modalities for peripheral post-traumatic osteomyelitis – a systematic review of the recent literature. Eur J Nucl Med Mol Imaging. Springer Berlin Heidelberg. 2017;44:1393–407.
28. Gotthardt M, Bleeker-Rovers CP, Boerman OC, Oyen WJG. Imaging of inflammation by PET, conventional scintigraphy, and other imaging techniques. J Nucl Med Technol. 2013;41(3):157–69.
29. Afzelius P, Nielsen OL, Schønheyder HC, Alstrup AKO, Hansen SB. An untapped potential for imaging of peripheral osteomyelitis in paediatrics using [18F] FDG PET/CT —the inference from a juvenile porcine model. EJNMMI Res. 2019;9:1–9.

Infection Mimics: Differential Diagnoses of Musculoskeletal Infections

5

Yushane Celestine Shih and Mihir M. Thacker

Introduction

"Biopsy what you culture and culture what you biopsy" is an age-old surgical principle that still holds true today. Overlapping clinical, laboratory, and imaging findings may cloud the diagnostic picture and challenge the orthopedic surgeon to differentiate bone infection from trauma, tumor, infarct, or autoimmune disease. Inability to appropriately diagnose these conditions that mimic osteomyelitis (summarized in Table 5.1), septic arthritis (summarized in Table 5.2), and pyomyositis (summarized in Table 5.3) may result in significant morbidity and occasionally mortality.

Overlapping Clinical Features

Children with acute osteomyelitis typically report focal pain as the most prevalent symptom (up to 80%), followed by localized erythema or swelling (70%), fever (61.7%), reduced range of movement (50.3%), and difficulty weight-bearing (49.3%) [1, 2]. The overall presentation is less pronounced in subacute or chronic osteomyelitis and in infants [3]. However, these signs are not specific to infection. Chronic nonbacterial osteomyelitis (CNO) represents a spectrum of autoinflammatory bone disease and may begin as mild bone pain, with or without local swelling and warmth or develop more acutely as severe pain, malaise, sometimes fever, and even fractures [4, 5]. Children with sickle cell disease frequently prompt the question of vaso-occlusive crisis versus osteomyelitis as both conditions present with localized bone pain, tenderness, swelling, and fever [6–9]. In benign and malignant bone tumors, pain is a frequent presenting symptom [3, 10–15]. This is often accompanied by local swelling and sometimes by an enlarging soft tissue mass or pathologic fracture. Several retrospective case series suggest that acute leukemia or malignant lymphoma should be suspected in a limping child with an irritable hip or knee, bone pain, and fever [16–18]. Nocturnal pain is found in both infectious and oncologic processes and may result in misdiagnosis of the former for the latter [13, 19]. Systemic symptoms classically associated with malignancy – such as weight loss, anorexia, fatigue, or night sweats – have been known to occur in osteomyelitis (especially tubercular osteomyelitis) as well [10, 19]. A history of trauma is reported in one-third of acute hematogenous osteomyelitis cases [20], but patients with an underlying bone tumor sometimes also attribute the onset of their pain to trauma or a sports injury [10, 21]. Bony stress injuries will present with similar focal pain, minimal to mild swelling, and more likely a history of

Y. C. Shih · M. M. Thacker (✉)
Nemours Children's Hospital, Delaware, Department of Orthopedic Surgery, Wilmington, DE, USA
e-mail: mthacker@nemours.org

© Springer Nature Switzerland AG 2022
M. V. Belthur et al. (eds.), *Pediatric Musculoskeletal Infections*,
https://doi.org/10.1007/978-3-030-95794-0_5

Table 5.1 Mimics for osteomyelitis and their characteristics

Condition	Age (years)	Pain	Swelling	Fever	Sites	Radiographs	Advanced imaging	Pathology findings	Treatment
Osteoid osteoma	5–20	++	+/–	–		Sclerosis, nidus	CT-nidus	Nidus surrounded by fibrovascular tissue	Radiofrequency ablation
Leukemia/ lymphoma	3–20	++	+/–	+/–	Any	Metaphyseal bands, lytic lesions, periosteal reactions	Marrow replacement (loss of fat signal within marrow)	Leukemic infiltrates	Chemotherapy
Langerhans cell histiocytosis	Infants to teens	++	+/–	+/–	Any (may be multiple)	Lucent lesion	Surrounding edema/ inflammatory change	Eosinophils, Langerhans cells	Observation, surgery, chemotherapy
Ewing sarcoma	5–20	++	++	+	Around the knee, axial skeleton	Lucent, onion skin periosteal reaction	Often large soft tissue masses	Small, round blue cell lesion	Chemotherapy, surgery/radiation
Sickle cell disease	Any	++	+/–	+	Humerus, femur, hand, spine	Lucent/mixed lesion		Avascular necrosis	Hydration, pain management, supportive
Stress fracture/ reaction	Mostly teenagers	++	+/–	–	Lower extremity – tibia/femur, occasionally pelvis	Normal or sclerosis, incomplete fracture line may be seen occasionally	Hypointense (dark) line through cortex on T1-weighted images, surrounding edema, rarely soft tissue involvement	Remodeling bone	Rest, immobilization
Chronic nonbacterial osteomyelitis	5–20	++	+/–	–	Clavicle/shoulder girdle classic, can involve any bone, including spine, may be solitary or multiple bones	Periphyseal lucent lesions with surrounding sclerosis, sometimes aggressive appearing with osteolysis and periosteal reaction, can also be sclerotic	Full body MRI to look for distant involvement, perilesional edema common	Inflammatory lymphoplasmacytic infiltrate	NSAIDs, steroids, immunotherapy
Scurvy	Any age: 3–13, neurologic disorder, abnormal diet	+	++	+	Skin, gums, teeth, metaphyses, epiphyseal separations	Periosteal elevation, physeal separations, pencil thin cortex, white line of Fraenkel	Diffuse multifocal decreased signal on T1-weighted imaging and increased signal on T2-weighted imaging within bone marrow, predominantly within the metaphyses, a varying degree of bone marrow enhancement, and adjacent periosteal elevation and soft tissue signal abnormalities	Subperiosteal hemorrhages with poor formation of bone osteoid causing disruption in endochondral bone formation	Vitamin C supplementation

Key: *CT* computed tomography, *MRI* magnetic resonance imaging, *NSAIDs* nonsteroidal anti-inflammatory drugs, *RFA* radiofrequency ablation

Table 5.2 Mimics for septic arthritis and their characteristics

Condition	Onset	Features	Systemic signs/symptoms at onset	ESR/CRP	Synovial fluid cell count (WBCs/Cu mm)	Synovial fluid culture	Synovial fluid PCR	Radiographs	Advanced imaging
Septic arthritis	Acute	Usually monoarticular, polyarticular in 20%	Fever, pain with limited ROM	Usually elevated	50,000–200,000 >90% PMNs	Pos	Pos	Soft tissue swelling	MRI with/without contrast shows synovial thickening with enhancement, joint effusion, marrow edema signal on both sides of the articular surface
Transient synovitis	Acute	Monoarticular	h/o upper respiratory infection	Normal/mild elevation	5000–15,000 variable PMNs	Neg	Neg	Soft tissue swelling	
Reactive arthritis	Acute	Oligoarticular – lower limb (knee)	Enthesitis, extraarticular features	Marked elevation	2000–65,000 variable PMNs	Neg	Neg	Soft tissue swelling	
Tubercular arthritis	Insidious	Oligoarticular	Fever, fatigue, weight loss	Usually elevated	40,000–130,000 variable PMNs, lymphocytes	Pos for AFB	Pos	Soft tissue swelling, later joint space narrowing, bony erosion	MRI synovial thickening, joint effusion, articular erosions, subchondral bone destruction, and marrow changes
Traumatic hemarthrosis	Acute	Monoarticular	h/o trauma	Normal/mild elevation	Blood – RBCs	Neg	Neg	Soft tissue swelling	
Hemophilic hemarthrosis	Acute	Monoarticular	h/o hemophilia/family h/o	Normal/mild elevation	Blood – RBCs	Neg	Neg	Soft tissue swelling	
Lyme arthritis	Intermediate after rash	Oligoarticular	50% with migratory arthralgia, fever, fatigue	Usually modest elevation	500–100,000 (25,000) 75% PMNs	Neg	Pos	Soft tissue swelling	
Juvenile idiopathic arthritis	Insidious	Oligoarticular, lower limb	Unusual	Usually, elevated	2000–50,000 60% PMNs	Neg	Neg	Soft tissue swelling	

(continued)

Table 5.2 (continued)

Condition	Onset	Features	Systemic signs/ symptoms at onset	ESR/CRP	Synovial fluid cell count (WBCs/Cu mm)	Synovial fluid culture	Synovial fluid PCR	Radiographs	Advanced imaging
Juvenile rheumatoid arthritis	Insidious	Polyarticular, symmetric	Pain, fatigue, stiffness, occasionally fever	Usually, elevated	2000–50,000 variable PMNs	Neg	Neg	Soft tissue swelling, later joint space narrowing, periarticular erosions	
Charcot arthropathy	Insidious	Monoarticular	Painless, insensate limb, unstable	May be elevated	2000–5000	Neg	Neg	Bone destruction, joint instability, loose bodies	MRI-large effusion, loose bodies, joint destruction
Pigmented villonodular synovitis	Insidious	Monoarticular	Recurrent effusions	May be elevated	Blood – RBCs	Neg	Neg	Soft tissue swelling	T2 W gradient echo MRI shows a large effusion with synovial thickening, heterogenous appearance with hemosiderin deposits
Synovial chondromatosis	Insidious	Oligoarticular	Recurrent effusions	Normal	2000–5000 variable PMNs	Neg	Neg	Multiple intraarticular calcifications with "ring and arc" chondroid mineralization	T2 W MRI shows multiple hypointense intraarticular calcifications with a large effusion

Key: *MRI* magnetic resonance imaging, *Neg* negative, *Pos* positive, *PMNs* polymorphonuclear neutrophils, *RBCs* red blood cells, *WBCs* white blood cells

Table 5.3 Mimics for pyomyositis and their characteristics

Condition	Pain	Swelling	Fever	Sites	Radiographs	Advanced imaging
Acute osteomyelitis	++	++	++	Usually femur/tibia	Normal/periosteal reaction	Contrast MRI will be diagnostic
Septic arthritis	++	+/–	++	Hip/knee	May be normal	Contrast MRI will show synovial thickening, joint effusion
Muscle contusion	+	+/–	–	Anywhere	Normal	MRI will show muscle edema without enhancement
Appendicitis	+	–	+	Abdomen	Normal	US/CT scan shows appendicitis and normal psoas muscle
Spondylodiscitis	+	–	+	Lower back, thoracic region	May be normal	MRI will show changes of infection in the vertebra
Hematoma	+	+	–	Anywhere	Normal	Ultrasound will show no involvement of underlying muscle
Thrombophlebitis	+	–	–	Lower extremities	Normal	Ultrasound/Doppler exam
Cellulitis	+	+/–	+/–	Lower extremities	Normal	Ultrasound/MRI will differentiate between muscle involvement and otherwise
Soft tissue sarcomas	+/–	+	–	Lower extremity	Normal	MRI will be diagnostic

repetitive activity instead of discrete preceding injury.

Given the clinical similarity of the aforementioned etiologies, it is essential to thoroughly question and examine the patient for any differentiating clues. Osteomyelitis and its corresponding pain most commonly occur in the metaphyses of long bones and "metaphyseal equivalents" of irregular bones [1, 15, 22]. "Metaphyseal equivalent" refers to bony-cartilaginous junctions like the sacroiliac joint, triradiate cartilage, calcaneal tuberosity apophysis, and spinal vertebral apophysis [23]. In children younger than 18 months, transphyseal vessels permit the extension of infection from the metaphysis to the epiphysis, hence the higher rate of epiphyseal damage and adjacent septic arthritis in infantile osteomyelitis [1, 20, 22]. Some metaphyses, such as the proximal radius and proximal femur, are intracapsular and allow direct seeding of the adjacent joint space [22].

Chronic nonbacterial osteomyelitis and its more severe form, chronic recurrent multifocal osteomyelitis (CRMO), also primarily affect the metaphyses and metaphyseal equivalents. Unlike hematogenous osteomyelitis, CNO often involves the shoulder girdle, notably the sternum or clavicle, and involvement is often multifocal [1, 4, 5, 24, 25]. It may present with other autoimmune conditions, such as inflammatory bowel disease (up to 10% of patients) or palmoplantar pustulosis, cystic acne, and psoriasis (up to 20%) [4, 5, 24]. Chronic nonbacterial osteomyelitis overlaps with synovitis, acne, pustulosis, hyperostosis, and osteitis (SAPHO) syndrome, which more frequently arises in adults [4, 5]. Other typical sites of CNO include the vertebral column and pelvis, and a third of patients develop noninfectious arthritis in joints distant from the bone lesion [4, 5, 25]. Uncommon in CNO and more likely in osteomyelitis are abscesses and deep vein thromboses, which are hallmarks of methicillin-resistant *Staphylococcus aureus* [26].

Compared with osteomyelitis in sickle cell disease, vaso-occlusive crises due to bone infarction tend to have shorter duration of pain and fever, more than one site of pain, and less swelling of the affected limb [1, 6]. The major challenge is that infarction and infection can coexist, and infection alone may lead to bone ischemia [9, 27]. When marrow infarction involves the epiphysis, the resultant joint effusion can mimic septic arthritis [9].

Tumors generally have a longer symptom duration, more gradual onset, and less systemic illness than acute osteomyelitis [1], although

20–28% of patients with Ewing sarcoma (ES) will have a fever [21]. Ewing sarcoma may be more likely than other malignant tumors to present with constitutional symptoms like fever, fatigue, and weight loss [28]. One retrospective cohort study determined that no clinical feature, other than ethnicity, improved the accuracy of discerning osteomyelitis from ES [29]. In one American cancer database, ES was most frequently diagnosed in Caucasians (91% of all patients) over a 30-year period [30]. Whereas ES tends to arise from the diaphysis or metadiaphysis, osteosarcoma usually originates in the metaphysis [21, 31]. Both sarcomas reach peak incidence during the adolescent growth spurt in the second decade of life [21, 31]. If an oncologic process is suspected, the peripheral lymph nodes, skin, and mucosal membranes should be examined. Although ES mainly metastasizes hematogenously, the lymphatic spread of skeletal ES is possible (though uncommon) [28]. Painless lymphadenopathy is classically associated with leukemia and lymphoma, especially cervical lymph node enlargement for Hodgkin lymphoma [17, 28, 32]. Leukemia can also result in pallor, fatigue, petechiae, and bleeding, depending on the degree of underlying anemia and thrombocytopenia [16]. Langerhans cell histiocytosis (LCH) has a predilection for the skeleton, cutaneous tissues, and central nervous system [33]; besides axial skeletal lesions, characteristic traits in children include papulosquamous granulomatous lesions in the scalp, mucosal lesions of the oral cavity and genitals, and endocrinopathies secondary to pituitary dysfunction [14, 33, 34]. Close attention should be paid to the neurologic status of patients with known or suspected cranial/spinal LCH involvement.

Initial Steps

The initial evaluation of osteomyelitis and its mimics consists of the same steps: comprehensive history and exam, laboratory studies, and plain radiographs. Only 36% of children with osteomyelitis will have an elevated white blood cell count (WBC) [35], but the combined use of erythrocyte sedimentation rate (ESR) and C-reactive protein (CRP) gives a 98% diagnostic sensitivity for infection if both markers are high [36]. C-reactive protein provides the additional benefit of monitoring recovery when serially trended, since it typically normalizes within 10 days [36, 37]. However, acute-phase reactants like CRP and ESR may also rise in the setting of autoinflammatory disease, malignant and benign tumors, and bone infarction [1–3, 8, 16, 18, 32, 38, 39]. Among patients who have CNO, half present with mild to moderately elevated CRP, and most have a normal WBC [5, 24, 40]. A high CRP without leukocytosis has been suggested to be strongly indicative of leukemia as well [16, 18]. Blast cells on peripheral smear are traditionally pathognomonic for leukemia, but they may only show in a third of patients, and thus their absence is not sufficient to exclude leukemia from the differential [16]. Because of this lack of specificity, research in recent years has shifted focus from the "traditional" markers of infection to other plasma and cellular acute-phase reactants. A few in particular – IL-6, procalcitonin, platelet count, and neutrophil-to-lymphocyte ratio – have demonstrated promise as more sensitive and specific predictors of musculoskeletal infection [37].

Imaging represents the next stage in the investigation, starting with plain radiographs. As a first-line modality, radiography helps to exclude other diagnoses such as fracture, but it has poor sensitivity (37%) and only moderate specificity (73%) for osteomyelitis [41–43]. Up to 80% of cases will have normal radiographs in the first 2 weeks of infection because bone marrow edema – the earliest pathological feature – does not show on plain film [41]. It takes an average of 15 days for periosteal reaction and 3–4 weeks for trabecular/cortical osteolysis to become visible on radiographs [15, 41]. After that time point, subacute osteomyelitis may develop a moth-eaten permeative appearance due to bone destruction or a well-circumscribed bony lucency representing an intraosseous Brodie's abscess [15, 22, 41]. A radiographic hallmark of chronic osteomyelitis is a sequestrum – a dense fragment of necrotic bone with surrounding clear space –

enclosed by a reactive shell of sclerotic bone known as an involucrum [15, 41, 42]. Soft tissue planes on radiography are historically thought to be blurred by infection and displaced by tumor [15].

Many of the radiographic findings are relatively nonspecific and better evaluated by other modalities [1, 15, 41]. Computed tomography (CT) clearly delineates any sequestrum, involucrum, or osteolysis and the presence of gas or fat-fluid levels in the bone marrow cavity, which can be very specific for osteomyelitis [15, 41]. Computed tomography (fine cuts) is the modality of choice for detection of the nidus in osteoid osteomas. Within the first 1–2 days of infection, magnetic resonance imaging (MRI) reveals bone marrow edema as hypointense (dark) to muscle on T1-weighted sequences and hyperintense (bright) on fluid-sensitive sequences like T2-weighted and short-tau inversion recovery (STIR) [1, 41, 42]. Abscesses similarly have hypointense T1 signal and hyperintense T2 or STIR signal at their center, with a discrete thin rim of granulation tissue that is isointense relative to muscle on T1-weighted, hypointense on T2-weighted, and highly enhanced on post-contrast fat-saturated (FS) T1-weighted images [12, 41, 44, 45]. This pattern of peripheral enhancement, called the penumbra sign, has been reported to be 73.3% sensitive and 99.1% specific for subacute infection [12, 45]. Intra- and extramedullary fat globules appear on T1-weighted images as small, rounded, hyperintense foci within the bone or subperiosteal space and increase the probability that a marrow-invading process is osteomyelitis [1, 41, 46, 47]. Either increased intramedullary pressure causes extrusion of medullary fat, or adipocyte lysis secondary to bacterial enzymes or local ischemia releases intracellular fat [1, 46]. Another distinctive trait of osteomyelitis is a sinus tract most visible on fluid-sensitive sequences that highlights the draining pus inside the cloaca [22, 41, 42, 48]. Intravenous gadolinium contrast adds diagnostic value to MRI in certain contexts: distinguishing an abscess from a phlegmon (solid inflammatory mass), suspected epiphyseal infection, and vertebral osteomyelitis with a possible epidural abscess [1, 41, 42, 49]. It is also quite useful in differentiating a fluid collection from a solid tumor, which may also be hyperintense on T2-weighted sequences. Solid tumors often show more diffuse enhancement with contrast administration. One diagnostic pitfall may be a rapidly growing tumor with central necrosis, which then may show only peripheral enhancement, like an abscess. Growth plate and epiphyseal cartilage involvement may sometimes only reveal itself on gadolinium-enhanced T1 sequences and be hard to appreciate on noncontrast MRI or bone scintigraphy [42, 49]. Scintigraphy does not require sedation, but it lacks specificity, has poor anatomical localization, generates substantial radiation, and hence is not routinely used [15, 20, 41, 42]. In cases with multifocal lesions, it may be helpful to select the sites that are easiest to biopsy. Scintigraphy's role in evaluating the extent of CNO lesions has been supplanted by full body MRI, which is more sensitive and involves much less radiation. Although positron emission tomography has better sensitivity (95%) and specificity (87%), it may not be able to differentiate tumor vs. infection, has limited availability, and delivers considerable radiation [20, 42]. It rarely is used for routine workup in these situations. Osteomyelitis remains a diagnostic dilemma despite recent advances in imaging, and any ambiguity that persists after the initial workup necessitates tissue biopsy and culture guided by careful review of the imaging. Potential differentials and their relevant details are discussed herein.

Classic Differential Diagnoses for Osteomyelitis

Stress Injuries

Stress injuries often present with pain and difficulty weight-bearing, similar to infections. There is rarely fever associated with these injuries. The imaging can be confusing as well, with edema within the affected bone. Bones undergoing repetitive stress may sustain bone marrow alterations, cortical striations, and irregular periosteal reaction that precede cortical fracture [50–53]. Magnetic resonance imaging is considered the gold standard for assessing stress injuries because of its ability to detect cortical lesions (disruption of hypointense cortex on T1 sequences) and periosteal and endosteal marrow edema (hyperintense marrow signal on T2 and STIR windows) [52]. In contrast to osteomyelitis, the abnormal signal is confined to the bone and poorly demarcated, normal fat is preserved throughout the marrow, and there are no inflammatory changes in adjacent soft tissue (Fig. 5.1) [41, 51]. Developing stress fractures may sometimes be confused for a pathologic fracture or lytic neoplasm (e.g., ES or primary lymphoma of bone) due to periosteal reaction and bone resorption as the bone attempts to heal itself (Fig. 5.2) [53, 54]. Interpretation of these findings needs to correlate with a clinical history of repetitive activity and mechanical pain. Stress reactions/fractures often show predilection for certain anatomic sites (tibial shaft, proximal tibial metaphysis, distal third of the fibula, femoral neck, femoral shaft, inferior pubic ramus, etc.), unlike infection that may affect any bone. Once the diagnosis is confirmed (usually on imaging, occasionally with a biopsy), the patient should immediately cease the activity and enter a period of "active" rest, exercising in a pain-free manner, while preventing muscle atrophy [55]. They then participate in general conditioning and strengthening specific to the injured extremity, and functional weight-bearing in the final phase allows gradual bone remodeling and return to the original level of the activity. Some authors have shown improved prediction of time to return to play by combining MRI grading, fracture location, and bone mineral density scores with dual-energy X-ray absorptiometry [50].

Chronic Noninfectious Osteomyelitis

Chronic noninfectious osteomyelitis/CRMO remains a diagnosis of exclusion with unknown pathophysiology; its hallmark is noninfectious activation of the innate immune system in the absence of autoreactive T cells or high-titer autoantibodies [4, 38]. Monocytes in CNO/CRMO

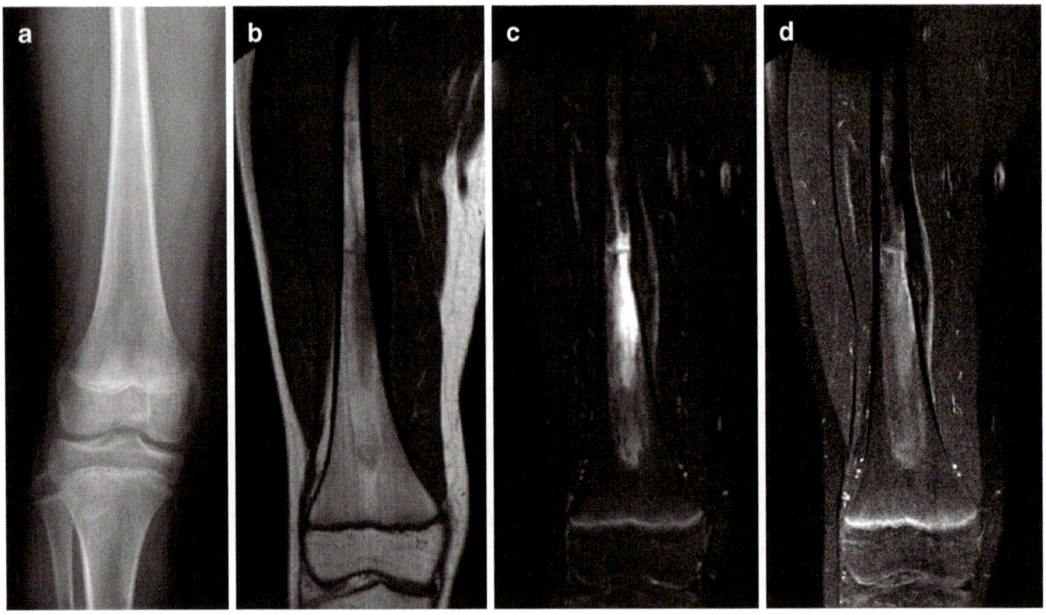

Fig. 5.1 Twelve-year-old male with atraumatic gradual onset of right distal thigh pain, activity-related, that self-resolved after 2 months. Radiographs (**a**) showed periosteal reaction in the femoral shaft, further delineated on MRI as a transverse fracture with surrounding periosteal reaction and marrow edema ((**b**) T1-weighted; (**c**) T2-weighted; (**d**) post-contrast T2-weighted). (Images printed with permission from Mihir Thacker, MD)

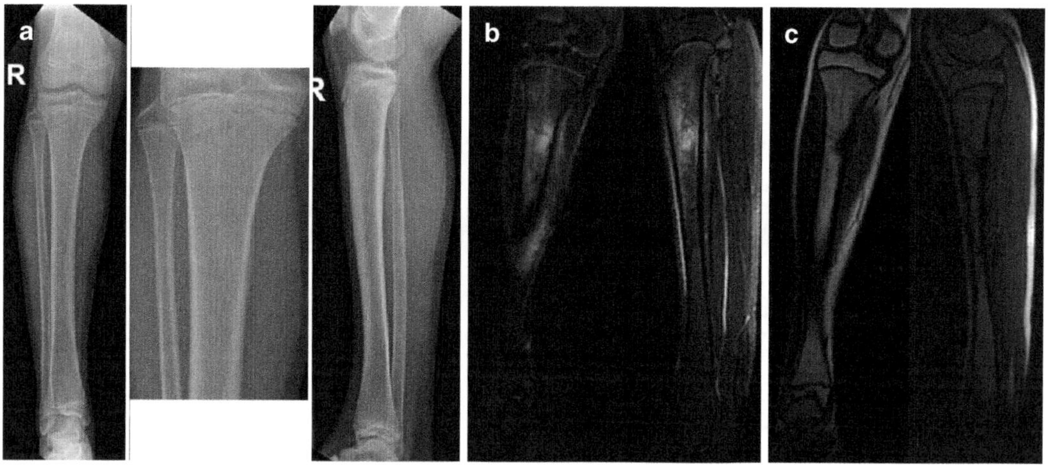

Fig. 5.2 Thirteen-year-old male with 2 weeks of atraumatic increasing right anteromedial proximal tibial pain, occurring mostly when weight-bearing and playing basketball. Ovoid lucency and subtle periosteal reaction within the proximal medial tibia on X-ray (**a**) corresponded to a transverse fracture line and adjacent marrow edema on MRI ((**b**) STIR-weighted; (**c**) T1-weighted). On both MRI windows, the abnormal marrow signal is confined to the bone and poorly demarcated; normal fat is preserved throughout the intramedullary space. There are no inflammatory changes in adjacent soft tissue. (Images printed with permission from Mihir Thacker, MD)

patients seem to exhibit a pro-inflammatory phenotype with increased expression of interleukin (IL)-1β, IL-6, and tumor necrosis factor (TNF)-α, resulting in chronic tissue inflammation, osteoclast activation, bone destruction, and in some cases hyperostosis and sclerosis [5, 38]. In the future, these serum proteins may act as biomarkers for CNO and help distinguish it from juvenile idiopathic arthritis and musculoskeletal infections [4]. The familial forms of CNO include Majeed syndrome (loss of function mutation in the LPIN2 gene), DIRA (deficiency of IL1 receptor antagonist), and PAP syndrome (pyogenic arthritis, pyoderma gangrenosum, and acne resulting from a mutation in the *PSTPIP1* gene). Fresh bone tissue requires testing for infectious agents, e.g., long-term cultures and microbial analysis, and reading by experienced pathologists to exclude neoplasm or infection [5]. The predominant histologic trait of CNO is chronic inflammation with lymphoplasmacytic infiltrates [24]. A clinical score has been proposed to help predict CNO/CRMO and reportedly has a positive predictive value of 97% and a sensitivity of 68% [40]. The parameters include normal WBC; symmetric bone lesions; lesions with marginal sclerosis and normal body temperature; lesions in the vertebra, clavicle, or sternum; more than one radiologically proven lesion; and CRP >1 mg/dL [40]. Inflammatory bone lesions may appear on plain film as radiolucent, osteolytic, or sclerotic but, overall, escape detection by radiography in the initial stages [4]. Whole body MRI is essential for diagnosing CNO/CRMO and detecting additional clinically silent lesions, especially in the pelvis and vertebral column [5, 25]. Chronic nonbacterial osteomyelitis in the spine affects the vertebrae itself, in contrast to osteomyelitis that centers on the intervertebral disc [54]. In the axial skeleton, CNO regularly manifests on strongly T2-weighted or post-contrast FS-T1 sequences as mild marrow edema without soft tissue edema, and nearly 90% of lesions in tubular bones involve periphyseal locations (Fig. 5.3) [1, 4, 25]. Serial whole body or regional MRIs can track the extent and distribution of lesions in response to treatment. Nonsteroidal anti-inflammatory drugs (NSAIDs) benefit most CNO patients if given on a regular schedule as many as 70% may achieve a pain-free state after 18 months [5]. Second-line options are corticosteroid "bursts" combined with disease-modifying antirheumatic drugs. Tumor necrosis factor inhibitors and IL-6 or IL-1 blocking agents hold promise in regulating the

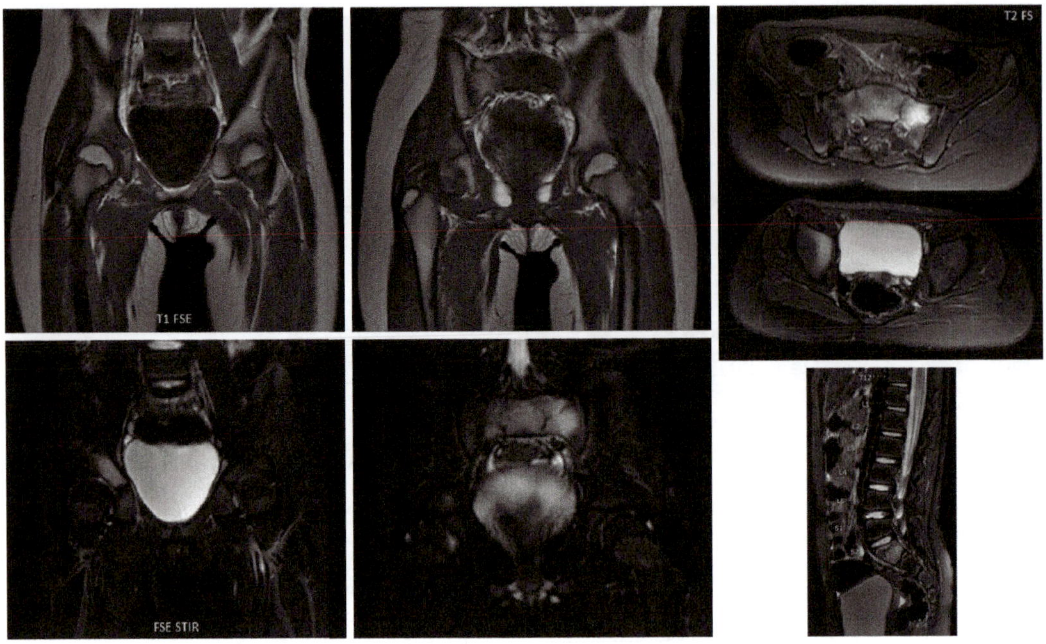

Fig. 5.3 Four-year-old female with 4 months of progressively worsening low back/sacral pain, inability to bear weight, and discomfort sitting on hard surfaces. Initial radiographs were unremarkable. Because her pain did not improve and she developed intermittent "fuzzy" feelings over her toes, neurology was consulted and ordered a spine MRI under sedation. This revealed abnormal infiltrative T2 hyperintensity and T1 hypointensity in the left S2 vertebrae and the right ilium. Bone marrow biopsy was negative. CT-guided core needle biopsy yielded extensive fibrosis and hypocellular fatty marrow on pathology, resulting in a diagnosis of CNO. (Images printed with permission from Mihir Thacker, MD)

imbalance between pro- versus anti-inflammatory cytokine expression [5, 24]. In hopes of preventing scoliosis secondary to osteolysis, TNF inhibitors and bisphosphonates have been recommended for vertebral involvement and severe CRMO [5].

Sickle Cell Crisis

It is exceedingly difficult to differentiate between infection and infarction (vaso-occlusive crisis) in sickle cell disease. The major challenges lie in the possible coexistence of infection with infarction and the skewed pretest probability of any imaging modality toward infarction; infarction is far more common than infection in patients with sickle cell disease [1, 7]. On radiographs, early osteonecrosis may create a poorly defined lucency simulating a tumor or calcifications resembling a chondroid lesion [9, 44]. On MRI, infarcts generally demonstrate a well-defined serpentine rim of hypointense T1 signal [44]. The rim may be hypointense, hyperintense, or both ("double line" sign) on T2-weighted images, sometimes accompanied by peripheral lobular calcifications with T2 hyperintensity [44]. Like infection, infarction can produce bone loss, subperiosteal fluid collections, and edema of the bone and surrounding soft tissues (Fig. 5.4) [8, 20]. On FS-T1 images, stagnant blood in an infarction is hyperintense, whereas infectious marrow edema is hypointense [1, 27]. A recent study attempted to use this sequence to separate the two etiologies but failed because the few cases of proven infection all arose in areas of infarction [27]. The same problem limits the diagnostic specificity of scintigraphy [1, 8, 9]. Ideally, ischemia demonstrates a lack of uptake on marrow scans, compared with increased bone scan uptake and normal marrow activity in infec-

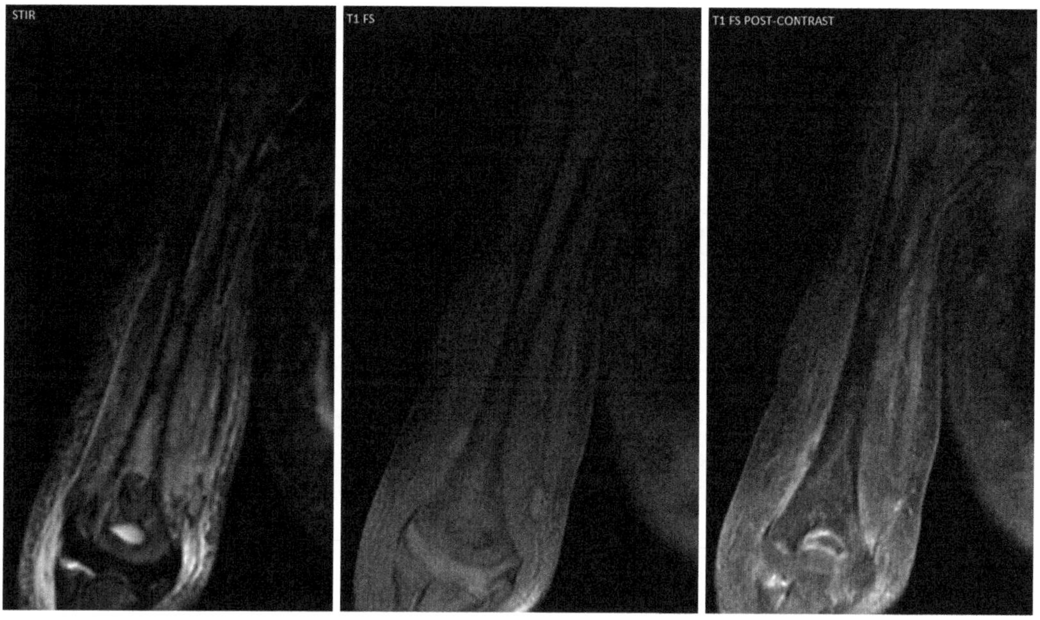

Fig. 5.4 Four-year-old male with right elbow pain/swelling and sporadic fevers (up to 38.5 ° C) in the setting of known sickle cell disease. Blood cultures were negative, and his inflammatory markers were elevated (WBC 20, ESR 52, CRP 8.5). X-rays showed soft tissue swelling and possible elbow joint effusion, but no fluid could be aspirated. MRI showed extensive edema and inflammatory changes centered around the right humerus metadiaphysis, but no drainable osseous abscesses. IV ceftriaxone was stopped, and his symptoms and inflammatory markers continued to improve, making avascular necrosis more likely than acute osteomyelitis. (Images printed with permission from Mihir Thacker, MD)

tions [1, 7]. However, this assumes that infection and infarction do not coexist, and this modality also involves significant radiation exposure [1]. Clinical judgment remains the primary method of distinguishing infarction from infection, and bone biopsy and culture are necessary if there is any doubt [9]. When sickle cell patients present with bone pain, localized swelling, and fever, intravenous hydration and empiric antibiotics are simultaneously initiated for vaso-occlusive crisis and osteomyelitis, respectively. Blood and stool cultures for *Salmonella* are drawn, and antibiotic therapy should be directed toward *S. aureus*, *H. influenzae*, pneumococcus, and meningococcus while waiting for results [8]. If the patient improves within 48 hours of fluid resuscitation and cultures are negative, the cause is most likely bone marrow ischemia [8]. A double-blind randomized controlled trial showed lower rates of painful crises, acute chest syndrome, and unscheduled blood transfusions in adults treated with hydroxyurea, and this was confirmed in another double-blind randomized controlled trial of hydroxyurea in young children with sickle cell disease [56]. Nearly half of the patients who experience one vaso-occlusive crisis are at risk for recurrent splenic sequestration that requires splenectomy [56].

Tumors

Ewing Sarcoma

Ewing sarcoma (ES) is a malignant tumor of bone and soft tissues hypothesized to be of neuroectodermal or mesenchymal stem cell derivation [21]. Pain is a common presenting feature and fever along with elevated leucocyte count may mimic infection. A lamellated ("onion skin") periosteal reaction, Codman triangle (ossified spur of elevated periosteum), may be suggestive but is not diagnostic of ES [15, 28, 31]. Ewing

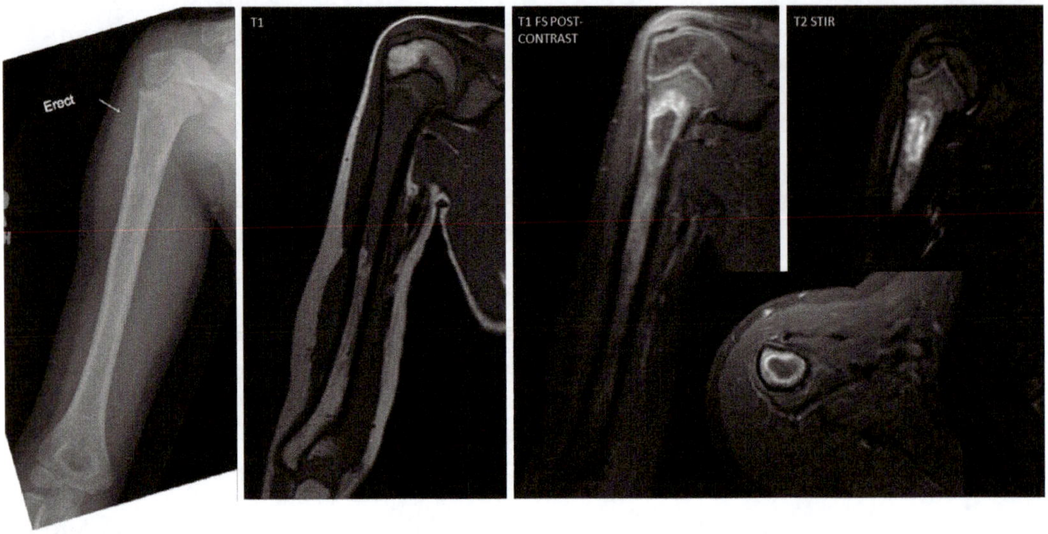

Fig. 5.5 Seven-year-old female with recurrent right shoulder pain that worsened with activity and would wake her from sleep at night. Inflammatory markers were normal. Radiographs demonstrated a permeative, lytic proximal humerus metaphyseal lesion, which was cystic on MRI and surrounded by diffuse inflammatory changes and multiple thin layers of periosteal reaction. During the open biopsy, the intraoperative frozen section contained neutrophils and plasma cells suggestive of an infective process. The lesion was irrigated and debrided, and antibiotics were started. No malignant cells were noted at that time on frozen section. Formal pathology later diagnosed her with small round blue cell neoplasm, consistent with Ewing sarcoma. (Images printed with permission from Mihir Thacker, MD)

sarcoma of the long bones usually looks like a permeative, moth-eaten, and destructive intramedullary lesion that favors the diaphysis or metadiaphysis [21, 28, 31]. On MRI, subacute and chronic osteomyelitis may form intra- and extraosseous granulation tissue, an indistinct border between normal and abnormal marrow that fades from the center of infection, and peripheral rim enhancement around abscesses (the "penumbra" sign) [41, 48]. Malignancies in contrast are characterized by an associated soft tissue mass that is solid and more discrete, a sharper and more defined margin between affected and unaffected marrow on T1-weighted images, and heterogenous enhancement on post-contrast FS-T1 sequences [21, 28, 29, 41, 42, 48, 57]. The "wraparound sign" – an intact, evenly T2 hypointense cortex despite a large soft tissue component wrapping around the bone – is a characteristic found in both ES and osseous lymphoma [28]. Several authors have suggested that the most unmistakable pattern of ES on MRI is a solid bone lesion (T1 hypointense and T2 hyperintense) with defined margins or a narrow transition zone (Fig. 5.5) [1, 57, 58]. The extent of the tumor is determined with the highest sensitivity on STIR sequences and the most specificity on T1-weighted sequences [58]. Staging workup depends on accurate imaging of the primary tumor and sites of metastasis, including chest radiographs, lung CT, bone scans, and bone marrow biopsy [21]. The MRI protocol must cover the entire bone and adjacent joints to check for skip lesions. Laboratory studies include complete blood count, ESR, serum lactate dehydrogenase, and baseline chemistry panels. Open biopsy provides a higher diagnostic yield than percutaneous biopsy (88% vs. 50%) but can still be inconclusive for cases of ES [29]. Histologically, the tumor contains densely packed round blue cells without matrix formation that express the antigen CD99, and break-apart fluorescence in situ hybridization confirms the translocation between chromosomes 11 and 22 on the *EWS* and *FLI1* genes [21]. Fourier-transformed infrared spectroscopy can differentiate osteomyelitis from ES

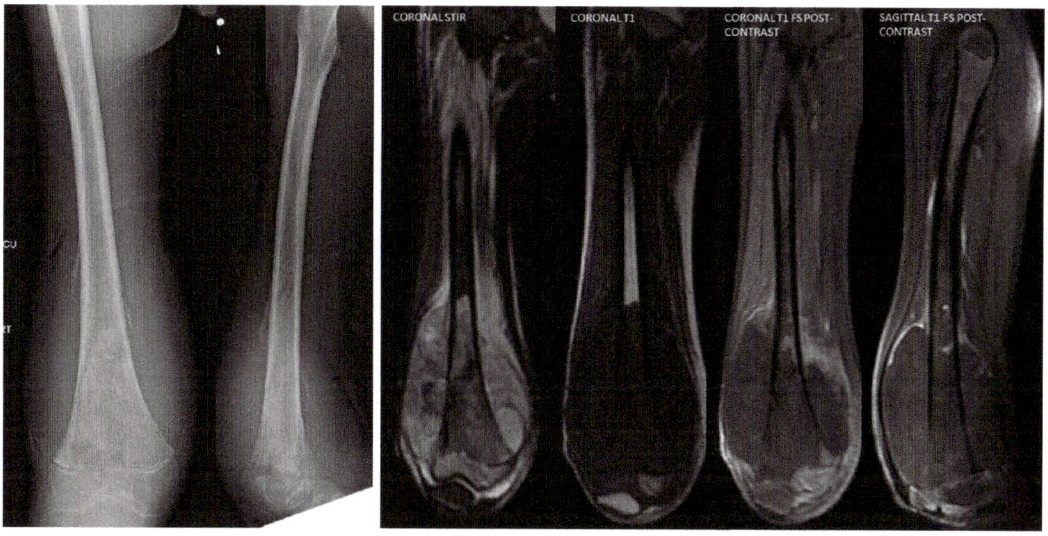

Fig. 5.6 Eleven-year-old male with right distal thigh mass and 3 months of pain limiting his weight-bearing, in the setting of acute respiratory distress. A mixed lucent/sclerotic lesion in the distal femur metadiaphysis was associated with cortical erosion, Codman triangles, and a large soft tissue mass on MRI that wrapped circumferentially around the femur. CT scan of the chest showed pleural effusions and pulmonary nodules, consistent with metastatic disease, and extremely elevated WBC (37.4), LDH (1246), and uric acid (6.3) suggested tumor lysis syndrome. CT-guided needle biopsy of the right femur mass yielded a pathologic diagnosis of conventional osteosarcoma. (Images printed with permission from Mihir Thacker, MD)

based on bone sample lipid and protein composition [59]. Chemotherapy agents carry their own risk of deleterious side effects, such as doxorubicin's cardiotoxicity, so additional scans (e.g., multigated acquisition scan) may be indicated before starting neoadjuvant chemotherapy [21, 60]. The standard of surgical care is wide/radical tumor resection because negative margins strongly correlate with better 5-year event-free survival and decreased rates of local recurrence [21]. Unfortunately, patients who have metastatic, refractory, or relapsed ES face a 5-year overall survival rate of 42% or less [59, 60].

Osteosarcoma

The most common primary malignant bone tumor in children, osteosarcoma, arises from primitive bone-forming mesenchyme and typically has a mixed appearance of bone destruction and bone formation [61]. Osteoid matrix proliferation is unique to the osteoblastic subtypes of osteosarcoma and is less likely seen in ES or osteomyelitis [48]. Like other malignant bone tumors, osteosarcoma may show cortical destruction, adjacent soft tissue mass, varying degrees of periosteal reaction, and hypointensity on T1-weighted images and hyperintensity on fluid-sensitive sequences (Fig. 5.6) [31, 61]. Conventional intramedullary osteosarcoma is associated with the "sunburst" pattern of periosteal reaction and prefers the metaphysis of the most rapidly growing bones in adolescence – distal femur, proximal tibia, proximal humerus, and distal radius [15, 21, 31]. These tumors can frequently cross the growth plate. Magnetic resonance imaging helps determine the transphyseal spread into the epiphysis and involvement of the neurovascular bundle [61]. There is usually a distinct margin between affected and unaffected marrow on T1-weighted images, compared with osteomyelitis, which has an ill-defined transition zone [1]. Staging and laboratory studies are like those described for ES (without the bone marrow biopsy). On histology, the presence of malignant osteoid and extensive pleomorphism define osteosarcoma, and it correlates with the retinoblastoma tumor-suppressor gene *RB1* [61]. Management consists of neoadjuvant chemotherapy and wide surgical resection, followed by additional adjuvant chemotherapy. Radiation rarely has a role except for palliative control [61]. Postoperative imaging follow-up depends on society recommendations and tumor grade, size, and site; chest CT is the recommended modality of monitoring lung metastases, and musculoskeletal surveillance intervals vary from every 3–6 months during the first 10 years to annually for up to 10 years [62].

Leukemia and Lymphoma

Leukemia is a malignant progressive disease in which the bone marrow and other hematopoietic organs generate increased numbers of immature or abnormal leukocytes, which then suppress the production of normal blood cells [63]. Many types exist; the most common form in children is acute lymphocytic leukemia (ALL), with a peak incidence between ages 2 and 6 years [18]. Children may often present with a limp and may be fussy and have tenderness to palpation over the extremities, mimicking infection. Radiographic findings in leukemia can be variable. If the lesion is osteolytic, it will frequently manifest in the long bone metaphysis or the pelvis. A specific finding of leukemia on radiography – a lucent metaphyseal band – may be seen in only 12% of patients [16]. The most often reported radiographic changes are multiple osteolytic foci in the metaphysis of long bones, with a noticeable absence of sclerosis [64]. Magnetic resonance imaging demonstrates marrow replacement rather than the marrow edema seen in osteomyelitis or CNO: the lesions appear hypointense on T1-weighted sequences and have sharp margins instead of blurred edges (Fig. 5.7) [26, 65]. The workup of leukemia incorporates a complete blood count, metabolic panel, liver function tests, uric acid levels, and coagulation panel, followed by peripheral blood smear and bone marrow aspiration/biopsy (especially for

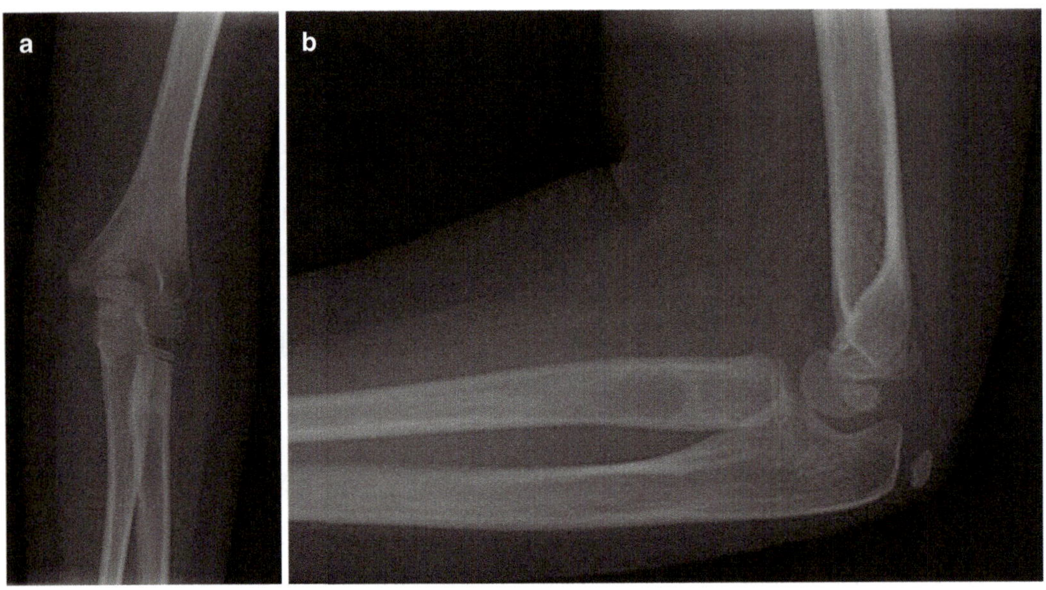

Fig. 5.7 Six-year-old female with 1 week of atraumatic left elbow pain and effusion. She had low-grade fevers, normal WBC (5.6), and high inflammatory markers (CRP 7.29 and ESR 93). The elbow was aspirated, and the synovial fluid showed no bacteria and a white cell count of 6000. Radiographs revealed permeative, lucent lesions in the proximal radius that enhanced on T2-weighted MRI (**a**–**d**). Antibiotics were started for presumed osteomyelitis. She returned a few days later with new left knee bony pain and recurrent low-grade fever. Bloodwork showed again normal WBC (4.0) and elevated inflammatory markers (CRP 11.9 and ESR 111), but this time with a low absolute neutrophil count (0.9) and extremely few blast cells (only 4%). X-rays found ill-defined lucencies in the distal femur diaphysis that enhanced on STIR and post-contrast sequences (**e**–**i**). Bone marrow biopsy returned positive for acute lymphoblastic leukemia. (Images printed with permission from Mihir Thacker, MD)

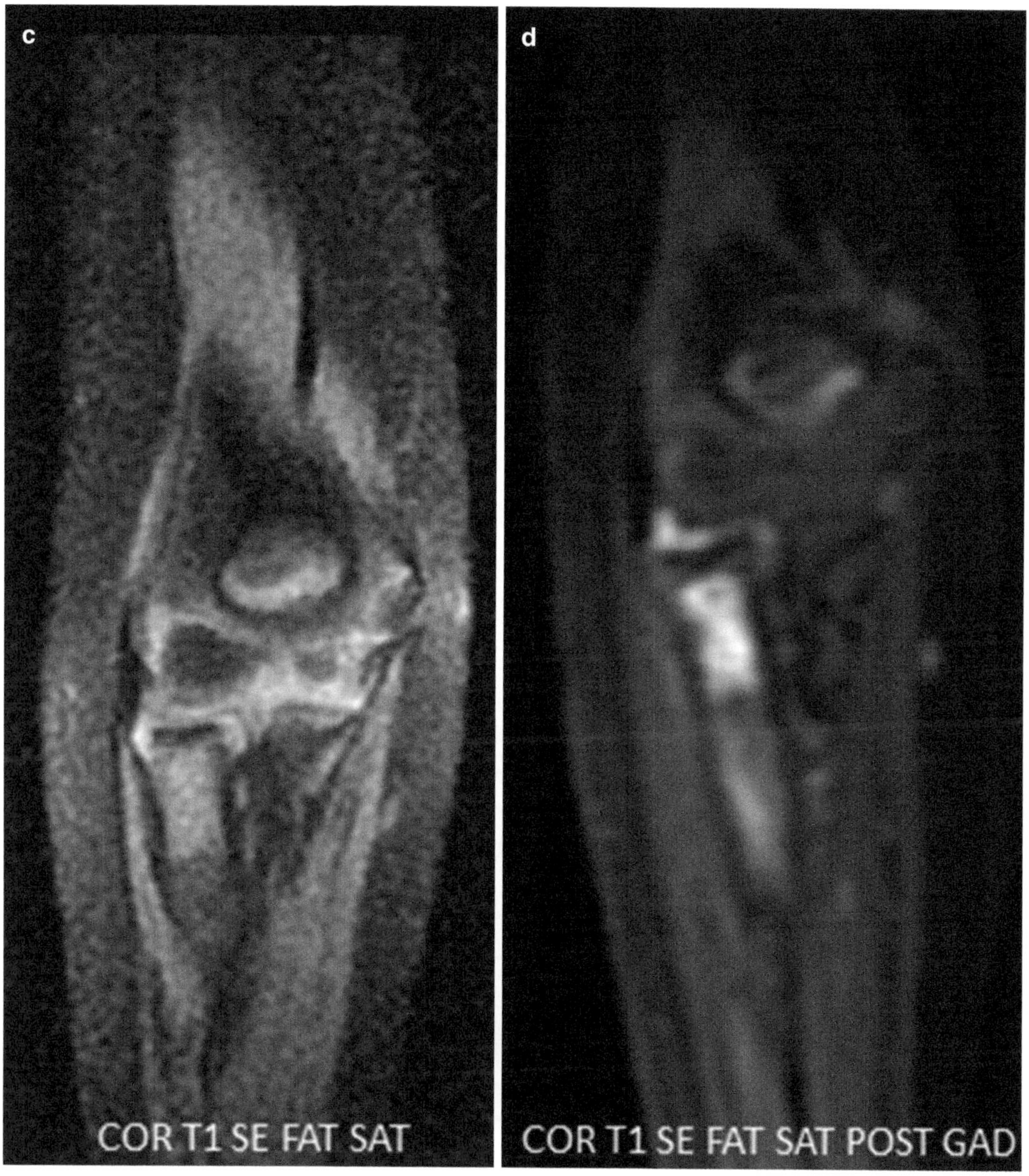

Fig. 5.7 (continued)

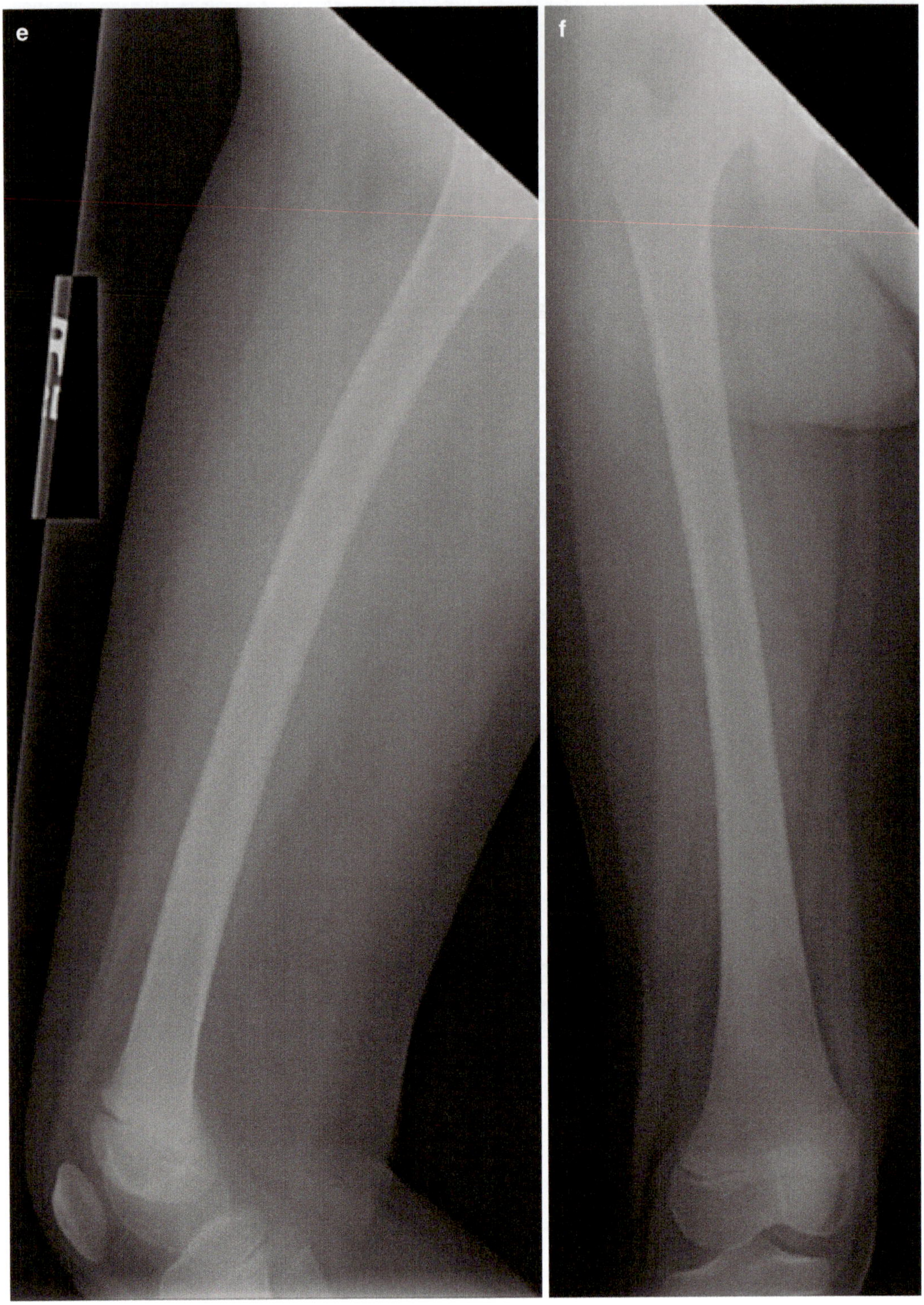

Fig. 5.7 (continued)

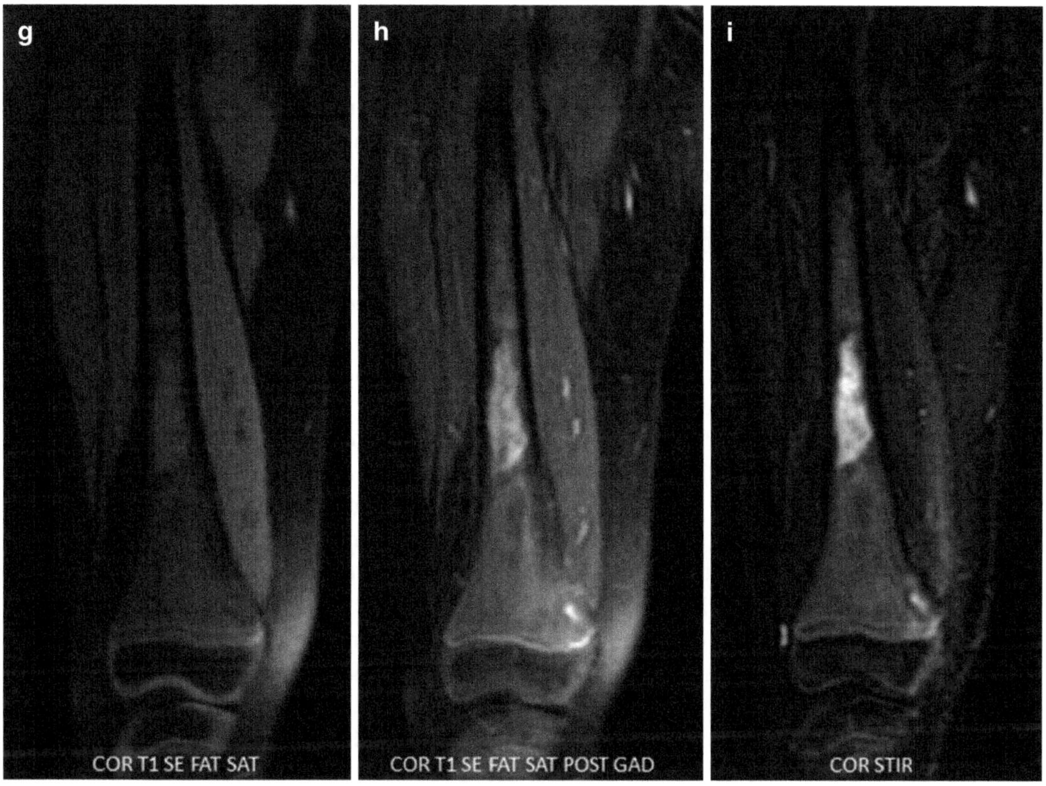

Fig. 5.7 (continued)

acute leukemias). Histologic features vary between different subtypes, and most cases require more detailed analyses (e.g., flow cytometry, cytogenetic testing) [66].

Lymphoma is a clonal proliferation of lymphoid cells that normally affects the lymph nodes, occasionally infiltrates the skeleton, and may be classified as Hodgkin's or non-Hodgkin's lymphoma [67]. Non-Hodgkin's lymphoma more commonly affects bone than Hodgkin's lymphoma, either as primary or secondary, with diffuse large B-cell lymphoma as the predominant subtype [28, 67]. Primary lymphoma of bone (PBL) is rare; it represents <1% of all non-Hodgkin's lymphoma and 3–5% of all malignant bone tumors [28]. Primary lymphoma of bone generally involves bones containing red marrow, with half localizing to the axial skeleton/skull and the other half in the long bones, notably the femur [28]. Like ES, PLB is found at the metaphysis (two-third of cases) or diaphysis (one-third of cases) [28] and seldom involves the epiphysis. The "wraparound" sign, previously described for ES, may also occur in PLB [28]. The cortex on T2-weighed sequence is regularly hypointense even though a large soft tissue component wraps around the bone, indicating that the slow permeative growth of the tumor has not destroyed much of the bone. Conversely, PLB can present aggressively as a destructive pattern of permeated cortical bone with intracortical linear signal hyperintensity on post-contrast MRI [16, 26, 28]. Radiographically, it presents as an osteolytic lesion without associated sclerosis, occasionally accompanied by a complex periosteal reaction of cortical breakthrough [26]. Incisional biopsy is crucial to establish a diagnosis since fine needle aspiration or core needle biopsy may yield an insufficient number of malignant cells and loss of tumor structure [32]. Specimens should be sent fresh, and not in formalin, to the pathologist to facilitate further testing (such as flow cytometry).

Under the microscope, nearly all lymphomas express common leukocyte antigen and B-cell markers like CD20 or CD30 [28, 68, 69]. Non-Hodgkin's lymphoma consists of diffuse round-cell infiltrates in its tumor stroma, and the hallmark of Hodgkin's lymphoma are Reed-Sternberg cells [68, 69]. Prognostic factors (e.g., extra nodal spread) guide the duration of chemotherapy and necessity of adjuvant radiation; radiation therapy is beneficial for early-stage disease in both Hodgkin's and non-Hodgkin's lymphoma but can be used for palliation in advanced cases [68, 69]. Surgery is only indicated for complications like pathologic fractures or spinal cord compression with neurologic deficits.

Osteoid Osteoma

Osteoid osteomas present as solitary, benign, and painful lesions that prefer the lower extremity long bones, posterior vertebral elements of the spine, and occasionally juxta-articular bone within a synovial cavity (intra-articular) [70]. Two-third of patients will experience severe pain that worsens at night and relieves with NSAIDs, due to an increased concentration of prostaglandins inside the lesion [70, 71]. Osteoid osteoma in the spine is the leading cause of painful scoliosis in children [70]. If the lesion is intra-articular, the resultant symptoms – joint effusion, decreased motion, and limping – may be mistaken for septic arthritis or other primary articular disorders [70, 71]. The radiographic signature in 85% of all cases is a nidus surrounded by thickened sclerotic cortex, usually located within the metaphyseal or diaphyseal cortices [70, 71]. Diagnosis becomes difficult for intramedullary, subperiosteal, or intra-articular lesions where there is limited reactive sclerosis [70, 71]. The nidus of an osteoid osteoma is close in appearance to a Brodie abscess, but it contains round calcified material in its center and is highly vascularized and ovoid, whereas a Brodie abscess is more elongated, avascular, and eccentrically filled by an irregular sequestrum [1, 15, 41, 70, 71]. Additionally, the inner wall is smooth in a nidus versus irregular in an intracortical abscess [71]. Computed tomography highlights these differences the best, especially on thin-section cuts and dynamic contrast enhancement (Fig. 5.8) [70, 71]. In osteoid osteoma, the vascular stroma within an unminer-

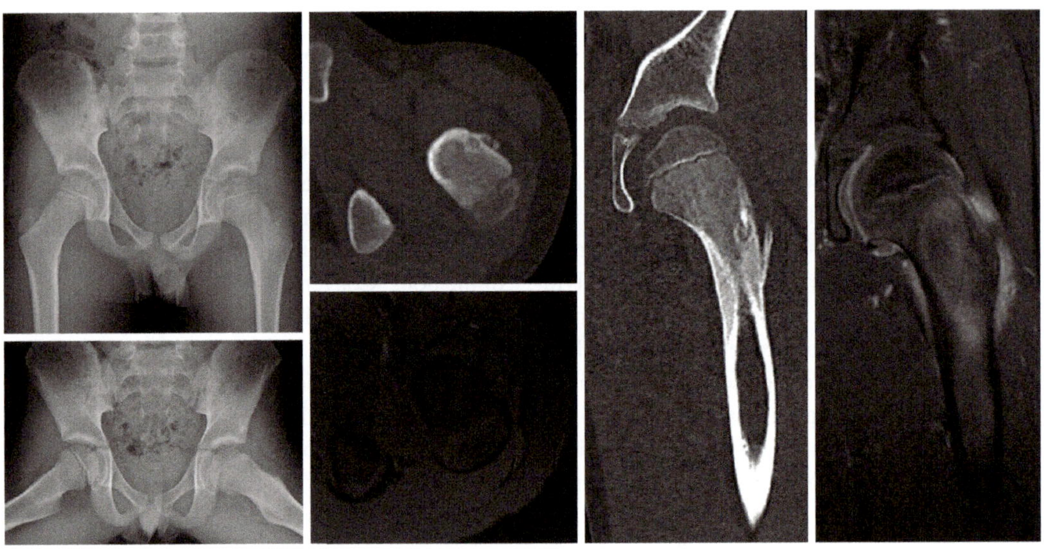

Fig. 5.8 Nine-year-old male with chronic left anterolateral hip pain that was more pronounced in the evening but did not wake him from sleep and was not responsive to nonsteroidal anti-inflammatories. MRI demonstrated post-contrast enhancement in the femoral neck and adjacent soft tissues. A lucent nidus with central ossification was definitively identified on CT, along with cortical thickening and hypertrophic spurring of the anterolateral femoral neck. The patient underwent radiofrequency ablation of the osteoid osteoma and his symptoms fully resolved. (Images printed with permission from Mihir Thacker, MD)

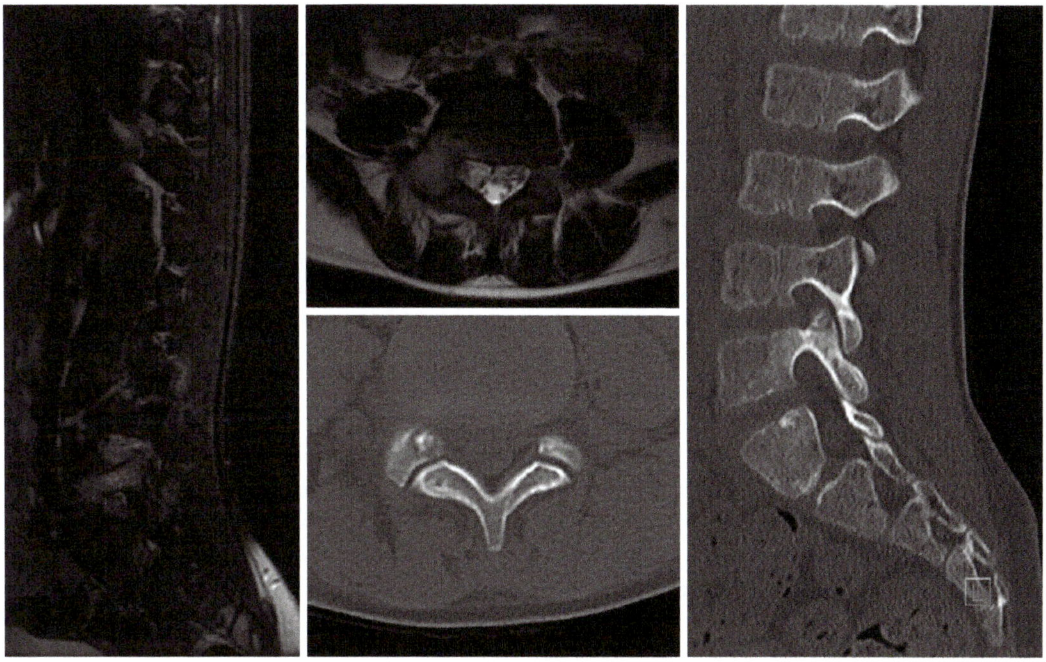

Fig. 5.9 Eight-year-old male with several weeks of increasing midline thoracolumbar pain that would awaken him at night and relieved with NSAIDs. MRI revealed bony edema localized to the L5 posterior elements. CT more clearly delineated the nidus within the right L5 superior articular facet. (Images printed with permission from Mihir Thacker, MD)

alized nidus will avidly enhance; in an intracortical abscess, the avascular center remains dark while the peripheral rim enhances on post-contrast images [41, 71]. Magnetic resonance imaging offers less utility than CT in nidus detection and could cloud the diagnostic picture by showing nonspecific marrow/soft tissue edema (Fig. 5.9) [70, 71]. Neither bone destruction nor soft tissue inflammation have been associated with osteoid osteomas [41]. Scintigraphy is another imaging modality to consider if the lesion is in an unusual location or lacks the usual reactive sclerosis. On technetium-99 bone scan, an osteoid osteoma accumulates radiopharmaceutical agents during the vascular, blood pool, and delayed phases; this double-density appearance is very specific and carries high diagnostic value [70]. Definitive management of osteoid osteoma ranges from percutaneous techniques (CT-guided radiofrequency ablation or excision) to open procedures (open or arthroscopic excision and laser ablation). High rates of success and similar recurrence rates are described for all these options, with shorter hospital stays reported for percutaneous techniques [72].

Langerhans Cell Histiocytosis

Langerhans cell histiocytosis – formerly known as "histiocytosis X" – is characterized by the infiltration and accumulation of abnormal histiocytes (Langerhans cells) within the bone marrow, skin, central nervous system, lung, liver, spleen, or lymph nodes [14, 33, 34]. It causes focal or systemic damage by excessive production of cytokines and prostaglandins [73]. Langerhans cell histiocytosis comprises a spectrum of clinical variants, previously thought to be three distinct syndromes: eosinophilic granuloma (unifocal solitary bone lesion), Hand-Schüller-Christian disease (multifocal with the classic triad of skull lesions, exophthalmos, and diabetes insipidus), and Letterer-Siwe disease (multisystem involvement) [34, 73]. Up to 80% of cases involve bone [14, 34]. In children, monostotic disease typically manifests in the vertebral bodies, long bones, and mandibles, whereas in adults, the cranium and ribs are most often affected [14, 26, 31]. In the acute phase, LCH routinely presents with aggressive features on radiography and MRI: permeative, lytic, poorly defined borders, periosteal reaction, endosteal scalloping, bone marrow edema, and post-contrast enhancement [14, 31, 39]. Lesions in the skull calvarium classically look "punched out" [34]. Formation of bony septa inside a lesion can give it a soap bubble-like appearance [14]. Eosinophilic granulomas may also contain a fragment of intact bone – a sequestrum – that could be mistaken for chronic osteomyelitis or the nidus of an osteoid osteoma [1, 31]. Osteomyelitis is associated with dramatic perilesional edema that extends along the marrow and into the soft tissues, and LCH in children may result in significant bone loss and perilesional edema as well [1, 39]. However, compared with osteomyelitis, which concentrates in the metaphysis, LCH is primarily diaphyseal (Fig. 5.10) [1]. If a metaphyseal lesion does occur, it rarely violates the growth plate [14]. A soft tissue mass may be associated with up to 70% of skeletal LCH [39]. As the lesions heal and regress, they eventually are enclosed by marginal sclerosis on radiographs and a hypointense endosteal rim on T1-weighted MRI [26, 31, 34]. Spinal involvement by LCH characteristically produces anterior wedging or complete collapse of the vertebral bodies (vertebra plana), while sparing end plates, disks, and posterior elements [14, 44]. Although pathognomonic in children, vertebra plana seldom occurs in adults [74]. Pediatric patients with multiple vertebral lesions are at risk for kyphoscoliosis, and some may develop progressive neurologic deficits that require surgical decompression and stabilization by instrumented fusion [14]. Fortunately, vertebral height is partially or almost completely regained upon healing of most lesions [14, 75]. Vertebral lesions predominantly appear in the cervical/thoracic

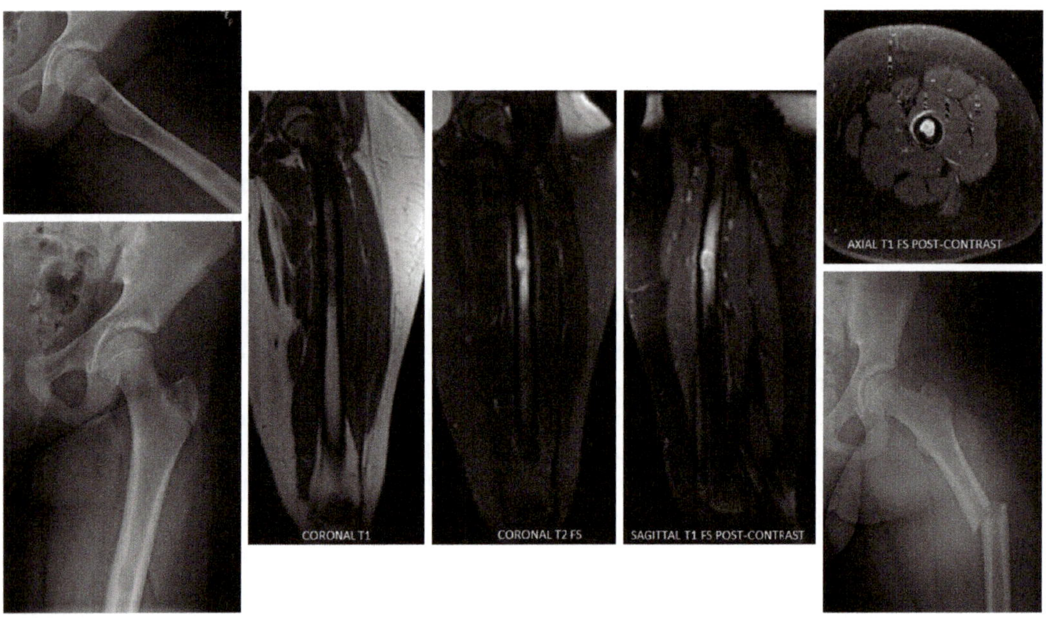

Fig. 5.10 Eleven-year-old female with gradual onset of left medial knee pain, aggravated by weight-bearing and motion, that also occurred at night. Radiographs showed a lucent lesion in distal femoral shaft with deep endosteal scalloping and periosteal reaction. This corresponded to a contrast-enhancing, T2 hyperintense lesion on MRI, along with extensive adjacent edema and thinning of the anterior femur cortex. A week after undergoing a needle biopsy, she fell off the monkey bars and sustained a pathologic left proximal third femur fracture. (Images printed with permission from Mihir Thacker, MD)

regions and should be evaluated by MRI to rule out intracanal compromise, which can be found in up to one-third of children and two-third of adults [34, 74]. If LCH targets the flat bones (e.g., skull base, pelvis, ribs, and scapula), CT is helpful for delineating the anatomy and location of lesions [31]. Suspicion for LCH should prompt a complete skeletal survey and chest radiograph to assess the extent of disease; whole-body MRI has gradually become the standard of care to map osseous, soft tissue, and nodal involvement without radiation [31, 34]. There is controversy over the benefits of biopsy in low-risk patients with a unifocal bone lesion, but in general, LCH is primarily a clinicopathological diagnosis because its imaging findings are non-specific [14, 33, 34, 73]. Only a core needle or open biopsy will provide enough tissue for histologic/immunohistochemical analysis [14]. Diagnostic criteria include positive staining for CD1a and/or Langerin (CD207) proteins and accumulation of Langerhans dendritic cells, which contain tennis racquet-shaped Birbeck granules on electron microscopy [14, 73]. In cases where the risks of biopsy outweigh the need for definitive diagnosis (such as a child with isolated upper cervical vertebral involvement), malignancy must be excluded by carefully monitoring the patient for at least the next 6 months [33]. No clear guidelines exist for the management of LCH; much depends on the extent and severity of LCH [33]. Unifocal bony lesions tend to be self-limited and may be closely observed or locally controlled (e.g., intralesional corticosteroid injection, curettage, or low-dose radiation therapy in surgically inaccessible areas) [14, 33]. In contrast, multifocal skeletal involvement and disseminated multisystem disease benefit from systemic regimens of chemotherapy and/or steroids [14, 33, 73]. Current guidelines do not recommend routine radiation therapy for multisystem disease [14]. The course of LCH is unpredictable since it may progress or spontaneously resolve, and routine imaging is necessary to check for recurrence [14, 73]. Positron emission tomography-CT could play a role in staging and monitoring treatment response for multifocal disease [31, 73].

Scurvy

Scurvy is caused by prolonged, severe dietary deficiency of vitamin C that results in a spectrum of dermatological, dental, bone, and systemic manifestations [76, 77]. Children with abnormal dietary habits, mental illness, or physical disabilities are prone to develop this disease. Vitamin C is an essential nutrient for humans and intimately concerned in the maintenance of intercellular connective tissues, osteoid, dentine, and collagen. Vitamin C plays an important role as a cofactor, enzyme complement, co-substrate, reducing agent, and an antioxidant in several biochemical reactions. Deficiency leads to fatigue, irritability, platelet dysfunction, petechiae, ecchymosis, gingival disease, poor teeth formation, subperiosteal hemorrhages, and physeal separations. Epiphyseal separation from the metaphysis occurs through the zone of calcified cartilage, known as "scorbutic lattice," which in the radiographs is represented as "the white line of Frankel." Other radiographic findings include osteopenia, subperiosteal hemorrhages, ring epiphysis, Pelkan spurs, a metaphyseal zone of rarefaction (Trummerfeld zone), and physeal separations. Characteristic MRI findings include diffuse multifocal decreased signal on T1-weighted imaging and increased signal on T2-weighted imaging within bone marrow, predominantly within the metaphyses, a varying degree of bone marrow enhancement, and adjacent periosteal elevation and soft tissue signal abnormalities. Diagnosis is confirmed by evaluating serum vitamin C levels (normal >23 μmol/L). Treatment involves supplementation with vitamin C. Treatment outcomes are very good [76, 77].

Charcot Arthropathy

Charcot neuropathic arthropathy in children is a rare condition which can be a part of the natural course and complicate surgical treatment of neuro-orthopedic disorders, like spinal dysraphism and hereditary sensory polyneuropathy. Predominant clinical features include a history of minor trauma, limited swelling, and progressive joint instability. Diagnosis is usually confirmed by imaging studies. Plain radiographs show bone destruction, joint instability, and loose bodies. MR imaging is significant for a large joint effusion, loose bodies, and joint destruction. Nonsurgical management is the treatment method of choice and includes total contact casts and orthotics. Reeducation of children and family is a crucial part of the treatment. Surgery should be used as a salvage procedure and should include thorough debridement, bone substitution, osteo-inductive supplement, and stable fixation [78, 79].

Classic Differential Diagnosis for Septic Arthritis

Monoarticular arthritis is a common presentation to the emergency department (ED) and major cause of disability in the world [80]. Monoarticular arthritis has a wide range of potential etiologies, ranging from benign to life-threatening. These include septic arthritis, transient synovitis, reactive arthritis, pyomyositis, tubercular arthritis, Lyme arthritis, traumatic hemarthrosis, hemophilic hemarthrosis, juvenile idiopathic arthritis, juvenile rheumatoid arthritis, pigmented villonodular synovitis, and synovial chondromatosis [78, 80–84]. These differential diagnoses, important clinical features, laboratory, and imaging findings are summarized in Table 5.2 and discussed in more detail in Chap. 12 "Septic Arthritis".

Classic Differential Diagnosis for Pyomyositis

Pyomyositis is an intramuscular infection caused by bacteria or other organisms. Pyomyositis presents with fever, pain, swelling, and refusal to walk and put weight on the affected extremity. The clinical presentation of pyomyositis is similar to osteomyelitis, septic arthritis, or several other conditions [85, 86]. The common sites of involvement are the pelvic musculature and lower extremity. Iliopsoas, obturator musculature, and gluteal muscle are the commonest muscles involved.[86] The differential diagnoses are summarized in Table 5.3 and are discussed in detail in Chap. 13 "Pyomyositis".

Conclusions

There are a multitude of conditions (benign and malignant) that can mimic infection. Awareness of these conditions and their presentations is critical in creating an appropriate list of differential diagnoses and initiating the correct workup. Laboratory studies and imaging findings, though very helpful, can frequently overlap. A biopsy (bone and/or soft tissue) or synovial fluid/tissue aspiration is frequently required, especially in borderline cases, to confirm the diagnosis. Possibility of a malignant tumor should be kept in mind when dealing with infection, and biopsy principles should be respected. The diagnosis and management of these infection mimics require good clinico-radiologic-pathologic correlation and a multidisciplinary team.

Box 5.1 Key Take Home Points

1. Infection mimics can delay diagnosis and appropriate treatment.
2. Always consider differential diagnosis when suspecting pediatric musculoskeletal infections.
3. Clinical features, laboratory, and imaging findings can overlap.
4. Always get samples before starting definitive treatment.
5. Bone and/or soft tissue samples and synovial fluid aspirate/tissue aspirate are essential.
6. Send samples for both microbiology and pathology.
7. Clinico-radiologic-pathologic correlation is essential in atypical or difficult cases.
8. Multidisciplinary team evaluation is essential.

References

1. Jaramillo D, Dormans JP, Delgado J, Laor T, St Geme JW. Hematogenous osteomyelitis in infants and children: imaging of a changing disease. Radiology. 2017;283(3):629–43.
2. Dartnell J, Ramachandran M, Katchburian M. Haematogenous acute and subacute paediatric osteomyelitis. J Bone Joint Surg Br. 2012;94-B(5):584–95.
3. Durbin M, Randall RL, James M, Sudilovsky D, Zoger S. Ewing's sarcoma masquerading as osteomyelitis. Clin Orthop Relat Res. 1998;357:176–85.
4. Hofmann SR, Kapplusch F, Girschick HJ, Morbach H, Pablik J, Ferguson PJ, Hedrick CM. Chronic recurrent multifocal osteomyelitis (CRMO): presentation, pathogenesis, and treatment. Curr Osteoporos Rep. 2017;15(6):542–54.
5. Hedrich CM, Morbach H, Reiser C, Girschick HJ. New insights into adult and paediatric chronic non-bacterial osteomyelitis CNO. Curr Rheumatol Rep. 2020;22(9):52.
6. Berger E, Saunders N, Wang L, Friedman JN. Sickle cell disease in children: differentiating osteomyelitis from vaso-occlusive crisis. Arch Pediatr Adolesc Med. 2009;163(3):251–5.
7. Buchanan GR. Differentiation of bone infarct from infection in a child in sickle cell disease. Pediatr Infect Dis J. 1996;15(8):725.
8. Wong AL, Sakamoto KM, Johnson EE. Differentiating osteomyelitis from bone infarction in sickle cell disease. Pediatr Emerg Care. 2001;17(1):60–3.
9. Almeida A, Roberts I. Bone involvement in sickle cell disease. Br J Haematol. 2005;129(4):482–90.
10. Kent PM, Trafton LW. Clinical presentation of bone tumors in children and young adults. Curr Probl Cancer. 2013;37(4):167–71.
11. Motamedi K, Seeger LL. Benign bone tumors. Radiol Clin N Am. 2011;49(6):1115–34, v.
12. Shimose S, Sugita T, Kubo T, Matsuo T, Nobuto H, Ochi M. Differential diagnosis between osteomyelitis and bone tumors. Acta Radiol. 2008;49(8):928–33.
13. Cottias P, Tomeno B, Anract P, Vinh TS, Forest M. Subacute osteomyelitis presenting as a bone tumour. Int Orthop. 1997;21(4):243–8.
14. DiCaprio MR, Roberts TT. Diagnosis and management of Langerhans cell histiocytosis. J Am Acad Orthop Surg. 2014;22(10):643–52.
15. Moser T, Ehlinger M, Chelli Bouaziz M, Fethi Ladeb M, Durckel J, Dosch J-C. Pitfalls in osteoarticular imaging: how to distinguish bone infection from tumour? Diagn Interv Imaging. 2012;93(5):351–9.
16. Kobayashi D, Satsuma S, Kamegaya M, Haga N, Shimomura S, Fujii T, Yoshiya S. Musculoskeletal conditions of acute leukemia and malignant lymphoma in children. J Pediatr Orthop B. 2005;14(3):156–61.
17. Tuten HR, Gabos PG, Kumar SJ, Harter GD. The limping child: a manifestation of acute leukemia. J Pediatr Orthop. 1998;18(5):625–9.
18. Chell J, Fernandes JA, Bell MJ. The orthopaedic presentation of acute leukaemia in childhood. Ann R Coll Surg Engl. 2001;83(3):186–9.
19. Huang P-Y, Wu P-K, Chen C-F, Lee F-T, Wu H-T, Liu C-L, Chen T-H, Chen W-M. Osteomyelitis of the femur mimicking bone tumors: a review of 10 cases. World J Surg Oncol. 2013;11:283.
20. Jaramillo D. Infection: musculoskeletal. Pediatr Radiol. 2011;41(Suppl 1):S127–34.
21. Maheshwari AV, Cheng EY. Ewing sarcoma family of tumors. J Am Acad Orthop Surg. 2010;18(2):94–107.
22. Horvai A. Bones, joints and soft tissue tumors. In: Kumar V, Abbas A, Aster J, editors. Robbins and Cotran pathologic basis of disease. 9th ed. Philadelphia: Elsevier Saunders; 2018. p. 1179–226.
23. Nixon GW. Hematogenous osteomyelitis of metaphyseal-equivalent locations. Am J Roentgenol. 1978;130(1):123–9.
24. Schnabel A, Range U, Hahn G, Berner R, Hedrich CM. Treatment response and longterm outcomes in children with chronic nonbacterial osteomyelitis. J Rheumatol. 2017;44(7):1058–65.
25. von Kalle T, Heim N, Hospach T, Langendörfer M, Winkler P, Stuber T. Typical patterns of bone involvement in whole-body MRI of patients with chronic recurrent multifocal osteomyelitis (CRMO). Rofo. 2013;185(7):655–61.
26. Sato TS, Watal P, Ferguson PJ. Imaging mimics of chronic recurrent multifocal osteomyelitis: avoiding pitfalls in a diagnosis of exclusion. Pediatr Radiol. 2020;50(1):124–36.
27. Delgado J, Bedoya MA, Green AM, Jaramillo D, Ho-Fung V. Utility of unenhanced fat-suppressed T1-weighted MRI in children with sickle cell disease—can it differentiate bone infarcts from acute osteomyelitis? Pediatr Radiol. 2015;45(13):1981–7.
28. Weber M-A, Papakonstantinou O, Nikodinovska VV, Vanhoenacker FM. Ewing's sarcoma and primary osseous lymphoma: spectrum of imaging appearances. Semin Musculoskelet Radiol. 2019;23(1):36–57.
29. McCarville MB, Chen JY, Coleman JL, Li Y, Li X, Adderson EE, Neel MD, Gold RE, Kaufman RA. Distinguishing osteomyelitis from Ewing sarcoma on radiography and MRI. AJR Am J Roentgenol. 2015;205(3):640–50.
30. Esiashvili N, Goodman M, Marcus RB Jr. Changes in incidence and survival of Ewing sarcoma patients over the past 3 decades: surveillance epidemiology and end results data. J Pediatr Hematol Oncol. 2008;30(6):425–30.
31. McCarville MB. The child with bone pain: malignancies and mimickers. Cancer Imaging. 2009;9(Spec No A):S115–21.
32. Majeed A, Chan O, Okolo O, Shponka V, Georgescu A, Persky D. Hodgkin lymphoma mimicking osteomyelitis. Case Rep Oncol. 2017;10(2):542–7.
33. Haupt R, Minkov M, Astigarraga I, Schäfer E, Nanduri V, Jubran R, Egeler RM, Janka G, Micic D, Rodriguez-Galindo C, Van Gool S, Visser J,

Weitzman S, Donadieu J, Euro Histio Network. Langerhans cell histiocytosis (LCH): guidelines for diagnosis, clinical work-up, and treatment for patients till the age of 18 years. Pediatr Blood Cancer. 2013;60(2):175–84.
34. Khung S, Budzik J-F, Amzallag-Bellenger E, Lambilliote A, Ares GS, Cotten A, Boutry N. Skeletal involvement in Langerhans cell histiocytosis. Insights Imaging. 2013;4(5):569–79.
35. Yeo A, Ramachandran M. Acute haematogenous osteomyelitis in children. BMJ. 2014;348:g66.
36. Pääkkönen M, Kallio MJT, Kallio PE, Peltola H. Sensitivity of erythrocyte sedimentation rate and C-reactive protein in childhood bone and joint infections. Clin Orthop Relat Res. 2010;468(3):861–6.
37. Moore-Lotridge S, Gibson B, Duvernay M, Martus J, Thomsen I, Schoenecker J. Pediatric musculoskeletal infection: an update through the four pillars of clinical care and immunothrombotic similarities with COVID-19. JPOSNA. 2020;2(2)
38. Hedrich CM, Hofmann SR, Pablik J, Morbach H, Girschick HJ. Autoinflammatory bone disorders with special focus on chronic recurrent multifocal osteomyelitis (CRMO). Pediatr Rheumatol Online J. 2013;11(1):47.
39. Samet J, Weinstein J, Fayad LM. MRI and clinical features of Langerhans cell histiocytosis (LCH) in the pelvis and extremities: can LCH really look like anything? Skelet Radiol. 2016;45(5):607–13.
40. Jansson AF, Müller TH, Gliera L, Ankerst DP, Wintergerst U, Belohradsky BH, Jansson V. Clinical score for nonbacterial osteitis in children and adults. Arthritis Rheum. 2009;60(4):1152–9.
41. Lee YJ, Sadigh S, Mankad K, Kapse N, Rajeswaran G. The imaging of osteomyelitis. Quant Imaging Med Surg. 2016;6(2):184–98.
42. Pugmire BS, Shailam R, Gee MS. Role of MRI in the diagnosis and treatment of osteomyelitis in pediatric patients. World J Radiol. 2014;6(8):530–7.
43. Tumeh SS, Aliabadi P, Weissman BN, McNeil BJ. Disease activity in osteomyelitis: role of radiography. Radiology. 1987;165(3):781–4.
44. Nascimento D, Suchard G, Hatem M, de Abreu A. The role of magnetic resonance imaging in the evaluation of bone tumours and tumour-like lesions. Insights Imaging. 2014;5(4):419–40.
45. Grey AC, Davies AM, Mangham DC, Grimer RJ, Ritchie DA. The "penumbra sign" on T1-weighted MR imaging in subacute osteomyelitis: frequency, cause and significance. Clin Radiol. 1998;53(8):587–92.
46. Davies AM, Hughes DE, Grimer RJ. Intramedullary and extramedullary fat globules on magnetic resonance imaging as a diagnostic sign for osteomyelitis. Eur Radiol. 2005;15(10):2194–9.
47. Hui CL, Naidoo P. Extramedullary fat fluid level on MRI as a specific sign for osteomyelitis. Australas Radiol. 2003;47(4):443–6.
48. Kan JH. Major pitfalls in musculoskeletal imaging–MRI. Pediatr Radiol. 2008;38(2):251–5.
49. Browne LP, Guillerman RP, Orth RC, Patel J, Mason EO, Kaplan SL. Community-acquired staphylococcal musculoskeletal infection in infants and young children: necessity of contrast-enhanced MRI for the diagnosis of growth cartilage involvement. AJR Am J Roentgenol. 2012;198(1):194–9.
50. Marshall RA, Mandell JC, Weaver MJ, Ferrone M, Sodickson A, Khurana B. Imaging features and management of stress, atypical, and pathologic fractures. RadioGraphics. 2018;38(7):2173–92.
51. Manaster B. Musculoskeletal imaging: the requisites. 3rd ed. Philadelphia: Mosby Elsevier; 2007. p. 545–64.
52. Moran DS, Evans RK, Hadad E. Imaging of lower extremity stress fracture injuries. Sports Med. 2008;38(4):345–56.
53. Stacy GS, Kapur A. Mimics of bone and soft tissue neoplasms. Radiol Clin N Am. 2011;49(6):1261–86, vii.
54. Fayad LM, Kamel IR, Kawamoto S, Bluemke DA, Frassica FJ, Fishman EK. Distinguishing stress fractures from pathologic fractures: a multimodality approach. Skelet Radiol. 2005;34(5):245–59.
55. Romani WA, Gieck JH, Perrin DH, Saliba EN, Kahler DM. Mechanisms and management of stress fractures in physically active persons. J Athl Train. 2002;37(3):306–14.
56. Meier ER, Miller JL. Sickle cell disease in children. Drugs. 2012;72(7):895–906.
57. Kasalak Ö, Overbosch J, Adams HJ, Dammann A, Dierckx RA, Jutte PC, Kwee TC. Diagnostic value of MRI signs in differentiating Ewing sarcoma from osteomyelitis. Acta Radiol. 2019;60(2):204–12.
58. Henninger B, Glodny B, Rudisch A, Trieb T, Loizides A, Putzer D, Judmaier W, Schocke MF. Ewing sarcoma versus osteomyelitis: differential diagnosis with magnetic resonance imaging. Skelet Radiol. 2013;42(8):1097–104.
59. Chaber R, Arthur CJ, Depciuch J, Łach K, Raciborska A, Michalak E, Cebulski J. Distinguishing Ewing sarcoma and osteomyelitis using FTIR spectroscopy. Sci Rep. 2018;8(1):15081.
60. Gaspar N, Hawkins DS, Dirksen U, Lewis IJ, Ferrari S, Le Deley M-C, Kovar H, Grimer R, Whelan J, Claude L, Delattre O, Paulussen M, Picci P, Hall KS, van den Berg H, Ladenstein R, Michon J, Hjorth L, Judson I, Luksch R, Bernstein ML, Marec-Berard P, Brennan B, Craft AW, Womer RB, Juergens H, Oberlin O. Ewing sarcoma: current management and future approaches through collaboration. J Clin Oncol. 2015;33(27):3036–46.
61. Chou A, Malek F. Osteosarcoma of bone. In: 3rd, editor. Orthopaedic knowledge update: musculoskeletal tumors. Rosemont: American Academy of Orthopaedic Surgeons; 2014. p. 159–70.
62. Tavare AN, Robinson P, Altoos R, LiMarzi GM, Scherer KF, Kransdorf MJ, Bancroft LW. Postoperative imaging of sarcomas. Am J Roentgenol. 2018;211(3):506–18.

63. Rogalsky RJ, Black GB, Reed MH. Orthopaedic manifestations of leukemia in children. J Bone Joint Surg Am. 1986;68(4):494–501.
64. Sinigaglia R, Gigante C, Bisinella G, Varotto S, Zanesco L, Turra S. Musculoskeletal manifestations in pediatric acute leukemia. J Pediatr Orthop. 2008;28(1):20–8.
65. Porter RP, Kaste SC. Imaging findings of recurrent acute lymphoblastic leukemia in children and young adults, with emphasis on MRI. Pediatr Radiol. 2004;34(5):400–8.
66. Vardiman JW, Harris NL, Brunning RD. The World Health Organization (WHO) classification of the myeloid neoplasms. Blood. 2002;100(7):2292–302.
67. Steffner RJ, Jang ES, Danford NC. Lymphoma of bone. JBJS Rev. 2018;6(1):e1.
68. Ansell SM. Hodgkin lymphoma: 2018 update on diagnosis, risk-stratification, and management. Am J Hematol. 2018;93(5):704–15.
69. Ansell SM. Non-Hodgkin lymphoma: diagnosis and treatment. Mayo Clin Proc. 2015;90(8):1152–63.
70. Lee EH, Shafi M, Hui JHP. Osteoid osteoma: a current review. J Pediatr Orthop. 2006;26(5):695–700.
71. Chai JW, Hong SH, Choi J-Y, Koh YH, Lee JW, Choi J-A, Kang HS. Radiologic diagnosis of osteoid osteoma: from simple to challenging findings. Radiographics. 2010;30(3):737–49.
72. May CJ, Bixby SD, Anderson ME, Kim YJ, Yen Y-M, Millis MB, Heyworth BE. Osteoid osteoma about the hip in children and adolescents. J Bone Joint Surg Am. 2019;101(6):486–93.
73. Kamal AF, Luthfi APWY. Diagnosis and treatment of Langerhans cell histiocytosis with bone lesion in pediatric patient: a case report. Ann Med Surg (Lond). 2019;45:102–9.
74. Huang WD, Yang XH, Wu ZP, Huang Q, Xiao JR, Yang MS, Zhou ZH, Yan WJ, Song DW, Liu TL, Jia NY. Langerhans cell histiocytosis of spine: a comparative study of clinical, imaging features, and diagnosis in children, adolescents, and adults. Spine J. 2013;13(9):1108–17.
75. Azouz EM, Saigal G, Rodriguez MM, Podda A. Langerhans' cell histiocytosis: pathology, imaging and treatment of skeletal involvement. Pediatr Radiol. 2005;35(2):103–15.
76. Agarwal A, Shaharyar A, Kumar A, Bhat MS, Mishra M. Scurvy in pediatric age group – a disease often forgotten? J Clin Orthopaed Trauma. 2015;6(2):101–7.
77. Pan T, Hennrikus EF, Hennrikus WL. Modern day scurvy in pediatric orthopaedics: a forgotten illness. J Pediatr Orthop. 2021;41(3):e279–84.
78. Nagarkatti D, Banta J, Thomson JD. Charcot arthropathy in spina bifida. J Pediatr Orthop. 2000;20(1):82.
79. Yalcin S, Kocaoglu B, Berker N, Erol B. Conservative treatment of Charcot artroparthy in a series of spina bifida patients: the experience of one center and review of the literature. J Pediatr Orthopaed B. 2007;16(5):373–9.
80. Long B, Koyfman A, Gottlieb M. Evaluation and management of septic arthritis and its mimics in the emergency department. West J Emerg Med. 2019;20(2):331–41.
81. Shuler FD, Buchanan GS, Stover C, Johnson B, Modarresi M, Jasko JJ. Pyomyositis mistaken for septic hip arthritis in children: the role of MRI in diagnosis and management. Marshall J Med. 2018;4(2):Article 5.
82. Lim W, Barras CD, Zadow S. Radiologic mimics of osteomyelitis and septic arthritis: a pictorial essay. Radiol Res Pract. 2021;2021:Article ID 9912257, 18 pages.
83. Willimon SC, Busch MT, Perkins CA. Pigmented villonodular synovitis of the knee: an underappreciated source of pain in children and adolescents. J Pediatr Orthop. 2018;38(8):e482–5.
84. Temponi EF, Mortati RB, Mortati GM, Mortati LB, Sonnery-Cottet B, de Carvalho Júnior LH. Synovial chondromatosis of the knee in a 2-year-old child. JBJS Case Connector. 2016;6(3) https://doi.org/10.2106/JBJS.CC.15.00284.
85. Elzohairy MM. Primary pyomyositis in children. Orthop Traumatol Surg Res. 2018; https://doi.org/10.1016/j.otsr.2017.12.005.
86. Vij N, Ranade AS, Kang P, Belthur MV. Primary bacterial pyomyositis in children: a systematic review. J Pediatr Orthop. 2021;41(9):e849–54. https://doi.org/10.1097/BPO.0000000000001944. PMID: 34411048.

MRSA and Virulent MSSA Infections

6

Stephanie N. Moore-Lotridge,
Monique R. Bennett, Cullen P. Moran,
Jonathan G. Schoenecker, and Isaac P. Thomsen

Staphylococcus aureus Basics

Staphylococcus aureus is a gram-positive, coccal bacterium that can be frequently found within the nose and on the skin of healthy individuals. In addition to acting as a commensal organism of the human microbiota, *S. aureus* can likewise be an opportunistic pathogen, leading to infections of the skin, bone, and muscle (Fig. 6.1). Once *S. aureus* enters the bloodstream, the pathogen utilizes multiple cellular programs to both hijack and evade the host acute-phase response (APR). As highlighted in Chap. 3, it has been established that "trauma" to musculoskeletal tissue is a major predisposing factor for establishment of an infection [1, 2]. Furthermore, normal bone and muscle growth during a child's development can mimic regenerative tissue following an injury, predisposing it to a similar relative risk of being targeted by bacteria. Within these sites, *S. aureus* binds to the matrix protein fibrinogen, triggering agglutination which subsequently restricts phagocytosis of the pathogen by host immune cells. In addition to steric hindrances, *S. aureus* expresses inhibitory factors that block the complement pathway and impede neutrophil function to protect the pathogen from the host's innate immune defense [3]. Together, these mechanisms allow *S. aureus* to stably colonize a host and distribute into the peripheral tissues.

Once established within peripheral tissues, *S. aureus* continues to hijack elements of the host APR, specifically fibrin and platelets, to support bacterial abscess formation [4]. Through the expression of virulence factors such as coagulase and von Willebrand factor binding protein (vWBP), *S. aureus* forms an abscess with two concentric structures: an inner pseudocapsule formed predominantly by coagulase and a thicker outer meshwork dependent on vWBP. Together, these redundant mechanisms generate a

S. N. Moore-Lotridge
Vanderbilt University Medical Center, Department of Orthopaedics, Nashville, TN, USA
e-mail: stephanie.n.moore.1@vumc.org

M. R. Bennett · I. P. Thomsen (✉)
Vanderbilt University Medical Center, Department of Pediatrics, Division of Infectious Diseases, and the Vanderbilt Institute for Infection, Immunology, and Inflammation, Nashville, TN, USA
e-mail: monique.r.bennett.1@vumc.org; isaac.thomsen@vumc.org

C. P. Moran
Vanderbilt University School of Medicine, Nashville, TN, USA
e-mail: cullen.p.moran@vanderbilt.edu

J. G. Schoenecker
Vanderbilt University Medical Center, Department of Orthopaedics, Department of Pediatrics, Department of Pathology Microbiology and Immunology, and Vanderbilt Center for Bone Biology, Nashville, TN, USA

Vanderbilt University, Department of Pharmacology, Nashville, TN, USA
e-mail: jon.schoenecker@vumc.org

© Springer Nature Switzerland AG 2022
M. V. Belthur et al. (eds.), *Pediatric Musculoskeletal Infections*,
https://doi.org/10.1007/978-3-030-95794-0_6

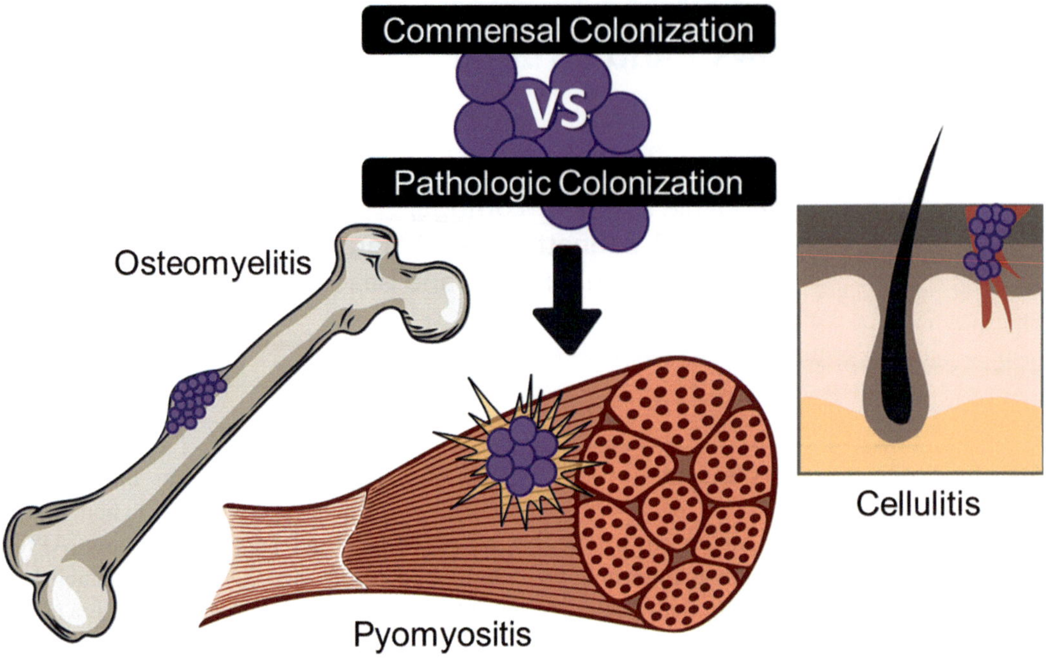

Fig. 6.1 Pathologic colonization of *Staphylococcus aureus* to musculoskeletal tissues such as the bone (osteomyelitis), muscle (pyomyositis), and skin (cellulitis). (Figure permission: Schoenecker Laboratory)

double-layered, fibrin-dependent protective barrier to prevent neutrophil access and clearance of the pathogen. Once protected from the host immune response, *S. aureus* can then proliferate until a quorum is reached. At this point, *S. aureus* activates the fibrinolytic system to dissolve the abscess, allowing the pathogen to disseminate to additional tissues and repeat this process.

> The acute-phase response (APR) is your bodies response to injury that activates proportionally to the severity of the infection. *S. aureus* hijacks elements of the host APR, specifically both coagulation and fibrinolysis, to evade the host immune response, allowing the infection to progress and subsequently disseminate.

Patient morbidity and risk of adverse outcomes following an MSKI are relative to the severity of the disease. Together, the virulence factors expressed by the pathogen, the rate of dissemination, and the level of the body's APR to the pathogen dictate disease severity (see Chap. 3: Pathology). While cases of isolated MSKI do occur, infections that are more severe and lead to adverse outcomes typically involve infection of multiple tissues (e.g., bone, muscle, and the intra-articular space) or systemic infections involving multiple body parts (e.g., bone and lung) following the rupture of an abscess [5–7]. Thus, to direct optimal treatment in patients with MSKI, physicians can utilize (1) the knowledge of a pathogen's antibiotic resistance to select an effective therapy and (2) knowledge of a pathogen's virulence factors to prognosticate disease severity and risk of adverse outcomes.

> Patient morbidity and risk of adverse outcomes following an MSKI are relative to the severity of the disease.

Evolution of Antibiotic Resistance in *Staphylococcus aureus*

Modern medicine has dramatically reduced the mortality from MSKI, which was estimated to be as high as 40% in the pre-antibiotic era [8, 9]. Along with the advent of surgical intervention, Alexander Fleming's discovery of penicillin marked the beginning of the antibiotic era. Shortly after the discovery of penicillin, other natural antibiotics including chloramphenicol, erythromycin, streptomycin, and tetracycline were identified. Together, these pharmacologic advancements drastically improved care for patients with infections previously considered to be fatal. Yet, this pharmacologic reprieve was short-lived as pathogens such as *S. aureus* quickly began to undergo a horizontal transfer of genes that facilitated antibiotic resistance [10]. For example, when introduced in the early 1940s, it was estimated that over 94% of *S. aureus* isolates were susceptible to penicillin [11, 12]. By the mid-1940s, marked penicillin resistance was already noted within hospitals and subsequently transitioned into the community, reaching pandemic levels by the 1950s [10, 11, 13, 14]. By the late 1960s, it was estimated that more than 80% of community or hospital-acquired *S. aureus* isolates were resistant to penicillin [13, 15]. Following a similar pattern, when other natural antibiotics were introduced into clinical practice in the early 1950s, *S. aureus* quickly gained resistance, such that by 1960 many hospitals had outbreaks of infections from strains of multiresistant *S. aureus*.

S. aureus resistance to penicillin was possible due to the pathogen acquiring a plasmid-encoded penicillinase, which hydrolyses the β-lactam ring that is essential for antimicrobial activity. To overcome this pharmacologic barrier, methicillin was introduced in the 1960s, possessing stability against degradation by staphylococcal penicillinase. However, much like antibiotics that had come before, *S. aureus* quickly gained resistance to methicillin through acquiring penicillin-resistant peptidoglycan transpeptidase, PBP-2′, encoded by *mec*A (Fig. 6.2). The transpeptidases in the cell wall of *S. aureus* strains with increased transcription of *mec*A exhibit a decreased affinity for methicillin, thereby making *S. aureus* resistant to nearly the entire β-lactam class of antibiotics, including penicillins, cephalosporins (with the exception of fifth-generation cephalosporins), and carbapenems [10]. From this point through the present day, methicillin-resistant staphylococcus aureus (MRSA) remains a major driver of invasive bacterial disease, including severe musculoskeletal infections.

Emergence of MRSA in the Community

Unlike methicillin-susceptible *Staphylococcus aureus* (MSSA), which has historically been found both in community and hospital-acquired settings, the majority of MRSA infections from the time of its emergence in the late 1960s until the early 1990s was hospital-acquired. While the incidence of MRSA strains varied throughout the 1970s [10, 16–20], by the mid-1980s, MRSA reached pandemic levels in hospitals and other institutional healthcare settings that continue through present time [10]. Although more limited with respect to potential treatment options, prior studies have suggested that hospital-acquired MRSA (HA-MRSA) infections are not more virulent than hospital-acquired MSSA (HA-MSSA) infections. The landscape of MRSA changed dramatically in the late 1990s, however, as the first truly community-acquired MRSA (CA-MRSA) infections were documented. In the years to follow, the prevalence of CA-MRSA infection markedly increased, such that the rate of hospitalizations between 1998 and 2007 due to CA-MRSA infections increased at least eight-fold, while the rate of hospitalization from HA-MRSA continued to increase by 1.5X during the same period [21]. By the late 2000s, in conjunction with national and local directives by health agencies, the rate of HA-MRSA and CA-MRSA infections both began to decrease annually, with a greater rate of decrease seen in HA-MRSA. Interestingly, during this same period, the rate of HA-MSSA infections did not significantly decrease, while the incidence of

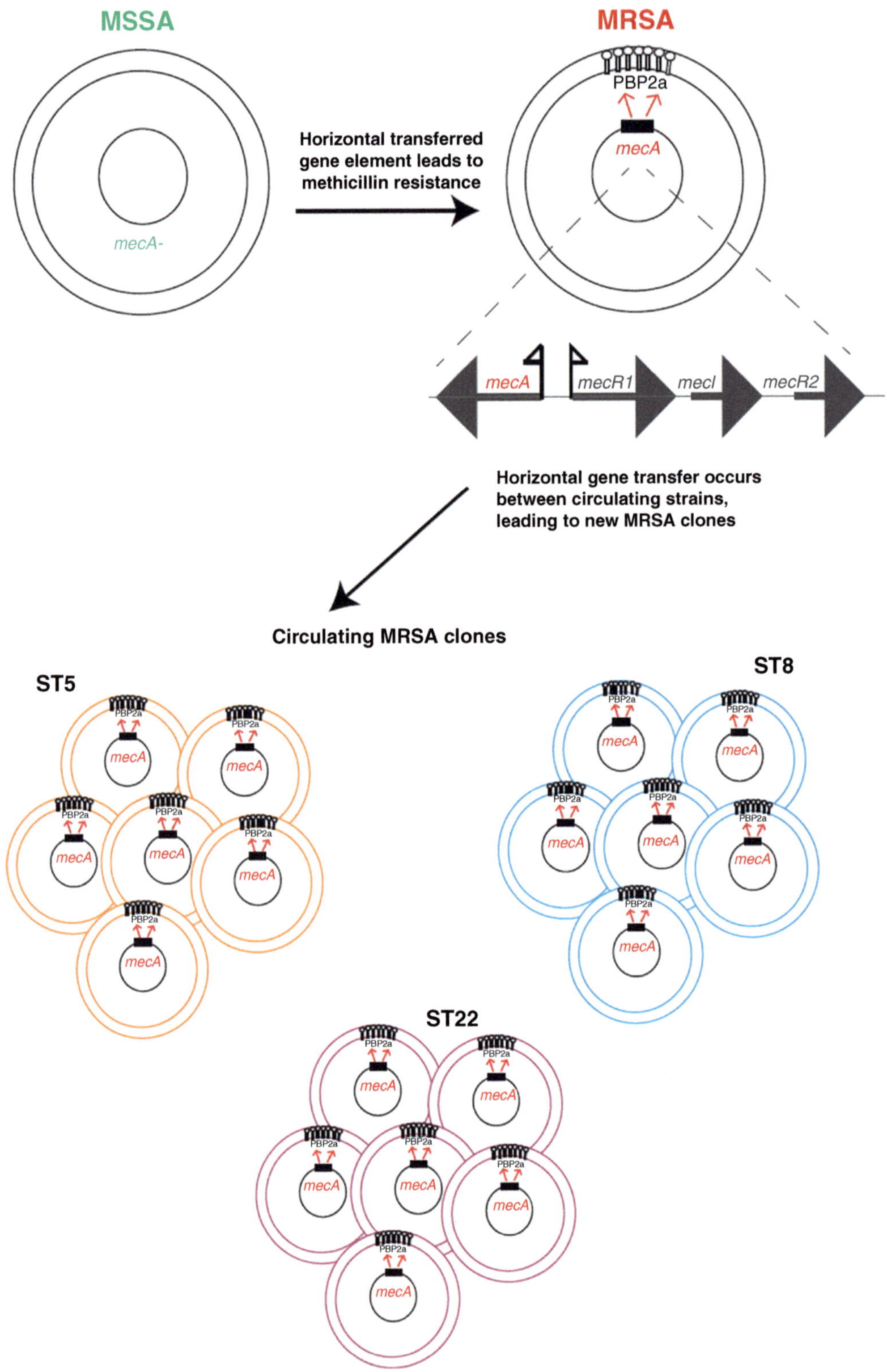

Fig. 6.2 Emergence of methicillin resistance in Staphylococcus aureus. The gene for methicillin resistance, mecA, is carried on a mobile gene element (SCCmec) and can spread between isolates in hospitals and the community. There are different types of genetic elements that circulate leading to distinct MRSA clones (e.g., ST5, ST8, and ST22). (Figure permission: Thomsen Laboratory)

Table 6.1 Comparison between cohorts of disease-causing *S. aureus*. There are inherent differences between MRSA and MSSA isolates including antibiotic susceptibility and disease type. (Table permission: Thomsen Laboratory)

	CA-MRSA	HA-MRSA	MSSA
Definition	Community-acquired strains of *S. aureus* that are resistant to methicillin antibiotics	Hospital-acquired strains of *S. aureus* that are resistant to methicillin antibiotics	Strains of *S. aureus* that are methicillin susceptible
Antibiotic susceptibility[a]	Resistant to β-lactams, clindamycin, and erthyromycin	Resistant to β-lactams, clindamycin, and ciprofloxacin	Methicillin sensitive, but similar rates of clindamycin resistance as MRSA
Type of infection	Skin and soft tissue; Occasionally invasive disease	Blood stream and respiratory; Surgical site infections	Skin and soft tissue, Invasive disease
Prevalence[b]	Declined ~7% between 2005–2016	Stable between 2013–2016	Increased ~4% from 2012–2017

[a]Peng et al. [22]
[b]Kourtis et al. [23]

CA-MSSA infections has continued to increase since 2012 (Table 6.1) [23].

What Sets CA-MRSA Apart?

CA-MRSA are unique and not merely variants of HA-MRSA that circulate in the community (Table 6.1). While many CA-MRSA and HA-MRSA isolates are erythromycin and clindamycin resistant (and these rates are gradually increasing), HA-MRSA strains have higher rates of multidrug resistance compared to CA-MRSA isolates [22, 24]. Furthermore, CA-MRSA and HA-MRSA can vary greatly in the virulence factors they express [22], as discussed in more detail below. These molecular differences can influence the severity and types of infections seen clinically, such that CA-MRSA is more commonly associated with skin and soft tissue infections, while HA-MRSA is commonly linked to the bloodstream, urinary tract, or respiratory tract infections [25]. Furthermore, the traditional risk factors for children acquiring HA-MRSA infections, such as recent hospitalization, invasive surgical procedures, indwelling catheters, endotracheal intubation, chronic illness, or prolonged or repeated exposure to antibiotics, are not relevant when assessing the risk of CA-MRSA [25–28]. A single-center, 14-year surveillance study reported that 89% of children with CA-MRSA infection had no identifiable risk factor for infection [29]. Additionally, it has been noted in a study from Texas Children's Hospital that there are no differences in risk factors between children who are infected with CA-MRSA to those with CA-MSSA [27]. Therefore, when assessing a pediatric patient for potential infection, clinical care teams must keep in mind that the absence of traditional risk factors does not imply the absence of risk for developing a CA-*S. aureus* infection [25].

Staphylococcus aureus Toxin-Mediated Virulence

S. aureus secretes several toxins that contribute to MSKI pathogenesis by allowing the bacterium to overcome the hostile host environment and secure nutrients for survival (Fig. 6.3). An important group of these toxins is the leukocidin family of toxins, which target host immune cells including phagocytes, lymphocytes, and natural killer cells. Leukocidins are highly lytic to neutrophils by dimerizing on their surface, forming a pore that leads to cell death.

The Panton-Valentine leukocidin (PVL) has garnered significant attention after being associated with the USA300 epidemic CA-MRSA clone in the late 1990s/early 2000s. The clinical importance of PVL is controversial, as while it is present in USA300 *S. aureus* strains, only about 5% of remaining clinical strains encode *pvl* [30]. PVL-producing isolates may be associated with necrotizing pneumonia, skin and soft tissue infections, or musculoskeletal infections, though again, these infections are also caused by PVL-negative strains of *S. aureus*. Several studies that investigated pediatric MSKI infections in the

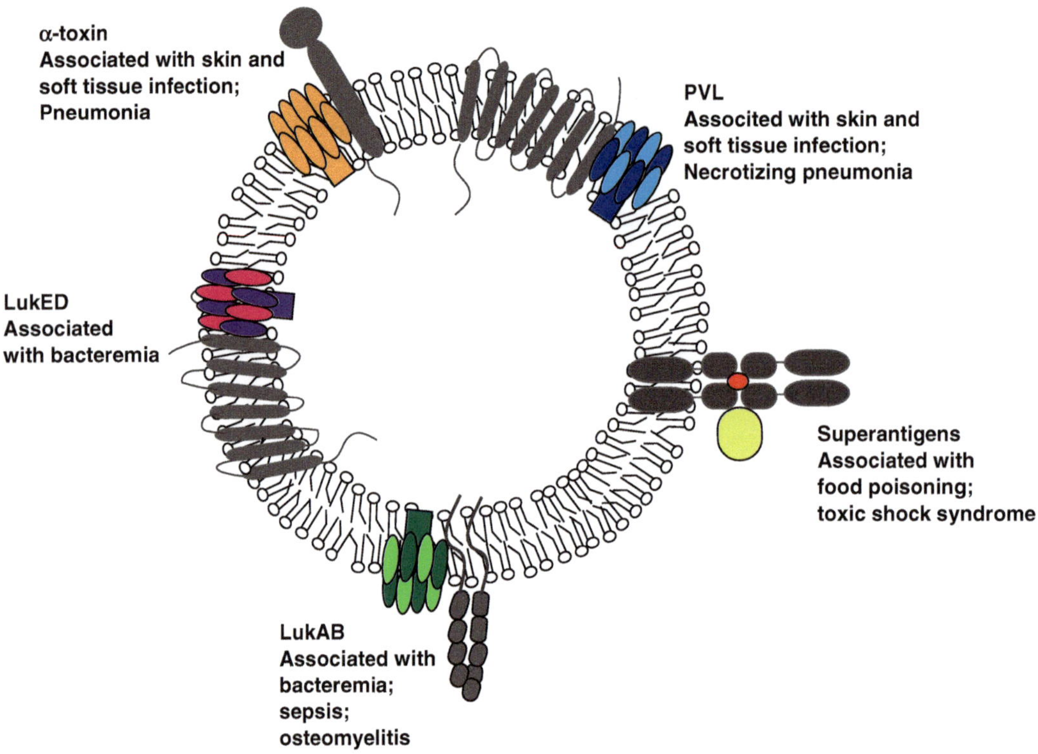

Fig. 6.3 *Staphylococcus aureus* toxin-mediated virulence. *S. aureus* toxins are associated with various forms of disease. Figure permission: Thomsen Laboratory

early 2000s found that PVL was more frequent in MRSA vs MSSA strains [31–35], though more recent data suggest this may no longer be the case [36, 37]. A recent 7-year retrospective study investigating invasive *S. aureus* infections at Texas Children's Hospital confirmed the findings of other, smaller studies that *pvl* is no longer restricted to the USA300 lineage. The majority (~85%) of invasive pediatric isolates (bloodstream or bone/joint infection) remains PVL-negative [38], indicating that this toxin is not required (or even common) for staphylococcal virulence.

The leukocidin LukAB, unlike PVL, has been shown to be present in all invasive pediatric clinical isolates assessed in numerous cohorts. LukAB targets neutrophils as well as monocytes and macrophages by binding to the integrin, CD11b on the surface of the cell. Several studies have reported that LukAB expression is conserved within clinical isolates of *S. aureus*, including both MRSA and MSSA, and contributes widely to invasive disease [39, 40]. A 5-year pediatric study typed 86 *S. aureus* isolates from 44 children, of which 64% were MSSA. The dominant clonotype from both was USA300 at 34%. Interestingly, every isolate investigated contained *lukAB,* highlighting the clinical relevance of this toxin [41]. A 2-year study specifically examining MSKI enrolled 42 children with 72% of the isolates being MSSA. Not only did all the *S. aureus* isolates investigated contain *lukAB*, but the patients mounted a robust anti-LukAB antibody response in the acute and convalescent phase [42]. The ubiquitous presence of LukAB in MSKI has even led some to propose a serological LukAB assay as a potential diagnostic tool for bacterial infections in the clinic [42, 43].

The bicomponent toxin LukED targets chemokine receptors such as CCR5 on the surface of neutrophils, macrophages, and T cells. Both *LukED* and *pvl* are often identified together in clinical *S. aureus* infections. For example, when investigating genes involved in MRSA strains associated with diabetic foot ulcers, *lukED* was found in 100% of the samples typed and *pvl* in 56.7% [44]. The presence of LukED has also been associated with biofilm production in *S. aureus* osteomyelitis-causing strains [45]. One hundred forty-three animal and human *S. aureus* isolates from China were obtained and typed from the Henan province, with only ~6% being MRSA. ~57% of the isolates from the study carried *lukED* and 6% carried *pvl* [46]. A study in Nigeria found similar results, with 100% of the investigated MRSA strains carrying *lukED* [47].

α-Toxin or Hla is a beta-barrel toxin that binds to the cellular receptor ADAM10 on the surface of its target cells before oligomerizing and forming a pore. Similar to the previous *S. aureus* toxins, Hla targets several host cell types including T cells, endothelial cells, and erythrocytes. Hla is secreted by ~95% clinical strains and is associated with the development of invasive *S. aureus* disease [48, 49]. Hla is prevalent in ~80–90% of both MRSA and MSSA isolates [50, 51], although clinically it has more closely linked to pneumonia rather than musculoskeletal infections.

Finally, superantigens are a large category of *S. aureus* toxins that act as T-cell mitogens by binding and cross-linking MHC class II and T-cell receptors, leading to an exuberant APR, cytokine storms, and T-cell proliferation [52] (Fig. 6.4). This perturbation of the host immune system can result in serious multisystem organ failure that is specific to the superantigen that caused it. For example, the staphylococcal enterotoxins are a distinct subset of superantigens that have strong emetic activity and are distinct from staphylococcal enterotoxin-like toxins. One of the most well-known superantigens,

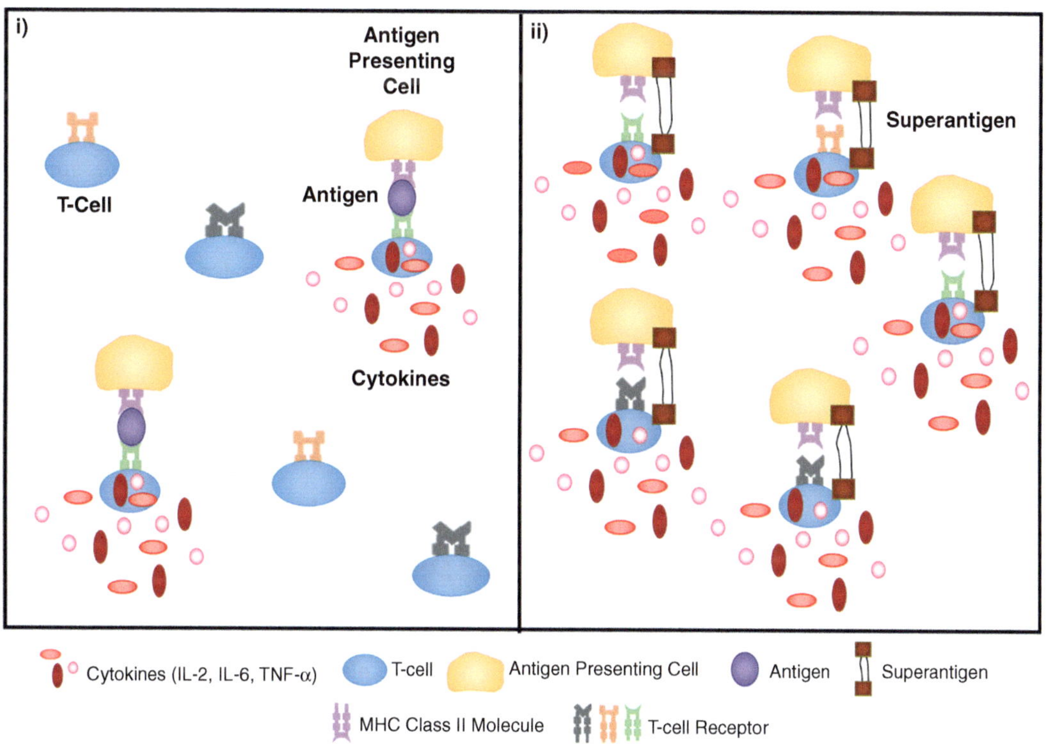

Fig. 6.4 Superantigens produced by *S. aureus* result in a massive release of cytokines (like TNF-α) into the systemic circulation. In the body's normal response to infection, MHC-II mediated presentation of antigens to T-cells results in the release of cytokines and bolsters the immune response (**i**). Bypassing MHC-restricted antigen processing in this manner, superantigens can activate an abnormally large fraction of host T-cells (up to 25%) and lead to an excessive inflammatory response (**ii**). These cytokines have a number of detrimental consequences including significant vasodilation, disruption of the vascular endothelium, and hypercoagulability. These systemic effects contribute to the septic shock and multi-organ failure that is often the cause of death in patients with severe infections. (Figure permission: Schoenecker Laboratory)

TSST-1, has been implicated in bone and joint infections. TSST-1 causes toxic shock syndrome, an illness that includes high fever, diarrhea, and potentially death. Furthermore, in addition to driving an exuberant APR, TSST-1 can likewise enhance osteoclastogenesis by stimulating osteoclasts and decreasing bone tissue strength during infection [53], leading to adverse patient outcomes. The prevalence of *tst-1* has been reported to be as high as 16.7% in MSSA isolates and 0.2% in MRSA ($n = 710$) [54]. A pediatric study in China found that 42.4% of the 125 typed *S. aureus* isolates were MRSA and ~97% contained a superantigen gene [55].

Current View of MRSA and MSSA in Pediatric MSKI

Epidemiology of MRSA and MSSA

While *S. aureus* remains the most common cause of pediatric MSKI [8, 56], the relative incidence of MRSA and MSSA varies with time, geographic region, and patient population. As highlighted above, the rate of MRSA and MSSA infections has varied over time, with increasing rates of MRSA in the early to mid-2000s, followed by a period of steady state and then decreased incidence in the late 2010s [57–59]. Across the same time period, the incidence of MSKI from MSSA has remained steady or has continued to rise. In a recent multicenter study of pediatric tertiary care centers conducted by the CORTICES group, it was found that S. *aureus* accounted for 65.1% of all culture-positive infections at the time of consultation by orthopedic providers across the United States, of which 37.4% were MRSA. Aligning with these findings, another large national study between 2009 and 2012 reported that 38% of pediatric osteomyelitis cases were caused by MRSA, with the remaining 62% being caused by MSSA [60].

In addition to variation over time, there are marked geographic differences in rates of MRSA and MSSA infections in the United States and Europe [61, 62]. Aligning with trends reported in the national CORTICES study, pediatric patients with MSKI in the Southern United States experienced a greater incidence of MSKI from MRSA compared to other regions [60, 63]. However, within the South, the CORTICES study reported variable MRSA and MSSA rates between institutions ranging from 13% to 42% of positive MRSA cultures at the consultation for a suspected MSKI. Comparable variability of MRSA to MSSA incidence was likewise observed in the West and Midwest, while the incidence in the Northeastern United States was consistent between institutions [64]. It has been hypothesized that the variance between regions and sites may be the product of variable antibiotic utilization patterns, varying patient demographics, or endemic bacteria [60, 65, 66]. Nevertheless, this variability calls into question the generalizability of prior clinical prediction algorithms aimed at differentiating MRSA infection from MSSA infection in children [67]. Given that such algorithms have been built from data of single institutions, this may explain the poor predictive capability when used at an institution with a different incidence of MRSA [68]. From the nationwide CORTICES assessment, an average MSSA/MRSA ratio of 1.84 was observed at the time of consultation for MSKI across 18 institutions [64]. This information can be used as a benchmark value for the anticipated rate of MRSA and MSSA, such that if an institution experiences a markedly greater ratio of MRSA at the time of consultation, this may indicate the need for an intervention to address a disproportionately higher relative rate.

Comparative Severity of MRSA and MSSA

To limit adverse outcomes in pediatric patients with MSKI, physicians caring for patients with suspected MSKI must continually assess the severity of the disease. The severity of an infection is a summation of the virulence and dissemination of the pathogen, combined with the level to which the body responds to the pathogen (see Chap. 3). As such, with the emergence of MRSA, numerous studies have focused on assessing the virulence of MRSA relative to MSSA, specifically in regard to disease severity and patient outcomes. To date, the relative severity of MSKI caused by MRSA compared to MSSA is not a settled matter.

> The severity of an infection is a summation of the virulence and dissemination of the pathogen, combined with the level to which the body responds to the pathogen.

Aligning with the emergence of MRSA in the early 2000s, reports began to demonstrate that pediatric patients with MSKI caused by MRSA exhibited different clinical presentations and outcomes than children with MSSA. For example, children with MRSA infections were reported to have higher temperatures, heart rates, and respiratory rates and were more commonly unable to bear weight upon presentation, compared to patients with MSSA [69, 70]. Likewise, studies reported that MRSA infections were associated with increased laboratory markers of inflammation on presentation, including higher levels of C-reactive protein (CRP), longer erythrocyte sedimentation rates, greater white blood cell (WBC) count, and greater absolute neutrophil counts [69–72]. From these results, clinical algorithms were developed to differentiate between MRSA and MSSA in pediatric MSKI upon presentation. Ju et al. used temperature >38 °C, hematocrit <34%, WBC >12,000 cell/μL, and CRP >13 mg/L as predictors of MRSA osteomyelitis in a logistic regression model with a predictive probability of 92% for MRSA when all 4 predictors were satisfied. A separate model developed by Dietrich et al. that used temperature, absolute neutrophil count, and CRP as predictive variables demonstrated 87% accuracy in predicting cases of MRSA and MSSA.

In addition to variable clinical presentation, multiple studies have reported that pediatric patients with MRSA infections experience higher levels of patient morbidity, with patients experiencing more febrile days, a longer length of hospital stay, a greater number of surgical interventions, and more frequent admissions to the ICU compared to patients with MSSA [33, 57, 71, 73]. Accordingly, patients with MRSA have also been reported to experience a greater rate of adverse outcomes, such as sepsis, respiratory distress or failure, thrombophlebitis, and pulmonary embolism compared to patients with MSSA infections [60]. Thus, patients with MRSA infections have also been shown to have worse long-term survival compared to patients with MSSA, resulting in a higher total cost of medical care [60].

While many reports from the previous decade found a clear difference in disease severity between MSSA and MRSA infections, it is important to note that this appears to be evolving over time and may no longer be the case as MSSA infection severity has increased. A large study of necrotizing pneumonia over 24 years in France found no difference in initial severity or management between MRSA and MSSA [74]. Further, a 2017 study of 91 MSKI cases reported similar clinical severity and outcomes for pediatric patients with MRSA or MSSA. Specifically, no difference in median hospital length of stay, febrile days, and antibiotic duration were noted. When an effective 2009 logistic regression model based on C-reactive protein, temperature, white blood cell count, pulse, and respiratory rate at presentation was applied in 2017, it no longer possessed the ability to effectively differentiate between MRSA and MSSA infection.

Furthermore, patients with MRSA or MSSA infections may have important underlying differences that confound these assessments. For example, pediatric patients with MRSA have been noted to possess a greater incidence of comorbid factors upon presentation and therefore worse prognoses compared to patients with MSSA [75]. Given this variance, it is therefore difficult to draw a causal relationship between the pathogen and adverse patient outcomes [76]. Aligning with this position, a study of 582 patients with MRSA or MSSA bacteremia found no statistically significant difference in infection-related hospital readmissions when adjusting for age, comorbidities, and other prognostic factors [76]. Taken together, these differing results maybe be a product of variable host factors, such as comorbidities between study populations, regional variation in pathogens, as well as a gradual evolution of pathogen virulence (with increased MSSA virulence) between the mid-2000s and late 2010s.

Pathogen type is but one factor that impacts MSKI severity and subsequently the risk of adverse patient outcomes. Given the variance in epidemiology by region and over time, physicians must not limit their assessment of disease severity to the identity of the pathogen. While pathogen identification is essential for applying antibiotic therapy, both MSSA and MRSA can drive the body's APR to exuberant levels, increasing the risk of adverse medical and musculoskeletal outcomes. Therefore, rather than relying on pathogen identification alone to determine disease severity, this information should be considered relative to laboratory measures of the APR when assessing MSKI disease severity and directing emergent treatment.

Pathogen type is but one factor that impacts MSKI severity and subsequently the risk of adverse patient outcomes. Therefore, rather than relying on pathogen identification alone to determine disease severity, this information should be considered relative to laboratory measures of the APR when assessing MSKI disease severity and directing emergent treatment.

Conclusions

Circulating clinical strains of *S. aureus* are continuously evolving as a result of gene transfer and dynamic mutations in the bacterial genome conferring virulence factors and antibiotic resistance. These changes, in addition to impacting which pharmacologic interventions will be efficacious, can markedly alter the severity of an MSKI and a child's risk of adverse outcomes. Thus, physicians should not rely on pathogen identification alone to determine disease severity; rather, this information should be considered relative to laboratory measures of the APR when assessing MSKI disease severity and directing emergent treatment.

Box 6.1 Key Learning Points

- *S. aureus* is continuously evolving in terms of acquired virulence factors and antibiotic resistance.
- While these changes will impact which antibiotics will be most effective at combating the pathogen, physicians should not rely on these designations alone to determine disease severity.
- Rather, this information should be considered relative to laboratory measures of the body's acute-phase response when assessing MSKI disease severity and directing emergent treatment.

References

1. Morrissy RT, Haynes DW. Acute hematogenous osteomyelitis: a model with trauma as an etiology. J Pediatr Orthop. 1989;9(4):447–56.
2. Whalen JL, Fitzgerald RH Jr, Morrissy RT. A histological study of acute hematogenous osteomyelitis following physeal injuries in rabbits. J Bone Joint Surg Am. 1988;70(9):1383–92.
3. Pietrocola G, Nobile G, Rindi S, Speziale P. Staphylococcus aureus manipulates innate immunity through own and host-expressed proteases. Front Cell Infect Microbiol. 2017;7:166.
4. An TJ, Benvenuti MA, Mignemi ME, Thomsen IP, Schoenecker JG. Pediatric musculoskeletal infection: hijacking the acute-phase response. JBJS Reviews. 2016;4(9):e4.
5. Mignemi ME, Benvenuti MA, An TJ, Martus JE, Mencio GA, Lovejoy SA, et al. A novel classification system based on dissemination of musculoskeletal infection is predictive of hospital outcomes. J Pediatr Orthop. 2018;38(5):279–86.
6. Amaro E, Marvi TK, Posey SL, Benvenuti MA, An TJ, Dale KM, et al. C-reactive protein predicts risk of venous thromboembolism in pediatric musculoskeletal infection. J Pediatr Orthop. 2019;39(1):e62–e7.
7. Copley LA, Barton T, Garcia C, Sun D, Gaviria-Agudelo C, Gheen WT, et al. A proposed scoring system for assessment of severity of illness in pediatric acute hematogenous osteomyelitis using objective

clinical and laboratory findings. Pediatr Infect Dis J. 2014;33(1):35–41.
8. Song KM, Sloboda JF. Acute hematogenous osteomyelitis in children. J Am Acad Orthop Surg. 2001;9(3):166–75.
9. Ciampolini J, Harding KG. Pathophysiology of chronic bacterial osteomyelitis. Why do antibiotics fail so often? Postgrad Med J. 2000;76(898):479–83.
10. Chambers HF, DeLeo FR. Waves of resistance: Staphylococcus aureus in the antibiotic era. Nat Rev Microbiol. 2009;7(9):629–41.
11. Livermore DM. Antibiotic resistance in staphylococci. Int J Antimicrob Agents. 2000;16 Suppl 1:S3–10.
12. Kirby WM. Extraction of a highly potent penicillin inactivator from penicillin resistant staphylococci. Science (New York, NY). 1944;99(2579):452–3.
13. Lowy FD. Antimicrobial resistance: the example of Staphylococcus aureus. J Clin Invest. 2003;111(9):1265–73.
14. Wentworth FH, Miller AL, Wentworth BB. Observations relative to the nature and control of epidemic staphylococcal disease. Am J Public Health Nations Health. 1958;48(3):287–98.
15. Rammelkamp CH, Maxon T. Resistance of staphylococcus aureus to the action of penicillin. Proc Soc Exp Biol Med. 1942;51(3):386–9.
16. Sabath LD, Laverdiere M, Wheeler N, Blazevic D, Wilkinson B. A new type of penicillin resistance of Staphylococcus aureus. Lancet. 1977;309(8009):443–7.
17. Mato R, Campanile F, Stefani S, Crisóstomo MI, Santagati M, Sanches SI, et al. Clonal types and multidrug resistance patterns of methicillin-resistant Staphylococcus aureus (MRSA) recovered in Italy during the 1990s. Microbial Drug Resistance (Larchmont, NY). 2004;10(2):106–13.
18. Peacock JE Jr, Marsik FJ, Wenzel RP. Methicillin-resistant Staphylococcus aureus: introduction and spread within a hospital. Ann Intern Med. 1980;93(4):526–32.
19. Barrett FF, McGehee RF, Finland M. Methicillin-resistant Staphylococcus aureus at Boston City Hospital. N Engl J Med. 1968;279(9):441–8.
20. Crisóstomo MI, Westh H, Tomasz A, Chung M, Oliveira DC, de Lencastre H. The evolution of methicillin resistance in Staphylococcus aureus: similarity of genetic backgrounds in historically early methicillin-susceptible and -resistant isolates and contemporary epidemic clones. Proc Natl Acad Sci. 2001;98(17):9865–70.
21. Mera RM, Suaya JA, Amrine-Madsen H, Hogea CS, Miller LA, Lu EP, et al. Increasing role of Staphylococcus aureus and community-acquired methicillin-resistant Staphylococcus aureus infections in the United States: a 10-year trend of replacement and expansion. Microb Drug Resist. 2011;17:321+.
22. Peng H, Liu D, Ma Y, Gao W. Comparison of community- and healthcare-associated methicillin-resistant Staphylococcus aureus isolates at a Chinese tertiary hospital, 2012–2017. Sci Rep. 2018;8(1):17916. https://doi.org/10.1038/s41598-018-36206-5.
23. Kourtis AP, Hatfield K, Baggs J, et al. Vital signs: epidemiology and recent trends in methicillin-resistant and in methicillin-susceptible Staphylococcus aureus bloodstream infections — United States. MMWR Morb Mortal Wkly Rep. 2019;68:214–9. https://doi.org/10.15585/mmwr.mm6809e1.
24. Wang X, Li X, Liu W, Huang W, Fu Q, Li M. Molecular characteristic and virulence gene profiles of community-associated methicillin-resistant Staphylococcus aureus isolates from pediatric patients in Shanghai, China. Front Microbiol. 2016;7:1818.
25. Nemerovski CW, Klein KC. Community-associated methicillin-resistant Staphylococcus aureus in the pediatric population. J Pediatr Pharmacol Ther. 2008;13(4):212–25.
26. Herold BC, Immergluck LC, Maranan MC, Lauderdale DS, Gaskin RE, Boyle-Vavra S, et al. Community-acquired methicillin-resistant Staphylococcus aureus in children with no identified predisposing risk. JAMA. 1998;279(8):593–8.
27. Sattler CA, Mason EO Jr, Kaplan SL. Prospective comparison of risk factors and demographic and clinical characteristics of community-acquired, methicillin-resistant versus methicillin-susceptible Staphylococcus aureus infection in children. Pediatr Infect Dis J. 2002;21(10):910–7.
28. Dietrich DW, Auld DB, Mermel LA. Community-acquired methicillin-resistant Staphylococcus aureus in southern New England children. Pediatrics. 2004;113(4):e347–52.
29. Purcell K, Fergie J. Epidemic of community-acquired methicillin-resistant Staphylococcus aureus infections: a 14-year study at Driscoll Children's Hospital. Arch Pediatr Adolesc Med. 2005;159(10):980–5.
30. Lina G, Piémont Y, Godail-Gamot F, Bes M, Peter MO, Gauduchon V, et al. Involvement of Panton-Valentine leukocidin-producing Staphylococcus aureus in primary skin infections and pneumonia. Clin Infect Dis. 1999;29(5):1128–32.
31. Ritz N, Curtis N. The role of Panton-Valentine leukocidin in Staphylococcus aureus musculoskeletal infections in children. Pediatr Infect Dis J. 2012;31(5):514–8.
32. Bocchini CE, Hulten KG, Mason EO Jr, Gonzalez BE, Hammerman WA, Kaplan SL. Panton-Valentine leukocidin genes are associated with enhanced inflammatory response and local disease in acute hematogenous Staphylococcus aureus osteomyelitis in children. Pediatrics. 2006;117(2):433–40.
33. Martínez-Aguilar G, Avalos-Mishaan A, Hulten K, Hammerman W, Mason EO Jr, Kaplan SL. Community-acquired, methicillin-resistant and methicillin-susceptible Staphylococcus aureus musculoskeletal infections in children. Pediatr Infect Dis J. 2004;23(8):701–6.
34. Sdougkos G, Chini V, Papanastasiou DA, Christodoulou G, Tagaris G, Dimitracopoulos G, et al. Methicillin-resistant Staphylococcus aureus

producing Panton-Valentine leukocidin as a cause of acute osteomyelitis in children. Clin Microbiol Infect. 2007;13(6):651–4.
35. Carrillo-Marquez MA, Hulten KG, Hammerman W, Mason EO, Kaplan SL. USA300 is the predominant genotype causing Staphylococcus aureus septic arthritis in children. Pediatr Infect Dis J. 2009;28(12):1076–80.
36. Albiński MK, Lutz N, Ceroni D, N'Dele D, Zambelli PY, Bregou A. Paediatric musculoskeletal infections with Panton-valentine leucocidin. Swiss Med Wkly. 2018;148:w14669.
37. Prista-Leão B, Abreu I, Duro R, Silva-Pinto A, Ceia F, Andrade P, et al. Panton-valentine leukocidin-producing Staphylococcus aureus infection: a case series. Infect Dis Rep. 2020;12(3):61–9.
38. Crandall H, Kapusta A, Killpack J, Heyrend C, Nilsson K, Dickey M, et al. Clinical and molecular epidemiology of invasive Staphylococcus aureus infection in Utah children; continued dominance of MSSA over MRSA. PLoS One. 2020;15(9):e0238991.
39. Thomsen IP, Dumont AL, James DB, Yoong P, Saville BR, Soper N, et al. Children with invasive Staphylococcus aureus disease exhibit a potently neutralizing antibody response to the cytotoxin LukAB. Infect Immun. 2014;82(3):1234–42.
40. Bennett MR, Thomsen IP. Epidemiological and clinical evidence for the role of toxins in S. aureus human disease. Toxins. 2020;12(6):408.
41. Thomsen IP, Kadari P, Soper NR, Riddell S, Kiska D, Creech CB, et al. Molecular epidemiology of invasive Staphylococcus aureus infections and concordance with colonization isolates. J Pediatr. 2019;210:173–7.
42. Wood JB, Jones LS, Soper NR, Xu M, Torres VJ, Buddy Creech C, et al. Serologic detection of antibodies targeting the Leukocidin LukAB strongly predicts Staphylococcus aureus in children with invasive infection. J Pediatric Infect Dis Soc. 2019;8(2):128–35.
43. Muthukrishnan G, Soin S, Beck CA, Grier A, Brodell JD Jr, Lee CC, et al. A bioinformatic approach to utilize a patient's antibody-secreting cells against Staphylococcus aureus to detect challenging musculoskeletal infections. ImmunoHorizons. 2020;4(6):339–51.
44. Kananizadeh P, Ohadian Moghadam S, Sadeghi Y, Rahimi Foroushani A, Adibi H, Pourmand MR. Molecular characteristics of methicillin-resistant Staphylococcus aureus (MRSA) isolated from diabetic foot infection. Iran J Pathol. 2019;14(4):329–37.
45. Yu S, Jiang B, Jia C, Wu H, Shen J, Hu X, et al. Investigation of biofilm production and its association with genetic and phenotypic characteristics of OM (osteomyelitis) and non-OM orthopedic Staphylococcus aureus. Ann Clin Microbiol Antimicrob. 2020;19(1):10.
46. Liu B, Sun H, Pan Y, Zhai Y, Cai T, Yuan X, et al. Prevalence, resistance pattern, and molecular characterization of Staphylococcus aureus isolates from healthy animals and sick populations in Henan Province, China. Gut Pathogens. 2018;10:31.
47. Enwuru NV, Adesida SA, Enwuru CA, Ghebremedhin B, Mendie UE, Coker AO. Genetics of bi-component leukocidin and drug resistance in nasal and clinical Staphylococcus aureus in Lagos, Nigeria. Microb Pathog. 2018;115:1–7.
48. Busche T, Hillion M, Van Loi V, Berg D, Walther B, Semmler T, et al. Comparative secretome analyses of human and zoonotic Staphylococcus aureus isolates CC8, CC22, and CC398. Mol Cell Proteomics: MCP. 2018;17(12):2412–33.
49. Suryadevara M, Clark AE, Wolk DM, Carman A, Rosenbaum PF, Shaw J. Molecular characterization of invasive Staphylococcus aureus infection in Central New York children: importance of two clonal groups and inconsistent presence of selected virulence determinants. J Pediatric Infect Dis Soc. 2013;2(1):30–9.
50. Tabor DE, Yu L, Mok H, Tkaczyk C, Sellman BR, Wu Y, et al. Staphylococcus aureus alpha-toxin is conserved among diverse hospital respiratory isolates collected from a global surveillance study and is neutralized by monoclonal antibody MEDI4893. Antimicrob Agents Chemother. 2016;60(9):5312–21.
51. Mir Z, Nodeh Farahani N, Abbasian S, Alinejad F, Sattarzadeh M, Pouriran R, et al. The prevalence of exotoxins, adhesion, and biofilm-related genes in Staphylococcus aureus isolates from the main burn center of Tehran, Iran. Iran J Basic Med Sci. 2019;22(11):1267–74.
52. Hysong AA, Posey SL, Blum DM, Benvenuti MA, Benvenuti TA, Johnson SR, et al. Necrotizing fasciitis: pillaging the acute phase response. J Bone Joint Surg Am. 2020;102(6):526–37.
53. Flammier S, Rasigade JP, Badiou C, Henry T, Vandenesch F, Laurent F, et al. Human monocyte-derived osteoclasts are targeted by staphylococcal pore-forming toxins and Superantigens. PLoS One. 2016;11(3):e0150693.
54. Parrish KL, Wylie KM, Reich PJ, Hogan PG, Wylie TN, Kennedy CR, et al. Carriage of the toxic shock syndrome toxin gene by contemporary community-associated Staphylococcus aureus isolates. Journal of the Pediatric Infectious Diseases Society. 2019;8(5):470–3.
55. Sun C, Wang Q, Li WT, Wen DN, Chen CH, Yang X, et al. Molecular characteristics and antimicrobial susceptibility of Staphylococcus aureus among children with respiratory tract infections in Southwest China. World J Pediatrics: WJP. 2020;16(3):284–92.
56. Blyth MJ, Kincaid R, Craigen MA, Bennet GC. The changing epidemiology of acute and subacute haematogenous osteomyelitis in children. J Bone Joint Surg Br. 2001;83(1):99–102.
57. Sarkissian EJ, Gans I, Gunderson MA, Myers SH, Spiegel DA, Flynn JM. Community-acquired methicillin-resistant Staphylococcus aureus musculoskeletal infections: emerging trends over the past decade. J Pediatr Orthop. 2016;36(3):323–7.
58. Weiss L, Lansell A, Figueroa J, Suchdev PS, Kirpalani A. Declining prevalence of methicillin-resistant Staphylococcus aureus septic arthritis and

osteomyelitis in children: implications for treatment. Antibiotics (Basel). 2020;9(3):101.
59. Dukic VM, Lauderdale DS, Wilder J, Daum RS, David MZ. Epidemics of community-associated methicillin-resistant Staphylococcus aureus in the United States: a meta-analysis. PLoS One. 2013;8(1):e52722.
60. Davis WT, Gilbert SR. Comparison of methicillin-resistant versus susceptible Staphylococcus aureus pediatric osteomyelitis. J Pediatr Orthop. 2018;38(5):e285–91.
61. Voss A, Milatovic D, Wallrauch-Schwarz C, Rosdahl VT, Braveny I. Methicillin-resistant Staphylococcus aureus in Europe. Eur J Clin Microbiol Infect Dis. 1994;13(1):50–5.
62. Sutter DE, Milburn E, Chukwuma U, Dzialowy N, Maranich AM, Hospenthal DR. Changing susceptibility of Staphylococcus aureus in a US pediatric population. Pediatrics. 2016;137(4):e20153099.
63. Kuehnert MJ, Hill HA, Kupronis BA, Tokars JI, Solomon SL, Jernigan DB. Methicillin-resistant-Staphylococcus aureus hospitalizations, United States. Emerg Infect Dis. 2005;11(6):868–72.
64. Schoenecker JG, The Children's Orthopaedic T, Infection Consortium for Evidence Based Study G. Defining the volume of consultations for musculoskeletal infection encountered by pediatric orthopaedic services in the United States. PLoS One. 2020;15(6):e0234055.
65. Schneider-Lindner V, Quach C, Hanley JA, Suissa S. Antibacterial drugs and the risk of community-associated methicillin-resistant Staphylococcus aureus in children. Arch Pediatr Adolesc Med. 2011;165(12):1107–14.
66. Hicks LA, Bartoces MG, Roberts RM, Suda KJ, Hunkler RJ, Taylor TH Jr, et al. US outpatient antibiotic prescribing variation according to geography, patient population, and provider specialty in 2011. Clin Infect Dis. 2015;60(9):1308–16.
67. Ju KL, Zurakowski D, Kocher MS. Differentiating between methicillin-resistant and methicillin-sensitive Staphylococcus aureus osteomyelitis in children: an evidence-based clinical prediction algorithm. J Bone Joint Surg Am. 2011;93(18):1693–701.
68. Wade Shrader M, Nowlin M, Segal LS. Independent analysis of a clinical predictive algorithm to identify methicillin-resistant Staphylococcus aureus osteomyelitis in children. J Pediatr Orthop. 2013;33(7):759–62.
69. Dietrich LN, Reid D, Doo D, Fineberg NS, Khoury JG, Gilbert SR. Predicting MSSA in acute hematogenous osteomyelitis in a setting with MRSA prevalence. J Pediatr Orthop. 2015;35(4):426–30.
70. Ju KL, Zurakowski D, Kocher MS. Differentiating between methicillin-resistant and methicillin-sensitive Staphylococcus aureus osteomyelitis in children: an evidence-based clinical prediction algorithm. JBJS. 2011;93(18):1693–701.
71. Hawkshead JJ 3rd, Patel NB, Steele RW, Heinrich SD. Comparative severity of pediatric osteomyelitis attributable to methicillin-resistant versus methicillin-sensitive Staphylococcus aureus. J Pediatr Orthop. 2009;29(1):85–90.
72. Saavedra-Lozano J, Mejías A, Ahmad N, Peromingo E, Ardura MI, Guillen S, et al. Changing trends in acute osteomyelitis in children: impact of methicillin-resistant Staphylococcus aureus infections. J Pediatr Orthop. 2008;28(5):569–75.
73. Erdem G, Salazar R, Kimata C, Simasathien T, Len KA, Bergert L, et al. Staphylococcus aureus osteomyelitis in Hawaii. Clin Pediatr. 2010;49(5):477–84.
74. Sicot N, Khanafer N, Meyssonnier V, Dumitrescu O, Tristan A, Bes M, et al. Methicillin resistance is not a predictor of severity in community-acquired Staphylococcus aureus necrotizing pneumonia--results of a prospective observational study. Clin Microbiol Infect. 2013;19(3):E142–8.
75. Hamdy RF, Dona D, Jacobs MB, Gerber JS. Risk factors for complications in children with Staphylococcus aureus bacteremia. J Pediatr. 2019;208:214–20.e2.
76. Yaw LK, Robinson JO, Ho KM. A comparison of long-term outcomes after methicillin-resistant and methicillin-sensitive Staphylococcus aureus bacteraemia: an observational cohort study. Lancet Infect Dis. 2014;14(10):967–75.

7 Systemic Effects of Musculoskeletal Infections and ICU Management

Rudolph Wong, Michael Lintner Rivera,
Vishal Gunnala, Shilpa Kalane, and David Tellez

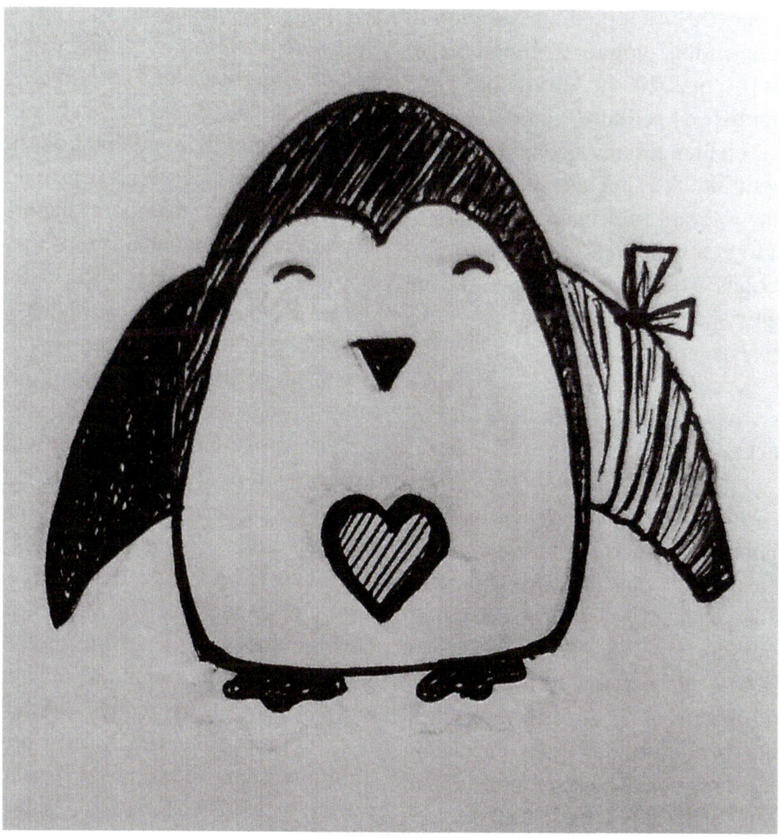

R. Wong · M. Lintner Rivera · V. Gunnala · D. Tellez (✉)
Department of Critical Care, Phoenix Children's Hospital, Phoenix, AZ, USA

Department of Child Health, University of Arizona College of Medicine, Phoenix, AZ, USA
e-mail: rwong3@phoenixchildrens.com; vgunnala1@phoenixchildrens.com; Dtellez@phoenixchildrens.com

S. Kalane
Deenanath Mangeshkar Hospital, Pune, India

© Springer Nature Switzerland AG 2022
M. V. Belthur et al. (eds.), *Pediatric Musculoskeletal Infections*,
https://doi.org/10.1007/978-3-030-95794-0_7

Introduction

Sepsis remains among the leading causes of childhood mortality worldwide [1, 2]. Once diagnosed, the global case fatality rate from pediatric sepsis is estimated to be 25% [3]. Analysis of large databases in high-income countries indicates only moderate achievements in outcome improvement in children with sepsis over the past several decades [4, 5]. Further, sepsis-related mortality remains disproportionately elevated in low- and middle-income countries (LMIC). In this context, the World Health Assembly in May 2017 adopted a resolution to improve the prevention, diagnosis, and management of sepsis [6]. In 2020, the Surviving Sepsis Campaign published pediatric guidelines to help meet the challenges in managing severe sepsis and septic shock [7]. This chapter serves to highlight the relevant information and strategies pertinent to treating children with musculoskeletal infections who have developed severe sepsis and septic shock requiring admission to a pediatric intensive care unit.

Case Vignette

A previously healthy 8-year-old boy with no history of trauma or infection presents to the emergency department with 3 days of worsening fever and malaise along with left knee pain and swelling with worsening limp. Upon presentation he has a temperature of 40.2 °C, heart rate of 150 beats per minute, blood pressure of 72/40, and respiratory rate of 30 breaths per minute. On exam, the patient is ill-appearing, uncomfortable, somnolent, and flushed appearing and holds his left knee in moderate flexion. The knee is red and swollen, warm, and tender to palpation. There is pain with passive and active extension and decreased range of motion. Initial laboratory studies are notable for white blood cell (WBC) count of 35,000 cells/uL, elevated CRP of 10 mg/dL, and ESR of 60 mm/hr. Initial venous blood gas is notable for pH of 7.25, pCO_2 of 36 mmHg, and HCO_3^- of 10 mmol/L with a lactate of 4 mmol/L. He has evidence of end-organ dysfunction with complete metabolic panel notable for creatinine of 2.0 mg/dl, AST of 150 IU/L, ALT of 120 IU/L, and an anion gap of 21 mmol/L. Ultrasound of the knee reveals increased blood flow on color Doppler and confirms effusion. MRI of the knee is obtained and confirms moderate effusion with surrounding synovial enhancement and abnormal signal within the distal femoral epiphysis and metaphysis, confirming septic arthritis (Fig. 7.1a–c). Orthopedic surgery is consulted and performs arthrocentesis. Synovial fluid is notable for WBC of 65,000 cells/uL with 94% polymorphonuclear leukocytes and gram-positive cocci in clusters seen on Gram stain.

While the diagnostic workup is ongoing, the patient receives three crystalloid boluses of Ringer lactate, but the blood pressure improves only slightly to 80/52. Immediately after blood cultures and joint fluid are obtained, he is started on empiric antibiotics with ceftriaxone, vancomycin, and nafcillin. Due to ongoing hypotension, an epinephrine drip is initiated at 0.04 mcg/kg/min with improvement in blood pressure to 98/60, and he is admitted to the pediatric intensive care unit (PICU) for further care and is scheduled for an imminent left knee arthrotomy and drainage of subperiosteal abscess by orthopedic surgery.

The above patient presents with sepsis with progression to septic shock secondary to bacterial septic arthritis and concurrent distal femur osteomyelitis. He demonstrates multi-organ dysfunction and a need for ongoing hemodynamic resuscitation. This patient is critically ill and requires ICU level of care. He ultimately will need a combination of antibiotics and source control to recover. After arthrotomy which confirms septic arthritis, broad-spectrum antibiotics are continued. The microbiology returns as MRSA (Fig. 7.2) and the patient continues IV vancomycin. With continued care from the intensive care team, orthopedic surgery and the infectious disease service, the patient quickly improves and is transferred out of the ICU. This chapter focuses on the epidemiology and pathophysiology of pediatric sepsis and septic shock and the systemic manifestations of musculoskeletal infections with an emphasis on care and management in the pediatric intensive care unit.

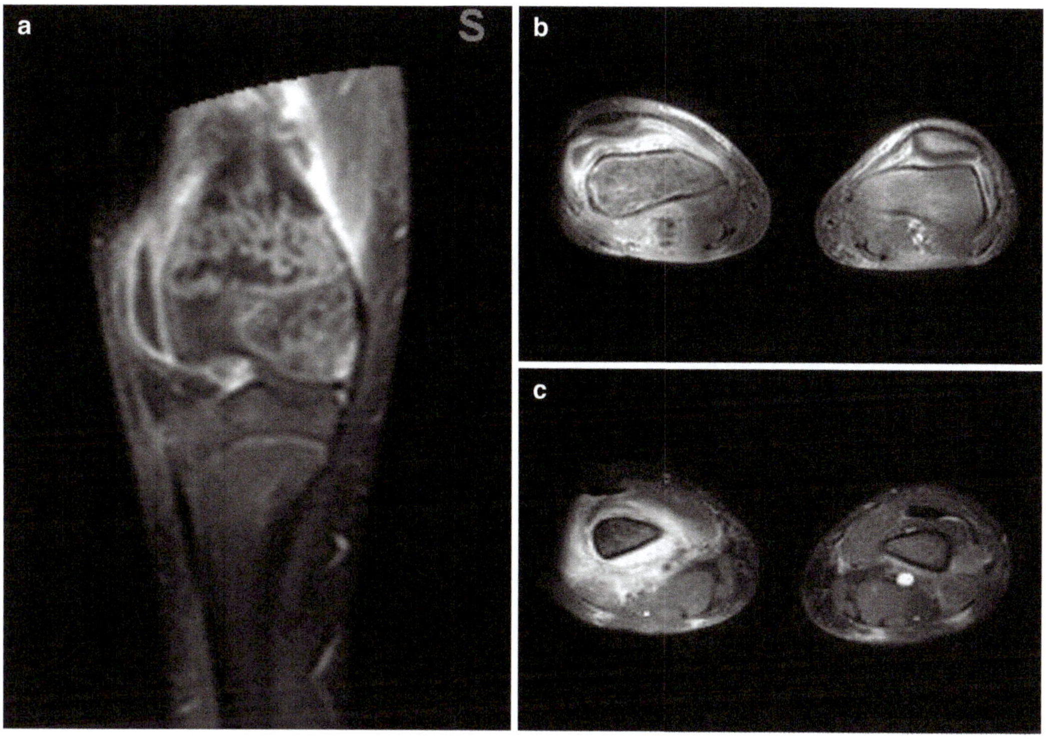

Fig. 7.1 (**a**–**c**) MRI of the right knee with distal femur. T1-weighted coronal and axial images of right knee post-contrast showing moderate effusion with surrounding synovial enhancement and abnormal signal within the distal femoral epiphysis and metaphysis, confirming septic arthritis with concurrent osteomyelitis

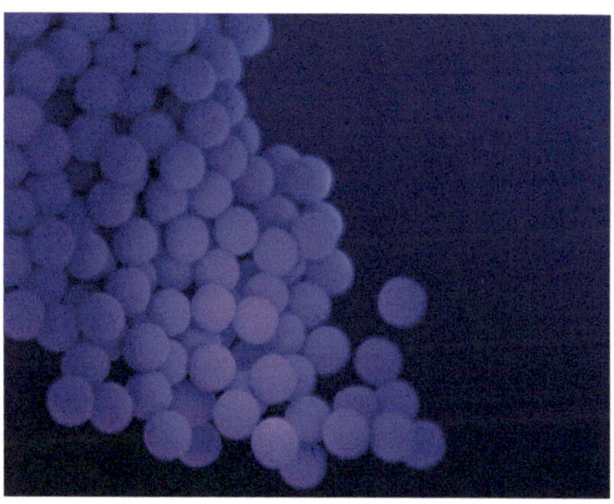

Fig. 7.2 Medical illustration of methicillin-resistant *Staphylococcus aureus*. (Source: ID # 23234/2019/ Medical Illustrator: Meredith Newlove/Center for Disease Control and Prevention, Atlanta, Georgia. (From the CDC public domain with permission, https://phil.cdc.gov/Details.aspx?pid=23234))

Definitions: Sepsis, Septic Shock

Although the first mention of sepsis dates to ancient Greece, a gold standard definition continues to elude clinicians and researchers [8]. Advances in the understanding of the pathophysiology of sepsis in recent decades have informed the current framework for defining sepsis.

The original definition of sepsis was put forth by Bone et al. in 1992 [9]. The authors defined sepsis as the "systemic inflammatory response to the presence of infection." The group also introduced the term *systemic inflammatory response syndrome* (SIRS) and laid the groundwork for standardizing nomenclature such as *severe sepsis*, *septic shock*, and *multi-organ dysfunction* (MOD) [9]. For the next quarter of a century, sepsis would be defined as the combination of SIRS with a proven or suspected infection.

In 2016, Sepsis 3 was published, revising the definitions of sepsis and septic shock in adults. In particular the authors eliminated the use of SIRS, and sepsis became defined as a "life-threatening organ dysfunction caused by a dysregulated response to infection" [10]. Organ dysfunction was categorized using the Sequential Organ Failure Assessment (SOFA) score, and the authors recommended the use of qSOFA (quick SOFA) for detecting patients at risk of poor outcomes outside of the ICU setting.

The first definition for pediatric sepsis stems from the International Consensus Conference on Pediatric and Organ Dysfunction in 2002. The resulting guideline published in 2005 provided the first consensus definitions of pediatric SIRS, sepsis, severe sepsis, and septic shock [11] (Table 7.1). Sepsis was defined using age-specific SIRS criteria in the presence of a proven or suspected infection (Tables 7.2 and 7.3). The authors recognized the poor specificity of the original definition and recognized that its use was more for research rather than for clinical purposes [12]. However, the definitions put forth by Goldstein et al. in 2005 for pediatric sepsis have yet to be modified and continue to inform how we define sepsis in children. At the

Table 7.1 Original definitions of pediatric sepsis

Systemic inflammatory response syndrome (SIRS)
Two or more of the following:
Temperature abnormality (less than 36 °C or greater than 38.5 °C)[a]
Tachycardia (or bradycardia for patients less than 1 year of age)
Tachypnea
Leukocytosis or leukopenia or bandemia[a]
Sepsis and severe sepsis and septic shock
Sepsis: above criteria in the setting of infection (definitive or likely)
Severe sepsis: sepsis in addition to cardiovascular instability, acute respiratory distress syndrome (ARDS), or multi-organ dysfunction
Septic shock: severe sepsis with cardiovascular dysfunction

[a]Either temperature abnormality or white count abnormality must be present to meet criteria

Table 7.2 Original criteria used to define organ dysfunction in pediatric sepsis

Cardiovascular
Hypotension
Need for vasoactive infusion for treatment of hypotension
Two or more of the following
Unexplained metabolic acidosis
Lactate elevation
Decreased urine output (Oliguria)
Prolonged capillary refill
Respiratory
PF ratio <300
$PaCO_2$ > 65 torr or >20 torr above baseline
Need for >50% FIO_2 to maintain SpO_2 >92%
Need for invasive or noninvasive mechanical ventilation
Neurologic
Glassgow Coma Score (GCS) <11
Acute mental status change with 3 more or point decrease in GCS
Hematologic
Thrombocytopenia
International normalized ratio (INR) >2
Renal
Creatinine greater than 2 times upper limit of normal for age or doubling of baseline creatinine
Hepatic
Total bilirubin ≥4 mg/dL
ALT greater than two times upper limit for age

Table 7.3 Age-specific pediatric vital sign criteria for SIRS

Age	Tachycardia	Bradycardia	Respiratory rate	White blood cell count	Systolic blood pressure
<1 week	>180	<100	>50	>34	<65
1 week to 1 month	>180	<100	>40	>19.5 or <5	<75
1 month to 1 year	>180	<90	>34	>17.5 or <5	<100
2–5 years	>140	–	>22	>15.5 or <6	<94
6–12 years	>130	–	>18	>13.5 or <4.5	<105
13–18 years	110	–	>14	>11 or <4.5	<117

Units: Tachycardia and bradycardia – beats per minute. Respiratory rate – breaths per minute. White blood cell (WBC) count – WBC × $10^3/mm^3$. Systolic blood pressure – mm Hg. Note that bradycardia is only a criteria for patients under 1 year of age time of this publication, the Society of Critical Care Medicine's Pediatric Sepsis Definition Taskforce is collaborating to develop criteria to identify children with sepsis and sepsis-associated organ dysfunction [13].

For the purposes of this chapter, we define sepsis as a life-threatening infection leading to organ dysfunction. Further, we define septic shock according to the 2020 Pediatric Surviving Sepsis Campaign guidelines as severe infection leading to cardiovascular dysfunction, including hypotension, need for treatment with a vasoactive medication, or impaired perfusion [14].

Risk Factors for the Development of Sepsis

The precise mechanisms which increase a host's risk factors for developing sepsis remain incompletely understood. Susceptibility to develop and succumb to sepsis appears multifactorial and related to host conditions (e.g., age, genetics, and immunocompromised state), environmental factors (indwelling catheters), and microorganisms and their virulence [15, 16].

A recent study by Prout et al. revealed that *Staph. aureus* remains the most common pathogen (9.4%) isolated from previously healthy children admitted with sepsis, followed by *E. coli* (7.1%) and *Streptococcus* species other than *S. pneumoniae* (6.3%) [17]. However, in children with at least one chronic disease, although *S. aureus* remains the most common organism (11%), it is followed closely by *Candida* species (9.8%) and *P. aeruginosa* (8.1%). This difference is noteworthy as recent research demonstrated that the majority (68%) of pediatric patients admitted to US hospitals with sepsis has at least one chronic condition [18].

Regarding pediatric musculoskeletal infections, the most frequent causative organisms remain *S. aureus* strains [(both methicillin-sensitive *Staph. aureus* (MSSA) and methicillin-resistant *Staph. aureus* (MRSA)] and *Strep. pyogenes*, which account for 95% of cases of osteomyelitis [19]. However, the age of the patient and suspected mechanism must be considered. For example, group B *Streptococcus* remains the most frequent cause of osteomyelitis in neonates, while puncture wounds increase the risk of *Pseudomonas aeruginosa* [20].

Epidemiologic data suggest cases related to MRSA are increasing. In a single-center retrospective study, MRSA was the causative organism in 12% of osteomyelitis and septic arthritis cases and 30% of pediatric musculoskeletal infections overall. In addition, children with MRSA were more likely to develop deep venous thrombosis and required more surgical interventions [21]. In comparison, a similar study from the same center done 20 years prior revealed no cases of osteomyelitis or septic arthritis due to MRSA [16].

Practitioners caring for children with musculoskeletal infections must remain aware of the risk factors that predispose their patients to develop sepsis and septic shock. Similarly, providers must maintain vigilance with regard to the prevalent infectious organisms in their communities and the associated antibiotic susceptibilities.

Pathophysiology: Sepsis and Septic Shock

Advances in our understanding of immunity have provided insight into how sepsis and the resultant immune dysregulation lead to tissue damage. An in-depth review of the host's immune response to sepsis is beyond the scope of this chapter. We refer the reader to the references provided in this section and to Chaps. 3, 10, and 28 in this book for a better understanding of the pathology of

MSK infections and interaction between the organism with host's immune system.

Innate and Adaptive Immunity

The inflammatory response elicited by severe infection is dependent on host factors as well as virulence factors of the causative microorganisms. Invading pathogens initiate an inflammatory response by activating the host's innate immune system (macrophages, monocytes, dendritic cells, natural killer cells, and granulocytes). "Pathogen-associated molecular patterns" (PAMPs), such as lipopolysaccharide (LPS), are recognized by innate immune cells via pattern recognition receptors (PRR), such as Toll-like receptor (TLRs) [16, 22–24]. The interaction between these cell-surface receptors and the foreign particles activates the immune cells initiating transcription and release of inflammatory cytokines such as TNF-α, IL-1, and IL-6. These inflammatory signals serve to attract other immune cells to the site of host damage. Interaction between the innate and adaptive immune system (T and B lymphocytes) results in a more targeted and specific immune response to the invading microorganism and initiation of a counteracting anti-inflammatory response [16, 22, 25]. The balance between pro- and anti-inflammatory mediators may depend on the injured host cells' release of "damage-associated molecular patterns" (DAMPs). These endogenous molecules, which include extracellular RNA, DNA, and ATP, can activate the same PRRs on innate immune cells and perpetuate a cycle characterized by the release of pro-inflammatory mediators and overactive inflammation. This exaggerated inflammatory response can lead to endothelial and epithelial injury, coagulopathy, and organ dysfunction [16, 22–25].

Multi-organ Dysfunction

One of the hallmarks of sepsis and septic shock is poor vascular tone and permeability. Central to this alteration is the endothelial and epithelial dysfunction provoked by inflammatory mediators in sepsis [16, 26–28]. The injury to both endothelial and epithelial layers lead to disruption in permeability, tissue edema, and organ damage. In the lung, for example, interstitial edema and extravasation of protein-rich fluid into the alveoli lead to poor compliance and are features of ARDS (acute respiratory distress syndrome) [16].

Normal interactions between the inflammatory and coagulation pathways are disrupted in sepsis. Endothelial and innate immune cell activation in response to invading pathogens leads to an imbalance between pro- and anti-inflammatory mediators resulting in a procoagulant state, microthrombi, impaired blood supply, and organ dysfunction [16, 22, 26]. The resultant microvascular ischemia seen in the tissue level can generate reactive oxygen species (ROS) and lead to mitochondrial damage. This mitochondrial injury may explain the impaired oxygen utilization seen in sepsis and likely contributes to end-organ damage, including cardiac, renal, CNS, and hepatic dysfunction [16, 22, 29, 30].

Septic Shock

Shock can be classified according to its etiology, such as hypovolemic, cardiogenic, obstructive, or distributive. Septic shock is considered to have features of both cardiogenic and distributive shock. Regardless of its etiology, shock leads to a life-threatening state that results when the body is unable to meet its oxygen and metabolic demands [29, 31]. The delivery of oxygen is dependent on both the cardiac output (L/min) and the arterial oxygen content (ml 3/dL):

$$DO_2 = CO \times CaO_2 \tag{7.1}$$

where DO_2 is oxygen delivery, CO is cardiac output, and CaO_2 is arterial oxygen content [32].

Cardiac output is determined by the stroke volume and heart rate. Arterial oxygen content is dependent on the amount of oxygen bound to hemoglobin, the fractional hemoglobin saturation, and the amount of oxygen dissolved in blood. The oxygen delivery equation thus becomes:

$$DO_2 = (HR \times SV) \times [(1.34 \times SaO_2 \times Hgb) + (PaO_2 \times 0.003)] \quad (7.2)$$

Arterial oxygen content is the amount of O_2 bound to hemoglobin plus the dissolved O_2 in the blood. The constant 1.34 is derived from the amount of oxygen (in mL) bound to 1 g of hemoglobin. The dissolved oxygen in the blood is equal to the solubility constant of oxygen in the blood (0.003) multiplied by the partial pressure of oxygen in arterial blood. As can be seen, the amount of dissolved oxygen has minimal contribution in oxygen delivery under normal circumstances.

Under physiologic conditions, the amount of oxygen delivered to the tissues (DO_2) is well above the amount utilized (VO_2). This physiologic reserve means that oxygen consumption is independent of oxygen delivery, as can be seen in Fig. 7.3. However, with decreased oxygen delivery or increased oxygen demand as commonly seen in sepsis, a critical point will be reached where oxygen utilization becomes dependent on delivery. At this critical point, lactic acidosis develops. Further, it is postulated that in certain pathogenic states such as sepsis, tissue oxygen consumption increases while oxygen utilization increases [33]. This results in a shift upward and to the right of the DO_2-VO_2 graph as seen in Fig. 7.4.

As mentioned previously, sepsis is a life-threatening condition. Alterations in vascular tone and permeability lead to a relative hypovolemic state as the vascular beds become more permeable and increase their capacitance. Furthermore, although sympathetic stimulus leads to tachycardia, there is evidence of depressed cardiac function in sepsis [32]. Simultaneously, hypoxia from lung injury impairs hemoglobin saturation.

Thus, for clinicians treating patients with septic, or any other form of shock, it is important to understand the determinants of oxygen delivery. Figure 7.5 is a visual representation of the determinants of oxygen delivery the clinician may be able to manipulate when treating patients in shock.

Clinical Presentation

Given the life-threatening nature of severe sepsis and septic shock, an expedited evaluation assessing for SIRS, source of infection, evidence of end-organ dysfunction, and signs of shock/

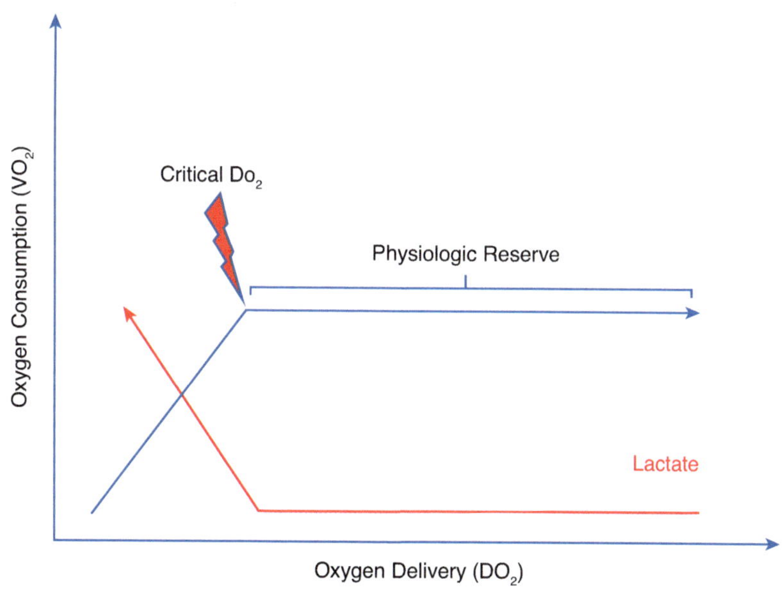

Fig. 7.3 Physiologic balance of DO_2 and VO_2. Below the critical DO_2 level, a shift occurs to anaerobic metabolism with a corresponding increase in lactate levels

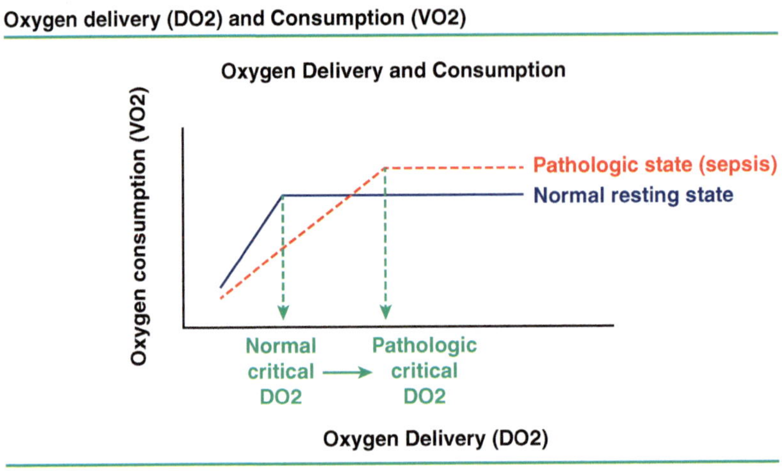

Fig. 7.4 In the normal state (blue line), oxygen consumption is constant over a range of Do_2, and decreases only when DO_2 falls below a critical level (critical Do_2). Pathologic changes caused by sepsis or systemic inflammatory responses (red line) cause increased VO_2 and impaired peripheral oxygen utilization, resulting in an elevation in critical DO_2. (Adapted from Rosen et al., *UpToDate* [33])

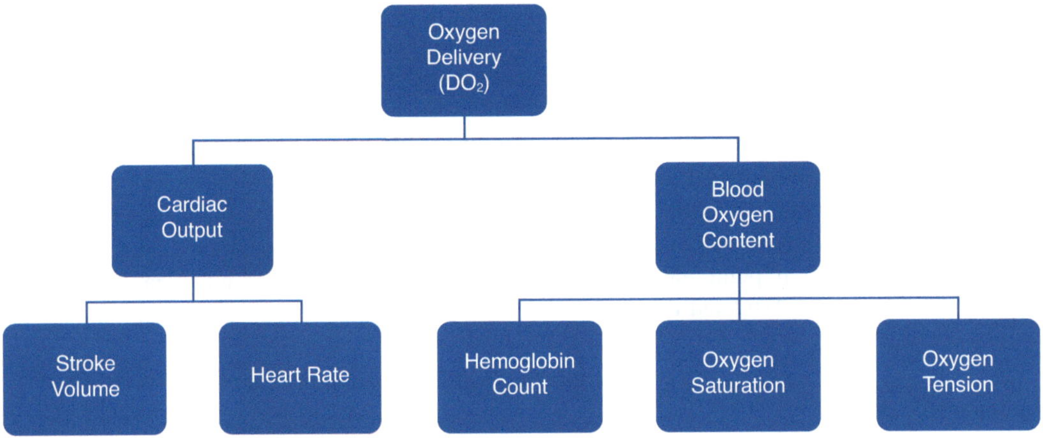

Fig. 7.5 Determinants of oxygen delivery. Oxygen delivery is determined by cardiac output and arterial oxygen content. Variation in contributing components results in corresponding changes in net oxygen delivery

altered perfusion is imperative for successful outcomes.

Children with sepsis have significant alterations in vital signs (hypothermia/hyperthermia, tachycardia/bradycardia, tachypnea). These clinical derangements, in conjunction with white blood cell count abnormalities (leukocytosis/leukopenia), are indicative of a SIRS response (Table 7.1) [11, 34].

The physical exam should be directed toward identifying possible sources of infection and the presence of shock. Signs of infection are largely organ specific. For instance, rales may be heard in the patient with lobar pneumonia, or costovertebral angle tenderness may be elicited in the patient with pyelonephritis. For musculoskeletal infections, in addition to the common signs of bone or joint infection (localized edema, erythema, warmth, pain), other manifestations of systemic inflammation are noteworthy such as macular erythema (e.g., toxic shock syndrome), petechiae, or purpura (e.g., meningococcemia, disseminated intravascular coagulation) [35].

Clinical signs of shock include altered mental status, oliguria/anuria, and/or perfusion abnormalities. Classic signs of "warm" shock include erythroderma, bounding pulses, and flash capillary refill (<1 second), while signs of "cold" shock include mottled skin, diminished pulses, and delayed capillary refill (>2 seconds) [19, 35]. It is important to emphasize that hypotension is not necessary for the clinical diagnosis of septic shock; however, its presence in a patient with suspected sepsis is usually confirmatory [35].

Diagnostic evaluation should include laboratory tests such as complete metabolic panel, complete blood count with differentiation, coagulation panel, blood lactate, and markers of inflammation such as C-reactive protein (CRP), erythrocyte sedimentation rate (ESR), and procalcitonin. Imaging should be guided by the location of the suspected infection and also obtained when signs or symptoms of organ dysfunction develop. For instance, chest radiographs may be indicated for respiratory distress or hypoxemia and echocardiograms obtained in the setting of cardiovascular dysfunction or shock [36].

A practical framework for evaluating a patient with suspected sepsis involves assessing for end-organ dysfunction using objective clinical and diagnostic data (Table 7.2) [11, 37]. For reasons related to the ease with which organ function can be measured, six organ systems are commonly evaluated in clinical practice and have been the most widely studied: cardiovascular, respiratory, neurological, renal, hepatic, and hematologic [37]. Importantly, dysfunction of a single organ in isolation is uncommon given the existence of "interorgan cross talk," and the failure of one organ usually leads to dysfunction in other organs simultaneously [38, 39]. This pattern of organ failure is the most important predictor of outcomes as mortality increases as the number of organs affected increases [39].

Numerous pediatric organ failure scoring tools have been created, largely for research purposes, to quantify the degree of organ dysfunction and estimate mortality [40]. Two of these that have been internally and independently validated include the Pediatric Logistic Organ Dysfunction (PELOD-2) score and the pediatric Sequential Organ Failure Assessment (pSOFA) [41, 42].

ICU Monitoring in Pediatric Severe Sepsis and Septic Shock

The patient with sepsis and severe musculoskeletal infections warrants close monitoring of hemodynamics, markers of cardiac output and oxygen delivery, markers of end-organ dysfunction, and early detection of clinical deterioration. ICU monitoring typically requires higher nurse to patient staffing ratios (e.g., 1 nurse to 2 patients) than typically available outside of the intensive care setting [43]. Frequent vital sign checks, at minimum every 1 hour, are also the standard in ICU monitoring. Close monitoring of urine output, typically with an indwelling Foley catheter, provides information on renal perfusion and therefore cardiac output and may alert staff of progression to renal failure. In the patient with a severe musculoskeletal infection in which limb perfusion or viability may be compromised, frequent neurovascular checks are also provided by the nursing staff. Frequent neurological checks are also indicated to monitor for altered sensorium, a concerning marker of central nervous system end-organ dysfunction. Both noninvasive and invasive technologies, when appropriate, augment bedside assessments and are detailed below.

Continuous Electrocardiographic (ECG) Monitoring

Continuous ECG monitoring, also known as telemetry, relies on cutaneous electrodes to detect underlying myocardial electrical activity [44]. In the critically ill patient with sepsis, continuous ECG monitoring generates trends in heart rate that can indicate improvement or worsening of hemodynamics and also allows for rapid detection of dysrhythmias that may be likely to occur in the setting of inotrope use or poor renal function with resultant electrolyte abnormalities.

Pulse Oximetry

Pulse oximetry utilizes red and infrared light in conjunction with a photodetector to provide a noninvasive continuous estimation of arterial oxyhemoglobin saturation (i.e., the percentage of hemoglobin bound to oxygen) [45]. In the patient with septic shock, pulse oximetry provides an indicator of adequacy of blood oxygenation, a particularly crucial factor given the underlying pathophysiology of shock being inadequate oxygen delivery, and should be used to titrate FiO_2 requirements. Additionally, pulse oximetry can also reveal heart rate trends and variations in perfusion such as pulsus paradoxus in the volume depleted patient or poor perfusion in a patient with dysrhythmias.

Near-Infrared Spectroscopy

Near-infrared spectroscopy (NIRS) utilizes technology similar to that in pulse oximetry, again using variation in near-infrared light absorption to estimate hemoglobin oxygenation status. NIRS, unlike pulse oximetry, analyzes nonpulsatile venous regional blood flow and estimates the saturation of deoxyhemoglobin rather than oxyhemoglobin, as in pulse oximetry [44]. Therefore, NIRS provides a noninvasive real-time continuous approximation of tissue venous oxygen saturation and can be used to trend changes in cardiac output. Of note, the trend of data tends to be more valuable than absolute values given technical and practical limitations (body habitus, poor sensor contact, variations in regional blood flow).

Blood Pressure Monitoring

Although hypotension is a late manifestation of shock, close blood pressure monitoring is crucial in the ICU setting. Noninvasive oscillometric arterial pressure monitoring with the blood pressure cuff may be employed at an increased frequency, but in the critically ill child with septic shock, invasive monitoring is frequently indicated. Invasive arterial pressure monitoring requires placement of a catheter into either a peripheral (e.g., radial) or central (e.g., femoral) artery, followed by connection to a transducer. Invasive arterial pressure monitoring provides real-time continuous blood pressure monitoring with ability for waveform analysis and also arterial blood sampling.

Additional ICU Considerations

ICU monitoring also typically involves frequent laboratory draws to trend markers of end-organ dysfunction, with a particular emphasis on renal (BUN and creatinine), gastrointestinal (LFTs and bilirubin), and hematologic (platelets, PT/PTT/INR, fibrinogen, and D-dimer) function. Other essential laboratory tests include markers of tissue perfusion (blood gasses and lactate levels), oxygen-carrying capacity (hemoglobin), and inflammation (CRP, ESR, procalcitonin, WBC). Many additional monitoring technologies also exist that may be implemented when clinically appropriate but are outside the scope of this text. For example, the mechanically ventilated patient typically benefits from capnography, and the neurologically impaired patient likely warrants continuous EEG monitoring. Of note, special attention must be paid to mitigating the risk of hospital acquired infections such as central line associated bloodstream infections (CLABSI), ventilator-associated pneumonia, and catheter-associated urinary tract infections (CAUTI) in the patient with multiple points of invasive monitoring. Please refer to additional critical care texts for further discussion.

Management of Septic Shock

As demonstrated in the clinical vignette, care for the pediatric patient suffering systemic manifestations of a musculoskeletal infection typically begins in the emergency department. Timely management of septic shock begins in the ED and continues in the PICU. Generally, proto-

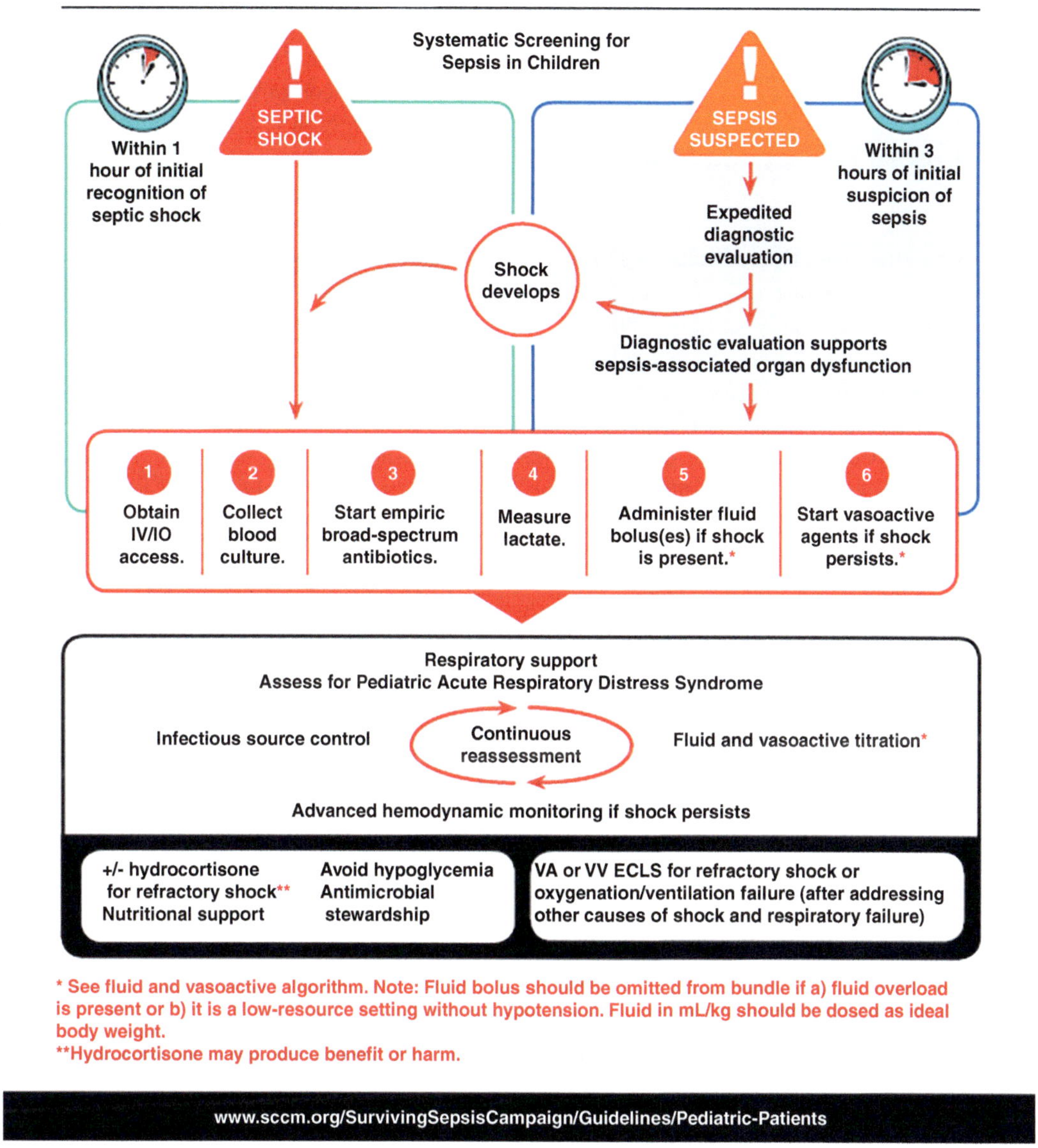

Fig. 7.6 Surviving Sepsis Campaign initial resuscitation algorithm for children

colized management of severe sepsis is associated with improved outcomes (viz., organ dysfunction and mortality) [14, 46, 47]. The below guidelines for management of septic shock are largely drawn from the 2020 Surviving Sepsis Campaign International Guidelines for the Management of Septic Shock and Sepsis-Associated Organ Dysfunction in Children (Fig. 7.6) [14]. Of note, the general level of evidence is weak for many aspects of pediatric care of septic shock. Nonetheless, the guidelines represent the current state of knowledge on management of pediatric septic shock and are reviewed below.

Initial Management

Within 1 hour of initial recognition of septic shock or within 3 hours of initial suspicion of sepsis, vascular access should be obtained, blood cultures obtained, antibiotics administered, lactate measured, and hemodynamic resuscitation begun. Frequent reassessments of hemodynamic and respiratory status are necessary to guide continued care [48].

Antimicrobial Therapy and Source Control

Addressing the underlying cause of sepsis remains the cornerstone of sepsis and septic shock management. Early antimicrobial therapy, initiated within 1 hour of recognition of septic shock or within 3 hours of sepsis in the absence of shock, is associated with reduced mortality in pediatric sepsis [14, 46, 49]. Evidence for the exact time interval before which antimicrobials should be administered remains weak though the general justification for earlier, rather than late, administration is sound (Fig. 7.7). See Chap. 2 in this book for in-depth discussion of antimicrobial therapy. In brief, initial empiric antibiotic therapy should be broad spectrum with adequate coverage of all likely pathogens with multiple agents potentially employed for the purposes of coverage of additional pathogens, decreasing likelihood of resistance or for synergy for particular pathogens [14, 49]. Antimicrobials should be tailored to organism susceptibility if such information is available. Additional consideration is warranted for the immunocompromised patient, neonate, or patient with high risk of multidrug-resistant pathogens.

Intervention to address the underlying source of infection such as abscess drainage, wound debridement, and infected hardware or catheter removal should take place as soon as possible and should not be delayed while awaiting clinical stability [14]. Rather, eradication of the source may be necessary for reversal of the shock state and delays in source control are associated with deterioration in clinical status and potentially increased mortality [5, 14, 51].

Hemodynamic Resuscitation

Fluids and Volume Resuscitation

Availability of intensive care guides fluid management in septic shock (Fig. 7.8) [52]. In health care settings where intensive care and mechanical ventilation are available, in the absence of signs of fluid overload and in the presence of abnormal perfusion with or without hypotension, fluid boluses of up to 40–60 mL/kg of crystalloid

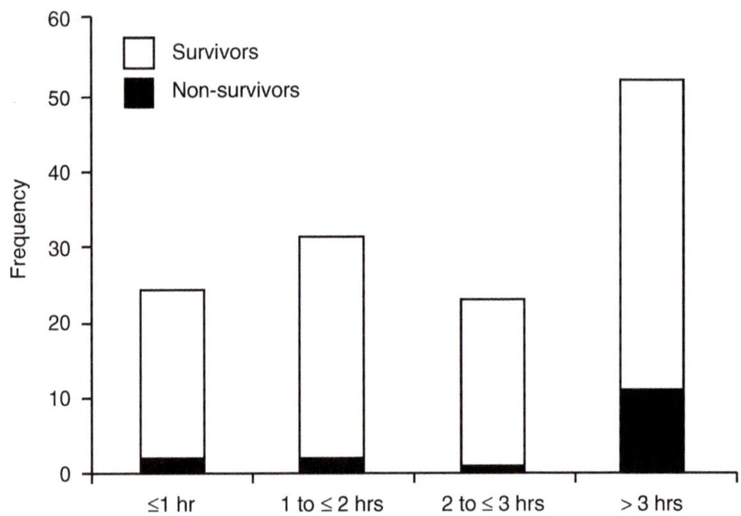

	≤1 hr	1 to ≤ 2 hrs	2 to ≤ 3 hrs	> 3 hrs
N	24	31	23	52
Mortality	8.3%	6.5%	4.3%	21.2%

Fig. 7.7 Time from sepsis recognition to initial antimicrobial administration with survival fraction. (Adapted from Weiss et al. [50])

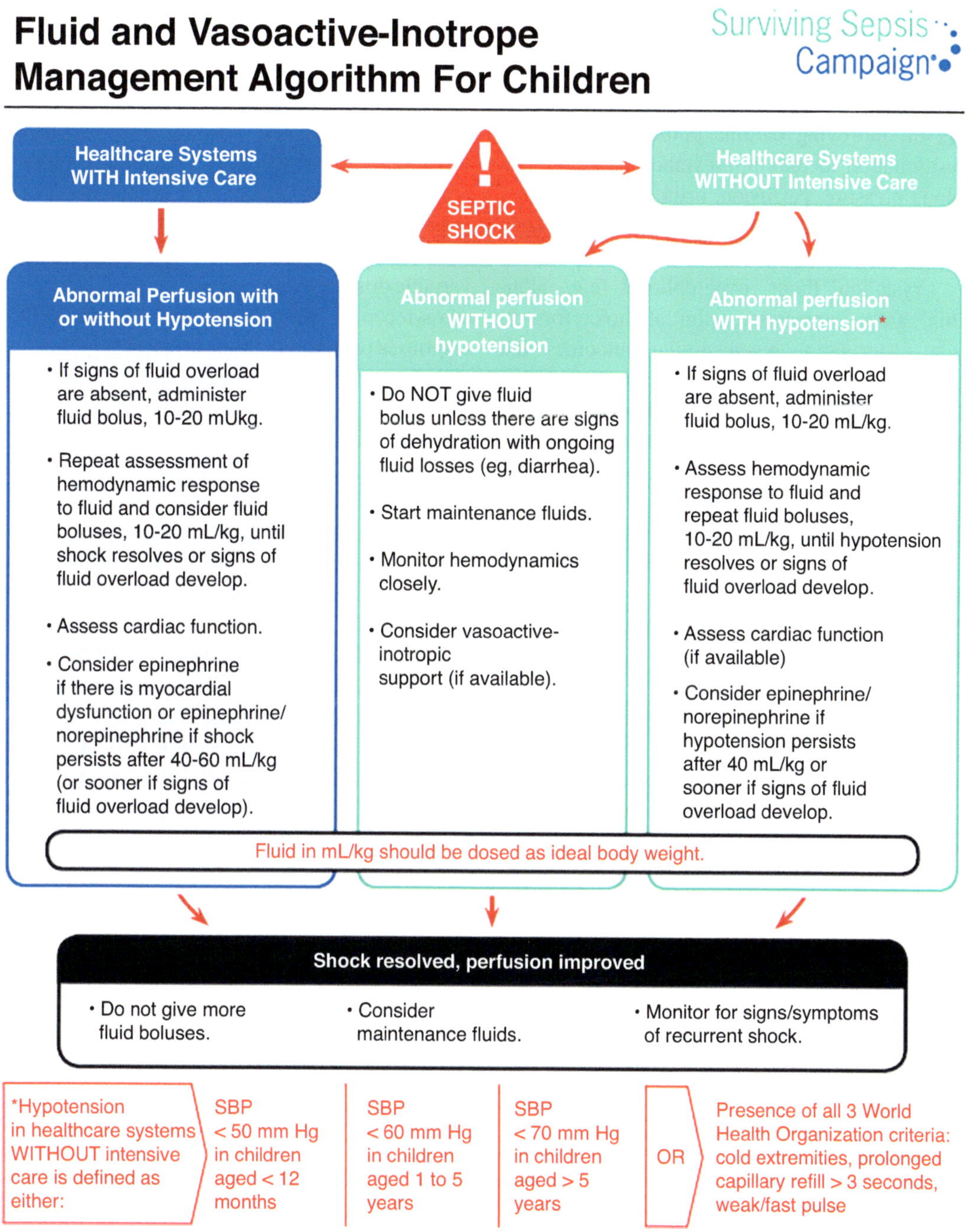

Fig. 7.8 Algorithm for volume and inotropic use per Surviving Sepsis Campaign

fluid should be administered [14, 53, 54]. The boluses should be administered in 10–20 mL/kg increments with frequent reassessment of effect and given until markers of cardiac output improve (Fig. 7.5) or signs of fluid overload develop [14, 53, 54]. Administration of fluid boluses restores cardiac preload and addresses effective volume depletion caused by capillary leak, vasodilation, or increased insensible losses [14]. Signs of fluid overload may manifest as tachypnea, rales on auscultation secondary to pulmonary edema, or hepatomegaly on abdominal exam. Early markers of improving cardiac output and effective resuscitation include improvement in heart rate, blood pressure, perfusion, urine output, level of consciousness, end-organ laboratory markers, and down-trending lactate levels [14, 43].

Crystalloid fluids, over colloids (e.g., albumin), are recommended as initial choice for volume resuscitation given similar outcomes and their favorable cost, availability, and low infection risks compared with colloids [14, 52]. Increasing evidence suggests decreased mortality and decreased acute kidney injury with use of balanced crystalloid fluids (e.g., Ringer lactate, Plasmalyte) over normal saline [55–57].

Inotropic/Vasoactive Agents

In the setting of fluid-refractory shock, as evidenced by persistent poor cardiac output (e.g., hypotension, delayed capillary refill, oliguria) after 40–60 mL/kg of fluid boluses, initiation of inotropic or vasoactive agents is appropriate (Fig. 7.8) [14]. Survival benefit and increased organ failure-free days have been demonstrated with epinephrine or norepinephrine over dopamine [57, 58]. Insufficient evidence is available to recommend epinephrine or norepinephrine over the other, and clinical judgement can guide the initial choice of agent. Historically, clinicians would attempt to differentiate between cold and warm shock by physical exam. However, several observational studies demonstrated poor quality of assessment and lack of correlation with cardiac index or measurements of systemic vascular resistance [59].

The primary targets of inotropic or vasoactive therapy are adrenergic receptors that, upon stimulation, augment cardiac output and blood pressure. Extensive discussion of the pharmacology of vasoactive and inotropic medications is outside the scope of this chapter. In brief, agonism of beta-1 adrenergic receptors, which are located most abundantly in the myocardium, results in inotropy (increased contractility) and chronotropy (increased rate). As a result, beta-1 agonism increases cardiac output (a product of stroke volume and heart rate) [60]. Agonism of alpha-1 adrenergic receptors, located in vasculature walls, results in vasoconstriction, increasing systemic vascular resistance and potentially blood pressure [60]. Epinephrine and norepinephrine both stimulate beta-1 and alpha-1 receptors with variable dose-response curves, various degrees of cross-receptor interactions, and various reflex responses [60]. Epinephrine is classically thought to have predominantly beta-1 activity at lower doses, with a primary effect of increasing cardiac output, whereas at higher doses, an alpha-adrenergic receptor effect predominates with a primary effect of systemic vasoconstriction. Norepinephrine is a potent alpha-1 and beta-1 agonist that exhibits a strong effect on systemic vascular resistance while also providing some inotropic effect. Vasopressin is an additional agent to consider in the setting of high-dose catecholamine use that may have additional positive effects on systemic vascular resistance via agonism of the vasopressin receptor [14]. All of the above agents are ideally administered via a central line but may be infused via peripheral IVs or intraosseous route while in the process of obtaining more suitable access [61].

Inotropic agents should be titrated to effect, with frequent reassessment of markers of cardiac output and perfusion (Fig. 7.9). Point of care ultrasound or formal cardiac echocardiography can also assist in hemodynamic resuscitation.

Additional Support Modalities

In the setting of refractory shock and progressive clinical deterioration and organ dysfunction, various therapies may be considered. Detailed discussion is beyond the scope of this text but a brief overview of occasionally considered and utilized technologies and treatment modalities is provided below.

Therapeutic endpoints for the ongoing management of septic shock in children* [1]

▪ Capillary refill ≤ 2 seconds
▪ Within threshold heart rate for age (beats/minute):
• Newborn to <2 years: 110 to 160
• Infant to preschool (2 to 6 years): 90 to 160
• Child (7 to 12 years): 70 to 150
▪ Normal pulses (central and peripheral pulses equal)
▪ Warm extremities
▪ Urine output >1 mL/kg/hour
▪ Normal mental status
▪ Normalization of laboratory studies including lactate and anion gap
▪ For patients without invasive monitoring: Normal blood pressure for age
▪ For patients with invasive monitoring (CVP and intraarterial pressure monitors):
Cardiac index 3.3 to 6.0 L/minute/m^2 (if monitoring available)
$ScVO_2$ > 70% ¶
▪ Normalization of glucose and calcium

$ScVO_2$: central venous oxygen saturation; MAP: mean arterial pressure; CVP: central venous pressure.
* Septic shock is being adequately treated when all therapeutic endpoints are achieved.
¶ Not applicable to patients with congenital heart disease with mixing lesions.
Δ The MAP goal is based upon the estimated formula for 50th percentile MAP for a child with 50th percentile height in the healthy population with an expected CVP = 0 mmHg. When the CVP is greater than zero, then the goal MAP should be adjusted accordingly to achieve adequate perfusion pressure. Although suggested by many experts as a therapeutic endpoint, evidence is lacking to guide the optimal target perfusion pressure.

Reference:
1. *Davis AL, Carcillo JA, Aneja RK, et al. American College of Critical Care Medicine Clinical Practice Parameters for Herrodynamic Support of Pediatric and Neonatal Septic Shock. Crit Care Med 2017; 45:1061.*

UpToDate®

Fig. 7.9 Therapeutic endpoints UpToDate

Renal Replacement Therapies

Renal replacement therapy may be indicated in the setting of fluid overload and renal dysfunction secondary to septic shock that is refractory to fluid restriction or diuretics. Fluid overload is associated with increased mortality in critically ill children [62]. Continuous renal replacement therapy (CRRT) is better tolerated in the hemodynamically tenuous patient and allows for control of fluid overload, improvement in acid-base status, normalization of electrolytes, and possibly cytokine clearance [63]. Early initiation of CRRT may be associated with mortality benefit but further studies are needed [64].

Extracorporeal Membrane Oxygenation

Extracorporeal membrane oxygenation (ECMO) provides the ability to externally support gas exchange (venovenous ECMO) or both gas exchange and cardiac output (venoarterial ECMO). Severe ARDS with refractory hypoxemia and gas exchange inadequately supported by conventional therapies may be an indication for venovenous ECMO [14]. Persistent refractory shock may be an indication for venoarterial ECMO. Specific evidence for candidacy and survival benefit is inadequate at this time and the decision to utilize ECMO must be carefully weighed against the risks (e.g., infection, hemorrhage, thromboembolic events) [65].

Immunoglobulins

Evidence for administration of intravenous immunoglobulins (IVIG) is lacking. IVIG theoretically may be beneficial by providing passive immunity and by neutralizing bacterial toxins and inflammatory mediators. However, evidence for mortality benefit is inadequate currently [14]. Of note, IVIG may be of more benefit for the specific patient with toxic shock syndrome with meta-analyses of adult studies noting mortality benefit [66].

Plasma Exchange (PLEX)

Plasma exchange (PLEX) is not routinely indicated for pediatric patients with septic shock in the absence of specific indications such as thrombocytopenia-associated multi-organ failure [67]. Theoretically PLEX aids in removal of inflammatory mediators and restoration of homeostasis, but evidence of mortality benefit in pediatric patients with septic shock is lacking [68].

Other ICU Considerations

Nutrition

Inadequate evidence exists for particular feeding or nutrition regimens for pediatric patients with septic shock. However, enteral feeding does not need to be held once hemodynamic stability is achieved and inotropic or vasoactive agents are no longer being increased. Commonly, enteral feeding may be initiated within 48 hours of admission for septic shock [14].

Glycemic Control

Hyperglycemia is associated with increased morbidity and mortality in critically ill pediatric patients, but the risk of hypoglycemia must be carefully weighed when considering tight glycemic control with insulin. Episodes of severe hypoglycemia may be associated with poor long-term developmental outcomes. Inadequate evidence exists for precise glucose targets. In practice and in accordance with guidelines for adults, an upper limit of glucose levels of 180 mg/dL may be appropriate [14]. Lower limits should not be below 140 mg/dL given the risk of hypoglycemia, but precise targets have not yet been defined [14].

Special Considerations for Low and Middle Income Countries

Sepsis is one of the leading causes of death globally, with the great majority of sepsis-related deaths occurring in low- and middle-income countries (LMIC) [69]. Furthermore, resource constraints in LMICs hinders delivery of critical care in many parts of the world [70]. The following section is intended not only to acknowledge the unfortunate disparity with regard to sepsis

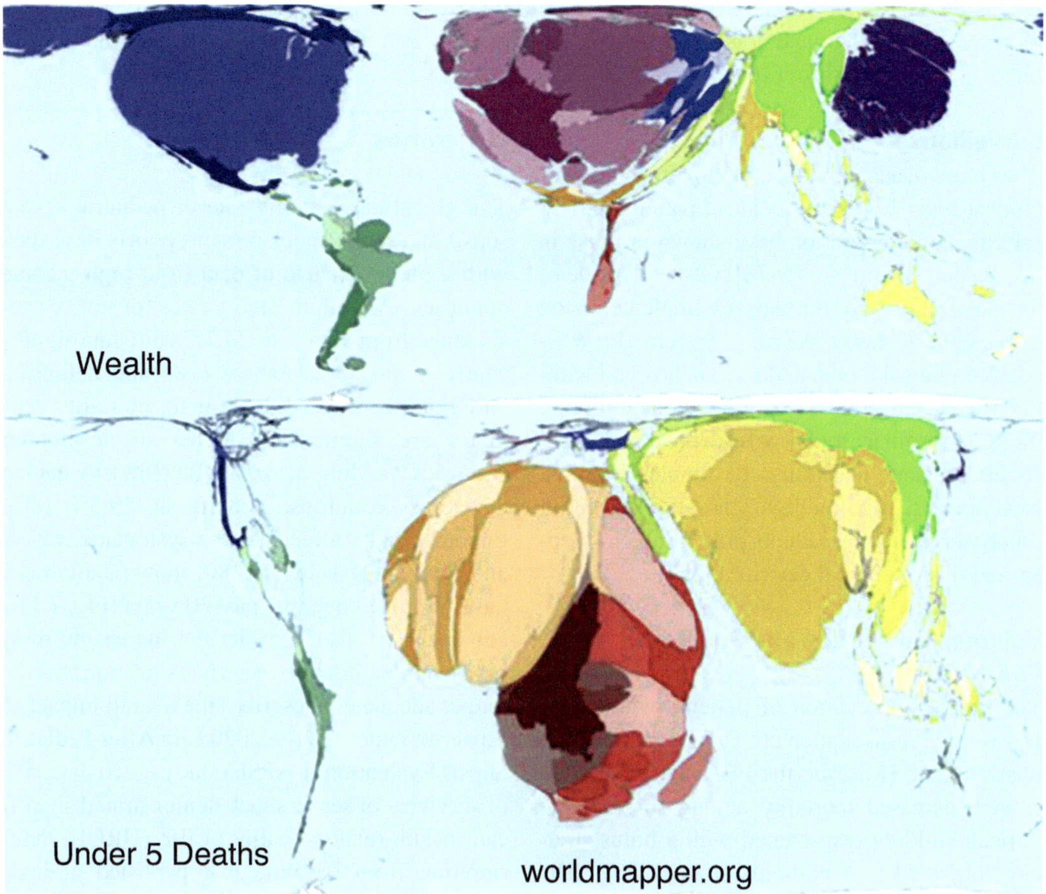

Fig. 7.10 World map comparison of wealth and under-5 deaths. (Adapted from Kissoon et al. [73]). Legend: Death from sepsis in pediatric patients under the age of 5 occur disproportionally in low-wealth countries. For example, the continent of Africa is small in the wealth section but is large in the "Under 5 Deaths" section

burden and mortality but to provide summarized recommendations applicable to LMICs, as well as references for further reading.

Global Sepsis Burden

The recent Global Burden of Disease study in sepsis highlighted gross regional and economic disparities with regard to sepsis burden: 85.0% of sepsis cases and 84.8% of related deaths worldwide occurred in countries with low, low-middle, or middle sociodemographic indices (SDI), particularly in sub-Saharan Africa and South-East Asia [71]. The three most common causes of sepsis-related deaths among children were infections related to neonatal disorders, lower respiratory infections, and diarrheal diseases. Furthermore, although the global case fatality for sepsis-related deaths appears to be improving, the disparities in outcomes are worsening. Children under 5 years of age in LMICs are now more than 18 times more likely to die, compared to 14 times more likely 30 years ago [72, 73]. Figure 7.10 highlights the distribution of wealth as compared to under-5 childhood mortality.

Applicability of Society Guidelines

Unfortunately, current definitions for sepsis were developed in high-income countries and may not be applicable to low-resource settings [73]. Similarly, recommendations from current sepsis guidelines may not be implementable where resources are limited, and epidemiology and etiology of sepsis may differ [69, 74].

Surveillance

The creation, adaptability, and implementation of clinical tools to detect pediatric patients at risk for clinical deterioration have shown promise in low-resource settings [75–78]. Olson et al. demonstrated improved mortality by implementation of a Pediatric Early Warning System (PEWS)-adapted clinical tool in a Malawian hospital without PICU capability [78]. The applicability of these or similar tools will depend on local resources and feasibility of implementation. Nevertheless, we highlight the importance of timely screening for patients presenting with sepsis and risk of clinical deterioration.

Volume, Antibiotics, and Source Control

The rapid identification of patients with sepsis and volume resuscitation are at the core of sepsis management. However, the FEAST trial demonstrated increased mortality among sub-Saharan African children resuscitated with a bolus strategy compared to a no-bolus strategy [52]. The recent Surviving Sepsis guidelines recommend against bolus administration in the absence of hypotension for settings lacking intensive care and mechanical ventilation [14] (Fig. 7.8). Thus, clinicians should exercise caution with regard to bolus administration, particularly in settings without critical care support. Early use of vasopressors or inotropic agents may be warranted to avoid fluid overload. Similarly, the timely administration of antibiotics and source control are essential components of the current standard of care in sepsis management as highlighted in previous sections (Fig. 7.6).

Sepsis is the leading cause of death in children worldwide and has been declared a serious global health issue. The challenges in managing pediatric septic patients are highlighted in LMICs where delivery of critical care is resource dependent and thus subject to unequal availability. A concerted effort to enhance our understanding of sepsis and further research into cost-effective interventions is required to address the global disparities of sepsis burden and outcomes.

Outcomes

The global case fatality rate of pediatric severe sepsis and septic shock remains poorly described with a predominance of data from high-income countries. Overall, mortality rates for severe sepsis range from 14.4% to 24.7% with data significantly limited by database code and definition variation [3, 5, 45, 79]. Of note, mortality estimates are significantly higher in developing countries, pooling at 32%, compared to that in developed countries, pooling at 19.3% [80]. Encouragingly, a recent large systematic review and meta-analysis by Tan [80] show fatality rates have improved over the past 30 years (Fig. 7.11), but one must also consider the increasing morbidity burden borne by survivors as mortality no longer adequately describes the overall impact of sepsis on children. The 2020 Life After Pediatric Sepsis Evaluation (LAPSE) study noted that 35% of survivors of septic shock demonstrated significant health-related quality of life (HRQL) deterioration from baseline that persisted at least 1 year following their hospitalization [81, 82]. Multiple studies have demonstrated correlation between severity of organ dysfunction and frequency of moderate to severe disability at discharge [83–85]. More specifically, several recent studies correlating classification scores with functional outcomes in children presenting with musculoskeletal infections confirmed the relationship of severity (dissemination) of infection with poor functional outcomes [86, 87].

Several risk factors related to the host characteristics, site of infection, and microbiology have been identified as predictors of morbidity and mortality. Case fatality rates (CFRs) are highest in infants under 1 year of age and across all age groups for children with comorbidities such as cancer or HIV [88, 89]. The site of infection also determines outcome as children with endocarditis, central nervous system infection, and primary bacteremia have the highest CFRs at 15–20% [88]. Pneumococcal and fungal infections, as

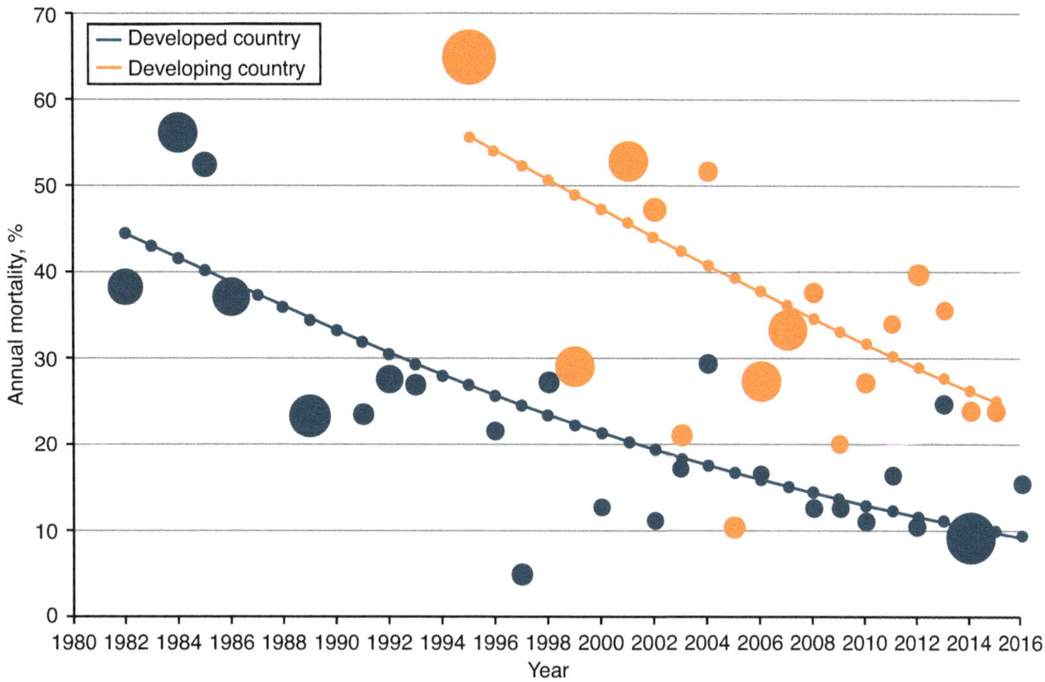

Fig. 7.11 Pooled weighted case-fatality rates (Tan). (From Tan et al.)

well as infections with multidrug-resistant organisms, are associated with higher CFRs [88]. Mortality increases with higher organ dysfunction scores with estimated mortality ranging from 0% to 7% with only one organ affected and up to 20–50% with two or more failing organ systems [88–91]. The need for multiple vasoactive infusions is also associated with higher CFRs in patients with severe sepsis and septic shock [89].

Conclusion

Pediatric sepsis is a global health problem with LMICs bearing the burden of sepsis cases and sepsis-related deaths. Providers caring for children with MSK infections should remain vigilant for early signs and symptoms of sepsis. The early diagnosis and treatment of sepsis and septic shock with volume resuscitation and antibiotics are associated with improved outcomes. Patients with sepsis and septic shock require close monitoring, ideally in an intensive care unit. Though the case fatality rates have improved over the past several decades, morbidity from organ injury is an increasing burden borne by survivors.

Box 7.1: Key Learning Points

- Sepsis is a global public health problem, with LMICs bearing the burden of sepsis cases and sepsis-related deaths.
- Sepsis is a dysregulated immune response to infection leading to organ dysfunction and potentially death.
- Dysregulation of host immunity is one of the primary contributors in developing sepsis, multi-organ dysfunction, and septic shock.
- Septic shock is defined as severe infection leading to cardiovascular dysfunction. The fundamental pathophysiology of shock is an imbalance between oxygen demand and delivery.
- Early diagnosis and treatment of sepsis and septic shock are associated with improved outcomes.

- Critically ill patients with sepsis and septic shock warrant admission to the PICU for monitoring.
- Monitoring for and treatment of end-organ dysfunction are key to management of sepsis and septic shock.
- Treatment of patients with sepsis and septic shock should include respiratory support, hemodynamic resuscitation, antimicrobial therapy, and source control.
- Though case fatality rates have improved over the past several decades, morbidity from organ injury is an increasing burden borne by survivors.

Box 7.2: Pitfalls to Avoid

- Children with sepsis may decompensate quickly. One must be cognizant of their risk of morbidity and mortality and avoid being lulled into a false sense of security.
- Hypotension may be a late finding in pediatric septic shock. Avoid delaying diagnostic workup and interventions solely because of normal blood pressure.
- Although obtaining blood and tissue cultures before initiating antibiotics is ideal, antibiotics should not be significantly delayed as delayed antibiotic administration is associated with increased mortality.

References

1. Kissoon N, et al. Sepsis in children: global implications of the world health assembly resolution on sepsis. Pediatr Crit Care Med. 2017;18:e625–7.
2. de Souza DC, et al. Epidemiology of pediatric septic shock. J Pediatr Intensive Care. 2019;8:3–10.
3. Weiss SL, et al. Global epidemiology of pediatric severe sepsis: the sepsis prevalence, outcomes and therapy study. Am J Resp Crit Care Med. 2015;191(10):1147–56.
4. Hartman ME, et al. Trends in the epidemiology of pediatric severe sepsis. Pediatric Crit Care Med. 2013;14:686–93.
5. Schlapbach LJ, et al. Mortality related to invasive infections, sepsis, and septic shock and critically ill children in Australia and New Zealand, 2002– – 13: a multi center retrospective cohort study. Lancet Infect Dis. 2015;15:46–54.
6. Reinhardt K, et al. Recognizing sepsis as a global health priority-a WHO resolution. N Engl J Med. 2017;377:414–7.
7. Weiss SL, et al. Surviving Sepsis campaign international guidelines for the management of septic shock and sepsis associated organ dysfunction in children. Intensive Care Med. 2020;46(1):510–67.
8. Funk DJ, Parrillo JE, Kumar A. Sepsis and septic shock: a history. Crit Care Clin. 2009;25(1):83–101., viii. https://doi.org/10.1016/j.ccc.2008.12.003.
9. Bone RC, Balk RA, Cerra FB, et al. Definitions for sepsis and organ failure and guidelines for the use of innovative therapies in sepsis. Chest. 1992;101(6):1644–55. https://doi.org/10.1378/chest.101.6.1644.
10. Singer M, Deutschman CS, Seymour CW, et al. The third international consensus definitions for sepsis and septic shock (sepsis-3). JAMA. 2016;315(8):801–10. https://doi.org/10.1001/jama.2016.0287.
11. Goldstein B, Giroir B, Randolph A, Sepsis M of the ICC on P. International pediatric sepsis consensus conference: definitions for sepsis and organ dysfunction in pediatrics*. Pediatr Crit Care Med. 2005;6(1):2–8. https://doi.org/10.1097/01.PCC.0000149131.72248.E6.
12. Brilli RJ, Goldstein B. Pediatric sepsis definitions: past, present, and future. Pediatr Crit Care Med. 2005;6(3 Suppl):S6–8. https://doi.org/10.1097/01.PCC.0000161585.48182.69.
13. Menon K, Schlapbach LJ, Akech S, et al. Pediatric sepsis definition—A systematic review protocol by the pediatric sepsis definition taskforce. Crit Care Explor. 2020;2(6) https://doi.org/10.1097/CCE.0000000000000123.
14. Weiss SL, Peters MJ, Alhazzani W, et al. Surviving sepsis campaign international guidelines for the management of septic shock and sepsis-associated organ dysfunction in children. Pediatr Crit Care Med. 2020;21(2):e52–e106. https://doi.org/10.1097/PCC.0000000000002198.
15. Thomas N, Tamburro R, Rajasekaran S, Fitzgerald J, et al. Bacterial sepsis. In: Nichols DG, Shaffner DH, et al., editors. Roger's textbook of pediatric intensive care. 5th ed. Wolters Kluwer: Philadelphia; 2016.
16. Gotts JE, Matthay MA. Sepsis: pathophysiology and clinical management. BMJ. 2016;353:1585. https://doi.org/10.1136/bmj.1585.
17. Prout AJ, Talisa VB, Carcillo JA, Decker BK, Yende S. Bacterial and fungal etiology of sepsis in children in the United States: reconsidering empiric therapy. Crit Care Med. 2020;48(3):e192–9. https://doi.org/10.1097/CCM.0000000000004140.
18. Prout AJ, Talisa VB, Carcillo JA, et al. Children with chronic disease bear the highest burden of pediatric sepsis. J Pediatr. 2018;199:194–199.e1. https://doi.org/10.1016/j.jpeds.2018.03.056.

19. Dhar AV, Huang CJ, Sue PK, et al. Team approach: pediatric musculoskeletal infection. JBJS Rev. 2020;8(3):e0121. https://doi.org/10.2106/JBJS.RVW.19.00121.
20. Dolitsky R, DePaola K, Fernicola J, Collins C. Pediatric musculoskeletal infections. Pediatr Clin N Am. 2020;67(1):59–69. https://doi.org/10.1016/j.pcl.2019.09.001.
21. Gafur OA, Copley LAB, Hollmig ST, Browne RH, Thornton LA, Crawford SE. The impact of the current epidemiology of pediatric musculoskeletal infection on evaluation and treatment guidelines. J Pediatr Orthop. 2008;28(7):777–85. https://doi.org/10.1097/BPO.0b013e318186eb4b.
22. Angus DC, van der Poll T. Severe sepsis and septic shock. N Engl J Med. 2013;369(9):840–51. https://doi.org/10.1056/NEJMra1208623.
23. Nguyen TC, Carcillo JA. Phenotyping sepsis-induced multiple organ dysfunction syndrome. In: Goswami EA, Bhalala US, editors. Current concepts in pediatric critical care. Society of Critical Care Medicine: Mount Prospect; 2020.
24. Gyawali B, Ramakrishna K, Dhamoon AS. Sepsis: the evolution in definition, pathophysiology, and management. SAGE Open Med. 2019;7 https://doi.org/10.1177/2050312119835043.
25. Agbeko RS, Klein NJ, Peters MJ. The immune system. In: Nichols DG, Shaffner DH, et al., editors. Roger's textbook of pediatric intensive care. 5th ed. Wolters Kluwer: Philadelphia; 2016.
26. Aird WC. The role of the endothelium in severe sepsis and multiple organ dysfunction syndrome. Blood. 2003;101(10):3765–77. https://doi.org/10.1182/blood-2002-06-1887.
27. Vallet B. Bench-to-bedside review: endothelial cell dysfunction in severe sepsis: a role in organ dysfunction? Crit Care. 2003;7(2):130–8.
28. Deutschman CS, Tracey KJ. Sepsis: current dogma and new perspectives. Immunity. 2014;40(4):463–75. https://doi.org/10.1016/j.immuni.2014.04.001.
29. Zingarelli B. Shock, ischemia, and reperfusion injury. In: Nichols DG, Shaffner DH, et al., editors. Roger's textbook of pediatric intensive care. 5th ed. Wolters Kluwer: Philadelphia; 2016.
30. Sato R, Nasu M. A review of sepsis-induced cardiomyopathy. J Intensive Care. 2015;3 https://doi.org/10.1186/s40560-015-0112-5.
31. Yager P, Noviski N. Shock. Pediatr Rev. 2010;31(8):311–8.; quiz 319. https://doi.org/10.1542/pir.31-8-311.
32. Roberts JK, Disselkamp M, Yataco AC. Oxygen delivery in septic shock. Ann Am Thorac Soc. 2015;12(6):952–5. https://doi.org/10.1513/AnnalsATS.201501-069CC.
33. Rosen I, Manaker S. Oxygen delivery (DO2) and consumption (VO2). UpToDate. 2021; https://www.uptodate.com/contents/oxygen-delivery-and-consumption?search=oxygen%20delivery%20and%20consumption&source=search_result&selectedTitle=1~150&usage_type=default&display_rank=1
34. Pavare J, Grope I, Gardovska D. Prevalence of systemic inflammatory response syndrome (SIRS) in hospitalized children: a point prevalence study. BMC Pediatr. 2009;9:25. https://doi.org/10.1186/1471-2431-9-25.
35. Davis A, Carcillo JA, Aneja RK, et al. America College of Critical Care Medicine clinical practice parameters for hemodynamic support of pediatric and neonatal septic shock. Crit Care Med. 2017;5:6. https://doi.org/10.1097/CCM.0000000000002425.
36. Ranjit S, Aram G, Kissoon N, et al. Multimodal monitoring for hemodynamic categorization and management of pediatric septic shock: a pilot observational study. Pediatr Crit Care Med. 2014;15:1. https://doi.org/10.1097/PCC.0b013e3182a5589c.
37. Lelubre C, Vincent JL. Mechanisms and treatment of organ failure in sepsis. Nat Rev Nephrol. 2018;14:7. https://doi.org/10.1038/s41581-018-0005-7.
38. Vincent JL, Sakr Y, Sprung CL, et al. Sepsis in European intensive care units: results of the SOAP study. Crit Care Med. 2006;34:2. https://doi.org/10.1097/01.ccm.0000194725.48928.3a.
39. Sakr Y, Lobo SM, Moreno RP, et al. Patterns and early evolution of organ failure in the intensive care unit and their relation to outcome. Crit Care Med. 2012;16:6. https://doi.org/10.1186/cc11868.
40. Hsu HE, Abanyie F, Agus MS, et al. A national approach to pediatric sepsis surveillance. Pediatrics. 2019;144:6. https://doi.org/10.1542/peds.2019-1790.
41. Matics TJ, Sanchez-Pinto LN. Adaptation and validation of a pediatric sequential organ failure assessment score and evaluation of the Sepsis-3 definitions in critically ill children. JAMA Pediatr. 2017;171:10. https://doi.org/10.1001/jamapediatrics.2017.2352.
42. Leteurtre S, Duhamel A, Salleron J, Grandbastien B, Lacroix J, Leclerc F, Groupe Francophone de Réanimation et d'Urgences Pédiatriques (GFRUP). PELOD-2: an update of the pediatric logistic organ dysfunction score. Crit Care Med. 2013;41(7) https://doi.org/10.1097/CCM.0b013e31828a2bbd.
43. Shaffner DH. Rogers' textbook of pediatric intensive care. Chapter 71. [VitalSource Bookshelf]. 2015. Retrieved from https://bookshelf.vitalsource.com/#/books/9781469888392/.
44. Shaffner DH. Rogers' textbook of pediatric intensive care. Chapter 45. [VitalSource Bookshelf]. 2015. Retrieved from https://bookshelf.vitalsource.com/#/books/9781469888392/.
45. Balamuth F, Weiss SL, Fitzgerald JC, Hayes K, Centkowski S, Chilutti M, Grundmeier RW, Lavelle J, Alpern ER. Protocolized treatment is associated with decreased oOrgan dysfunction in pediatric severe sepsis. Pediatr Crit Care Med. 2016;17(9):817–22. https://doi.org/10.1097/PCC.0000000000000858. PMID: 27455114; PMCID: PMC5008999.
46. Fitzgerald JC, Weiss SL, Kissoon N. 2016 update for the Rogers' textbook of pediatric intensive care: recognition and initial management of shock. Pediatr Crit Care Med. 2016;17(11):1073–9. https://doi.org/10.1097/PCC.0000000000000942. PMID: 27749512; PMCID: PMC5389123.

47. Schlapbach LJ. Paediatric sepsis. Curr Opin Infect Dis. 2019;32(5):497–504. https://doi.org/10.1097/QCO.0000000000000583. PMID: 31335441.
48. Society of Critical Care Medicine. Initial Resuscitation Algorithm for Children. 2020. https://www.sccm.org/getattachment/SurvivingSepsisCampaign/Guidelines/Pediatric-Patients/Initial-Resuscitation-Algorithm-for-Children.pdf?lang=en-US
49. Weiss SL, Fitzgerald JC, Balamuth F, Alpern ER, Lavelle J, Chilutti M, Grundmeier R, Nadkarni VM, Thomas NJ. Delayed antimicrobial therapy increases mortality and organ dysfunction duration in pediatric sepsis. Crit Care Med. 2014;42(11):2409–17. https://doi.org/10.1097/CCM.0000000000000509. PMID: 25148597; PMCID: PMC4213742.
50. Weiss SL, Fitzgerald JC, Balamuth F, et al. Delayed antimicrobial therapy increases mortality and organ dysfunction duration in pediatric sepsis. Crit Care Med. 2014;42(11):2409–17. https://doi.org/10.1097/CCM.0000000000000509.
51. Martínez ML, Ferrer R, Torrents E, Guillamat-Prats R, Gomà G, Suárez D, Álvarez-Rocha L, Pozo Laderas JC, Martín-Loeches I, Levy MM, Artigas A, Edusepsis Study Group. Impact of source control in patients with severe sepsis and septic shock. Crit Care Med. 2017;45(1):11–9. https://doi.org/10.1097/CCM.0000000000002011. PMID: 27611975.
52. Maitland K, Kiguli S, Opoka RO, Engoru C, Olupot-Olupot P, Akech SO, Nyeko R, Mtove G, Reyburn H, Lang T, Brent B, Evans JA, Tibenderana JK, Crawley J, Russell EC, Levin M, Babiker AG, Gibb DM, FEAST Trial Group. Mortality after fluid bolus in African children with severe infection. N Engl J Med. 2011;364(26):2483–95. https://doi.org/10.1056/NEJMoa1101549. Epub 2011 May 26. PMID: 21615299.
53. Carcillo JA, Davis AL, Zaritsky A. Role of early fluid resuscitation in pediatric septic shock. JAMA. 1991;266(9):1242–5. PMID: 1870250.
54. American Heart Association. Highlights of the 2020 American Heart Association Guidelines for CPR and ECC. Eccguidelines.heart.org. 2020.
55. Emrath ET, Fortenberry JD, Travers C, McCracken CE, Hebbar KB. Resuscitation with balanced fluids is associated with improved survival in pediatric severe sepsis. Crit Care Med. 2017;45(7):1177–83. https://doi.org/10.1097/CCM.0000000000002365. PMID: 28437373.
56. Semler MW, Self WH, Wanderer JP, Ehrenfeld JM, Wang L, Byrne DW, Stollings JL, Kumar AB, Hughes CG, Hernandez A, Guillamondegui OD, May AK, Weavind L, Casey JD, Siew ED, Shaw AD, Bernard GR, Rice TW, SMART Investigators and the Pragmatic Critical Care Research Group. Balanced crystalloids versus saline in critically ill adults. N Engl J Med. 2018;378(9):829–39. https://doi.org/10.1056/NEJMoa1711584. Epub 2018 Feb 27. PMID: 29485925; PMCID: PMC5846085.
57. Ventura AM, Shieh HH, Bousso A, Góes PF, de Cássia FO, Fernandes I, de Souza DC, Paulo RL, Chagas F, Gilio AE. Double-blind prospective randomized controlled trial of dopamine versus epinephrine as first-line vasoactive drugs in pediatric septic shock. Crit Care Med. 2015;43(11):2292–302. https://doi.org/10.1097/CCM.0000000000001260. PMID: 26323041.
58. Ramaswamy KN, Singhi S, Jayashree M, Bansal A, Nallasamy K. Double-blind randomized clinical trial comparing dopamine and epinephrine in pediatric fluid-refractory hypotensive septic shock. Pediatr Crit Care Med. 2016;17(11):e502–12. https://doi.org/10.1097/PCC.0000000000000954. PMID: 27673385.
59. Walker SB, Conlon TW, Zhang B, Mensinger JL, Fitzgerald JC, Himebauch AS, Glau C, Nishisaki A, Ranjit S, Nadkarni V, Weiss SL. Clinical signs to categorize shock and target vasoactive medications in warm versus cold pediatric septic shock. Pediatr Crit Care Med. 2020;21(12):1051–8. https://doi.org/10.1097/PCC.0000000000002481. PMID: 32740190.
60. Shaffner DH. Rogers' textbook of pediatric intensive care. Chapter 22. [VitalSource Bookshelf]. 2015. Retrieved from https://bookshelf.vitalsource.com/#/books/9781469888392/.
61. Patregnani JT, Sochet AA, Klugman D. Short-term peripheral vasoactive infusions in pediatrics: where is the harm? Pediatr Crit Care Med. 2017;18(8):e378–81. https://doi.org/10.1097/PCC.0000000000001230. PMID: 28617763.
62. Sutherland SM, Zappitelli M, Alexander SR, Chua AN, Brophy PD, Bunchman TE, Hackbarth R, Somers MJ, Baum M, Symons JM, Flores FX, Benfield M, Askenazi D, Chand D, Fortenberry JD, Mahan JD, McBryde K, Blowey D, Goldstein SL. Fluid overload and mortality in children receiving continuous renal replacement therapy: the prospective pediatric continuous renal replacement therapy registry. Am J Kidney Dis. 2010;55(2):316–25. https://doi.org/10.1053/j.ajkd.2009.10.048. Epub 2009 Dec 30. PMID: 20042260.
63. Palevsky PM. Indications and timing of renal replacement therapy in acute kidney injury. Crit Care Med. 2008;36(4 Suppl):S224–8. https://doi.org/10.1097/CCM.0b013e318168e3fb. PMID: 18382198.
64. Gulla KM, Sachdev A, Gupta D, Gupta N, Anand K, Pruthi PK. Continuous renal replacement therapy in children with severe sepsis and multiorgan dysfunction – A pilot study on timing of initiation. Indian J Crit Care Med. 2015;19(10):613–7. https://doi.org/10.4103/0972-5229.167044. PMID: 26628828; PMCID: PMC4637963.
65. Chang TH, Wu ET, Lu CY, Huang SC, Yang TI, Wang CC, Chen JM, Lee PI, Huang LM, Chang LY. Pathogens and outcomes in pediatric septic shock patients supported by extracorporeal membrane oxygenation. J Microbiol Immunol Infect. 2018;51(3):385–91. https://doi.org/10.1016/j.jmii.2017.07.012. Epub 2017 Aug 4. PMID: 28821378.
66. Parks T, Wilson C, Curtis N, Norrby-Teglund A, Sriskandan S. Polyspecific intravenous immunoglobulin in clindamycin-treated patients with streptococ-

cal toxic shock syndrome: a systematic review and meta-analysis. Clin Infect Dis. 2018;67(9):1434–6. https://doi.org/10.1093/cid/ciy401. PMID: 29788397; PMCID: PMC6186853.
67. Lima LM, McCracken CE, Fortenberry JD, Hebbar KB. Use of plasma exchange in pediatric severe sepsis in children's hospitals. J Crit Care. 2018;45:114–20. https://doi.org/10.1016/j.jcrc.2018.01.028. Epub 2018 Feb 3. PMID: 29433093.
68. Rimmer E, Houston BL, Kumar A, Abou-Setta AM, Friesen C, Marshall JC, Rock G, Turgeon AF, Cook DJ, Houston DS, Zarychanski R. The efficacy and safety of plasma exchange in patients with sepsis and septic shock: a systematic review and meta-analysis. Crit Care. 2014;18(6):699. https://doi.org/10.1186/s13054-014-0699-2. PMID: 25527094; PMCID: PMC4318234.
69. Dünser MW, Festic E, Dondorp A, et al. Recommendations for sepsis management in resource-limited settings. Intensive Care Med. 2012;38(4):557–74. https://doi.org/10.1007/s00134-012-2468-5.
70. Murthy S, Adhikari NK. Global health care of the critically ill in low-resource settings. Annals ATS. 2013;10(5):509–13. https://doi.org/10.1513/AnnalsATS.201307-246OT.
71. Rudd KE, Johnson SC, Agesa KM, et al. Global, regional, and national sepsis incidence and mortality, 1990–2017: analysis for the global burden of disease study. Lancet. 2020;395(10219):200–11. https://doi.org/10.1016/S0140-6736(19)32989-7.
72. Chan M, Lake A. Towards ending preventable child deaths. Lancet. 2012;379(9832):2119–20. https://doi.org/10.1016/S0140-6736(12)60908-8.
73. Kissoon N, Carapetis J. Pediatric sepsis in the developing world. J Infect. 2015;71(Suppl 1):S21–6. https://doi.org/10.1016/j.jinf.2015.04.016.
74. Huynh B-T, Padget M, Garin B, et al. Burden of bacterial resistance among neonatal infections in low income countries: how convincing is the epidemiological evidence? BMC Infect Dis. 2015;15:127. https://doi.org/10.1186/s12879-015-0843-x.
75. Agulnik A, Mora Robles LN, Forbes PW, et al. Improved outcomes after successful implementation of a pediatric early warning system (PEWS) in a resource-limited pediatric oncology hospital. Cancer. 2017;123(15):2965–74. https://doi.org/10.1002/cncr.30664.
76. Nielsen KR, Aronés Rojas R, Tantaleán da Fieno J, Huicho L, Roberts JS, Zunt J. Emergency department risk factors for serious clinical deterioration in a paediatric hospital in Peru. J Paediatr Child Health. 2018;54(8):866–71. https://doi.org/10.1111/jpc.13904.
77. George EC, Walker AS, Kiguli S, et al. Predicting mortality in sick African children: the FEAST Paediatric Emergency Triage (PET) Score. BMC Med. 2015;13(1):174. https://doi.org/10.1186/s12916-015-0407-3.
78. Olson D, Preidis GA, Milazi R, et al. Task shifting an inpatient triage, assessment and treatment programme improves the quality of care for hospitalised Malawian children. Tropical Med Int Health. 2013;18(7):879–86. https://doi.org/10.1111/tmi.12114.
79. Ruth A, et al. Pediatric severe sepsis: current trends and outcomes from the pediatric health information systems database. Pediatr Crit Care Med. 2014;15(9):828–38.
80. Tan B, et al. Global case fatality rate in pediatric severe sepsis and septic shock: a systematic review and meta-analysis. JAMA Pediatr. 2019;173:352–61.
81. Zimmerman J, et al. Critical illness factors associated with long term mortality and health related quality-of-life morbidity following community acquired pediatric septic shock. Crit Care Med. 2020;4(83):319–28.
82. Zimmerman J, et al. Trajectory of mortality and health related quality-of-life morbidity following community acquired pediatric septic shock. Crit Care Med. 2020;48(3):329–37.
83. Nadal S, et al. Researching severe sepsis and organ dysfunction in children: a global perspective RESOLVE study group: Drotrecogin alpha in children with severe sepsis: a multi center phase 3 randomized controlled trial. Lancet. 2007;369:836–43.
84. Farris RW. Functional outcomes in pediatric severe sepsis: further analysis of the researching severe sepsis and organ dysfunction in children: a global perspective trial. Pediatr Crit Care Med. 2013;14:835–42.
85. Lin JC, et al. Sepsis pPrevalence, outcomes, and therapy study investigators: new or progressive multiple organ dysfunction syndrome in pediatric severe sepsis: a sepsis phenotype with higher morbidity and mortality. Pediatr Crit Care Med. 2017;18:8–16.
86. Mignemi ME, Benvenuti MA, An TJ, Martus JE, Mencio GA, Lovejoy SA, et al. A novel classification system based on dissemination of musculoskeletal infection is predictive of hospital outcomes. J Pediatr Orthop. 2018;38(5):279–86.
87. Vorhies JS, Lindsay EA, Tareen NG, Kellum RJ, Jo CH, Copley LA. Severity adjusted risk of long-term adverse sequelae among children with osteomyelitis. Pediatr Infect Dis J. 2019;38(1):26–31.
88. Watson RS, et al. The epidemiology a severe sepsis in children in the United States. Am J Respir Crit Care Med. 2003;167:695.
89. Kutko MC, et al. Mortality rates in pediatrics septic shock with and without multiple organ system failure. Pediatr Crit Care Med. 2003;4:333.
90. Prouix F, et al. Epidemiology of sepsis and multiple organ dysfunction syndrome in children. Chest. 1996;109:1033.
91. Graciano AL, et al. The pediatric multiple organ dysfunction score P-MODS: dDevelopment and validation of an objective scale to measure the severity of multiple organ dysfunction in critically ill children. Crit Care Med. 2005;33:1484.

Local Antibiotic Drug Delivery Systems for Musculoskeletal Infections

8

Jessica Burns, Martin McNally, and Janet Conway

Introduction and Epidemiology

Pediatric musculoskeletal infection often requires treatment with prolonged antibiotics in order to eradicate the infection [1–3]. The development of penicillin in the 1940s revolutionized the treatment of pediatric acute hematogenous osteomyelitis, reducing the morbidity and mortality of the disease itself, as well as the morbidity associated with extensive and repeat surgery [4–7]. Over time, inappropriate use of antibiotics has caused the development of and amplified the prevalence of extensively drug-resistant and multidrug-resistant organisms. Multidrug-resistant organisms are defined as microbes with resistance to at least three antibiotic classes that the organism would typically be susceptible to. This transformation is due to transmission of genetic materials that lead to resistance [8, 9].

Multidrug resistance in infections is a major global public health burden, estimated to lead to ten million deaths globally in 2050, surpassing the rates of cancer death [10, 11]. The presence of these organisms has been shown to result in poorer outcomes in patients with bone infection [12]. In addition to the burden secondary to multidrug-resistant organisms, musculoskeletal infection is further complicated by the formation of biofilms. Two-thirds of human infections are thought to be related to biofilm formation [13]. Biofilms evade the host immune system and systemic antimicrobial treatment due to their complex three-dimensional communities that produce extracellular polysaccharides (EPSs). This structure allows for facile transmission of genetic material that can incur resistance to antimicrobials. Furthermore, the EPSs allow for adherence to a surface with the ability to avoid penetration of antibiotics or the host immune system [14–16]. In children, biofilms form on surfaces without significant biologic activity, which is most commonly necrotic bone, orthopedic implants, or both. The treatment options for these challenging infections include surgical debridement and extended antimicrobial therapy [14, 16]. These treatment options have limitations, since prolonged systemic antibiotic therapy is associated with increased complications [17, 18]. The potential for locally delivered treatment has

J. Burns (✉)
Department of Child Health, The University of Arizona College of Medicine – Phoenix, Phoenix, AZ, USA

Phoenix Children's Hospital, Phoenix, AZ, USA
e-mail: jburns@phoenixchildrens.com

M. McNally
Oxford Bone Infection Unit, Oxford University Hospitals, Oxford, UK
e-mail: Martin.Mcnally@ouh.nhs.uk

J. Conway
International Center for Limb Lengthening, Rubin Institute for Advanced Orthopaedics, Sinai Hospital of Baltimore, Baltimore, MD, USA
e-mail: JConway@lifebridgehealth.org

© Springer Nature Switzerland AG 2022
M. V. Belthur et al. (eds.), *Pediatric Musculoskeletal Infections*,
https://doi.org/10.1007/978-3-030-95794-0_8

implications to improve the outcome for the patient, while potentially reducing cost [19].

In the cases of challenging infections with biofilm formation, local delivery vehicles can be utilized to dispense a high concentration of antimicrobial directly into the infected area. Tissues that are chronically infected or have the presence of an implant have poor perfusion, making systemic therapy ineffective treatment [20]. The concentration of the antibiotic delivered systemically that would be necessary to eradicate the infection would cause significant adverse reactions. Biofilms can only be eradicated once the minimum eradication concentration has been reached (MBEC), which is harder to achieve than the standard minimum inhibitory concentration (MIC) for planktonic bacteria. Local antimicrobial delivery devices have the ability to achieve high concentrations of antimicrobials without the complications associated with systemic administration. Furthermore, local delivery can be utilized when the biofilm has formed over a large surface area that complete surgical debridement would lead to severe bone and soft tissue loss, create a large void or dead space, or a dysfunctional limb [19, 21–25].

The most common local delivery vehicle is antimicrobial loaded poly(methyl methacrylate) (PMMA). Biodegradable ceramics have become increasingly popular, as they do not require surgical removal but are still biocompatible, are capable of elution of high concentration of antimicrobials, and provide some mechanical strength to fill dead space. These biodegradable ceramics are based on either calcium sulfate, calcium phosphate, or both [24].

The indications for incorporation of local delivery vehicles in pediatric musculoskeletal infection are controversial. Published indications include acute hematogenous osteomyelitis (AHO) [26] and chronic osteomyelitis with and without fracture or bone defects [21, 23, 27]. The literature is further weakened by the lack of prospective studies in pediatrics. There are many variables and controversies in indications that limit the ability to study these applications broadly.

Pathology

Chronic Osteomyelitis

Chronic osteomyelitis can develop after acute hematogenous osteomyelitis, open fractures, or septic arthritis in children. The persistence of infection beyond 6–12 weeks or the development of dead bone defines chronicity and occurs most commonly secondary to delay in presentation or suboptimal initial treatment of the acute infection (Fig. 8.1). Chronic osteomyelitis often results in bone necrosis, called sequestrum with new bone formation around this area, called involucrum. The sequestrum has no associated blood supply and becomes isolated from host immune response and penetration of antibiotics. While acute osteomyelitis may be treatable with antibiotics alone, the presence of sequestrum mandates surgical intervention. Dead bone must be removed, leaving only well perfused, viable bone [28–33]. The combination of pathogen and host factors contributes to the development of chronic osteomyelitis. Patients with underlying malnutrition, diabetes, chronic steroid use, immunocompromised status, or presence of malignancy are at increased risk for persistence of disease despite appropriate treatment [32–34]. Furthermore, specific gene expression, particularly in *Staphylococcus aureus*, leads to a more virulent and adherent form, leading to biofilm formation [29].

Treatment of chronic osteomyelitis is challenging and costly [28, 32, 33]. In pediatric patients, the combination of surgery and pathogen-specific antimicrobials are recommended. Surgery is necessary for debridement of necrotic bone and biofilm, sequestrectomy, and implant or foreign body removal. This is requisite for the penetration of systemic antimicrobials to the remaining planktonic bacteria. Additionally, surgery may be required to stabilize associated fracture deformity associated with infected non-union of fracture. After surgical debridement, dead space management is critical to lessen the morbidity and to promote healing. Dead space is a void in the anatomic structure of bone that pre-

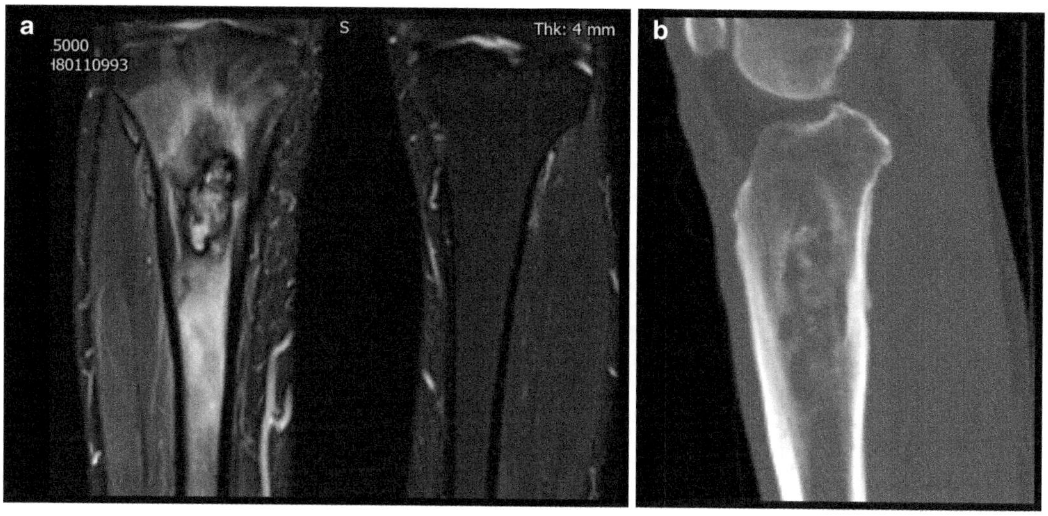

Fig. 8.1 A patient initially presented with knee pain, which was treated with oral antibiotics for several weeks. He later presented with fever, pain, redness, and swelling around the proximal tibia. An MRI (**a**) obtained shows the typical features of chronic osteomyelitis with medullary edema, periosteal reaction, and central dead bone with necrosis. The CT scan (**b**) demonstrates fragments of dead bone (sequestra) within the proximal metadiaphysis. There is also new bone formation posteriorly (involucrum). (Imaging courtesy of the Oxford Bone Infection Unit, UK)

vents the body's innate ability to heal. Options for dead space management include local delivery vehicles. Poly(methyl methacrylate) (PMMA) has been used for this purpose since the 1970s with the ability to fill voids, provide limited mechanical structure, and elute antibiotics [19, 30]. However, PMMA prevents the growth of normal tissue into the void and so can only be regarded as a temporary void filler, which needs to be removed and often replaced with bone graft [35, 36]. More recently, bioceramics may allow a single-stage treatment by filling the dead space, delivering antimicrobials, and allowing bone ingrowth [37, 38].

Biofilms

It is estimated that two-thirds of all human infections are related to biofilm formation, with a huge economic, social, and clinical burden in regard to musculoskeletal infections [39]. Biofilms are a complex, highly organized, three-dimensional accumulation of microorganisms that can consist of one or more species. Although most commonly formed by Gram-positive bacteria in musculoskeletal infections, Gram-negative bacteria and fungi can establish biofilms. Compared to planktonic microorganisms, they are less metabolically active and do not replicate rapidly.

The classic biofilm model formation includes adhesion, production of extracellular polymeric substances (EPSs) and cellular aggregation, maturation into microcolonies, and finally dissemination of the biofilm (Fig. 8.2). They are able to adhere to host tissue and to implants but are also found as floating aggregates. Adherence is facilitated by microorganism matrix components such as fibronectin and sialoproteins. Once adhesion has occurred, the microorganisms become more sessile and form extracellular polymeric substances (EPSs). There is a high density of microorganisms in biofilms at this stage, which facilitates horizontal transfer of genetic material, which can increase their resistance patterns. If a foreign implant is present, fewer cells are needed to establish an infection and less virulent organ-

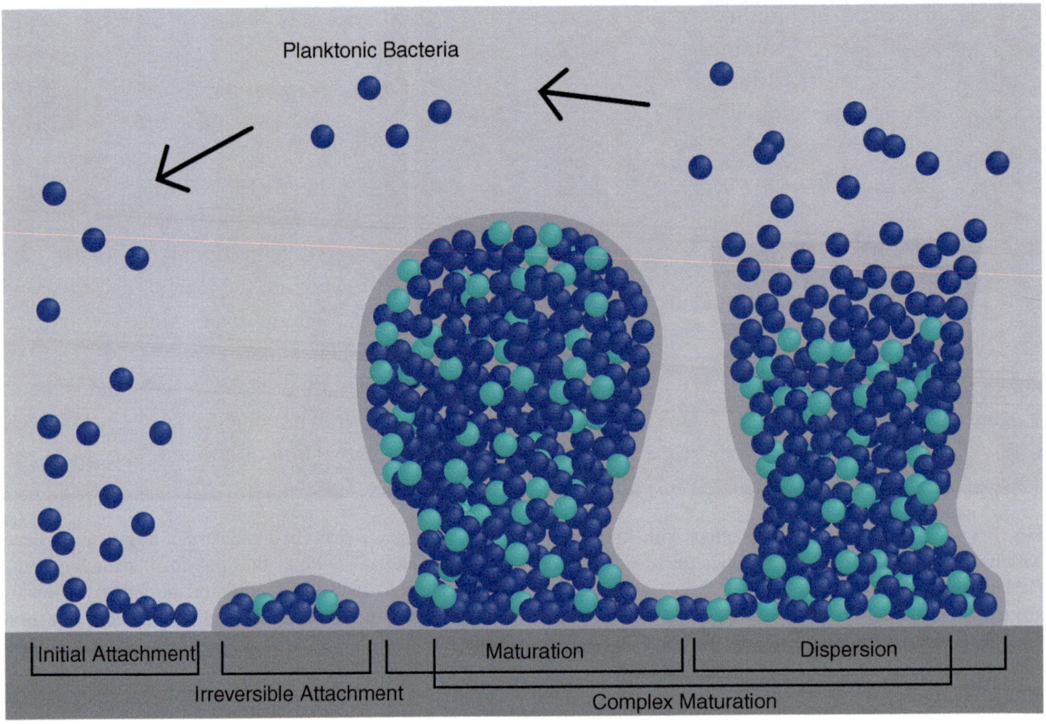

Fig. 8.2 Stages of biofilm development. Planktonic microorganisms adhere to a surface and can invade host cells. This stage is reversible. The bacteria then begin to form microcolonies with aggregation of cells and formation of extracellular polysaccharides (EPSs). The colonies begin to mature and form a three-dimensional structure formation. As the complexity of the structure increases, the biofilm maturates and is able to disperse planktonic bacteria systemically. (Illustration courtesy of Carlie Brooks, BS, USA)

isms, such as *Staphylococcus epidermidis*, and fungi can survive and colonize. The colonies then mature, remodel, and even form towers. There is then dispersal of the microorganism, which can return to its planktonic state, disseminate, and cause systemic infection [13–16]. Fungal osteomyelitis is rare but is a highly problematic and difficult condition to treat and can present up to 3 years after inoculation. Although traditionally thought to be limited to immunocompromised patients, the incidence of fungal osteomyelitis is increasing in immunocompetent patients. Biofilm formation by *Candida* spp. and *Aspergillus* spp. make treatment in orthopedic infections challenging to manage. Treatment usually necessitates surgical debridement in conjunction with prolonged systemic antifungal therapy secondary to biofilm formation [40, 41].

A defining feature that makes biofilms difficult to treat is the ability to evade the host immune system and conventional antimicrobial therapy. One method utilized to accomplish this is the invasion of host cells, such as osteoblasts with as little as 2 hours of exposure. This invasion allows the microorganisms to avoid systemic antimicrobial therapy and then can colonize the area by inducing apoptosis. Furthermore, a mature biofilm has a dense polymeric matrix that prevents some leukocyte phagocytosis. If leukocytes are able to penetrate the biofilm, they are impaired in their function, with reduced ability to clear the biofilm [14]. This has been termed “frustrated phagocytosis.” Antibiotics can be utilized to clear biofilms, but conventional therapy is ineffective unless concentrations are around 1000 times traditional doses. Local delivery vehicles have the ability to deliver high concentrations of antimicrobials at the site of biofilm formation, but it must be able to reach the minimum biofilm eradication concentration (MBEC) of that particular microorganism. The elution of antimicrobials from drug delivery vehicles, most commonly PMMA, has been studied in regard to MBEC and can be utilized clinically to assist in treatment of the biofilm formation [42].

Delivery Vehicles

PMMA

Poly(methyl methacrylate) (PMMA) is a synthetic acrylic that was first utilized industrially in airplane canopies and periscopes under the trade name Plexiglass in the 1930s. It was inadvertently found to be biocompatible and was initially used to make contact lenses and dentures. Dr. John Charnley first applied this acrylic to orthopedics for hip arthroplasty in the 1950s but modified it to improve its characteristics, labeling it "bone cement." Commercially available PMMA has solid and liquid components. The solid powder contains the polymer, the catalyst, and a radio-opaque material, while the liquid portion contains the monomer, a reaction accelerator, and a stabilizer [43].

PMMA has the ability to be modified to include antibiotics, which is also termed antibiotic-loaded bone cement (ALBC). This was first developed in the 1970s for the treatment and prevention of periprosthetic joint infection. Antibiotics elute from PMMA in a dose-dependent fashion. The antibiotic elution also depends on many factors, including the porosity of the PMMA used, the surface area of the ALBC, the solubility of the antibiotic, and the dose of the antibiotic. Generally, ALBC with PMMA will elute high levels of antibiotic for several days after implantation. Beyond 3 weeks, the carrier should not be retained as it will elute subtherapeutic levels of antimicrobials which can induce resistance [44]. The dose of antibiotics that are loaded into PMMA depends on the type of antibiotic and whether the antibiotic will be used for treatment or for prophylaxis. The surgeon has the option to mix antibiotics in during the surgical preparation or use commercially prepared ALBC [27] (Fig. 8.3).

Aminoglycosides (gentamicin or tobramycin) are generally recommended for culture-negative infections, due to their activity against both Gram-positive and Gram-negative bacteria, with favorable elution properties from PMMA. It should be noted that PMMA cures in a highly exothermic reaction (70 °C), so only heat-stable antibiotics can be added. In the case of fungal implant or bone infection, locally delivered high concentration antifungals have been proposed for treatment. PMMA can be loaded with either amphotericin B or voriconazole, but each has limitations in elution and subsequent reduction in PMMA biomechanical properties, respectively. Alternative antifungals, such as caspofungin, have been proposed, but there is limited published data on the matter [40, 41, 45–48].

The clinical application of PMMA has several limitations. The biomechanical properties of ALBC are changed due to the addition of antibiotics which further change after the elution of the antibiotic. The well-described reduction in compressive strength limits how long the PMMA can be retained and can even lead to fracture of the cement. In addition to changes in the biomechanics, PMMA is not bioabsorbable. When fashioned as a spacer or beads for treatment of osteomyelitis, PMMA requires a subsequent operation for removal [19, 30, 43, 49].

Bioabsorbable Ceramics

An increasingly popular alternative to PMMA are bone graft substitutes loaded with antibiotics, which have the advantage of being bioabsorbable [50]. Additionally, they are osteoconductive, encouraging new bone growth in bone defects. Bone graft substitutes commonly include calcium sulfates (CS), calcium phosphates, and combinations. CS has specifically been commer-

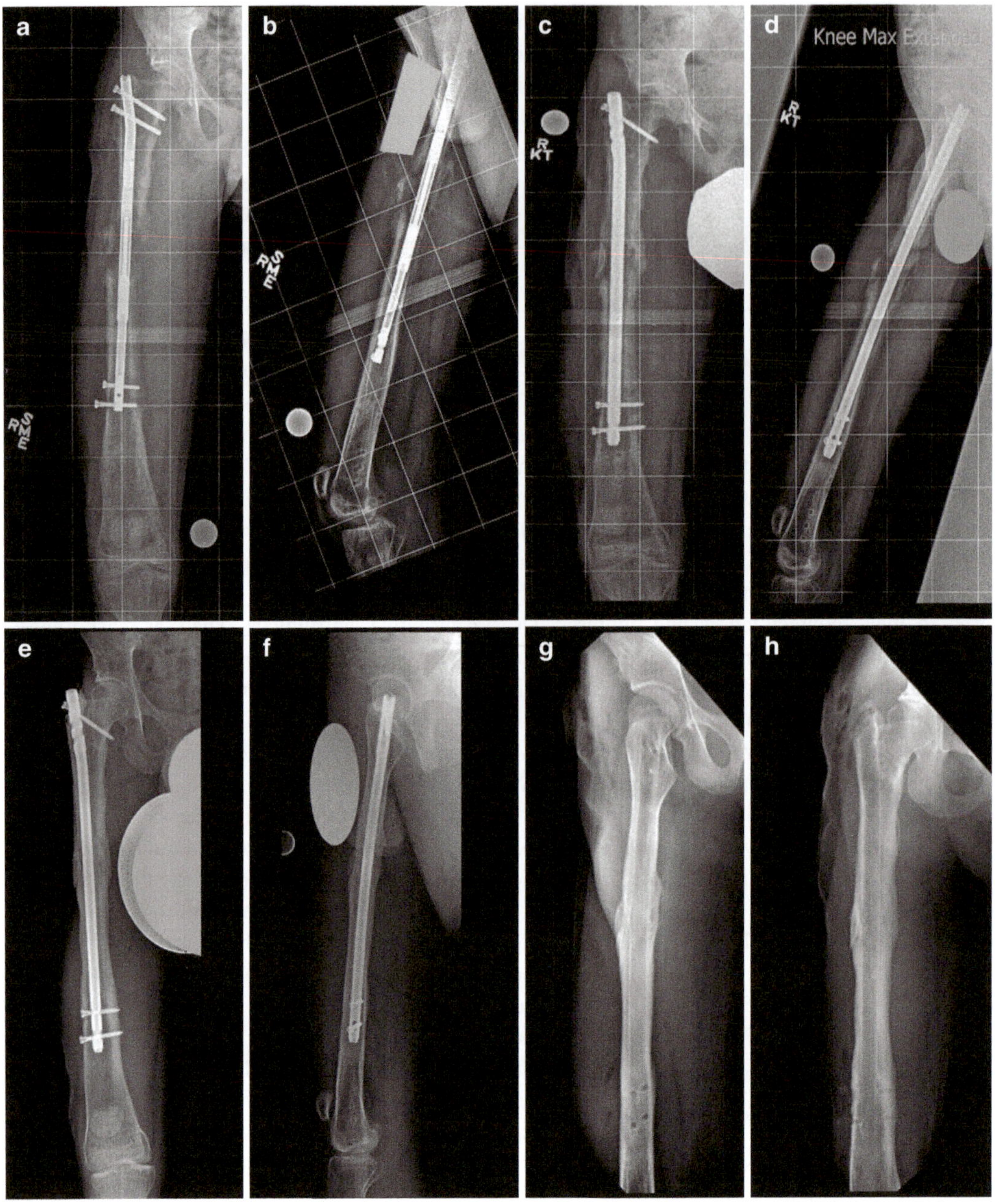

Fig. 8.3 A 15-year-old male with leg length discrepancy who underwent lengthening over an intramedullary nail. He presented postoperatively with wound drainage and radiographic appearance of osteomyelitis (**a**, **b**). The patient underwent rod exchange with an antibiotic-loaded cement coated intramedullary nail (**c**, **d**). Four years later, he had union of the osteotomy site and was symptom-free (**e**, **f**). He subsequently had removal of the antibiotic-coated nail 5 years after initial placement of the lengthening intramedullary nail (**g**, **h**)

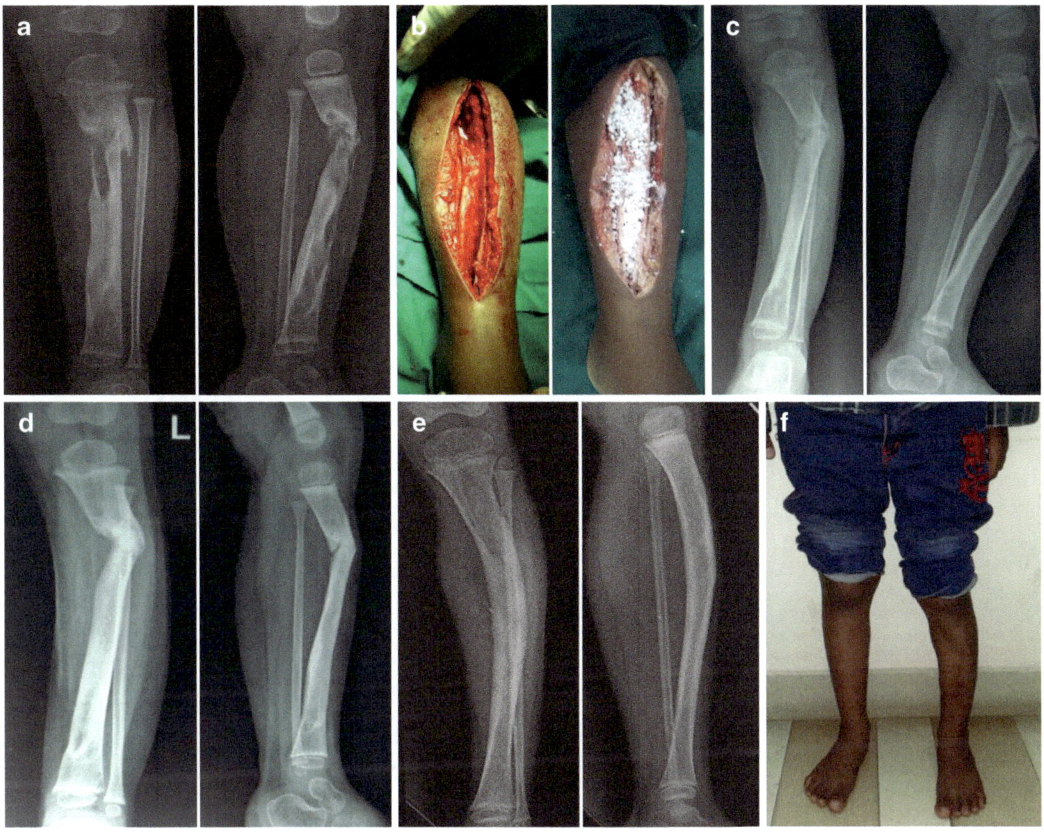

Fig. 8.4 An 18-month-old male who developed chronic osteomyelitis of the left tibia (**a**). The patient underwent extensive debridement with placement of calcium sulfate pellets loaded with vancomycin and gentamicin (**b**). Three months post-op, the diaphysis is consolidating with fracture present in the proximal tibia (**c**). Eleven months post-op, the patient has procurvatum and varus deformity of the tibia (**d**). Three years post-op, the patient is remodeling, has no recurrence of disease, and is pain-free (**e**, **f**). (Case courtesy of Jayanth Sampath, MD, FRCS Bangalore, India)

cially manufactured to include tobramycin and gentamicin but can also be fashioned to elute the antibiotic of the surgeon's choice (Figs. 8.4 and 8.5). A systematic review evaluating the effectiveness of these ceramics in skeletally mature patients showed that infection eradication varied from 80% to 100%, bone ingrowth ranged from 87.5% to 100%, and it had near 100% absorption of the graft material [51]. The addition of hydroxyapatite to calcium sulfate with gentamicin has been shown to increase bone formation in infected defects after surgical resection [52] (Fig. 8.6).

There has been one randomized controlled trial comparing PMMA to calcium sulfate, both commercially preloaded with tobramycin. Thirty skeletally mature patients that needed surgical intervention for chronic long bone osteomyelitis or infected non-union were randomized to surgical debridement and either calcium sulfate or PMMA to fill the bone void. Infection was eradicated in 86% of both groups. Union was achieved in seven of eight of the calcium sulfate group and six of eight of the PMMA group. Five patients required more surgery in the calcium sulfate group, compared to nine in the PMMA

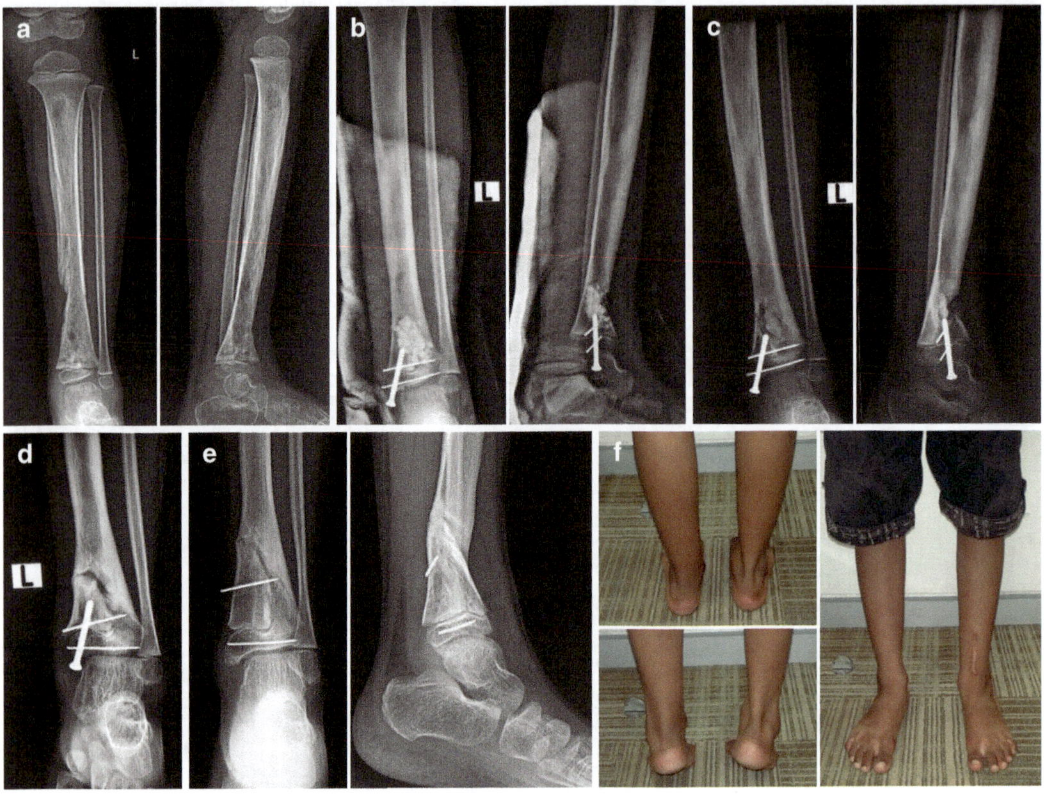

Fig. 8.5 A 4-year-old male with chronic osteomyelitis and associated lateral distal tibia physeal bar causing valgus deformity at the ankle (**a**). The patient had a single-stage surgical debridement, bar excision, and distal tibia medial screw for growth modulation. Calcium sulfate pellets loaded with vancomycin and gentamicin were placed in the bony defect (**b**). One month post-op, the bone graft substitute is visualized in the distal tibia metaphysis with defect seen anteriorly (**c**). Eleven months postoperatively, the patient shows improvement in valgus alignment but has incomplete union of the bony defect (**d**). Four years postoperatively, the patient has no significant coronal plane or clinical deformity, has no recurrence of disease, and is pain-free (**e**, **f**). (Case courtesy of Jayanth Sampath, MD, FRCS Bangalore, India)

group. The repeat operations in the PMMA group were also of greater magnitude. The authors concluded that the outcomes between the two local antibiotic delivery systems are similar, with the exception of reoperation rate in the PMMA group [53]. CS has the limitation of increased rate of wound discharge, which is usually aseptic but can be associated with recurrence of infection. This has been observed in up to 20% of cases. Discernment between the commonly observed fluid discharge of the wound and infection recurrence can be challenging [54].

Other Delivery Vehicles

Other types of delivery vehicles include polyurethane scaffolds (PUR), which are also capable of drug elution and are bioabsorbable. Patient-specific scaffolds can be 3D printed from the combination of polycaprolactone (PCL) and poly(lactic-co-glycolic acid) (PLGA) that can be shaped specifically for a patient while eluting antibiotics. Microspheres are an additional local delivery vehicle that contains a polymer shell surrounding an antibiotic. These can be utilized

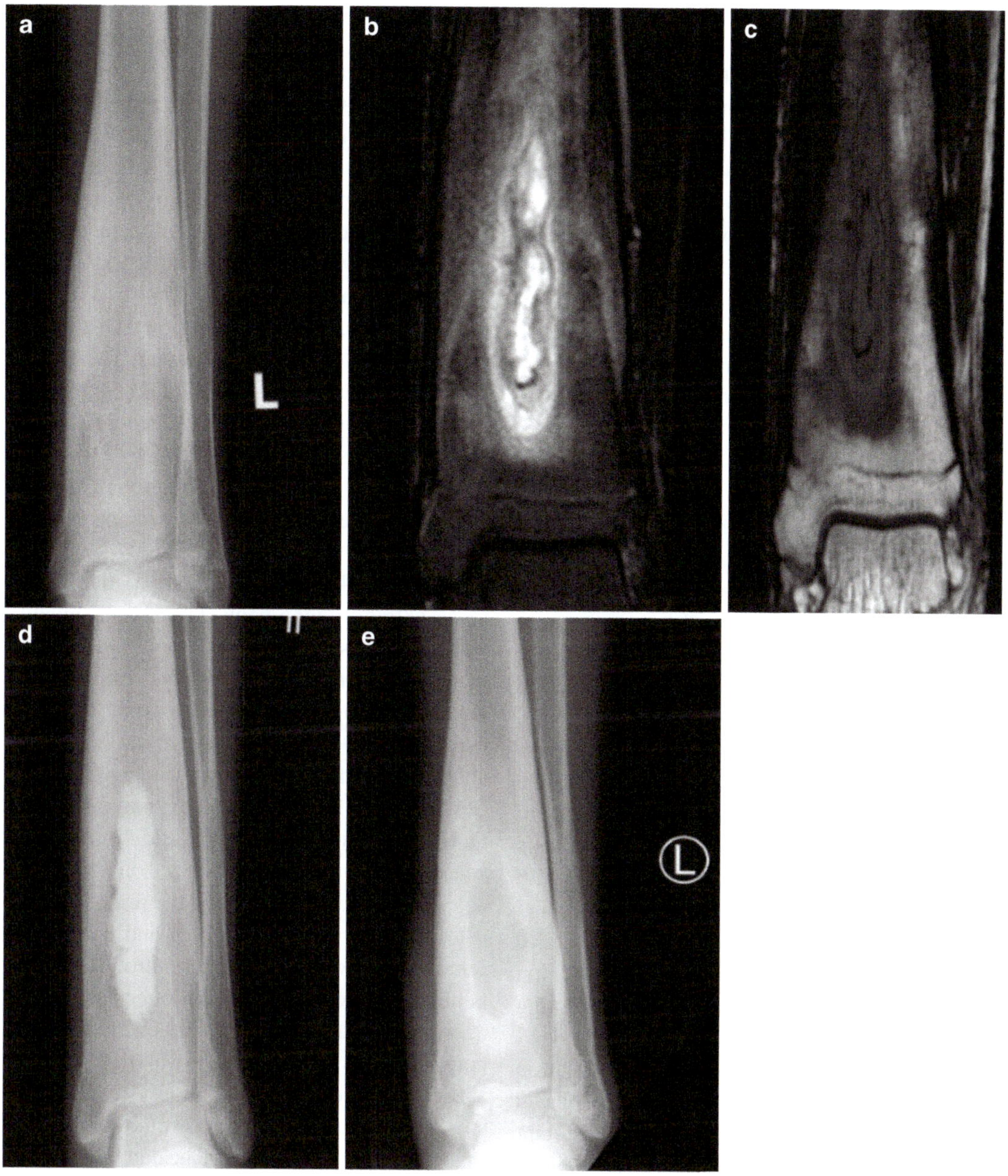

Fig. 8.6 The patient presented with 7 months of pain and ankle swelling without history of trauma or constitutional symptoms. Plain radiographs (**a**) showed widening of the tibial metaphysis due to involucrum formation and central bone lysis. The diagnosis of a Brodie's abscess was suspected (sub-acute medullary hematogenous osteomyelitis). MRI obtained confirmed this diagnosis (**b**, **c**). The infected dead bone was excised, and the dead space was filled with calcium sulfate and hydroxyapatite with gentamicin and vancomycin (Cerament G and V, Bonesupport AB, Lund, Sweden) (**d**). The cultures speciated with *Staphylococcus aureus* and he was given oral flucloxacillin for 6 weeks. Two years after surgery, he had a well healed limb with no pain and good new bone formation in the distal tibia (**e**). (Imaging courtesy of the Oxford Bone Infection Unit, UK)

in combination with polymeric scaffolds [19]. Additionally, water-based hydrogels, such as alginate, chitosan, silk, gelatin, and keratin, have been utilized for drug elution. The gels are able to be customized to optimize the elution properties of the antibiotic. Sponges composed of collagen and chitosan have been used to locally deliver antibiotics and are bioabsorbable and have shown to be able to clear biofilms [55].

Local Antimicrobials in Pediatric Musculoskeletal Infections

Osteomyelitis

Acute bone infections in children can often be managed with systemic antibiotics alone, and there is rarely an indication for local therapy [56]. Chronic osteomyelitis is the most frequent indication for the use of local antibiotic delivery systems in pediatric orthopedics. Although PMMA and bioabsorbable ceramics loaded with antibiotics have been reported for use in pediatrics in the literature, specific indications for the use of these delivery vehicles are not clearly defined. In a study by Ellur et al., 34 patients with chronic osteomyelitis were treated with sequestrectomy, wide surgical debridement, and extensive lavage with saline, hydrogen peroxide (3%), and aqueous povidone-iodine. Antibiotic impregnated pellets were prepared by mixing dry calcium sulfate with 1 g of vancomycin powder and combining it with gentamicin solution (240 mg/6 mL) to create a paste that was placed into a mold mat to form pellets. The resultant dead space was filled with the antibiotic pellets. At an average of 42 month follow-up in 31 of the 34 patients, all patients had been cured of the disease. All patients had resorption of the pellets and radiographic bone healing at an average of 3 months. Three patients did experience serous discharge from the surgical wound, which was managed with local wound care [22] (Figs. 8.4 and 8.5).

In a study by Andreacchio et al., 12 pediatric patients with chronic osteomyelitis of the long bones were treated with single-stage surgery including resection of necrotic bone, soft tissue debridement, curettage and reaming of the intramedullary canal, and placement of prepackaged 3.3-mm calcium sulfate pellets imbedded with 4% tobramycin. The pellets were utilized to fill the associated bone defect after debridement of necrotic bone, ranging from 10 to 30 mL without the use of internal fixation. All patients were treated with systemic antibiotics for 14–90 days. No patients had recurrence, pathologic fracture, nephrotoxicity, ototoxicity, or growth disturbance at a minimum of 2-year follow-up. The authors conclude that the results are encouraging but limited by lack of a control group, single surgeon, and relatively small numbers [57].

Traditional antibiotic-loaded bone cement (ALBC) has been studied in the pediatric population in limited case series. In a study by Bar-On et al., four skeletally immature patients with lower extremity long bone chronic osteomyelitis were treated surgically with thorough debridement, including intramedullary reaming, and extensive lavage. Cement rods were fashioned using gentamycin-impregnated PMMA in a 28G chest tube with a 1.2-mm Kirschner wire in the center, bent to 90 degrees at the proximal and distal ends to aid in later removal. Additional cement beads were formed into a necklace on nonabsorbable suture and placed around the primary site of osteomyelitis. The cement rods and beads were removed 16 to 62 days after introduction. All patients also received IV antibiotics for an average of 6 weeks. All four patients had soft tissue complications after rod removal that required subsequent procedures or surgery. One patient sustained a fracture after rod removal that was treated in a cast. The fracture healed with significant recurvatum that was subsequently treated with osteotomy and external fixation. All patients had clinical and radiographic resolution of disease in an average of 6 months. At a mean follow-up of 41 months from rod removal, all patients continued to have full function without symptoms of infection and C-reactive protein (CRP) within normal limits. The authors conclude that this method is a relatively safe and effective method of treating chronic osteomyelitis of the long bones in pediatric patients.

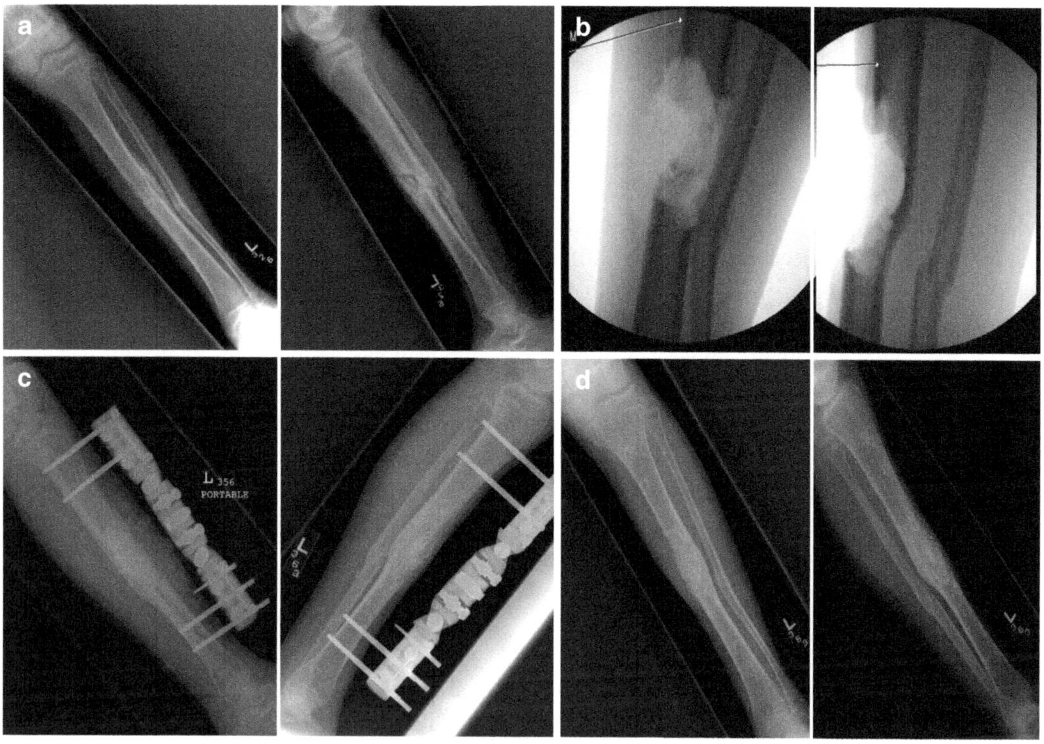

Fig. 8.7 A 15-year-old male with chronic osteomyelitis after a closed midshaft tibia fracture treated with closed reduction and percutaneous pinning (**a**). He underwent sequestrectomy and debridement of devitalized bone (**b**). He was treated with an antibiotic-loaded bone cement spacer and external fixator, per the Masquelet technique (**c**). He subsequently had removal of the cement spacer and external fixator with bone grafting within the induced membrane. He had successful union of his bone defect (**d**)

Infected Non-Union

In the case of chronic osteomyelitis in the setting of a non-union or large bone defect, an antibiotic-loaded cement spacer can be utilized after debridement for periosteal membrane induction prior to reconstruction with bone graft and fixation (Fig. 8.7). This technique, first described by Masquelet in 1986 [58], has been studied in pediatric patients with bone defect secondary to trauma, tumor, and congenital pseudarthrosis and was shown in meta-analysis to have excellent success, with a union rate of 91% [59]. Recent analysis suggests that this technique is less successful when there is an associated infection [60]. In regard to application in pediatric patients with chronic osteomyelitis, a case series of eight patients by Rousset et al. has described their technique and results. Pediatric patients underwent a two-stage surgical approach to chronic osteomyelitis with and without non-union. In the first stage, the patients underwent extensive debridement and lavage with application of ALBC spacer. The ALBC was prepared using 0.5 g of gentamicin per 40-g of methyl methacrylate powder mixed with liquid monomer. The cement was shaped into the patient-specific bone defect with the intent of forming a bioactive membrane. A Kirschner wire was utilized to make small pits in the cement spacer to aid in antibiotic elution. The cement spacer was retained until the normalization of inflammatory markers. In the second stage, the cement spacer was removed, and the induced membrane was filled with either beta-tricalcium phosphate or bone graft. At a minimum of 1-year follow-up, all patients had returned to functional activities without pain, and inflammatory markers were within normal limits [61].

The first report of utilizing ALBC in pediatric patients with osteomyelitis was a case series by Paley and Herzenberg of nine patients, four of whom were aged 16 or younger with intramedullary infections after placement of intramedullary nails. The initial surgery of the four pediatric patients was performed for deformity correction. Two of the pediatric patients underwent nailing for deformity correction related to fibrous dysplasia with fixator-assisted nailing. The other two pediatric patients underwent lengthening over an intramedullary nail. Once the infection was identified, these patients were treated with removal of the intramedullary implant with extensive debridement and lavage of the intramedullary canal with placement of an intramedullary cement rod. The ALBC was prepared by mixing 2.4 g of tobramycin and 2 g of vancomycin per 40-g bag of methyl methacrylate. Additional liquid monomer is required due to the addition of antibiotic powder. A cement rod was prepared by injecting the ALBC into chest tube with an inner diameter similar in size the outer diameter of the removed intramedullary implant. A 3-mm beaded intramedullary guide wire was placed in the center and left proud, looped on either end to aid in removal. The duration of cement rod retention ranged from 59 to 212 days for the pediatric patients. Three of the four pediatric patients had the cement rod removed with a new intramedullary rod placed. All of the pediatric patients in this series achieved union and infection eradication, which was sustained at a minimum of 3-year follow-up [62].

Treatment of acute hematogenous osteomyelitis (AHO) with local delivery of antibiotics has been studied less. In a case series by Zhang et al., 22 infants (age <12 months) with AHO and an associated bone lesion were treated with debridement of the lesion and application of resorbable calcium sulfate (CS) mixed with 0.5 g of vancomycin into the bone defect. The delivery vehicle was prepared by mixing the diluent with the calcium sulfate and antibiotic powders to a dough-like consistency. The CS was then molded into pellets and placed into the bone defect once dried. Seven patients had complications, including limb length difference, avascular necrosis of the femoral head, and pathologic subluxation of the hip. Complications were more likely to occur in patients who had associated septic arthritis. Fifteen patients had good outcome without complication. The authors conclude that CS is a viable adjunct to surgical debridement in infants with AHO [26].

Conclusion

Local antibiotic delivery systems can be used as an adjunct to surgical management of complex chronic infections in pediatrics (Fig. 8.8). PMMA loaded with antibiotics have been used the most historically; however, they are limited by the requirement for subsequent surgical removal. Bone graft substitutes loaded with antibiotics are gaining popularity due to their osteoconductive properties and ability to be resorbed, negating a second-stage operation. CS with antibiotics has been observed to have associated wound drainage, which can be confused for recurrent infection. Application in pediatric infections is optimized in long bone infections, including chronic osteomyelitis and infected non-union. Appropriate techniques include debridement of necrotic bone with placement of PMMA beads or calcium sulfate pellets, PMMA cement rod for intramedullary infection, or the Masquelet membrane-inducing technique for infected non-unions.

Study	Country	Cases (n)	Mean age	Avg length of follow up (years)	Indication	Surgical treatment method	Results	Complications
Paley and Herzenberg **J Orthop Trauma** **2002**	USA	4 pediatric (9 total)	13.5 yrs	3.4	Chronic osteomyelitis, infectednon-union in previously nailed long bones	Two-stage surgery with removal of implant and placement of PMMA loaded with 2 g vancomycin and 2.4 g tobramycin per 40 g bag of methyl methacrylate Second stage removal and reimplantation of rod if needed	Union and resolution of osteomyelitis in all patients	Stitch abscess in 1 patient
Bar-On, et al. **J Pediatr Orthop** **2010**	Isreal	4	9.3 yrs	3.4	Chronic osteomyelitis	Two-stage surgery with intramedullary gentamicin loaded PMMA rods and beads Removal of cement at second stage	Resolution of disease in all patients	Soft tissue abscess or defect in all 4 patients Deformity and pathologic fracture in 1 patient
Rousset, et al. **Int J Orthop Sci** **2017**	France	8	13 yrs	2.4	Chronic osteomyelitis, infected non-union	Two-stage surgery for biomembrane induction, (Masquelet technique) 0.5 g gentamicin PMMA spacer in bone defect Cement spacer removed and bone graft or substitute placed within the biomembrane	Resolution of disease in all patients	10 cm LLD in 1 patient
Zhang, et al. **J Orthop Surg Res** **2018**	China	22	6.3 months	3.0	Acute hematogenous osteomyelitis, chronic osteomyelitis 10 patients with concomitant septic arthritis	Bone defect filled with calcium sulfate mixed with 0.5 g vancomycin molded into into pellets	Resolution of disease in all patients	LLD in 4 patients AVN in 3 patients Pathologic hip subluxation in 1 patient
Andreacchio, et al. **J Pediatr Orthop B** **2019**	Italy, Switzerland, France	12	10.3 yrs	3.4	Chronic osteomyelitis	Single stage surgery with debridement, defect filled with commercially prepared 4% tobramycin-infused calcium sulfate pellets	Resolution of disease in all patients	None reported
Ellur, et al. **J Pediatr Orthop** **2020**	India	34	7.1 yrs	3.5	Chronic osteomyelitis	Single stage surgery with debridement, void filled with calcium sulfate combined with 1 g vancomycin and 240 mg gentamicin	Resolution of disease in the 31 patients that followed up	Serous drainage in 3 patients LLD in 2 patients Procurvatum in 1 patient

Fig. 8.8 Literature review of application of local delivery vehicles in pediatric orthopedic infections. (*PMMA* poly(methyl methacrylate), *LLD* limb length difference, *AVN* avascular necrosis)

Box 8.1

Antibiotic eluting local delivery vehicles

- **Poly (methyl methacrylate) (PMMA)**
- **Bioabsorbable bone graft substitutes**
  - Calcium sulfate
  - Calcium phosphate
- **Others**
  - Scaffolds (polyurethane, polycaprolactone, poly (lactic-co-glycolic acid)
  - Microspheres
  - Sponges
  - Hydrogels

Antibiotic-loaded bone cement (ALBC)

- **Surgeon prepared ALBC targeted toward cultures**
- **Aminoglycoside (tobramycin or gentamicin) if culture negative**
- **Commercially prepared ALBC (37)**
  - Palacos ® Biomet Inc. (0.5 g Gentamicin)
  - Depuy 1 DepuyOrthopaedics, Inc. (1 g gentamicin)
  - Cemex ® Genta, Exactech, Inc. (0.5 g gentamicin)
  - VersaBond™AB, Smith & Nephew, Inc. (1 g gentamicin)
  - Simplex™ P, Stryker ® Orthopaedics(1 g tobramycin)

Antibiotic-loaded bone graft substitutes

- **Calcium sulfate (CS)**
  - Osteoset ®, Wright Medical Technology Inc. (4% gentamicin)
  - Stimulan®, BiocompositesLtd (gentamicin, vancomycin, tobramycin added)
- **Calcium phosphate**
  - Surgeon prepared with aminoglycoside (tobramycin, gentamicin)
- **Combination**
- **Cerament ® G, Bone Support AB (60% CS, 40% hydroxyapatite, gentamicin)**
  - Herafill® beads G, Heraeus Medical GmbH (72% CS, 18% calcium carbonate, 9% hydrogenated triglyceride, gentamicin)

Acknowledgements Jayanth Sampath, MD, FRCS for contributing case examples.

Mohan V Belthur, MD for contributing case example.

Carlie Brooks, BS for illustration contribution.

References

1. Funk SS, Copley LAB. Acute Hematogenous osteomyelitis in children: pathogenesis, diagnosis, and treatment. Orthop Clin North Am. 2017;48(2):199–208.
2. Arnold JC, Bradley JS. Osteoarticular infections in children. Infect Dis Clin N Am. 2015;29(3):557–74.
3. Donaldson N, Sanders J, Child J, Parker S. Acute Hematogenous bacterial Osteoarticular infections in children. Pediatr Rev. 2020;41(3):120–36.
4. Beekman F. Acute Hematogenous osteomyelitis. Bull N Y Acad Med. 1930;6(12):792–807.
5. Crossan ET. Conservative treatment of acute Hematogenous osteomyelitis. Ann Surg. 1936;103(4):605–12.
6. Compere EL, Schnute WJ, Cattell LM. The use of penicillin in the treatment of acute hematogenous osteomyelitis in children. Ann Surg. 1945;122:954–62.
7. Gillespie WJ, Mayo KM. The management of acute haematogenous osteomyelitis in the antibiotic era: a study of the outcome. J Bone Joint Surg Br. 1981;63-B(1):126–31.
8. Yusef D, Shalakhti T, Awad S, Algharaibeh H, Khasawneh W. Clinical characteristics and epidemiology of sepsis in the neonatal intensive care unit in the era of multi-drug resistant organisms: A retrospective review. Pediatrics & Neonatology. 2018;59(1):35–41.
9. Aira A, Fehér C, Rubio E, Soriano A. The intestinal microbiota as a reservoir and a therapeutic target to fight multi-drug-resistant bacteria: A narrative review of the literature. Infect Dis Ther. 2019;8(4):469–82.
10. de Kraker MEA, Stewardson AJ, Harbarth S. Will 10 million people die a year due to antimicrobial resistance by 2050? PLoS Med. 2016;13(11):e1002184.
11. World Health Organization. Antimicrobial resistance: global report on surveillance. Geneva, Switzerland: World Health Organization; 2014. p. 232.
12. Hotchen AJ, Dudareva M, Corrigan RA, Ferguson JY, McNally MA. Can we predict outcome after treatment of long bone osteomyelitis? Bone Joint J. 2020;102-B(11):1587–96.
13. Saeed K, McLaren AC, Schwarz EM, Antoci V, Arnold WV, Chen AF, et al. 2018 international consensus meeting on musculoskeletal infection: summary from the biofilm workgroup and consensus on biofilm related musculoskeletal infections. J Orthop Res. 2019;37(5):1007–17.
14. Arciola CR, Campoccia D, Montanaro L. Implant infections: adhesion, biofilm formation and immune evasion. Nat Rev Microbiol. 2018;16(7):397–400.
15. Zimmerli W, Moser C. Pathogenesis and treatment concepts of orthopaedic biofilm infections. FEMS Immunol Med Microbiol. 2012;65(2):158–68.
16. Zimmerli W, Sendi P. Orthopaedic biofilm infections. APMIS. 2017;125(4):353–64.
17. Ceroni D, Dayer R, Steiger C. Are we approaching the end of pediatric culture-negative osteoarticular infections? Future Microbiol. 2019;14(11):917–9.
18. Spyridakis E, Gerber JS, Schriver E, Grundmeier RW, Porsch EA, St Geme JW, et al. Clinical features and outcomes of children with culture-negative septic arthritis. J Pediatric Infect Dis Soc. 2019;8(3):228–34.
19. Ford CA, Cassat JE. Advances in the local and targeted delivery of anti-infective agents for management of osteomyelitis. Expert Rev Anti-Infect Ther. 2017;15(9):851–60.
20. Jensen LK, Koch J, Henriksen NL, Bue M, Tøttrup M, Hanberg P, et al. Suppurative inflammation and local tissue destruction reduce the penetration of cefuroxime to infected bone implant cavities. J Comp Pathol. 2017;157(4):308–16.
21. Bar-On E, Weigl DM, Bor N, Becker T, Katz K, Mercado E, et al. Chronic osteomyelitis in children: treatment by intramedullary reaming and antibiotic-impregnated cement rods. J Pediatr Orthop. 2010;30(5):508–13.
22. Ellur V, Kumar G, Sampath JS. Treatment of chronic Hematogenous osteomyelitis in children with antibiotic impregnated calcium Sulphate. J Pediatr Orthop. 2020;4.
23. Canavese F, Corradin M, Khan A, Mansour M, Rousset M, Samba A. Successful treatment of chronic osteomyelitis in children with debridement, antibiotic-laden cement spacer and bone graft substitute. Eur J Orthop Surg Traumatol. 2017;27(2):221–8.
24. Ferguson J, Diefenbeck M, McNally M. Ceramic biocomposites as biodegradable antibiotic carriers in the treatment of bone infections. J Bone Jt Infect. 2017;2(1):38–51.
25. Ruppen C, Hemphill A, Sendi P. In vitro activity of gentamicin as an adjunct to penicillin against biofilm group B streptococcus. J Antimicrob Chemother. 2017;72(2):444–7.
26. Zhang Z, Li H, Li H, Fan Q, Yang X, Shen P, et al. Clinical experience of debridement combined with resorbable bone graft substitute mixed with antibiotic in the treatment for infants with osteomyelitis. J Orthop Surg Res. 2018;13(1):218.
27. Metsemakers W-J, Fragomen AT, Moriarty TF, Morgenstern M, Egol KA, Zalavras C, et al. Evidence-based recommendations for local antimicrobial strategies and dead space Management in Fracture-Related Infection. J Orthop Trauma. 2020;34(1):18–29.

28. Parsons B, Strauss E. Surgical management of chronic osteomyelitis. Am J Surg. 2004;188(1, Supplement 1):57–66.
29. Nasser A, Azimi T, Ostadmohammadi S, Ostadmohammadi S. A comprehensive review of bacterial osteomyelitis with emphasis on Staphylococcus aureus. Microb Pathog. 2020;148:104431.
30. Nandi SK, Bandyopadhyay S, Das P, Samanta I, Mukherjee P, Roy S, et al. Understanding osteomyelitis and its treatment through local drug delivery system. Biotechnol Adv. 2016;34(8):1305–17.
31. Masters EA, Trombetta RP, de Mesy Bentley KL, Boyce BF, Gill AL, Gill SR, et al. Evolving concepts in bone infection. Bone Res. 2019;15:7.
32. Ostrea ACM, Ramos MDR, Frez RV. Pediatric chronic fibular Pandiaphyseal osteomyelitis: case report with literature review. Asian Journal of Orthopaedic Research. 2020;17:18–28.
33. Panteli M, Giannoudis PV. Chronic osteomyelitis: what the surgeon needs to know. EFORT Open Rev. 2016;1(5):128–35.
34. Beard LJ, Ferris L, Ferrante A. Immunoglobulin G subclasses and lymphocyte subpopulations and function in osteomyelitis and septic arthritis. Acta Paediatr Scand. 1990;79(6–7):599–604.
35. McNally M, Nagarajah K. Osteomyelitis. Orthopaedics Trauma. 2010;24(6).
36. Cierny G, DiPasquale D. Treatment of chronic infection. J Am Acad Orthop Surg. 2006;14(10 Spec No.):S105–110.
37. McNally MA, Small JO, Tofighi HG, Mollan RA. Two-stage management of chronic osteomyelitis of the long bones. The Belfast technique. J Bone Joint Surg Br. 1993;75(3):375–80.
38. McNally MA, Ferguson JY, Lau ACK, Diefenbeck M, Scarborough M, Ramsden AJ, et al. Single-stage treatment of chronic osteomyelitis with a new absorbable, gentamicin-loaded, calcium sulphate/hydroxyapatite biocomposite: a prospective series of 100 cases. Bone Joint J. 2016;98-B(9):1289–96.
39. Lamagni T. Epidemiology and burden of prosthetic joint infections. J Antimicrob Chemother. 2014;69(Suppl 1):i5–10.
40. Henry MW, Miller AO, Walsh TJ, Brause BD. Fungal musculoskeletal infections. Infect Dis Clin N Am. 2017;31(2):353–68.
41. Ramage G, Rajendran R, Sherry L, Williams C. Fungal Biofilm Resistance. Int J Microbiol. 2012;2012:1–14.
42. Roy R, Tiwari M, Donelli G, Tiwari V. Strategies for combating bacterial biofilms: a focus on anti-biofilm agents and their mechanisms of action. Virulence. 2018;9(1):522–54.
43. Sa Y, Yang F, Wang Y, Wolke JGC, Jansen JA. Modifications of Poly(Methyl Methacrylate) cement for application in orthopedic surgery. In: Chun HJ, Park CH, Kwon IK, Khang G, editors. Cutting-edge enabling technologies for regenerative medicine. (Advances in Experimental Medicine and Biology). Singapore: Springer; 2018. p. 119–34.
44. Stravinskas M, Horstmann P, Ferguson J, Hettwer W, Nilsson M, Tarasevicius S, et al. Pharmacokinetics of gentamicin eluted from a regenerating bone graft substitute: in vitro and clinical release studies. Bone Joint Res. 2016;5(9):427–35.
45. Cunningham B, McLaren AC, Pauken C, McLemore R. Liposomal formulation increases local delivery of amphotericin from bone cement: a pilot study. Clin Orthop Relat Res. 2012;470(10):2671–6.
46. Goss B, Lutton C, Weinrauch P, Jabur M, Gillett G, Crawford R. Elution and mechanical properties of antifungal bone cement. J Arthroplast. 2007;22(6):902–8.
47. Kweon C, McLaren AC, Leon C, McLemore R. Amphotericin B delivery from bone cement increases with porosity but strength decreases. Clin Orthop Relat Res. 2011;469(11):3002–7.
48. McCormack PL, Perry CM. Caspofungin: a review of its use in the treatment of fungal infections. Drugs. 2005;65(14):2049–68.
49. Wentao Z, Lei G, Liu Y, Wang W, Song T, Fan J. Approach to osteomyelitis treatment with antibiotic loaded PMMA. Microb Pathog. 2017;102:42–4.
50. Oliver RA, Lovric V, Christou C, Walsh WR. Comparative osteoconductivity of bone void fillers with antibiotics in a critical size bone defect model. J Mater Sci Mater Med. 2020;31(9).
51. van Vugt TAG, Geurts J, Arts JJ. Clinical application of antimicrobial bone graft substitute in osteomyelitis treatment: A systematic review of different bone graft substitutes available in clinical treatment of osteomyelitis. Biomed Res Int. 2016;2016.
52. Ferguson J, Athanasou N, Diefenbeck M, McNally M. Radiographic and histological analysis of a synthetic bone graft substitute eluting gentamicin in the treatment of chronic osteomyelitis. J Bone Jt Infect. 2019;4(2):76–84.
53. McKee MD, Li-Bland EA, Wild LM, Schemitsch EH. A prospective, randomized clinical trial comparing an antibiotic-impregnated bioabsorbable bone substitute with standard antibiotic-impregnated cement beads in the treatment of chronic osteomyelitis and infected nonunion. J Orthop Trauma. 2010;24(8):483–90.
54. Menon A, Soman R, Rodrigues C, Phadke S, Agashe VM. Careful interpretation of the wound status is needed with use of antibiotic impregnated biodegradable synthetic pure calcium sulfate beads: series of 39 cases. J Bone Jt Infect. 2018;3(2):87–93.
55. Cobb LH, McCabe EM, Priddy LB. Therapeutics and delivery vehicles for local treatment of osteomyelitis. J Orthop Res. 2020;38(10):2091–103.
56. Peltola H, Pääkkönen M. Acute osteomyelitis in children. N Engl J Med. 2014;370(4):352–60.
57. Andreacchio A, Alberghina F, Paonessa M, Cravino M, De Rosa V, Canavese F. Tobramycin-impregnated calcium sulfate pellets for the treatment of chronic osteomyelitis in children and adolescents. J Pediat Orthopaed B. 2019;28(3):189–95.

58. Masquelet AC, Fitoussi F, Begue T, Muller GP. Reconstruction of the long bones by the induced membrane and spongy autograft. Ann Chir Plast Esthet. 2000;45(3):346–53.
59. Morelli I, Drago L, George DA, Romanò D, Romanò CL. Managing large bone defects in children: a systematic review of the 'induced membrane technique'. J Pediat Orthopaed B. 2018;27(5):443–55.
60. Mathieu L, Durand M, Collombet J-M, de Rousiers A, de l'Escalopier N, Masquelet A-C. Induced membrane technique: a critical literature analysis and proposal for a failure classification scheme. Eur J Trauma Emerg Surg. 2020;23.
61. Rousset M, Walle M, Cambou L, Mansour M, Samba A, Pereira B, et al. Chronic infection and infected non-union of the long bones in paediatric patients: preliminary results of bone versus beta-tricalcium phosphate grafting after induced membrane formation. International Orthopaedics (SICOT). 2018;42(2):385–93.
62. Paley D, Herzenberg JE. Intramedullary infections treated with antibiotic cement rods: preliminary results in nine cases. J Orthop Trauma. 2002;16(10):723–9.

9 Evidence-Based Management of Pediatric Musculoskeletal Infections

Scott B. Rosenfeld, Kishore Mulpuri, and Lawson A. Copley

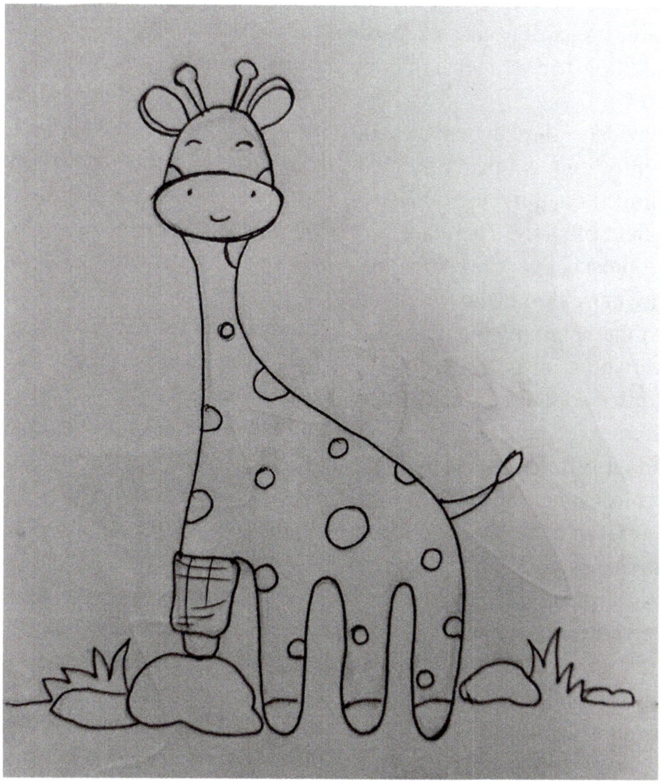

S. B. Rosenfeld
Department of Orthopaedic Surgery, Texas Children's Hospital, Baylor College of Medicine, Houston, TX, USA
e-mail: sbrosef@texaschildrens.org

K. Mulpuri
Department of Orthopaedic Surgery, BC Children's Hospital, University of British Columbia, Vancouver, BC, Canada
e-mail: kmulpuri@cw.bc.ca

L. A. Copley (✉)
Department of Orthopaedic Surgery, Texas Scottish Rite Hospital for Children and Children's Health System of Texas, University of Texas Southwestern, Dallas, TX, USA
e-mail: lawson.copley@childrens.com

© Springer Nature Switzerland AG 2022
M. V. Belthur et al. (eds.), *Pediatric Musculoskeletal Infections*,
https://doi.org/10.1007/978-3-030-95794-0_9

Introduction and Epidemiology in Brief

There is a wide range of conditions included under the topic of musculoskeletal infection in children. The primary categories include osteomyelitis, septic arthritis, and infectious myositis as deep infection subtypes. While some would not include skin and skin structure infections under the heading of musculoskeletal infection, many pediatric orthopedic surgeons are obligated to evaluate and treat these conditions whenever they involve the upper or lower extremities of children. It is therefore necessary to review the evidence and guidelines regarding these superficial infections in addition to the deep infection varieties.

The concept of evidence-based management of musculoskeletal infections is inherently challenging, given the limited quantity and quality of publications in this field of study. There are very few randomized, prospective investigations devoted to pediatric musculoskeletal infection. This is partly due to the nature of the disease in which substantial variation exists at the time of hospital admission; affected children range from mild to severe extremes of disease. However, there are also important differences between the experiences of musculoskeletal infection at institutions in separated geographic regions that would limit the generalizability of published data, even if it were carefully controlled and executed as a study of a specific condition. Another important challenge is that treatment alternatives are not easily compared against options in which they would be withheld or substantially modified, such as antibiotic treatment or surgical intervention. Within the past two decades, the Infectious Diseases Society of America has published guidelines on a variety of conditions with the intention of systematically weighting the strength of recommendations and quality of evidence using the Grading of Recommendations, Assessment, Development, and Evaluation (GRADE) system [1, 2]. While less than perfect, these guidelines have an anchoring effect which allows providers to frame decision-making on an externally validated thought process and literature review. Another benefit is the recognition of gaps in the evidence and opportunities for future studies that may help close these gaps.

Evidence-based management is ideally intended to minimize the randomness introduced when providers and institutions take a case-by-case approach to care [3]. While no two cases are alike, the ability to learn from cumulative experience is severely truncated when no two treatment methods are alike either. More importantly, the evaluation process involved in assessing these conditions, which are inherently uncertain, must be standardized to avoid skipping essential processes of care by simply failing to follow guidelines. An example is the indispensable nature of blood cultures which should be acquired in all cases of deep infection evaluation, prior to antibiotic administration [4]. Failing to do so may eliminate the one opportunity to identify the causative organism without resorting to more invasive techniques.

Recently the Children's Orthopaedic Trauma and infection Consortium for Evidence-Based Study (CORTICES) Group published multicenter data from 18 tertiary pediatric medical centers in the United States and reported the rate of consultations for musculoskeletal infection (Fig. 9.1) [5]. The principal investigators at each center subsequently participated in a survey to understand the practice patterns for joint aspiration in the evaluation of pediatric septic arthritis [6]. This type of study is valuable in understanding the essential and non-essential pathways that may help confirm a diagnosis and initiate appropriate, and timely, therapy. The purpose of this chapter is to review the current evaluation and treatment guidelines for the key subtypes of deep and superficial infection of the musculoskeletal system in children.

Pathology and Microbiology

Acute Hematogenous Osteomyelitis

Bone infection in immunocompetent children is predominantly due to *Staphylococcus aureus* which is isolated in over 90% of culture-positive

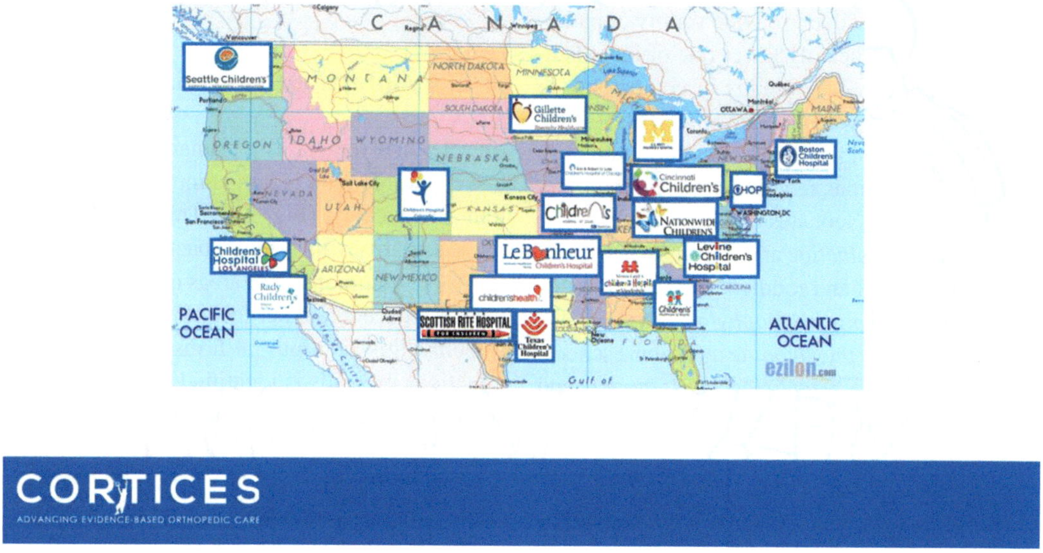

Fig. 9.1 Map of tertiary pediatric medical center participating in the original charter group formulating the Children's Orthopaedic Trauma and Infection Consortium for Evidence-Based Studies (CORTICES) group. Participating centers include Ann & Robert H. Lurie Children's Hospital; Boston Children's Hospital; Children's Healthcare of Atlanta; Children's Hospital Los Angeles; Children's Hospital of Philadelphia; Cincinnati Children's Hospital; Colorado Children's Hospital; Gillette Children's Hospital; Le Bonheur Children's Hospital; Levine Children's Hospital; Nationwide Children's Hospital; Rady Children's Hospital; Seattle Children's Hospital; Texas Children's Hospital; Texas Scottish Rite Hospital for Children; University of Michigan; Vanderbilt; Washington University in St. Louis

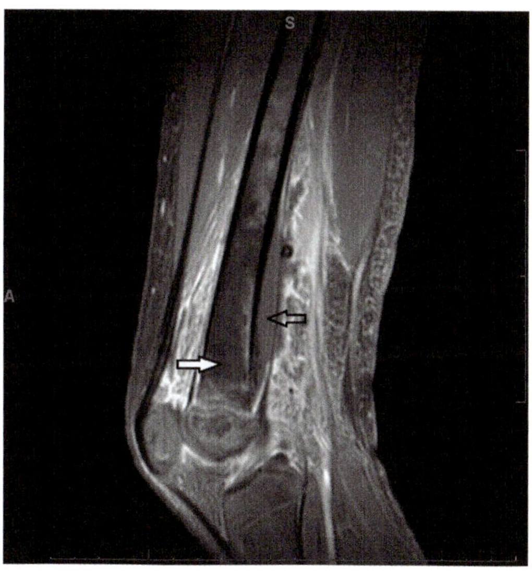

Fig. 9.2 Post-contrast, fat saturation, T1 weighted, sagittal MRI image demonstrating acute hematogenous osteomyelitis of the right distal femur with extensive intra-osseous (white arrow) and subperiosteal (opposite arrow) abscess in a 6-year-old girl

cases (Fig. 9.2) [4]. There is a moderately high rate of bacteremia among children with acute osteomyelitis, ranging from 30% to 50% [7–9]. When bone aspiration or debridement procedures are performed, the rate of culture-positive identification of the pathogen may be over 90% if carefully obtained [4]. There has been a progressive evolution of antibiotic resistance displayed by this pathogen which was initially treatable with penicillin. In the modern era, methicillin-resistant strains are emerging in communities [2–5, 7]. Moreover, clindamycin resistance and vancomycin intermediate susceptibility are creating challenges to antibiotic selection [2, 10, 11]. Because bone infections may mimic other conditions, it is appropriate to send samples for pathology evaluation whenever a biopsy or debridement is performed. The typical histologic features are that of acute bone inflammation with neutrophil infiltration of the cancellous architecture.

Primary Septic Arthritis

Joint infections are due to a wide variety of pathogens, with a significantly lower rate of identification of *Staphylococcus aureus* in comparison to that which is seen with osteomyelitis (Fig. 9.3) [4, 12]. The bacteria identified among children with joint space infections tend to aggregate into age-based groupings. Neonates (up to 6 months) have *Streptococcus agalactiae* and *Enterobacteriaceae* infections; infants and toddlers (6 to 48 months) have *Kingella kingae*, *Staphylococcus aureus*, and *Streptococcus pneumoniae* infections; school-age children have *Staphylococcus aureus* and *Streptococcus pyogenes* infections; and adolescents and teens have *Staphylococcus aureus* and *Streptococcus pyogenes* and *Neisseria gonorrhoeae* infections. The rate of culture positivity is substantially lower for joint fluid specimens than for bone specimens [4, 12]. Septic arthritis is microbiologically confirmed in approximately 35% of children who are believed to have infection based on their clinical features and response to treatment [4, 12]. This low rate is thought to be due to the inhibitory effect of joint fluid on bacterial growth in culture. In order to successfully identify the causative pathogen in children with septic arthritis, increasingly molecular diagnostic tests are being utilized with a rate of positivity above 50% [12]. This is most helpful in the age group in which *Kingella kingae* predominates, 6–48 months, as this organism is difficult to grow in clinical laboratories.

Primary Infectious Myositis

Muscle involvement as a primary site of musculoskeletal infection is less common than bone or joint involvement (Fig. 9.4). This may be due to the vascularity which limits bacterial deposition. It is more common to see areas of muscle inflammation adjacent to other foci of infection, such as osteomyelitis or septic arthritis. When primary infectious myositis is identified, it is often in the suppurative state, which leads to greater clinical illness and abscess formation. Pericapsular/obturator pyomyositis is an important consideration in the workup of infections about the hip. Its presentation is very similar to that of septic arthritis of the hip, and advanced imaging is required to make the diagnosis and avoid aspiration of the hip through this abscess which could seed an otherwise sterile joint [29] (Fig. 9.5). Growing bacteria from a drained abscess of the deep tissues (muscle or bone) is usually successful, so the culture positivity rate of pyomyositis is as high as seen in osteomyelitis [4]. The most common pathogen confirmed in muscle infections is *Staphylococcus aureus* (about 85%) followed by *Streptococcus pyogenes* [4]. Because the muscle is largely displaced and disrupted by the local infection and

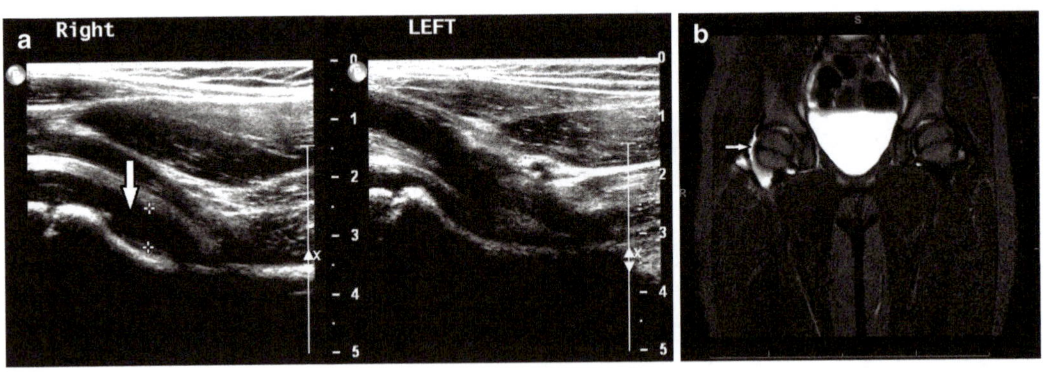

Fig. 9.3 Comparison hip ultrasound (**a**) coronal short tau inversion recovery (STIR) MRI image (**b**) sequences demonstrating an isolated right hip effusion (white arrows) in a 4-year-old girl with primary septic arthritis of the right hip

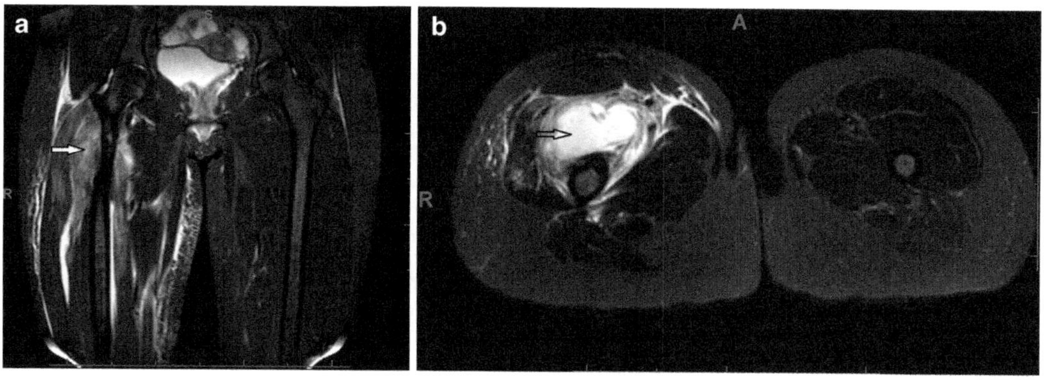

Fig. 9.4 Depiction of primary infectious myositis of the right vastus intermedius muscle (white arrow) in a 16-year-old female as seen on coronal STIR (**a**) and sagittal STIR (**b**). The sagittal imaging illustrates a large intramuscular abscess (arrow) which is clearly defined, even without contrast

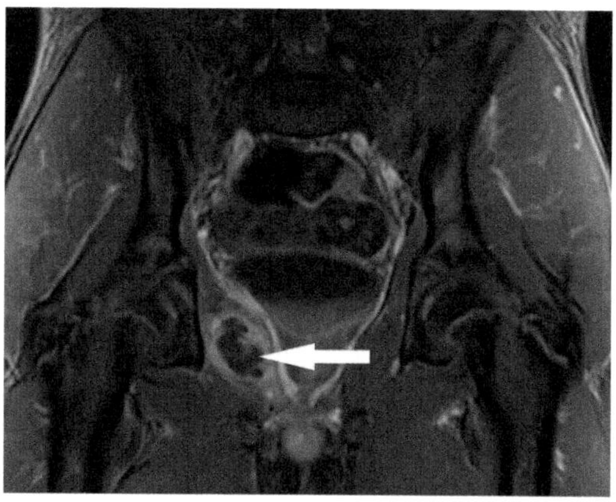

Fig. 9.5 Coronal post-contrast T1-weighted image of pericapsular pyomyositis located in the right obturator internus muscle (white arrow)

inflammation, there is seldom any motivation to send a separate pathology specimen.

Skin and Skin Structure Infections

Two general categories of skin and skin structure infections make up the majority of these conditions. These include abscesses, typically caused by *Staphylococcus aureus*, and cellulitis, fasciitis, lymphangitis, and lymphadenitis, typically caused by *Streptococcus pyogenes* [1]. Because abscesses generally yield pus that may be easily obtained and submitted for culture and susceptibility, the pathogen is almost always confirmed when this is done [4]. In contrast, cellulitis is not generally aspirated or pursued for a confirmed pathogen. Necrotizing fasciitis is extremely rare in children (Fig. 9.6). Over nine decades, there have been 298 cases from 195 reports, indicating that most of the experience is reported in case reports and small case series [13]. The experience of recognizing this serious condition is largely generated from adult orthopedic care as the affected individuals typically present in extremis. Aggressive surgical management, inclusive of obtaining tissue for pathology to confirm the diagnosis, frequently leads to amputation in an effort to save the life of the patient. Fortunately, this occurrence and the case fatality rate are substantially lower in children [13].

Investigations/Workup

The evaluation of children with suspected musculoskeletal infection should be systematic and detailed [3, 14]. Musculoskeletal infection evaluations begin with a clinical concern or suspicion that the child being evaluated may have an infection of the musculoskeletal system. There is inherent uncertainty involved in this process given the wide spectrum of infectious, inflammatory, and neoplastic disorders which may have a similar clinical presentation at the onset of evaluation. There are also varying degrees of inflammation along a continuum of severity at the time of presentation of the affected children, which may fur-

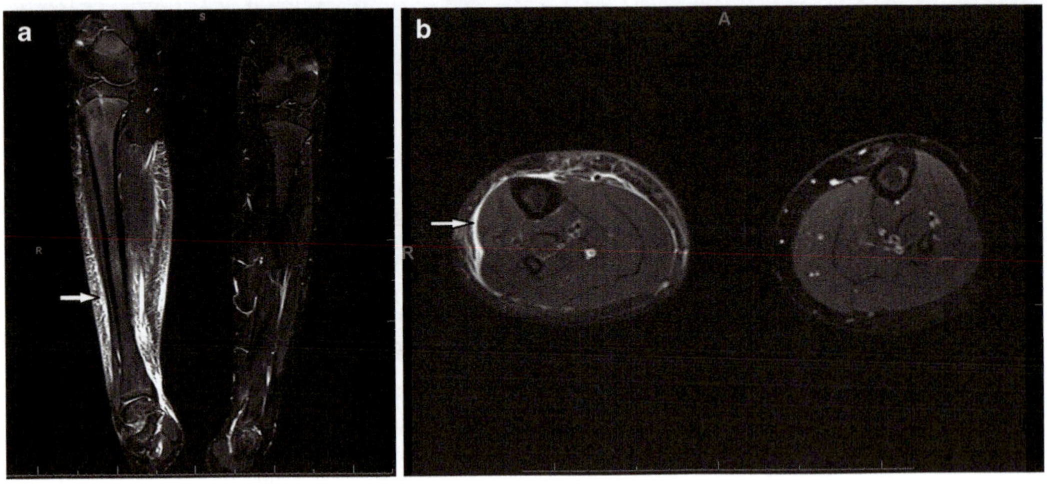

Fig. 9.6 Coronal (**a**) and sagittal (**b**) STIR images of the right leg of a 15-year-old male with cellulitis and fasciitis (white arrows). There is no subfascial or osseous involvement

ther cloud the clinical picture and make it difficult to differentiate between mild infectious and advanced non-infectious processes. Therefore, the process of evaluation of children with suspected musculoskeletal infection requires judgment and decision-making under uncertainty. To mitigate against this challenge, institutions are increasingly adopting clinical practice algorithms to delineate the essential workflows involved in the evaluation of specific forms of musculoskeletal infection (Fig. 9.7) [1–3, 14]. Implementation of these algorithms has been shown to impact the efficiency of processes and improve the short-term and intermediate-term outcomes of treatment [15, 16]. Although implementation of guidelines and continuous surveillance to ensure they are followed correctly is a labor-intensive endeavor, a multidisciplinary, guideline-directed approach appears to be beneficial [14].

The appropriate location for an evolving musculoskeletal infection evaluation has bearing on the services involved and the manner of interdisciplinary communication. Common locations include ambulatory clinic, urgent/first care, emergency room, inpatient ward, and intensive care. Determinants of the most appropriate setting to perform the workup include the acuity of presentation, the initial impression of the appearance of the child which may invoke a sense of concern or worry, and the availability of the resources devoted to this purpose at any given institution.

In general, there are three types of evaluation which can be encapsulated categorically for the purposes of the initial assessment of a child who presents with signs or symptoms of possible musculoskeletal infection: (1) Outpatient evaluation is appropriate and may be performed when benign self-limited conditions such as transient synovitis or post-viral reactive inflammation are considered to be more likely than infection. These may be referred for an early (2–4 days) outpatient "second look," either to ensure spontaneous resolution or to identify progression of symptoms or inflammatory marker elevation suggestive of the increasing possibility of infection; (2) inpatient evaluation is necessary when infection or a clinically important neoplastic or inflammatory process is considered more likely than benign, self-limited conditions. These evaluations frequently require additional input from subspecialist consultants, advanced imaging with magnetic resonance imaging (MRI), and supplemental laboratory studies to reach a diagnosis; and (3) intensive care unit (ICU) resuscitation and evaluation are necessary in children with evolving sepsis and hemodynamic compromise. These children should be admitted to the ICU for concurrent resuscitation with fluid, inotropic medication, and broad spectrum bactericidal antibiotic therapy [14].

Historically, there have been efforts made to develop a limited set of risk factors intended to

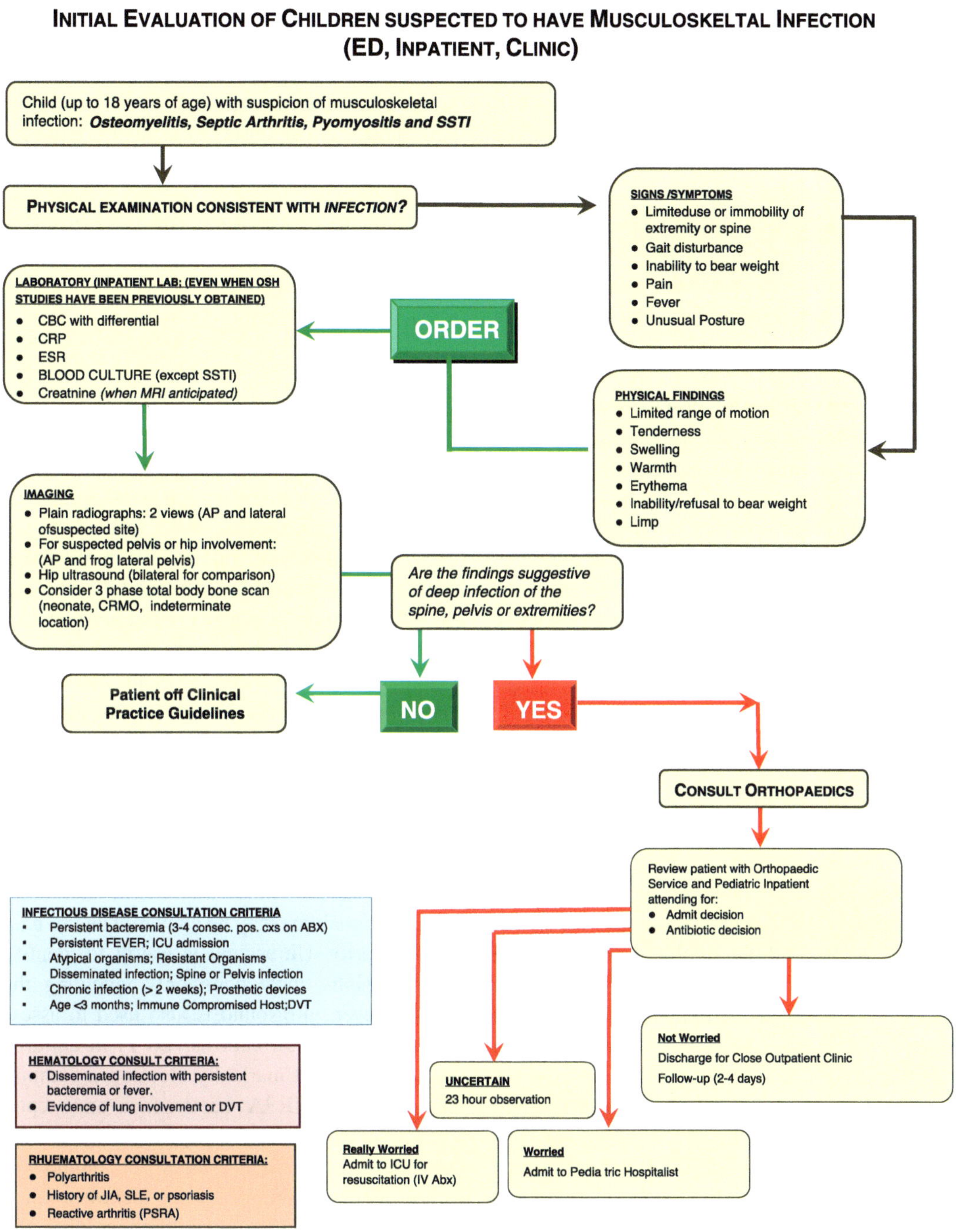

Fig. 9.7 Flow chart depicting initial evaluation of children suspected to have musculoskeletal infection. ED emergency department, OSH outside hospital, MRI magnetic resonance imaging, Y yes, N no

distinguish the conditions of musculoskeletal infection from similar appearing non-infectious conditions [17, 18]. The Kocher criteria and Boston Children's septic arthritis of the hip algorithm were established, for example, to help providers differentiate between transient synovitis and septic arthritis involving the hip joint in children who are at risk of having either condition

[17]. While helpful in establishing a mental framework in evaluating the relative degree of concern, application of these predictive algorithms has limitations as is evident by the lack of consistent generalizability to other geographic regions or patient populations [19]. There is also difficulty of accurately detecting infections caused by less virulent organisms, such as *Kingella kingae* or *Borrelia burgdorferi*, which may present with minimal acute findings. Similarly, non-infectious conditions with advanced degrees of inflammation at the initial presentation, such as occasional presentations of transient synovitis, post-streptococcal reactive arthritis, or Kawasaki's disease may appear similar to bacterial infection. Such examples appear to break the rules and lead to diagnostic delay of septic arthritis on one hand or invasive procedures for non-infectious conditions on the other. While it is appealing for providers to have objective cutoff values to apply using predictive algorithms, there is potential for mis-categorization of infectious conditions as non-infectious, and vice-versa.

Laboratory Studies

The initial workup of suspected musculoskeletal infection should include the systematic acquisition of the following: complete blood cell count (CBC) with differential; C-reactive protein (CRP); erythrocyte sedimentation rate (ESR); and aerobic blood culture (when deep infection is suspected). Septic arthritis evaluation should additionally include a joint fluid sample for nucleated cell count and segmented neutrophil differential; aerobic joint fluid culture; and 16S polymerase chain reaction (PCR) or multi-plex PCR [12]. When bone infection is suspected, evaluation should include a biopsy and culture by trocar (often using an 11-gauge biopsy needle) to obtain an aspiration of bone for aerobic culture and a core needle biopsy for histopathology of bone. If the ultimate goal is to achieve absolute certainty for musculoskeletal infection diagnoses, there may be increased costs, invasiveness, and inconvenience of care. Some of this may be unnecessary if initiation of empiric antibiotic treatment results in appropriate clinical and laboratory improvement within a short timeframe while under direct observation in the inpatient setting. Trending of the markers of inflammation, with or without treatment, is also valuable in guiding the thought process. This is a reasonable approach when there is an overall impression that the condition has a high probability of being viral or reactive.

Radiographic Studies

The initial workup of suspected musculoskeletal infection should be limited to plain radiographs of the symptomatic body area. In the vast majority of cases, musculoskeletal infection is mono-focal. Multi-focal symptoms should be carefully assessed for inflammatory or reactive conditions, unless they are accompanied by signs or symptoms of septic shock or bacteremia. Plain radiographs should be inspected for joint effusions, deep soft tissue swelling adjacent to bone, or metaphyseal lucent lesions. Plain X-rays may help identify other conditions including neoplasms, fractures, or superficial soft tissue swelling suggestive of skin and skin structure infection.

It is after the initial assessment that other imaging modalities may be contemplated to gain greater clarity. Ultrasound is useful to identify joint effusions, most commonly involving the hip. However, ultrasound is also used to assess for deep venous thrombosis (DVT) in children who present with markedly elevated inflammatory markers, MRSA bacteremia, and septic shock with an appearance of patchy infiltrates on chest X-ray, consistent with septic pulmonary emboli [9]. This form of pattern identification is useful for ICU-admitted children so that the ultrasound may be obtained before MRI and surgery so that surgical dressings and drains do not interfere with the ease of acquiring the ultrasound to evaluate for DVT after the fact [9, 14].

MRI acquisition should be conducted in a multidisciplinary, coordinated manner, as children with infection frequently need general anesthesia in order to keep still during the imaging acquisition process [14, 16]. The best evidence suggests that when MRI is orchestrated through careful, interdisciplinary communication and coordination, it is possible to reduce the number of MRIs obtained, the number of sequences per scan, the use of contrast material, the scan duration, the utilization of anesthesia, and the duration of anesthesia when utilized [16]. The MRI will illustrate the anatomic and spatial extent of the infection and provide guidance regarding surgical indications and the best approach to adequately address the foci of infection [20–22].

Severity of Illness

Recent evidence suggests that acute hematogenous osteomyelitis may be differentiated into categorically differentiated phenotypes of disease based on a relatively easy to calculate severity of illness score which may be determined within the first few days of inpatient hospitalization [23]. This score correlates with long-term clinical outcomes and has implications for decision-making as to which children are likely to require additional resources, including surgeries, readmissions, and long-term follow-up to identify complications [15, 22]. Additional focus is currently being directed toward the initial and subsequent platelet counts for children in the highest severity category; the coagulation cascade, which appears to be overexpressed and upregulated by MRSA infections, may result in the consumption of platelets, DVTs, and the occurrence of a disseminated intravascular coagulation phenomenon [9, 24]. Many of these children have an initial thrombocytopenia and then develop a lower platelet count (referred to as a platelet nadir) within the first couple of days of intensive care admissions. These children are among the sickest children and require the greatest amount of resources for care with prolonged hospitalizations and extended antibiotic treatment courses [14, 15, 25].

Differential Diagnoses

Acute Hematogenous Osteomyelitis

Fortunately, due to the high rate of culture positivity and the high rate of initial bacteremia, children with acute primary bone infections are seldom mistakenly perceived as having other conditions. However, in atypical cases, including culture negative, subacute onset, multi-focal, epiphyseal location, with the appearance of a neoplastic process, or immunocompromise, consideration should be given to Ewing's sarcoma, osteosarcoma, chronic non-bacterial osteomyelitis (formerly referred to as chronic recurrent multi-focal osteomyelitis), or atypical organisms (other than *Staphylococcus aureus*).

Primary Septic Arthritis

The evaluation of children suspected to have primary septic arthritis is inherently uncertain. This is due not only to a variety of inflammatory and reactive conditions that mimic infection but also due to a high rate of culture-negative septic arthritis [4, 12, 19]. Historically, investigators have sought to differentiate septic arthritis from non-infectious conditions through prediction algorithms based on a limited number of parameters or risk factors [17, 18]. There is considerable challenge involved in using these algorithms for gray area cases that occasionally contradict the prediction rules [19]. Consideration typically turns to joint aspiration to help guide decision-making, but there is also uncertainty involved in this endeavor. Culture negativity is reported in up to 65% of cases, even when nucleated cell counts are above 50,000 cells/mL [12]. Among the conditions that mimic septic arthritis are viral processes, including transient synovitis and Kawasaki's disease; reactive arthritis, including post-streptococcal reactive arthritis (PSRA); inflammatory arthritis, including juvenile idiopathic arthritis (JIA) and systemic lupus erythematosus (SLE); and rarely hematologic disorders, including the initial presentation of hemophilia.

Primary Infectious Myositis

Similar to osteomyelitis, the ability to grow bacteria easily from infected muscle minimizes the likelihood to mistake other conditions for primary infectious myositis. Additionally, the diagnosis is relatively straightforward on the merit of history, physical examination, laboratory, and imaging findings. Rarely, a muscle hematoma may present with an appearance of infection, but there is often a compelling history of trauma in those cases. Neoplastic processes, such as rhabdomyosarcoma are sufficiently rare to minimize concern, but these cases would often be deciphered relatively easily with MRI and biopsy.

Treatment Options

Antibiotic Therapy

The treatment for children with musculoskeletal infection inevitably requires antibiotic administration in a sequential parenteral to oral manner [1, 2]. The initiation of antibiotics should always be withheld until a blood culture has been obtained. Ideally, antibiotics should also be withheld until after tissue cultures are obtained from the suspected focus of infection (joint fluid, bone aspiration, or pus acquired from the bone, muscle, or soft tissue abscess) [4]. This is most important for children suspected to have primary septic arthritis, as the administration of antibiotic therapy may minimize the return of positive culture results. The other reason to avoid this is that the initiation of antibiotics to children who have inflammatory, reactive, or viral processes may confuse the clinical evaluation when a brief period of observation may have allowed downward trending of the inflammatory markers without intervention. An obvious exception to the guidance to withhold antibiotics is when there is the need for resuscitation of children with septic shock [14]. Blood cultures before antibiotics are still indispensable, but these are easily obtained while starting the intravenous line through which the antibiotic will be given [4].

Selection of empiric antibiotics should be guided by knowledge of the local microbiome within any community but should be specifically focused on the component of the microbiome that causes invasive musculoskeletal infection. In many cases, the hospital microbiome data is inclusive of all pathogens, regardless of source, and may imply a higher antibiotic resistance rate than actually occurs in bone, joint, or muscle source specimens. The CORTICES group has shown that the rate of specific pathogens varies substantially between regions of the United States, but also that the differences are not so great that a framework of empiric antibiotic recommendation may still be feasible [5].

After the pathogen is identified, antibiotic therapy should be more specifically focused on the causative organism based on susceptibility data. This is increasingly relevant given the rising incidence of MRSA and the occurrence of clindamycin resistance among MRSA and MSSA isolates [2]. When treating children in septic shock who have bacteremia, there are now available molecular diagnostic studies which help to identify whether the bacteria is MRSA or MSSA before antibiotic susceptibility results are returned. This new technology makes it possible to know this information within hours of a positive gram stain and allows the transition from vancomycin to a more appropriate and safer bactericidal drug using a semisynthetic penicillin or a first-generation cephalosporin. This reduces the risk of acute kidney injury which is common among ICU-admitted children with musculoskeletal infection who are treated with vancomycin [26].

Duration of antibiotic treatment is generally 4–6 weeks for osteomyelitis. There is evidence to support as few as 20 days of antibiotic treatment, but the data is generated from Scandinavia where there is no MRSA or USA300 *Staphylococcus aureus* which are frequently isolated in the United States [27]. The Finnish study group has also published data which suggests that primary septic arthritis may be successfully treated with as few as 10 days of antibiotics [28]. However, given the potential for unrecognized foci of osteomyelitis in children with septic arthritis, it is reasonable to cover for a minimum of 3 weeks [20–22]. Pyomyositis responds well to 3–4 weeks of antibiotic therapy. It should be noted that some children who have severe illness due to osteomyelitis may not resolve their infection with only 4 weeks of antibiotic treatment. While there is no published data to prove that they require the longer duration, one long-term outcome study showed that the children with high severity of illness scores did receive over 2 months of treatment during their course to normalize the ESR, which may be the only guide to determine the end point of therapy [15].

Surgical Treatment

Decision-making for surgery as a component of the treatment for children with musculoskeletal infection is based on the motivation to minimize long-term adverse outcomes. The importance of surgical source control during care for some children is seldom disputed. However specific indications for surgery have not been studied as it would be challenging to do so. In the United States, most children with septic arthritis undergo arthroscopic or open irrigation and drainage procedures. Despite the majority of these procedures being done open, there is ample evidence to support arthroscopy as a safe and effective alternative to open decompression [29, 30]. There is also limited support of serial aspiration treatment for septic arthritis [31].

Bone infections may be treated with or without surgery depending on the amount of inflammation within or adjacent to the bone that may accumulate to a volume of purulent material sufficient to merit from open debridement. Some evidence suggests that there may be a gradient of infection severity that corresponds to the occurrence of surgery or multiple surgeries during the care of children with osteomyelitis [22]. Children with the highest severity of illness scores undergo significantly more surgical intervention among a higher rate of children when compared to children with mild or moderate illness severity [15, 22]. However, there is a gap of knowledge as to the most appropriate surgical techniques for specific indications that may best influence outcomes.

Complications

Regardless of antibiotic or surgical measures taken to treat children with osteomyelitis, it appears that the greatest driver of long-term clinical outcomes for children with acute hematogenous osteomyelitis is likely to be the severity of illness at the time of the initial hospitalization [15, 23]. Motivation to minimize the occurrence of osteonecrosis, chondrolysis, joint destruction, growth disturbance, deformity, recurrent or chronic infection, and progression of the infection to more severe states including septic shock creates discussion as to whether these conditions should be treated as emergency conditions. However, in clinical practice, there is tremendous challenge in mobilizing all of the coordinated services which would be required to do this effectively [14]. A more common approach is to work as a team to organize sedated imaging with MRI and a procedure to immediately follow [14, 16]. The team approach to MRI acquisition involves interdisciplinary communication and coordination on the day of the scan. The leader of the team (typically the orthopedic surgeon) ensures that all stakeholders (pediatric hospitalist, radiologist, anesthesiologist, operating room charge nurse, and family) are informed about the decision to obtain the MRI, the anticipated need for sedation, the body area to be imaged, the desired imaging sequences, and the potential for a procedure to follow the MRI while under continued sedation. When the scan is obtained, the orthopedic surgeon is available to review images (real time) with the radiologist and MRI technician to be able to make a decision as to the need for surgery. If surgery is undertaken, the surgeon communicates this plan with the operating room charge nurse and transport team so that there is a smooth transition from the MRI scanner to the operating room. This practice minimizes confusion and increases the efficiency of imaging which results in shorter scan duration and less anesthetic exposure while avoiding contrast use.

One matter that has yet to be clarified in the literature is whether primary septic arthritis is as prone to complications as is septic arthritis with contiguous osteomyelitis. This is an important distinction and the potential subject of future research.

Overall, children with acute hematogenous osteomyelitis with or without septic arthritis have excellent long-term outcomes. One study determined that 92.1% of children had no further need for follow-up [14]. Even the 7.9% of children with adverse outcomes had good patient-reported outcome measures as rated by the Pediatric Outcomes Data Collection Instrument (PODCI) and Pediatric Quality of Life Inventory (PedsQL) questionnaires [14]. This has implications for the decision as to how long children with musculoskeletal infection should be followed. With the rising cost of healthcare and limited access to subspecialty clinics, which may be remote from the family and primary care physician's community, it is helpful to have evidence to suggest that not all children require extensive long-term follow-up. This is particularly true for children with mild or moderate severity of illness. However, even children with severe illness who are prone to adverse outcomes may be identified relatively early during the follow-up period, as radiographic changes of osteonecrosis, chondrolysis, joint destruction, and complex pathologic fractures with the potential for non-union tend to declare themselves within a few months of hospital discharge (Boxes 9.1 and 9.2).

Box 9.1 Key Learning Points

- Bone infection in immunocompetent children is predominantly due to *Staphylococcus aureus* [4].
- Blood culture is indispensable to help identify the causative pathogen in osteomyelitis [4, 12].
- Primary joint infections are due to a wide variety of pathogens [4, 12].
- Molecular diagnostic tests (e.g., PCR) are helpful to identify the pathogens, particularly *Kingella kingae* [12].
- MRI acquisition should ideally be conducted in a multidisciplinary, coordinated manner [14, 16].

Box 9.2 Pitfalls to Avoid

- Clinical prediction algorithms have limitations and should be applied with caution [17–19].
- MRI acquisition performed without multidisciplinary communication may lead to prolonged scan duration, prolonged anesthesia, unnecessary use of contrast, and repeated anesthetic inductions [16].

References

1. Stevens DL, Bisno AL, Chambers HF, Dellinger EP, Goldstein EJC, Gorbach SL, Hirschman JV, Kaplan SL, Montoya JG, Wade JC. Practice guidelines for the diagnosis and management of skin and soft tissue infections: 2014 update by the Infectious Diseases Society of America. Clin Infect Dis. 2014;59(2):e10–52.

2. Liu C, Bayer A, Cosgrove SE, Daum RS, Fridkin SK, Gorwitz RJ, Kaplan SL, Karchmer AW, Levine DP, Murray BE, Rybak J, M, Talan DA, Chambers HF. Clinical practice guidelines by the Infectious Diseases Society of America for the treatment of methicillin-resistant *Staphylococcus aureus* infections in adults and children. Clin Infect Dis. 2011;52(3):e18–55.
3. Copley LA, Kinsler A, Gheen T, Shar A, Sun D, Browne R. The impact of evidence-based clinical practice guidelines applied by a multidisciplinary team for the care of children with osteomyelitis. J Bone Joint Surg. 2013;95(8):686–93.
4. Section J, Gibbons SE, Barton T, Greenberg DE, Jo CH, Copley LA. Microbiological culture methods in pediatric musculoskeletal infection: a guideline for optimal use. J Bone Joint Surg. 2015;97(6):441–9.
5. Schoenecker JG, The Children's Orthopaedic Trauma and Infection Consortium for Evidence Based Study (CORTICES) Group* (includes Copley LA). Defining the volume of consultations for musculoskeletal infection encountered by pediatric orthopaedic services in the United States. PLoS One. 2020;15(6):e0234055. https://doi.org/10.1371/journal.pone.0234055.
6. Shaw KA, Sanborn R, Shore B, Truong W, Murphy JS, CORTICES Study Group. Current variation in joint aspiration practice for the evaluation of pediatric septic arthritis. J Am Acad Orthop Surg. 2020;4(9):1–7.
7. McNeil JC, Kaplan SL, Vallejo JG. The influence of the route of antibiotic administration, methicillin susceptibility, vancomycin duration and serum trough concentration on outcomes of pediatric *Staphylococcus aureus* bacteremic osteoarticular infection. Pediatr Infect Dis J. 2017;36(6):572–7.
8. Chiappini E, Camposampiero C, Lazzeri S, Indolfi G, De Martino M, Galli L. Epidemiology and management of acute haematogenous osteomyelitis in a tertiary paediatric center. Int J Environ Res Public Health. 2017;14(5):pii: E477. https://doi.org/10.3390/ijerph14050477.
9. Ligon JA, Journeycake JM, Josephs SC, Tareen NG, Lindsay EA, Copley LAB. Differentiation of deep venous thrombosis among children with or without osteomyelitis. J Pediatr Orthop. 2018;38(10):e597–603.
10. Kishk OA, Lardieri AB, Heil EL, Morgan JA. Vancomycin AUC/MIC and corresponding troughs in a pediatric population. J Pediatr Pharmacol Ther. 2017;22(1):41–7.
11. Bradley JS, Arrieta AC, Digtyar VA, Popejoy MW, Grandhi A, Bokesch P, Hershberger E, Dorr MB, Tan CM, Murata Y, Wolf DJ, Bensaci M. Daptomycin for pediatric gram-positive acute hematogenous osteomyelitis. Pediatr Infect Dis J. 2020;39(9):814–23.
12. Carter K, Doern C, Jo CH, Copley LA. Clinical usefulness of polymerase chain reaction as a supplemental diagnostic tool in the evaluation and treatment of children with septic arthritis. J Pediatr Orthop. 2016;36(2):167–72.
13. Schröder A, Gerin A, Firth GB, et al. A systematic review of necrotizing fasciitis in children from its first description in 1930 to 2018. BMC Infect Dis. 2019;19:317. https://doi.org/10.1186/s12879-019-3941-3.
14. Dhar AV, Huang CJ, Sue PK, Patel K, Farrow-Gillespie AC, Hammer MR, Zia AN, Mittal VS, Copley LA. Team approach: pediatric musculoskeletal infection. JBJS Rev. 2020;8(3):e0121. https://doi.org/10.2106/JBJS.RVW.19.00.00121.
15. Vorhies JS, Lindsay EA, Tareen NG, Kellum RJ, Jo CH, Copley LA. Severity adjusted risk of long-term adverse sequelae among children with osteomyelitis. Pediatr Infect Dis J. 2019;38(1):26–31.
16. Ojeaga PO, Hammer MR, Lindsay EA, Tareen NG, Jo CH, Copley LA. Quality improvement of magnetic resonance imaging for musculoskeletal infection in children results in decreased scan duration and decreased contrast use. J Bone Joint Surg Am. 2019;101:1679–88.
17. Caird MS, Flynn JM, Leung YL, Millman JE, D'Italia JG, Dormans JP. Factors distinguishing septic arthritis from transient synovitis of the hip in children. A prospective study. J Bone Joint Surg Am. 2006;88(6):1251–7.
18. Kocher MS, Mandiga R, Zurakowski D, Barnewolt C, Kasser JR. Validation of a clinical prediction rule for the differentiation between septic arthritis and transient synovitis of the hip in children. J Bone Joint Surg Am. 2004;86(8):1629–35.
19. Luhmann SJ, Jones A, Schootman M, Gordon JE, Schoenecker PL, Luhmann JD. Differentiation between septic arthritis and transient synovitis of the hip in children with clinical prediction algorithms. J Bone Joint Surg Am. 2004;86(5):956–62.
20. Rosenfeld S, Bernstein DT, Daram S, Dawson J, Zhang W. Predicting the presence of adjacent infections in septic arthritis in children. J Pediatr Orthop. 2016;36(1):70–4. https://doi.org/10.1097/BPO.0000000000000389.
21. Monsalve J, Kan JH, Schallert EK, Bisset GS, Zhang W, Rosenfeld SB. Septic arthritis in children: frequency of coexisting unsuspected osteomyelitis and implications on imaging work-up and management. Am J Roentgenol. 2015;204(6):1289–95.
22. Tuason D, Gheen T, Sun D, Huang R, Copley L. Clinical and laboratory parameters associated with multiple surgeries in children with acute hematogenous osteomyelitis. J Pediatr Orthop. 2014;34(5):565–70.
23. Athey A, Mignemi ME, Gheen WT, Lindsay EA, Jo CH, Copley LA. Validation and modification of a severity of illness score for children with acute hematogenous osteomyelitis. J Pediatr Orthop. 2019;39(2):90–7.
24. Gaviria-Agudelo C, Carter K, Tareen N, Pascual V, Copley LA. Gene expression analysis of children with acute hematogenous osteomyelitis caused by methicillin-resistant Staphylococcus aureus: cor-

relation with clinical severity of illness. PLoS One. 2014;9(7):e103523.
25. Mignemi ME, Benvenuti MA, An TJ, Martus JE, Mencio GA, Lovejoy SA, Copley LA, Williams DJ, Thomsen IP, Schoenecker JG. A novel classification system based on dissemination of musculoskeletal infection is predictive of hospital outcomes. J Pediatr Orthop. 2018;38(5):279–86.
26. Aljefri DM, Avedissian SN, Rhodes NJ, Postelnick MJ, Nguyen K, Scheetz MH. Vancomycin area under the curve and acute kidney injury: a meta-analysis. Clin Infect Dis. 2019;69(11):1881–7.
27. Peltola H, Pääkkönen M, Kallio P, Kallio MJ, Osteomyelitis-Septic Arthritis Study Group. Short-versus long-term antimicrobial treatment for acute hematogenous osteomyelitis of childhood: prospective, randomized trial on 131 culture-positive cases. Pediatr Infect Dis J. 2010;29(12):1123–8. https://doi.org/10.1097/INF.0b013e3181f55a89.
28. Peltola H, Pääkkönen M, Kallio P, Kallio MJ, Osteomyelitis-Septic Arthritis (OM-SA) Study Group. Prospective, randomized trial of 10 days versus 30 days of antimicrobial treatment, including a short-term course of parenteral therapy, for childhood septic arthritis. Clin Infect Dis. 2009;48(9):1201–10. https://doi.org/10.1086/597582.
29. Ellis HB, Copley L, Pennock A, Nepple JJ, Willimon C, Mayer SW, Yen YM. Tractionless hip arthroscopy for septic arthritis in children. Arthrosc Tech. 2021;10(3):e659–67. https://doi.org/10.1016/j.eats.2020.10.079. eCollection 2021 Mar. PMID: 33738199.
30. Sanpera I, Raluy-Collado D, Sanpera-Iglesias J. Arthroscopy for hip septic arthritis in children. Orthop Traumatol Surg Res. 2016;102(1):87–9. https://doi.org/10.1016/j.ostr.2015.008. PMID: 26725213.
31. Givon U, Liberman B, Schindler A, et. al. Treatment of septic arthritis of the hip joint by repeated ultrasound-guided aspirations. J Pediatr Orthop. 2004;24:266–70.

10 Paediatric Musculoskeletal Infections: A LMIC Perspective

Loro Antonio, Horn Anria, Franceschi Fulvio, and Mohan V. Belthur

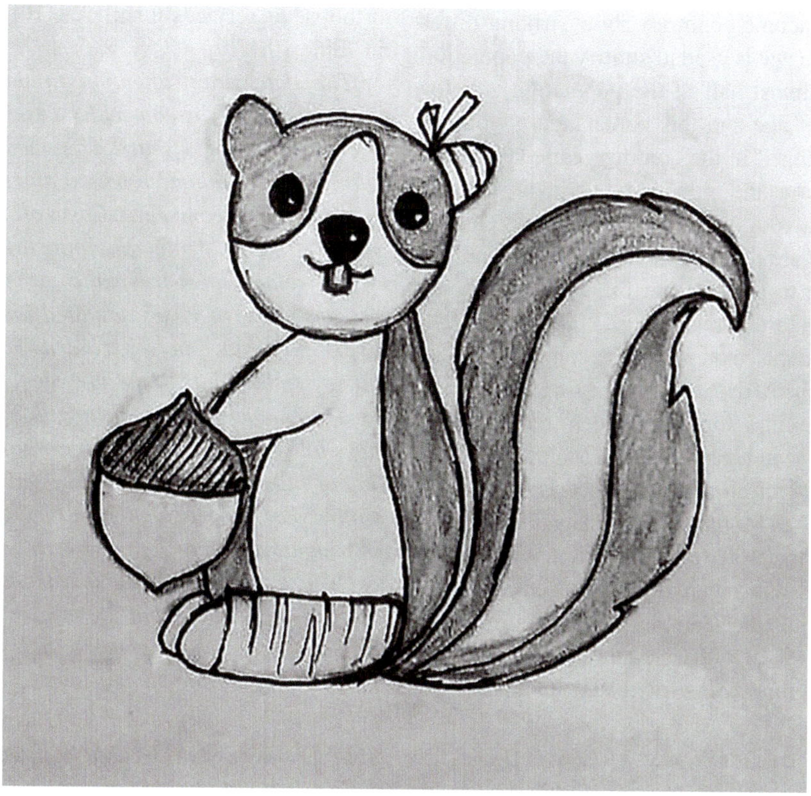

L. Antonio (✉)
Department of Orthopedic Surgery, CoRSU Rehabilitation Hospital, Kisubi, Uganda

H. Anria
Division of Orthopaedic Surgery, University of Cape Town, South Africa, Cape Town, South Africa

Red Cross War Memorial Children's Hospital, Cape Town, South Africa
e-mail: anria.horn@uct.ac.za

F. Fulvio
Consultant Paediatric Orthopaedic Surgeon, Trento, Italy

M. V. Belthur
Department of Child Health & Orthopedics, University of Arizona College of Medicine, Phoenix, AZ, USA

Department of Orthopedics, Phoenix Children's Hospital, Phoenix, AZ, USA
e-mail: mbelthur@phoenixchildrens.com

© Springer Nature Switzerland AG 2022
M. V. Belthur et al. (eds.), *Pediatric Musculoskeletal Infections*,
https://doi.org/10.1007/978-3-030-95794-0_10

Introduction

Epidemiology and Burden of Disease

In low- and middle-income countries (LMICs), paediatric musculoskeletal (MSK) infections are so common that in every surgical department there is a ward, or a cubicle, dedicated to the "septic cases", osteomyelitis in primis.

In his paper about the global burden of paediatric MSK diseases, Schwend estimated that 12 million affected children with paediatric MSK infections live in the least developed countries of the world [1]. Demographic data comparing low- and high-income countries show striking differences when age is used to stratify the population. In LICs, almost half of the population is below 18 years of age and this percentage is going to stay unchanged in the coming years, taking into consideration the population growth rates of countries across Africa and Asia. Since children of any age are the target of MSK infections, it is reasonable to assume that the above-mentioned number is close to reality.

Papers focused on paediatric conditions across sub-Saharan Africa underline how MSK infections represent a common burden to all of them. Studies done in Uganda [2] and Malawi [3] found that 3–3.5% of all surgical procedures were for osteomyelitis. Moreover, in the Ugandan study, it was found that 10% of all out-patient visits in five selected hospitals were done for osteomyelitis.

In Banjul, the Gambia, osteomyelitis represented 15.4% of 1726 paediatric surgical admissions in a time frame of 2 and half years [4]. Reports from hospitals located in Togo [5], Nigeria [6], and Burkina Faso [7] further emphasize the importance of osteomyelitis as a frequent cause for admission and its impact on the health systems.

The incidence of acute MSK infections is also higher in LMIC than in the developed world. Although accurate epidemiological data is scarce, studies from Malawi demonstrated an incidence of 5–20/100000 [8] for paediatric septic arthritis, whereas the incidence in the USA is as low as 1/100000 [9].

Data collected from the primary author's base hospital in Uganda, where paediatric plastic and orthopaedic services are offered [10], are reported in Table 10.1.

The data draw attention to the increasing number of new osteomyelitis cases per annum *over a period of 8 years. The numbers refer to surgical cases admitted with a diagnosis of haematogenous osteomyelitis. Cases of osteomyelitis-septic arthritis, isolated septic arthritis, spine osteomyelitis, post-traumatic or post-surgical osteomyelitis, or cases admitted for reconstructive surgery have been excluded. The column at the far right points to the prevalence of tuberculous osteomyelitis in our setting. It is a diagnostic possibility to keep in mind when working in areas where tuberculosis is endemic and poorly controlled. For this reason, it is our policy to perform intraoperative biopsy for tuberculosis culture in each case of haematogenous osteomyelitis.*

It is well known that the eradication of bone infections may require more than one surgery, particularly in the management of multi-focal

Table 10.1 Data from CoRSU Hospital in Uganda, representing the burden of MSK infections in their total patient population

Year	Total number of procedures in our hospital/year (n)	Number of new cases of osteomyelitis/year (n)	Number of TB osteomyelitis, as a percentage of all new osteomyelitis cases (%) (n)
2009	1309	100	12% (12)
2010	1632	122	4.1% (5)
2011	1651	136	6.9% (7)
2012	2014	175	6.8% (12)
2013	2368	257	8.5% (22)
2014	2485	264	14.4% (38)
2015	2284	260	13.5% (35)
2016	2464	305	7.9% (24)
Total	16,207	1658	9.3% (155)

disease, or when bone-soft tissue reconstruction is required. It is when all the procedures for MSK infections are counted that they have represented 18% of our surgical burden in this time span.

Challenges to Optimal Treatment in LMIC

MSK infections preferentially target poor and disadvantaged children living in remote areas or in decayed slums around the big cities. The reasons why children living in LMIC are so prone to infections are still debated; walking barefoot, poor sanitation, and unbalanced nutrition have all been thought to be responsible [11]. MSK infections in these settings are further complicated by poverty, local beliefs, limited access to struggling health facilities, and inappropriate or untimely treatment (Table 10.2).

Acute osteomyelitis and septic arthritis are often misdiagnosed or undiagnosed in developing countries for several reasons.

Firstly education, or lack thereof. Parents often do not immediately react to a painful or swollen limb and do not seek medical attention as rapidly as in developed countries. Access to resources like the Internet is also limited. Furthermore, health-care workers are not adequately trained to identify MSK infections early, resulting in missed diagnoses. This is compounded by the tendency of patients living in rural areas to seek advice from traditional healers as a first option. Management mostly consists of unconventional treatments such as herbal remedies and scarification, and modern medical advice is only sought once the initial treatment has been proven ineffective.

Table 10.2 Differences in osteomyelitis between LMIC and high-income countries

Low- and middle-income country	High-income country
Common	Uncommon
Poor living conditions and nutrition	Good nutrition and hygiene
Neglect, superstition	Early presentation
Mismanagement, under-treatment	Awareness
Late presentation	Early treatment, antimicrobial agents available
Limited laboratory techniques and imaging techniques (X-ray)	Advanced laboratory technique and diagnostic imaging (bone scan, CT, MRI, PET)
Limited number of qualified centres and specialists	Multidisciplinary teams in dedicated centres
Operative treatment	*Nonoperative treatment*

Secondly, access to care. Most patients living in LMIC are poor. Transport to health facilities is expensive or simply not available, and parents may choose to adopt the "watch-and-wait" approach. Local clinics in the outlying areas are often staffed by nurses only with no access to simple investigations such as radiographs and basic blood tests.

Thirdly, the frequent confounding history of trauma. Many patients presenting with acute MSK infections have a history of a minor injury followed by pain and/or swelling of the affected limb. X-rays will be taken and will inevitably be normal, and the patient is dismissed as having a minor soft tissue injury.

Consequently, mismanagement in the early stages of the disease is common, and at the time of presentation to qualified centres, surgery is commonly the only option for the eradication of the infection. This is in line with the findings reported from a study done in a tertiary referral centre in Tanzania [12]. We fully agree with the statement that early osteomyelitis is "one of the worst treated diseases in primary care" [13].

One such example is that of a 12-year-old male who presented to the casualty department at his local hospital with a swollen, painful ankle. He fell off his skateboard 2 days previously and the pain has been getting worse. He was diagnosed with an ankle sprain and told to return the next day for X-rays to exclude a fracture, as there were none available after hours on a Sunday. The patient duly returned the next day; X-rays were taken and were normal. He was given a bandage and some analgesia and discharged.

Three day later, his parents took him to a private doctor as the pain and swelling was getting worse and he had developed a fever. The GP immediately diagnosed an infection and referred

him to the regional hospital. Appropriate treatment was administered there including several debridements in theatre and targeted antibiotics. His cultures initially demonstrated a sensitive staphylococcus, but subsequent cultures grew resistant Klebsiella. He furthermore developed extensive wound breakdown and tissue loss. Bone necrosis and ankle joint arthritis rendered the limb unsalvageable, and a below-knee amputation was performed.

The family has filed a lawsuit against the provincial Department of Health; the case was found to be indefensible and was settled out of court for a large sum.

Impact

MSK infections represent a heavy burden on health systems and on the society at large in LMICs. Resources for their eradication and management are often needed but rarely available, especially in national health systems that can allocate, more or less, $50/per year/per person. According to a study performed in China, the cost of treating traumatic and non-traumatic osteomyelitis was $10,504 and $2819, respectively [14]. There are many ways one can decrease these costs, and surgeons in LMICs are no strangers to finding innovative ways to reduce costs but still deliver first-class care. Nonetheless, the costs of treating neglected MSK infections remain significant.

The social burden of neglected infections affects the patients themselves as well as their families. Children can miss years of education, and social reintegration may be extremely difficult, considering the permanent disability that severe MSK infections can cause. In a study from South Africa, children with complicated osteomyelitis were admitted to hospitals as long as 65 weeks [15]. In addition, it has been shown that prolonged hospital admission during childhood is associated with behavioural problems, delinquency, and even unstable job patterns in adulthood [16]. Parents must spend extended periods away from work and may even lose their jobs as a result of the child's condition.

One such example is that of a 7-year-old girl who was brought in by her mother with a 6 months' history of a swollen, painful, and pus-discharging leg. She reported that the disease started quite suddenly, with swelling, pain, and fever. A few days after, a boil burst, and pus began to drain. She brought her to the nearby practitioner in the village where local massage, smearing of the skin, and scarification using a razor blade were administered. However, due to worsening of the condition, she decided to borrow some money for the trip to a hospital in the capital city.

At presentation to this hospital, the child was in pain, ill looking, and using a walking stick. The leg was swollen, several sinuses were present, sequestra were visible through skin breaches, and the knee was held in flexion. The radiographs showed a large tibial sequestrum with poor involucrum formation and damage to the upper tibial physis. The girl was started on adequate nutrition and, as first step, a sequestrectomy was performed and the resulting bone defect was stabilized with an external fixator. The knee joint was also mobilized in extension. A few weeks later, after healing of the soft tissues, a bone transport technique was employed to reconstruct the bone. It took 6 months for this girl to recover.

Pathology and Microbiology

MSK infections are caused by haematogenous spread in about 80% of cases, with the remaining 20% being post-traumatic or post-surgical [17, 18]. A history of minor trauma is reported in over 30% of cases, days to weeks prior to the onset of symptoms.

The bones of the lower limbs are more likely to be involved, with the tibia topping the list, followed by the femur, humerus, fibula, radius, and ulna. The clavicle, calcaneus, metatarsals, and metacarpals are less frequently involved [18].

Staphylococcus aureus is the responsible bacteria in most cases with rates ranging from 57 to

93% of organisms cultured in cases presenting with acute septic arthritis or osteomyelitis (25,27,28). Rates of methicillin resistance are lower in LMIC than those reported in the developed world, as low as 0% in some studies, probably due to relatively limited access to antibiotics [15, 19, 20]. Interestingly, the presence of the Panton-Valentine leukocidin (PVL) does not appear to be associated with methicillin resistance in the few studies available from LMICs [21, 22]. This is contrary to the situation in the developed world. Despite this, the presence of PVL is certainly associated with a more severe disease. Unfortunately, PVL is not routinely tested for in laboratories in LMIC, and in most countries, the test is not available.

In neonates, group B streptococcus (*S. agalactiae*) and *Escherichia coli* are common pathogens, as are other *Enterobacter* species [23, 24]. There is a disproportionately high rate of *Salmonella* septic arthritis in low-income countries, with rates ranging from 40% to 60% according to studies from sub-Saharan Africa. This is associated with poverty, sickle cell anaemia, and malnutrition and appears to be due to a high rate of *Salmonella* bacteremia in these children [25–27].

Tuberculosis is endemic in many LMIC, and routine testing should be performed on all samples taken from infected bones or joints to rule out concomitant tuberculous infection.

How the pathogens enter the blood stream is still unclear. History of pharyngitis, otitis, or other infections is rarely reported. In neonates, history of infection involving the umbilical cord should be looked for. A source of infection was found in 67% of patients in a study performed in Namibia [11]. Barefoot walking is the norm in LMIC, and skin lesions might be the entry point; thorn pricks are often reported, and infected insect bites are another common source. Jiggers, a parasitic infestation caused by *Tunga penetrans* and spread by the chigoe flea, is very common in sub-Saharan Africa and South America. Poor nutrition and poor hygiene are commonly reported in history taking.

Clinical Presentation and Examination

Chronic or neglected osteomyelitis may present in a variety of ways depending on the duration of the disease, the number of sites affected, established complications, and treatment given. It is not uncommon for children to receive some form of treatment before presentation, such as scarification of the skin, manipulations, smearing, and bandaging the site with herbal concoctions. In LMICs, you must expect the unexpected.

Pain, swelling, purulent discharge, and loss of function are the main presenting complaints, although, quite surprisingly, pain may not be a major symptom in longstanding cases. Fever is not a presenting sign in normal circumstances. It may be recorded in case of an abscess or pyomyositis, disseminated infection, or at an early stage of the disease.

An accurate and systematic clinical examination represents the cornerstone of the management plan. The attention must be directed not only to the obvious site of infection, but to every possible site of infection, as other active or quiescent sites must be looked for, especially in the hip and shoulder girdles. In an unpublished series by the primary author, another site of infection was found in 1 out of 10 to 15 children.

Foul smelling wounds are typical. Discharging sinuses are often present, several at times, and the skin in between, mainly in the leg and forearm, can be of poor status. Look for sinuses in covered parts of the body, mainly around the pelvic bones, genital areas, upper third of the thigh, axilla, and scapula. Sinuses around the ilium and upper third of the thigh may be the only findings hinting to an underlying tuberculosis infection of the spine (Fig. 10.1).

Protruding sequestra are commonly encountered, and the exposed sequestrum may be brown or greenish in colour. When massive in size, they are associated with pathological fracture, axial deformity, and limb shortening. Consequently, limping is a common feature, more so when joint involvement is present (Fig. 10.2).

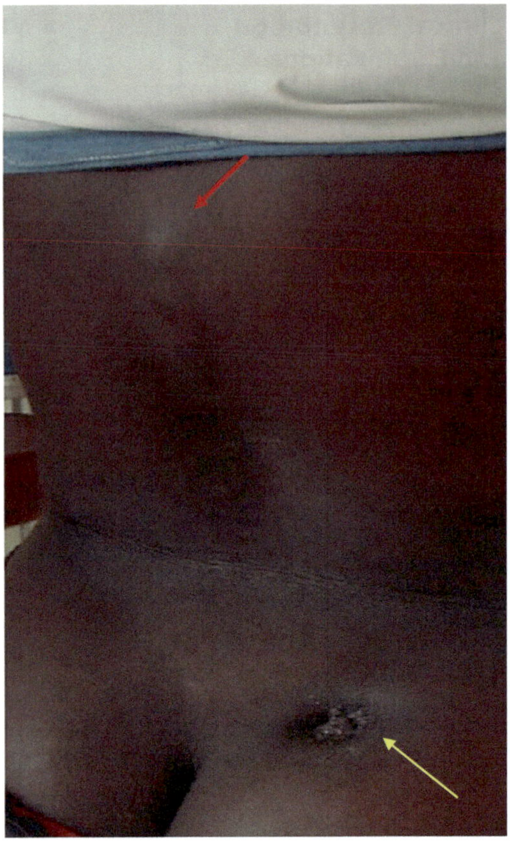

Fig. 10.1 Tuberculosis of the spine (Pott's disease). A sinus over the ilium that was overlooked for quite a while (yellow arrow), delaying the diagnosis of thoracolumbar TB indicated by the clinically evident gibbus (red arrow)

Pseudoparalysis is another important presenting feature, especially in neonates and young children. Several cases of septic arthritis of the hip present with fever, irritability, and pseudoparalysis of the affected limb, yet they can go undetected because of poor clinical judgement.

Multiple site localization can be found in 6% of cases, while in 8% of children, active septic arthritis or its sequelae may be observed at presentation (Unpublished data, AL), with up to eight bones or joints being infected at the same time. There are cases where other localizations follow months or years after the eradication of the first one.

At presentation, children may present with one of the following clinical entities:

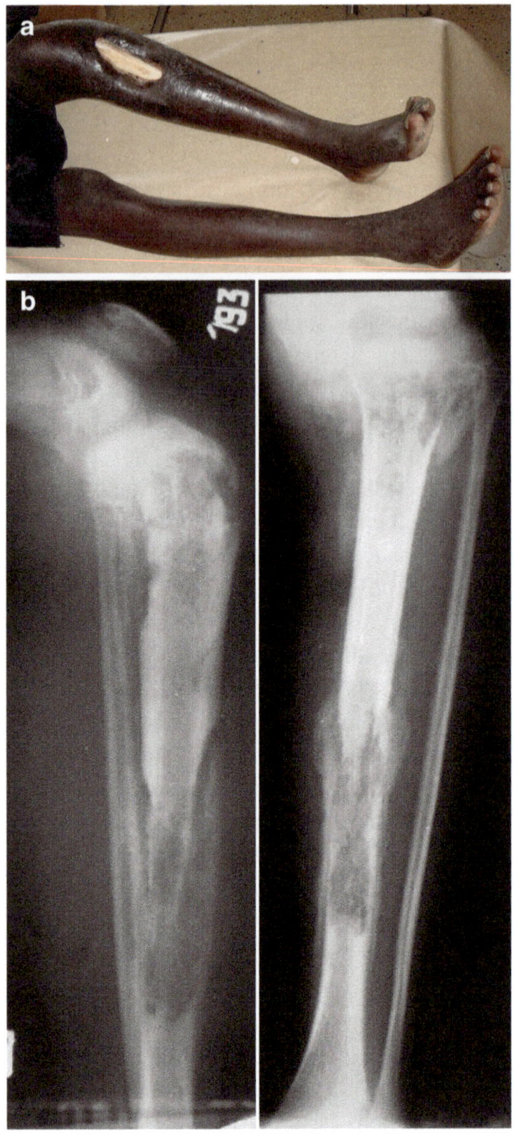

Fig. 10.2 (**a**) Clinical photograph and (**b**) X-rays of a left tibial osteomyelitis in an 11-year-old girl. The onset of the infection was a year prior to presentation. The presence of a pathological fracture, bone and soft tissue loss, and a knee contracture required multidisciplinary management by orthopaedic and plastic surgical specialists

- Single site osteomyelitis (sometimes with pyomyositis)
- Single site septic arthritis
- Single site osteomyelitis-septic arthritis (Fig. 10.3)

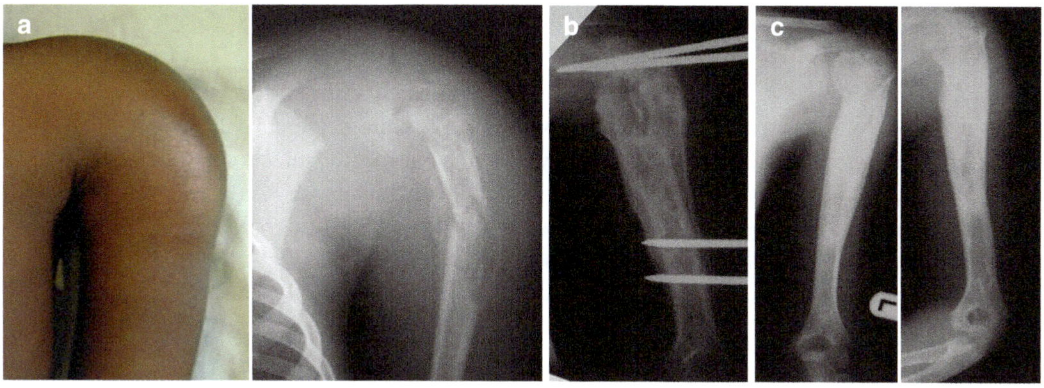

Fig. 10.3 (**a**) Clinical photograph and X-ray of an 8-year-old boy who presented with fever, pseudoparalysis and severe pain, and a diagnosis of osteomyelitis-septic arthritis of left shoulder. (**b**) Emergency joint debridement and simple external fixation was performed, favouring resizing of the sequestrum, involucrum formation, and union of the fracture. (**c**) Radiographs taken 1 year after surgery. Excellent bone reconstruction is seen, reflected clinically in a good shoulder function. Surgery must always enhance the excellent healing potential so typical of children, while maintaining good alignment and stability

- Floating sequestra in a peri-osseous abscess
- Multiple site infections
- Post-infectious complications

These clinical presentations, coupled with radiographic features, represent the elements on which our management plans must be based.

Tips and tricks: initial assessment

- Fever is not a presenting sign in chronic osteomyelitis
- Do a thorough clinical examination and look for other possible sites of infection
- Request recent, up-to-date radiographs
- Have a high index of suspicion for Tuberculosis

Special Investigations and Work-Up

Laboratory Investigations

In the rare instance that patients present with acute infections, simple clinical signs, such as fever and signs of inflammation, and blood tests may be utilized to confirm or exclude a diagnosis of MSK infection. A full blood count and erythrocyte sedimentation rate (ESR) should be requested, as well as a c-reactive protein (CRP) if this test is available. Kocher [28] developed a set of criteria (a history of fever, inability to weight bear, ESR >40 mm/Hr, white cell count (WCC) >12x10^9/l), published in 1999, to help differentiate between transient synovitis of the hip and septic arthritis in patients presenting with an irritable hip. Although not originally described for this purpose, the Kocher criteria remain a useful method of distinguishing between MSK infection and other causes of MSK pain. The erythrocyte sedimentation rate can be measured using nothing more than a test tube and anti-coagulated blood.

In chronic or neglected cases, a full blood count and albumin levels should be requested. A moderate anaemia is usually found. Leukocytosis can be found in cases of disseminated infection or pyomyositis. Erythrocyte sedimentation rate (ESR) is not helpful in longstanding cases, and it is not a routine test in our facility; it may be useful in evaluating the clinical course in disseminated infections or in tuberculous foci. The albumin level is a crude indication of nutritional status and may guide nutritional support and optimization in the per-operative period.

Imaging Studies

Acute MSK Infection

In acute osteomyelitis, radiographs are typically normal. In the case of septic arthritis, there may be displacement of the soft tissue planes surrounding the joint, suggesting an effusion. Rarely, there is subluxation or dislocation of the hip. Nonetheless, plain radiographs of the affected bone or limb should be obtained in the first instance.

Advanced imaging such as MRI is seldom available, but ultrasound may be helpful to identify collections or large joint effusions. Clinical suspicion is the mainstay of diagnosing acute infections, and intervention should not be delayed while awaiting special investigations.

Chronic or Neglected MSK Infections

Plain radiographs of the affected segment must be taken, including the adjacent joints. Digital radiographs offer better details but are still unavailable in most of the health structures.

It is advisable to repeat the radiographs when the original ones, brought by the patients, are hazy or older than 1 month. Infected bone changes rapidly, particularly in small children. Sequestra may revascularize, may reduce in size or may have been expelled before presentation. Recent radiographs must be at hand before undertaking any surgical procedure.

MRI and CT scan are requested only in particular cases, such as in pelvic or mandibular infections, to identify and properly locate sequestra that may not be clearly seen in plain radiographs. CT or MRI scan is sometimes required to confirm the diagnosis when radiographic findings could suggest a bone sarcoma. MRI can be useful for the localization of an intramedullary abscess or to detect joint infections in early phases. It is useful when soft tissues must be studied. Routinely, they are not necessary to reach a proper diagnosis and their cost and availability must be kept in mind.

Tissue Sampling

Deep bone and tissue specimens for culture and sensitivity are preferably taken intraoperatively to rule out specific infections and to help with the differential diagnosis. As a rule, all specimens must be sent for microbiology and histopathology. Microscopic investigations should include a gram stain and Ziehl-Neelsen stain for acid-fast bacilli. Cultures for aerobic and anaerobic bacteria, tuberculosis, and fungi should be performed. Microbiology results may be misleading when they are taken from the sinuses or exposed sequestra; therefore, deep tissue specimens are mandatory.

Differential Diagnosis

Sometimes it is necessary to exclude other diagnoses, and this can be difficult preoperatively. In areas where sickle cell disease is endemic, it might be difficult to differentiate a bone infarction from an early osteomyelitis. Bone pain is present in both situations, often with fever. The blood test can be misleading since leukocytosis is a common finding in sickle cell anaemia. Surgical exploration is the best way to reach a definitive diagnosis.

Bone tumours may also mimic bone infection. Ewing's sarcoma or Burkitt's lymphoma, although rare, may be tricky to differentiate without an open biopsy. Osteosarcomas, mainly around the knee, may be radiographically confused with bone infection, especially when there is huge involucrum formation, with a sunburst appearance, and open biopsy is mandatory.

Decision-Making and Classification

Acute MSK Infection In the acute setting, if the patient has three or more Kocher criteria for infection, or if there is significant clinical suspicion, surgery in the form of arthrotomy or incision and drainage of an abscess is recommended [24]. If surgical facilities are unavailable, joint aspiration may be performed as an alternative. Open surgery affords one the opportunity to obtain deep tissue samples for culture and histopathology, and a negative arthrotomy is preferential to delay in treatment of a true septic arthritis. We do not recommend waiting for advanced imaging in the presence of high clinical suspicion.

Chronic or Neglected MSK Infection The eradication of the infection and the restoration of the function of the affected site are the goals of treatment. There are cases for which the priority is the eradication of the infection, others for which the eradication must be associated with corrective and reconstructive surgery. Furthermore, there are cases in which, with quiescent infection, the priority is the reconstruction of the site to re-establish or improve the impaired function.

In the last two decades, classifications have been proposed from African practitioners, based on different parameters. Meier et al. in 1993 [6], Solagberu et al. in 2003 [29], Thomas et al. in 2007 [30], and Wynn Jones et al. in 2009 [31] focused their classifications on haematogenous osteomyelitis, taking into consideration duration, clinical findings, and radiological features. We found them difficult to use in daily practice and unable to accommodate all the variable clinical presentations seen in LMICs. In the last few years, we have started to utilize a different classification.

The following classification system, as elaborated in the following sub-sections, is the first step in the proper management of the condition. It has been developed to aid surgeons in the decision-making process regarding possible referral to qualified centres. This should help minimize inappropriate surgical procedures that, in some contexts, might result in worsened outcomes for the patients. Clinical findings, radiologic features, surgeon's skills, and equipment available are the factors on which any management plan should be grounded.

Osteomyelitis Type 1 (Uncomplicated Osteomyelitis)

In osteomyelitis type 1, or uncomplicated osteomyelitis, the function of the affected segment is not in jeopardy, the bone is clinically stable, and the adjacent joints are not compromised. Radiographically, the infection site and the sequestra are clearly defined, and the growth plates are spared (Figs. 10.4 and 10.5). The clinical priority here is the eradication of the infection. Surgery is quite straightforward, relying on basic surgical skills and orthopaedic sets. It can

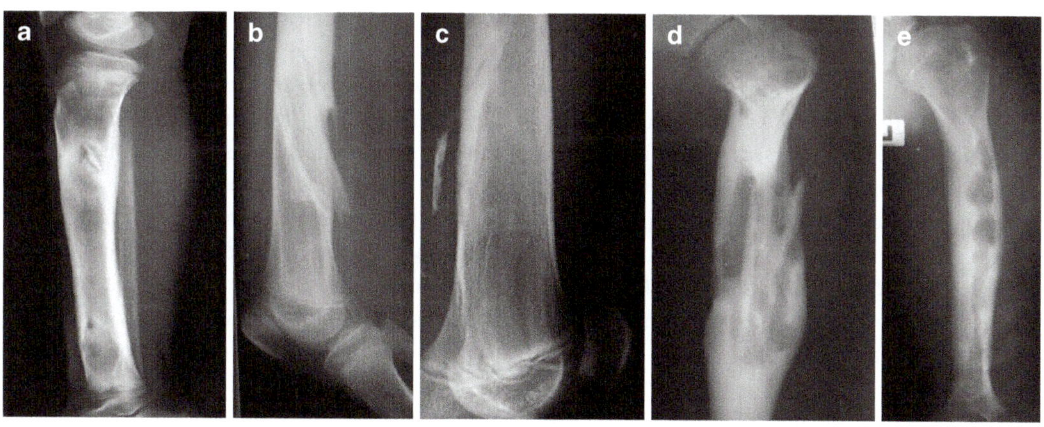

Fig. 10.4 (**a–e**) Radiographs illustrating cases of type 1 osteomyelitis. (**c**) The so-called floating sequestrum. (**e**) The typical appearance of intramedullary abscesses

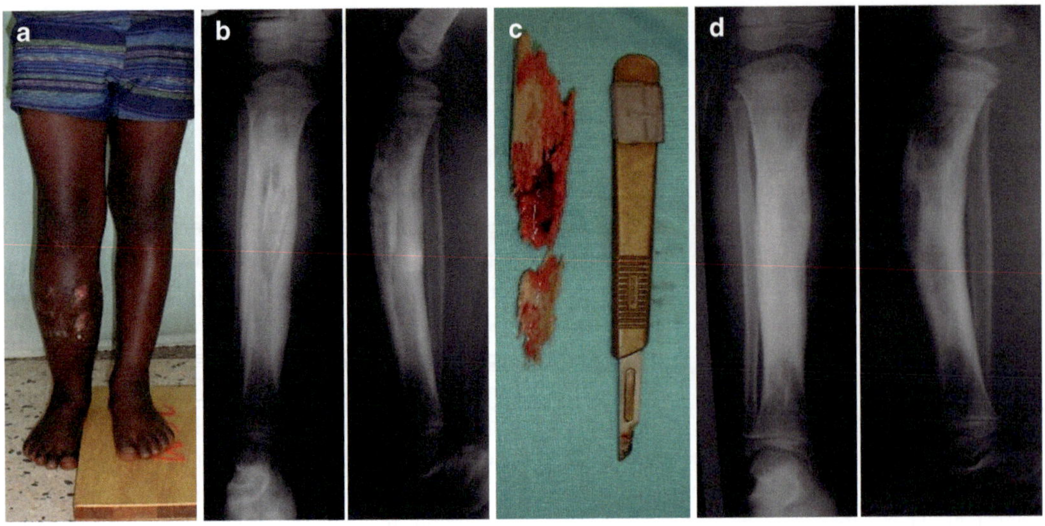

Fig. 10.5 (**a**, **b**) A typical case of uncomplicated osteomyelitis in a 6-year-old boy. The infection started 12 months before, apparently following a trivial trauma. The main concern was the continuous purulent discharge, with little discomfort. (**c**) Sequestrectomy was followed by a rapid recovery. (**d**) Radiographs taken 12 months after surgery, showing advanced bone remodelling

be carried out in departments of general surgery, with no need for referral to qualified centres. The risk of intraoperative and post-operative complications is low. With a combination of appropriate medical and surgical treatment, good outcome and normal limb function are likely, and recurrence is rare. Good outcomes have been reported without the use of antibiotics as adjuvant treatment, but this remains controversial [6].

Osteomyelitis Type 2 (Complicated Osteomyelitis)

In osteomyelitis type 2, or complicated osteomyelitis, the function of the segment(s) is compromised or in jeopardy. Pathological fractures, bone loss, soft tissue defects, shortening, joint contractures, septic joints, and multiplicity of sites (as for TB and sickle cell anaemia) may be present. Cases of involvement of an entire bone, with a multicystic appearance on X-ray, are also included here, considering the surgical skill required to eradicate the infection (Fig. 10.6). Surgery requires expertise, skills, and proper equipment. Ancillary services must be at hand such as C-arm, external fixators, blood for transfusion, and good laboratory services. The likelihood of recurrence is higher since complete eradication of infection may be difficult to obtain, especially when a tourniquet cannot be employed. These cases should be referred to qualified centres, if available, in the country.

Osteomyelitis Type 3 (Cases for Reconstruction)

Osteomyelitis type 3 focuses on cases which need reconstruction. This group includes the complications of MSK infections such as bone defects, angular deformities, limb shortening or overgrowth, joint fusions, or neglected dislocations. Corrective and reconstructive surgery can be really challenging and can put an expert surgeon to the test, even in presence of proper equipment and facilities. These cases must be managed in a specialized centre with appropriate facilities and surgical expertise present.

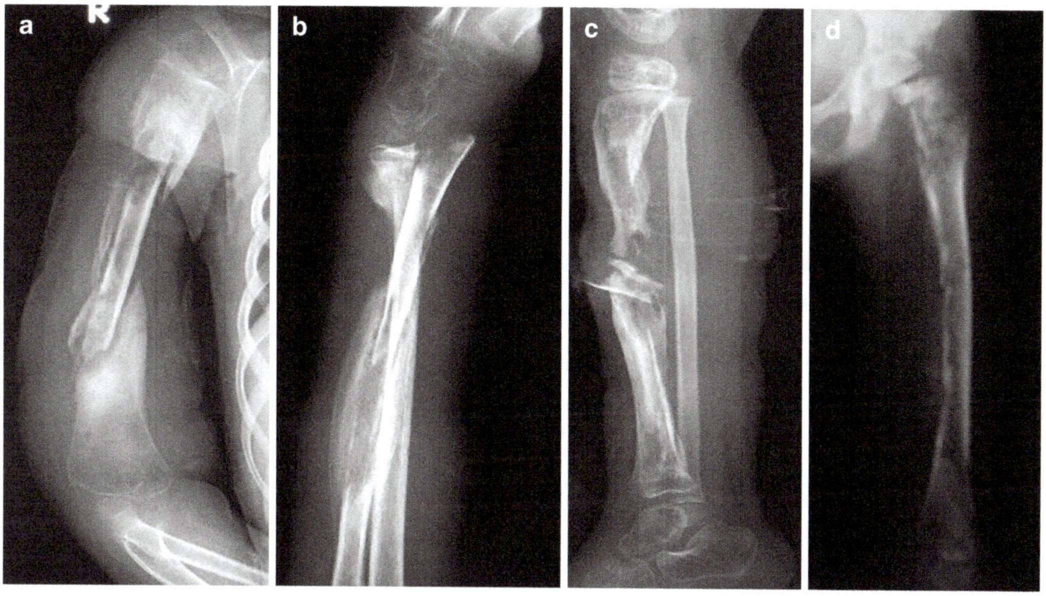

Fig. 10.6 (**a**–**d**) Radiographic examples of type 2 osteomyelitis showing pan-diaphyseal involvement with pathological fracture and bone loss. (**d**) This is a case of osteomyelitis-septic arthritis, not a multicystic one

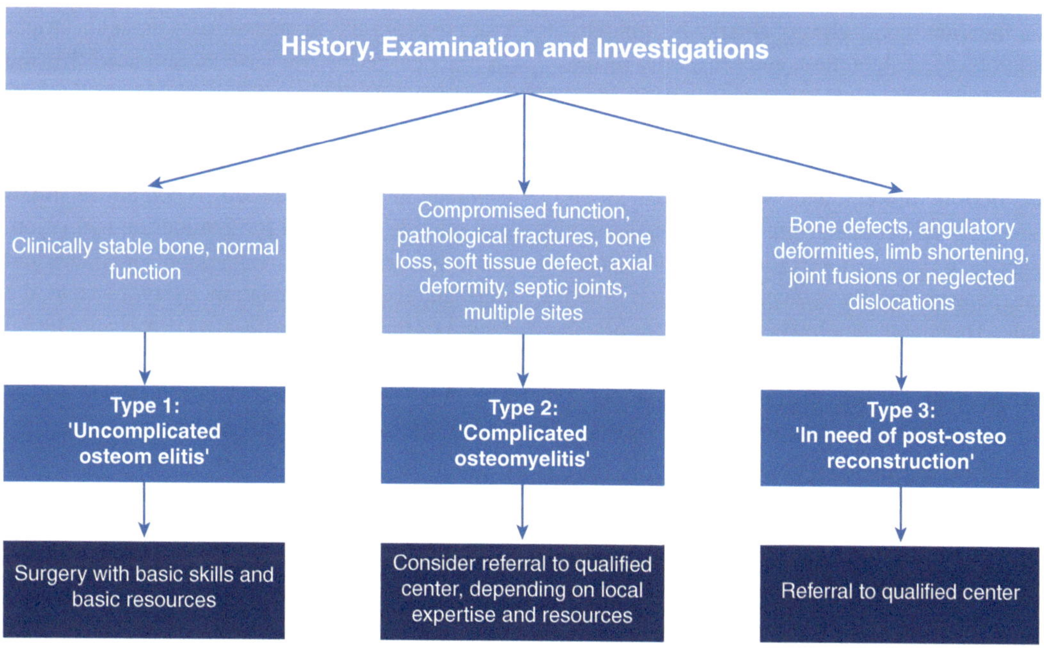

Medical Treatment

The medical treatment is based on two major elements: antibiotics and nutrition. There is an abuse of antibiotics in the pre-surgical phase of the disease, often given in combinations and predisposing patients to develop resistant infections. In the presence of sequestra, antibiotics alone are never indicated, can be dangerous, and can cause a heavy financial burden to the family. The role of antibiotics post-operatively is controversial, especially if surgery is judged to have been radical and accurate [32]. However, most surgeons would still administer a 4- to 6-week course of targeted antibiotics, based on deep tissue culture results, post-operatively.

Antibiotics are employed in type 2 osteomyelitis, in presence of large abscesses, disseminated infection, and septic arthritis. They are used for 1 or 2 weeks after surgery. Antibiotic therapy should be guided by local guidelines. Further antibiotic choice should be guided by microbiological, culture, and sensitivity results.

Nutrition is especially important during the pre- and post-operative phases. It should be considered a drug in these settings. The diet should be rich in protein and hypercaloric, possibly using cheap products that are available in the region. In Uganda, for example, this diet includes inexpensive, locally sourced foods such as silver fish, groundnuts, sunflower oil, maize flour, eggs, sugar, milk, and fresh fruit, such as avocado and bananas. An adequate diet is a must, especially in disseminated cases, and in patients with sickle cell anaemia or tuberculosis.

Recovery is associated with improvement of the laboratory parameters and body weight, in addition to local healing, in terms of sinus closure and reduced pain. The psychological change is an important sign as well. It is difficult to describe in words, but we all know what a smile and willingness to play mean in clinical terms. It is the mother, usually, who reports how her child relates and interacts in a vastly different way.

Surgery and MSK Infections

Before undertaking surgery, factors to be considered include the surgeon's self-assessment, the aforementioned classification, and the surgical facility. There are big differences in what hospitals located in LMICs can offer to patients. Many are poorly equipped, with extremely limited financial resources. This section on surgical management is directed to these facilities. The healing potential of children, especially below the age of 5 years, must always be enhanced by the surgery. In surgical planning, the first question should always be: is this infected bone, at this stage of the disease, ready for surgery? If yes, which type of surgery? (Fig. 10.7).

Timing of surgical intervention is controversial [30, 32], yet it is essential to prevent serious complications. There are authors who see the sequestrum as a stimulus for involucrum formation, while other authors think that the involucrum formation is independent of the sequestrum. In practical terms, we have experienced that the sequestrum itself has to be considered an exploitable, useful foreign body, provided it is not completely devascularized, floating free in the segment, or widely exposed. When left in situ, it can provide a scaffold for involucrum formation, it can be a useful anchorage point for screws and pins, and it can help maintain, to some extent, the length of the bone (Fig. 10.8). It gives an internal stability to the infected segment, and, in small children, it may be completely resorbed in a short time [33].

Management of the soft tissues is a critical step, particularly in the leg. Unhealthy, scarred, and poorly vascularized skin requires great attention when choosing the surgical approach. Plastic procedures are often needed, preceded by vacuum-assisted closure, where available. Local flaps are elegant solutions in the leg, but expertise is required. Free vascularized flaps may be considered in facilities with the required expertise [34].

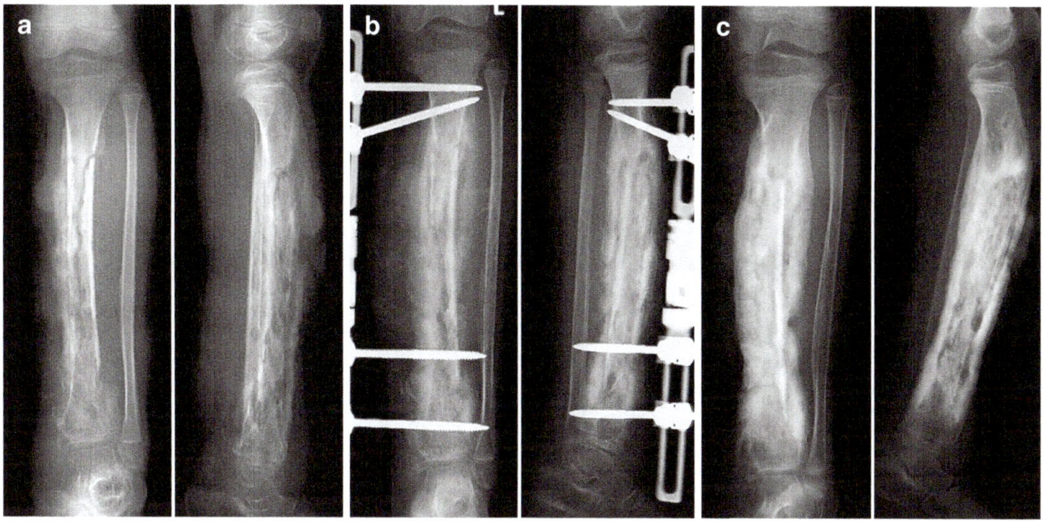

Fig. 10.7 (**a**) A case of impending pathological fracture, with no clear demarcation of the sequestered shaft. (**b**) Stabilization of the segment with a simple external fixator allows involucrum formation and increases stability of the bone while maintaining alignment. (**c**) Four months later, sufficient structural involucrum has formed to allow for sequestrectomy without any further reconstructive procedures

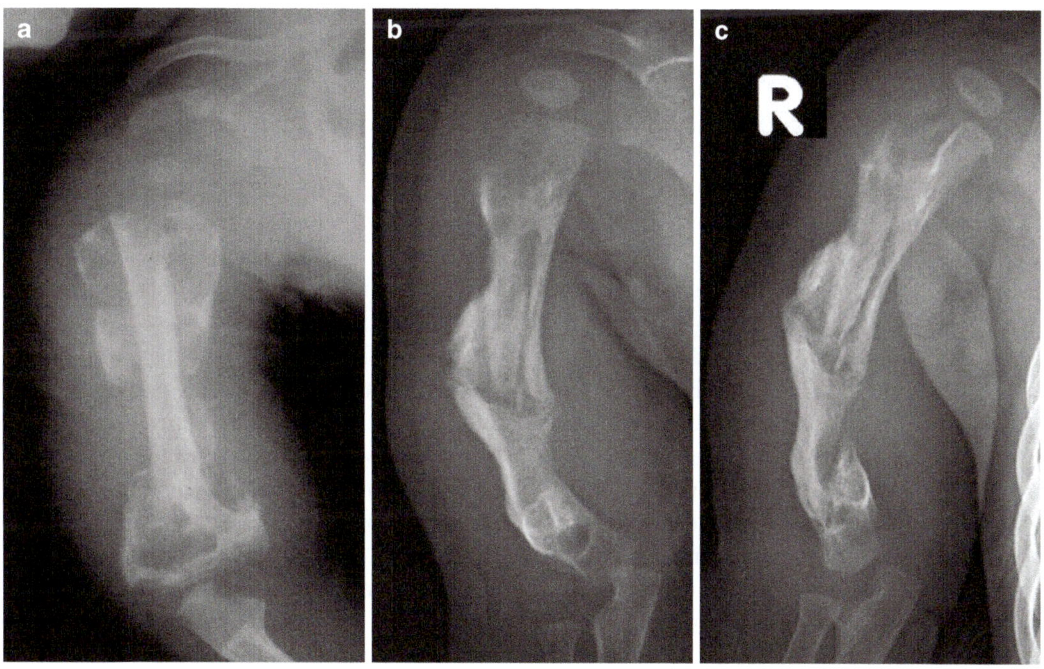

Fig. 10.8 (**a**–**c**) In very young children, the sequestrum may be partially or totally reintegrated, stimulating involucrum formation at the same time

> **Stop and Think before surgery:**
>
> 1. Is this infected bone, at this stage of the disease, ready for surgery?
> 2. Does the surgeon have the skills and expertise for the type of surgery needed?
> 3. Does this facility have the appropriate resources to deal with the surgery, post-operative care and the possible complications?
>
> If any of the answers to the questions above is a NO, reconsider your management plan and consider referral

Treatment Options and Surgical Procedures

Osteomyelitis

Sequestrectomy and decompression of pus are the main priorities, preceded or followed by proper segment stabilization. Segment stabilization can be achieved by means of a simple external fixator construct, using either a monolateral construct (Orthofix™, Verona, Italy), a modular external fixator such as the Hoffman fixator (Stryker™, Michigan, USA) or AO external fixator (DePuy Synthes, Massachusetts, USA), or a circular fixator. Whereas these implants are strictly single use in the developed world, the external components can, and is, used repeatedly in the developing world with minimal complications related to re-use. The surgical implant cost is therefore limited to the half-pins, and even these can be re-used if necessary. Advanced soft tissue reconstruction is often required, ranging from skin, fasciocutaneous, gastrocnemius, and osteocutaneous flaps, and should be performed under tourniquet to ensure a bloodless field.

In case of sequestrectomy, look for sequestra in the bone, soft tissues, and sinuses. Compare what is removed with the corresponding radiographic images. Explore the sinuses and cloacae that are visible in the field. Be aware of intracortical sequestra, they can be fully hidden in the thick cortices or involucrum. Rarely, in endemic areas, caseous necrosis can be found in bone cavities, leading to a prompt diagnosis of tuberculous osteomyelitis.

In cases of protruding or exposed sequestra, sequestrectomy inevitably results in a bone defect with poor soft tissue cover. Techniques to address large bone defects and dead space are discussed later in the chapter.

In cases of sequestra in the soft tissues, the bone is usually not actively infected at the time of surgery. Sequestra are most commonly found in the thigh, followed by the arm and axilla. They can be small and difficult to locate and remove. It is usually the discharging sinus tract that helps in their location and removal. Look for them in the pyogenic membranes and pus that you remove from the site.

The canoeing technique may be useful when a long fenestration is required for proper exposure and debridement of the medullary space (Fig. 10.9). We recommend creating a 5–10-mm-diameter rectangular slot of appropriate length that allows for good vision and accurate debridement without putting the bone stability at risk. A multiple windows technique is extremely useful in preventing iatrogenic fractures. Should a fracture occur, an external fixator should be applied during the same surgical session [33] (Box 10.1).

In the presence of an intramedullary abscess, bone windowing is preferred to drill holes, since it allows for better drainage and inspection of the medullary canal (Boxes 10.2 and 10.3).

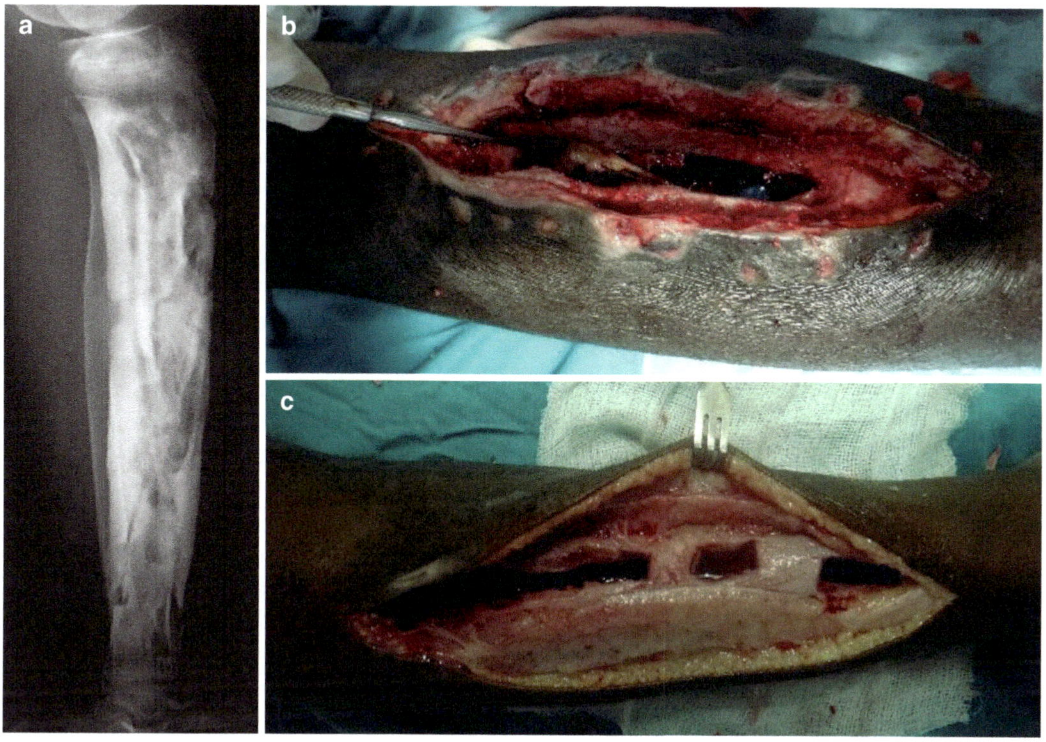

Fig. 10.9 Canoeing may be required when infection is involving the entire bone (**a**). A long segment of cortex is removed, transforming the shape of the bone to that resembling a canoe (**b**). To avoid intraoperative fracture bridges of bone may be carved out, connecting the two sides of the bone window (**c**)

Box 10.1 Key Learning Points

- Haematogenous osteomyelitis in developing countries is a common clinical problem. Clinical acumen and radiological features lead to a correct diagnosis in most of the cases.
- Infections are usually seen in late stages making surgery the key element of treatment.
- Septic arthritis, even when suspected, needs urgent surgical attention.
- Adequate management plan must be laid down from admission day. Choosing the right timing in the surgical plan is a fundamental step for healing.
- Untreated or mistreated HO is an important cause of permanent disability in children.

Box 10.2 Tips and Tricks

- Intraoperative biopsy is strongly recommended in regions where TB is poorly controlled.
- Adequate surgical equipment must be at hand. External fixation may be required in complicated cases.
- Sequestra must be looked for in soft tissues, sinuses, and involucrum.
- Recent, clear radiographs must be available at the time of surgery.
- Look for other sites of active or quiescent infection, particularly in the hip and shoulder girdles.
- When possible, use the pneumatic tourniquet or Esmarch's bandage.

Box 10.3 Pitfalls to Avoid

- Untimely extensive debridement and periosteal elevation in cases without clear demarcation of the sequestered segment.
- Missing a diagnosis of septic arthritis, particularly of the hip in small children. Not every fever is caused by malaria.
- Rely on long period of systemic antibiotics in presence of clear sequestra.
- Undertaking surgery without being ready for intervening complications.
- Avoiding aggressive surgery in small children since sequestra may be spontaneously reabsorbed.

Septic Arthritis

In case of early septic arthritis, immediate arthrotomy must be carried out, even on simple suspicion that the hip joint is at risk. Unfortunately, septic hips are often seen very late, leaving the surgeon with limited salvage options including excision arthroplasty (if the femoral head has not been resorbed completely (Fig. 10.10) or arthrodesis (Fig. 10.11)). In late septic arthritis of the knee, knee fusion is advised, in association with limb lengthening, simultaneously or staged. Fusion is also the choice for the ankle and wrist joints. In long-standing monoarticular infection, in the presence of a "perplexing" joint as described by Sharrard [35], tuberculosis must be always suspected. Caseation is rarely found in the joint cavity, so biopsy is the only way to reach a proper diagnosis. Occasionally, draining sinus is found surrounding the joint and an immediate diagnosis can be made (Fig. 10.12).

Dead Space Management

Radical debridement and sequestrectomy leave behind a dead space, at times exceptionally large. For larger defects, a variety of techniques exist and are discussed elsewhere. It is important to be aware that large bone defect management is time-consuming and costly and should not be attempted in the absence of adequate skills and resources.

For smaller defects, in the presence of bone continuity and proper skin cover, a simple and inexpensive solution is to fill the dead space with dry gauze, leaving one end outside through the pre-existing sinuses or through loose, interrupted sutures. The gauze is removed 24–36 hours after surgery, during the first dressing change, using a ketamine cocktail for pain management. Dead spaces fill well in children, rather quickly in those below 5 years of age, accompanied by bone remodelling [17, 36].

In selected cases, Papineau's excision-graft technique may offer an elegant solution to handle infected sites, where other techniques have failed [37, 38]. This must be considered in small defects

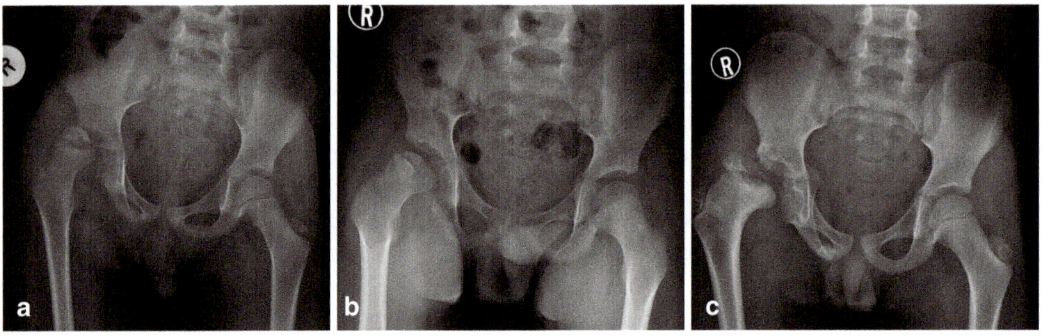

Fig. 10.10 (**a**) A 5-year-old boy presented late with septic arthritis of the right hip and subluxation. (**b**) The hip was reduced and placed in a spica and subsequently developed AVN. (**c**) Latest radiographs show near complete resorption of the femoral head

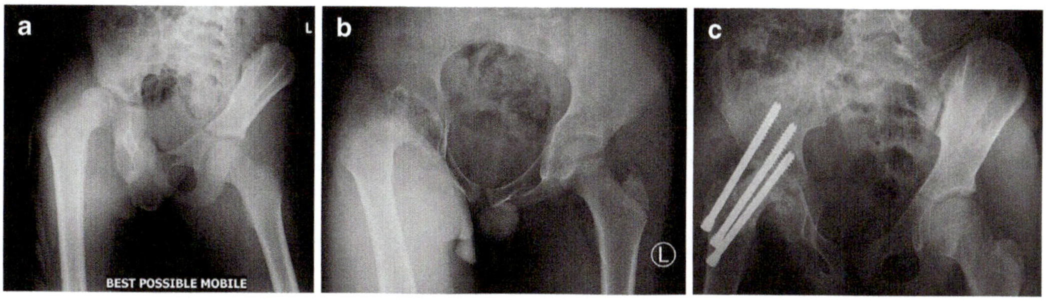

Fig. 10.11 (**a**) An 11-year male, poorly managed septic arthritis of the right hip with ongoing infection and hip subluxation. (**b**) Joint destruction and deformity ensued, accompanied by extreme pain. (**c**) An open debridement and arthrodesis were performed correcting the deformity and alleviating the pain

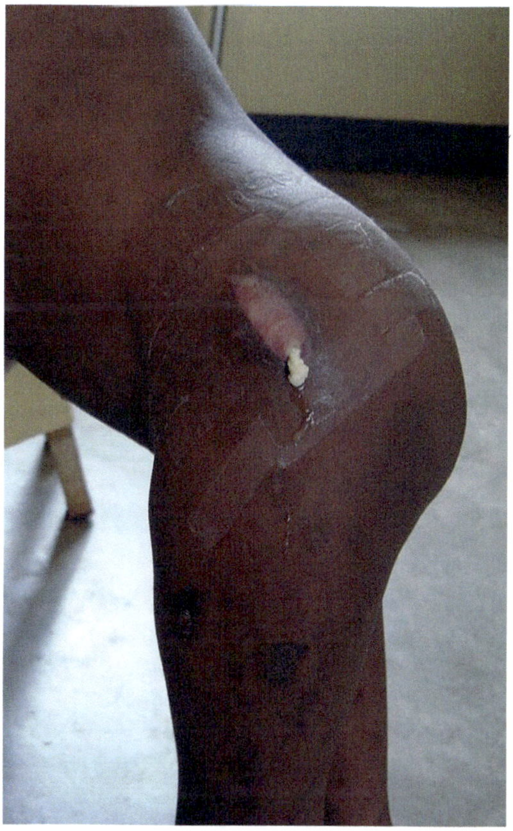

Fig. 10.12 Caseous discharge from a previous arthrotomy wound in tuberculosis of the hip

located in the middle or distal third of the leg in the presence of bone stability (Fig. 10.13).

The dead space can be temporarily filled with antibiotic-loaded cement or with polymethylmethacrylate antibiotic beads [37]. Availability and cost of these treatments limit their use in poorer countries, and they are not suitable when large open wounds are present. Locally made beads impregnated with antibiotic may be an option, and the technique is still performed by some surgeons. Local muscle and fasciocutaneous flaps can be utilized, usually in soft tissue defects in the leg and forearm, followed by bone reconstruction techniques.

Autogenous bone graft, gradual and immediate bone transport [39], non-vascularized fibula, and vascularized fibula grafts [40] are all techniques in the surgeon's armamentarium (Fig. 10.14). They are all reviewed by Rasool in his paper concerning tibial defects following osteomyelitis [41] and elsewhere in this text.

Complications

Bleeding is one of the most dreaded post-surgical complications, especially in small children. It may follow simultaneous surgery for multiple site infections, extensive canoeing (technique previously described), or surgery around the pelvis. Although severe bleeding is uncommon, close care must be taken in the first 48 hours postoperatively. If emergency blood or transfusion services are not readily available, patients should be optimized prior to surgery. This can be achieved by nutritional support and oral iron, folic acid, and vitamin C supplements following a strict regime preoperatively [42]. Measures to limit intraoperative bleeding should always be employed.

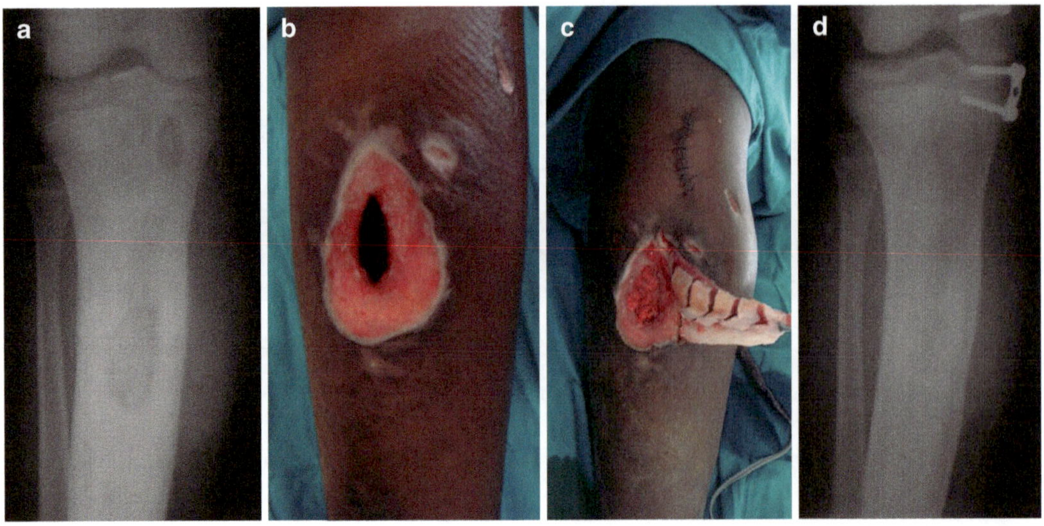

Fig. 10.13 (**a**, **b**) X-rays and post-debridement clinical picture of a 13-year-old patient who presented with long-standing osteomyelitis of the right tibia and two previous surgeries. She had a draining sinus over the site of infection, surrounded by poorly vascularized, invaginated skin and scar tissue. Following debridement of all necrotic and scar tissue, simple dressings are applied until granulation tissue covers the entire defect. (**c**) The defect is then filled with cancellous bone chips and the wound is covered with a gastrocnemius flap. (**d**) Perfect integration and eradication of the infection is seen 3 years later. Guided growth was employed to correct a residual valgus deformity

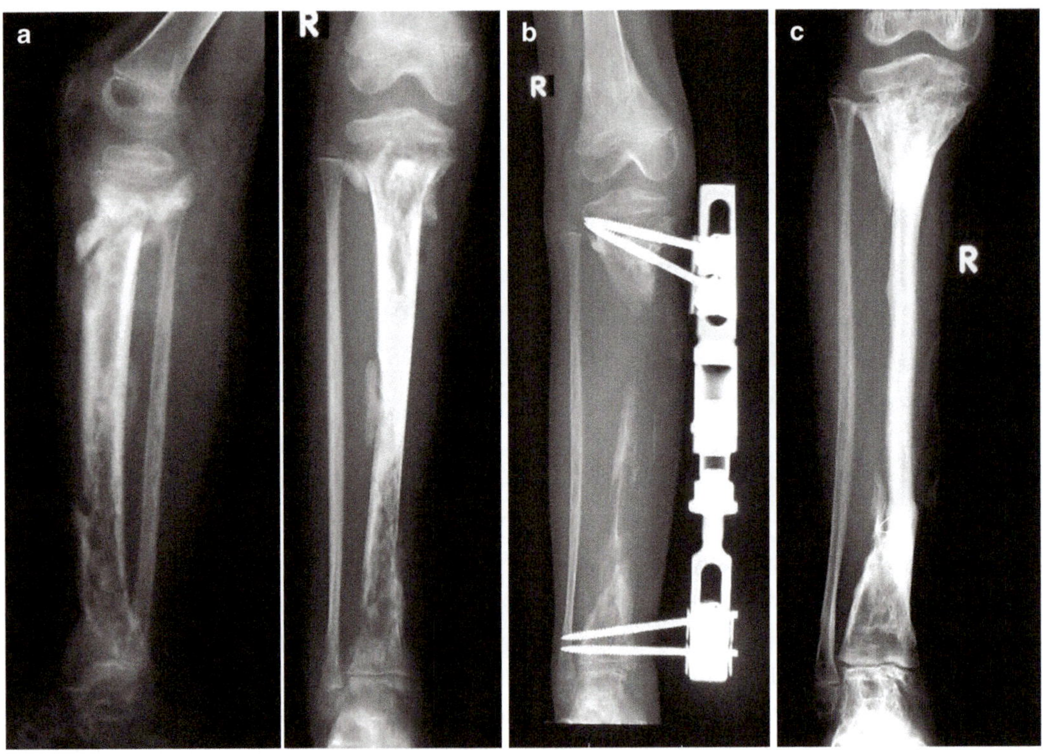

Fig. 10.14 (**a**) Sequestration of the entire diaphysis of the right tibia, with loss of soft tissue envelope, in a 6-year-old girl. (**b**) Following eradication of the infection, bone and soft tissue defects were both addressed using a vascularized osteocutaneous fibula flap with external fixation. (**c**) Integration of the graft and restoration of function 1 year following surgery

Nerve palsy, mainly involving the radial nerve, may follow an application of elastic bandage in the axilla or arm during surgery. It is important to pad the axilla properly and to leave the bandage in situ for no more than 30–35 minutes. Foot drop can follow surgery for fibula or hip infections.

Iatrogenic fractures can happen intraoperatively, as a complication of bone windowing in sclerotic or eburnated bones, or post-operatively, following sequestrectomy performed days or weeks before. In both cases, the site should be stabilized, preferably by use of an external fixator, and if radiographic signs of healing do not appear in 2–3 months, the site should be opened and debrided and external fixation applied.

Skin necrosis can follow surgery in presence of unhealthy or scarred skin, mainly in the medial aspect of the leg. If possible, the skin incision should be curvilinear, over the anterolateral compartment and minimal exposure obtained. Windowing on the lateral cortex of the tibia may be helpful in cases of poor skin cover. Local fasciocutaneous or gastrocnemius flaps may be required in the days following the surgery.

Relapse of the bone infection is not rare. The surgeon's experience reduces the rate of relapse significantly. Recurrence can follow inadequate debridement, with sequestra left in situ or not looked for, or if non-viable bone segments are not removed due to the surgeon's uncertainty. When infection persists, especially after revision surgery, the cause for recurrence may be a tuberculous osteitis. In addition, excessive periosteal stripping may lead to iatrogenic devascularization of bony segments that might require further debridement weeks or months later.

In longstanding cases a limb length discrepancy may occur, either due to bone overgrowth due to increased local metabolism, or physeal damage caused either by the infection itself, or the surgical interventions offered. For the same reason, angular deformities are commonly observed in the long run [43].

Sadly, in some cases, limb salvage is not possible, either due to complete bone and joint destruction and/or extensive soft tissue loss. In these cases, amputation remains a feasible option to eradicate the infection and restore some degree of function by means of prosthetic reconstruction.

One such patient, an 8-year-old boy, presented with chronic, neglected osteomyelitis of his right leg. The entire tibial diaphysis was sequestered, extruded in toto. *Radiographs confirmed a pyogenic diaphysectomy, with loss of the ankle joint. The boy also had a dislocation of his left hip joint, likely a sequela of an untreated pyogenic arthritis. Sequestrectomy was performed with associated management of the soft tissue loss followed by a vascularized fibula flap a few months later. Unfortunately, the flap failed due to vascular problems. The relatives refused any further reconstructive procedures, so a through-knee disarticulation was suggested as salvage procedure (*Fig. 10.15*).*

Surgery in a Resource-Challenged Environment

Providing care is the real meaning of the medical profession, in every corner of the world. The question is: what quality of surgical care can be provided in the LMIC countries, where health facilities are so different in terms of human resources and equipment? What is described in chapters one and two of *Primary Surgery* [13] is a must-read for every surgeon working in LMICs, as the social and economic situation in these countries has not changed much over the last 30 years and is unlikely to do so in the foreseeable future.

A typical example is a surgeon working in a district hospital, often alone with perhaps the assistance of a couple of orthopaedic officers, overwhelmed by complex surgical requests, yet asked to share the only operating room, to take care of his basic surgical sets and to assure himself that the system in place will allow him to work. Surgical skills aside, patient outcomes are inevitably related to the working environment.

It is the security and consistency that health care systems should provide that is often missing, clearly having repercussions on the quality-of-service delivery and on the staff morale. It may be hard to believe that surgeons in LMICs must still reckon with the lack of basic equipment like

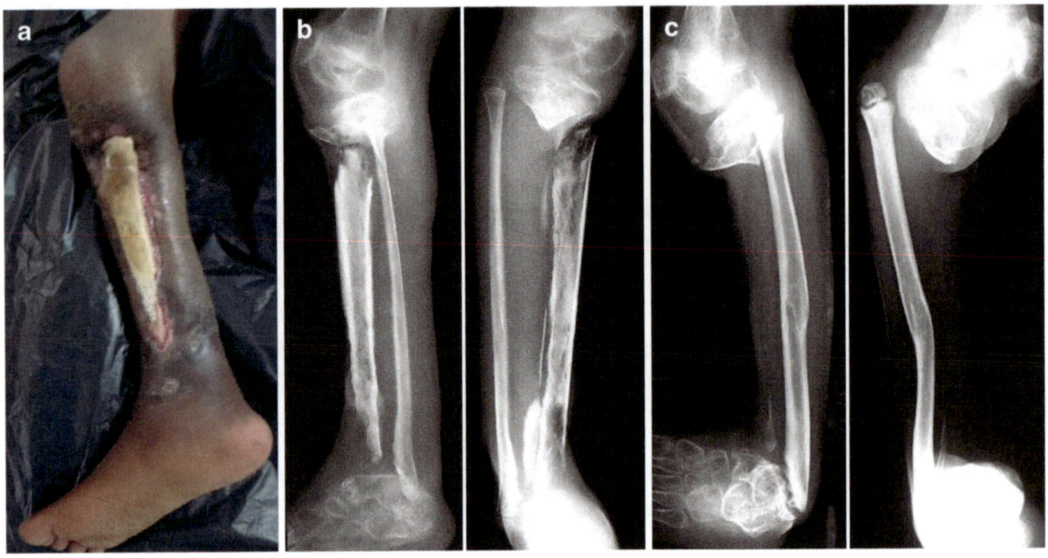

Fig. 10.15 (**a**) Clinical and (**b**) radiographic images showing an extruded diaphyseal sequestrum of the right tibia and ankle joint loss. (**c**) Following failed vascularized fibula transfer, the boy was bearing wait on the deformed, shortened leg with no pain. Fibular transfer was proposed as a final reconstructive attempt, but the patient's relatives refused any further surgery

gloves, gowns, anaesthetic drugs, and sutures. Not to mention erratic water and electric supply, relying on the standby generator to not let you down when you need it most.

Maintenance of the equipment is another thorny issue. Many theatres in LMICs depend on ageing equipment that are poorly maintained. When this equipment inevitably fails, surgery may be stopped for weeks on end while awaiting repairs or replacements. Typical examples are anaesthetic machines, theatre lights, autoclaves, and suction units.

Staff burn-out and frustration, related to inability to do your work, professional isolation, and poor remuneration in a failing health system, further compromises service delivery to this most desperate and vulnerable population.

As alluded to previously, there are many ways to circumvent these difficulties and reduce costs. Nelson and Watts [44], in their chapter on working in resource-challenged environments, cover this topic comprehensively and have many useful tips and tricks to boot. The reader is also referred to the text, "Global Orthopaedics: Caring for Musculoskeletal Conditions and Injuries in Austere Settings" [45], for more information on working in this challenging environment.

Future Directions

Improving the care of children with MSK infections in LMICs will require a public health approach, which includes three main categories elaborated on below:

1. *Education and Building Awareness.*

The key to improving the care of children with MSK infections in LMIC is education, starting with healthcare professionals. We see too many children who did seek medical attention during the acute phase of the disease, who were treated suboptimally or not at all. Medical and nursing students should be educated regarding the presenting features of MSK infections and the devastating consequences of untreated infections. At the author's institution, it is emphasized to all medical students that no limping child, or a child with unexplained limb pain or pseudoparalysis, should be discharged without actively excluding infection.

Awareness campaigns focusing on MSK conditions have been successful in the past, for instance, back-carrying to reduce the incidence of DDH in the Southern Chinese population [46]. However, campaigns like these rely heavily on charitable organisations' involvement, access to the most rural of communities, and ease of communication. The success of these interventions are difficult, if not impossible to assess due to confounding factors such as participant reactivity [47] (also known as the Hawthorne effect) and lack of long-term follow-up. In the author's experience, interventions that are not imbedded in the culture of the population do not stand the test of time.

2. *Building Capacity and Developing Referral Mechanisms to Specialized Centres.*

In rural or peripheral regions, where most children live and become sick, there are very few orthopaedic centres and even less orthopaedic surgeons. However, most LMICs have at least one central referral centre where specialist services are available.

With the increased availability of the Internet and other technologies that allow for the electronic transmission of data and images, early consultation and appropriate, timely referral are becoming more feasible.

Furthermore, the increasing number of orthopaedic and plastic surgeons, at least in some regions, coupled with up-to-date equipment, has expanded the treatment options and, ultimately, the long-term prognosis for thousands of children [10]. The supply of these services is, however, still widely insufficient when compared to the demand, considering the high population growth rate in most countries. The establishment of at least one dedicated bone sepsis unit in each country, with clear referral pathways, would go a long way to providing the specialist care that these patients require. "One Country-One Septic Unit". In addition, in the coming decade, we should be able to see the setting up of a properly equipped and staffed Regional Septic Unit where the most challenging cases could be referred. Even here, "One Region-One Septic Unit".

3. *Build Effective Review Mechanisms to Learn from Experience and Mistakes.*

Many surgeons in LMICs work in isolation with no peer review and no support. This may lead to apathy and lack of professional development. The current Covid-19 pandemic has normalized video conferencing and non-traditional mechanisms of communication, introducing a new way of thinking and knowledge translation. Regular meetings, be it virtual or physical, where complicated cases are discussed, advice is sought, and mistakes are shared and learnt from, is invaluable to the rural and urban surgeon alike. Another format to be exploited is instant messaging. A WhatsApp group (or similar) where cases can be discussed and results shared is extremely beneficial and accessible to most.

Creating a multicentre support group of teams across the world, caring for children with paediatric MSK infections to discuss cases, share results and collect data on the functional outcomes of different modalities of treatment would facilitate knowledge transfer and collaboration to improve quality of life for these children.

Conclusions

MSK infections and socio-economic conditions are strictly connected. In LMICs, these infections are usually seen late, or very late in their natural history. Consequently, they are one of the top causes of permanent disability in children. The unique situation in LMICs requires an adapted approach to treating these infections, including knowledge of local disease factors and optimal utilization of limited resources (Box 10.1).

Managing neglected MSK infections are challenging and costly, but highly rewarding. Internal and international solidarity has been on the frontline for footing bills and covering transport costs to access health institutions in many regions.

International aid, in terms of equipment and surgical items, has significantly helped in changing the prognosis for children in LMICs and will hopefully continue in the coming years. It is however not a sustainable solution, and governments and health department need to develop systems that are culturally appropriate for the respective regions.

MSK infections are as old as mankind and will remain a challenge for the foreseeable future. A comprehensive knowledge of the disease and its manifestations, as well as an armamentarium of strategies and solutions to address these various manifestations, is therefore essential to any orthopaedic surgeon.

References

1. Schwend RM. The burden of pediatric musculoskeletal diseases worldwide. Orthopedic Clinics. 2020;51(2):207–17.
2. Stanley CM, et al. Estimating the healthcare burden of osteomyelitis in Uganda. Trans R Soc Trop Med Hyg. 2010;104(2):139–42.
3. Lavy C, et al. Surgery in Malawi–a national survey of activity in rural and urban hospitals. The Annals of The Royal College of Surgeons of England. 2007;89(7):722–4.
4. Bickler SW, Sanno-Duanda B. Epidemiology of paediatric surgical admissions to a government referral hospital in the Gambia. Bull World Health Organ. 2000;78:1330–6.
5. Tekou H, Foly A, Akue B. Le profil actuel des ostéomyelites hématogènes de l'enfant au centre hospitalier universitaire de Tokoin, Lomé, Togo, à propos de 145 cas. Med Trop. 2000;60(4):365–8.
6. Meier D, et al. Hematogenous osteomyelitis in the developing world: a practical approach to classification and treatment with limited resources. Contemp Orthop. 1993;26:495.
7. Nacoulma S, et al. Ostéomyélites chroniques au CHU de Ouagadougou (Burkina Faso). Étude rétrospective de 102 cas (1996–2000). Bull Soc Pathol Exot. 2007;100(4):264–8.
8. Lavy C, Peek A, Manjolo G. The incidence of septic arthritis in Malawian children. Int Orthop. 2005;29(3):195–6.
9. Gafur OA, et al. The impact of the current epidemiology of pediatric musculoskeletal infection on evaluation and treatment guidelines. J Pediatr Orthop. 2008;28(7):777–85.
10. CoRSU Rehabilitation Hospital. Annual report. 2017.
11. Lauschke F, Frey C. Hematogenous osteomyelitis in infants and children in the northwestern region of Namibia. Management and two-year results. J Bone Joint Surg Am. 1994;76(4):502–10.
12. Ali AM, Maya E, Lakhoo K. Challenges in managing paediatric osteomyelitis in the developing world: analysis of cases presenting to a tertiary referral Centre in Tanzania. Afr J Paediatr Surg. 2014;11(4):308.
13. King M, BP, Cairns J, Thornton J. Non-Trauma. In: Primary surgery. Oxford, UK: Oxford university press; 1993. p. 83–103.
14. Jiang N, et al. Health care costs of post-traumatic osteomyelitis in china: current situation and influencing factors. J Surg Res. 2020;247:356–63.
15. Horn A, Wever S, Hoffman E. Complications following acute severe haematogenous osteomyelitis of the long bones in children. SA Orthopaedic J. 2019;18(3):23–9.
16. Bonn M. The effects of hospitalisation on children: a review. Curationis. 1994;17(2):20–4.
17. Wirbel R, Hermans K. Surgical treatment of chronic osteomyelitis in children admitted from developing countries. Afr J Paediatr Surg. 2014;11(4):297.
18. Mantero E, et al. Diagnosis and treatment of pediatric chronic osteomyelitis in developing countries: prospective study of 96 patients treated in Kenya. Musculoskelet Surg. 2011;95(1):13–8.
19. Robertson AJ, et al. Epidemiology of acute osteoarticular sepsis in a setting with a high prevalence of pediatric HIV infection. J Pediatr Orthop. 2012;32(2):215–9.
20. Knudsen C, Hoffman E. Neonatal osteomyelitis. J Bone Joint Surg Br Vol. 1990;72(5):846–51.
21. Breurec S, et al. Epidemiology of methicillin-susceptible Staphylococcus aureus lineages in five major African towns: high prevalence of Panton-valentine leukocidin genes. Clin Microbiol Infect. 2011;17(4):633–9.
22. Oosthuysen W, et al. Population structure analyses of Staphylococcus aureus at Tygerberg hospital, South Africa, reveals a diverse population, a high prevalence of Panton–valentine leukocidin genes, and unique local methicillin-resistant S. aureus clones. Clin Microbiol Infect. 2014;20(7):652–9.
23. Lavy CB. Septic arthritis in Western and sub-Saharan African children-a review. Int Orthop. 2007;31(2):137–44.
24. Visser HF, et al. Paediatric septic arthritis in a tertiary setting: a retrospective analysis. SA Orthopaedic J. 2010;9(2):92–6.
25. Lavy C, Lavy V, Anderson I. Salmonella septic arthritis of the shoulder in Zambian children. J R Coll Surg Edinb. 1996;41(3):197–9.
26. Molyneux E, French G. Salmonella joint infection in Malawian children. J Infect. 1982;4(2):131–8.
27. Nduati RW, Wamola I. Bacteriology of acute septic arthritis. J Trop Pediatr. 1991;37(4):172–5.
28. Kocher MS, Zurakowski D, Kasser JR. Differentiating between septic arthritis and transient synovitis of the hip in children: an evidence-based clinical prediction algorithm. JBJS. 1999;81(12):1662–70.

29. Solagberu B. A new classification of osteomyelitis for developing countries. East Afr Med J. 2003;80(7):373–8.
30. Thomas D, Sanchez P, Hoffman E. Chronic haematogenous osteomyelitis in children. In Orthopaedic proceedings. Br Editorial Soc Bone Joint Surg. 2005.
31. Jones HW, et al. Radiologic classification of chronic hematogenous osteomyelitis in children. J Pediatr Orthop. 2009;29(7):822–7.
32. Spiegel DA, Penny JN. Chronic osteomyelitis in children. Tech Orthop. 2005;20(2):142–52.
33. Tetsworth K, Cierny G III. Osteomyelitis debridement techniques. Clin Orthopaed Relat Res (1976–2007). 1999;360:87–96.
34. Panteli M, Giannoudis PV. Chronic osteomyelitis: what the surgeon needs to know. EFORT Open Reviews. 2016;1(5):128–35.
35. Sharrard WJW. Paediatric orthopaedics and fractures. In: Paediatric orthopaedics and fractures; 1971. p. ix, 1126.
36. Peltier LF. The orr method in osteomyelitis, compound fractures and other infections. Clin Orthopaed Relat Res. 1999;360:3–5.
37. Pelser P. Management of septic non-unions. SA Orthopaed J. 2009;8(2):29–34.
38. Perry CR. Bone repair techniques, bone graft, and bone graft substitutes. Clin Orthopaed Relat Res. 1999;360:71–86.
39. Cruickshank JA, Graham SM, Harrison WJ. Immediate bone transport: a novel technique for the management of bone defects after chronic osteomyelitis in children. Trop Dr. 2018;48(1):64–6.
40. Zalavras CG, et al. Reconstruction of large skeletal defects due to osteomyelitis with the vascularized fibular graft in children. JBJS. 2007;89(10):2233–40.
41. Rasool M. The treatment of tibial defects following chronic pyogenic haematogenous osteomyelitis in children. SA Orthopaed J. 2008;7(1):34–43.
42. Muñoz M, et al. International consensus statement on the peri-operative management of anaemia and iron deficiency. Anaesthesia. 2017;72(2):233–47.
43. Ilharreborde B. Sequelae of pediatric osteoarticular infection. Orthop Traumatol Surg Res. 2015;101(1):S129–37.
44. Nelson SC, Watts HG. Working in resource-challenged environments. In: Pediatric lower limb deformities. Springer; 2016. p. 215–28.
45. Gosselin RA, Spiegel DA, Foltz M. Global orthopedics: caring for musculoskeletal conditions and injuries in austere settings. Springer; 2019.
46. Graham SM, et al. Back-carrying infants to prevent developmental hip dysplasia and its sequelae: is a new public health initiative needed? J Pediatr Orthop. 2015;35(1):57–61.
47. Paradis E, Sutkin G. Beyond a good story: from Hawthorne effect to reactivity in health professions education research. Med Educ. 2017;51(1):31–9.

Part II

Acute Musculoskeletal Infections

Acute Hematogenous Osteomyelitis

11

Scott B. Rosenfeld and Lawson A. Copley

Introduction and Epidemiology in Brief

Acute hematogenous osteomyelitis (AHO) is a bacterial infection of bone that occurs in otherwise healthy children and adolescents, who typically have open growth plates. There is an incidence of approximately 8 cases per 100,000 children from birth to age 18 years (average 8 years) per year with a male-to-female ratio of approximately 1.9 to 1 [1, 2]. The occurrence of AHO varies regionally and seasonally suggesting that the underlying pathophysiology may be impacted by differences in local microbiota and regional weather systems [3]. Evaluation and treatment of AHO is amenable to institutional guideline development and implementation with favorable long-term outcomes for children who are expeditiously diagnosed and effectively treated [1, 2]. However, adverse outcomes appear to be associated with the most severe clinical phenotypes of disease as calculated by a recently developed and validated severity of illness score which is assessed early in the course of the initial hospitalization [2, 4]. Illness severity may be driven by the genomic virulence armamentarium encoded by the causative organism with a significantly greater number of virulence genes identified within the genome of methicillin-resistant *Staphylococcus aureus* (MRSA) isolates than that found in methicillin-sensitive *Staphylococcus aureus* (MSSA) isolates [5]. Because the severity of illness score is largely established prior to substantial treatment or intervention, it seems that adverse outcomes of children with severe forms of osteomyelitis are not entirely controllable by the treating team. Fortunately, adverse outcomes occur in less than eight percent of children with osteomyelitis, and they predominantly occur in children with the greatest severity of illness, so they are somewhat predictable [2]. Chronic osteomyelitis is probably the result of inadequate recognition and treatment of acute hematogenous osteomyelitis. This is extremely rare in the United States and other developed countries. Lack of recognition and insufficient antibiotic treatment of AHO in developing countries likely contribute to the occurrence of this challenging problem which requires complex solutions in order to achieve resolution. Other long-term adverse outcomes, including osteonecrosis, joint destruction, limb length inequality, and deformity necessitate close orthopedic outpatient follow-up for those at

S. B. Rosenfeld
Department of Orthopaedic Surgery, Texas Children's Hospital, Baylor College of Medicine, Houston, TX, USA
e-mail: sbrosef@texaschildrens.org

L. A. Copley (✉)
Department of Orthopaedic Surgery, Texas Scottish Rite Hospital for Children and Children's Health System of Texas, University of Texas Southwestern, Dallas, TX, USA
e-mail: lawson.copley@childrens.com

© Springer Nature Switzerland AG 2022
M. V. Belthur et al. (eds.), *Pediatric Musculoskeletal Infections*,
https://doi.org/10.1007/978-3-030-95794-0_11

greatest risk to ensure recognition and allow for intervention or delayed reconstruction if necessary [2].

Pathology and Microbiology

AHO commonly occurs in the cancellous bone of the metaphyseal region near the growth plate. The posterior tuberosity of the calcaneus, inferior pubic rami of the pelvis, triradiate cartilage of the acetabulum, and endplates of the vertebral bodies are long-bone equivalent sites that may also be affected with AHO. Diaphyseal and epiphyseal osteomyelitis may rarely occur but should be considered atypical and promote consideration of other etiologies or evaluation for unusual pathogens (Fig. 11.1).

The pathophysiology of AHO is believed to be initiated when, without a known or obvious point of entry, such as scratch, scrape, puncture, or other penetrating inoculation, the causative organism enters the blood stream, creating a transient bacteremia. *Staphylococcus aureus* is the predominate pathogen of AHO, responsible for over 90% of culture-confirmed cases. *Streptococcus pyogenes* is isolated from about 4% of affected children [6]. The remainder of culture-positive osteomyelitis is due to a wide variety of atypical organisms that may affect children with comorbid conditions, such as sickle cell disease associated with *Salmonella* species, or within specific age groups, such as neonates with *Streptococcus agalactiae* or preschool children with *Kingella kingae* or *Streptococcus pneumoniae* [6]. The causative organism presumably circulates until it leaves the blood stream and deposits at the site of eventual infection within the bone. The metaphyseal bone in children contains sinusoidal, hairpin turn vascular networks that create a relative slowing of blood flow. This sluggish blood flow can lead to increased potential for bacterial organisms to exit the vascular channels and adhere to, and propagate within, the metaphysis. A history of minor trauma in the area of subsequent infection preceding the onset of AHO occurs in over 65% of cases, suggesting that increased blood flow to, and vascular permeability within, the affected region may play a role in local bacterial deposition. After initiation of infection, the child then becomes symptomatic with fever, pain, bone tenderness, and limited use of the affected body region. Approximately 20% of children with AHO develop adjacent joint space infections (Fig. 11.2) [7, 8]. Once osteomyelitis develops, bacteria can then be intro-

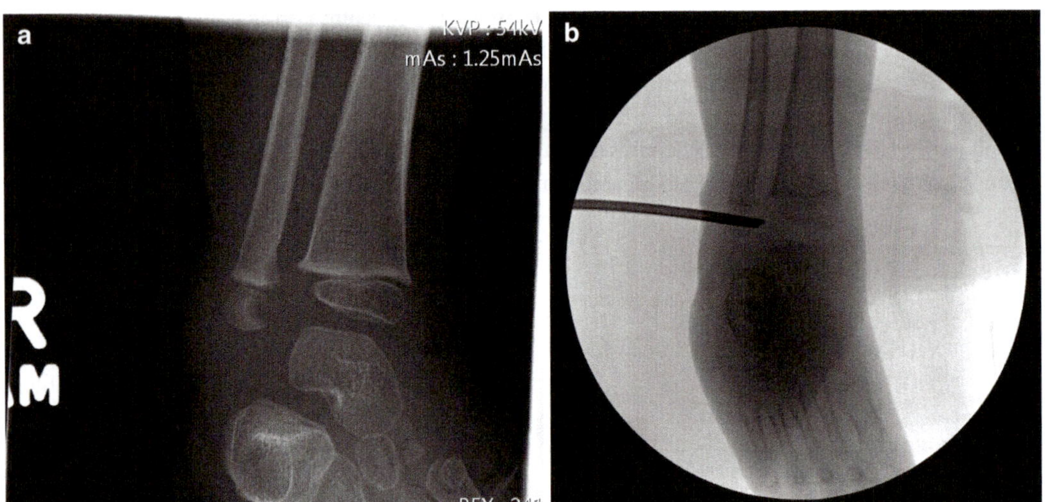

Fig. 11.1 Anterior to posterior radiograph (**a**) of the right ankle of a 22-month-old girl demonstrating a lytic lesion of the distal fibula appearance. She had fever, pain, and limping for 3 weeks prior to admission. She had a mildly elevated erythrocyte sedimentation rate (ESR) of 24 mm/hr. Biopsy and culture by trocar with an 11 gauge bone biopsy needle (**b**) identified *Kingella kingae* as the causative organism

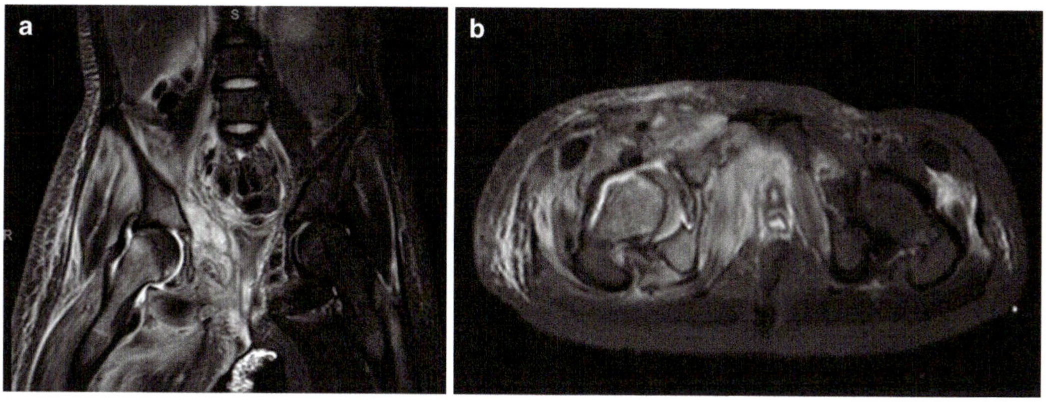

Fig. 11.2 Coronal (**a**) and axial (**b**) short tau inversion recovery (STIR) MRI images of a 12-year-old female with acute hematogenous osteomyelitis of the proximal femur and acetabulum with contiguous septic arthritis of the right hip and adjacent infectious myositis of the pelvic musculature. The infection was due to MRSA and was associated with deep venous thrombosis and septic pulmonary emboli. She underwent five surgeries during a 6-week hospitalization, including 3 weeks in the intensive care unit

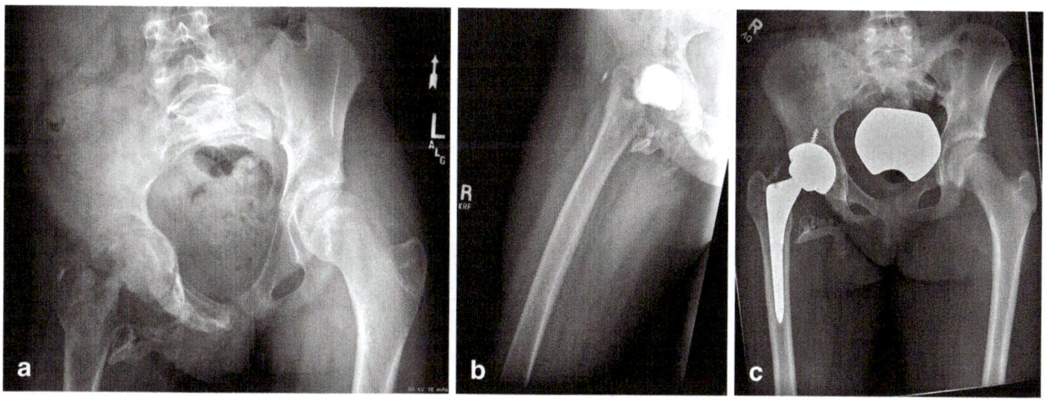

Fig. 11.3 Devastating complication of a pathologic fracture of the femoral neck (**a**) 4 ½ months after hospital discharge following the treatment of osteomyelitis with contiguous septic arthritis. She underwent resection of the femoral head with placement of a methyl-methacrylate antibiotic spacer (**b**) followed by total hip arthroplasty (**c**) at 13 years of age

duced into the joint through intraosseous or subperiosteal abscess formation and subsequent decompression into the joint or through migration through transphyseal vessels which are unique to young children. Several joints including the proximal femur, proximal humerus, distal fibula, and proximal radius have intra-articular metaphyses and are thus more prone to adjacent septic arthritis since the sinusoidal network that predisposes to osteomyelitis is already within the joint capsule. Contiguous septic arthritis is considered an independent risk factor for the occurrence of adverse outcomes (Fig. 11.3) [2].

Staphylococcus aureus AHO has a moderately high rate of bacteremia identified with the initial blood culture. Persistence of the bacteremia beyond the initiation of antibiotic treatment also occurs commonly due to this pathogen because of its ability to survive in the bloodstream for prolonged periods despite antibiotic administration. The potential for *Staphylococcus aureus* to cause a wide spectrum of illness among children with AHO is thought to be due to the virulence behavior of the specific bacteria that caused the infection [5]. Genomic heterogeneity of clinical isolates within a single community and virulence gene annotation of these pathogens support the theory that the invasiveness and proclivity to potentiate severe illness may be due to the variety and quantity of virulence genes which are expressed by the specific strain of *Staphylococcus aureus* that gained entry to the bloodstream of an otherwise healthy child [5, 9, 10].

Investigations/Work-Up

Due to the rapid onset of signs and symptoms, children with AHO are often evaluated in the emergency department. The initial work-up should include a complete blood count (CBC) with differential of the white blood cell (WBC) component and inflammatory markers, including C-reactive protein (CRP) and erythrocyte sedimentation rate (ESR). All children who are suspected to have AHO should have an aerobic blood culture obtained prior to administration of antibiotics. The high rate of *Staphylococcus aureus* bacteremia (SAB) among children with AHO provides an excellent opportunity to identify the causative organism without an invasive procedure, provided a blood culture is obtained prior to antibiotic administration. Antibiotic pretreatment, either prior to hospitalization or within the institution, has a negative impact on the rate of bacteremia [6]. Therefore, community and institutional awareness of antimicrobial stewardship and the need to follow guidelines should be actively promoted to improve the yield of blood cultures for children with AHO.

The guidance of the initial laboratory evaluation goes beyond establishing the diagnosis as this data also initiates an understanding of the relative severity of illness of the child with an evolving infection [4]. Parameters involved in assessment of illness severity include initial and subsequent CRP values and the band percentage of the WBC [4]. Children with AHO who have markedly elevated CRP values and high band percentages fit a pattern of disease that commonly is associated with ICU admission, patchy infiltrates on chest X-ray suggestive of septic pulmonary emboli (SPE), and methicillin-resistant *Staphylococcus aureus* (MRSA) bacteremia [11]. Such children are more likely to have venous thromboembolism (VTE) than those with methicillin-sensitive *Staphylococcus aureus* (MSSA) infections [12]. They can be expected to have prolonged fever, several days of bacteremia, and the occurrence of surgery which often is repeated [2, 13]. Additional laboratory patterns which often occur in these children include anemia and thrombocytopenia with a platelet nadir within the first couple of days of hospitalization due to the rapid consumption of blood products. Gene expression analysis of children with MRSA AHO performed within 3–4 days of hospitalization has demonstrated an overexpression of the innate immune response and upregulation of the coagulation cascade concurrent with an underexpression of adaptive immunity [10].

Imaging of children with AHO inevitably begins with plain radiographs of the symptomatic region. In most children, these X-rays demonstrate no focal bone abnormality, but there often is a finding of deep soft tissue swelling adjacent to the bone (Fig. 11.4). Metaphyseal lucent areas

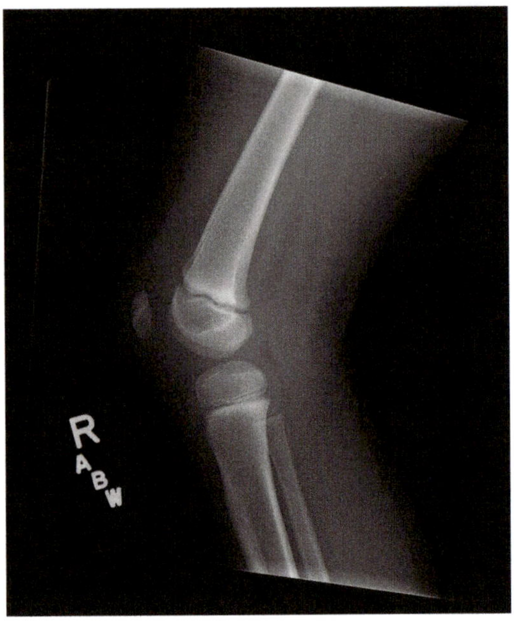

Fig. 11.4 Lateral X-ray of the right knee demonstrating deep soft tissue swelling posterior to the distal femur with otherwise normal appearing bone architecture in a 6-year-old girl with acute hematogenous osteomyelitis of the right distal femur

or cortical disruption may be seen if there is substantial delay from symptom onset to clinical presentation (Fig. 11.5). It is increasingly recognized that advanced imaging with magnetic resonance imaging (MRI) offers value during the work-up of children with AHO by defining the anatomic and spatial extent of the inflammation and guiding decision for surgical approach and extent of exposure or debridement [14]. Institutional process improvements have been shown to substantially improve the workflow and resource utilization of sedated MRI acquisition [14]. Children with AHO who require anesthesia for MRI may have complete imaging performed with minimal use of contrast, shortened anesthesia duration, and post-MRI diagnostic and/or surgical procedures accomplished using a well-orchestrated team approach [11, 14]. This improves safety and outcomes while minimizing exposure to contrast and anesthetic agents which are thought to persist in the brain or be neurotoxic for the young, developing brain.

Pattern recognition should lead to an awareness that a high rate of deep venous thrombosis (DVT) identification occurs in children with high severity of illness scores [12]. An ultrasound to assess for DVT should be performed early in the hospitalization and ideally before MRI and surgery [11, 12]. This allows identification of the DVT before surgical intervention when dressings and drains may preclude unimpeded access to the extremities for ultrasound assessment.

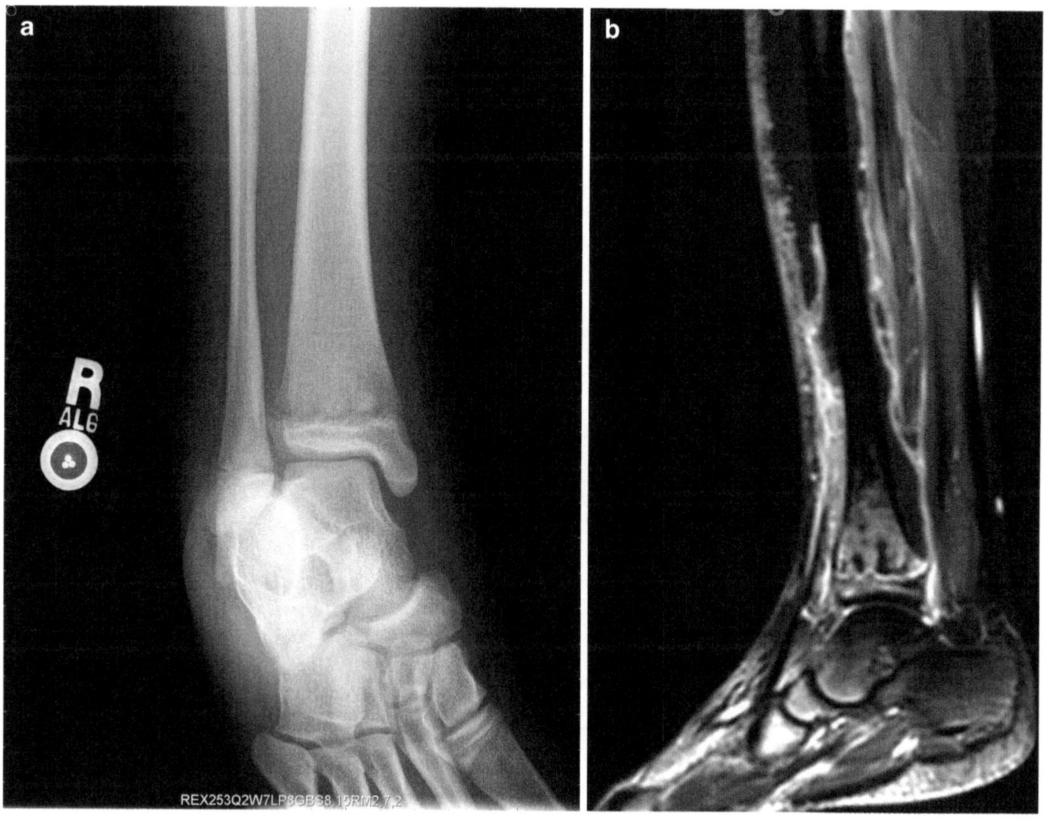

Fig. 11.5 Anterior to posterior X-ray of the ankle (**a**) of an 8-year-old girl with 2 weeks of pain and swelling which started after a minor trauma. She had fever at home and worsening pain. Her CRP was 3.5 mg/dL and ESR was 83 mm/hr. at the time of admission. The sagittal T1-weighted fat saturation view (**b**) demonstrated the osteomyelitis of the right distal tibia with intraosseous and subperiosteal abscesses of the distal tibia. The abscess extends proximally and becomes a subcutaneous collection anterior to the tibia in the mid-leg

Differential Diagnoses

Fortunately, children with AHO present with predictable and well-defined clinical and laboratory findings. The uncertainty which makes primary septic arthritis difficult to assess in children, due to the long list of conditions in the realistic differential, is not often present during the work-up of children suspected to have AHO. The high rate of bacteremia, pattern of elevation of the inflammatory markers, and findings on plain X-ray and MRI usually support the diagnosis of AHO. Leukemia and Ewing's sarcoma are the most relevant conditions to include within the realistic differential. Leukemia tends to affect the CBC findings with impact on all three cell lines which may include leukopenia or leukocytosis, anemia, and thrombocytopenia. The peripheral smear visually depicts the blast cells and commonly prompts a hematology/oncology consultation and bone marrow biopsy that establishes the diagnosis. MRI findings of children with leukemia tend toward extensive bone marrow changes which are patchy and disseminated. MRI sequences should include extended field of view short tau inversion recovery (STIR) and T1 techniques. Whenever the pelvis or lower extremities are visualized, it is recommended to always image bilaterally (Fig. 11.6). These images capture the bone marrow irregularities common to leukemia. Children with Ewing's sarcoma often have plain radiograph features that are atypical for AHO as the location is often diaphyseal and the visible osseous infiltrative changes and periosteal new bone formation suggest neoplasm as opposed to infection. However, the principle to biopsy every culture and culture every biopsy will serve as a safety measure to ensure that Ewing's sarcoma or any other neoplastic condition is not inadvertently treated as AHO.

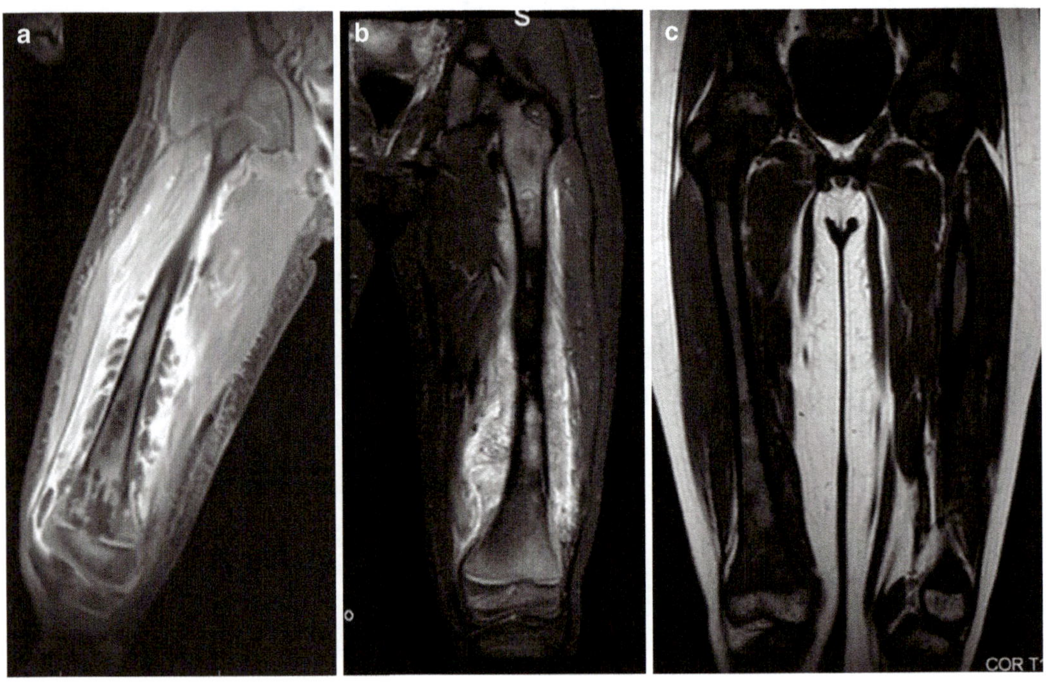

Fig. 11.6 (**a**) Post-contrast coronal T1 FS MRI demonstrating osteomyelitis and subperiosteal abscess of the right femur. (**b**) Coronal STIR MRI demonstrating Ewing's sarcoma with large soft tissue component surrounding the left femur. (**c**) Coronal T1 MRI demonstrating leukemic infiltration of bilateral femoral diaphyses and epiphyses

Treatment Options

Antibiotic treatment is the mainstay of therapy for AHO. This should be guided by culture identification and antimicrobial susceptibility of the causative organism [6]. Increasingly, communities are reporting a variety of antibiotic resistance patterns which may wax and wane over years of surveillance. This includes the potential for resistance to methicillin, clindamycin, and vancomycin. As such, there is a need to know, which has progressively increased over time, that should motivate providers to take steps to identify the causative pathogen whenever possible. This is based on principles which should be embedded into institutional guidelines and workflows [1]. First, an aerobic blood culture must be obtained in every child who has history, physical, and laboratory findings to suggest a possible deep infection of bone, muscle, or joint space. Second, no child who meets this criterion should be administered antibiotics, at any institution, without first drawing an aerobic blood culture.

If a sedated MRI is being obtained in a child suspected to have AHO and the blood culture is no growth so far, there should be an attempt to obtain a biopsy and culture by trocar, with a bone marrow biopsy needle, while the child is still under anesthesia immediately following the MRI. This is a relatively simple procedure to perform and may often be done by anatomic landmarks in the MRI anesthesia recovery unit or, briefly, in the operating room with C-arm fluoroscopy guidance for difficult to reach locations. The procedure may be done taking as briefly as a few minutes, and the results are quite valuable in guiding therapy.

If the child is old enough to have a non-sedate MRI, or the coordination of sedated MRI with immediate biopsy under the same anesthesia is not possible, then the options will exist after the diagnosis of AHO to consider whether a biopsy and culture are indicated, which would require additional sedation, or if initiation of empirical antimicrobial therapy with assessment of clinical and laboratory response to treatment are preferred. Regional or institutional microbiome data, specific to deep musculoskeletal infections, should be used to guide empiric antibiotic selections [6]. Recently the Children's Orthopaedic Trauma and Infection Consortium for Evidence-Based Study (CORTICES) group investigated the rate and spectrum of culture-positive bone infections at 18 tertiary pediatric medical centers in the United States [15]. While there is some regional variation in pathogens, particularly the relative rate of MRSA versus MSSA, knowing that *Staphylococcus aureus* is responsible for most childhood osteomyelitis, the antibiotic selection may be tailored to the methicillin or clindamycin susceptibility patterns within the local communities [15].

Antibiotic Treatment

Antimicrobial treatment is commonly enacted in a sequential, parenteral to oral, manner with intravenous administration until there is sufficient clinical and laboratory improvement to minimize concern about the likelihood that the child will require additional procedural intervention or hospital readmission [16]. This is often guided by temperature trend to an afebrile state, resolution of bacteremia for at least 48 hours, and downward trending of inflammatory markers, particularly the CRP. There is no absolute CRP value that must be reached prior to discharge provided there is downward progression. Overall, there should be a strong sense that the child is improving in overall appearance with increasing mobility and use of the affected region of the musculoskeletal system and a sense that the child is "becoming themself" again, in the eyes of the parent(s). After discharge and transition to oral therapy, the common pattern of progress is for resolution or normalization of the CRP within a week or two of hospital discharge. The ESR is often the remaining abnormal finding that helps guide decisions about completion of the antibiotic course. In general, uncomplicated cases of AHO may be treated with as few as 3 weeks of antibiotic duration 17. This has been shown in a prospective, randomized trial to be effective but in a region that does not contend with MRSA or USA300 *Staphylococcus aureus* [17]. In the United States, the guidance has generally been to target therapy for approximately 4 weeks, provided there is clinical and laboratory normalization within that timeframe. Given that ESR is the last element to reach normalization, this may be the only useful test to guide decision-making at the late follow-up visit. For children with the highest severity of illness, treatment may need to be extended for more than 2 months to reach this end of therapy measurement [2].

Some children will present in septic shock and require immediate resuscitation in the intensive care unit. These children will be treated with broad spectrum empiric antibiotics during the resuscitation, often including vancomycin for gram-positive bactericidal coverage and ceftriaxone for the potential of gram-negative endotoxemia [11]. With modern laboratory molecular diagnostic tools, there is the potential for early detection of the pathogen, even prior to laboratory susceptibility testing. As soon as MRSA or MSSA is identified by these techniques, the gram-negative coverage may be discontinued and the antibiotic focus directed toward the *Staphylococcus aureus*. MSSA should be treated with a first-generation cephalosporin or semisynthetic penicillin to provide therapy that is more rapidly bactericidal and less nephrotoxic than vancomycin [18]. Because vancomycin is slowly bactericidal, with limited penetration into infected bone, and is associated with nephrotoxicity, children with MRSA AHO must be carefully monitored for renal function and response to treatment so that a transition to alternative antibiotics may be made as soon as possible.

Surgical Treatment

Surgical decision-making has not been standardized for children with AHO [13, 19, 20]. Some children undergo multiple surgeries in the effort to attain source control [13]. Generally, children who are admitted to the ICU and who have markedly elevated inflammatory markers undergo surgery with the potential to continue raising sufficient concern after the index procedure that they have subsequent MRIs and surgical procedures. On the other end of the spectrum are children who do not have any surgical procedures during their care for AHO. They respond to antibiotic treatment and resolve their infection solely with medical treatment. From the available literature, it appears that surgical intervention may merit from a sliding scale approach based on the severity of illness of the affected child with AHO [2, 13]. Indications for surgical intervention are often based on the presence and size of abscess identified on MRI and the existence of contiguous septic arthritis. Children with large abscesses and/or joint effusions pose minimal controversy in the decision for surgery. However, there may be substantial variation as to whether the surgeon will choose to drain a subperiosteal abscess without debridement of the cancellous bone at the epicenter of the infection. Some will only drain the abscess, others may drill the bone without creating a cortical window, and some will create a bone window to remove most of the cancellous bone while sparing the growth plate (Fig. 11.7).

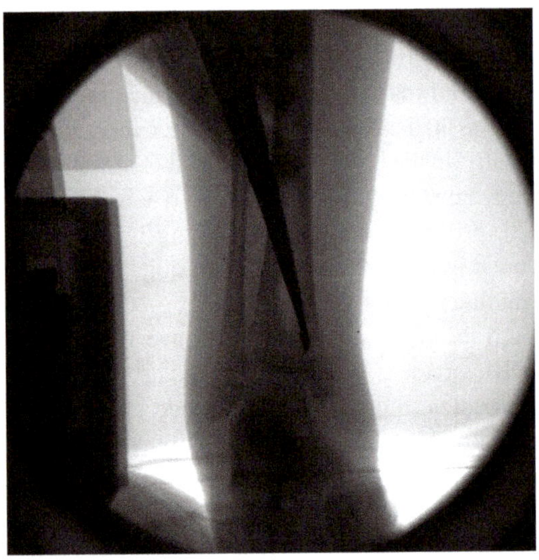

Fig. 11.7 Curettage of the metaphyseal cancellous bone of the distal tibia through an anterior cortical window. C-arm fluoroscopy is used to ensure there is a safe margin from the distal tibial physis

Complications

Children with AHO have excellent long-term clinical outcomes. A study of 195 children with AHO found an 8% long-term complication rate that was mostly isolated to children with high severity of illness scores (7 to 10 out of 10) [2]. At 2 ½ years of average follow-up with a 71.3% rate of return for evaluation, the general findings of children were normal radiographs and physical exam (41%); minor radiographic findings but normal clinical exam (51.1%); and abnormal radiographs and exam with the need for further orthopedic surveillance or intervention (7.9%) [2]. The outcome measures of the Pediatric Outcomes Data Collection Instrument (PODCI) (92.7 vs 96.7 vs 96.6) and Pediatric Quality of Life Inventory (PedsQL) (86.6 vs 92.4 vs 94.3) questionnaires were lowest among children with severe illness compared to those of children with moderate or mild illness, respectively [2]. Overall, however, there was no evidence of chronic osteomyelitis for children in the study. The adverse long-term outcomes included osteonecrosis, joint destruction, deformity, and limb length inequality. These occurred in 32.0% of children with severe illness, 5.9% of children with moderate illness, and 1.3% of children in the mild illness cohort [2]. There was an interesting finding of central physeal tenting which was associated with a completely normal physical examination and normal Harris arrest lines on X-rays in 22.3% of children, regardless of the severity of illness (Fig. 11.8) [2]. Another common complication of children with AHO is the occurrence of pathologic fractures. This is attributed to altered architecture of the bone due to the infection and the surgical procedures which lead to insufficiency and fracture as activities are being increased, typically after the hospitalization (Fig. 11.9). The risk is greater in patients with subperiosteal abscess and sharp demarcation of enhancement on MRI [21].

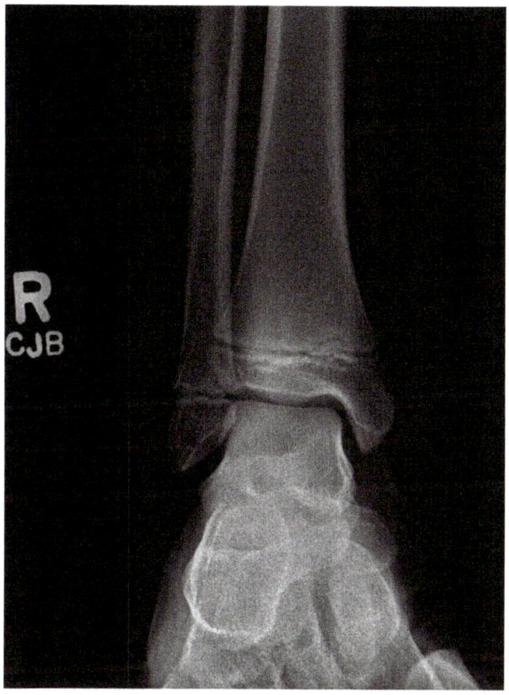

Fig. 11.8 Central physeal tenting of the distal tibial growth plate identified 2 ½ years after the treatment and resolution of acute hematogenous osteomyelitis of the distal tibia in a 10-year-old boy. He had a normal physical exam with no limb length discrepancy, no deformity, and full range of motion compared to the opposite ankle

Understanding the potential for complications and relative risk based on the severity of illness score of the child with AHO is important as it influences the decision-making about the follow-up duration following hospitalization. This is important to families and primary care physicians as they would otherwise be obligated to pursue long-distance travel and days off of work with expensive follow-up visits for subspecialty evaluations without the knowledge that this is rarely necessary except in cases of severe illness or when there is a high index of suspicion that they are at risk for adverse sequelae. Given the risk of pathologic fractures, it is important to provide supplemental immobilization and weight-bearing restrictions for a period of time following surgical treatment. Generally, there will be substantial healing and remodeling during the first 3 months after surgery sufficient to allow progression toward normal activities. Casting or brace support along with limited weight-bearing may be prudent for the first 4 to 6 weeks after surgery.

Flow Charts

Fig. 11.10

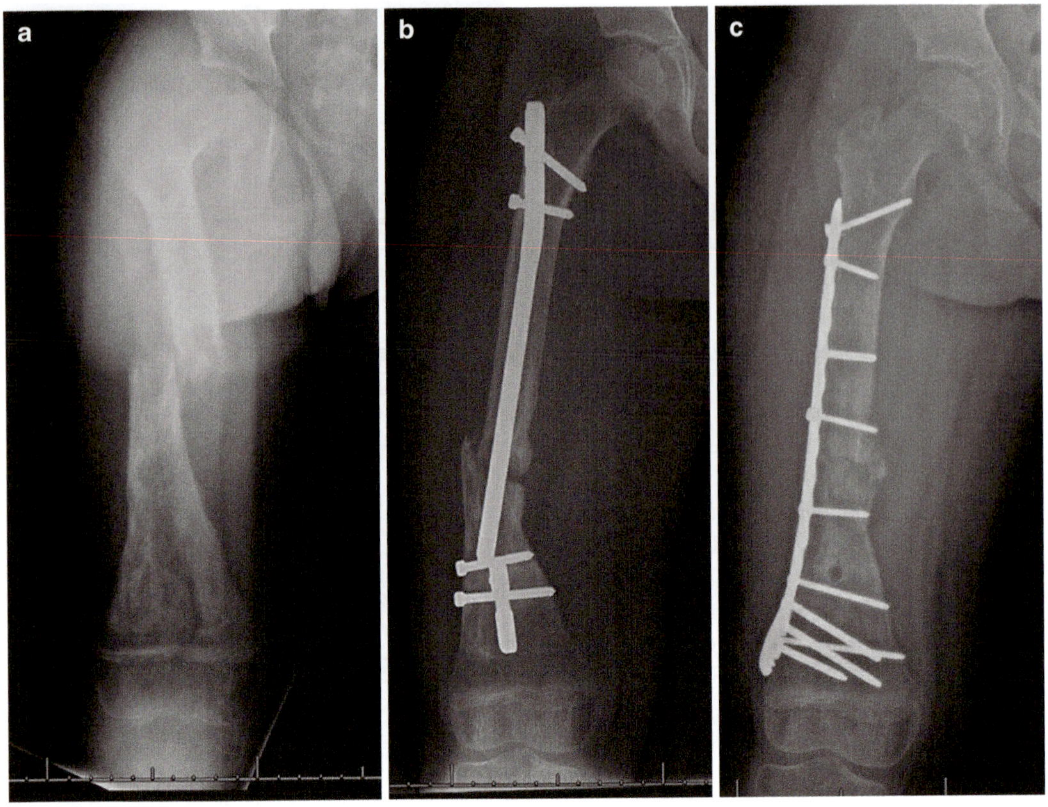

Fig. 11.9 (**a**) Pathologic fracture of the right femoral diaphysis as a complication of acute hematogenous osteomyelitis. (**b**) Persistent nonunion with implant failure after intramedullary fixation. (**c**) Revision ORIF after debridement of devitalized bone

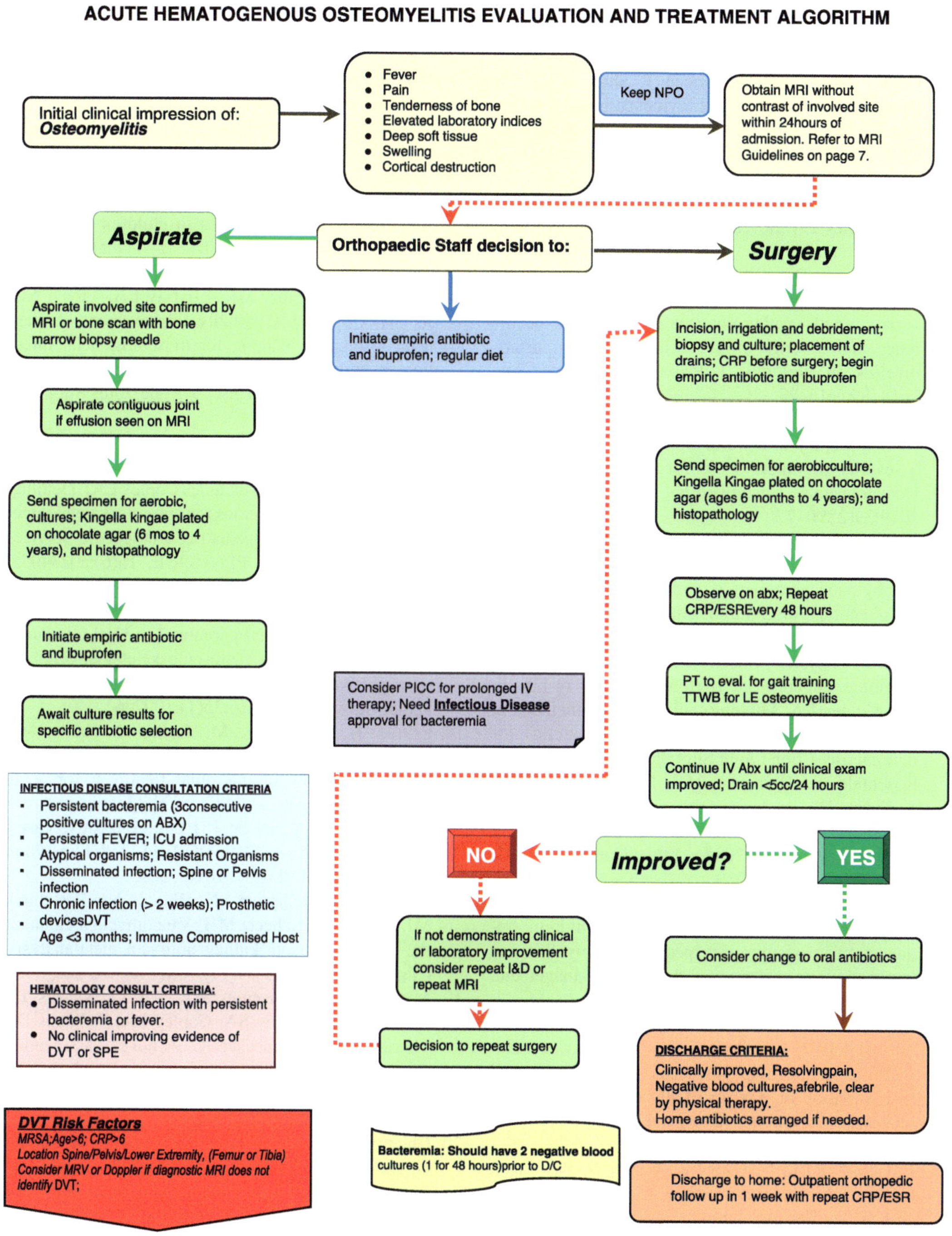

Fig. 11.10 Flow diagram of an evaluation and treatment algorithm for acute hematogenous osteomyelitis in children

References

1. Copley LA, Kinsler A, Gheen T, Shar A, Sun D, Browne R. The impact of evidence-based clinical practice guidelines applied by a multidisciplinary team for the care of children with osteomyelitis. J Bone Joint Surg. 2013;95(8):686–93.
2. Vorhies JS, Lindsay EA, Tareen NG, Kellum RJ, Jo CH, Copley LA. Severity adjusted risk of long-term adverse sequelae among children with osteomyelitis. Pediatr Infect Dis J. 2019;38(1):26–31.
3. Lindsay EA, Tareen N, Jo CH, Copley LA. Seasonal variation and weather changes related to the occurrence and severity of acute hematogenous osteomyelitis in children. J Pediatr Infect Dis Soc. 2018;7(2):e16–23.
4. Athey A, Mignemi ME, Gheen WT, Lindsay EA, Jo CH, Copley LA. Validation and modification of a severity of illness score for children with acute Hematogenous osteomyelitis. J Pediatr Orthop. 2019;39(2):90–7.
5. Collins A, Wakeland EK, Raj P, Kim MS, Kim J, Tareen NG, Copley LAB. The impact of Staphylococcus aureus genomic variation on clinical phenotype of children with acute hematogenous osteomyelitis. Heliyon. 2018;e00674. https://doi.org/10.1016/j.heliyon.2018.e00674.
6. Section J, Gibbons SE, Barton T, Greenberg DE, Jo CH, Copley LA. Microbiological culture methods in pediatric musculoskeletal infection: a guideline for optimal use. J Bone Joint Surg. 2015;97(6):441–9.
7. Rosenfeld S, Bernstein DT, Daram S, Dawson J, Zhang W. Predicting the presence of adjacent infections in septic arthritis in children. J Pediatr Orthop. 2016;36(1):70–4. https://doi.org/10.1097/BPO.0000000000000389.
8. Monsalve J, Kan JH, Schallert EK, Bisset GS, Zhang W, Rosenfeld SB. Septic arthritis in children: frequency of coexisting unsuspected osteomyelitis and implications on imaging work-up and management. Am J Roentgenol. 2015;204(6):1289–95.
9. Gaviria-Agudelo C, Aroh C, Tareen N, Wakeland EK, Kim M, Copley LA. Genomic heterogeneity of methicillin resistant Staphylococcus aureus associated with variation in severity of illness among children with acute Hematogenous osteomyelitis. PLoS One. 2015;10(6):e0130415.
10. Gaviria-Agudelo C, Carter K, Tareen N, Pascual V, Copley LA. Gene expression analysis of children with acute Hematogenous osteomyelitis caused by methicillin-resistant Staphylococcus aureus: correlation with clinical severity of illness. PLoS One. 2014;9(7):e103523.
11. Dhar AV, Huang CJ, Sue PK, Patel K, Farrow-Gillespie AC, Hammer MR, Zia AN, Mittal VS, Copley LA. Team approach: pediatric musculoskeletal infection. JBJS Rev. 2020;8(3):e0121. https://doi.org/10.2106/JBJS.RVW.19.00.00121.
12. Ligon JA, Journeycake JM, Josephs SC, Tareen NG, Lindsay EA, Copley LAB. Differentiation of deep venous thrombosis among children with or without osteomyelitis. J Pediatr Orthopaed. 2018;38(10):e597–603.
13. Tuason D, Gheen T, Sun D, Huang R, Copley L. Clinical and laboratory parameters associated with multiple surgeries in children with acute Hematogenous osteomyelitis. J Pediatr Orthop. 2014;34(5):565–70.
14. Ojeaga PO, Hammer MR, Lindsay EA, Tareen NG, Jo CH, Copley LA. Quality improvement of magnetic resonance imaging for musculoskeletal infection in children results in decreased scan duration and decreased contrast use. J Bone Joint Surg Am. 2019;101:1679–88.
15. Schoenecker JG, The Children's Orthopaedic Trauma and Infection Consortium for Evidence Based Study (CORTICES) Group* (includes Copley LA). Defining the volume of consultations for musculoskeletal infection encountered by pediatric orthopaedic services in the United States. PLoS ONE. 15(6):e0234055. https://doi.org/10.1371/journal.pone.0234055.
16. Erickson C, Sue P, Stewart K, Jo CH, Lindsay E, Copley LA. Sequential parenteral to Oral clindamycin dosing in pediatric musculoskeletal infection: a retrospective review of 30mg/kg/day vs 40mg/kg/day. Pediatr Infect Dis J. 2016;35(1):1092–6.
17. Peltola H, Pääkkönen M, Kallio P. Kallio MJ; osteomyelitis-septic arthritis study group. Short-versus long-term antimicrobial treatment for acute hematogenous osteomyelitis of childhood: prospective, randomized trial on 131 culture-positive cases. Pediatr Infect Dis J. 2010;29(12):1123–8. https://doi.org/10.1097/INF.0b013e3181f55a89.
18. Aljefri DM, Avedissian SN, Rhodes NJ, Postelnick MJ, Nguyen K, Scheetz MH. Vancomycin area under the curve and acute kidney injury: a meta-analysis. Clin Infect Dis. 2019;69(11):1881–7.
19. Mignemi ME, Benvenuti MA, An TJ, Martus JE, Mencio GA, Lovejoy SA, Copley LA, Williams DJ, Thomsen IP, Schoenecker JG. A novel classification system based on dissemination of musculoskeletal infection is predictive of hospital outcomes. J Pediatr Orthop. 2018;38(5):279–86.
20. Chiappini E, Camposampiero C, Lazzeri S, Indolfi G, De Martino M, Galli L. Epidemiology and management of acute haematogenous osteomyelitis in a tertiary paediatric center. Int J Environ Res Public Health. 2017;14(5):477–88.
21. Belthur M. Birchansky, Sherri, Verdugo, Alejandro, et al. pathologic fractures in children with acute Staphylococcus aureus osteomyelitis. J Bone Joint Surg Am. 2012;94(1):34–42. https://doi.org/10.2106/JBJS.J.01915.

Septic Arthritis

12

Sreeharsha V. Nandyala, Martin J. Herman,
and Mininder S. Kocher

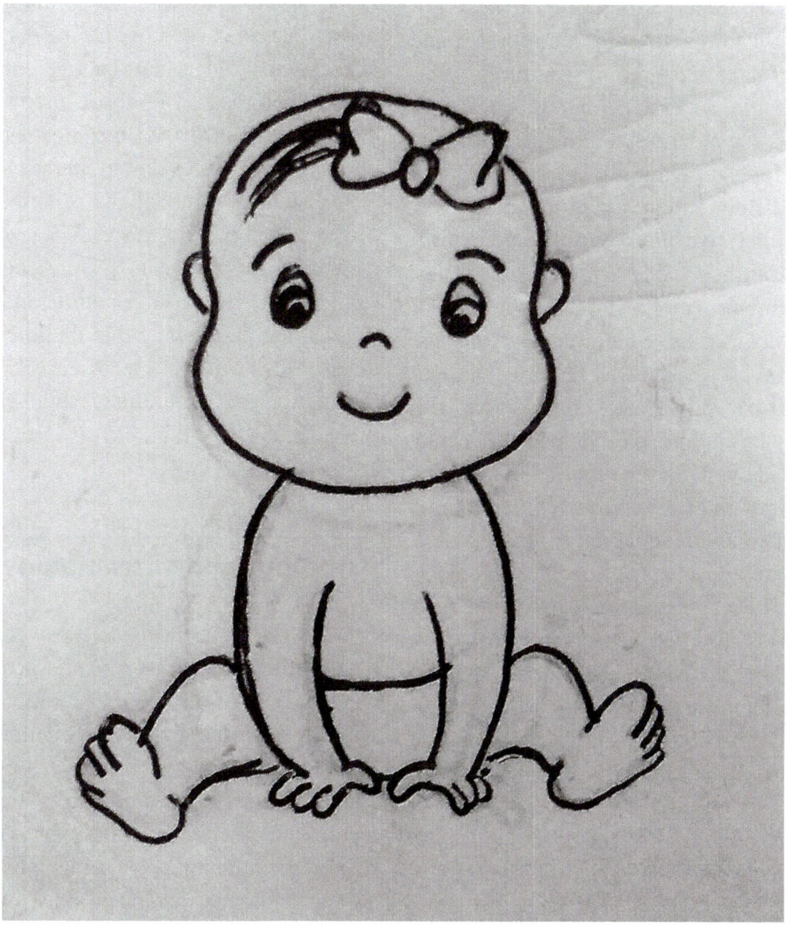

S. V. Nandyala
Boston Children's Hospital, Harvard Medical School,
Boston, MA, USA

M. J. Herman
Drexel University College of Medicine, Philadelphia,
PA, USA

Orthopedic Surgery, St. Christopher's Hospital for
Children, Philadelphia, PA, USA

M. S. Kocher (✉)
Department of Orthopaedic Surgery, Boston
Children's Hospital, Harvard Medical School,
Boston, MA, USA
e-mail: mininder.kocher@childrens.harvard.edu

© Springer Nature Switzerland AG 2022
M. V. Belthur et al. (eds.), *Pediatric Musculoskeletal Infections*,
https://doi.org/10.1007/978-3-030-95794-0_12

Introduction and Epidemiology

Osteoarticular infections are a source of significant morbidity within the pediatric population. Expeditious diagnosis and multidisciplinary management are of paramount importance in an effort to mitigate complications and disability. Pediatric osteoarticular infections manifest as osteomyelitis and septic arthritis. Septic arthritis is defined as an acute infection of the synovial joints leading to inflammation and destruction of the affected joint structures, cartilage, and potential for extension to the metaphysis leading to secondary osteomyelitis in some joints. Therefore, mitigation of these complications is predicated upon judicious diagnosis, expeditious operative intervention, and antibiotic administration.

The literature provides a variable incidence of pediatric septic arthritis, which ranges from 4 to 12 per 100,000 [1–8]. The vast majority of these studies are retrospective case-control series with relatively small sample sizes [1–8] which may explain the wide variation in reported incidences. In contrast, Safdieh et al. reported epidemiologic data from a nationwide inpatient database analysis by querying hospital billing and diagnosis coding [6]. The authors demonstrated an incidence of 5.2 per 100,000 for septic arthritis [6]. This was similar to another inpatient database analysis that demonstrated a septic arthritis incidence of 4.2 per 100,000 [5]. The majority of studies suggest a static trend in the incidence of pediatric septic arthritis over time [1–8]. In resource-poor regions, the incidence of septic arthritis has been reported to be higher up to 20 per 100,000 [9].

Several risk factors and demographic associations have been noted in the literature. Okubo et al. demonstrated that pediatric septic arthritis was more prevalent among children who are male, white or black, and between ages 0 and 4 years [5]. In addition, low socioeconomic status seems to be associated with an increased prevalence of septic arthritis [5]. Furthermore, older children (10–14 years of age) were associated with increased rate of complications and sequelae such as osteomyelitis and bacteremia/septicemia [5]. The vast majority of septic arthritis cases involve the hip, knee, and ankles, although septic arthritis can be manifested in any synovial joint. Other risk factors for septic arthritis include immunodeficiency syndromes, sickle cell disease, prematurity, respiratory distress syndrome, and low birth weight [10].

Lyme disease is also a common entity that can cause infectious arthritis in pediatric patients. Lyme disease is classically a multisystem tick-borne disease caused by the spirochete, *Borrelia burgdorferi*, and is particularly common in the northeastern region of the United States. Lyme disease is noted to be the most common tick-borne disease in the United States [11]. It is associated with a bimodal age distribution among pediatric patients from ages 5–9 years and adults from ages 55–59 years [11]. According to the Centers for Disease Control and Prevention (CDC), the geographic distribution of high incidence areas with Lyme disease appears to be expanding and, therefore, should be a more prominent differential diagnosis alongside septic arthritis [11].

Pathology and Microbiology

Primary septic arthritis is most commonly the result of hematogenous spread. Local inoculation can also occur from joint penetration and trauma. An array of inflammatory biochemical processes is elicited following bacterial joint infection. Intra-articular bacteria release toxins that trigger a cytokine cascade from the synovial tissue. The resulting inflammatory acute phase response attracts leukocytes which produce a viscous cycle of cytokine-induced damaged via the release of collagenases and peptidases that can lead to cartilage damage within 8 hours of infection [12–16]. This aggressive response represents an orthopedic surgical emergency and can be quelled with expeditious source control via surgical intervention and antibiotic administration.

Secondarily, septic arthritis can occur from bacterial translocation from an adjacent source. The synovial joint capsule of the shoulders, elbows, hips, and ankles also contain the metaphysis. In these joints, extra-cortical extension of a metaphyseal osteomyelitis can seed the capsular joint space. Conversely, primary septic arthritis can cause a metaphyseal osteomyelitis via spread through the transphyseal network of vessels. This latter mode of metaphyseal spread is more common during the first 18 months of age [17]. Merlini et al. reviewed contrast-enhanced MRI studies and demonstrated that the transphyseal network of vessels can potentiate translocation of bacteria and cause concomitant hip osteomyelitis and septic arthritis in patients less than 18 months of age, which was a previous hypothesis proposed by Alderson et al.'s animal model study [17, 18].

Across all age groups, *Staphylococcus aureus* is the most commonly found bacterial cause of septic arthritis, with increasing rates of community-acquired *methicillin-resistant Staphylococcus aureus* (MRSA) [17] (Figs. 12.1 and 12.2). MRSA genotypes with two genes, *Panton-Valentine leukocidin (pvl)* and *fibronectin-binding factor (fnbB)*, produce an aggressive form of septic arthritis [19]. MRSA genotypes that stem from an USA300 clone often carry both of these genes. Carrillo-Marquez et al. demonstrated that MRSA-USA300 is the predominant MRSA genotype that causes septic arthritis in children – 81% of MRSA infections [20]. This genotype is associated with longer duration of fever, higher incidence of bacteremia, osteomyelitis, thrombophlebitis, pulmonary embolism, and longer hospital stay [19, 20]. The severity of infection associated with MRSA-USA300 is linked to the gene products of *pvl and fnbB*. *Pvl* cytotoxin fenestrates the leukocyte cell membrane and instigates cell lysis, which releases more cytokines and fuels the inflammatory viscous cycle. This is aided by the function of *fnbB*, which encodes proteins that facilitate enhanced bacterial invasion, adhesion, and biofilm formation [19, 20].

Certain pediatric populations are associated with other types of bacterial septic arthritis (Table 12.1). Namely, in infants, Group B Streptococcus is prevalent and is a common cause of many osteoarticular infections [21, 22]. *Neisseria gonorrhoeae* must be considered in sexual assault victims or in sexually active adolescents presenting with signs of septic arthritis. In addition, *Kingella kingae* is increasingly found in culture and polymerase chain reaction (PCR) analysis in septic arthritis cases in children younger than 4 years of age [23, 24]. Furthermore, *Salmonella* associated septic arthritis is more frequent in countries such as Zambia, Kenya, and Malawi

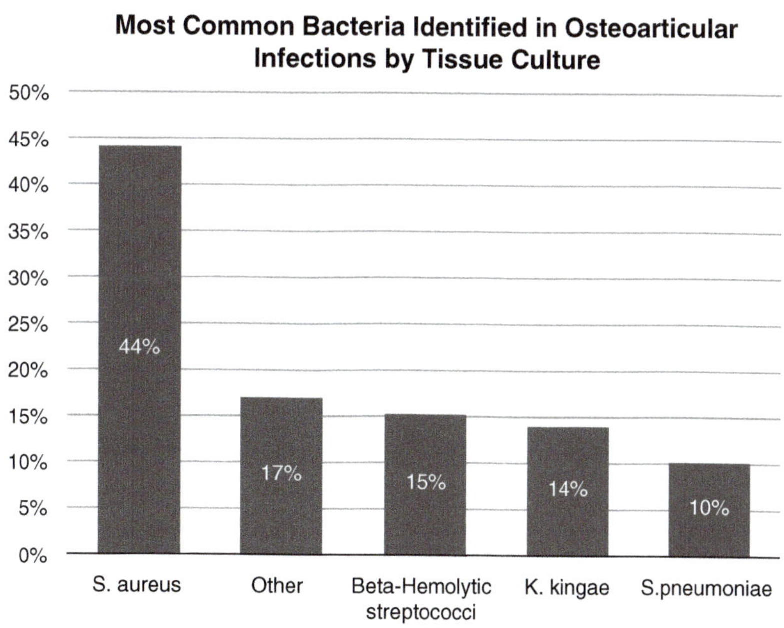

Fig. 12.1 Bacterial causes of osteoarticular infection [17]

where there is a higher prevalence of sickle cell disease and malaria [9].

The pathophysiology of Lyme arthritis has been extensively studied. Arthritis is the most prominent feature of Lyme disease [11]. Following a deer tick bite, *B. burgdorferi* modifies surface lipoproteins that promote infection to the synovial tissue and facilitate inflammation of the joint [25] (Fig. 12.3a, b). Acutely, arthritis results from synovial inflammation, preponderance of neutrophils, immune complex accumulation, and cytokine release [25]. Several host genetic factors have been studied that may predispose and facilitate progressive and refractory arthritis [26]. Following antibiotic treatment for acute Lyme arthritis, some patients can have recurrent polyarticular disease. Steere et al. have elucidated three main theories for this phenomenon: T-cell epitope mimicry, persistent or recurrent infection, and bystander activation (persistent immune reactivity despite eradication of *B. burg-*

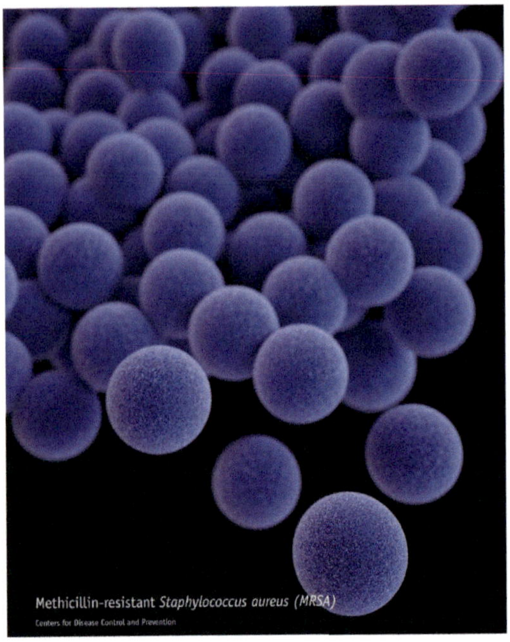

Fig. 12.2 This illustration depicts a three-dimensional (3D) computer-generated image of a group of methicillin-resistant *Staphylococcus aureus* (MRSA) bacteria, which were arranged in a cluster. ID # 19059, Center for Disease Control USA 2013/Antibiotic Resistance Coordination and Strategy Unit/Courtesy Jennifer Oosthuizen - Medical Illustrator. (With permission)

Table 12.1 Other causative organisms of septic arthritis

Organism	Circumstance
Group B streptococcus	Infants
Neisseria gonorrhoeae	Sexual abuse victims, sexually active adolescents
Salmonella typhi	Sickle cell disease or trait
Kingella kingae	Young children below 4 years of age
Pseudomonas aeruginosa	Penetrating foot trauma
Pasteurella sp.	Animal bite
Haemophilus influenzae	Unimmunized patient

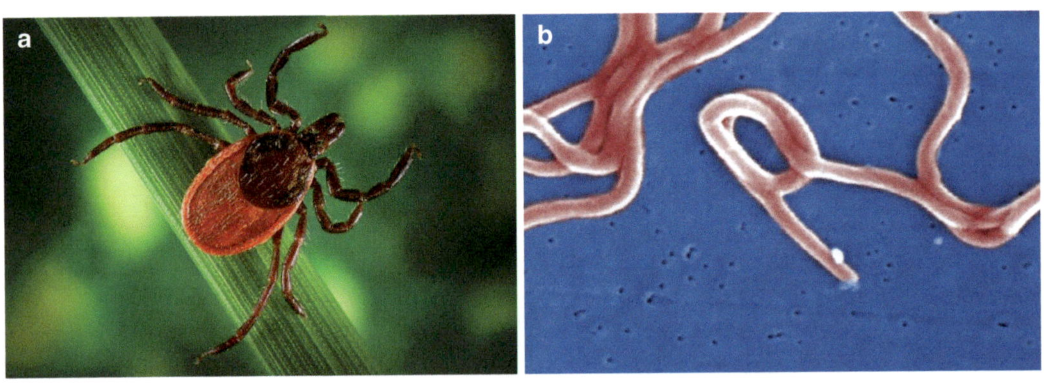

Fig. 12.3 (**a**) Photograph showing the blacklegged tick, *Ixodes pacificus*, known vector for the zoonotic spirochetal bacteria, *Borrelia burgdorferi*, which is the pathogen responsible for causing Lyme disease. ID # 7663/Center for Disease Control USA 2005/Courtesy James Gathany; William L. Nicholson, Ph.D. (With permission). (**b**) This digitally colorized scanning electron microscopic (SEM) image depicts a grouping of gram-negative, anaerobic, *Borrelia burgdorferi* bacteria, which had been derived from a pure culture. ID # 13176/Center for Disease Control USA 2011/Claudia Molins/Courtesy: Janice Haney Carr. (With permission)

dorferi) [25]. Even after antibiotic treatment, *B. burgdorferi* can remain intracellular and be detected with culture and PCR testing [27, 28].

Clinical Presentation and Examination

Septic arthritis is most commonly a monoarticular disease characterized by acute onset of pain, swelling, and joint immobility (pseudoparalysis). In general, fever is also reported. Initially, each patient must be assessed for associated life-threatening systemic conditions. Patients with fever, tachycardia, tachypnea, and hypotension should be investigated for sepsis. In addition, patients with nuchal rigidity should be concomitantly evaluated for meningitis. Similarly, auscultation of the heart and lungs may prompt evaluation for pneumonia, if there are abnormal breath sounds, or infectious endocarditis, if a cardiac murmur is present.

Initial diagnosis of septic arthritis in the emergency department is difficult. Vardiabasis et al. demonstrated that the initial emergency department diagnosis of septic arthritis was consistent only 42% of the time with the final definitive diagnosis [29]. This is particularly true in younger children who are non-ambulatory and/or nonverbal. Infants can have general malaise, distress, and pain upon moving the affected joint. Infants may not have fever or other systemic signs of infection. In the young child, diagnosis is also difficult as they can have distress with diaper changes, refusal to eat, and persistent crying. Patients of ambulatory age may refuse to bear weight and favor the contralateral extremity.

On examination, the affected joint may have swelling, effusion, warmth, and erythema (Fig. 12.4). Any attempt with short arc range of motion will produce pain and distress. In cases with septic hip arthritis, the child will present with pain and limp. In addition, capsular accumulation of fluid or abscess will prompt the child to place the hip joint in flexion, abduction, and external rotation in an effort to maximize intracapsular volume and limit stretching of the joint capsule, which triggers pain. In some instances,

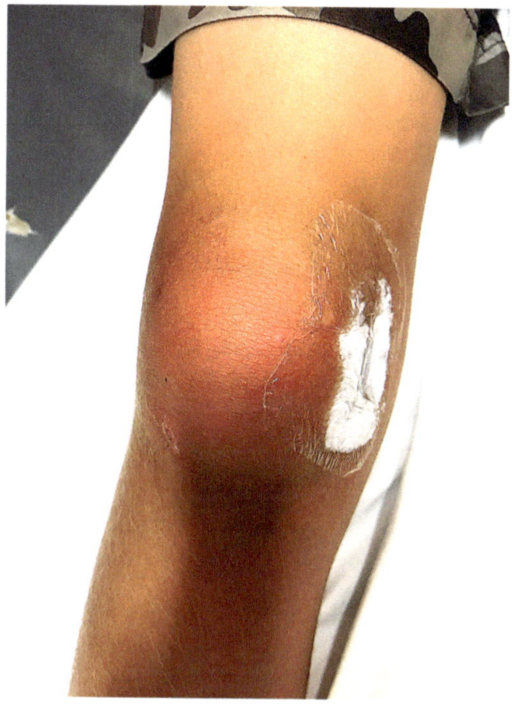

Fig. 12.4 A 10-year-old male who presented with a warm, swollen, erythematous, and painful left knee with an obvious effusion. Topical analgesia cream applied before knee joint arthrocentesis

hip pain can be referred to the knee – which may be the chief presenting complaint. This is due to nerve innervation of the hip joint by articular branches of the obturator nerve that refer pain to the dermatomal distribution along the anteromedial thigh via cutaneous nerve branches. If increased intracapsular pressure causes a capsular tear, fluid collections can develop in the surrounding musculature, and hip joint instability should be considered.

In addition to septic arthritis, Lyme disease is an important consideration in a child who presents with joint pain and limp, particularly in endemic regions. It must be noted that Lyme can present many months after the initial tick bite and pain can be recurrent [30]. The Centers for Disease Control has provided criteria for clinical case definition along with laboratory diagnostic criteria (Table 12.2) [11]. Aiyer et al. reported on the distribution of joint involvement in patients with Lyme disease and demonstrated that the knee is most commonly involved

Table 12.2 CDC clinical and diagnostic criteria for Lyme disease [1]

Clinical case criteria
Erythema migrans, or
One advanced manifestation, as defined below, and laboratory confirmation of infection
Recurrent, brief attacks (lasting weeks or months) of objective joint swelling in one or a few joints, sometimes followed by chronic arthritis in one or a few joints
Manifestations not considered criteria for diagnosis include chronic progressive arthritis, not preceded by brief attacks, and chronic symmetrical polyarthritis
Arthralgia, myalgia, or fibromyalgia syndromes alone are not criteria for musculoskeletal involvement
Laboratory criteria
Positive culture for *B. burgdorferi* from clinical specimen, or
Demonstration of diagnostic levels of IgM and IgG antibodies to the spirochetes in serum
Two-tier testing interpreted using established criteria, where:
Positive IgM is sufficient only when B30 days from system onset
Positive IgG is sufficient at any point during illness
Single-tier IgG immunoblot seropositivity using established criteria, or
CSF antibody positive for *B. burgdorferi* by enzyme immunoassay (EIA) or immunofluorescence assay (IFA), when the titer is higher than it was in serum

[1] Information adapted from CDC [11] and table adapted from Aiyer et al. [31]

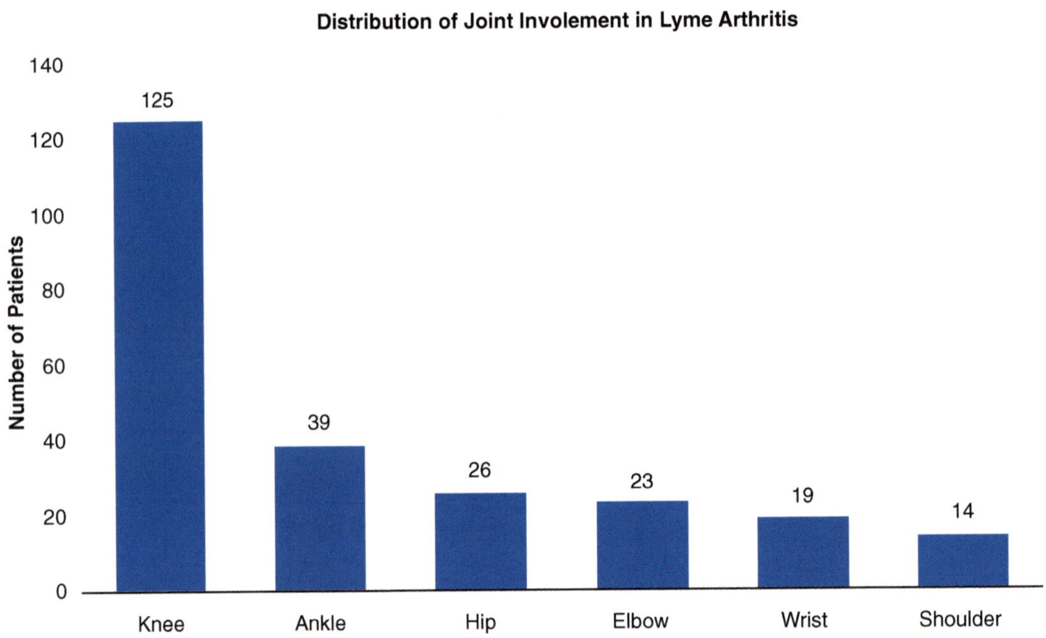

Fig. 12.5 Adapted from case series from Aiyer et al. [31] Distribution of joints involved with Lyme arthritis in 155 patients

in vast majority of cases, followed by the ankle (Fig. 12.5) [31]. Steere et al. demonstrated that 80% of patients diagnosed with Lyme disease had arthritis of some degree [32]. Symptoms were migratory and were noted, on average, 2 weeks after the onset of erythema migrans [32] (Fig. 12.6). This was associated with recurrent fatigue which lasted as long as 6 years [32]. The relapsing and remitting nature of these symptoms can distinguish Lyme from that of septic arthritis.

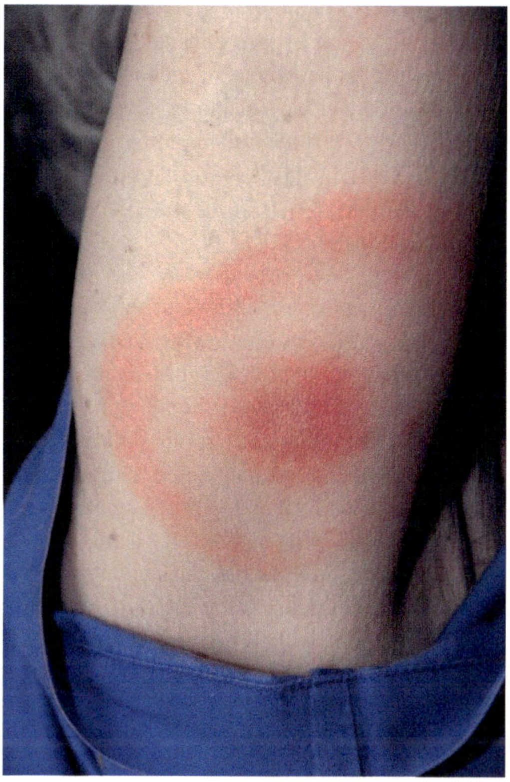

Fig. 12.6 This clinical photograph depicts the pathognomonic erythematous rash in the pattern of a bull's-eye, referred to as erythema migrans. The rash manifested at the site of a tick bite, signifies a case of Lyme disease, caused by the bacterium *Borrelia burgdorferi*, and transmitted to humans, by the bite of infected blacklegged ticks. ID # 9875 / Center for Disease Control 2007/ James Gathany / Courtesy: James Gathany. (With permission)

Investigations and Differential Diagnosis

Septic arthritis is a clinical diagnosis with laboratory and imaging studies utilized in an adjunctive fashion in an effort to corroborate a high pre-test probability.

Laboratory Studies

In addition to a white blood cell (WBC) count and polymorphonuclear cell-type predominance (left-shift) on the peripheral complete blood count (CBC) study, serum inflammatory markers are elevated in the setting of septic arthritis. Most centers test for acute phase reactants such as C-reactive protein (CRP) and the erythrocyte sedimentation rate (ESR). The standard values for the ESR are dependent upon the testing laboratory and generally peak at 3–5 days within the onset of infection and normalize within 7–10 days after treatment (up to 4–6 weeks). An elevated CRP signifies an acute inflammatory response and peaks within 48 hours of onset of the infection and starts declining within 6 hours of treatment initiation. Pääkkönen et al. demonstrated that if both studies remain normal after a 3-day hospital stay, then septic arthritis is a low probability [33]. However, CRP elevation may not be apparent in some circumstances, particularly in *K. kingae* infections. Basmaci et al. demonstrated that in 10% of septic arthritis cases with *S. aureus* or *K. kingae*, the CRP was less than 10 mg/L [34]. Similarly, Ceroni et al. developed a diagnostic laboratory criterion to differentiate *K. kingae* septic arthritis from that of *S. aureus* [35]. The authors demonstrated that the CRP was consistently decreased in the setting of *K. kingae* infections [35]. CRP is not acutely elevated in cases of osteomyelitis or other chronic infections.

Table 12.3 Kocher criteria [42]

Non-weight-bearing on affected side
Erythrocyte sedimentation rate >40 mm/hr
Fever >38.5 °C (101.3 °F)
White blood cell count >12,000 cells/mm^3

Many diagnostic algorithms have been developed to aid in the diagnosis of septic arthritis and distinguish this entity from transient synovitis [36–42]. The Kocher criteria was originally described to differentiate hip septic arthritis from transient synovitis of the hip (Table 12.3) [42]. The positive predictive probability was <0.2% for zero variables, 3% for one variable, 40% for two variables, 93.1% for 3 variables, and 99.6% for four variables. When applied to other patient populations, the Kocher criteria demonstrated diminished but good diagnostic positive predictive probabilities [41]. This criterion has been broadly applied to diagnose infections of other joints [42]. Other investigators have studied the utility of CRP and its role within diagnostic algorithms for septic arthritis [36–40]. Caird et al. performed a prospective randomized controlled trial to distinguish pediatric septic arthritis from transient synovitis of the hip and demonstrated that CRP >20 mg/L was a strong independent risk factor and the second-best predictor of septic arthritis [38]. This prospective trial reaffirmed the role of CRP in the diagnostic armamentarium for septic arthritis, as published by previous retrospective literature [36, 37]. CRP can also be utilized to trend the patient's clinical response to antibiotic treatment and need for additional surgical intervention.

In addition to inflammatory markers, blood cultures should also be drawn prior to the administration of antibiotics to rule out bacteremia.

Imaging

Plain radiographs should be obtained as an initial test for patients who present with joint pain, inability to bear weight, and weakness. Plain radiographs serve to rule out trauma and neoplastic bone or soft tissue disorders. In the setting of septic arthritis, plain radiographs can demonstrate signs of joint space expansion with fluid, i.e., effusion, fat pad signs, or medial joint space widening in the setting of hip or shoulder septic arthritis [40]. The role of plain radiography in the setting of septic arthritis is to rule out other co-existing pathology such as fracture or subacute-chronic osteomyelitis.

Ultrasound has become widely adopted and utilized to diagnose joint effusions in a child suspected of septic arthritis. Most centers have become reliant upon ultrasound to diagnose deep joint effusions such as in the hip or shoulder as a prerequisite to joint aspiration [43]. Ultrasound is expeditious, readily available, and without radiation. In addition, in infants, ultrasound is a reliable imaging modality to assess the status of deep joint structures, such as the cartilaginous ossific nucleus, which cannot be visualized on radiographs in infants. If both hips are imaged, a difference in joint fluid volume >5 mm compared with the contralateral side is considered an indication for aspiration [44] (Fig. 12.7). Ultrasound

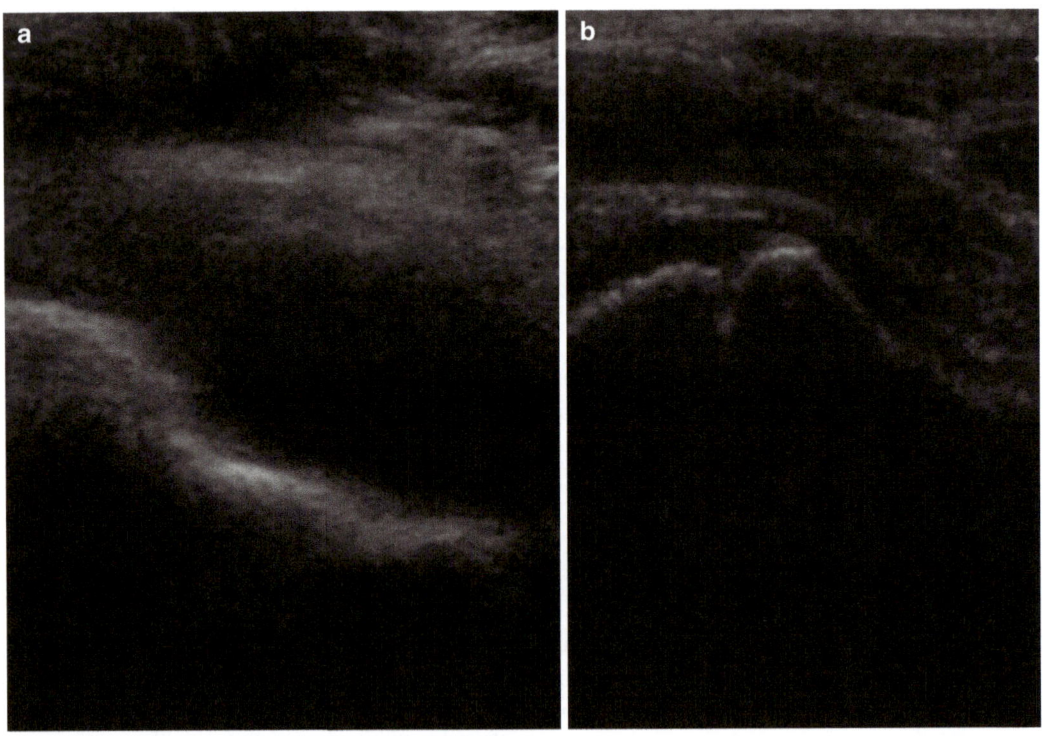

Fig. 12.7 Ultrasound of pediatric hip. (**a**) is long ultrasound cut of the hip with a large effusion. (**b**) is example of normal hip ultrasound

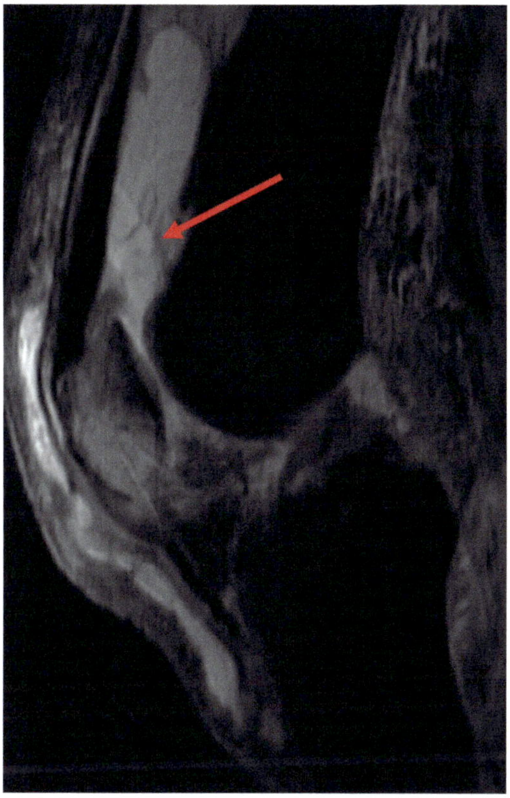

Fig. 12.8 MRI sagittal T2 image of patient with large joint effusion in setting of knee septic arthritis

is associated with a 5% false-negative rate and is suggested to be less reliable in patients with symptoms less than 24-hours or those with polyarticular involvement [45]. A negative ultrasound considerably lowers the probability of septic arthritis [46]. However, adjacent infections such as osteomyelitis and intramuscular infections must be ruled out with magnetic resonance imaging (MRI) if clinical suspicion for an osteoarticular infection is high [46]. In the setting of positive ultrasound findings, along with concerning clinical and laboratory studies, arthrocentesis is warranted. It should be noted that an ultrasound cannot differentiate fluid density between joint purulence and sterile effusions, as seen in the setting of inflammatory arthropathies.

To characterize the full extent of an osteoarticular infection, an MRI is an extremely valuable and indispensable tool (Fig. 12.8). MRI can also be utilized if there is a diagnostic quandary with equivocal ultrasound or laboratory results with high clinical suspicion and pre-test probability. Furthermore, an MRI is effective at identifying concomitant unsuspected adjacent osteoarticular infections [47, 48]. Monsalve et al. reviewed MRI studies of patients with septic arthritis of which 68% had concomitant unsuspected osteomyelitis [47]. As such, some authors have recommended routine MRI studies in patients suspected of septic arthritis in an effort to detect these related adjacent infections [47, 49]. However, other authors have expressed caution and developed algorithms to ensure appropriate use of cross-sectional imaging [50]. Rosenfeld et al. demonstrated that age above 3.6 years, CRP >13.8 mg/L, duration of symptoms >3 days, platelets <314 × 10 cells/μL, and ANC >8.6 × 10 cells/μL were risk factors for adjacent infection in the setting of pediatric septic arthritis [50]. Patients with three or more of these risk factors were associated with an 80% positive predictive value for adjacent osteoarticular infection [50].

In the setting of Lyme disease, Ecklund et al. identified three characteristic MRI findings – myositis, adenopathy, and lack of subcutaneous edema. These findings along with a consistent clinical picture of Lyme arthritis may prevent unnecessary surgical intervention [51].

Arthrocentesis

If the clinical picture and the serum laboratory and radiology studies are concerning for septic arthritis, the next best step in diagnosis is a joint aspiration. The sample should be obtained prior to the initiation of antibiotics. In most cases, aspiration of a superficial joint, such as the knee or elbow, can be performed at bedside with relative ease and accuracy with proper pain control for the child. For deep joints, such as the hip, an ultrasound-assisted arthrocentesis is often helpful and necessary. The joint aspirate sample should be sent to the laboratory expeditiously to evaluate, at a minimum, for gram stain/culture and synovial fluid cell count with differential. If an ultrasound-guided arthrocentesis fails to yield synovial fluid for laboratory analysis, a surgical arthrocentesis is recommended in the operating room under anesthesia. This sample should be sent for immediate analysis to aid in surgical decision-making.

The role of gram stain has been questioned. In a systematic review of the English literature, Kang et al. demonstrated that gram stain alone is only positive for approximately 30% of cases, which increased when the tissue was also cultured [10, 52]. Furthermore, Bram et al. demonstrated that gram stain is a poor screening tool for the detection of septic arthritis and the sensitivity further drops for the detection of gram-negative organisms [52]. As such, a negative gram stain must be taken into clinical context and further work-up must be performed if suspicion for septic arthritis remains high.

PCR studies of synovial fluid or tissue can expedite the identification of the causal organism and is an area of further research [53]. PCR studies are of particular utility if antibiotics were initiated prior to joint fluid aspiration, in which case, gram staining and culture become less worthwhile. In addition, PCR studies for the detection of *K. kingae* have garnered increased attention and practice [54]. In endemic regions, Lyme titer and PCR should also be obtained.

Synovial fluid total nucleated cell count ≥50,000/mm^3 with increased percentage of polymorphonuclear cells (>90%) is classically associated with septic arthritis [55]. Margaretten et al. demonstrated the likelihood ratios for septic arthritis as a function of synovial fluid total nucleated cell count (Table 12.4) [55]. For counts ≥50,000/mm^3, the likelihood ratio for septic arthritis is 2.9 (confidence interval (CI), 2.5–3.4) [55]. Despite these findings, the evidence for diagnostic cell count thresholds remains debated and the clinical picture must be given greater weight [56]. For example, Heyworth et al. demonstrated that hip septic arthritis was associated with synovial fluid cell counts of 25,000 to 75,000/mm^3 [56]. In 17% of their cases, the synovial fluid WBC values were <50,000/mm^3 [56].

Table 12.4 Synovial WBC count stratified by likelihood for septic arthritis [55]

Synovial WBC count	Likelihood ratio for septic arthritis	95% confidence interval for likelihood ratio
<25,000/μL	0.32	0.23–0.43
≥25,000/μL	2.9	2.5–3.4
≥50,000/μL	7.7	5.7–11.0
≥100,000/μL	28.0	12.0–66.0

Adapted from Margaretten et al. [55]

Lyme Arthritis

Lyme arthritis and inflammatory arthritis may be polyarticular and migratory and accompany dermatologic findings. Titers for Lyme must be obtained if the patient resides in endemic areas and if the clinical suspicion is high. The CDC provides a diagnostic laboratory algorithm for Lyme disease (Fig. 12.9) [11]. A modified two-stage serologic test is utilized [57]. The initial ELISA or immunofluorescence assay is confirmed with a Western blot analysis. Negative IgG titers rule out Lyme disease [57]. PCR testing of Lyme from synovial fluid has a sensitivity of 80–85%; however, active infection is difficult to determine as the PCR can detect DNA from past infection with persistent *B. burgdorferi* genetic material [57]. In addition, there is no agreed upon threshold for synovial fluid total nucleated cell counts that define Lyme arthritis. Some authors have noted an average of 25,000 cells/mm^3 but can be up to 100,000 cells/ [3, 58].

Differential Diagnosis

Trauma, neoplastic processes, and other osteoarticular infections must be considered in patients who present with joint pain consistent with septic arthritis. For hip pain specifically, Legg-Calve-Perthes disease, slipped capital femoral epiphysis, transient synovitis, osteomyelitis, and local intramuscular abscess can mimic signs of septic arthritis. Furthermore, conditions such as cellulitis, inflammatory arthritis, and hemarthroses must be assessed. To rule out adjacent

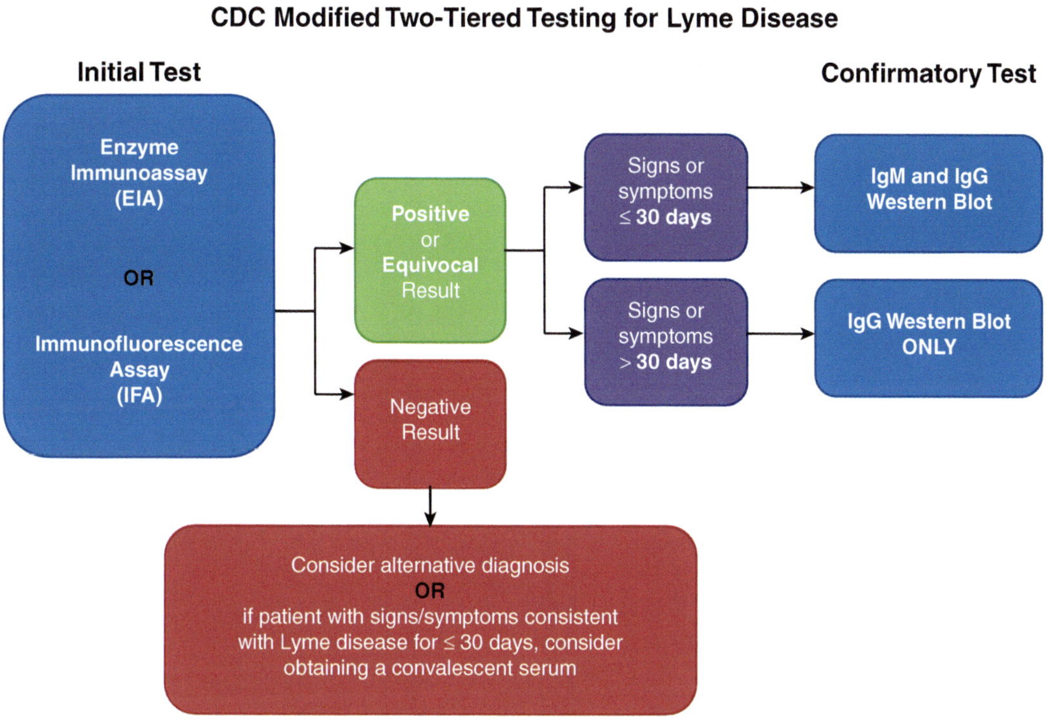

Fig. 12.9 The CDC recommended modified two-step diagnostic process for Lyme disease

osteomyelitis in the hip, some authors have recommended ilium and femoral neck bone marrow aspiration during surgical intervention, particularly if the MRI is equivocal [59]. Transient synovitis typically follows a history of an upper respiratory tract infection and is less likely to present with high fever and chills.

Clinical diagnostic rules, such as the Kocher criteria, have been developed and validated to help distinguish septic arthritis from other similar processes such as transient synovitis [42]. In addition, the range of the synovial fluid total nucleated cell count can be indicative of the disease process. In a systematic review of the literature with meta-analysis, Cruz et al. stratified synovial fluid cell counts with 95% confidence intervals (CI) as 5644–15,388 cells/mm^3 for transient synovitis, 47,533–64,242 cells/mm^3 for Lyme arthritis, and 105,432–260,214 cells/mm^3 for septic arthritis [60].

Bockenstedt et al. provide an excellent comparison of various types of arthritis seen pediatric patients (Table 12.5).

Treatment

After establishing a diagnosis of septic arthritis, treatment is twofold and is optimized with multidisciplinary management and coordination with general pediatrics, orthopedic surgery, and infectious disease specialists. Adequate source control of the infection with joint irrigation and debridement is paramount. In addition, determination of the causal organism and subsequent antibiotic sensitivity is necessary for definitive antibiotic treatment. Prior to this, empiric antibiotics should be prescribed based upon evidence-based recommendations with regard to the most causal organism, patient's age, microbiome of the region, and the patient's clinical state. Typically, antibiotics should be held until a synovial fluid or tissue culture is obtained in an effort to tailor antibiotics to the causal bacteria – except in situations of sepsis and hemodynamic instability, where empiric broad spectrum antibiotics may be life-saving and should not be delayed.

Table 12.5 Comparison of common arthritides in pediatric patients [58]

	Lyme arthritis	Bacterial septic arthritis	Gonococcal arthritis	Reactive arthritis	Oligoarticular juvenile inflammatory arthritis	Rheumatoid arthritis
Onset	Intermediate, months (average 6 months) after rash	Acute (days–2 weeks)	Acute, within 1 month of initial infection	Acute, 2–4 weeks post initial viral infection	Insidious	Insidious
Arthritis features	Oligoarticular, especially knee; may be migratory (<5 joints)	Usually monoarticular	Usually monoarticular	Oligoarticular, lower limb, especially knee	Oligoarticular, lower limb	Classically symmetric, polyarticular pain, stiffness
Systemic signs/ symptoms at arthritis onset	50% with antecedent migratory arthralgia; fatigue; occasionally fever	Fever in 60%	Migratory polyarthralgia, often fever, rash, tenosynovitis	Enthesitis, extra-articular features	Unusual	Fatigue
ESR/CRP	Usually modest elevation, but occasionally normal or very elevated	Usually elevated	Usually elevated	Marked elevation in acute phase	Usually elevated	Usually elevated
Synovial fluid cell count (white blood cells/mm^3)	500–>100,000 (average 25,000) 75% PMNs	2000–>100,000 >90% PMNs	15,000–>100,000 >90% PMNs	2000–64,000 variable PMNs	2000–50,000 (ave 20,000) 60% PMNs	2000–50,000 (mean 15,000) variable PMNs
Synovial fluid culture	Negative	Positive in 70–90%	Positive in <50%	Negative	Negative	Negative
Synovial fluid PCR for bacterial DNA	Positive	Data not available	Positive	Negative	Negative	Negative

Adapted from Bockenstedt et al. [58]

Medical Intervention

Optimal empiric antibiotic selection for pediatric septic arthritis is predicated mainly upon the age of the patient, the patient's immunization status (*H. influenza*), and the prevalence rate of MRSA in the local population. Regions with MRSA prevalence ≥10%, ICU patients, or immunocompromised hosts should be treated empirically for MRSA [61]. It should be noted that if vancomycin and gentamycin are prescribed, a target trough level must be monitored regularly and the antibiotic dosing be adjusted accordingly. In addition, the patient's blood cell counts and hepatorenal function must be monitored in the setting of antibiotic therapy to assess for toxicity.

The empiric antibiotic treatment plan for children less than 3 months of age is typically vancomycin and gentamicin combination therapy [62, 63]. This regimen will cover MRSA, Group B Streptococcus, and gram-negative pathogens. The optimal dosing, frequency, and monitoring can vary, and a multidisciplinary dosing protocol should be discussed with infectious disease specialists and pharmacy. For older children, a first-generation cephalosporin is generally prescribed – or vancomycin if there is high rate of community-acquired MRSA. It is important to note that cephalosporins also covers *K. kingae*, whereas vancomycin does not. As such, if both MRSA and *K. kingae* are prevalent, a cephalosporin should be added along with vancomycin [24]. This is similar for *N. gonorrhoeae* as well along with the alternative, doxycycline. Following synovial fluid or tissue culture and antibiotic sensitivity, the antibiotics should be tailored appropriately.

The duration of antibiotic treatment is dependent upon how the patient performs clinically. In most cases, a short course of intravenous antibiotic treatment followed by 3 weeks of oral therapy is sufficient for septic arthritis [64]. Complicated septic arthritis may warrant longer intravenous antibiotic treatment. Several studies have assessed the optimal time to switch from intravenous to oral therapy [65–69]. Chou et al. demonstrated good clinical outcomes when oral antibiotics were initiated when a 50% reduction in CRP is observed with intravenous antibiotics [67]. Arnold et al. recommended that a CRP less than 2 mg/DL is an indicator of stopping antibiotic treatment [65]. Ultimately, the patient's clinical picture will dictate optimal transition time and duration of treatment. The expediated switch to oral therapy is a departure from historic practices of keeping patients on intravenous antibiotics for several weeks, as similar outcomes were noted with both regimens alongside lesser complication profile with oral therapy [68, 69].

In addition to antibiotics, the role of corticosteroids has been assessed as an adjunctive method to reduce morbidity [70, 71]. Farrow et al. performed a systematic review and meta-analysis of both human and animal model trials in the setting of septic arthritis and demonstrated an overall consensus with regard to a reduction in duration of symptoms and inflammatory markers with corticosteroid therapy [70]. In addition, in the animal model data, corticosteroid plus antibiotic therapy was associated with a protective effect on cartilage. These findings were similar to another meta-analysis reported by Qin et al. [71]

For Lyme disease, adequate antibiotic therapy at the time of diagnosis is associated with good outcomes and can mitigate the risk for recurrent migratory arthritis [72]. Lyme arthritis is treated with antibiotics, and surgical intervention is typically not needed. It should be noted, as above, that persistent joint inflammation may be seen for several weeks or months after treatment. Clinical guidelines from the Infectious Diseases Society of America recommend 28 days of one of several oral antibiotics, typically doxycycline or a cephalosporin such as cefuroxime [73]. Dosing, need for intravenous antibiotics, and additional duration of therapy should be evaluated by infectious disease specialists [73].

Surgical Intervention

Septic arthritis represents a true orthopedic surgical urgency for which an irrigation and debridement of the infected joint is the cornerstone of treatment. After diagnosis and imaging to characterize the extent of infection, surgical intervention should be performed expeditiously. In the setting of hemodynamic instability, emergent surgical intervention is necessary for source control.

The type of surgical intervention, either an open arthrotomy or arthroscopic decompression, should be based upon surgeon comfort and the patient's clinical status. Arthroscopic procedures can be performed in nearly all large joints, including the hip in young patients [74, 75]. Arthroscopic hip decompression with irrigation and debridement is typically performed utilizing lateral portals although medial portal arthroscopy has been theoretically proposed [76]. Open hip arthrotomy is more commonly performed. This is achieved utilizing a direct anterior or modified anterolateral approach. Care must be taken to avoid neurovascular structures, maintain perfusion to the hip, and avoid damage to chondral surfaces.

Arthroscopic knee irrigation and debridement is popular and performed readily by most trained orthopedic surgeons. Compared to open arthrotomy, arthroscopic knee decompression is associated with less need for repeat procedures, earlier knee range of motion, and weight-bearing [77]. In addition, arthroscopic knee irrigation and debridement can be performed if a repeat procedure is indicated. In the setting of a septic knee, the risk for revision decompression is associated with bacteremia, older children, and those with late presentation [77–79]. Revision surgery is indicated if the inflammatory markers do not improve after postoperative day two, continued wound drainage, or if the patient is clinically deteriorating.

Following surgical treatment, antibiotics should be prescribed with consultation from infectious disease specialists as detailed above. Surgical follow-up should be maintained for at least a year.

Complications

Timely diagnosis, surgical decompression, and antibiotics are typically associated with favorable outcomes for septic arthritis. However, late presentation, misdiagnosis, or delay in treatment can lead to significant morbidity and even mortality. Modern data from developed regions suggest that the 1-year rate of clinical dysfunction is 10%, compared with greater than 50% in resource-poor settings and historical data [80–82]. Advancements in diagnostic capabilities, testing, imaging, and care delivery were touted as reasons for this difference [81]. Misdiagnosis is associated with delay to arthrotomy as many culture-negative cases were attributed to juvenile inflammatory arthritis or other pathology that did not necessitate antibiotics or surgical intervention [80, 82]. In the study by Howard-Jones et al., limb-length discrepancy, hip instability, reduced range of motion, and recurrence of septic arthritis were the complications noted at 1 year [81].

Complications associated with septic arthritis of the lower extremity include limp, decreased range of motion, osteonecrosis of the femoral head in the hip or femoral condyle of the knee, limb-length discrepancy, hip instability, osteomyelitis, destruction of the epiphyseal plate, progressive ankylosis, chondral injury leading to early arthritis, and ankylosis leading to long term gait abnormalities [83–85]. Complications in the upper extremity include limb-length discrepancy, angular deformity, pain, and loss of motion. Prematurity and greater severity of illness is correlated with increased rate of long-term sequelae [80, 84]. For the hip specifically, classification systems have been reported in an effort to guide treatment [86–89]. Choi et al. proposed a modified radiographic classification based upon findings of Hunka et al. and proposed treatment regimens for each category [87–89].

Reconstructive options for deformity associated with sequelae of septic arthritis varied and complex. Goals should be aimed to optimize joint range of motion, pain control, and clinical function. Spiegel et al. proposed several treatment options for various sequelae of septic arthritis [90]. Leg length discrepancies can be addressed with epiphysiodesis, guided growth, osteotomies, or soft tissue releases. Hip instability can benefit from open reduction, pelvic support osteotomy, or arthroplasty depending upon the degree of arthritis. Contracture and loss of motion will often necessitate soft tissue releases. In the hip, abductor insufficiency from greater trochanter growth arrest may benefit from greater trochanteric transfer, pelvic support osteotomy, or hip arthrodesis [90]. Each treatment must be tailored to the patient's functional demands, cultural expectations, and resources available to the surgeon and caretakers.

In an effort to minimize variation in care, clinical practice guidelines have been established at various institutions to prevent delay and optimize outcomes for pediatric patients with suspected septic arthritis [91–93]. Standard order sheets that reflect multidisciplinary consensus opinions have been established [91–93]. Kocher et al. demonstrated that the utilization of a clinical guideline at their institution was associated with lower follow-up inflammatory markers, radiation from imaging, presumptive drainage rate along with faster time to discharge, transition to oral antibiotic therapy, and greater compliance of recommended antibiotic therapy [93]. As such, adoption of institution-specific multidisciplinary clinical care guidelines can provide efficiency and optimize outcomes in the setting of pediatric septic arthritis.

Conclusion

Septic arthritis demands a multidisciplinary approach for diagnosis and management (Box 12.1). It is a diagnostic challenge and remains a true orthopedic surgical emergency. Timely diagnosis, surgical decompression, and antibiotic administration are crucial to optimize outcomes. Rates of complication and long-term sequelae from septic arthritis have diminished due to advancements in diagnostic capabilities, broad recognition, and heighted awareness among various providers. However, long-term morbidity, need for additional surgeries, and disability pose a significant challenge and is a realm of significant research and improvement.

Box 12.1 Key Learning Points

1. Septic arthritis is a true orthopedic emergency.
2. A multidisciplinary approach is key for diagnosis and management.
3. Early diagnosis, surgical decompression, and antibiotics are essential for good outcome.
4. Delayed diagnosis and inappropriate and inadequate treatment are associated with long-term sequela.

Disclosure No funds were received in support of this work. No benefits in any form have been or will be received from any commercial party related directly or indirectly to the subject of this manuscript

References

1. Christiansen P, Frederiksen B, Glazowski J, Scavenius M, Knudsen FU. Epidemiologic, bacteriologic, and long-term follow-up data of children with acute hematogenous osteomyelitis and septic arthritis: a ten-year review. J Pediatr Orthop B. 1999;8(4):302–5. Epub 1999/10/08.
2. Welkon CJ, Long SS, Fisher MC, Alburger PD. Pyogenic arthritis in infants and children: a review of 95 cases. Pediatr Infect Dis. 1986;5(6):669–76. Epub 1986/11/01.
3. Jackson MA, Nelson JD. Etiology and medical management of acute suppurative bone and joint infections in pediatric patients. J Pediatr Orthop. 1982;2(3):313–23. Epub 1982/08/01.
4. Gafur OA, Copley LA, Hollmig ST, Browne RH, Thornton LA, Crawford SE. The impact of the current epidemiology of pediatric musculoskeletal infection on evaluation and treatment guidelines. J Pediatr Orthop. 2008;28(7):777–85. Epub 2008/09/25.
5. Okubo Y, Nochioka K, Marcia T. Nationwide survey of pediatric septic arthritis in the United States. J Orthop. 2017;14(3):342–6, Epub 2017/07/15.
6. Safdieh G, Silberman J, Nguyen J, Doyle SM, Blanco JS, Scher DM, et al. Pediatric septic arthritis and osteomyelitis in the USA: a national KID database analysis. HSS J. 2019;15(2):159–66. Epub 2019/07/23.
7. Malcius D, Trumpulyte G, Barauskas V, Kilda A. Two decades of acute hematogenous osteomyelitis in children: are there any changes? Pediatr Surg Int. 2005;21(5):356–9. Epub 2005/04/19.
8. Gillespie WJ. Epidemiology in bone and joint infection. Infect Dis Clin N Am. 1990;4(3):361–76. Epub 1990/09/01.
9. Lavy CB, Peek AC, Manjolo G. The incidence of septic arthritis in Malawian children. Int Orthop. 2005;29(3):195–6. Epub 2005/04/05.
10. Kang SN, Sanghera T, Mangwani J, Paterson JM, Ramachandran M. The management of septic arthritis in children: systematic review of the English language literature. J Bone Joint Surg. 2009;91(9):1127–33. Epub 2009/09/02.
11. Prevention CfDCa. Lyme Disease. Recent Surveillance Data; 2019 [cited 2020]; Available from: https://www.cdc.gov/lyme/datasurveillance/recent-surveillance-data.html#:~:text=In%202018%2C%20a%20total%20of,Disease%20Surveillance%20System%20(NNDSS).
12. Benvenuti M, An T, Amaro E, Lovejoy S, Mencio G, Martus J, et al. Double-edged sword: musculoskeletal infection provoked acute phase response in children.

Orthop Clin North Am. 2017;48(2):181–97. Epub 2017/03/25.
13. Papathanasiou I, Malizos KN, Poultsides L, Karachalios T, Oikonomou P, Tsezou A. The catabolic role of toll-like receptor 2 (TLR-2) mediated by the NF-kappaB pathway in septic arthritis. J Orthop Res. 2011;29(2):247–51. Epub 2010/08/27.
14. Oronsky A, Ignarro L, Perper R. Release of cartilage mucopolysaccharide-degrading neutral protease from human leukocytes. J Exp Med. 1973;138(2):461–72. Epub 1973/08/01.
15. Harris ED Jr, Parker HG, Radin EL, Krane SM. Effects of proteolytic enzymes on structural and mechanical properties of cartilage. Arthritis Rheum. 1972;15(5):497–503. Epub 1972/09/01.
16. Smith RL, Schurman DJ, Kajiyama G, Mell M, Gilkerson E. The effect of antibiotics on the destruction of cartilage in experimental infectious arthritis. J Bone Joint Surg Am. 1987;69(7):1063–8. Epub 1987/09/01.
17. Merlini L, Anooshiravani M, Ceroni D. Concomitant septic arthritis and osteomyelitis of the hip in young children; a new pathophysiological hypothesis suggested by MRI enhancement pattern. BMC Med Imaging. 2015;15:17. Epub 2015/05/20.
18. Alderson M, Speers D, Emslie K, Nade S. Acute haematogenous osteomyelitis and septic arthritis--a single disease. An hypothesis based upon the presence of transphyseal blood vessels. J Bone Joint Surg. 1986;68(2):268–74. Epub 1986/03/01.
19. Dohin B, Gillet Y, Kohler R, Lina G, Vandenesch F, Vanhems P, et al. Pediatric bone and joint infections caused by Panton-valentine leukocidin-positive Staphylococcus aureus. Pediatr Infect Dis J. 2007;26(11):1042–8. Epub 2007/11/07.
20. Carrillo-Marquez MA, Hulten KG, Hammerman W, Mason EO, Kaplan SL. USA300 is the predominant genotype causing Staphylococcus aureus septic arthritis in children. Pediatr Infect Dis J. 2009;28(12):1076–80. Epub 2009/10/13.
21. Sankaran G, Zacharia B, Roy A, Purayil SP. Current clinical and bacteriological profile of septic arthritis in young infants: a prospective study from a tertiary referral Centre. Eur J Orthop Surg Traumatol. 2018;28(4):573–8. Epub 2018/02/11.
22. Branson J, Vallejo JG, Flores AR, Hulten KG, Mason EO, Kaplan SL, et al. The contemporary microbiology and rates of concomitant osteomyelitis in acute septic arthritis. Pediatr Infect Dis J. 2017;36(3):267–73. Epub 2016/11/22.
23. Williams N, Cooper C, Cundy P. Kingella kingae septic arthritis in children: recognising an elusive pathogen. J Child Orthop. 2014;8(1):91–5. Epub 2014/02/04.
24. Arnold JC, Bradley JS. Osteoarticular infections in children. Infect Dis Clin N Am. 2015;29(3):557–74. Epub 2015/08/28.
25. Steere AC, Glickstein L. Elucidation of Lyme arthritis. Nat Rev Immunol. 2004;4(2):143–52. Epub 2004/03/26.
26. Guerau-de-Arellano M, Huber BT. Chemokines and toll-like receptors in Lyme disease pathogenesis. Trends Mol Med. 2005;11(3):114–20. Epub 2005/03/12.
27. Nocton JJ, Dressler F, Rutledge BJ, Rys PN, Persing DH, Steere AC. Detection of Borrelia burgdorferi DNA by polymerase chain reaction in synovial fluid from patients with Lyme arthritis. N Engl J Med. 1994;330(4):229–34. Epub 1994/01/27.
28. Girschick HJ, Huppertz HI, Russmann H, Krenn V, Karch H. Intracellular persistence of Borrelia burgdorferi in human synovial cells. Rheumatol Int. 1996;16(3):125–32. Epub 1996/01/01.
29. Vardiabasis NV, Schlechter JA. Definitive diagnosis of children presenting to a pediatric emergency department with fever and extremity pain. J Emerg Med. 2017;53(3):306–12. Epub 2017/10/11.
30. Smith BG, Cruz AI Jr, Milewski MD, Shapiro ED. Lyme disease and the orthopaedic implications of Lyme arthritis. J Am Acad Orthop Surg. 2011;19(2):91–100. Epub 2011/02/05.
31. Aiyer A, Hennrikus W, Walrath J, Groh B, Ostrov B. Lyme arthritis of the pediatric lower extremity in the setting of polyarticular disease. J Child Orthop. 2014;8(4):359–65. Epub 2014/07/24.
32. Steere AC, Schoen RT, Taylor E. The clinical evolution of Lyme arthritis. Ann Intern Med. 1987;107(5):725–31. Epub 1987/11/01.
33. Paakkonen M, Kallio MJ, Kallio PE, Peltola H. Sensitivity of erythrocyte sedimentation rate and C-reactive protein in childhood bone and joint infections. Clin Orthop Relat Res. 2010;468(3):861–6. Epub 2009/06/18.
34. Basmaci R, Ilharreborde B, Bonacorsi S, Kahil M, Mallet C, Aupiais C, et al. Septic arthritis in children with normal initial C-reactive protein: clinical and biological features. Arch Pediatr. 2014;21(11):1195–9. Epub 2014/10/06.
35. Ceroni D, Cherkaoui A, Combescure C, Francois P, Kaelin A, Schrenzel J. Differentiating osteoarticular infections caused by Kingella kingae from those due to typical pathogens in young children. Pediatr Infect Dis J. 2011;30(10):906–9. Epub 2011/04/16.
36. Singhal R, Perry DC, Khan FN, Cohen D, Stevenson HL, James LA, et al. The use of CRP within a clinical prediction algorithm for the differentiation of septic arthritis and transient synovitis in children. J Bone Joint Surg. 2011;93(11):1556–61. Epub 2011/11/08.
37. Sultan J, Hughes PJ. Septic arthritis or transient synovitis of the hip in children: the value of clinical prediction algorithms. J Bone Joint Surg. 2010;92(9):1289–93. Epub 2010/08/28.
38. Caird MS, Flynn JM, Leung YL, Millman JE, D'Italia JG, Dormans JP. Factors distinguishing septic arthritis from transient synovitis of the hip in children. A prospective study. J Bone Joint Surg Am. 2006;88(6):1251–7. Epub 2006/06/08.
39. Luhmann SJ, Jones A, Schootman M, Gordon JE, Schoenecker PL, Luhmann JD. Differentiation between septic arthritis and transient synovitis of the hip in children with clinical prediction algorithms.

J Bone Joint Surg Am. 2004;86(5):956–62. Epub 2004/05/01.
40. Jung ST, Rowe SM, Moon ES, Song EK, Yoon TR, Seo HY. Significance of laboratory and radiologic findings for differentiating between septic arthritis and transient synovitis of the hip. J Pediatr Orthop. 2003;23(3):368–72. Epub 2003/05/02.
41. Kocher MS, Mandiga R, Zurakowski D, Barnewolt C, Kasser JR. Validation of a clinical prediction rule for the differentiation between septic arthritis and transient synovitis of the hip in children. J Bone Joint Surg Am. 2004;86(8):1629–35. Epub 2004/08/05.
42. Kocher MS, Zurakowski D, Kasser JR. Differentiating between septic arthritis and transient synovitis of the hip in children: an evidence-based clinical prediction algorithm. J Bone Joint Surg Am. 1999;81(12):1662–70. Epub 1999/12/23.
43. Plumb J, Mallin M, Bolte RG. The role of ultrasound in the emergency department evaluation of the acutely painful pediatric hip. Pediatr Emerg Care. 2015;31(1):54–8. quiz 9-61. Epub 2015/01/07.
44. Moss SG, Schweitzer ME, Jacobson JA, Brossmann J, Lombardi JV, Dellose SM, et al. Hip joint fluid: detection and distribution at MR imaging and US with cadaveric correlation. Radiology. 1998;208(1):43–8. Epub 1998/07/01.
45. Gordon JE, Huang M, Dobbs M, Luhmann SJ, Szymanski DA, Schoenecker PL. Causes of false-negative ultrasound scans in the diagnosis of septic arthritis of the hip in children. J Pediatr Orthop. 2002;22(3):312–6. Epub 2002/04/19.
46. Montgomery NI, Epps HR. Pediatric septic arthritis. Orthop Clin North Am. 2017;48(2):209–16. Epub 2017/03/25.
47. Monsalve J, Kan JH, Schallert EK, Bisset GS, Zhang W, Rosenfeld SB. Septic arthritis in children: frequency of coexisting unsuspected osteomyelitis and implications on imaging work-up and management. AJR Am J Roentgenol. 2015;204(6):1289–95. Epub 2015/05/23.
48. Schallert EK, Kan JH, Monsalve J, Zhang W, Bisset GS 3rd, Rosenfeld S. Metaphyseal osteomyelitis in children: how often does MRI-documented joint effusion or epiphyseal extension of edema indicate coexisting septic arthritis? Pediatr Radiol. 2015;45(8):1174–81. Epub 2015/02/24.
49. Mignemi ME, Menge TJ, Cole HA, Mencio GA, Martus JE, Lovejoy S, et al. Epidemiology, diagnosis, and treatment of pericapsular pyomyositis of the hip in children. J Pediatr Orthop. 2014;34(3):316–25. Epub 2013/11/01.
50. Rosenfeld S, Bernstein DT, Daram S, Dawson J, Zhang W. Predicting the presence of adjacent infections in septic arthritis in children. J Pediatr Orthop. 2016;36(1):70–4. Epub 2015/01/13.
51. Ecklund K, Vargas S, Zurakowski D, Sundel RP. MRI features of Lyme arthritis in children. AJR Am J Roentgenol. 2005;184(6):1904–9. Epub 2005/05/24.
52. Bram JT, Baldwin KD, Blumberg TJ. Gram stain is not clinically relevant in treatment of pediatric septic arthritis. J Pediatr Orthop. 2018;38(9):e536–e40. Epub 2018/07/24.
53. El Houmami N, Bzdrenga J, Durand GA, Minodier P, Seligmann H, Prudent E, et al. Molecular tests that target the RTX locus do not distinguish between Kingella kingae and the recently described Kingella negevensis species. J Clin Microbiol. 2017;55(10):3113–22. Epub 2017/08/11.
54. Carter K, Doern C, Jo CH, Copley LA. The clinical usefulness of polymerase chain reaction as a supplemental diagnostic tool in the evaluation and the treatment of children with septic arthritis. J Pediatr Orthop. 2016;36(2):167–72. Epub 2015/04/19.
55. Margaretten ME, Kohlwes J, Moore D, Bent S. Does this adult patient have septic arthritis? JAMA. 2007;297(13):1478–88. Epub 2007/04/05.
56. Heyworth BE, Shore BJ, Donohue KS, Miller PE, Kocher MS, Glotzbecker MP. Management of pediatric patients with synovial fluid white blood-cell counts of 25,000 to 75,000 cells/mm(3) after aspiration of the hip. J Bone Joint Surg Am. 2015;97(5):389–95. Epub 2015/03/06.
57. Aguero-Rosenfeld ME, Wang G, Schwartz I, Wormser GP. Diagnosis of Lyme borreliosis. Clin Microbiol Rev. 2005;18(3):484–509. Epub 2005/07/16.
58. Bockenstedt LK, Wormser GP. Review: unraveling Lyme disease. Arthritis Rheumatol. 2014;66(9):2313–23. Epub 2014/06/27.
59. Schlung JE, Bastrom TP, Roocroft JH, Newton PO, Mubarak SJ, Upasani VV. Femoral neck aspiration aids in the diagnosis of osteomyelitis in children with septic hip. J Pediatr Orthopedics. 2018;38(10):532–6. Epub 2016/09/08.
60. Cruz AI Jr, Anari JB, Ramirez JM, Sankar WN, Baldwin KD. Distinguishing pediatric Lyme arthritis of the hip from transient synovitis and acute bacterial septic arthritis: a systematic review and meta-analysis. Cureus. 2018;10(1):e2112. Epub 2018/03/28.
61. Bachra BN. Calcification of connective tissue. Int Rev Connect Tissue Res. 1970;5:165–208. Epub 1970/01/01.
62. Kabak S, Halici M, Akcakus M, Cetin N, Narin N. Septic arthritis in patients followed-up in neonatal intensive care unit. Pediatr Int. 2002;44(6):652–7. Epub 2002/11/08.
63. Samora JB, Klingele K. Septic arthritis of the neonatal hip: acute management and late reconstruction. J Am Acad Orthop Surg. 2013;21(10):632–41. Epub 2013/10/03.
64. Castellazzi L, Mantero M, Esposito S. Update on the Management of Pediatric Acute Osteomyelitis and Septic Arthritis. Int J Mol Sci. 2016;1:17(6). Epub 2016/06/04.
65. Arnold JC, Cannavino CR, Ross MK, Westley B, Miller TC, Riffenburgh RH, et al. Acute bacterial osteoarticular infections: eight-year analysis of C-reactive protein for oral step-down therapy. Pediatrics. 2012;130(4):e821–8. Epub 2012/09/12.
66. Paakkonen M, Kallio MJ, Peltola H, Kallio PE. Antibiotic treatment and surgery for acute Hematogenous calcaneal osteomyelitis of child-

hood. J Foot Ankle Surg. 2015;54(5):840–3. Epub 2015/04/29.
67. Chou AC, Mahadev A. The use of C-reactive protein as a guide for transitioning to Oral antibiotics in pediatric Osteoarticular infections. J Pediatr Orthop. 2016;36(2):173–7. Epub 2015/05/02.
68. Keren R, Shah SS, Srivastava R, Rangel S, Bendel-Stenzel M, Harik N, et al. Comparative effectiveness of intravenous vs oral antibiotics for postdischarge treatment of acute osteomyelitis in children. JAMA Pediatr. 2015;169(2):120–8. Epub 2014/12/17.
69. Peltola H, Paakkonen M. Acute osteomyelitis in children. N Engl J Med. 2014;370(4):352–60. Epub 2014/01/24.
70. Farrow L. A systematic review and meta-analysis regarding the use of corticosteroids in septic arthritis. BMC Musculoskelet Disord. 2015;16:241. Epub 2015/09/08.
71. Qin YF, Li ZJ, Li H. Corticosteroids as adjunctive therapy with antibiotics in the treatment of children with septic arthritis: a meta-analysis. Drug Des Devel Ther. 2018;12:2277–84. Epub 2018/08/09.
72. Dattwyler RJ, Luft BJ, Kunkel MJ, Finkel MF, Wormser GP, Rush TJ, et al. Ceftriaxone compared with doxycycline for the treatment of acute disseminated Lyme disease. N Engl J Med. 1997;337(5):289–94. Epub 1997/07/31.
73. Wormser GP, Dattwyler RJ, Shapiro ED, Halperin JJ, Steere AC, Klempner MS, et al. The clinical assessment, treatment, and prevention of Lyme disease, human granulocytic anaplasmosis, and babesiosis: clinical practice guidelines by the Infectious Diseases Society of America. Clin Infect Dis. 2006;43(9):1089–134. Epub 2006/10/10.
74. Sanpera I, Raluy-Collado D, Sanpera-Iglesias J. Arthroscopy for hip septic arthritis in children. Orthop Traumatol Surg Res. 2016;102(1):87–9. Epub 2016/01/05.
75. Thompson RM, Gourineni P. Arthroscopic treatment of septic arthritis in very young children. J Pediatr Orthop. 2017;37(1):e53–e7. Epub 2015/09/24.
76. Edmonds EW, Lin C, Farnsworth CL, Bomar JD, Upasani VV. A medial portal for hip arthroscopy in children with septic arthritis: a safety study. J Pediatr Orthop. 2018;38(10):527–31. Epub 2016/09/08.
77. Johns B, Loewenthal M, Ho E, Dewar D. Arthroscopic versus open treatment for acute septic arthritis of the knee in children. Pediatr Infect Dis J. 2018;37(5):413–8. Epub 2017/09/26.
78. Telleria JJ, Cotter RA, Bompadre V, Steinman SE. Laboratory predictors for risk of revision surgery in pediatric septic arthritis. J Child Orthop. 2016;10(3):247–54. Epub 2016/05/14.
79. Agout C, Lakhal W, Fournier J, de Bodman C, Bonnard C. Arthroscopic treatment of septic arthritis of the knee in children. Orthop Traumatol Surg Res. 2015;101(8 Suppl):S333–6. Epub 2015/10/01.
80. Nunn TR, Cheung WY, Rollinson PD. A prospective study of pyogenic sepsis of the hip in childhood. J Bone Joint Surg Br. 2007;89(1):100–6. Epub 2007/01/30.
81. Howard-Jones AR, Isaacs D, Gibbons PJ. Twelve-month outcome following septic arthritis in children. J Pediatr Orthop B. 2013;22(5):486–90. Epub 2013/03/28.
82. Newman JH. Review of septic arthritis throughout the antibiotic era. Ann Rheum Dis. 1976;35(3):198–205. Epub 1976/06/01.
83. Fabry G, Meire E. Septic arthritis of the hip in children: poor results after late and inadequate treatment. J Pediatr Orthop. 1983;3(4):461–6. Epub 1983/09/01.
84. Wang CL, Wang SM, Yang YJ, Tsai CH, Liu CC. Septic arthritis in children: relationship of causative pathogens, complications, and outcome. J Microbiol Immunol Infect. 2003;36(1):41–6. Epub 2003/05/14.
85. Lunseth PA, Heiple KG. Prognosis in septic arthritis of the hip in children. Clin Orthop Relat Res. 1979;139:81–5. Epub 1979/03/01.
86. Forlin E, Milani C. Sequelae of septic arthritis of the hip in children: a new classification and a review of 41 hips. J Pediatr Orthop. 2008;28(5):524–8. Epub 2008/06/27.
87. Choi IH, Yoo WJ, Cho TJ, Chung CY. Operative reconstruction for septic arthritis of the hip. Orthop Clin North Am. 2006;37(2):173–83, vi. Epub 2006/04/28.
88. Choi IH, Shin YW, Chung CY, Cho TJ, Yoo WJ, Lee DY. Surgical treatment of the severe sequelae of infantile septic arthritis of the hip. Clin Orthop Relat Res. 2005;434:102–9. Epub 2005/05/03.
89. Hunka L, Said SE, MacKenzie DA, Rogala EJ, Cruess RL. Classification and surgical management of the severe sequelae of septic hips in children. Clin Orthop Relat Res. 1982;171:30–6. Epub 1982/11/01.
90. Spiegel DPJ, Banskota A, Shrestha O. Sequelae of septic arthritis of the hip. HELP Organization; 2007. p. 22.
91. Spruiell MD, Searns JB, Heare TC, Roberts JL, Wylie E, Pyle L, et al. Clinical care guideline for improving pediatric acute musculoskeletal infection outcomes. J Pediatric Infect Dis Soc. 2017;6(3):e86–93. Epub 2017/04/19.
92. Quick RD, Williams J, Fernandez M, Gottschalk H, Cosgrove P, Kahlden K, et al. Improved diagnosis and treatment of bone and joint infections using an evidence-based treatment guideline. J Pediatr Orthop. 2018;38(6):e354–e9. Epub 2018/05/05.
93. Kocher MS, Mandiga R, Murphy JM, Goldmann D, Harper M, Sundel R, et al. A clinical practice guideline for treatment of septic arthritis in children: efficacy in improving process of care and effect on outcome of septic arthritis of the hip. J Bone Joint Surg Am. 2003;85(6):994–9. Epub 2003/06/05.

Pyomyositis

13

Ashish S. Ranade, Nirmal Raj Gopinathan,
Neeraj Vij, and Mohan V. Belthur

Introduction

Pyomyositis is a bacterial or rarely nonbacterial intramuscular infection. Pyomyositis can be difficult to diagnose due to considerably variable presentations. Pyomyositis is more common in the tropics. However, there have been several reports of pyomyositis in non-tropical areas [1–5]. The pediatric population makes up a third of pyomyositis cases. Pyomyositis is often omitted from the initial differential diagnosis given its nonspecific symptoms. A high degree of suspicion is necessary for diagnosing pyomyositis. Early diagnosis leads to timely treatment and avoids complications and sequelae. Pyomyositis differentiated from the intramuscular abscess by an initial stage which consists of intramuscular bacterial infection leading to inflammation which leads to abscess formation.

Pyomyositis can be classified as primary or secondary pyomyositis depending on the source of the pathogen. The primary pyomyositis ensues due to the hematogenous spread of bacteria from an occult source, and in the secondary pyomyositis, the bacteremia is secondary to nearby infectious sources such as septic arthritis or osteomyelitis.

In this chapter, we discuss the epidemiology, clinical features, and the management principles of pyomyositis.

Primary Pyomyositis

Epidemiology

Pyomyositis is more common in tropical geographical areas [6–10] and is often referred to as tropical pyomyositis. Pyomyositis was traditionally thought to be uncommon in temperate areas. However, there have been several reports of pyomyositis in non-tropical areas [1–5, 11–13]. Pyomyositis constitutes 2.2% to 4% of all surgical admissions in tropical countries [2]. The number of admissions is much lower in the USA and other non-tropical regions. In the USA, in the

A. S. Ranade (✉)
Blooming Buds Centre for Pediatric Orthopaedics, Deenanath Mangeshkar Hospital, Pune, Maharashtra, India
e-mail: ranadea2@gmail.com

N. R. Gopinathan
Division of Paediatric Orthopaedics, Department of Orthopaedic Surgery, Post Graduate Institute of Medical Education and Research, Chandigarh, India

N. Vij
University of Arizona College of Medicine – Phoenix, Phoenix, AZ, USA
e-mail: neerajvij@email.arizona.edu

M. V. Belthur
Department of Child Health & Orthopedics, University of Arizona College of Medicine, Phoenix, AZ, USA

Department of Orthopedics, Phoenix Children's Hospital, Phoenix, AZ, USA

© Springer Nature Switzerland AG 2022
M. V. Belthur et al. (eds.), *Pediatric Musculoskeletal Infections*,
https://doi.org/10.1007/978-3-030-95794-0_13

decade 2004–2015, increasing numbers were noted by Maravelas [5]. There is seasonal variation in incidence, and peak incidence has been reported during the months of July to October [14]. Usually, a single muscle is involved; however, although rare, multifocal involvement can also happen [15].

The most commonly involved muscles are the pelvic muscles such as the obturator internus, iliopsoas, and quadriceps femoris muscles. Pyomyositis involving gluteus medius and minimus, adductor longus, piriformis, external oblique, internal oblique, transverse abdominis, and paraspinal muscles has also been reported [16–20]. Also, in countries endemic for tuberculosis, it is important to rule out spinal tuberculosis in a child presenting with iliopsoas abscess.

The burden of pyomyositis is greater in low-middle income countries (LMICs) as financial constraints serve as a barrier to medical and surgical management [8]. Further, the attitude that pyomyositis is a benign condition not only disregards the high morbidity associated with this condition but also further inhibits the delivery of care [9].

Pathology and Microbiology

Although pyomyositis may affect individuals with malignancy or hematological disorder, it has also been described to affect patients with chronic renal failure, diabetes, and immunodeficiencies [21]. It is thought that uninjured skeletal muscles are resistant to infection. Prior history of trauma has been shown to predispose the muscle to develop pyomyositis [22]. After trauma, the muscle gets hematogenous invasion by bacteria which can lead to abscess formation. The causative organism is *Staphylococcus aureus* in more than 75% of cases. Community-acquired *S. aureus* is also common [1, 3, 23, 24]. MRSA forms approximately 10% of the pelvic pyomyositis [23–26]. The second common organism to cause pyomyositis is *Streptococcus*. It forms approximately 10–15% of cases. Mycobacterium tuberculosis, *Streptococcus pyogenes*, and anaerobic bacteria can also cause pyomyositis [26–28]. There are reports of pseudomonas pyomyositis [29].

Nonbacterial organisms could cause pyomyositis. Various viral, parasitic, and fungal pathogens have been reported to cause pyomyositis. The commonest cause of viral pyomyositis in children is influenza viruses [30].

The pathogens express various virulence factors which contribute to the pathogenesis of pyomyositis. The acute phase inflammatory response plays a pivotal role in initiating the body's response to tissue injury. The virulence factors expressed by pathogens modulate and hijack the acute phase response. The excessive inflammatory response may lead to tissue injury and systemic toxicity and many other complications [31, 32].

The disease consists of three stages: stage 1 being inflammation and edema of the muscle, stage 2 consists of abscess formation in the muscle. In stage 3, there might be abscesses at distant sites, and there is a systemic spread of the infection. Although it can affect any muscle, commonly affected muscles are the muscles of the pelvis and lower extremity. Psoas muscle is a frequent site of involvement. In some patients, it may be associated with osteomyelitis and septic arthritis [33–35]. Pyomyositis has been reported to involve uncommon sites such as the gluteal muscles, triceps, biceps, anterior tibialis, gastrocnemius, levator scapulae, and paraspinal muscles [16–20].

Clinical Presentation

Pyomyositis has varied clinical presentation. It may present with fever, swelling, and limp with pain in the affected extremity. These symptoms could be presenting symptoms of many musculoskeletal infective conditions and make it difficult to diagnose pyomyositis based on clinical presentation. Pyomyositis may be misdiagnosed as septic arthritis of the hip, appendicitis, or gastrointestinal infection [1]. In stage 1 of the disease (inflammatory stage), the child may present with localized pain, fever, and malaise. There might be a history of trauma, and the child may limp or may refuse to walk. The involved muscle is inflamed and tender on palpation. In stage 2 (suppurative stage), there may be local swelling if the muscle is superficial and is associated with severe pain and fever. Aspiration will reveal purulent material. The third stage involves systemic effects of septicemia, multifocal abscess formation, and septic shock.

Sometimes pyomyositis may present as nonspecific abdominal pain if the pyomyositis involves muscles of the abdominal wall [36].

Younger children may present with symptoms like excessive crying, poor feeding, reduced movements of the limb, and refusal to bear weight on one extremity. Fever and systemic signs and symptoms may be absent in neonates.

In pyomyositis involving pelvic muscles, patients will present with hip pain. Hip movements are restricted and the child refuses to bear weight on the affected extremity. In a study by Mignemi et al., 32% of patients who were initially diagnosed to have septic arthritis of the hip were subsequently diagnosed to have pericapsular pyomyositis [37].

Evaluation

A high index of suspicion is necessary to diagnose pyomyositis. There could be a delay of few days to reach the diagnosis considering nonspecific symptoms, which may point toward several conditions in a child. In a study by Zyulunoy et al., an average delay of 12 days has been reported [38].

Radiographs should be obtained as the first line of investigation. But they may not show signs of bone or muscle involvement. They may rule out other differential diagnoses such as a bone tumor and osteomyelitis. The radiographs may show a soft tissue shadow but are not diagnostic of pyomyositis.

Ultrasonography is the first line of investigation and can be used in an emergency situation as well. Ultrasonography is inexpensive and is easily available without the risk of radiation. However, it needs a trained professional and can be operator-dependent. In the initial stages, sonography demonstrates muscle edema, generalized hyperemia, disrupted hyperechoic muscle fibers, and hypoechoic septa [6]. In the late suppurative stage, fluid collection or abscess can be seen [6]. The fluid can be aspirated under ultrasonic guidance. However, when there are concerns of coexisting osteomyelitis or spondylodiscitis, MRI is the modality of choice. Ultrasound can be a valuable imaging modality in the diagnosis and follow-up especially in settings when MRI has limited availability [39].

CT scan has also been used in the evaluation of pyomyositis. CT scan may not diagnose the pyomyositis in stage 1 (inflammatory stage). CT scan can be highly sensitive but is less specific for intramuscular abscess as the hypointensity may not differentiate between other differentials such as necrotic neoplasms and chronic hematomas [27]. There are concerns of increased radiation dose with the CT scan. CT scan is useful for aspiration of the abscess under image guidance [11]. Currently, the role of CT scans has been limited to performing diagnostic or therapeutic aspirations. Bone scans have a limited role in the evaluation of pyomyositis. Radioisotope bone scan lacks sensitivity but may show associated bony involvement.

MRI is the modality of choice to diagnose pyomyositis. MRI has high sensitivity and specificity and is considered the preferred modality [6, 7]. In the first stage, muscle enlargement with loss of definition and heterogeneous increased T2-weighted signal abnormalities are seen. In stage 2, T2-weighted images show hyperintensity with corresponding hypointense T1 signal. Post-contrast T1-weighted images with fat saturation show rim-enhancing fluid collection, a typical finding of an abscess. MRI will also show other areas of involvement such as the bone or joints [40]. The disadvantages of obtaining an MRI scan are cost, availability, longer duration to complete the scan, and need for sedation/anesthesia.

The evaluation also includes laboratory investigations such as complete blood count which may show anemia and leukocytosis. Inflammatory parameters like ESR and CRP are also checked. Serial blood counts are necessary to monitor the response to the treatment and to monitor the disease course. Muscle enzymes are normal which differentiates it from polymyositis.

Blood culture should be obtained in the case of suspected pyomyositis. Pus culture should be done to identify the organism and start the appropriate antibiotic. Pus culture positivity rates are high and blood culture positivity rates are lower [14] (Fig. 13.1).

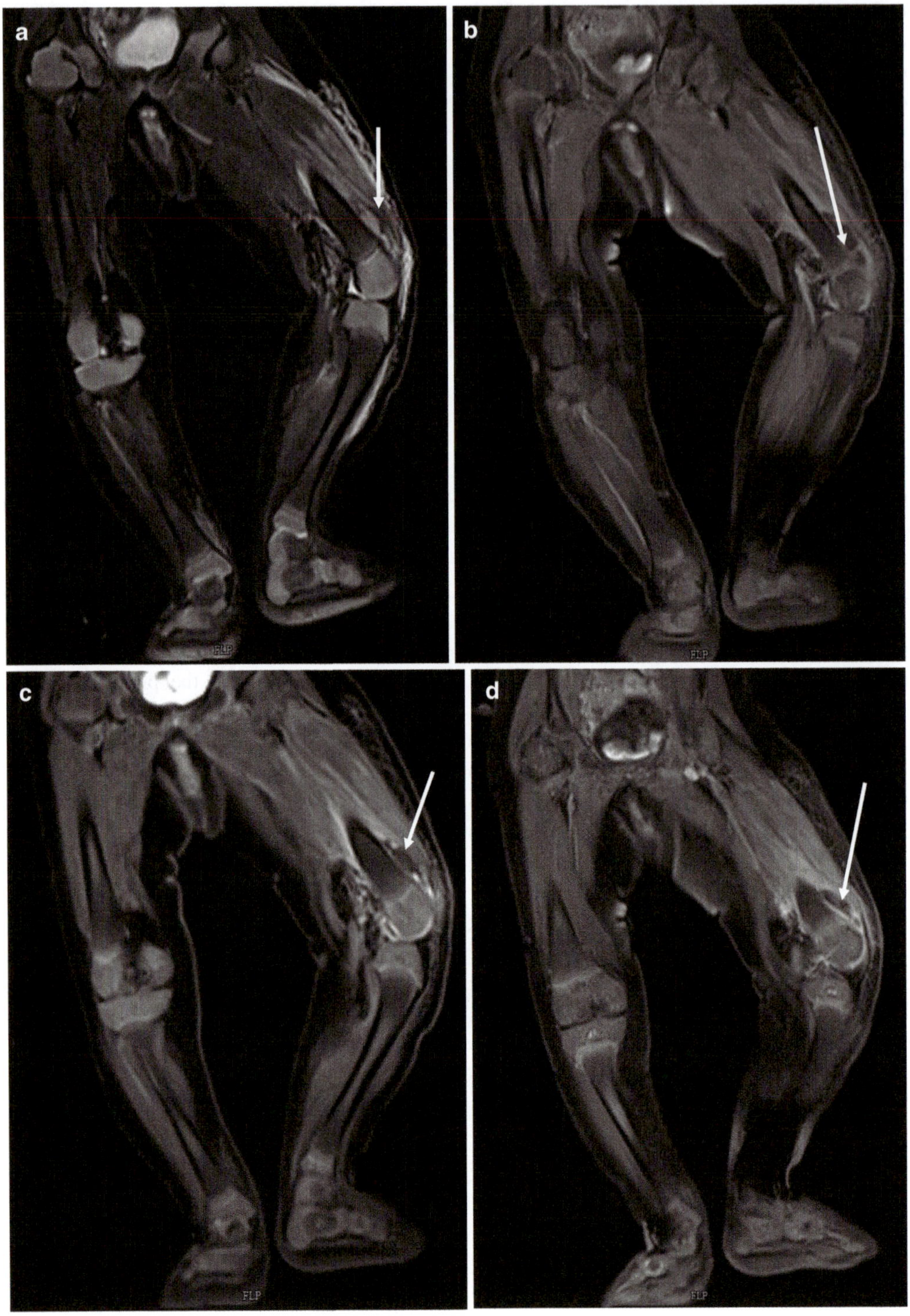

Fig. 13.1 (**a**, **b**) A 15-month-old girl with left quadriceps pyomyositis. Coronal STIR and T1 fat suppression images of the left lower limb show diffuse reactive muscle edema and abscess. There is no bony involvement. (**c**, **d**) Post-contrast T1FS images show heterogeneous enhancement in the left mid and lower thigh muscles with pockets of peripherally enhancing fluid collections (abscesses). There is no bony involvement or involvement of the knee joint. (**e**) Axial T2W image through left mid-thigh shows muscle edema

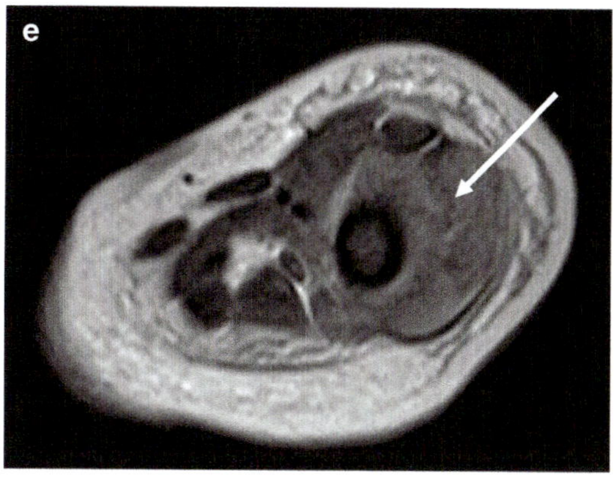

Fig. 13.1 (continued)

Differential Diagnoses

Differential diagnoses include conditions like osteomyelitis, septic arthritis, appendicitis, spondylodiscitis, contusion, muscle strain, hematoma, thrombophlebitis, cellulitis, and soft tissue sarcoma.

Treatment

Pyomyositis is not a difficult disease to manage provided it is diagnosed early and treated by the appropriate modality. There could be difficulty in diagnosing pyomyositis, especially in cases involving the pelvic musculature.

Medical Treatment

Antibiotics constitute the foundation of the treatment of pyomyositis. After diagnosis, the treatment is appropriate antibiotic therapy and possibly abscess drainage depending on the stage of the disease. Once a localized and sizeable abscess is noted on imaging, abscess drainage is recommended [28, 41]. Pyomyositis may be managed by medical treatment alone if the abscess has not yet formed. Systemic antibiotics prevent the spread of infection and also prevent abscess formation [42]. The choice of antibiotics depends on the local bacteriological, epidemiological, and susceptibility factors. Typically, an antibiotic to cover *Staphylococcus aureus* is started. Nafcillin, oxacillin, and cloxacillin are the common first-line drugs. Typical antibiotic regimen is a second- or third-generation cephalosporin with addition of anaerobic coverage through amoxicillin and clindamycin [4, 7, 43]. Notably, Unnikrishnan reported a 100% successful medical management rate with this medical approach [43]. There are also reports on the addition of penicillin or aminoglycosides to the cephalosporin-based regimen [4, 12, 44]. There are no studies regarding the optimal duration, route of antibiotics, or the choice of antibiotic. Intravenous antibiotics are given until clinical improvement is seen. Clinical improvement and laboratory investigations showing a downward trend in the CRP and ESR values are the pointers to switch to oral antibiotics. Oral medications are given for further 1 to 2 weeks after stopping IV antibiotics. A review has shown that medical management was successful in 60% of patients [45].

Surgical Treatment

Indication for surgery is the formation of an abscess. In a review, slightly less than half of the patients with pyomyositis (40%) are required to undergo surgical treatment. Of these, a majority (90%) had undergone open abscess drainage, and the remaining 10% had percutaneous image-guided drainage of the abscess [45]. In pelvic pyomyositis, surgical abscess drainage and washout is indicated for abscess confirmed on MRI which is not responding to antibiotics and abscess causing mass effect on solid organs and neurovascular structures [23, 46].

Pelvic pyomyositis poses a challenge to treat the pelvis abscess. Peculiar anatomy of the pelvis makes the treatment of pelvic pyomyositis challenging. Abscess drainage can be open or percutaneous with or without image guidance. Traditionally, pelvic pyomyositis is drained through an ilioinguinal approach or the Pfannenstiel approach. These approaches need longer incisions and extensive dissection around the neurovascular structures and pose a risk of neurovascular damage and iatrogenic injury to the corona mortis [47]. In the last few years, two new approaches have been described to drain the obturator abscesses: the Vanderbilt medial approach

[23] and the posterior transgluteal approach [24]. The medial approach is through the adductor brevis and follows obturator nerve proximally into obturator foramen. This approach is done in the supine position. The trans-gluteal approach avoids damage to the obturator nerve. In this approach, obturator muscles are approached by splitting the gluteus maximus along the medial side of the ischial tuberosity to drain obturator internus pyomyositis. This approach is performed in the lateral or prone position.

Open drainage may not be possible for certain pelvic abscess locations or the patient's general condition may preclude the open surgical abscess drainage. The percutaneous drainage is an alternative to open drainage. Percutaneous drainage procedure is done by interventional radiology. It can be done under ultrasound guidance, or it has also been described under CT guidance [11, 48, 49].

Outcomes: Most children do well when pyomyositis is diagnosed early and is treated with appropriate antibiotics and timely surgical drainage of the intramuscular abscess. A systematic review reported good outcomes in 90% of children with no complications. The average duration of hospital stay was 12 +/−4.6 days [45]. Long-term outcomes of treatment of pyomyositis are not available (Fig. 13.2).

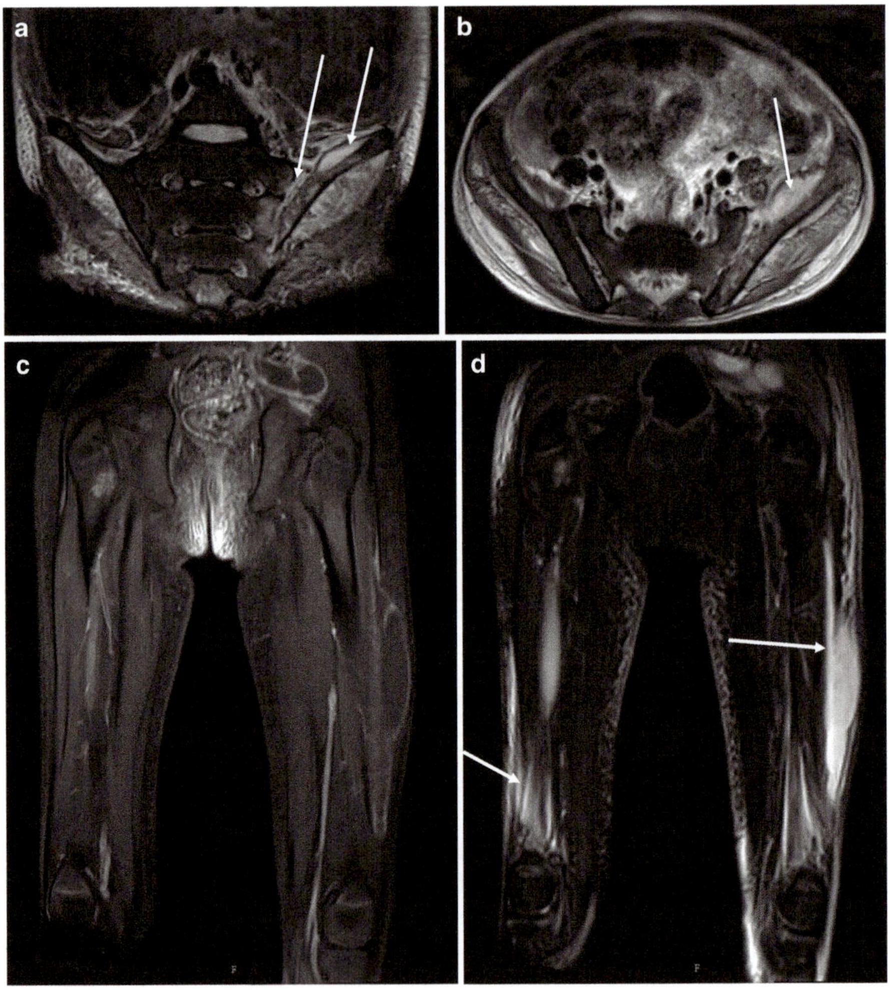

Fig. 13.2 (**a**, **b**) Coronal and axial STIR images of an 8-year-old boy show iliacus abscess and sacroiliac joint involvement. (**c**, **d**) Coronal fat suppression and post-contrast T1FS images show altered marrow signals and enhancement on both sacroiliac joints along with joint effusion and left-sided extra-osseous soft tissue abscess consistent with infective arthropathy. A peripherally enhancing subcutaneous collection along the lateral aspect of mid-thigh on the left side. Edematous changes are also seen in bilateral lower thigh muscles

Complications

Most children do well; however, approximately 10% may develop complications [45].

Late diagnosis is associated with complications. Frequently reported complications are septic arthritis, pneumonia, venous thromboembolism, and osteomyelitis. *S. aureus* with PVL was associated with longer hospital stay and more complications [14, 34].

Other uncommon complications are spinal epidural abscess [50], protrusio acetabuli [51], and compartment syndrome [35, 52]. Mortality after pyomyositis is rare but has been reported [53].

Box 13.1 Key Learning Points

- Pyomyositis may present with nonspecific symptoms.
- Consider pyomyositis as a differential diagnosis of bone and joint infection.
- Pyomyositis may coexist with osteomyelitis or septic arthritis.
- Consider obtaining an MRI at an early stage to differentiate between bone/joint, and soft tissue involvement.
- Most children do well (90%) and a few have complications.

Box 13.2 Pelvic Pyomyositis - Pitfalls to Avoid

- Pericapsular pyomyositis may present as septic arthritis of the hip.
- Early diagnosis is the key to a good outcome.
- An abscess may need open drainage via medial or posterior transgluteal approach.
- CT-guided aspiration may be an option.
- Antibiotic therapy constitutes one of the main pillars of the treatment of pyomyositis and is essential in addition to surgical treatment.

Secondary Pyomyositis

Introduction Secondary pyomyositis is conventionally a contiguous extension of infection from an underlying primary pathology or can result from direct inoculation from penetrating trauma. It differs from primary pyomyositis by the fact that primary pyomyositis results from hematogenous seeding of striated muscle due to transient bacteremia from an occult source. The most common presentation of secondary pyomyositis in the literature is iliopsoas abscess, and many of the findings enumerated here are from these studies on secondary pyomyositis of iliopsoas [46].

Etiology Secondary psoas abscesses are due to the extension of organisms directly to retrofascial space from pathologies in adjacent structures. The commonest source is gastrointestinal disorders notably Crohn's disease. Other pathologies of the gastrointestinal tract enlisted are appendicitis, colonic inflammation or neoplasm, and intra-abdominal/retroperitoneal infections [54]. Other etiologies are infections of the perinephric space, reproductive organs, pleural space, adjacent bone and joint, etc. It is important for the attending physician to be aware of the relationship between Crohn's disease and secondary psoas suppuration as it is the commonest cause for these secondary abscesses [55]. Psoas abscess with bowel organism originates secondary to gastrointestinal disease unless proven otherwise [54]. Driver et al. reported three cases of psoas abscess secondary to an underlying renal pathology [56].

The secondary abscess may develop from primary osseous pathology in the spine, ilium, and sacroiliac joint and may extend anteriorly to the thigh or hip through the femoral or obturator canal and to the buttock or hip through the greater or lesser sciatic foramen.

Another mechanism of acquiring secondary pyomyositis is penetrating trauma. Brook et al. over a period of 16 years came across six patients with anaerobic pyomyositis and three of them had a history of penetrating trauma (tibialis anterior, biceps, and gluteal region, respectively). The authors highlight the significance of the possibility of anaerobic secondary pyomyositis in children with penetrating trauma or injections and discussed the higher incidence of anaerobic suppurations in adults with parenteral drug abuse [57].

Clinical Features The diagnosis of psoas abscess remains a clinical challenge even in the era of advanced imaging techniques due to the nonspecific presentation. The triad of limp, fever, and pain although common may not be the presenting complaint in all cases. In secondary abscesses, the primary pathology that incites the muscular suppuration can mask the presence of abscess and can make timely diagnosis difficult especially in conditions like Crohn's disease which requires a high element of suspicion. Pain in the back, flank, or abdomen is the commonest presenting complaint. Also, there might be tenderness in the flank or a tender mass palpable over the flank or just below the inguinal ligament. In secondary iliopsoas abscesses, the hip is kept flexed and externally rotated and any attempt to extend or internally rotate the hip is resisted. The findings may be confused with septic arthritis of the hip, but here further flexion and external rotation of the hip joint is possible, whereas septic arthritis causes global restriction of movements [58].

Investigations A high index of suspicion is warranted when the clinical picture is less revealing especially in conditions like Crohn's disease. Blood investigation parameters are similar to the primary pyomyositis cases. Conventional radiography is neither specific nor sensitive except in cases with gas-forming abscesses where mottled gas shadows are seen in retroperitoneum in KUB. Ultrasonography is useful for diagnosing the abnormalities of the psoas compartment as well as the renal tract. CT scan is more sensitive and is of help in confirming the diagnosis and also can define the extension of the abscess [58].

Although USG is useful for visualizing the retroperitoneal space and aspiration, it may not be of much help in a small lesion, overlying gas, obesity, or significant scoliosis. CT scan is better in defining pathologies, and MRI is undoubtedly more accurate in localization and assessment of extension. It is important to be highly vigilant and utilize appropriate imaging to diagnose the secondary abscesses so that they can be managed in a timely manner [55].

Treatment

Medical Management

Delayed or inadequate treatment is the main cause of mortality and a high index of suspicion is necessary especially in cases suspected to have developed secondary abscesses. Antibiotics are adjunctive to surgical management and have been recommended according to the geographical location, age, and possible etiology. There is no confusion regarding psoas abscess in developing nations which is considered primary, and a single agent against *Staphylococcus* is the preferred primary agent. In Europe, the predominance of secondary bowel etiology warrants use of the agents effective against aerobic and anaerobic bowel flora. In the USA and Canada, the occurrence of both primary and secondary warrants combining both the abovementioned agents that are directed against *Staphylococcus* and enteric flora [54]. In countries like Taiwan where urological pathology is the common primary etiology, coverage should be directed against *Enterobacteriaceae* species (*E. coli* and *Klebsiella* species). The duration of therapy is according to the response and is at least 2 to 3 weeks after deference or after surgical drainage [58].

Percutaneous Drainage (PCD) Primary abscess usually responds to ultrasound or CT-guided percutaneous drainage (PCD) and may obviate the need for open surgical drainage. The criteria that are not favorable for PCD are coexistent underlying pathology of adjacent structures like bowel lesions, diffuse muscle inflammation without liquefaction, multi-loculations, tenacious thick collection, etc. In a hemodynamically stable patient when a secondary psoas abscess is suspected, further evaluation is indicated so that a definitive procedure can be planned for management of the primary pathology as well as the psoas abscess itself. The surgery for emergent management of secondary abscess is drainage which can be an image-guided PCD but is rarely definitive/curative. When definitive pathology is localized, it can be managed along with the abscess as a single-stage procedure [54].

Surgical Intervention Secondary abscesses required intervention directed at the primary pathology along with drainage. For example, drainage along with bowel resection or diversion resolved abscess in many of the Crohn's disease patients, appendectomy in patients with appendicitis, etc. [54]. Definitive therapy depends upon primary etiology in secondary cases. PCD alone may not be effective in secondary cases. In bowel pathologies like Crohn's disease, resection of the diseased bowel segment is required along with drainage or after drainage depending upon the individual's general condition. Huang et al. insisted that surgical drainage is indicated in patients with abscess concurrent with obstruction of the urinary tract, and patients might require radical procedures like nephrectomy in cases where PCD alone fails [58]. Surgical drainage or even radical procedures like nephrectomy is necessary in cases of urological origin with a fulminant course or those refractory to percutaneous drainage, due to the associated higher morbidity and mortality when compared to primary cases [56].

Mortality in these cases resulted mainly from sepsis followed by pulmonary embolism, etc.

Pyomyositis and Osteoarticular Infections Pannaraj PS in a study on admissions spread over 6 years in a non-tropical region identified 182 patients admitted for pyomyositis or myositis. Of them, there were 5 with an open wound or a medical procedure and 85 of them had either concurrent osteomyelitis, septic arthritis, or both [34]. Spiegel et al. reported 7 of the 12 patients with signal abnormalities in the neighboring osseous and articular tissues in MRI but the plain radiography films failed to reveal bony changes [49] (Fig. 13.3).

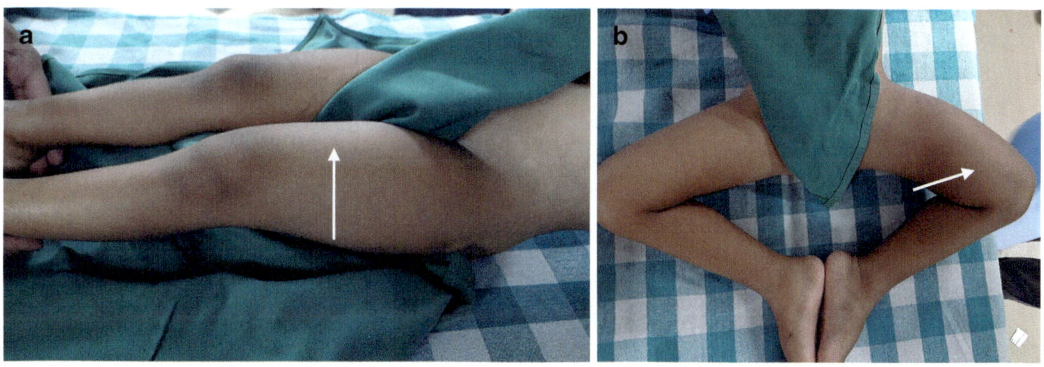

Fig. 13.3 (**a**, **b**) A 2-year-old with left thigh pyomyositis and distal femur osteomyelitis. Left thigh swelling is seen with symmetrical hip movements. (**c**, **d**, and **e**) show minimal left hip joint effusion on the ultrasound scan and soft tissue swelling of the left thigh on the radiographs. The patient had treatment at an outside facility and was referred after 5 days in view of no response to IV antibiotics. (**f**, **g**) Coronal and axial fat suppression images show abscess formation along the anterior, medial, and posterior aspects of the left thigh. (**h**, **i**) T2 sagittal and FS coronal images show abscess formation in the left thigh. (**j**) Post-contrast T1 FS image shows enhancement in the muscles as well as distal femur suggestive of osteomyelitis with intramedullary abscess formation. (**k**) Intra-operative photograph showing pus which grew MRSA

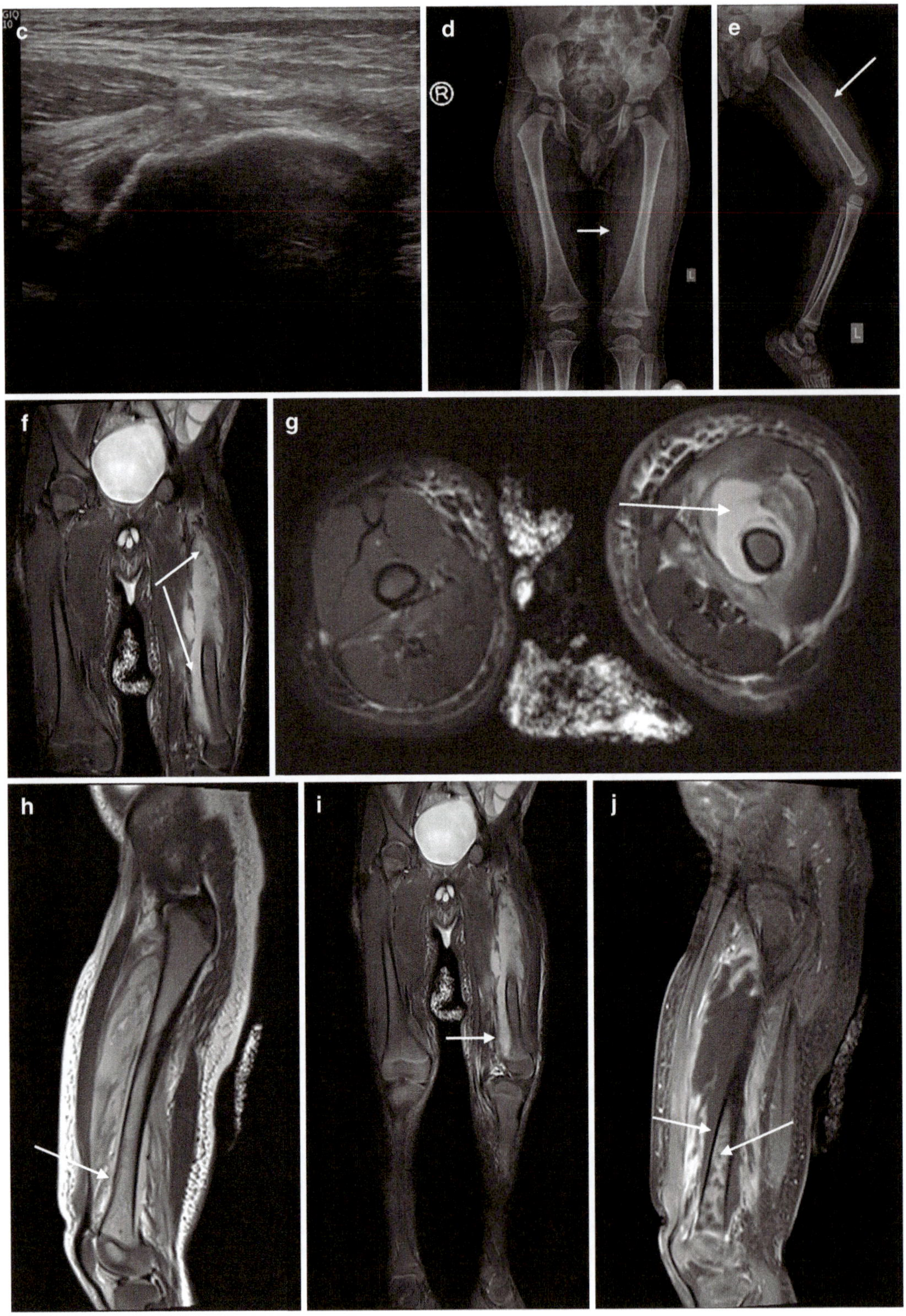

Fig. 13.3 (continued)

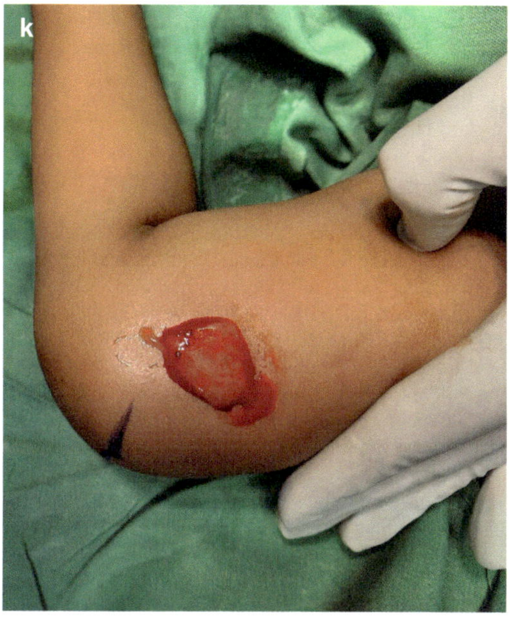

Fig. 13.3 (continued)

With the cases diagnosed late, the authors opined that if osteoarticular involvement was primary etiology, it would have been revealed in plain films and hence could be because of secondary reactive changes induced by long-standing muscle suppuration or early osteomyelitis from the contiguous extension. It has been repeatedly emphasized in the literature that the osseous changes revealed by MRI in a majority of patients denote the reactive changes to an adjacent inflammatory process rather than primary osteomyelitis [46]. The role of contrast MRI remains unknown in differentiating these reactive changes and osteomyelitis.

Acknowledgement The authors would like to thank Sanjay Desai, MD FRCR, Pune, India for helping with the description of the MRI images.

References

1. García-Mata S, Hidalgo-Ovejero A, Esparza-Estaun J. Primary obturator-muscle pyomyositis in immunocompetent children. J Child Orthop. 2012; https://doi.org/10.1007/s11832-012-0418-y.
2. Comegna L, Guidone PI, Prezioso G, Franchini S, Petrosino MI, Di Filippo P, Chiarelli F, Mohn A, Rossi N. Pyomyositis is not only a tropical pathology: a case series. J Med Case Rep. 2016; https://doi.org/10.1186/s13256-016-1158-2.
3. Moriarty P, Leung C, Walsh M, Nourse C. Increasing pyomyositis presentations among children in Queensland. Australia Pediatr Infect Dis J. 2015; https://doi.org/10.1097/INF.0000000000000470.
4. Nithin Unnikrishnan P, Perry DC, George H, Bassi R, Bruce CE. Tropical primary pyomyositis in children of the UK: An emerging medical challenge. Int Orthop. 2010; https://doi.org/10.1007/s00264-009-0765-6.
5. Maravelas RK, Melgar T, Sadarangani S, Lima N, Rich Z, Vos D. 765. Pyomyositis in the United States: trends and associations from the healthcare utilization project Nationwide inpatient sample database. Open Forum Infect Dis. 2019; https://doi.org/10.1093/ofid/ofz360.833.
6. Trusen A, Beissert M, Schultz G, Chittka B, Darge K. Ultrasound and MRI features of pyomyositis in children. Eur Radiol. 2003; https://doi.org/10.1007/s00330-002-1585-x.
7. Renwick SE, Ritterbusch JF. Pyomyositis in children. J Pediatr Orthop. 1993; https://doi.org/10.1097/01241398-199311000-00016.
8. Okeniyi JAO, Olubanjo OO, Ogunlesi TA, Oyelami OA. Comparison of healing of incised abscess wounds with honey and EUSOL dressing. J Altern Complement Med. 2005; https://doi.org/10.1089/acm.2005.11.511.
9. Aderele WI, Osinusi K. Pyomyositis in childhood. J Trop Med Hyg. 1980;
10. Borgesálvaro HD, Faragher B, Lalloo DG. Pyomyositis in the upper negro river basin. Brazilian Amazonia Trans R Soc Trop Med Hyg. 2012; https://doi.org/10.1016/j.trstmh.2012.06.008.
11. Elzohairy MM. Primary pyomyositis in children. Orthop Traumatol Surg Res. 2018; https://doi.org/10.1016/j.otsr.2017.12.005.
12. Arkader A, Brusalis C, Warner WC, Conway JH, Noonan K. Update in pediatric musculoskeletal infections: when it is, when it Isn't, and what to do. J Am Acad Orthop Surg. 2016; https://doi.org/10.5435/JAAOS-D-15-00714.
13. Hsieh MC, Chiu NC, Chi H, Huang FY. Clinical characteristics of pyomyositis in children: 20-year experience in a medical center in Taiwan. J Microbiol Immunol Infect. 2009.
14. Verma S, Singhi SC, Marwaha RK, Singhi P, Singh S, Singh M. Tropical pyomyositis in children: 10 years experience of a tertiary care hospital in northern India. J Trop Pediatr. 2013; https://doi.org/10.1093/tropej/fmt005.
15. Harrington P, Scott B, Chetcuti P. Multifocal streptococcal pyomyositis complicated by acute compartment syndrome: case report. J Pediatr Orthop Part B. 2001; https://doi.org/10.1097/00009957-200104000-00008.
16. Hiddema J, Hassan S, Mangat N, Siddiqui N. Pyomyositis of the pectineus muscle in an adolescent male. Ann R Coll Surg Engl. 2017; https://doi.org/10.1308/rcsann.2017.0142.

17. Siddiq MAB, Rasker JJ. Piriformis pyomyositis, a cause of piriformis syndrome—a systematic search and review. Clin Rheumatol. 2019; https://doi.org/10.1007/s10067-019-04552-y.
18. Fountoukis T, Tsatsanidis N, Tilkeridou M, Konstantinou I, Fytas P, Skandalos I. Abdominal rectus muscle pyomyositis: report of a case and review of the literature. Infect Dis Rep. 2018; https://doi.org/10.4081/idr.2018.7522.
19. Hassan FOA, Shannak A. Primary pyomyositis of the paraspinal muscles: a case report and literature review. Eur Spine J. 2008; https://doi.org/10.1007/s00586-007-0507-7.
20. Ray S, Iyer A, Avula S, Kneen R. Acquired torticollis due to primary pyomyositis of the paraspinal muscles in an 11-year-old boy. BMJ Case Rep. 2016; https://doi.org/10.1136/bcr-2015-213409.
21. Shittu A, Deinhardt-Emmer S, Vas Nunes J, Niemann S, Grobusch MP, Schaumburg F. Tropical pyomyositis: an update. Trop Med Int Heal. 2020; https://doi.org/10.1111/tmi.13395.
22. Chiedozi LC. Pyomyositis. Review of 205 cases in 112 patients. Am J Surg. 1979; https://doi.org/10.1016/0002-9610(79)90158-2.
23. Menge TJ, Cole HA, Mignemi ME, Corn WC, Martus JE, Lovejoy SA, Stutz CM, Mencio GA, Schoenecker JG. Medial approach for drainage of the obturator musculature in children. J Pediatr Orthop. 2014; https://doi.org/10.1097/BPO.0000000000000118.
24. White S, Stopka S, Nimityongskul P, Jorgensen D. Transgluteal approach for drainage of obturator internus abscess in pediatric patients. J Pediatr Orthop. 2017; https://doi.org/10.1097/BPO.0000000000000681.
25. Amari R, Yokoi H. Pyomyositis of the obturator internus muscle extending to septic arthritis of the hip in a child: a case report. J Pediatr Orthop Part B. 2014; https://doi.org/10.1097/BPB.0b013e328365295d.
26. Bertrand SL, Lincoln ED, Prohaska MG. Primary pyomyositis of the pelvis in children: a retrospective review of 8 cases. Orthopedics. 2011; https://doi.org/10.3928/01477447-20111021-07.
27. Viani RM, Bromberg K, Bradley JS. Obturator internus muscle abscess in children: report of seven cases and review. Clin Infect Dis. 1999; https://doi.org/10.1086/515080.
28. Stevens DL, Bisno AL, Chambers HF, Dellinger EP, Goldstein EJC, Gorbach SL, Hirschmann JV, Kaplan SL, Montoya JG, Wade JC. Practice guidelines for the diagnosis and management of skin and soft tissue infections: 2014 update by the infectious diseases society of America. Clin Infect Dis. 2014; https://doi.org/10.1093/cid/ciu296.
29. Migliarino V, Naviglio S, Barbi E, Rabusin M. Pseudomonas aeruginosa Pyomyositis in a child with acute lymphoblastic leukemia. J Pediatr Hematol Oncol. 2020; https://doi.org/10.1097/mph.0000000000002029.
30. Crum-Cianflone NF. Nonbacterial myositis. Curr Infect Dis Rep. 2010; https://doi.org/10.1007/s11908-010-0118-z.
31. Benvenuti M, An T, Amaro E, Lovejoy S, Mencio G, Martus J, Mignemi M, Schoenecker JG. Double-edged sword: musculoskeletal infection provoked acute phase response in children. Orthop Clin North Am. 2017; https://doi.org/10.1016/j.ocl.2016.12.009.
32. An TJ, Benvenuti MA, Mignemi ME, Thomsen IP, Schoenecker JG. Pediatric musculoskeletal infection: hijacking the acute-phase response. JBJS Rev. 2016; https://doi.org/10.2106/JBJS.RVW.15.00099.
33. Mitsionis GI, Manoudis GN, Lykissas MG, Sionti I, Motsis E, Georgoulis AD, Berisa AE. Pyomyositis in children: early diagnosis and treatment. J Pediatr Surg. 2009; https://doi.org/10.1016/j.jpedsurg.2009.02.053.
34. Pannaraj PS, Hulten KG, Gonzalez BE, Mason EO, Kaplan SL. Infective pyomyositis and myositis in children in the era of community-acquired, methicillin-resistant Staphylococcus aureus infection. Clin Infect Dis. 2006; https://doi.org/10.1086/507637.
35. Ovadia D, Ezra E, Ben-Sira L, Kessler A, Bickels J, Keret D, Yaniv M, Wientroub S, Lokiec F. Primary pyomyositis in children: a retrospective analysis of 11 cases. J Pediatr Orthop Part B. 2007; https://doi.org/10.1097/BPB.0b013e3280140548.
36. Fujiwara M, Abe Y, Kodera A, Araki T. Pyomyositis and osteomyelitis: An unusual cause of abdominal pain. BMJ Case Rep. 2018; https://doi.org/10.1136/bcr-2017-223871.
37. Mignemi ME, Menge TJ, Cole HA, Mencio GA, Martus JE, Lovejoy S, Stutz CM, Schoenecker JG. Epidemiology, diagnosis, and treatment of pericapsular pyomyositis of the hip in children. J Pediatr Orthop. 2014; https://doi.org/10.1097/BPO.0000000000000106.
38. Zvulunov A, Gal N, Segev Z. Acute hematogenous osteomyelitis of the pelvis in childhood: diagnostic clues and pitfalls. Pediatr Emerg Care. 2003; https://doi.org/10.1097/00006565-200302000-00008.
39. Shahid M, Holton C, O'Riordan S, Kraft JK. Sonography of musculoskeletal infection in children. Ultrasound. 2020; https://doi.org/10.1177/1742271X20901736.
40. Wasserman PL, Way A, Baig S, Gopireddy DR. MRI of myositis and other urgent muscle-related disorders. Emerg Radiol. 2020; https://doi.org/10.1007/s10140-020-01866-2.
41. Lorenz JM, Al-Refaie WB, Cash BD, et al. ACR appropriateness criteria radiologic Management of Infected Fluid Collections. J Am Coll Radiol. 2015; https://doi.org/10.1016/j.jacr.2015.04.025.
42. Miller NJK, Duncan RDD, Huntley JS. The conservative management of primary pyomyositis abscess in children: case series and review of the literature. Scott Med J. 2011; https://doi.org/10.1258/smj.2011.011131.
43. Tanir G, Tonbul A, Tuygun N, Aydemir C, Ertan U. Soft tissue infections in children: a retrospective

analysis of 242 hospitalized patients. Jpn J Infect Dis. 2006.
44. Gubbay AJ, Isaacs D. Pyomyositis in children. Pediatr Infect Dis J. 2000; https://doi.org/10.1097/00006454-200010000-00015.
45. Vij N, Ranade AS, Kang P, Belthur MV. Primary bacterial Pyomyositis in children: a systematic review. J Pediatr Orthop. 2021;41(9):e849–54. https://doi.org/10.1097/BPO.0000000000001944.
46. Bickels J, Ben-Sira L, Kessler A, Wientroub S. Primary pyomyositis. J Bone Jt Surg – Ser A. 2002; https://doi.org/10.2106/00004623-200212000-00024.
47. Teague DC, Graney DO, Routt MLC. Retropubic vascular hazards of the Ilioinguinal exposure: a cadaveric and clinical study. J Orthop Trauma. 1996; https://doi.org/10.1097/00005131-199604000-00002.
48. Chuprin A, Beavers NT, Fong V, Vingan H, Aggarwal A. Percutaneous transgluteal computed tomography-guided aspiration of obturator internus pyomyositis in adolescent athlete: a case report and literature review. Radiol Case Reports. 2018; https://doi.org/10.1016/j.radcr.2018.08.007.
49. Spiegel DA, Meyer JS, Dormans JP, Flynn JM, Drummond DS. Pyomyositis in children and adolescents: report of 12 cases and review of the literature. J Pediatr Orthop. 1999; https://doi.org/10.1097/01241398-199903000-00002.
50. Boulyana M, Kilani MS. Nontropical pyomyositis complicated with spinal epidural abscess in a previously healthy child. Surg Neurol Int. 2014; https://doi.org/10.4103/2152-7806.130718.
51. Gupta G, Rabbi Q, Bohra V, Shah MM. Protrusio acetabulae as a sequel to septic arthritis of the hip with obturator internus pyomyositis. J Pediatr Orthop B. 2020; https://doi.org/10.1097/bpb.0000000000000823.
52. Park S Do, Shatsky JB, Pawel BR, Wells L (2007) Atraumatic compartment syndrome: a manifestation of toxic shock and infectious pyomyositis in a child - a case report. J Bone Jt Surg – Ser A https://doi.org/10.2106/00004623-200706000-00024.
53. Ameh EA. Pyomyositis in children: analysis of 31 cases. Ann Trop Paediatr. 1999; https://doi.org/10.1080/02724939992347.
54. Ricci MA, Rose FB, Meyer KK. Pyogenic psoas abscess: worldwide variations in etiology. World J Surg. 1986; https://doi.org/10.1007/BF01655254.
55. Bresee JS, Edwards MS. Psoas abscess in children. Pediatr Infect Dis J. 1990; https://doi.org/10.1097/00006454-199003000-00011.
56. Driver CP, Renshaw PR, Youngson GG. Psoas abscess associated with renal pathology in children. Pediatr Surg Int. 1997; https://doi.org/10.1007/s003830050112.
57. Brook I. Pyomyositis in children, caused by anaerobic bacteria. J Pediatr Surg. 1996; https://doi.org/10.1016/S0022-3468(96)90745-9.
58. Huang JJ, Ruaan MK, Lan RR, Wang MC. Acute pyogenic iliopsoas abscess in Taiwan: clinical features, diagnosis, treatments and outcome. J Infect. 2000; https://doi.org/10.1053/jinf.2000.0643.

14 Musculoskeletal Infections in the Neonate

Atul R. Bhaskar and Ashok N. Johari

Introduction

Bone and joint infections in the neonate are considered a systemic emergency and can have serious consequences if left untreated. The incidence of neonatal skeletal infections (NSK) varies in different regions globally. Ho et al. reported an incidence of 0.12/1000 live births and 0.67/1000 for all nursery admissions in Singapore [1]. Narang et al., from India, reported an incidence of 1/1500 live births [2]. The incidence increases to 3–8/1000 live births in premature and immunocompromised babies that required prolonged care in the neonatal intensive care unit (NICU) [3, 4, 5, 6].

The ability of the foetus to adapt to the intrauterine environment, its passage through the birth canal and final exposure to the external environment is an innate or a natural process. Despite this, musculoskeletal infections in the newborn can occur in the prenatal period due to direct maternal transmission such as HIV, syphilis and viral organisms or after birth (postnatal) [7]. Infections can also occur in the birth canal due to aspiration of amniotic fluid into the lungs or gastrointestinal tract. Postnatal infection largely occurs due to colonization of umbilical stump or secondary to involvement of other systems, usually following respiratory, urinary or gastrointestinal tract infections (RTI, UTI, GTI) or skin infections [6, 8, 9]. This susceptibility further increases in the hostile environment of the NICU due to a changing microbial environment and increasing resistance of pathogens to available antibiotics.

Infections in the neonatal period may be classified as early acute, late acute and delayed or chronic based on the time of onset of symptoms [10]. If a child is febrile or listless in the first 48 hours after birth, the infection is labelled as immediate onset or early acute. Any onset of symptoms between 48 hours and 7 days is classified as late acute. Infection that is acquired after 7 days and up to 28 days is labelled as delayed or chronic infection (Table 14.1). The initial diagnosis is often delayed or missed due to paucity or vagueness of signs and symptoms in the neonatal period. The impact of this delay can cause catastrophic damage to the immature skeleton [11].

A. R. Bhaskar (✉)
RN Cooper Hospital - HBT Medical College, Bombay Hospital Institute of Medical Sciences, Mumbai, Maharashtra, India

A. N. Johari
Children's Orthopaedic Centre, Mahim, Mumbai, India

© Springer Nature Switzerland AG 2022
M. V. Belthur et al. (eds.), *Pediatric Musculoskeletal Infections*, https://doi.org/10.1007/978-3-030-95794-0_14

Table 14.1 Microbiology of neonatal infections related to onset of signs and symptoms

Intrauterine infection	Organisms
	Syphilis
	Candida albicans
	Neisseria gonorrhoeae
Early acute (Birth–48 hours)	*Staphylococcus aureus*
	Group B Streptococci
	Klebsiella pneumoniae
Late acute (48 hours–7 days)	*Staphylococcus aureus*
	Group B streptococci
	Klebsiella pneumoniae
	Haemophilus influenzae
Delayed or chronic (After 7 days)	*Staphylococcus aureus*
	Klebsiella pneumoniae
	Escherichia coli
	Pseudomonas aeruginosa
	Group B streptococci
	Haemophilus influenzae

Table 14.2 Typical spectrum of microbiology in 66 neonates with bone and joint sepsis [6]

Organism	Number of cases	Percentage
S. aureus	37	56
Gram-negative bacilli	16	24.3
K. pneumoniae	8	
Pseudomonas aeruginosa	3	
Others[a]	5	
Streptococcus agalactiae	10	15.2
Staphylococcus epidermidis	2	3
Haemophilus influenzae type b	1	1.5
Total	**66**	**100**

[a]Others Serratia marcescens, *Proteus mirabilis*, *Acinetobacter baumannii*, *Enterobacter cloacae*, *Escherichia coli* (**one each**)

Microbiology and Risk Factors for Neonatal Infections

Staphylococcus aureus (*S. aureus*), group β streptococci (GBS – *Streptococcus agalactiae*) and gram-negative organisms (*Escherichia coli*, *Klebsiella pneumoniae*) are the predominant cause of NSK (Table 14.2). *S. aureus* account for over 70% of culture-positive cases [9, 12, 13, 14]. A study from Finland reported that GBS accounts for 77% of cases of bacteraemia but only 2% of cases of NSK infections [15]. Fungal infection due to *Candida albicans* and *Aspergillus aeruginosa* are seen in immunocompromised host and in babies with prolonged intensive care [16, 17]. As the immune system is also immature in neonates, less virulent organisms that colonize the skin or the nasal passage can give rise to severe infection [18]. The microbiology varies if the neonate acquires infection from the community/nursery or due to in-hospital stay. Neonates that present with late infection between 7 days and 28 days after uncomplicated delivery usually have community-acquired *S. aureus*, while some may acquire nosocomial infection. In a study from Edmonton, methicillin-resistant *S. aureus* (MRSA) or methicillin-sensitive *S. aureus* (MSSA) infections accounted for 60% of hospital-acquired or nosocomial infections, 15% were gram-negative, and 17% infections were caused by *Candida* species [19, 20, 21]. Community-acquired arthritis was caused most often by streptococci (52%), followed by staphylococci (26%) and gonococci (17%) (Table 14.2).

In an institutional study of 15 neonates in Mumbai with septic arthritis (SA) and osteomyelitis (OM), the spectrum of organisms cultured from the pus/fluid was as follows: 33% gram-negative, 7% fungal, and 20% gram-positive. No organism was found in 6 cases (40%) [22]. The aspiration of amniotic fluid in the birth canal or soon after birth can cause primary infection with *E. coli* or *Klebsiella pneumoniae* (KPN), both gram-negative organisms. The ensuing GTI or RTI can spread to the MSK system. Thus, gram-negative infection is on the rise even in hospital-acquired infections [23, 24].

Risk Factors for Neonatal Skeletal Infections

Prematurity, low birth weight, neonatal jaundice and systemic or local organ sepsis are the leading risk factors for NSK [25, 26] (Table 14.3). Liao et al. listed chorioamnionitis due to prolonged rupture of membranes and perinatal birth

Table 14.3 Risk factors for neonatal infections

Maternal factors/natal factors	Post-natal factors
High-risk pregnancy, multiple gestation	Prematurity
Ruptured membrane >24 hours	Low birth weight <1500g
Maternal fever >38°C	Poor Apgar score <5 at 1 min
Chorioamnionitis	Respiratory distress
Foul smelting liquor	Neonatal jaundice
	Mechanical ventilation
	Central lines, catheterization

asphyxia as the two main causative factors for infection [27]. Extended hospitalization caused by the abovementioned conditions, with a concomitant need for invasive clinical monitoring, provides fertile ground of seeding of bacteria. Urinary catheters, intravenous lines, gastrointestinal tubes and endotracheal tubes for ventilatory assistance are all potential causes of transgressions in the neonates that may lead to iatrogenic infections. Umbilical cord catheterization is also a common route for spread of infection. Rapid colonization of these devices can act as the focus of infection; *S. epidermidis*, coagulase negative *Staphylococcus* and *S. hominis* and GBS are the main culprits in these types of nosocomial infection [28]. Ish-Horowicz et al. looked at the risk factors in 22 NICU babies that had resistant *S. aureus* osteomyelitis. In 11 babies with infections, the weight was less than 1500 g, and in 14 children (70%) with infections, an intravascular device was the primary site of infection [29].

Neonatal host immunity is tenuous, especially for the preterm child, and opportunistic infections due to fungi, histoplasma species and *Cryptococcus* are some uncommon causes of NSK in the relatively immunocompromised neonate [30]. *Klebsiella pneumoniae* causing long bone osteomyelitis has also been implicated in a Spanish study of 35 children, 68% of whom had a previous history of neonatal sepsis [31]. *Pseudomonas aeruginosa* causing septic arthritis of the knee in premature infants has also been reported [32].

Haemophilus influenzae type b was a common pathogen in the neonatal period before the advent of the conjugated vaccine. In one study, it was responsible for 5% of culture-positive osteomyelitis and 41% of culture-positive septic arthritis in unvaccinated neonates [33]; cases now are extremely rare and seen mostly in the unvaccinated.

Pathophysiology of Neonatal Skeletal Infections

Haematogenous spread from any foci – heel puncture, umbilical vein catheterization, urinary tract, etc. – is the primary route of infection. Direct inoculation can occur after abscess formation following intramuscular injection or vaccination.

The epiphysis that forms the ends of long bones, the physis (or growth plate) and the metaphysis, which is the most dynamic region for bone growth, are all vulnerable to infection; the metaphysis, however, is the most common site for bone infections. Metaphyseal spongy bone with its sinusoidal vascular system, sluggish blood flow and paucity of white cells serves as the perfect environment for bacterial seeding [34]. The presence of transphyseal vessels in children younger than age 2 years can also lead to rapid transmission of infection from the diaphyseal marrow and metaphysis into the joint [35]. As the epiphysis, physis and metaphysis are intracapsular in the shoulder, elbow, hip and ankle in neonates, osteomyelitis and septic arthritis can be indistinguishable in this age group, and in 76% of cases both bone and joint infection occur concurrently [35, 36, 37]. The joint and bone are also sensitive to tamponade secondary to inflammatory fluid. Even a small volume of pus (2 ml to 3 ml) can cause avascular necrosis of bone, as well as damage to the overlying cartilage, leading to devastating sequelae.

Site of Involvement

The most common site of involvement for NSK is hip/proximal femur, shoulder/proximal humerus, knee/distal femur, elbow/distal humerus and distal tibia/ankle joint [38]. Spine involvement is rare in neonates. Narang et al. reported on involvement of 33 joints in 35 neonates. Hip and knee were the most commonly involved (48% each), followed by shoulder and elbow (4%) [2]. Multifocal joint or bone involvement is also common in neonates due to rapid systemic spread in small babies [39]. In an Australian study involving 22 babies with osteomyelitis, 11 (50%) had multifocal involvement, with the long bones, particularly of the upper limb, commonly affected [29].

Infections have also been reported from unusual sites such as the acromioclavicular joint, the temporomandibular joint and the skull secondary to an infected cephalhaematoma [40, 41, 42]. Septic arthritis of shoulder with proximal humerus osteomyelitis and soft tissue abscess can also cause brachial plexus palsy [43].

Constitutional symptoms of bone infection and sepsis are variable in neonates. Fever as a presenting symptom is present in only 50% of neonates. Persistent high fever (greater than 39 degrees C) is common with *S. aureus* infection [37]. Other symptoms include excessive crying, listlessness, lethargy, poor feeding, abdominal distension, diarrhoea and decreased or painful movements of the involved extremity as noticed by caregivers. The most common clinical finding are local swelling of the involved limb, cellulitis and asymmetry in joint movement, regional tenderness of the bone or joint and pseudoparalysis [44, 45, 46, 47] (Table 14.4) (Fig. 14.1).

A thorough general examination must be carried out to assess the umbilical stump, signs of thrombophlebitis and other skin and scalp infections to ascertain the primary source.

Systemic signs of respiratory distress, tachycardia and fluctuating blood pressure may occur

Table 14.4 Signs and symptoms of NSK infections

Symptoms	Signs
Refusal of feeds	Local erythema, swelling
Paucity of movement of affected limb	Localized tenderness
Listlessness	Resting position of limb
Fever (frequently not present)	Pain with joint movement
Irritability	Pseudo-paralysis

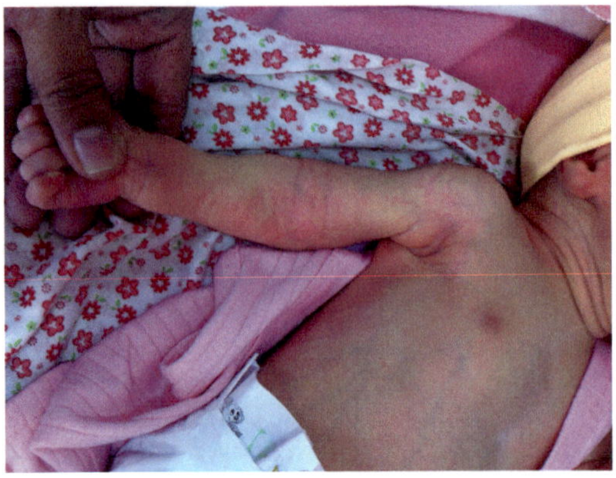

Fig. 14.1 Septic arthritis of the elbow in the neonate. Overlying skin redness and cellulitis are tell-tale signs of underlying infection in the neonate

with increasing sepsis. In a study by Narang, 19 of 25 babies (76%) had septicaemia [2].

Differential diagnosis can include child abuse, bone fragility syndromes with multiple fractures, congenital syphilis and blood dyscrasias, among other possible diagnoses.

Imaging in NSK Infections

The choice of imaging modality depends on availability, accessibility and the local resources of the institution where the child is being evaluated [48].

Plain Radiographs

Plain radiographs are non-specific in the first 48–72 hours. The suspected area of bone involvement may show rarefaction in the metaphysis, a soft tissue shadow over the cortex and an increase in joint width or space due to inflammatory fluid [49, 50]. Deshpande et al. reported soft tissue swelling on plain radiographs in 9 (58%) of the 17 children in their study. After about 4–5 days, radiographs often reveal the tell-tale signs of bone infection: lytic areas in the bone, cortical erosions and periosteal elevation, joint subluxation or dislocation and epiphyseal separation around the hip and shoulder [51]. Radiographic changes become apparent when more than 1/third of bone matrix is affected. Importantly plain radiographs are also extremely useful to assess the progress of bone healing or destruction in response to treatment.

Ultrasound

In reliable and experienced hands, if available, ultrasonography (USG) is perhaps the fastest, safest and best modality to diagnose osteomyelitis and septic arthritis. The classic findings of osteomyelitis (OM) include deep soft tissue oedema, periosteal elevation more than 2 mm and circumferential soft tissue abscesses [52] (Fig. 14.2). Pathological changes can be detected as early as 48 hours from the onset of infection. USG can also reveal metaphyseal cortical erosions, joint fluid collection and capsular distension of septic arthritis by the third or fourth day after onset of illness [52, 53]. USG-guided fluid or pus aspiration is useful to obtain a specimen for culture and can also be therapeutic in some cases. Follow-up scans can help in monitoring results of intervention.

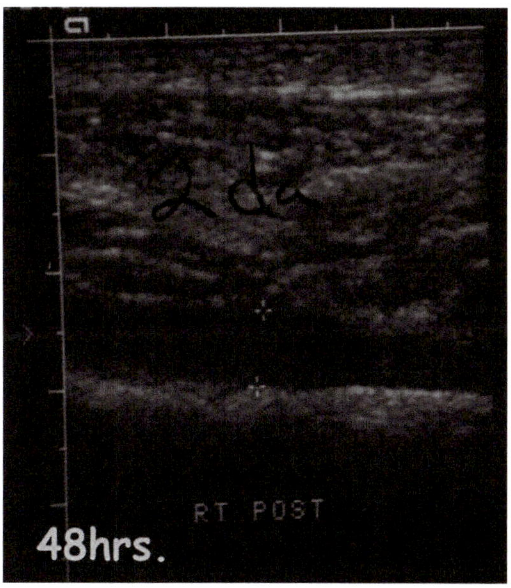

Fig. 14.2 Ultrasound of the hip after 48 hours of acute onset of septic arthritis showing distension of the anterior capsule due to infective fluid

Bone Scintigraphy

A three-phase total body technetium bone scan can show the classic markers of bone infection: hyperperfusion, vasodilatation and cold or hot spots in the affected bone – before it is evident on the plain radiographs. It can also detect multifocal involvement and infection in deep sites such as the pelvis or spine. In a study of 20 neonates, the sensitivity of bone scan was 90% in diagnosing focal skeletal involvement, whereas for plain radiographs the sensitivity was only 60% [54]. Other studies have shown that bone scan is unreliable and should not overshadow clinical judgement. Bone scintigraphy, however, is not easily available, and with added risk of radiation and difficulty with interpretation of images, it is not the preferred choice of investigation [55, 56]. In a study of 22 neonates, Frederiksen reported that plain radiographs were more efficient than bone scan in diagnosing osteomyelitis. As the neonatal bones are gracile, plain radiographs can reveal early bone destruction by 3–4 days as compared to young children where radiographs can be unreliable, and negative, up to 10–14 days [25].

MRI

MRI is the investigation of choice in the diagnosis of SA or OM in a neonate. For non-contrast scans, the sensitivity and a specificity rates are 91% and 96%, respectively (56). While USG has a lag of 4 days to detect early signs, an MRI can detect infective changes as early as 48 hours of onset of symptoms. These changes include early myositis, cellulitis, joint effusion, intraosseous and periosteal collections and small abscesses. Gadolinium-enhanced MRI is mainly used for spinal infections and for relapse cases after surgical intervention. MRI can also differentiate between psoas pyomyositis and hip infection, both of which present with a similar clinical picture. MRI can detect changes in the epiphysis, physis and the joint cartilage. Bone erosion, physeal damage and sequestrum formation are seen in late stages. Identifying these findings can help with planning of treatment and to determine prognosis [56, 57].

CT Scan

CT is less frequently used in neonates as it doesn't reveal the soft tissue changes and fluid in the bone and joint. It is often used in chronic cases to detect sequestrum and bony abnormality. It has been shown that early advanced imaging at the onset of infection can help in directing effective treatment and reduce untoward sequelae [57, 58].

Spectrum of Infection Unique to Neonates

The predilection for sepsis in the proximal femur (hip), knee, distal tibia and shoulder is due to the peculiar vascular anatomy unique to neonates [38]. The hip joint is the most vulnerable and, with delayed presentation or inadequate treatment, bears the brunt of the worst outcome – epiphyseal necrosis, joint subluxation or dislocation [59]. Multiple bone and joint involvement are typically seen in NICU patients with concurrent illness. Upper extremity, spine, pelvis and ribs are rarely involved. This is due to the presence of collateral spinal vessels that prevent vertebral infection in neonates.

Management of SA and OM in Neonates

The principles of management in neonatal bone and joint infections involve establishing a rapid diagnosis and early medical and surgical intervention. Antibiotics save lives and surgery saves the bone! In the pre-antibiotic era, and recently as the 1950s, the mortality rate due to neonatal sepsis was about 45%–50%. Advances in neonatal care, a multidisciplinary approach, and sound surgical principles have reduced this rate to less than 1% of cases. Often the treatment of bone and joint infection depends whether the event occurred in the NICU or hospital setting or after the baby had been discharged after an uneventful birth and then presented to the clinician with symptoms suggestive of skeletal infection; NICU-acquired infections have worse outcomes overall [19].

The treatment of bone and joint sepsis in a neonate is multidisciplinary. Irrespective of the type of presentation of infection, whether community-acquired or during a hospital stay, the key is to establish the severity of infection, localize the site and source of infection and then institute management appropriate to the clinical presentation [26].

Laboratory confirmation of sepsis by basic haematological investigations includes complete blood count (CBC), C reactive protein (CRP), erythrocyte sedimentation rate (ESR), serum procalcitonin (procal) and platelet count [60] (Table 14.5). A serum procal cut-off value of less than 0.5 ng/ml is more sensitive for osteomyelitis [61, 62]. Some neonates will have a normal WBC count but a high platelet count (thrombocytosis). Blood culture or bone biopsy has a high yield in systemic sepsis and must always be done before commencing antibiotic therapy. Plain radiographs, USG and MRI scans are useful to identify location and extent of infection. Thus, a high index of suspicion and thorough clinical examination is required for every child, especially for patients in NICU or for those seen in the community with known risk factors of NSK infection [63].

Aspiration of abscesses or the joint space may be done with USG; even deep-seated muscle abscesses, such as around the hip or pelvis, can be "tapped" and the pus sent for bacteriology and antibiotic sensitivity testing.

Table 14.5 Diagnostic parameters in bone and joint sepsis

Laboratory parameters in neonatal bone and joint sepsis	
Complete blood count (CBC)	>20,000/mm^3
ESR	>20
CRP	>20mg/L
Gram staining of aspirate	Gram negative or positive
Blood culture	Positive culture
CSF culture and Gram stain	For severe sepsis in NCIU

Management of Neonatal Bone and Joint Infection

The treatment of neonatal bone and joint infections involves both rapid administration of parenteral antibiotics and surgical intervention based on local signs, imaging and systemic parameters.

An objective grading system such as the HOMSA score (Haematogenous Osteomyelitis and Septic Arthritis Score) can be used to assess the severity of infection in neonates and also to guide surgical intervention (Table 14.6). The score uses both clinical and laboratory parameters with an imaging modality to confirm bone involvement. A score equal to or greater than 6, with radiological confirmation of bone infection, predicated surgical intervention in 92.8% cases in a study of 41 children, in which 50% of cases were neonates [63].

In mild to moderate infections, resolution of local swelling, cellulitis and painless recovery of joint range of motion within 48–72 hours of commencement of antibiotics indicates an adequate early response. Blood parameters such as decreasing WBC and CRP also mirror this improvement. In severe cases, the initial response to medical treatment may be inadequate or incomplete. Both systemic and local signs and symptoms continue to deteriorate despite intravenous antibiotics for 2–3 days. Persistent pyrexia, an increasing WBC count more than 20,000, and a CRP greater than 20 mg/L may indicate suppuration and mandate early surgical intervention.

Medical Management

The antibiotic regimen for each child depends on the prevalence and type of pathogens commonly encountered in the community and the hospital setting. An infectious disease (ID) specialist who has experience with neonatal infection protocols is ideally consulted before instituting medical therapy. Arbitrary and illogical antibiotic practice can cause more harm than good by delaying recovery and thereby increasing the risk of complications or leading to incomplete treatment with an increased risk of recurrence [64].

Parenteral antibiotics must commence as soon as there is suspicion of infection but after blood cultures and local aspirate have been sent for cytology and microbiology. In neonates with single joint involvement, a second-generation cephalosporin (cefuroxime) with an aminoglycoside such as amikacin, or gentamicin, will cover most pathogens [65, 66]. In severe infection secondary to visceral involvement, a third-generation cephalosporin (cefotaxime) will provide adequate cover against *S. aureus*, group B streptococci and gram-negative organisms [67, 68].

Neonates in the NICU or those with nosocomial infection should be commenced with vancomycin, nafcillin or tobramycin to cover MRSA as well as coagulase-negative *Staphylococcus aureus*. These can also be combined with an aminoglycoside to cover enterobacteria [69]. The imipenem group is efficacious against gram-negative infections caused by *Klebsiella* and *Pseudomonas* organisms.

Table 14.6 Clinical and laboratory score for septic arthritis

HOMSA SCORE (Haematogenous Osteomyelitis and Septic Arthritis Scoring System)				
Clinical	**Parameters**	**Variations of primary parameters**		**Score**
	Pain	Non-weight bearing/	Paucity of movements	**1**
	Fever	Local Warmth		**1**
	Swelling	Joint effusion		**1**
	ROM	Painful	Restricted	**1**
Labs		**Normal values**	**Value**	**Score**
	WBC count	>16,000 up to 2 yrs >14,000 2–18 yrs	Elevated	**1**
	Diff. count (polymorphs)		Elevated	**1**
	CRP	N – up to 10mg/L	Elevated	**1**
	ESR	(N – up to puberty 13mm)	Elevated	**1**
Total score				**8**

For *Candida* infection, amphotericin B and fluconazole are the drugs of choice. Fluconazole can be given orally once there is a response to the intravenous antifungal regimen.

The duration of parenteral antibiotic therapy in neonates is debatable. In uncomplicated cases of neonatal infection, 2 weeks of intravenous antibiotics followed by 2 weeks of oral medications is adequate, based on clinical and laboratory improvement. An early switch from intravenous to oral antibiotics is possible when there is rapid resolution of signs and symptoms, and the infection is caused by culture-positive gram-positive organisms with known drug sensitivity. In complicated cases associated with prolonged sepsis and osteomyelitis, intravenous antibiotics may be continued for a prolonged course, sometimes as long as 10–12 weeks [70, 71].

Surgical Approach to Neonatal Infections

Surgical decompression of the infection can be early, concomitant or late depending on the response to medical treatment of the rapidity or onset of infection. This is paramount to prevent permanent bone and joint damage especially for hip and shoulder involvement [59].

Due to the unique blood flow pattern in neonates, the pus fluid, rich in proteases and catalytic enzymes, can rapidly destroy the delicate skeletal structures in contiguity. Time is of the essence, as often the diagnosis is delayed, due to overwhelming systemic sepsis. A delay of more than 72 hours can lead to devastating sequelae, particularly around the hip and shoulder joints [39, 72, 73]. A critically ill NICU baby, who may not be stable enough for general anaesthesia, with infections involving knee, ankle and shoulder joint can undergo "arthrocentesis" and "joint lavage" in the NICU procedural area, to reduce the local bacterial load and to obtain sample for testing (Fig. 14.3). Fungal culture must always be obtained with multifocal involvement, and those that don't respond to conventional antibiotics. Surgery should be contemplated even for community-acquired infection if the clinical signs don't improve in 48 hours of empirical antibiotic therapy [39, 73, 74].

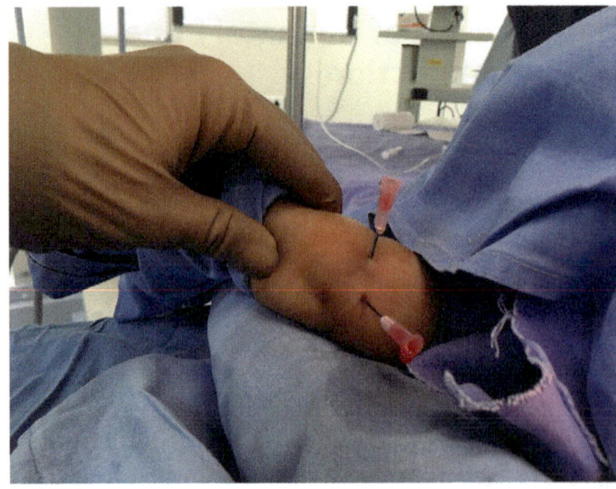

Fig. 14.3 Needle arthrocentesis with saline lavage can be done for the superficial joints like elbow and knee. One can repeat if the local signs are not improving

Hip and Proximal Femur

Surgical approach to the joint, bones and muscle will be dictated by the finding on imaging. The hip joint is usually exposed through the conventional anterior modified Smith-Petersen approach. If the proximal femur shaft is also involved, then a modified Watson-Jones approach is more appropriate. Once the muscle planes are separated, the distended capsule is pierced with an 18 G needle syringe to aspirate the thick pus or sero-purulent fluid. After the capsular incision, thorough saline wash is given to remove fibrinous and purulent material from the joint. The hip is moved in all directions to squeeze out any pus from posterior and inferior recesses of the joint. If there is metaphyseal osteomyelitis and intraosseous pus collection, drill holes are made with 1.5 mm "K" wires to decompress the bone. The joint stability is assessed at this stage. The capsule is left open and the muscle planes approximated over a drain. Joint immobilization after surgery is important to control pain and spasm. If the hip is stable, an abduction splint suffices, but in the presence of instability, a broom-stick plaster or hip spica is used for 3 to 4 weeks. Parsch et al. studied 24 neonatal septic hips, of which 18 underwent emergency arthrotomy and bone

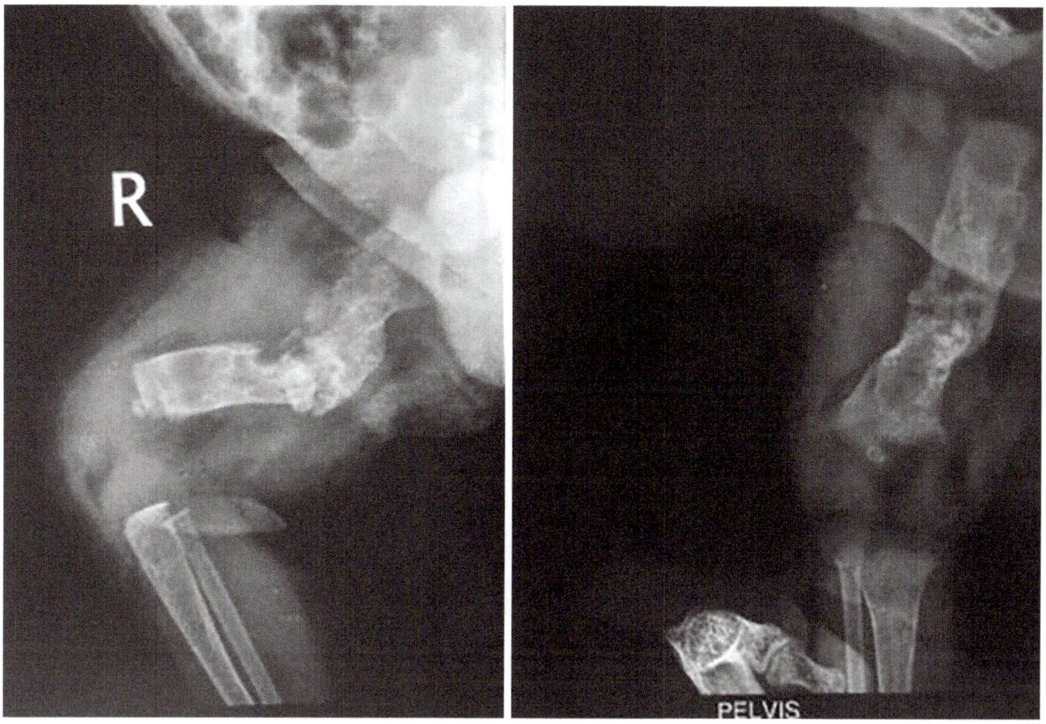

Fig. 14.4 A 10-day-old child in NICU with osteomyelitis of the femur and septic arthritis of the hip. He sustained pathological fracture after debridement and was splinted in a spica cast

decompression. The authors recommend USG for initial diagnosis and parenteral intravenous antibiotics until the CRP normalizes. Surgery instituted within 72 hours gave the best outcome with no residual bone defect [75, 76] (Fig. 14.4).

Knee

The knee joint is easily accessible; arthrocentesis and anterior open drainage each play a role in management. If there is bone involvement in the distal femur, the surgical approach is dictated by the site of involvement. Open knee joint decompression, joint lavage and bone debridement are essential to clear the infective material and enhance healing in cases of osteomyelitis with a knee sepsis; often drill holes are made in the metaphyseal bone to decompress the intraosseous purulent material. For isolated knee septic arthritis, arthrocentesis is useful to obtain a sample for culture and confirm the diagnosis, but knee open drainage is employed for severe or late infections.

Shoulder

For infections about the shoulder and proximal humerus, an anterior delto-pectoral approach is utilized to give optimal exposure. The axillary pouch has purulent remnants that must be sought and debrided to clear the shoulder joint. The extent of the incision is based on presence of infection in the proximal humerus. Often, there is a posterior or lateral swelling that will require a more direct approach (Figs. 14.5, 14.6, 14.7, and 14.8).

Elbow and Ankle

The elbow and ankle joints can be approached percutaneously, unless the extent of involvement is severe or synovial thickening dictates a formal incision. The principles of open drainage, however, remain consistent – open the capsule and expose joint, collect pus and send for microbiology, perform thorough lavage, look for extraneous pus pockets, remove dead or necrotic tissue, insert a drain if required and

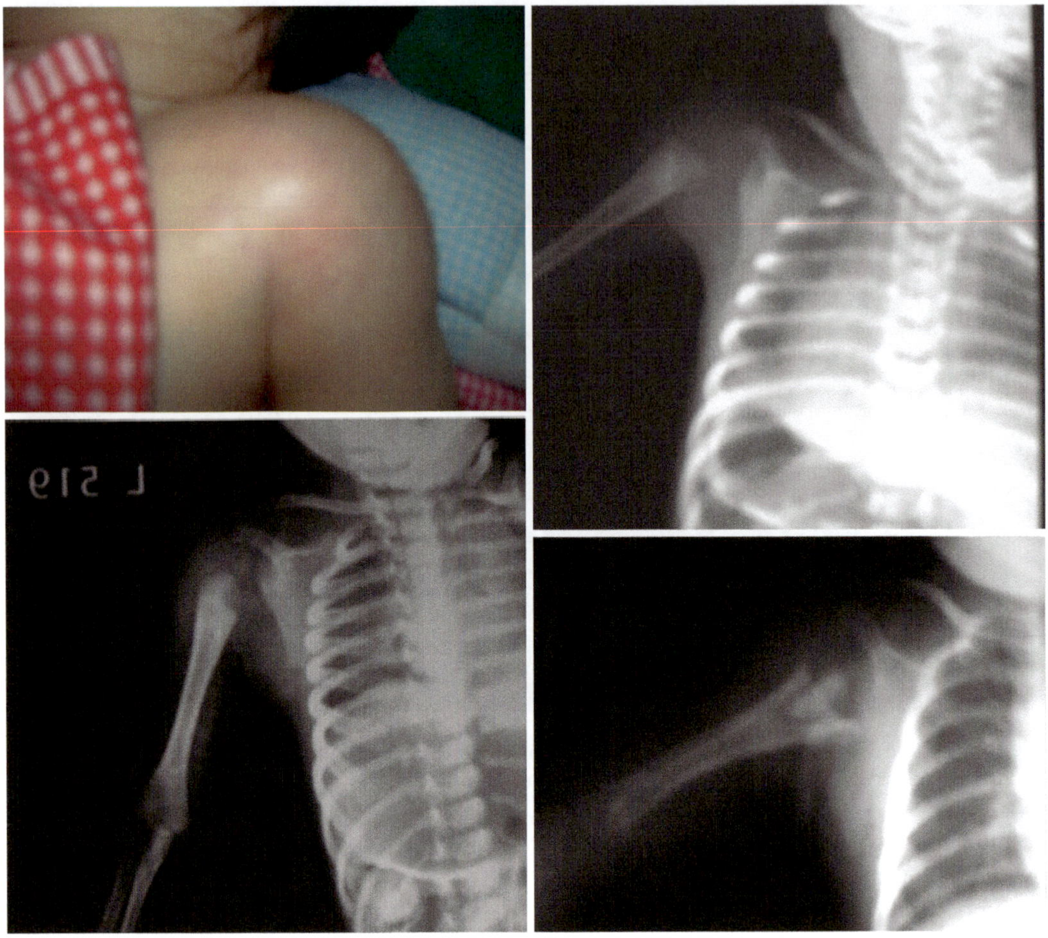

Figs. 14.5, 14.6, 14.7, and 14.8 Septic arthritis of the shoulder with redness and cellulitis over the joint. Radiograph at sixth and tenth day reveal early osteopenic patch and erosion. The child presented after 10 days and had septic necrosis of proximal epiphysis and osteomyelitis with sequestrum in the humeral shaft.

splint the joint post-operatively for comfort [74]. In certain cases, the response to surgical decompression and appropriate medical therapy is as dramatic as the onset of infection, with rapid recovery after decompression. Often, multiple sites need surgical drainage concurrently, especially in NICU babies [39].

Psoas

Psoas muscle pyomyositis can mimic septic hip, and often pyelonephritis can mimic psoas myositis; hence appropriate imaging must be undertaken in any neonate that presents with a flexed hip and abdominal signs (Fig. 14.9). Often, deep muscle abscesses can also mimic joint septic arthritis of the shoulder, knee and elbow joints. A negative joint exploration with persisting symptoms should alert the clinician to proceed with further imaging. Any cellulitis overlying the joint or abscess over a limb is a "sign of osteomyelitis" unless proven otherwise. The authors have seen several cases where the abscess is lanced, leading to a discharging sinus from a deeper focus of infection. Radiographs taken at this late stage shows an underlying bone destruction and a missed opportunity for early intervention.

Antibiotics After Surgery

The duration of post-operative parenteral antibiotic therapy is based on the improvement in

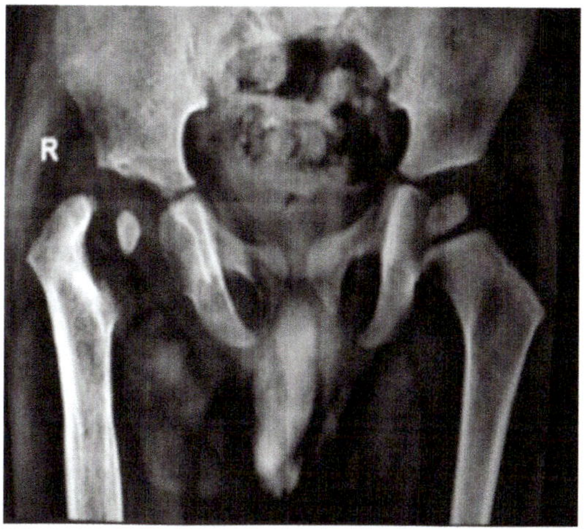

Fig. 14.9 Recurrence of sepsis 5 days after hip arthrotomy MRI reveals a large psoas abscess that required intervention (black and yellow arrow)

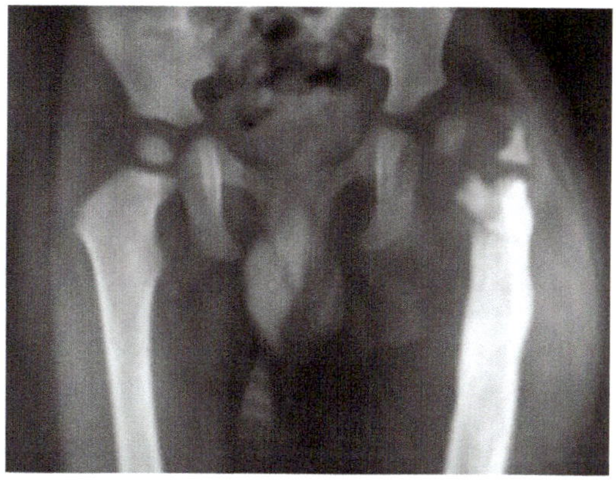

Figs. 14.10 Septic arthritis of the hip can lead to damaging sequelae depending on the severity of infection. Both these children underwent arthrotomy of the hip at 10 days and 16 days, respectively, and subsequent follow-up at 3 months revealed pseudarthrosis of the femoral neck

clinical and laboratory parameters and the microbiology report. At least 2–3 weeks of parenteral therapy is required to control bone and joint infection. Intravenous therapy helps overcome issues of poor adherence to prescribed therapy sometimes seen with oral regimens, as well as gastrointestinal-related absorption issues, to ensure optimal drug concentrations [14]. Drug regimens are discussed above but are individualized based on the extent of infection and the causative organism. In one study, Ecury-Gooseen et al. advised a 2-week course of intravenous antibiotics until clinical, microbial and radiological healing was observed in select preterm neonates, followed by 4 weeks of oral clindamycin [77].

Complications and Sequelae

Early Complications

Early complications typically follow inadequate treatment or delay in surgical intervention after 4–5 days. Bone and joint destruction, infective epiphysiolysis of the proximal femur and joint dislocation, especially of the hip due to purulent material, can lead to skeletal deformity [59, 78, 79]. Epiphyseal necrosis can also render the joint unstable (Figs. 14.10 and 14.11). Parsch reported that a delay of 5 weeks led to permanent bone and joint destruction in the majority of cases [75].

Late Complications

Growth abnormalities due to physeal involvement can manifest up to 9 years after the acute event. Hence all children with NSK infections should be monitored until skeletal maturity. Waters et al. reported that even children who had successful initial treatment can present later with physeal bar formation causing joint deformities [80] (Fig. 14.12a, b). In certain patients, sepsis can cause vascular damage that presents with delay in cartilage ossification. Singson et al. reported four neonates with a "missing femoral condyle"; arthrography revealed that the cartilaginous condyle was present but unossified, necessitating an osteotomy alone to achieve limb realignment [81]. Angular deformities and LLD are common following distal femoral osteomyelitis. Coxa vara, coxa breva and coxa valga can occur due to physeal damage of the proximal femur. Significant damage to the proximal humerus physis can cause marked shortening of the upper limb. Multiple sites of joint damage can be seen with polyarticular neonatal sepsis (Figs. 14.13).

The prognosis and outcome of neonatal septic arthritis depends on several factors, but delay in treatment more than 4 days, USG proven fluid collection and septic arthritis with concomitant osteomyelitis are factors that herald a poor prognosis [38, 78, 82].

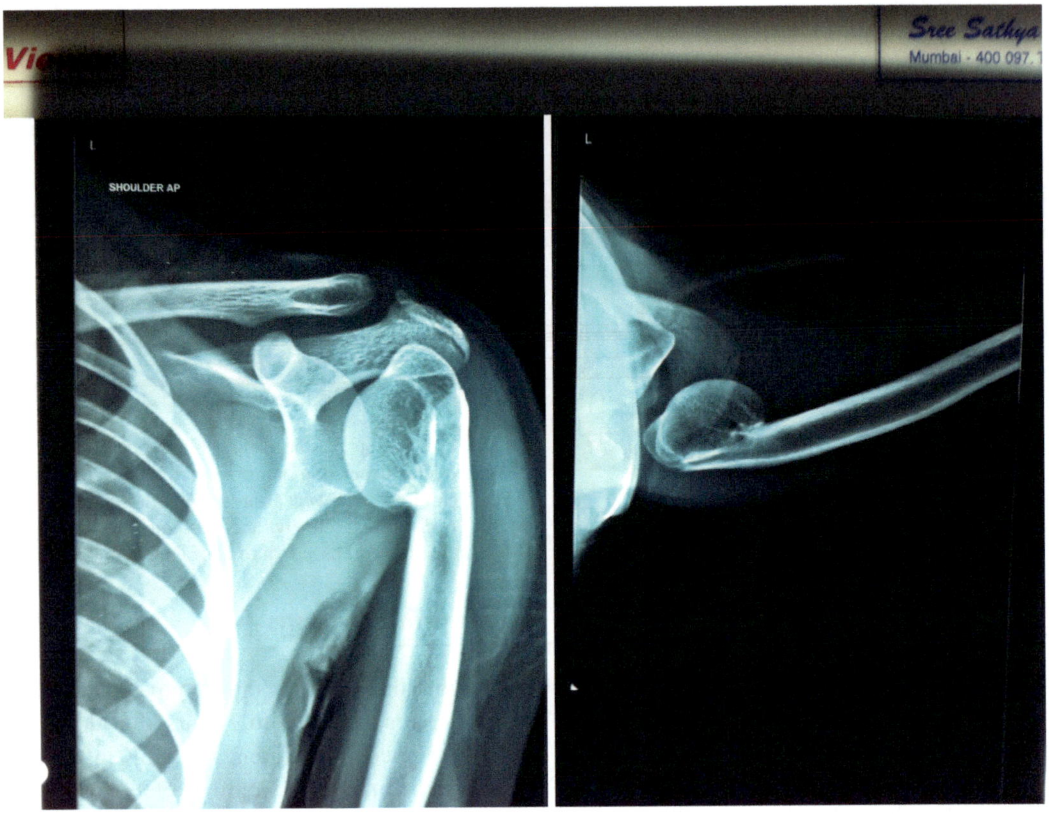

Fig. 14.11 Late sequelae of septic arthritis of the shoulder joint showing physeal arrest and varus deformity at skeletal maturity

Prognostic Factors affecting Outcome[82]

Birth weight < 1.5 kg

Time taken to present to medical facility> 4 days

Septic arthritis and osteomyelitis

Joint USG corroborative

Hip Joint

Previous intravenous cannulation

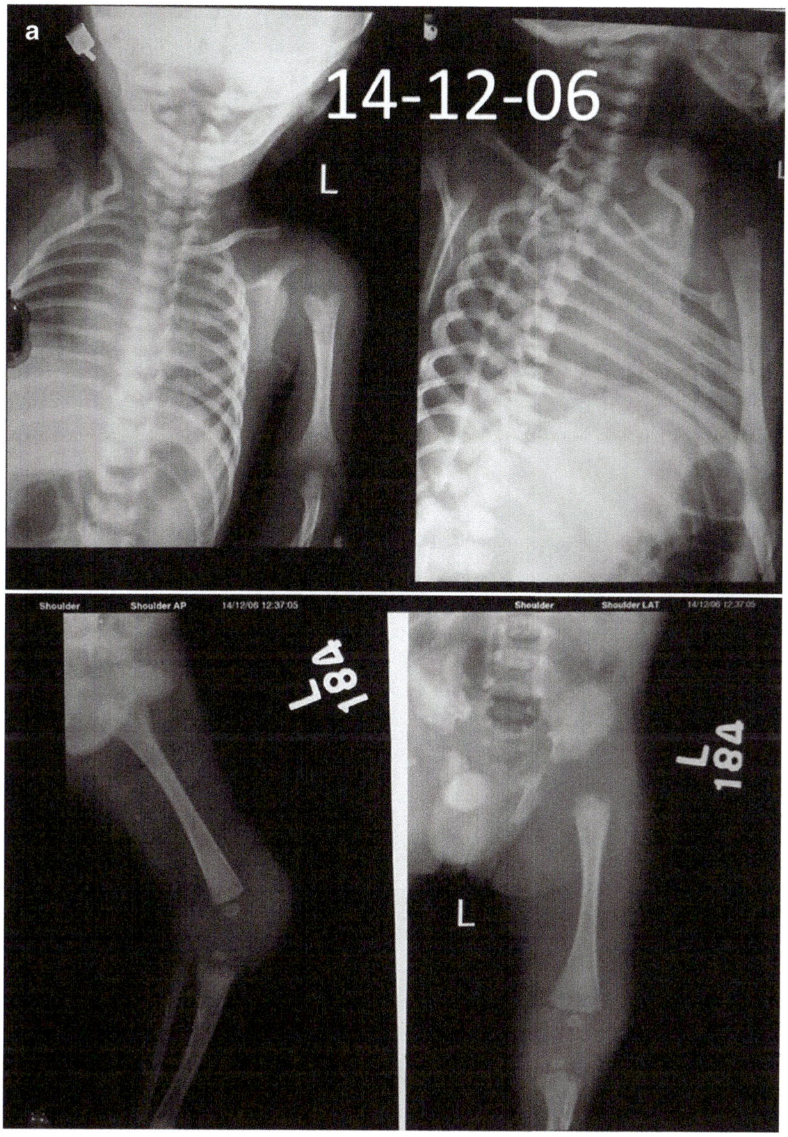

Fig. 14.12 (**a** and **b**) Neonate with septicaemia and multifocal osteomyelitis involving the left shoulder and knee, respectively, and bilateral hip involvement. Radiographs at 18 months reveal sequelae of infection: absent ossific nucleus of the hips and proximal humerus

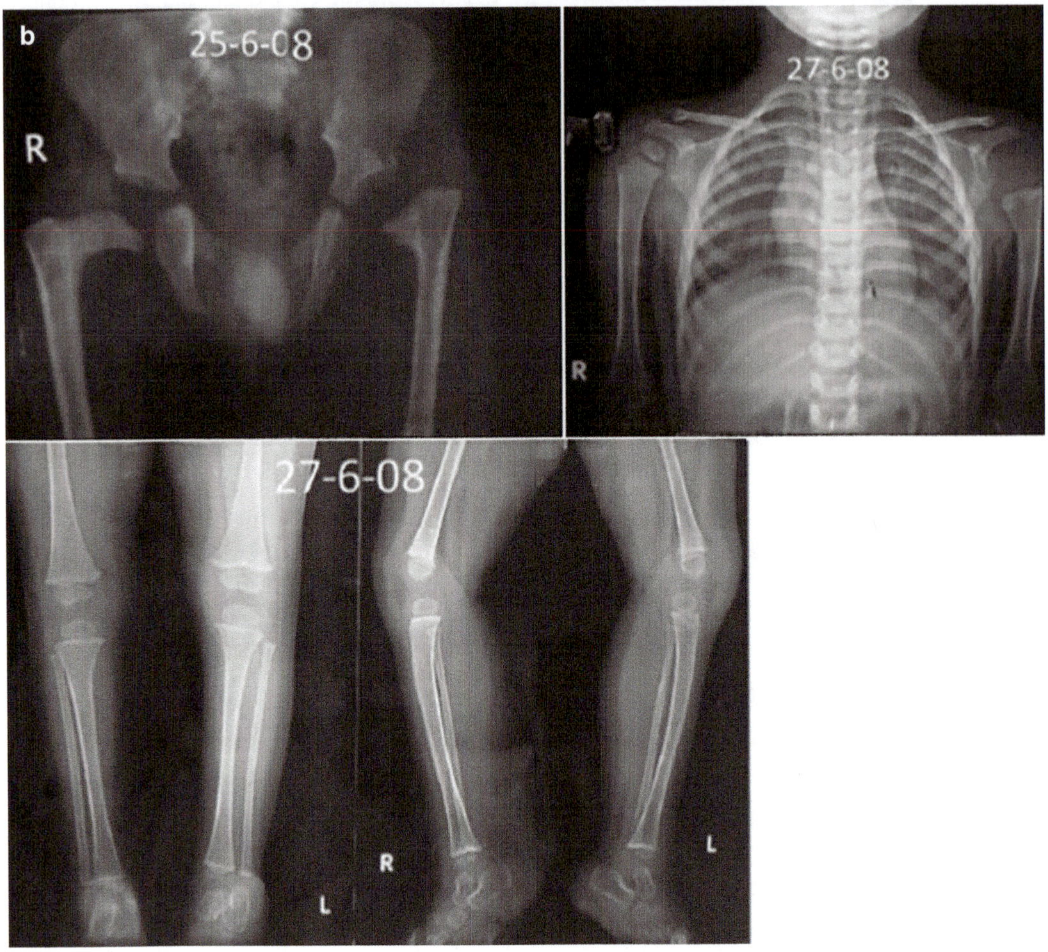

Fig. 14.12 (continued)

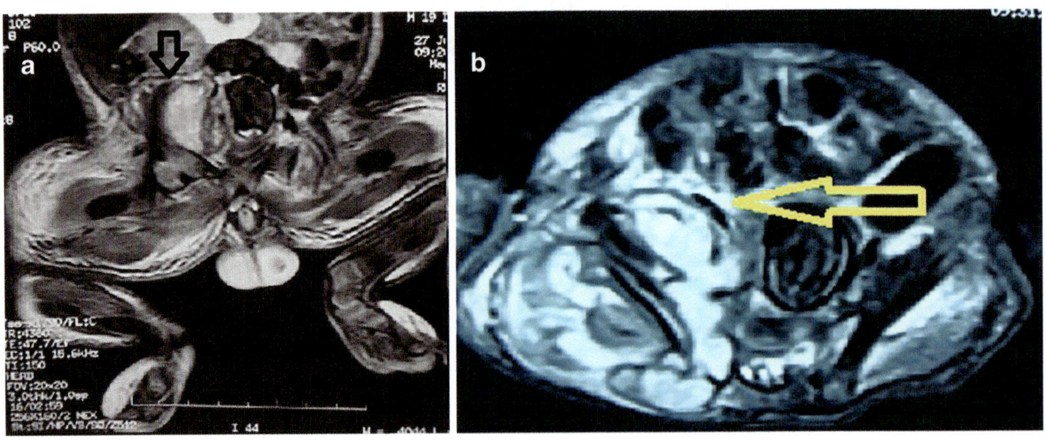

Fig. 14.13 Multifocal neonatal osteomyelitis showing involvement of the hip, knee and shoulder. Common with severe sepsis in an immunocompromised host

Box 14.1: Key Learning Points

- Neonatal osteomyelitis can present acutely in a healthy newborn.
- Premature infants (33 weeks), those with low birth weight and NICU babies with invasive interventions are at highest risk for neonatal sepsis secondary to bone and joint infections.
- An irritable NICU baby or neonate with limb pseudoparalysis or asymmetrical limb movements, abnormal swelling or cellulitis should raise suspicion for bone and joint infection.
- Laboratory tests as well as basic and advanced imaging should be performed concurrently and urgently to assess the severity of infection.
- Joint fluid aspirate and bone biopsy is imperative to identify the microbial pathogen.
- Empirical antibiotics should be commenced until the definitive antibiogram of the infection is available.
- Monitor clinical, haematological and radiological responses to treatment.
- The threshold for surgery should be low in the presence of pus in the joint, even if the clinical and haematological parameters are equivocal.
- Surgical intervention within 72 hours of onset of infection yields the best outcome.
- Appropriate investigations, including repeat aspirations for culture, and imaging, should be carried out to determine the cause for the failure of response to antibiotics.
- Protect and splint affected bones and joints during convalescence phase.
- Complications arise due to inadequate, inappropriate or incomplete treatments.
- Remember this when treating NSK infections: "Save the life and save bone".

References

Introduction

1. Ho NK, Low YP, See HF. Septic arthritis in the newborn--a 17 years' clinical experience. Singap Med J. 1989;30(4):356–8. PMID: 2814537.
2. Narang A, Mukhopadhyay K, Kumar P, Bhakoo ON. Bone and joint infection in neonates. Indian J Pediatr. 1998;65(3):461–4. https://doi.org/10.1007/BF02761144. PMID: 10771999.
3. Pittard WB 3rd, Thullen JD, Fanaroff AA. Neonatal septic arthritis. J Pediatr. 1976;88(4 Pt 1):621–4. https://doi.org/10.1016/s0022-3476(76)80022-4. PMID: 943494.
4. Kabak S, Halici M, Akcakus M, et al. Septic arthritis in patients followed up in neonatal intensive care unit. Pediatr Int. 2002;44:652–7.
5. Goldmann DA, Durbin WA Jr, Freeman J. Nosocomial infections in a neonatal intensive care unit. J Infect Dis. 1981;144(5):449–59.
6. Berberian G, Firpo V, Soto A, Lopez Mañan J, Torroija C, Castro G, Polanuer P, Espinola C, Piñeiro JL, Rosanova MT. Osteoarthritis in the neonate: risk factors and outcome. Braz J Infect Dis. 2010;14(4):413–8.
7. Ford-Jones E, Ryan G. Implications for the fetus of maternal infections in pregnancy. In: Armstrong D, Cohen J, Ronald A, editors. Infectious Diseases. London: Mosby International; 1999.
8. Lim MO, Gresham EL, Franken EA Jr, Leake RD. Osteomyelitis as a complication of umbilical artery catheterization. Am J Dis Child. 1977;131(2):142–4.
9. Dessì A, Crisafulli M, Accossu S, Setzu V, Fanos V. Osteo-articular infections in newborns: diagnosis and treatment. J Chemother. 2008;20(5):542–50.
10. Lauschke FH, Frey CT. Hematogenous osteomyelitis in infants and children in the northwestern region of Namibia. Management and two-year results. J Bone Joint Surg Am. 1994;76(4):502–10.
11. Choi IH, Pizzutillo PD, Bowen JR, Dragann R, Malhis T. Sequelae and reconstruction after septic arthritis of the hip in infants. J Bone Joint Surg Am. 1990;72(8):1150–65.

Microbiology

12. Castellazzi L, Mantero M, Esposito S. Update on the management of pediatric acute osteomyelitis and septic arthritis. Int JMol Sci. 2016;17:E855.
13. Perkins MD, Edwards KM, Heller RM, Green NE. Neonatal group B streptococcal osteomyelitis and suppurative arthritis. Outpatient therapy. Clin Pediatr (Phila). 1989;28(5):229–30. https://doi.org/10.1177/000992288902800506. PMID: 2495877.

14. Memon IA, Jacobs NM, Yeh TF, Lilien LD. Group B Streptococcal osteomyelitis and septic arthritis. Its occurrence in infants less than 2 months old. Am J Dis Child 1979;133(9):921–923. doi: https://doi.org/10.1001/archpedi.1979.02130090049009. PMID: 382837.
15. Kalliola S, Vuopio-Varkila J, Takala AK, Eskola J. Neonatal group B streptococcal disease in Finland: a ten-year nationwide study. Pediatr Infect Dis J. 1999;18(9):806–10. https://doi.org/10.1097/00006454-199909000-00012. PMID: 10493342.
16. Yousefzadeh DK, Jackson JH. Neonatal and infantile candidial arthritis with or without osteomyelitis: a clinical and radiographical review of 21 cases. Skelet Radiol. 1980;5(2):77–90. https://doi.org/10.1007/BF00347327. PMID: 6769164.
17. Ward RM, Sattler FR, Dalton AS Jr. Assessment of antifungal therapy in an 800-gram infant with candidial arthritis and osteomyelitis. Pediatrics. 1983;72(2):234–8. PMID: 6866610.
18. Goldmann D, Durbin W, Freeman J. Nosocomial infections in a neonatal intensive care unit. J Infect Dis. 1981;144:449–59.
19. Septic DM. Arthritis in young infants: clinical and microbiologic correlations and therapeutic implications. JO Rev Infect Dis. 1984;6(2):147–55. https://doi.org/10.1093/clinids/6.2.147.
20. Korakaki E, Aligizakis A, Manoura A, Hatzidaki E, Saitakis E, Anatoliotaki M, Velivasakis E, Maraki S, Giannakopoulou C. Methicillin-resistant Staphylococcus aureus osteomyelitis and septic arthritis in neonates: diagnosis and management. Jpn J Infect Dis. 2007;60(2–3):129–31. PMID: 17515648.
21. Rai A, Chakladar D, Bhowmik S, Mondal T, Nandy A, Maji B, et al. Neonatal septic arthritis: Indian perspective. Eur J Rheumatol. 2019; https://doi.org/10.5152/eurjrheum.2019.19052.
22. Deshpande PG, Wagle SU, Mehta SD, Bharucha BA, Irani SF. Neonatal osteomyelitis and septic arthritis. Indian Pediatr. 1990;27(5):453–7. PMID: 2276772.
23. Adeyemo AA, Akindele JA, Omokhodion SI. Klebsiella septicaemia, osteomyelitis and septic arthritis in neonates in Ibadan. Nigeria Ann Trop Paediatr. 1993;13(3):285–9. https://doi.org/10.1080/02724936.1993.11747661. PMID: 7505556.
24. Sreenivas T, Nataraj AR, Kumar A, Menon J. Neonatal septic arthritis in a tertiary care hospital: a descriptive study. Eur J Orthop Surg Traumatol. 2016;26(5):477–81. https://doi.org/10.1007/s00590-016-1776-9.

Risk Factors of NSK

25. Frederiksen B, Christiansen P, Knudsen FU. Acute osteomyelitis and septic arthritis in the neonate, risk factors and outcome. Eur J Pediatr. 1993;152(7):577–80. https://doi.org/10.1007/BF01954084. PMID: 8354317.
26. Devi RU, Bharathi SM, Anitha M. Neonatal septic arthritis: clinical profile and predictors of out¬come. Indian J Child Health. 2017;4:10–4.
27. Liao SL, Lai SH, Lin TY, Chou YH, Hsu JF. Premature rupture of the membranes: a cause for neonatal osteomyelitis? Am J Perinatol. 2005;22:63–6.
28. Knudsen FU, Petersen S. Neonatal septic osteoarthritis due to umbilical artery catheterisation. Acta Paediatr Scand. 1977;66(2):225–7. https://doi.org/10.1111/j.1651-2227.1977.tb07837.x. PMID: 842343.
29. Ish-Horowicz MR, McIntyre P, Nade S. Bone and joint infections caused by multiply resistant Staphylococcus aureus in a neonatal intensive care unit. Pediatr Infect Dis J. 1992;11:82–7.
30. Asmar BI. Osteomyelitis in the neonate. Infect Dis Clin N Am. 1992;6(1):117–32.
31. Coto-Cotallo G, Solis-Sanchez G, Crespo-Hernandez M, et al. Osteomielitis neonatal: studio de una serie de 35 casos. Ann Esp Pediatr. 1990;33:429.
32. Shahar E, Theodore R, Davidson S, Cohen BE. Neonatal Enterobacter Suppurative arthritis and osteomyelitis. Helv Paediatr Acta. 1981;36(6):573–7.
33. Howard AW, Viskontas D, Sabbagh C. Reduction in osteomyelitis and septic arthritis related to H. influenzae type b vaccination. J Pediatr Orthop. 1999;19:705–9.

Pathophysiology of NSK

34. Ogden JA. Pediatric osteomyelitis and septic arthritis: the pathology of neonatal disease. Yale J Biol Med. 1979;52(5):423–48. PMID: 524924; PMCID: PMC2595778.
35. Ogden JA. Changing patterns of proximal femoral vascularity. J Bone Joint Surg. 1974;56-A:941–50.
36. Ogden JA, Lister G. The pathology of neonatal osteomyelitis. Pediatrics. 1975;55:474–8.
37. Trueta J. Three types of acute haematogenous osteomyelitis. J Bone Joint Surg Br. 1959;41:671.

Sites of Involvement of NSK

38. Li Q, Zhou Q, Liu Y, Chen W, Li J, Yuan G, et al. Delayed treatment of septic arthritis in neonates: a review of 52 cases. Medicine. 2016;95(5):1–5.
39. Deshpande SS, Nagda T, Modi N, Singrakhia M. Changing epidemiology of neonatal septic arthritis treatment. J Orthop Surg (Hong Kong). 2004;12(1):10–3.
40. Levy HL, O'Connor JF, Ingall D. Bacteremia, infected cephalhematoma, and osteomyelitis of the skull in a newborn. Am J Dis Child. 1967;114(6):649–51. https://doi.org/10.1001/archpedi.1967.02090270105012.
41. Parmar J. Case report: septic arthritis of the temporomandibular joint in a neonate. Br J Oral Maxillofac Surg. 2008;46(6):505–6. https://doi.org/10.1016/j.

bjoms.2008.01.005. Epub 2008 Feb 20. PMID: 18282642.
42. Martini S, Tumietto F, Sciutti R, et al. Methicillin-resistant Staphylococcus aureus mandibular osteomyelitis in an extremely low birth weight preterm infant. Ital J Pediatr. 2015;41:54.
43. Wang YC, Lin FK, Hung KL, Wu DY. Brachial plexus neuropathy secondary to septic arthritis and osteomyelitis: report of two cases. Zhonghua Min Guo Xiao ErKe Yi Xue Hui Za Zhi. 1994;35(5):449–54. PMID: 7942033.

Signs and Symptoms

44. Omene JA, Odita JC, Okolo AA. Neonatal osteomyelitis in Nigerian infants. PediatrRadiol. 1984;14(5):318–22. https://doi.org/10.1007/BF01601884. PMID: 6472917.
45. Wong M, Isaacs D, Howman-Giles R, Uren R. Clinical and diagnostic features of osteomyelitis occurring in the first three months of life. Pediatr Infect Dis J. 1995;14:1047.
46. Sarlangue J, Castella C, Pontailler J, Chateil J. Neonatal infections of the bone and joints. Archives de Pediatrie. 2007:S108–12.
47. Morrey BF, Bianco AJ Jr, Rhodes KH. Septic arthritis in chil¬dren. Orthop Clin North Am. 1975;6(4):923–34.

Imaging

48. Jaramillo D, Treves ST, Kasser JR, Harper M, Sundel R, Laor T. Osteomyelitis and septic arthritis in children: appropriate use of imaging to guide treatment. AJR Am J Roentgenol. 1995;165(2):399–403.
49. Volberg FM, Sumner TE, Abramson JS, Winchester PH. Unreliability of radiographic diagnosis of septic hip in children. Pediatrics. 1984;73:118–20.
50. Kothari NA, Pelchovitz DJ, Meyer JS. Imaging of musculoskeletal infections. Radiol Clin N Am. 2001;39:653–71.
51. Deshpande SS, Nagda TV, Modi N, Singrakhia M. Changing epidemiology of neonatal septic arthritis. J Orthop Surg (Hongkong). 2004;12(1):10–3.
52. Mah ET, LeQuesne GW, Gent RJ, Paterson DC. Ultrasonic features of acute osteomyelitis in children. J Bone Joint Surg Br. 1994;76(6):969–74.
53. Steiner GM, Sprigg A. The value of ultrasound in the assessment of bone. Br J Radiol. 1992;65:589–93.
54. Aigner RM, Fueger GF, Ritter G. Results of three phase bone scintigraphy and radiography in 20 cases of neonatal osteomyelitis. Nucl Med Commun. 1996;17(1):20–28; 34. Ellefsen BK, Frierson MA, Raney EM, Ogden JA.
55. Mok PM, Reilly BJ, Ash JM. Osteomyelitis in the neonate. Clinical aspects and the role of radiography and scintigraphy in diagnosis and management. Radiology. 1982;145(3):677–82.
56. Jaramillo D, Dormans JP, Delgado J, Laor T. St. Gemme JW. Haematogenous osteomyelitis in infants and children: imaging of a changing disease. Radiology. 2017;283(3):629–43.
57. Pineda C, Espinosa R, Pena A. Radiographic imaging in osteomyelitis: the role of plain radiography, computed tomography, ultrasonography, magnetic resonance imaging, and scintigraphy. Semin Plast Surg. 2009;23:80–9.
58. Montgomery CO, Siegel E, Blasier RD, Suva LJ. Concurrent septic arthritis and osteomyelitis in children. J Pediatr Orthop. 2013;33:464–7.
59. Hunka L, Said S, Mac Kenzie D, et al. Classification and surgical management of the severe sequelae of septic hips in children. Clin Orthop. 1982;171:30–6.

Management Laboratory Investigation

60. Peltola H, Vahvanen V, Aalto K. Fever, C-reactive protein, and erythrocyte sedimentation rate in monitoring recovery from septic arthritis: a preliminary study. J Pediatr Orthop. 1984;4:170–4.
61. Butbul-Aviel Y, Koren A, Halevy R. Sakran W Procalcitonin as a diagnostic aid in osteomyelitis and septic arthritis. Pediatr Emerg Care. 2005;21(12):828–3.
62. Karthikeyan M, Patro DK, Menon J, Hariharan AP, Parija SC, Poduval M, et al. Serum Procalcitonin is a sensitive and specific marker in the diagnosis of septic arthritis and acute osteomyelitis. J Orthop Surg Res. 2013;8:19.
63. Harish P. Early surgical intervention in children with a suspected diagnosis of acute Septic arthritis or osteomyelitis: is it justified? Paediatr Orthop Relat Sci. 2017;3:43–50.

Antibiotic Regimen

64. Afghani B, Kong V, Wu FL. What would pediatric infectious disease consultants recommend for management of culture-negative acute hematogenous osteomyelitis? J Pediatr Orthop. 2007;27:805–9.
65. Peltola H, Paakkonen M, Kallio MI. Prospective, randomized trial of 10 days versus 30 days of antimicrobial treatment, including a short term course of parenteral therapy, for childhood septic arthritis. CID. 2009;48:1201–10.
66. Harik NS, Smeltzer MS. Management of acute hematogenous osteomyelitis in children. Expert Rev Anti-Infect Ther. 2010;8:175–81.
67. Nelson JD. The bacterial etiology an antibiotic management of septic arthritis in infants and children. Pediatrics. 1972;50:437–40.
68. Wang CL, Wang SM, Yand YJ, Tsai CH, Liu CC. Septic arthritis in children: relationship of causative pathogens, complications and outcomes. J Microbial Immunol Infect. 2003;36:41–6; 11. Scoor

RJ, Christofersen MR, Roberson WW Jr, Davidson RS, Rankin.
69. Kaplan SL, Mason EOJr, Feigin RD. Clindamycin versus nafcillin or methicillin in the treatment of Staphylococcus aureus osteomyelitis in children. South Med J. 1982;75:138–42.
70. Jagodzinski NA, Kanwar R, Graham K, Bache CE. Prospective evaluation of a shortened regimen of treatment for acute osteomyelitis and septic arthritis in children. J Pediatr Orthop. 2009;9:518–25.
71. Ceroni D, Regusci M, Pazos JM, et al. Risk and complications of prolonged parenteral antibiotic treatment in children with acute osteoarticular infections. Act Orthop Belg. 2003;69:400–4.

Surgical Approach and Prognosis

72. Ilharreborde B. Sequelae of pediatric osteoarticular infection. Orthop Traumatol Surg Res. 2015;101(1 suppl):S129–37.
73. Fabry G, Miere E. Septic arthritis of the hip in children: poor results after late and inadequate treatment. J Pediatr Orthop. 1983;3(4):461–6.
74. Agarwal A, Aggarwal AN. Bone and joint infections in children: septic arthritis. Indian J Pediatr. 2015:1–9.
75. Parsch K, Savvidis E. Die Koxitisbeim Neugeborenen und Säugling. Diagnose und Therapie [Coxitis in the newborn infant and infant. Diagnosis and therapy]. Orthopade. 1997;26(10):838–47. German. https://doi.org/10.1007/s001320050163. PMID: 9446091.
76. Singer P. Neonatal psoas pyomyositis simulating pyoarthrosis of the hip. Pediatr Emerg Care. 1993;9(2):87–9.
77. Bergdahl S, Ekengren K, Eriksson M. Neonatal hematogenous osteomyelitis: risk factors for long-term sequelae. J Pediatr Orthop. 1985;5:564–8.
78. Kaye JJ, Winchester PH, Freiberger RH. Neonatal septic "dislocation" of the hip: true dislocation or pathological epiphyseal separation. Radiology. 1975;114:671–4.
79. Waters P, Irving J, Letts M. Long-term effects of neonatal bone and joint infection on adjacent growth plates. J Pediatr Orthop. 1992;12(6):806–10.
80. R D Singson, W E Berdon, F Feldman, J R Denton, S Abramson, D H Baker. Missing femoral condyle: an unusual sequela to neonatal osteomyelitis and Septic Arthritis Radiology. 1986;161(2):359–61.
81. Rai A, Chakladar D, Bhowmik S, Mondal T, Nandy A, Maji B, et al. Neonatal septic arthritis: Indian perspective. Eur J Rheumatol. 2020;7(Suppl 1):S72–7.
82. Lee SC, Shim JS, Seo SW, Lee SS. Prognostic factors of septic arthritis of hip in infants and neonates: minimum 5-year follow-up. Clin Orthop Surg. 2015;7(1):110–9. https://doi.org/10.4055/cios.2015.7.1.110. Epub 2015 Feb 10. PMID: 25729527; PMCID: PMC4329523.

15 Subacute Osteomyelitis

Hitesh Shah and Benjamin Joseph

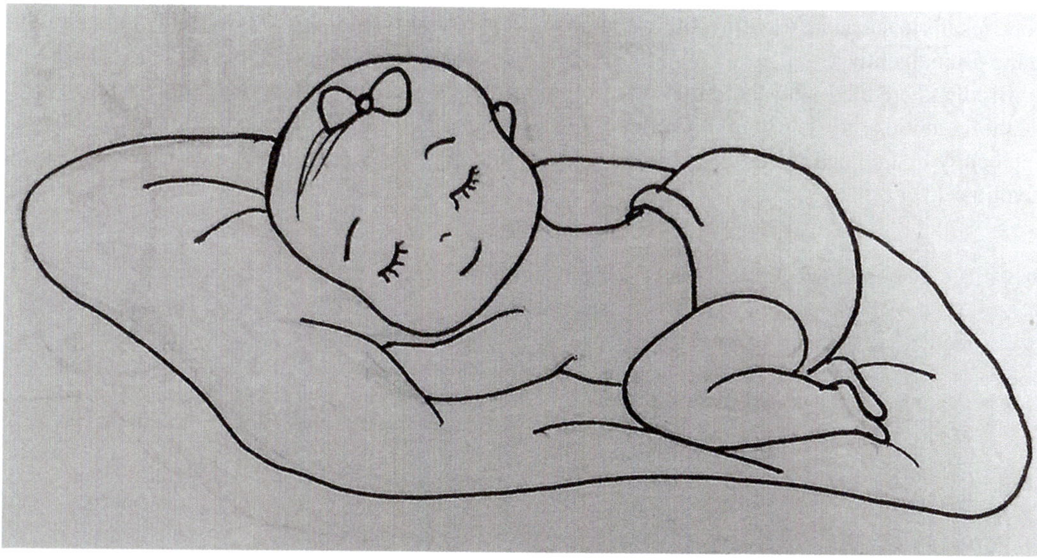

H. Shah (✉) · B. Joseph
Kasturba Medical College, Manipal Academy of Higher Education, Manipal, Karnataka, India

© Springer Nature Switzerland AG 2022
M. V. Belthur et al. (eds.), *Pediatric Musculoskeletal Infections*, https://doi.org/10.1007/978-3-030-95794-0_15

Introduction

Subacute osteomyelitis is an infection of bone with characteristics that distinctly differentiate it from both acute osteomyelitis and chronic osteomyelitis (Table 15.1). The cardinal features of subacute osteomyelitis are mild localized bone pain and tenderness usually of over 2 weeks' duration, absence of constitutional symptoms, a negative blood culture and presence of positive findings on plain radiographs [1].

It is assumed that either because the individual has good resistance or because the virulence of the organism is low, inoculation of bacteria in bone results in subacute osteomyelitis rather than acute osteomyelitis [2–5].

Brodie is credited with the initial description of the condition in 1836 and Billroth in 1881 apparently first coined the term "subacute osteomyelitis" [3].

Pathology and Microbiology

Subacute osteomyelitis usually results from haematogenous spread of the infective organism but may rarely occur by percutaneous inoculation [6].

The strong immune response of the host and low virulence of the organism result in the infection being localized to the site of bacterial inoculation without systemic spread. Frank suppuration often does not occur; instead inflammatory granulation tissue develops at the site of infection.

In conformity with other pyogenic osteoarticular infections, the commonest causative organism is methicillin-susceptible *Staphylococcus aureus* (MSSA) [7] Recently, methicillin-resistant *Staphylococcus aureus* (MRSA) infections are being reported more frequently [8]. *Haemophilus influenzae* type B, *Kingella kingae* and *Mycobacterium tuberculosis* have also been reported [1, 9]. *Kingella kingae* is usually

Table 15.1 Characteristics of acute, subacute and chronic haematogenous osteomyelitis in children

Characteristic	Acute osteomyelitis	Subacute osteomyelitis	Chronic osteomyelitis
Age	Young children	Older children	Older children
Site of infection	Metaphysis predominantly	Metaphysis frequently, epiphysis and diaphysis less frequently	Metaphysis and diaphysis
Onset	Acute	Insidious Does not follow acute osteomyelitis	Follows acute osteomyelitis
Pain	Severe	Mild	Mild
Systemic symptoms (e.g. fever)	Almost always present	Absent	Absent
Loss of function of limb	Present (e.g. unable to bear weight on the limb is lower limb bone is affected)	Absent	Absent
Laboratory investigations	Markedly elevated ESR, CRP	Mildly elevated ESR, CRP or normal occasionally	Moderately elevated ESR, CRP
Blood culture	May be positive	Negative	Negative
Plain radiographs	Normal for first few days	Abnormal at presentation	Abnormal at presentation
Propensity for complications	High	Low	High

encountered in children younger than 4 years of age [9]. *Kingella kingae* and *Mycobacterium tuberculosis* have been identified in subacute osteomyelitis involving the epiphysis [10]. Similarly, *Mycobacterium tuberculosis* may be the causative organism in cases where the lesion crosses the physis [11]. Cultures from lesions of one-fourth of cases are sterile without any organism being isolated; this could be partly due to the fact that 40% of children with subacute osteomyelitis have had an antibiotic for an unrelated infection prior to the onset bone related symptoms [1, 7].

Clinical Presentation and Examination

The mean age of onset of subacute osteomyelitis is greater than that of acute osteomyelitis [12]. The commonest site for subacute osteomyelitis is the metaphysis of long bones and as with acute osteomyelitis, the distal femur and proximal tibia are most frequently affected. Less frequently, it can occur in the epiphysis or the diaphysis of long bones. A few reports of subacute osteomyelitis of vertebrae, pelvis and tarsal bones have appeared in the literature [13].

The commonest symptom at presentation is pain but the pain is seldom severe enough to compromise function of the limb; children with subacute osteomyelitis of the lower limb bones continue to walk. Consequently, an orthopaedic opinion is often sought only after 2 weeks or more. Systemic features of infection are minimal or absent in children with subacute osteomyelitis.

Tenderness is often present at the site of involvement. Occasionally some swelling and warmth may be present. The range of motion of the adjacent joint is usually normal.

Investigations

The white cell count, erythrocyte sedimentation rate (ESR) and the C-reactive protein (CRP) may be mildly elevated or may even be normal [1–4]. Plain radiography is the most valuable investigation with a 96% positive predictive value in the diagnosis of subacute osteomyelitis [3–5, 14]. The radiologic features vary, and on the basis of the location of infection and the radiologic appearances, subacute osteomyelitis was first classified by Gledhill [3], and the classification was modified by Roberts et al. (Fig. 15.1) [4]. The cardinal feature that is common to all types is the presence an area of lucency; the characteristics of the surrounding bone are variable (Figs. 15.1 and 15.2), and they are the basis for these classifications (Table 15.2).

MRI is useful to differentiate subacute osteomyelitis from osteolytic benign and malignant lesions with similar plain radiographic appearances [1]. A characteristic sign, the "penumbra sign", may be seen on unenhanced T1-weighted MRI scans of children with subacute osteomyelitis [15, 16]. It is a discrete peripheral zone of higher signal intensity than the central bony abscess cavity (Fig. 15.3). A thin layer of granulation tissue lining the abscess cavity is responsible for this appearance. Surrounding this zone, there is a rim of lower signal intensity produced by oedema and reactive new bone.

Differential Diagnosis

Conditions other than subacute osteomyelitis that have an area of lucency on plain radiographs (Table 15.2) need to be excluded before embarking on treatment; these include both benign and malignant conditions (Figs. 15.4, 15.5, and 15.6).

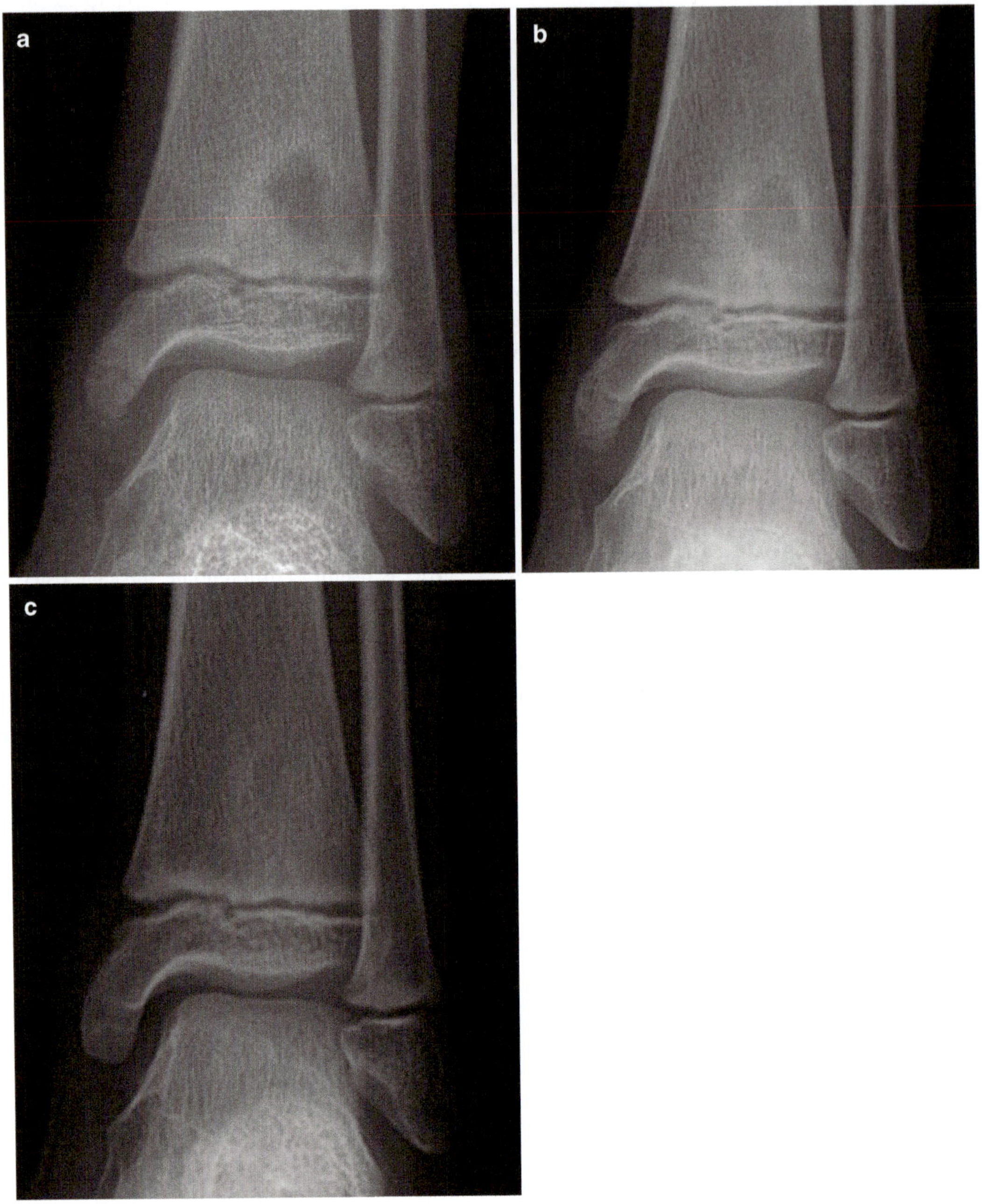

Fig. 15.1 Sequential plain radiographs of a child with subacute osteomyelitis (type II) of the distal tibia. A well-defined radiolucent area is surrounded by a zone of sclerotic bone (**a**) which is best appreciated in the second image (**b**). The lesion is healing and has reduced in size with antibiotics (**c**)

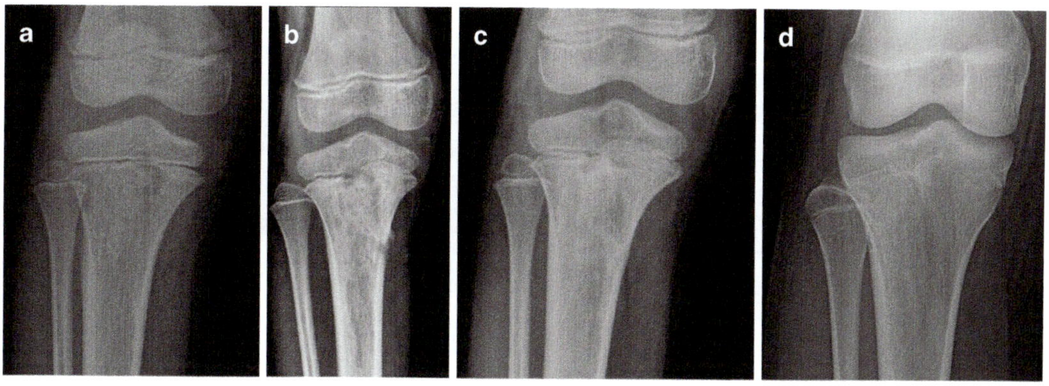

Fig. 15.2 Sequential plain radiographs of a child with subacute osteomyelitis of the proximal tibia. There is an ill-defined area of radiolucency with no surrounding sclerosis (**a**). Biopsy confirmed the diagnosis of osteomyelitis. The infection resolved overtime (**b–c**) without any complication. Nine years later, there is no evidence of previous infection and there is no growth arrest (**d**)

Table 15.2 Radiologic classification of subacute osteomyelitis

Type	Location	Radiologic features	Differential diagnosis
Type IA	Metaphysis	Area of lucency No marginal sclerosis	Eosinophilic granuloma
Type IB	Metaphysis	Area of lucency Reactive bone surrounds lucent area (classical Brodie's abscess)	
Type II	Metaphysis	Area of lucency (often eccentric) Cortical erosion[a]	Osteosarcoma
Type III	Diaphysis	Area of lucency Periosteal reaction[a]	Osteoid osteoma
Type IV	Diaphysis	Area of lucency Sub-periosteal new bone[a]	Ewing's sarcoma
Type V	Epiphysis	Area of lucency	Chondroblastoma
Type VI	Vertebra	Area of lucency	

[a]Biopsy indicated

Establishing the Diagnosis and Identifying the Causative Organism

Establishing the Diagnosis

Establishing the diagnosis in a child with a type IB lesion showing features of a classical Brodie's abscess (an area of lucency in the metaphysis surrounded by reactive sclerosis) and MRI scans demonstrating a penumbra sign is relatively straightforward. However, confirming the diagnosis in the other types may be a bit more challenging, and a biopsy may be needed to exclude a more sinister diagnosis. We recommend a biopsy if there is a cortical breach, periosteal reaction or periosteal new bone formation (see Table 15.2). A needle biopsy should be the technique of choice in all accessible sites and an

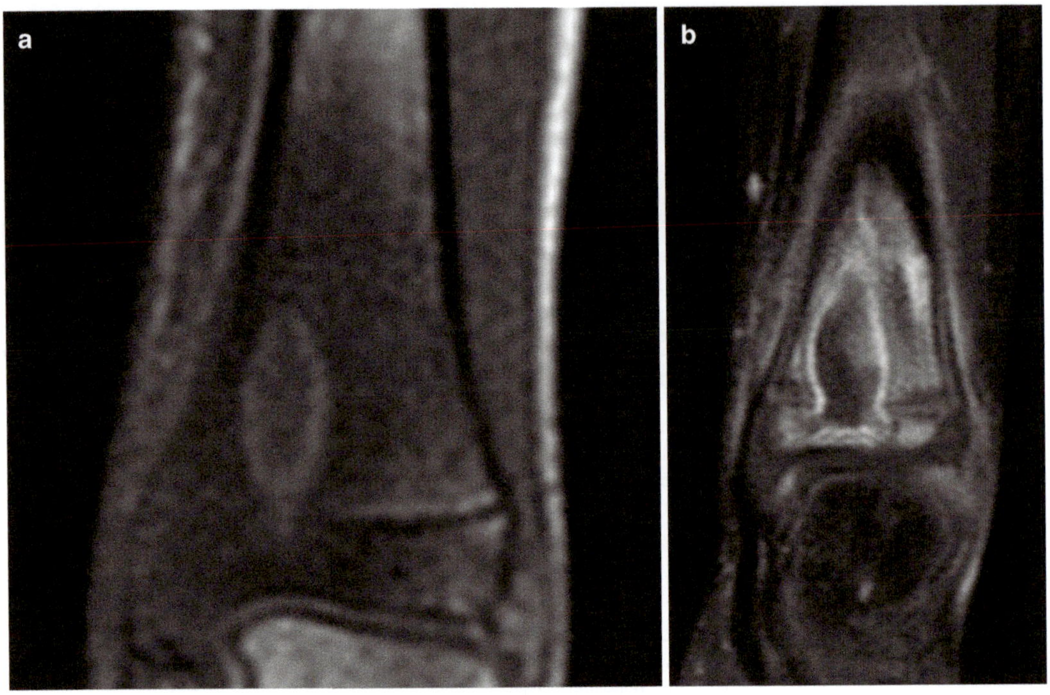

Fig. 15.3 MRI scans of two cases of subacute osteomyelitis of the distal tibia showing the "penumbra sign". (**a**) Involvement of metaphysis, and (**b**) metaphyseal lesion crosses the physis

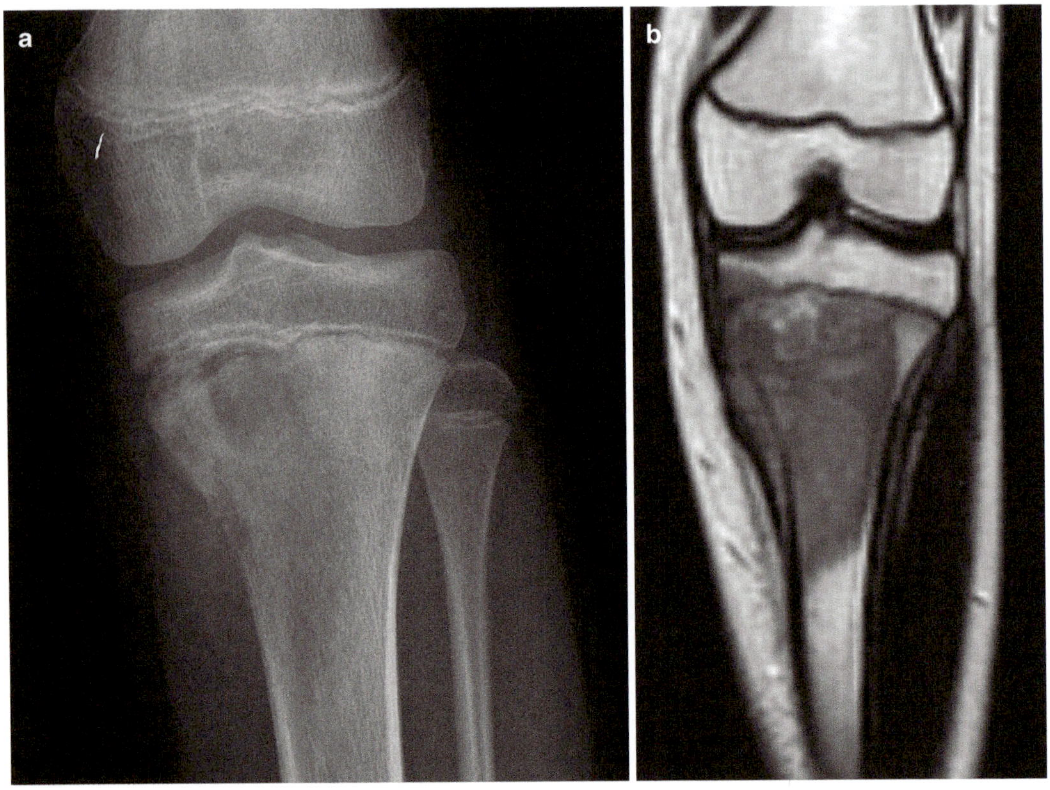

Fig. 15.4 Osteolytic lesion in the proximal tibial metaphysis with a breach of the cortex (**a**) that could be interpreted as osteomyelitis but the coronal T1-weighted MRI scan (**b**) clearly shows that it is an osteosarcoma

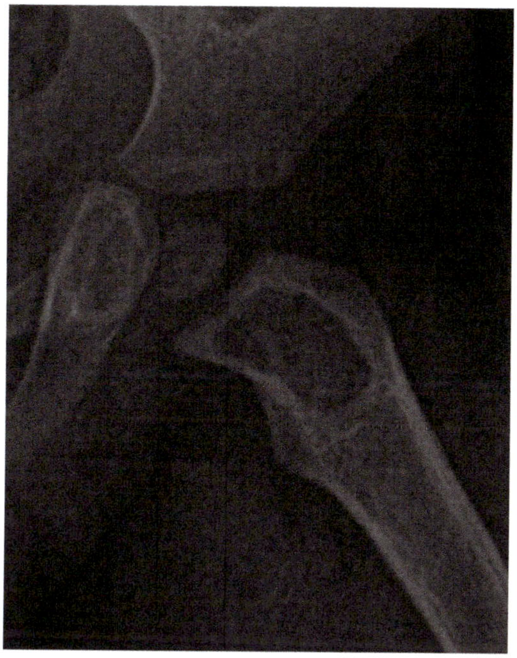

Fig. 15.5 Osteolytic lesion in the femoral neck of a young child. A rim of sclerosis surrounds the lucent area. The biopsy confirmed that the diagnosis of tuberculous osteomyelitis

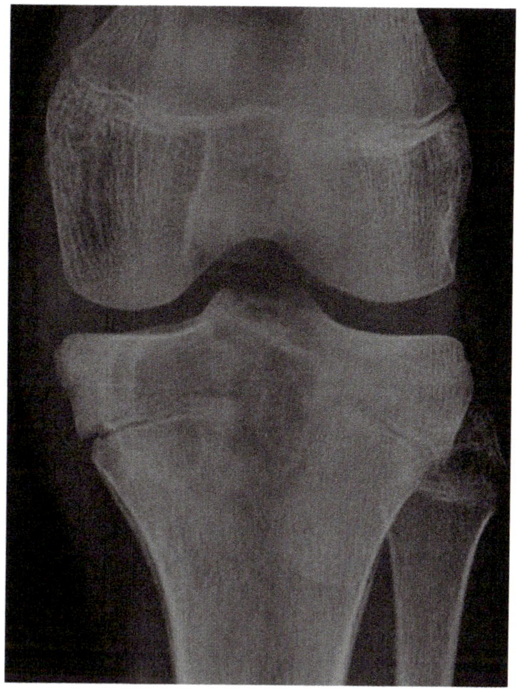

Fig. 15.6 Chondroblastoma presented with an osteolytic lesion involving the epiphysis and metaphysis of the proximal tibia

open biopsy reserved for the rare occasion of a vertebral lesion not amenable to a needle biopsy. A trephine biopsy will enable the culture of any fluid obtained from the area and also provide tissue for examination. The tissue obtained should be sent for both histopathologic examination and for microbiological studies to increase the likelihood of obtaining a positive culture. Despite this, in some cases, the organism may not be cultured.

Identifying the Causative Organism

Needle aspiration and culture of the fluid from the lesion offers the best chance of isolating the causative organism. Apart from routine cultures for pyogenic organisms, the surgeon must specifically request for appropriate special cultures to exclude *Mycobacterium tuberculosis* particularly if the lesion crosses the physis (Fig. 15.7) and culture for *Kingella kingae* if the lesion is located in the epiphysis [9, 17, 18].

Treatment Options

There is no consensus regarding the optimum treatment of subacute osteomyelitis; in particular, the role of surgery is not well defined [3–5, 7]. There are reports that show that a proportion of cases of subacute osteomyelitis can be cured with antibiotics alone [5], and it follows that a trial of antibiotic therapy may be instituted in children in whom an infection is proven and in children with classical features of a Brodie's abscess even without bacteriologic proof of infection. Surgical intervention should be reserved for children not responding to non-operative treatment and for children who have a high risk of a fracture as outlined in the flowchart (Fig. 15.8).

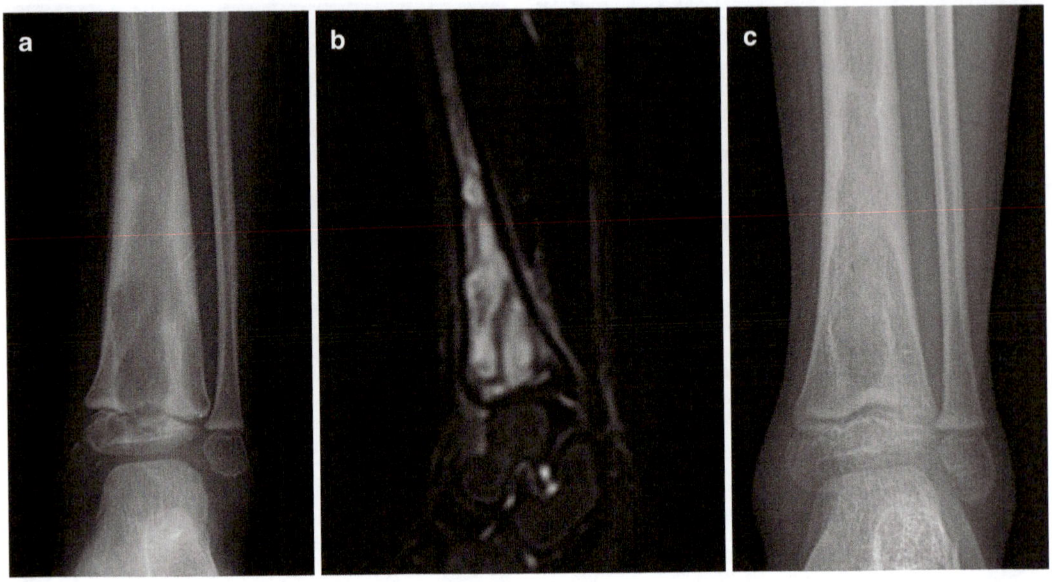

Fig. 15.7 Plain radiograph (**a**), CT scan (**b**) and MRI scan (**c**) of tuberculous osteomyelitis of the tibia. The lesion has crossed the physis but after treatment the lesion healed. The child needs to be followed up till skeletal maturity to monitor for growth arrest

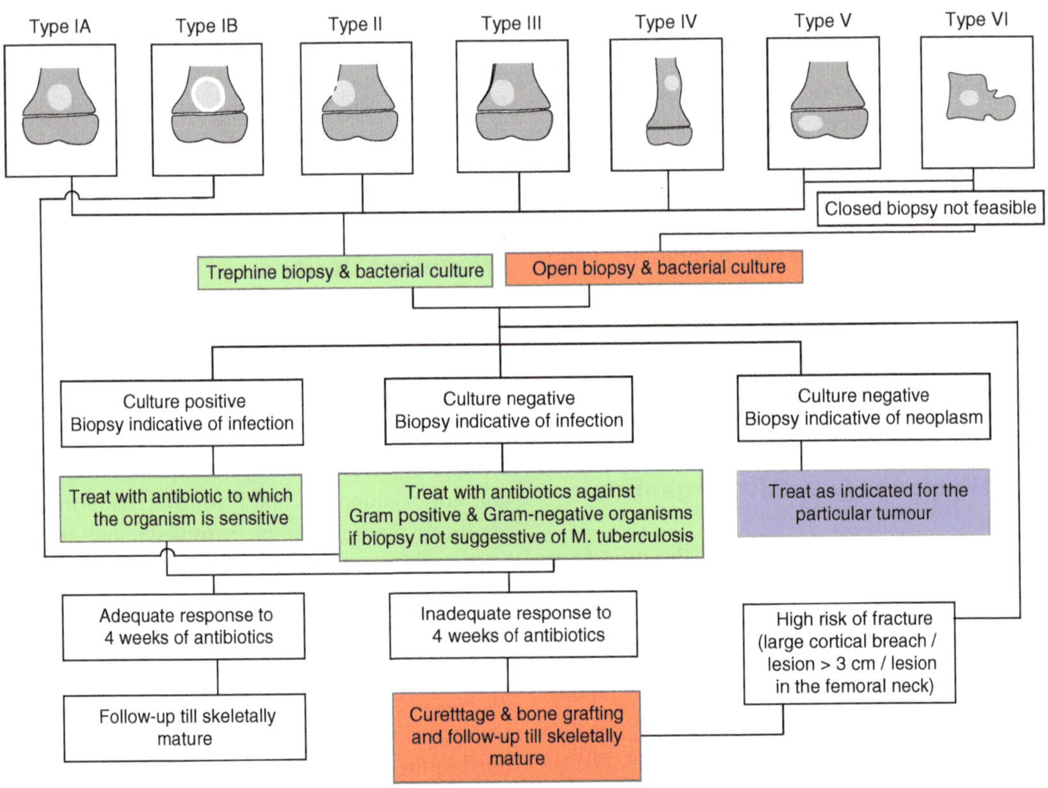

Fig. 15.8 Flow chart showing a summary of treatment of subacute osteomyelitis in children. The red boxes represent surgical intervention and the green boxes represent non-operative intervention

Complications

Complications are infrequent in subacute osteomyelitis [12], and when they occur, they are often not as severe in nature as those that may follow acute or chronic osteomyelitis. Stimulation of the growth plate with increased length of the affected bone and growth arrest with shortening have both been described [13, 19]. Consequently every child with subacute osteomyelitis should be followed till skeletal maturity with yearly weight-bearing long leg radiographs to detect growth abnormalities.

Box 15.1 Key Learning Points

- Subacute osteomyelitis is a low-grade infection of the bone without systemic manifestations.
- The most common site of involvement is the metaphysis of the long bones.
- The most typical symptom of presentation is pain of insidious onset.
- A well-demarcated osteolytic lesion with or without marginal sclerosis is the typical plain radiographic feature.
- Complications are few.

Box 15.2 Tips and Tricks for a Successful Outcome

- Osteolytic lesions suggestive of subacute osteomyelitis must be evaluated with biopsy and culture to confirm the diagnosis.
- A trial of conservative treatment is recommended in all children who are not candidates for surgery.
- Surgery is indicated in children who do not respond to 4 weeks of antibiotics.
- Bone grafting is recommended if the area of lucency exceeds 3 cm, if the lesion is in the femoral neck or if the cortex is severely breached.

Box 15.3 Pitfalls to Avoid

- Tumours and tumour-like conditions must be ruled out in every case of suspected subacute osteomyelitis.
- Every culture must include a biopsy, and every biopsy specimen must be cultured.
- In children with a negative culture for pyogenic organisms, special cultures for *Kingella* and *Mycobacterium* must be performed.
- Children with subacute osteomyelitis must be followed until skeletal maturity to detect subtle growth abnormalities.

References

1. Dartnell J, Ramachandran M, Katchburian M. Haematogenous acute and subacute paediatric osteomyelitis: a systematic review of the literature. J Bone Joint Surg Br. 2012;94(5):584–95.
2. Ezra E, Khermosh O, Assia A, Spirer L, Wientroub S. Primary subacute osteomyelitis of the axial and appendicular skeleton. J Pediatr Orthop B. 1993;1:148–52.
3. Gledhill RB. Subacute osteomyelitis in children. Clin Orthop. 1973;96:57–69.
4. Roberts JM, Drummond DS, Breed AL, Chesney J. Subacute hematogenous osteomyelitis in children: a retrospective study. J Pediatr Orthop. 1982;2:249–54.
5. Hamdy RC, Lawton L, Carey T, Wiley J, Marton D. Subacute hematogenous osteomyelitis: are biopsy and surgery always indicated? J Pediatr Orthop. 1996;16:220.
6. Rajakulendran K, Picardo NE, El-Daly I, Hussein R. Brodie's abscess following percutaneous fixation of distal radius fracture in a child. Strategies Trauma Limb Reconstr. 2016;11(1):69–73.
7. Foster CE, Taylor M, Schallert EK, Rosenfeld S, King KY. Brodie abscess in children: a 10-year single institution retrospective review. Pediatr Infect Dis J. 2019;38(2):e32–4.
8. Chiappini E, Krzysztofiak A, Bozzola E, Gabiano C, Esposito S, Lo Vecchio A, Govoni MR, Vallongo C, Dodi I, Castagnola E, Rossi N, Valentini P, Cardinale F, Salvini F, Bona G, Bossi G, Olivieri AN, Russo F, Fossali E, Bottone G, Dellepiane M, De Martino M, Villani A, Galli L. Risk factors associated with complications/sequelae of acute and subacute haematog-

enous osteomyelitis: an Italian multicenter study. Expert Rev Anti-Infect Ther. 2018;16(4):351–8.
9. Spyropoulou V, DhouibChargui A, Merlini L, Samara E, Valaikaite R, Kampouroglou G, Ceroni D. Primary subacute hematogenous osteomyelitis in children: a clearer bacteriological etiology. J Child Orthop. 2016;10(3):241–6.
10. Yoo WJ, Choi IH, Yun YH, Cho TJ, Cheon JE, Song MH, Chung CY, Park MS, Choi E, Lee HJ, Park KU. Primary epiphyseal osteomyelitis caused by mycobacterium species in otherwise healthy toddlers. J Bone Joint Surg Am. 2014;96(17):e145.
11. El Houmami N, Minodier P, Bouvier C, Seligmann H, Jouve JL, Raoult D, Fournier PE. Primary subacute epiphyseal osteomyelitis caused by mycobacterium species in young children: a modern diagnostic approach. Eur J Clin Microbiol Infect Dis. 2017;36(5):771–7.
12. Blyth MJ, Kincaid R, Craigen MA, Bennet GC. The changing epidemiology of acute and subacute haematogenous osteomyelitis in children. J Bone Joint Surg Br. 2001;83(1):99–102.
13. Pulido PG, Hotchen A, Gojanur A, Corbett J, Stohr KK. Brodie's abscesses can stimulate the growth plate in children. J Bone Jt Infect. 2019;4(6):264–7.
14. Lopes TD, Reinus WR, Wilson AJ. Quantitative analysis of the plain radiographic appearance of Brodie's abscess. Investig Radiol. 1997;32(1):51–8.
15. Grey AC, Davies AM, Mangham DC, Grimer RJ, Ritchie DA. The 'penumbra sign' on T1-weighted MR imaging in subacute osteomyelitis: frequency, cause and significance. Clin Radiol. 1998;53(8):587–92.
16. Davies AM, Grimer R. The penumbra sign in subacute osteomyelitis. Eur Radiol. 2005;15(6):1268–70.
17. Ezra E, Cohen N, Segev E, Hayek S, Lokiec F, Keret D, Wientroub S. Primary subacute epiphyseal osteomyelitis: role of conservative treatment. J Pediatr Orthop. 2002;22(3):333–7.
18. Shah MM, Gupta G, Makadia AS, Rabbi Q. Primary epiphyseal osteomyelitis (PEO) in 18 children: a rare entity with atypical features. J Pediatr Orthop. 2020;40(7):361–6.
19. Stephens MM, MacAuley P, Brodie's abscess. A long-term review. Clin Orthop Relat Res. 1988;(234):211–6.

Surgical Site Infections in Pediatric Orthopedic Surgery

16

Aditya Thandoni and Martin J. Herman

Introduction and Epidemiology

Surgical site infections (SSIs) involve the bacterial invasion of the anatomic space, surgical incision, or tissues and organs directly involved in an operative procedure. SSIs are significant healthcare-associated adverse events that present challenges in patient recovery and subsequently increase the morbidity and mortality rates in individuals undergoing surgical interventions. The US Centers for Disease Control and Prevention (CDC) estimates that 22% of all healthcare-associated infections are due to SSIs [1]. Despite current advances in infection control and treatment, an estimated 110,800 SSIs were associated with inpatient surgeries in all age groups, leading to a 3% mortality rate in 2015 [1, 2]. Seventy-five percent of those SSI-associated deaths are directly attributable to medical complications and sequelae of the primary post-surgical infection [2].

As such, SSIs generate implications in many aspects of healthcare, especially medical expenditures. SSIs are the most costly type of healthcare-associated infections, as they accrue an estimated cost of $3.3 billion annually [3]. Prior studies have shown that each case of SSI can lead to an increase of $27,288 in overall cost, ultimately leading to one million additional inpatient days annually in order to accommodate for therapeutic medical interventions [3]. To address this issue in the USA, the Health Reform Law of 2015 imposed a 1% payback for poor performance and Medicare reimbursement penalties for hospitals with high infection rates in adult patients. SSIs are deemed a persistent but preventable adverse healthcare event leading to difficulties in all aspects of both adult and pediatric care. Therefore, a focus on methodologies and practices that lead to the reduction of SSIs has become a topic of the utmost importance in the literature and current clinical practice [1–3].

This chapter will focus on infections occurring after pediatric orthopedic surgical procedures other than those involving the spine; postoperative infection after pediatric spinal surgery will be discussed in a separate chapter.

SSIs in Pediatric Orthopedic Surgery

The rate of SSIs in the adult orthopedic surgery patients is estimated to occur in about 11% of cases across all types of orthopedic surgery.

A. Thandoni
Drexel University College of Medicine, Philadelphia, PA, USA
e-mail: At978@drexel.edu

M. J. Herman (✉)
Drexel University College of Medicine, Philadelphia, PA, USA

Orthopedic Surgery, St. Christopher's Hospital for Children, Philadelphia, PA, USA

© Springer Nature Switzerland AG 2022
M. V. Belthur et al. (eds.), *Pediatric Musculoskeletal Infections*,
https://doi.org/10.1007/978-3-030-95794-0_16

However, SSIs have shown variability in the different pediatric surgical subspecialties, with reported infection rates between 2.5 and 20% [4]. This may be due to differences attributable to inherent risk factors specific to pediatric surgical patients including multiple comorbidities, congenital anomalies and syndromic diagnoses, hereditary immunodeficiency syndromes, behavioral diagnoses, and nutritional deficits. Even when comparing SSI rates related to specific surgical procedures, other factors, such as longer follow-up time, and hospital differences in pediatric care play a role in exacerbating SSI rates across pediatric sub-specialties [5].

Pediatric orthopedic surgery has its unique set of challenges that lead to SSIs, and wide variability in reported infection rates exists. A study conducted by Chagas et al. identified statistically significant differences for the incidence of SSI in pediatric orthopedic surgery for variables including implant placement (OR = 7.3; 95%CI 1.46–36.3), length of hospitalization (OR = 20.6; 95%CI 3.7–114.2), and postoperative period length (OR = 9.8; 95%CI 1.83–53.0), with an overall 2.88% infection rate [4]. Viquiera et al., in another review of SSIs in pediatric orthopedic patients, reported an overall SSI rate of 2.8%, in a population of 1079 surgical patients, with variation from 2.4 to 4% yearly over the study period [6]. By contrast, Kaabachi et al. described an SSI incidence of 8.3% in a patient population of 458 children [7]. The reported variability among institutions highlights the difficulties of studying SSIs in pediatric orthopedics. A wide variability in diagnoses, patient ages, perioperative factors, infection documentation and reporting, and infection site differences, among other factors, makes determining the precise incidence of SSIs in pediatric orthopedic surgery difficult [3, 4, 6, 7].

Microbiology of SSIs

Staphylococcus Species

The most common organism implicated in SSIs after pediatric orthopedic procedures is *Staphylococcus aureus*. *S. aureus* is a gram-positive aerobic bacterium that is a part of the normal skin biota, asymptomatically colonizing one third of the population. The most common location of inhabitance of both methicillin-sensitive *S. aureus* (MSSA) and methicillin-resistant *S. aureus* (MRSA) is the nares. The ability of *S. aureus* to form biofilms on orthopedic implants and develop resistance to antibiotics enhances the difficulty of eradication after orthopedic surgery [8–10].

S. aureus represents almost 40% of all SSI in pediatric orthopedic procedures with incidence seen most commonly after open reduction of fractures, hip reconstructions, limb amputations, and spinal fusions [8, 11]. While the resistance profile of staph species varies by geographic region, resistance to varying dosages of oxacillin, methicillin, and cefoxitin, among other antibiotics, has been reported in about 1/3rd of isolates across many regions globally [9, 10]. Coagulase-negative staphylococci, such as *Staphylococcus epidermidis*, represent another etiology of orthopedic SSIs, identified in 5–10% of cases in some reports [10].

Propionibacterium Acnes

Propionibacterium acnes is a gram-positive, facultative anaerobic bacteria that can be found in pilosebaceous skin follicles in areas such as the back, chest, and ear [12]. *P. acnes* is an indolent, slow-growing bacteria with low virulence and may play a pathological role in all types of orthopedic surgical infections, especially those that involve surgical implants [12]. *P. acnes*-associated surgical infections are most common when the surgical site is the shoulder or spine, related to the fact that, aside from the face, the dermis of the shoulder areas and back have a relatively high density of sebaceous follicles [13, 14]. Additionally, *P. acnes*, like some other SSI-causing bacteria, also has the ability to form an antibiotic-resistant polysaccharide matrix biofilm [12].

In an effort to reduce the risk of SSIs posed by *P. acnes*, to prevent SSIs, it has been our practice, based on published evidence, to take several steps (Box 16.1) for patients who present with acne, especially when it is visible on at the area of the planned incision [12–14].

Box 16.1 Tips to Reduce SSIs for Patients with Acne

Referral to a dermatologist who can prescribe and monitor a skin care plan, ideally 3–6 months prior to the elective surgery date
The use of chlorhexidine gluconate or other agents with efficacy against *P. acnes*, as a preoperative scrub of the region where the incision will be made for 1–3 days prior to the procedure
Administration of prophylactic antibiotics with effectiveness against *Propionibacterium acnes* 30–60 minutes prior to incision with re-dosing for long cases
Utilizing a fresh knife for deep dissection after the initial skin incision is made to avoid introducing skin flora into the deep soft tissues
Avoid touching of the skin after it is prepped, with glove exchange if concern that skin contamination or perforation has occurred

Other Bacterial Etiologies of SSIs

Other bacterial etiologies of SSIs in pediatric orthopedic surgery, based on a review of the National Ag Safety Database of over 1000 patients, include *Escherichia coli* (9.5%), *Pseudomonas aeruginosa* (10%), *Enterobacter* species (6.3%), and *Enterococcus faecalis* (3.1%). *Klebsiella pneumoniae* (4.8%), *Serratia* species (3.1%), *Viridans streptococci* (0.6%), and *Candida albicans* (0.6%) [11]. Antibiotic resistance of these less common organisms also may be found, especially with *Escherichia coli*, *Enterobacter* species, and *Pseudomonas* isolates. As with the more common staph species-related SSIs, identification of the organism and determining a sensitivity profile so that antibiotic treatment can be tailored to the organism is critical to eradication of the SSIs [11]. A list of the common pathogens that lead to SSIs in pediatric orthopedic surgery can be found in Table 16.1.

Table 16.1 Common pathogens for SSIs in pediatric orthopedic surgery (by order of occurrence)

Staphylococcus species (40%) [8, 9, 10]
MSSA (7.1%)
MRSA (29.3%)
Epidermidis (8%)
Propionibacterium acnes (10%) [12]
Escherichia coli (9.5%) [11]
Pseudomonas aeruginosa (10%) [11]
Enterobacter species (6.3%) [11]
Klebsiella pneumoniae (4.8%) [11]
Serratia species (3.1%) [11]
Enterococcus faecalis (3.1%) [11]
Viridans streptococci (0.6%) [11]
Candida albicans (0.6%) [11]

Refer to citations section for listed references [8–12]

Clinical Presentation and Exam

History

Making the diagnosis of SSIs in Pediatric Orthopedic Surgery may be challenging. These infections present in a myriad of ways based on the timing of diagnosis after surgery, the extent of the infection, and whether an implant is present. A detailed history and exam must include several key details in order to help establish the diagnosis and classify the SSI (Box 16.2).

Exam

The exam starts with obtaining vital signs and a general assessment of the patient's appearance, comfort, and mobility. Evaluation of the entire length of the wound must be performed, taking care to remove all dressings, casts, splints, or braces. Wound inspection for drainage, dehiscence and/or exposed hardware, erythema, and swelling is followed by careful palpation for tenderness, fluid collections, induration, or warmth at both the suture line and in the surrounding tissue [15]. For extremity wounds, the entire limb is examined, assessing for swelling, joint effusions and limited or painful motion, cellulitic streaking, and distant sites of tenderness. Additionally, the surgeon must document the affected limb's neurovascular status and assess for signs of deep vein thrombosis (Box 16.3).

Box 16.2 Key Patient Evaluation Questions

Key questions
1. When was the surgery?
2. Were implants placed? What type?
3. Have you had a fever, chills, or fatigue since surgery?
4. Have you experienced pain at the incision site?
5. Have you noticed any drainage, redness, or swelling at the wound site?.

Box 16.3 Keys to Wound Diagnosis

Key wound findings
1. Wound drainage
2. Wound dehiscence or exposed hardware
3. Tenderness, erythema, or induration around the incision
4. Visible or palpable soft tissue collections or abscess

Diagnostic Evaluation

Serum Markers and Cultures

For patients with a suspected infection, blood work is typically drawn to assist in making the diagnosis, including CBC with differential, ESR, and CRP most commonly. If signs of systemic illness are present, such as fever or chills, blood cultures are also obtained. Wound culture or aspiration after careful sterile skin preparation is also useful in some settings, understanding that superficial skin contaminants may be identified; cultures taken at the time of operative debridement or via image-guided aspiration after sterile prep and drape are more likely to yield positive cultures of the causative organism or organisms [16].

Diagnostic Imaging

X-rays of the site, including the entire limb and the full extent of the implant, are essential. Elevated deep soft tissue planes, bony changes such as lysis or periosteal reaction, delayed bone healing, and implant loosening or breakage are some indications of a potential SSI. Ultrasound is useful to assess for local fluid collections or abscesses. Advanced imaging such as CT, or more commonly MRI, can assess for soft tissue edema, abscess formation, and osteomyelitis, among other findings [15, 17]. Distinguishing superficial from deep incisional SSIs is sometimes difficult. Diagnostic imaging may be useful in distinguishing these types and may also serve as a guide for interventional radiologic techniques or operative planning.

Classification of SSIs

The various SSI subtypes and other differential diagnoses must be considered when evaluating a patient with signs or symptoms of an incisional wound infection. The US Centers for Disease Control defines several subtypes of SSI that are pertinent to Pediatric Orthopedic Surgery (Table 16.2) [1].

Table 16.2 Types of SSIs

1. *Immediate-onset SSI*: Superficial or deep SSIs are defined as those that occur within 90 days of surgery; the subtype is based on the depth of the infection (above vs below deep fascia) and the extent of deep tissue involvement (minimal tissue injury vs soft tissue necrosis or osteomyelitis)
2. *Delayed-onset SSI*: Surgical site infection defined as those that occur between 90 days and 1 year after surgery. These often are seen in conjunction with implants
3. *Late-onset SSI*: Surgical site infection defined as those diagnosed 1 year after surgery. These infections are typically insidious in onset, representing either activation of bacteria that colonized the surgical wound or implants at the time of surgery or a new infection from seeding of the wound bed or implants longer than 1 year after the procedure. Late-onset SSIs are most commonly seen after spinal surgery with implants

Differential Diagnosis

Differential diagnoses include:

1. Sterile wound dehiscence
2. Inflammatory reaction at the wound site related to sutures, (stitch abscess), implants, or dressing materials
3. Subacute osteomyelitis without abscess or soft tissue inflammation
4. Sterile hardware failure (Fig. 16.1)
5. Sterile nonunion

Treatment Options: The Authors' Preferred Methods

Treatment of SSIs is dependent upon the overall medical stability of the patient, the type of infection, and the presence of implants.

Immediate-Onset Superficial Infections

Immediate-onset superficial infections are those SSIs diagnosed within 90 days of the index surgery that are determined to be above the deep fascia and associated with no deep soft tissue injury or deep tissue purulence [1]. For patients with no systemic symptoms, these types of infections may be managed with local wound care and oral antibiotic therapy that covers predominantly staph species, regardless of the presence of implants. Dressing changes with an antibiotic ointment, or other wound care product, can be used for minor dehiscence and drainage. For larger superficial wound separations, or those with drainage, placement of a temporary incisional wound VAC for 4–7 days often obviates the need for surgical wound management (Fig. 16.2). Surgical wound exploration and revi-

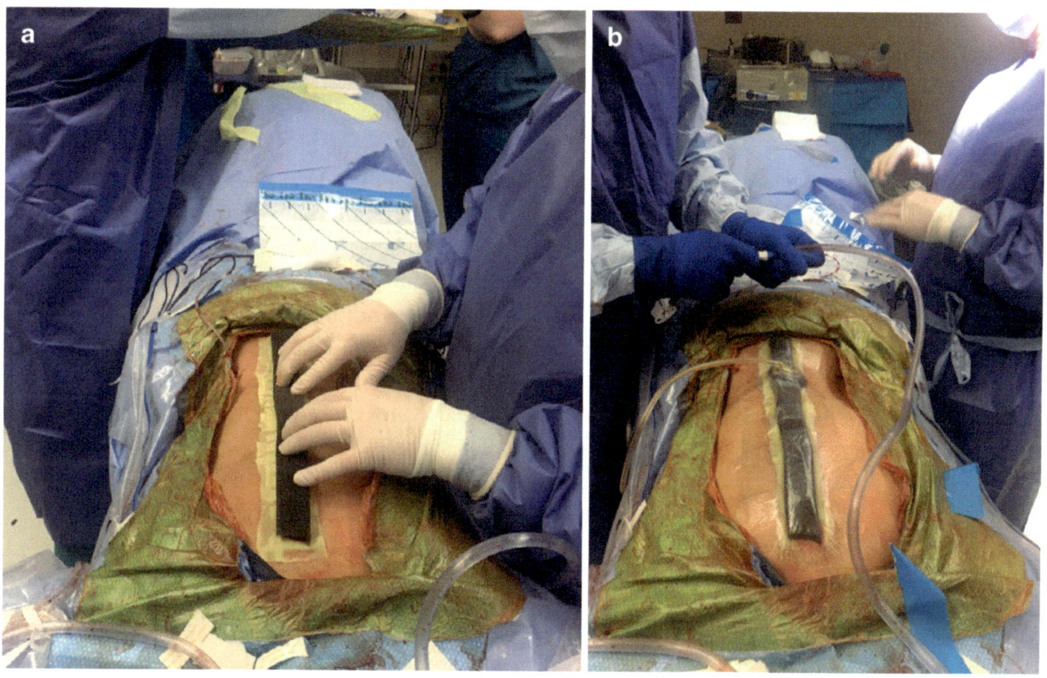

Fig. 16.1 (**a**) An incisional VAC dressing applied to an immediate-onset superficial SSI after spinal fusion. (**b**) Application of the wound sponge to the non-occlusive dressing and sealing of the sponge

sion closure is indicated if VAC therapy is not appropriate due to wound size or availability or if non-surgical means have failed to achieve adequate wound healing [18].

Immediate-Onset Deep Infections

Immediate-onset deep infections are those that are diagnosed within 90 days of the index surgery but are determined to extend below the deep fascia with soft tissue abscesses, tissue necrosis, osteomyelitis, and implant encroachment all possible [1]. Distinguishing this type from its superficial counterpart may be difficult clinically and often demands imaging and surgical exploration to diagnosis. Surgical exploration (I and D) of the wound, evacuation of pus or collections, debridement of necrotic or devitalized tissue, and critical assessment of the extent of the infection at the level of the implant are all components of the surgical procedure. In many instances, implants are salvageable and may be retained. After I and D, closure over drains or use of a VAC device facilitate wound healing. A prolonged course of antibiotic therapy, sometimes as long as 3–6 months, may be indicated if the implant is retained or osteomyelitis was suspected (Figs. 16.1, 16.2, and 16.3).

Delayed- and Late-Onset Deep Infections

Delayed- and late-onset deep infections may be challenging to diagnose because of the delay of symptom onset and the vagueness of the early signs such as fatigue, low-grade fever, or aches [2]. These types of SSIs are approached similarly with a stepwise surgical approach (Fig. 16.4a–c and Flowchart 16.1).

Step 1: Wound Exploration and Debridement

Surgical wound exploration includes obtaining deep tissue cultures, drainage of collections, and debridement of soft tissue necrosis or osteomyelitis as described for the immediate SSI subtypes.

Step 2: Implant Decision-Making

Implant removal, revision, and retention are all options based on the clinical situation. The surgeon ideally makes this decision preoperatively so that the appropriate equipment for removal or revision are available at the time of the debridement. Obviously infected, loose, or broken implants are removed. Implants placed for fracture management, fusions, or osteotomies are also removed if adequate bone healing has been achieved. Revision of implants is indicated when adequate bone healing has not been achieved. Replacement of the infected implant with a sterile implant or alternative fixation choices such as external fixation are the considerations. Retention of implants is occasionally the only option. Implant irrigation and debridement of obvious debris attached to the implant is performed in this scenario. Retention of an implant demands a prolonged course of suppressive antibiotic therapy after surgery. In the face of a serious infection, the surgeon should have an ultimate plan to revise the implants or remove them [19].

Fig. 16.2 (**a**, **b**) Radiographs of a 12-year-old male who presented with an unstable Rt proximal tibia metadiaphyseal displaced fracture following a MVA. (**c**, **d**): Radiographs of Rt tibia showing ORIF Rt proximal tibia. (**e**, **f**) Development of wound infection and skin necrosis 10 x10 cms 5 weeks later, resulting in wound debridement, medial gastrocnemius flap (MGF), and split-thickness skin grafting (STSG). Implants were retained. Infection was not controlled. Clinical photographs 2 weeks later showing persisting infection under the MGF and a discharging sinus. (**g**, **h**) Clinical photographs showing wound debridement, removal of hardware, and a spanning external fixator Rt knee/tibia with application of a wound VAC. He grew coagulase-negative *S. aureus*, *E. faecalis*, and *Peptoniphilus asaccharolyticus*. He was treated with Augmentin and Unasyn for 6 weeks. (**i**) Clinical photographs 3 days later showing soft tissue reconstruction with a gracilis Free flap, STSG, and a spanning external fixator. (**j**) Radiographs after placement of knee spanning external fixator. (**k**) Clinical photograph showing healed soft tissue defect. (**l**) Radiographs after removal of spanning Exfix with healed fracture with good alignment

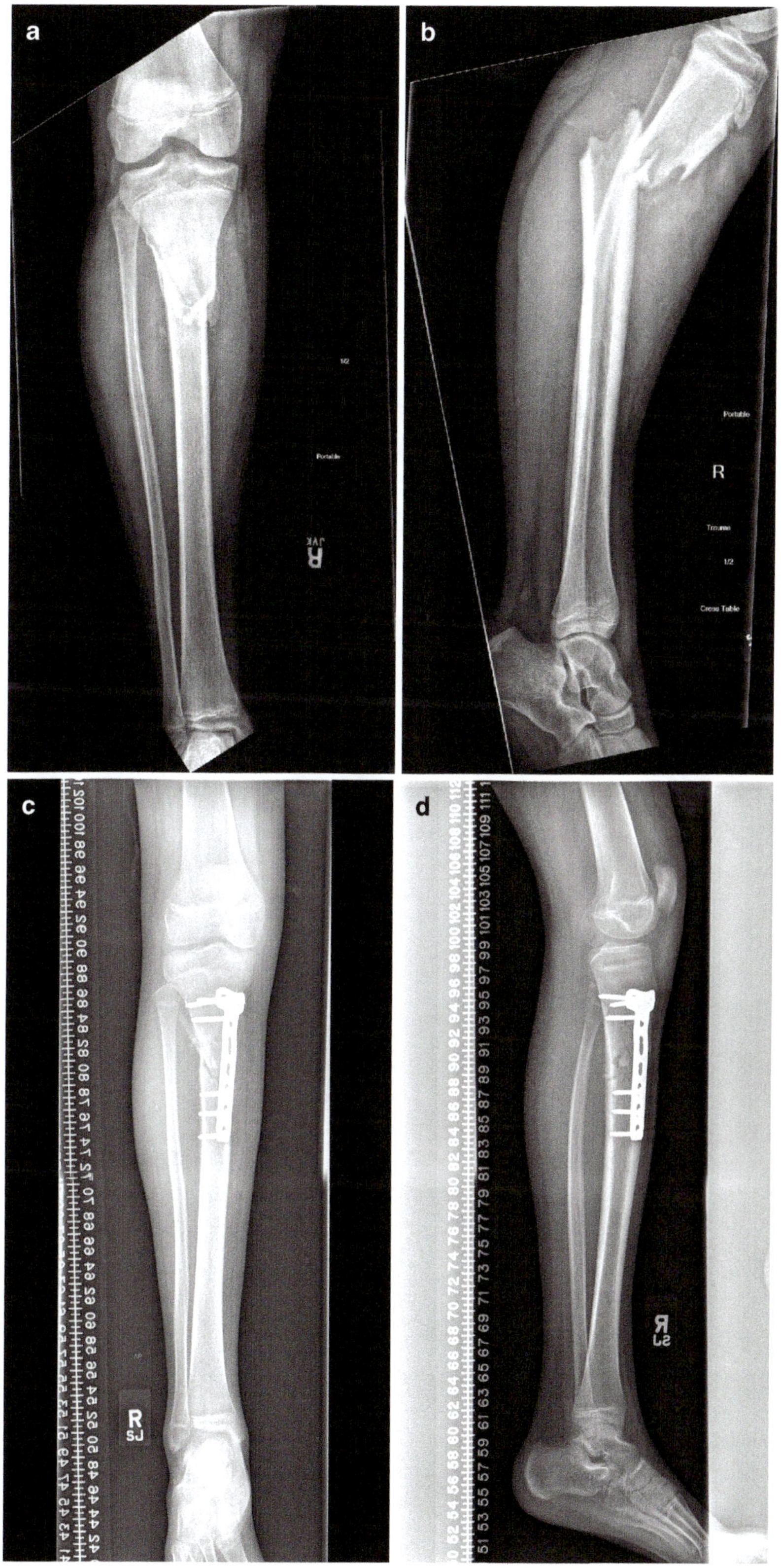
a
b
c
d
Portable
R
R
SJ

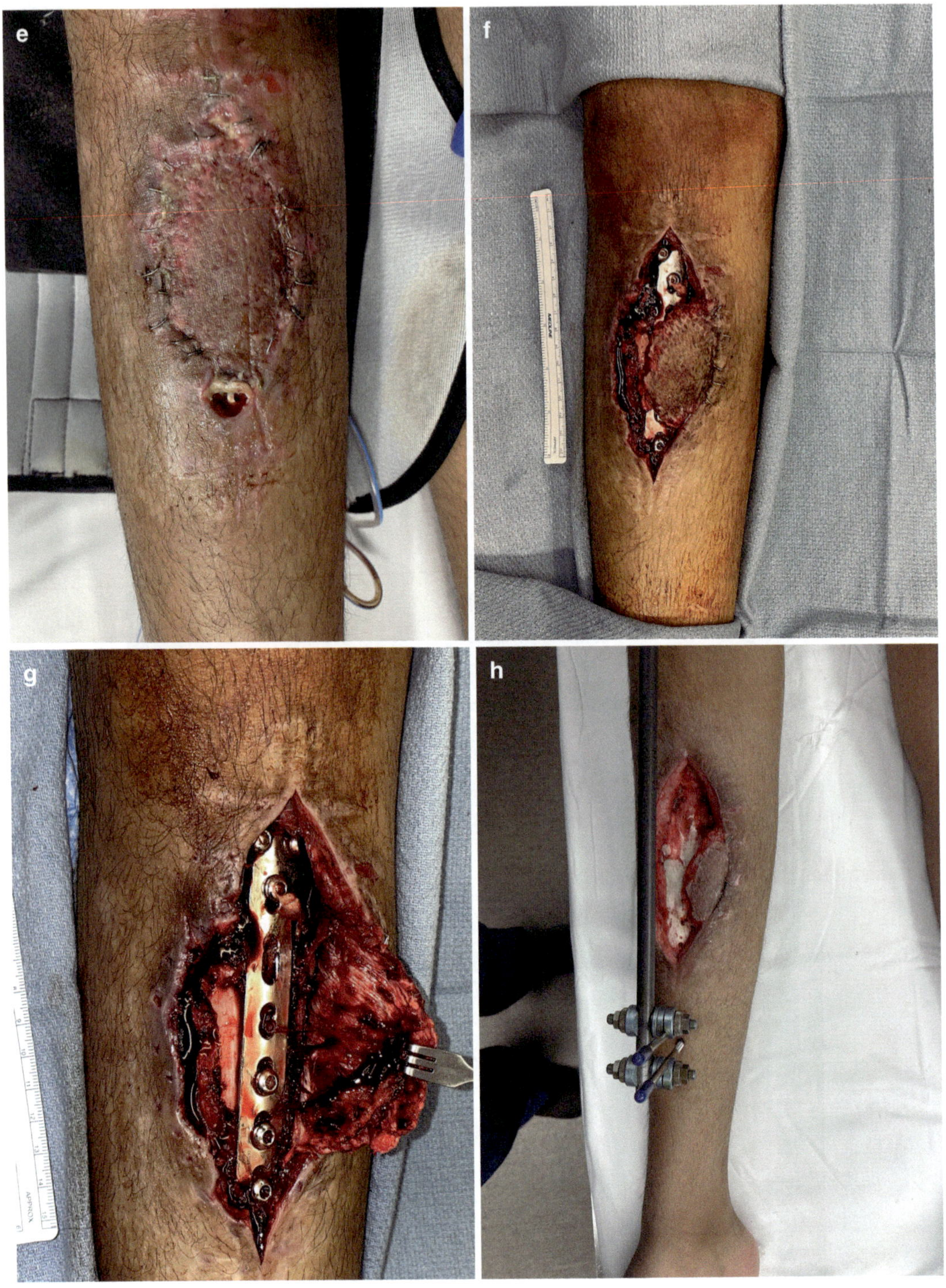

Fig. 16.2 (continued)

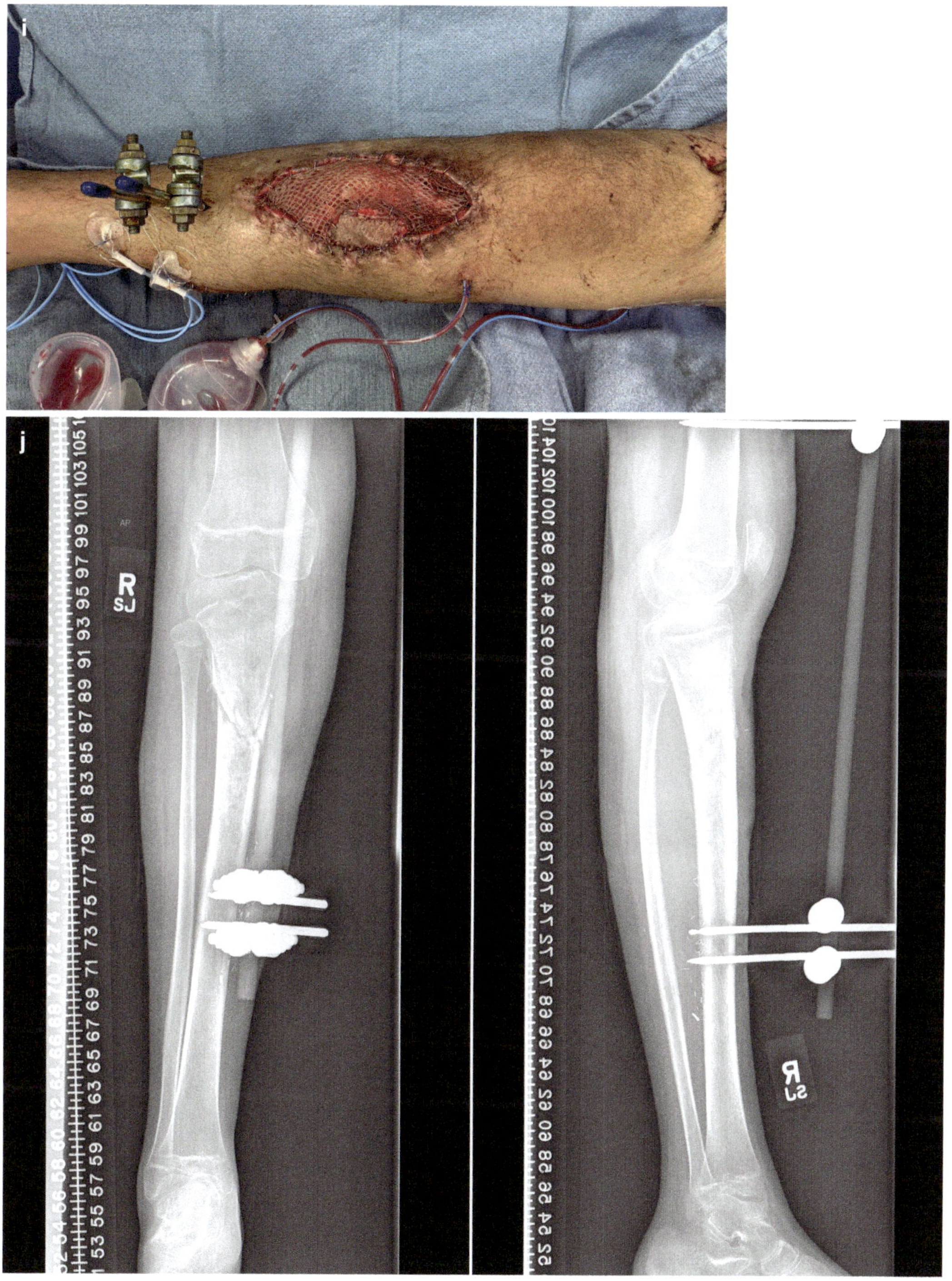

Fig. 16.2 (continued)

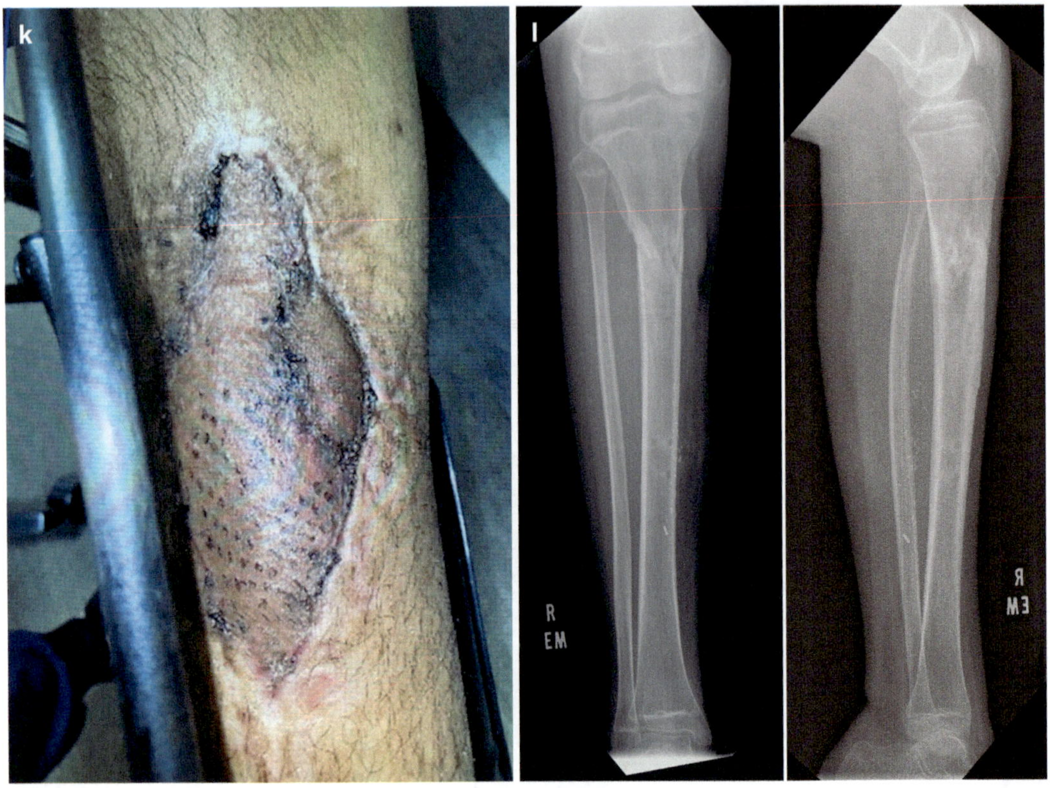

Fig. 16.2 (continued)

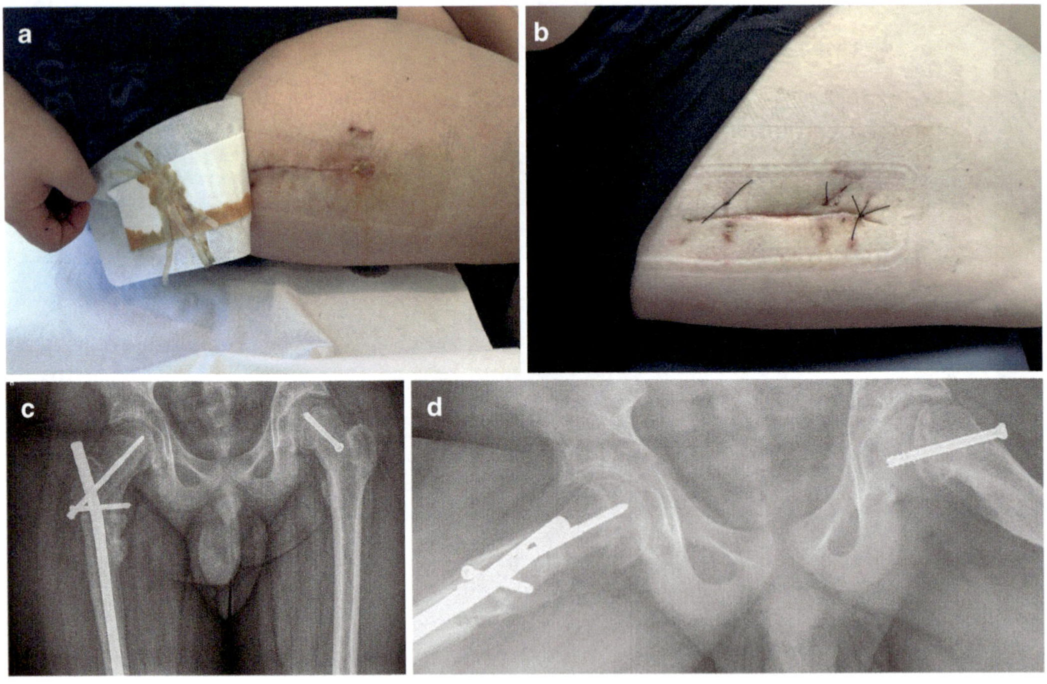

Fig. 16.3 (**a**) Clinical photograph of SSI of nailing a subtrochanteric fracture. (**b**) Post debridement, washout, and VAC treatment. (**c, d**) SSI after nailing with healing callus on AP and lateral radiographs

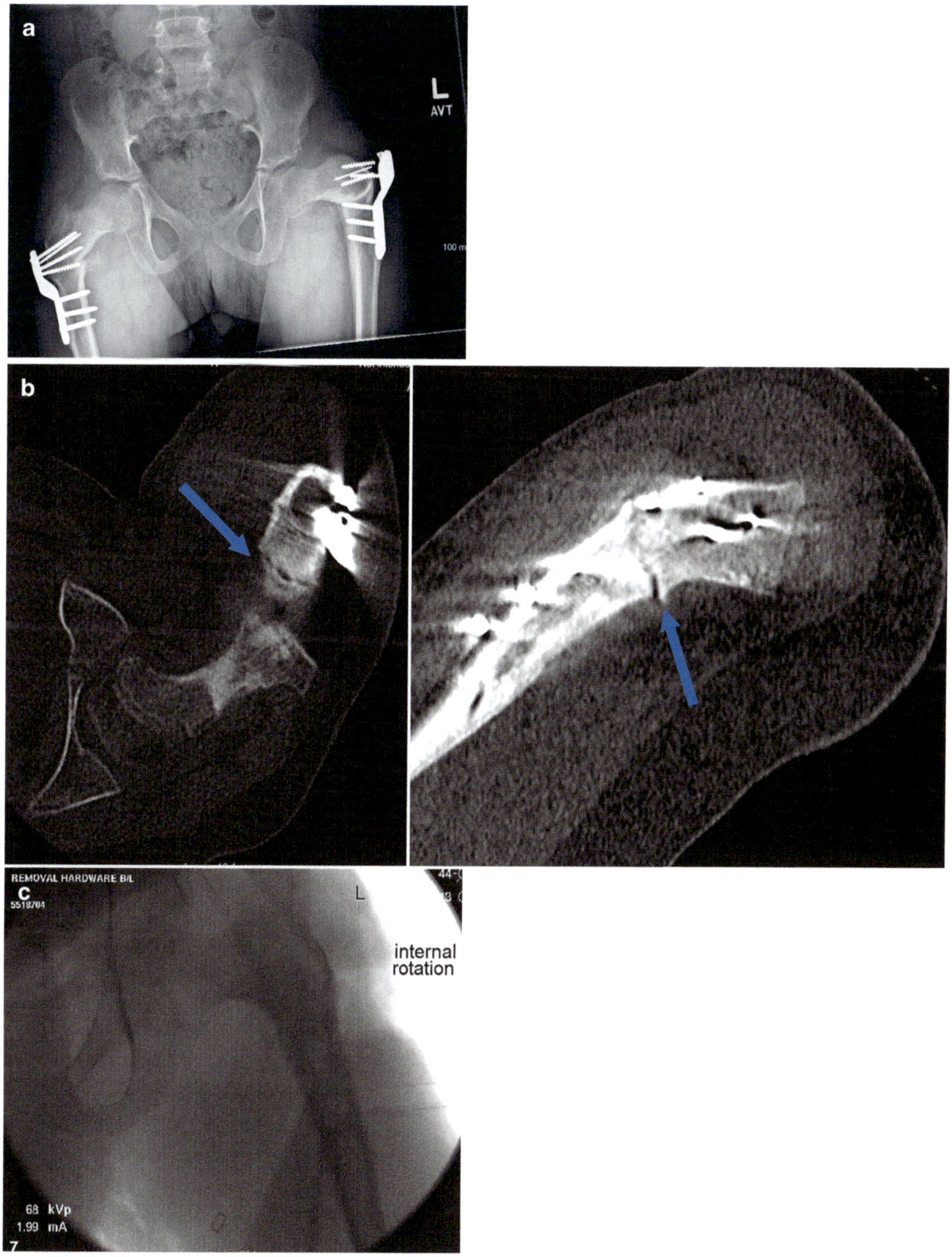

Fig. 16.4 (**a**) AP pelvis radiograph of an 8-year-old boy 1 year after varus osteotomies for spastic hip dysplasia. (**b**) CT scan images in the coronal (**b**.1) and lateral (**b**.2) planes reveal a nonunion. Image-guided aspiration of the site identified no soft tissue collections, and a bone biopsy was negative for infection. The diagnosis of sterile nonunion was made. The patient had a revision of the implant and bone grafting. (**c**) AP fluoroscopic image of the hip during implant removal at 16 months after revision surgery of the nonunion. The osteotomy was healed

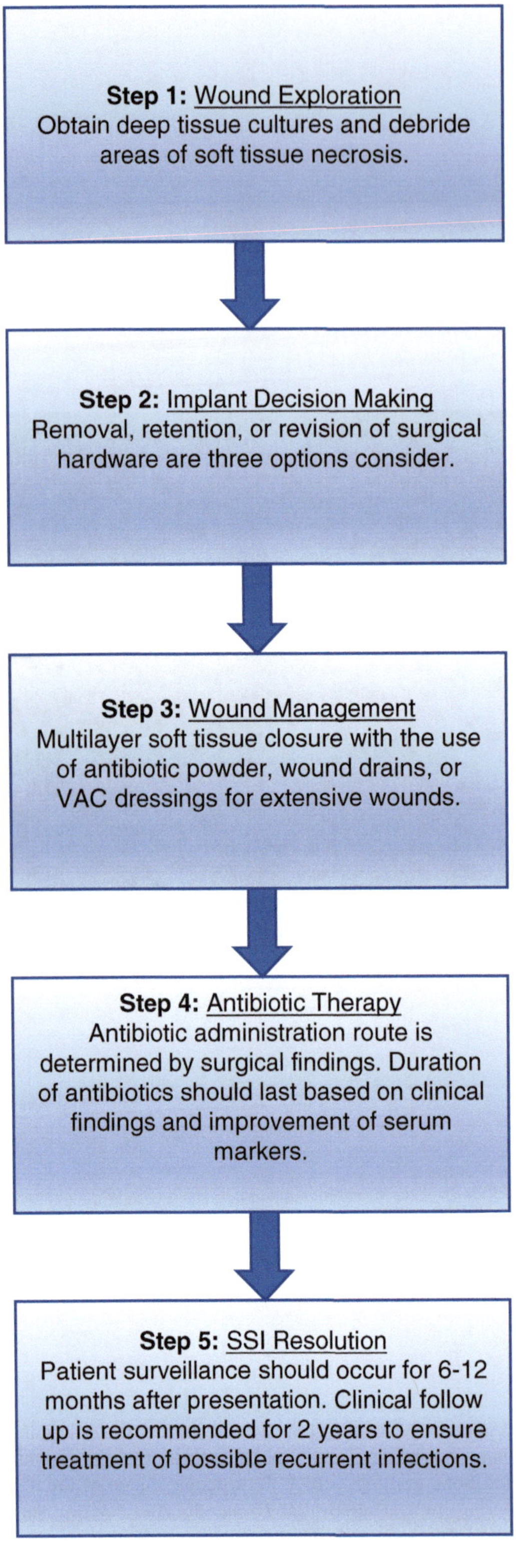

Flowchart 16.1 Stepwise surgical approach to SSIs

Step 3: Wound Management

Meticulous multilayer closure of the soft tissues is critical. The use of antibiotic powder, or placement of antibiotic-coated beads, is controversial and, in our practice, indicated only for managing underlying severe osteomyelitis associated with the infection [20, 21]. Wound drains or VAC dressings are applied after wound closure, depending on the depth and extent of the wounds.

Step 4: Antibiotic Therapy

Empiric intravenous antibiotics are initiated postoperatively, until culture and sensitivities are determined. Duration and route of administration (oral versus intravenous) are ultimately determined by surgical findings, the patient's clinical response, and the improvement of serum inflammatory markers, notably CRP and ESR [2]. In our institution, complex SSIs are managed using a team approach that includes pediatric infectious disease specialists, primary care physicians, nutritionists, and physical therapists, based on patient needs.

Step 5: SSI Resolution

Careful surveillance for recurrent infection or incomplete infection resolution for 6–12 months after the SSI presentation is crucial to successful outcomes. Serial clinical examinations, wound inspection, and trending of inflammatory markers are all aspects of surveillance after SSI treatment. It is our experience that diagnostic imaging can be sometimes difficult to interpret, especially within 3–6 months after surgical debridement because of the secondary changes related to the debridement and subsequent healing; MRI is especially difficult to interpret in these scenarios. Clinical and radiographic follow-up for a minimum of 2 years is recommended to ensure that recurrent infections may be identified and managed in a timely fashion.

SSI Prevention Strategies

It remains controversial if it is possible to make SSIs the so-called never events, i.e., to achieve a zero percent infection rate. The goal for all orthopedic surgeons, however, should be to take all steps possible to avoid postoperative infections, especially for elective cases. Strategies to prevent SSIs fall into two broad categories:

1. Patient modifiable factors:

Health-related variables that can be optimized prior to surgery, many of which are unique to pediatric orthopedic patients owing to their many complex diagnoses and comorbidities.

2. Surgical factors:

Aspects of perioperative management and the intraoperative environment that may reduce SSI risks. These are factors not necessarily unique to the care of pediatric orthopedic patients.

Patient-Modifiable Risk Factors

Nutritional Status

Obesity

Pediatric patients who are obese, characterized by a body mass index (BMI) greater than 30, have an increased risk of SSIs after all types of orthopedic procedures. Blackwood et al. demonstrated that pediatric patients who are obese or overweight, defined as a BMI between 25 and 30, have a 1.23 times increased risk of developing infections after surgery [22]. The most important factors that contribute to increased SSI rates in obese patients include increased operative time, increased wound complications such as dehiscence, drainage and delayed healing, and postoperative difficulties in patient mobilization.

Underweight

Children who are underweight are also at increased risk of SSI. Cies et al. showed that children who were underweight, classified as a BMI less than 18.5, also had a higher risk for SSIs compared to some children who are normal weight or obese [23]. Factors that contribute to SSIs in underweight patients include delayed wound healing and wound breakdown, especially at the site of prominent implants, and the potential for decubiti to develop, which may lead secondarily to infection at the surgical wound.

Nutritional Optimization Prior to Surgery

Obesity

Optimizing nutritional status and achieving a more normal BMI may help to reduce the risk of developing SSIs [24, 25]. Referral of obese patients to a certified nutritionist or a pediatric gastroenterologist for evaluation and preoperative weight reduction is recommended prior to elective pediatric orthopedic surgery. Setting attainable weight goals prior to surgery may be helpful for minimizing postoperative complications, understanding that data to support the success of this strategy is limited, as many obese patients are unable to achieve and maintain weight reduction [26]. Because of this fact, it is our practice for patients undergoing elective surgery to attempt weight reduction strategy but within a finite time limit, typically 3–6 months, such that the pathology we are managing does not progress to a great degree during the process.

Underweight

The significantly underweight or malnourished patient also is at increased risk for SSIs. Wound healing complications can arise in patients who have laboratory abnormalities secondary to malnutrition. For patients who will require implants, while subjective, it is worthwhile to assess the soft tissue coverage at the area of implantation, for example, the skin, fat, and muscle tissue overlying the greater trochanter for a child who is to undergo hip reconstruction with a blade plate. Laboratory studies are also indicated preoperatively. A total lymphocyte counts under 1500, serum albumin levels less than 3.5 g/dl, and a transferrin level below 226 mg/dl are all associated with wound healing impairment after surgical intervention. Individualized nutrition plans should, therefore, be implemented for these patients when elective surgery is planned, with a focus on normalizing markers of nutritional deficiency and achieving weight gain [26]. It is our practice to refer patients who are underweight, or who appear malnourished, to pediatric gastroenterology for evaluation and treatment 3–4 months prior to a planned surgery. Options to consider, in addition to medical management of potential causes of poor intake such as inadequate swallow function or reflux, are adjunctive feeding via supplements to regular meals and temporary or permanent placement of a feeding tube. The decision to proceed with the planned procedure is made after multidisciplinary medical discussion, including the child's caregivers in the decision-making.

Chronic Pediatric Diseases

Patients who are at risk for surgical complications, including SSIs, secondary to medical conditions such as seizure disorders, malignancies, genitourinary disorders, and other illnesses should undergo thorough evaluation prior to any operation. It is our practice to obtain a preoperative clearance and a perioperative management plan from all specialists caring for patients with chronic disease. Many with chronic childhood diseases that require medications with potentially adverse effects on nutritional status and weight, wound healing, or predispose to infection because of secondary effects on the immune response are at increased risk for SSIs. For example, patients with juvenile inflammatory arthritis (JIA) on corticosteroids or disease-modifying anti-rheumatic (DMARDs) medications, who ideally are to continue his or her medications in the perioperative period, must be followed closely for development of wound complications. Corticosteroid use in particular increase the risk of SSIs and impairs wound healing, making it crucial for surgeons weigh the benefit of surgery against the risk of SSI [26]. Diabetes poses an especially challenging problem, especially if it is not well-controlled. Counseling about the importance of tight glycemic control is critical perioperatively so that complications such as poor wound healing and SSIs may be minimized [24–26] Common pediatric diseases that often have treatments and/or disease sequelae that present an increased risk for SSIs are listed in Table 16.3.

Table 16.3 Pediatric conditions with an increased SSI risk

Obesity
Underweight (GI and feeding disorders)
Chronic medical conditions including:
Juvenile inflammatory arthritis (JIA)
Insulin-dependent diabetes mellitus (IDDM)
Seizure disorder
Sickle cell anemia
Genetic immunological conditions
Malignancy
Dental disease
Urinary incontinence

Dental Disease

Pediatric patients with a history of dental disease or oral surgery ideally undergo preoperative dental evaluation as oral bacteria can hematogenously spread and lead to implant infections. This is especially important for children with intellectual disabilities who are unable to perform dental self-care. Proper oral hygiene prior to surgery via dental referrals and patient education can limit this source of infection [26]. In our practice, oral rehabilitation by a pediatric dentist is a component of our preoperative checklist prior to surgery that involves implants such as hip osteotomies or spinal fusion.

Urinary Incontinence

Patients with urinary incontinence who are diapered or require regular straight catheterization, such as the child with spastic quadriplegic cerebral palsy or spina bifida, are at risk for urinary tract colonization or active urinary tract infections. Organisms that thrive in the urinary tract, such as *E. coli*, may be etiologic of an SSI. For these patients, it is recommended that preoperative evaluation includes a urinalysis and clean catch urine specimen for culture/sensitivity analysis. Surgery may proceed in scenarios in which bacteriuria is present without symptoms of urinary irritation or obstruction, the urinalysis is negative for infection, or if patients with bacteriuria present with colony counts of less than 10^3/mL. Patients with count greater than 10^3 should be treated with a postoperative course of an appropriate oral antibiotic [26].

Surgical Factors

Factors controlled by the surgeon also play a crucial role in decreasing the risk of SSIs after pediatric orthopedic surgery. Preoperative considerations such as skin preparation and choice of prophylactic antibiotics, intraoperative factors, and surgical practices and postoperative management choices, such as dressing type, among other things, must be considered in prevention strategies [27–29]. The list of considerations is daunting because so many factors must be taken into consideration, and no standardization exists for even the most routine procedures; a complete discussion is beyond the scope of this chapter [30–33]. Table 16.4 lists some of the surgeon-controlled factors to consider in the prevention of SSIs [18, 19, 34, 35]. Evidence-based decision-making is not possible for many of these variables because adequate studies have not been executed, and therefore controversy exists. It is our recommendation that each surgeon review each step of the perioperative process and make decisions that are best for your patients and care for the environment.

Complications

The sequelae from SSIs vary dramatically in their impact on the patient. Most immediate-onset superficial infections are successfully treated with no sequelae. Immediate-onset deep infections and delayed- or late-onset infections generally present some morbidity and mortality, with these details determined by the extent of the SSI [36–38]. Unplanned repeat surgeries and antibiotic therapy are common to nearly all patients who develop these more serious SSIs. The potential list of complications is included in Table 16.5.

Table 16.4 Perioperative factors to consider for SSI prevention

Preoperative considerations
Skin preparation prior to surgery: Use either chlorhexidine scrub or povidone-iodine [19] hair clipping or shaving: Clipping hair carries only 3.1% of infection risk [18, 21, 22] antibiotic prophylaxis: Given 60 minutes prior to incision [23, 24]
Sterile preparation and draping: Perform adequately in every surgical setting
OR environment
Air quality
Room traffic
Hand scrubbing and gloving
Surgical variables
OR time
Irrigation fluid
Implant types
Antibiotic powder
Post-op dressings
Pediatric orthopedic surgical "bundles"

Table 16.5 Complications of SSIs in Pediatric Orthopedic Surgery

1. Unplanned surgeries
2. Prolonged antibiotic therapy
3. Chronic osteomyelitis
4. Nonunion/pseudarthrosis
5. Limb deformity 2° to growth disturbance
6. Amputation
7. Sepsis
8. Death

References

1. CDC. National Healthcare Safety Network, Centers for Disease Control and Prevention. Surgical Site Infection (SSI) event. CDC: 2022:1–39. https://www.cdc.gov/nhsn/pdfs/pscmanual/9pscssicurrent.pdf. Accessed 01/10/2022.
2. Berriós-Torres SI, Umscheid CA, Bratzler DW, et al. Centers for disease control and prevention guideline for the prevention of surgical site infection, 2017. JAMA Surg. 2017;152:784–91.

3. Schriefer J, Sanders J, Michels J, Wolcott K, Ruddy C, Hanson Jan Schriefer J, Professor of Pediatrics A, of Orthopaedics P, Hanson J implementation of a pediatric orthopaedic bundle to reduce surgical site infections. Orthop Nurs. 36:49.
4. Chagas M, Costa A, PM-RP. Analysis of surgical site infections in pediatric patients after orthopedic surgery: a case-control study. Rev Paul Pediatr. 2017;35(1):18–24.
5. Jones S, Shepherd J, Robinson K, Khandekar SA. Surgical site infection following elective non-spinal pediatric orthopedic surgery: a prospective review. J Pediatr Orthop B. 2019;28(1):89–93.
6. Viqueira AQ, Caravaca GR, Quesada Rubio JA, Francés VS. Surgical site infection rates and risk factors in orthopedic pediatric patients in Madrid, Spain. Pediatr Infect Dis J. 2014;33(7):693–6.
7. Kaabachi O, Letaief I, Nessib MN, Jelel C, Ben Abdelaziz A, Ben Ghachem M. Prevalence and risk factors for postoperative infection in pediatric orthopedic surgery: a study of 458 children. Rev Chir Orthop Reparatrice Appar Mot. 2005;91(2):103–8.
8. Chen AF, Wessel CB, Rao N. Staphylococcus aureus screening and decolonization in orthopaedic surgery and reduction of surgical site infections infection. Clin Orthop Relat Res. 2013;471:2383–99.
9. Garcia DR, Deckey D, Haglin JM, Emanuel T, Mayfield C, Eltorai AEM, Spake CS, Jarrell JD, Born CT. Commonly encountered skin biome-derived pathogens after orthopedic surgery. Surg Infect. 2019;20:341–50.
10. Walrath JJ, Hennrikus WL, Zalonis C, Dyer AM, Latorre JE. The Prevalence of MRSA Nasal Carriage in Preoperative Pediatric Orthopaedic Patients. Adv Orthop. 2016;5646529:1–6.
11. Lake JG, Weiner LM, Milstone AM, Saiman L, Magill SS, See I. Pathogen Distribution and Antimicrobial Resistance among Pediatric Healthcare-Associated Infections Reported to the National Healthcare Safety Network, 2011-2014. Infect Control Hosp Epidemiol. 2018;39(1):1–11.
12. Portillo ME, Corvec S, Borens O, Trampuz A. Propionibacterium acnes: an underestimated pathogen in implant-associated infections. Biomed Res Int. 2013;804391:1–10.
13. Saltzman MD, Nuber GW, Gryzlo SM, Marecek GS, Koh JL. Efficacy of surgical preparation solutions in shoulder surgery. J Bone Joint Surg Am. 2009;91(8):1949–53.
14. Swarup I, Gruskay J, Price M, Yang J, Blanco J, Perlman S, Widmann R. Propionibacterium acnes infections in patients with idiopathic scoliosis: a case-control study and review of the literature. J Child Orthop. 2018;12:173–80.
15. Ruzic A, Gadepalli SK, Gish JS. Surgical Infection. Waldhausen J, Powell D, Hirschl R, (eds). Surgical Infection; Copyright © 2020 American Pediatric Surgical Association. https://www.pedsurglibrary.com/apsa/view/Pediatric-Surgery-NaT/829027/all/Surgical_Infection. Accessed 01/15/2022.
16. Goldstein B, Giroir B, Randolph A; International Consensus Conference on Pediatric Sepsis. International pediatric sepsis consensus conference: definitions for sepsis and organ dysfunction in pediatrics. Pediatr Crit Care Med. 2005;6(1):2–8.
17. Ranson M. Imaging of pediatric musculoskeletal infection. Semin Musculoskelet Radiol. 2009;13:277–99.
18. Halvorson J, Jinnah R, Kulp B, Frino J. Use of vacuum-assisted closure in pediatric open fractures with a focus on the rate of infection. Orthopedics. 2011;7;34(7):e256–60.
19. Foster CE, Lamberth LB, Kaplan SL, Hulten KG. Clinical Characteristics and Outcomes of Staphylococcus aureus Implant-associated Infections in Children. Pediatr Infect Dis J. 2019;38(8):808–811.
20. Kanj W, Flynn J, Spiegel D, Orthopedics JD. 2013 Vancomycin prophylaxis of surgical site infection in clean orthopedic surgery. healio.com. https://doi.org/10.3928/01477447-20130122-10.
21. Prasarn ML, Zych G, Ostermann PA. Wound management for severe open fractures: use of antibiotic bead pouches and vacuum-assisted closure. Am J Orthop (Belle Mead NJ). 2009;38(11):559–63.
22. Cies JJ, Chan S, Hossain J, Brenn BR, Di Pentima MC. Influence of body mass index and antibiotic dose on the risk of surgical site infections in pediatric clean orthopedic surgery. Surg Infect (Larchmt). 2012;13(6):371–6.
23. Cies St Christopher JJ, Chan S, Hossain J, Randall Brenn B, Cecilia Di Pentima M, Randall B, Pentima D, Cecilia M, Digital Commons Jefferson Digital Commons J. Influence of body mass index and antibiotic dose on the risk of Influence of body mass index and antibiotic dose on the risk of surgical site infections in pediatric clean orthopedic surgery. Surgical site infections in pediatric clean orthopedic surgery. liebertpub.com. 2012;13:371–5.
24. Greene K, Wilde A, Arthroplasty BS-TJ of. 1991 preoperative nutritional status of total joint patients: relationship to postoperative wound complications. Elsevier.
25. Dreblow DM, Anderson CF, Moxness K. Nutritional assessment of orthopedic patients. Mayo Clin Proc. 1981;56(1):51–4.
26. Moucha CS, Clyburn TA, Evans RP, Prokuski L. Modifiable risk factors for surgical site infection. Instr Course Lect. 2011;60:557–64.
27. Darouiche RO, Wall MJ, Itani KMF, et al. Chlorhexidine–alcohol versus povidone–iodine for surgical-site antisepsis. N Engl J Med. 2010;362:18–26.
28. Spencer M, Barnden M, Johnson HB, Fauerbach LL, Graham D, Edmiston CE. Perioperative hair removal: a review of best practice and a practice improvement opportunity. journals.sagepub.com. 2018;28:159–66.
29. Iwakiri K, Kobayashi A, Seki M, Ando Y, Tsujio T, Hoshino M, Nakamura H. Waterless Hand Rub Versus Traditional Hand Scrub Methods for Preventing the Surgical Site Infection in Orthopedic Surgery. Spine (Phila Pa 1976). 2017;15;42(22):1675–1679.

30. Al-Habdan I, Corea JR, Sadat-Ali M. Double or single gloves: which is safer in pediatric orthopedic surgery. J Pediatr Orthop. 2006;26(3):409–11.
31. Al-Habdan I, Sadat-Ali M. Glove perforation in pediatric orthopedic practice. J Pediatr Orthop. 2003;23(6):791–3.
32. Nguyen S, McDowell M, Schlechter J. Casting: Pearls and pitfalls learned while caring for children's fractures. World J Orthop. 2016;18;7(9):539–45.
33. Kokavec M, Fristáková M. Efficacy of antiseptics in the prevention of post-operative infections of the proximal femur, hip and pelvis regions in orthopedic pediatric patients. Analysis of the first results. Acta Chir Orthop Traumatol Cech. 2008;75(2):106–9.
34. Parikh SN, Grice SS, Schnell BM, Salisbury SR. Operating room traffic: is there any role of monitoring it? J Pediatr Orthop. 2010;30(6):617–23.
35. Hardy A, Sabatier V, Rosello O, Salauze B, Barbut F, Vialle R. More than just teddy bears: Unconventional transmission agents in the operating room. Arch Pediatr. 2018;25(7):416–420.
36. Tosti R, Foroohar A, Pizzutillo PD, Herman MJ. Kirschner wire infections in pediatric orthopaedic surgery. J Pediatr Orthop. 2015;35(1):69–73.
37. Combs K, Frick S, Kiebzak G. Multicenter Study of Pin Site Infections and Skin Complications Following Pinning of Pediatric Supracondylar Humerus Fractures. Cureus. 2016;3;8(12):e911.
38. Kao HK, Chen MC, Lee WC, Yang WE, Chang CH. A prospective comparative study of pin site infection in pediatric supracondylar humeral fractures: daily pin care vs. no pin care. Arch Orthop Trauma Surg. 2014;134(7):919–23.

Surgical Site Infection in Spine Surgery

17

Anthony A. Catanzano Jr and Vidyadhar V. Upasani

Introduction and Epidemiology

Despite advances in surgical technique, preoperative optimization, and peri-operative protocols in pediatric spine surgery, surgical site infections (SSIs) remain a challenging complication for patients and caregivers and place a substantial burden on the healthcare system. Once diagnosed, SSIs result in hospital readmissions with prolonged stays and require IV antibiotics or multiple revision surgeries and overall hospital charges up to US $10 billion dollars annually across the healthcare system nationally [1–3].

The Center for Disease Control (CDC) has outlined criteria for SSIs, defining a superficial SSI as occurring within 30 days of surgery and involving *only* the skin and subcutaneous tissue of the incision, while a deep SSI may occur within 90 days of surgery and involves tissue layers deeper than the subcutaneous tissue (fascia, muscles, etc.). Patients must either present with systemic symptoms of infection (e.g., fever), or purulent drainage, or have culture or imaging-proven evidence of an abscess or infection [4]. While superficial SSIs may only require a course of antibiotics and local wound care, deep SSIs, especially when there are implants present, require more significant interventions that will be covered in this chapter.

SSIs have been reported throughout all pediatric patient populations, not only those with severe comorbidities and neuromuscular conditions but also in healthy adolescents with idiopathic scoliosis undergoing spinal fusion. In a report from the Scoliosis Research Society (SRS) Morbidity and Mortality Committee reviewing 25,432 pediatric spine surgeries, the overall infection rate was 2.7%; however, other large cohort studies have reported rates as high as 8.5%. Among the different surgical procedures, SSI rates were similar within the pediatric cohort, with the exception of an increased rate in procedures for kyphosis (5.5%) and primary tumors (3.3%) [5, 6]. More recent reports of single institutions with large cohorts have reported consistent rates of deep SSI at 3.6–4.2% [7, 8]. These studies have stratified patients undergoing spinal arthrodesis by underlying etiology. While those with adolescent idiopathic scoliosis had rates of 1.0–2.7%, those with genetic/syndromic scoliosis had rates of infection of 4.2–5.3%, with neuromuscular patients having the highest rate of 10–14.3%.

Surgical characteristics must also be considered, such as surgical approach and instrumentation levels. Posterior-based surgery typically has higher rates of infection when compared to anterior procedures. In 20 years of experience, Janik et al. reported no deep infections associated with an anterior approach, nor has the Harms Study

A. A. Catanzano Jr (✉) · V. V. Upasani
Rady Children's Hospital, San Diego, San Diego, CA, USA

© Springer Nature Switzerland AG 2022
M. V. Belthur et al. (eds.), *Pediatric Musculoskeletal Infections*, https://doi.org/10.1007/978-3-030-95794-0_17

Group, while other reports such as that by Grossfeld et al. reported a deep infection rate of just 1.2% [9–11]. Regarding instrumentation, Mackenzie et al. reported an odds ratio of 3.05 (1.83 to 5.09) of developing an SSI when instrumentation extended to the pelvis [12].

It is critical to note that these numbers do not reflect the rates of those undergoing growth-friendly surgeries, such as magnetically controlled or traditional growing rods, or vertical expandable prosthetic titanium ribs (VEPTR). This population is of particular importance due to the need for multiple planned repeat surgeries, but also the potential for *unplanned* returns to the operating room. Smaller series have quoted a 72–81% rate of at least 1 unplanned return to the operating room, with higher rates among those with syndromic or neuromuscular etiologies. With all factors considered, SSI rates in this young population may be as high as 40%, with the individual risk for infection increasing with each subsequent surgery [13–15].

Pathology and Microbiology

While acute SSIs are theorized to result from bacterial seeding at the index procedure, infections presenting later are more often the result of hematogenous seeding or possibly re-activation of previously seeded organisms incited by local inflammation related to the instrumentation. Mackenzie et al., in reviewing 1347 procedures, found 67% of infections occurred within the first 30 days postoperatively, and 90% were identified within the first 6 months [12]. Either way, once an SSI has been recognized, identifying the causative bacteria is valuable to providing effective treatment.

Specific bacterial species may not only guide antibiotic choices and treatment duration but also indicate an overall prognosis for patients. Both Gram-negative and Gram-positive aerobic and anaerobic bacteria have been described in pediatric spinal SSIs. However, while some studies report culture positivity in >90% of cases, cultures may only be positive in 50% of cases. It has become increasingly important to understand local and regional bacteriograms, including the increasing incidence of resistant strains, in order to better predict potential bacterial sources. In addition to environmental factors, the underlying medical conditions and diagnoses may also play a role in the potential types of causative bacteria. For purposes of this portion of the text, it may be easier to discuss idiopathic, non-idiopathic, and neuromuscular etiologies independently.

Idiopathic Etiologies (See Boxes 17.1 and 17.2 for Case Examples of Idiopathic Etiology)

The most common inciting bacteria reported are *Staphylococcus epidermidis, methicillin-susceptible Staphylococcus aureus (MSSA), Propionibacterium acnes, and Escherichia coli*, with nearly 80% of SSIs in idiopathic etiologies being Gram-positive organisms. Methicillin-resistant *Staphylococcus aureus* (MRSA) was found in ~15–20% of cultures, which is a 100% increase when comparing reviewed cases between 2000–2006 and 2007–2012, demonstrating the increasing burden of resistant bacterial strains which require more aggressive treatment and prolonged courses of antibiotics [8]. It is important to note that while a majority of patients with idiopathic scoliosis had monomicrobial infections, up to 14% of infections may have polymicrobial cultures.

Box 17.1: Case 1: Acute Infection in AIS with Retained Implants

Clinical Scenario: A 13-year-old female with progressive AIS, resistant to bracing efforts, underwent posterior spinal fusion from T4-L2 and was discharged on POD3 with no complications. She presented at 2 weeks for a wound check notable for drainage from her surgical incision.

- Diagnostic Work-up
  - Laboratory work-up: ***CRP 7.1, ESR 83, WBC 12.1***
  - Plain radiographs demonstrated no acute changes to initial correction and implantation.
- Surgical Decision-Making
  - Given the ***wound drainage*** and ***elevated inflammatory markers***, the patient was indicated for irrigation and debridement ***with implant retention*** due to the acute nature and immature fusion mass.
  - Intraoperative tissue cultures obtained, with ***Pseudomonas Aeruginosa*** isolated
- Medical Management
  - Infectious disease specialists were consulted and began treatment with ***clindamycin and cefepime*** while awaiting final culture data.
  - Final culture and sensitivity results showed AmpC-inducible ***beta lactamase resistance*** which may increase the risk of developing resistance to cefepime over time.
  - Given culture data, recommendation was ***IV meropenem for 6 weeks with weekly CRP to monitor response.***
- Overall Outcome
  - Patient is now at 3-year follow-up and recovered well, with no further operative intervention or additional concern and a well healed surgical scar. (Fig. 17.1)

Box 17.2: Case 2: Chronic Deep Infection

Clinical Scenario: A 34-year-old female who is 20 years status post-posterior spinal fusion for adolescent idiopathic scoliosis. Over the previous year, she developed ***left-sided thoracic and lower extremity radicular pain*** and intermittent swelling over her lower-thoracic back.

- Diagnostic Work-up
  - Laboratory tests: a ***CRP of < 0.50 and an ESR of < 10***
  - Radiographs: Intact posterior instrumentation and maintenance of deformity correction
  - ***CT scan (coronal, sagittal, axial images seen in*** Fig. 17.2): Demonstrates findings suspicious for infection including "halo" formation around the T11 pedicle screw. The arrows in Fig. 17.1 images highlight the cystic bony changes, with a sclerotic ring around the pedicle and vertebral body indicative of potential infection.
- Surgical Decision-Making
  - Patient underwent irrigation and debridement and removal of implants
    - Intraoperative tissue cultures: ***P. acnes***
    - Fusion mass assessed intraoperatively and again postoperatively with imaging demonstrating ***pseudoarthrosis and defect within the caudal portion of the previous fusion***.
    - The remainder of the fusion mass was intact, and the patient was treated with implant removal.
- Medical Treatment
  - Infectious disease specialist consulted, and after final cultures and sensitivities, 6 weeks of ***clindamycin*** were recommended with eventual repeat instrumentation and bone grafting.
- Overall Outcome
  - Patient re-instrumented from original levels (T2-L2) with bone grafting (Fig. 17.3)

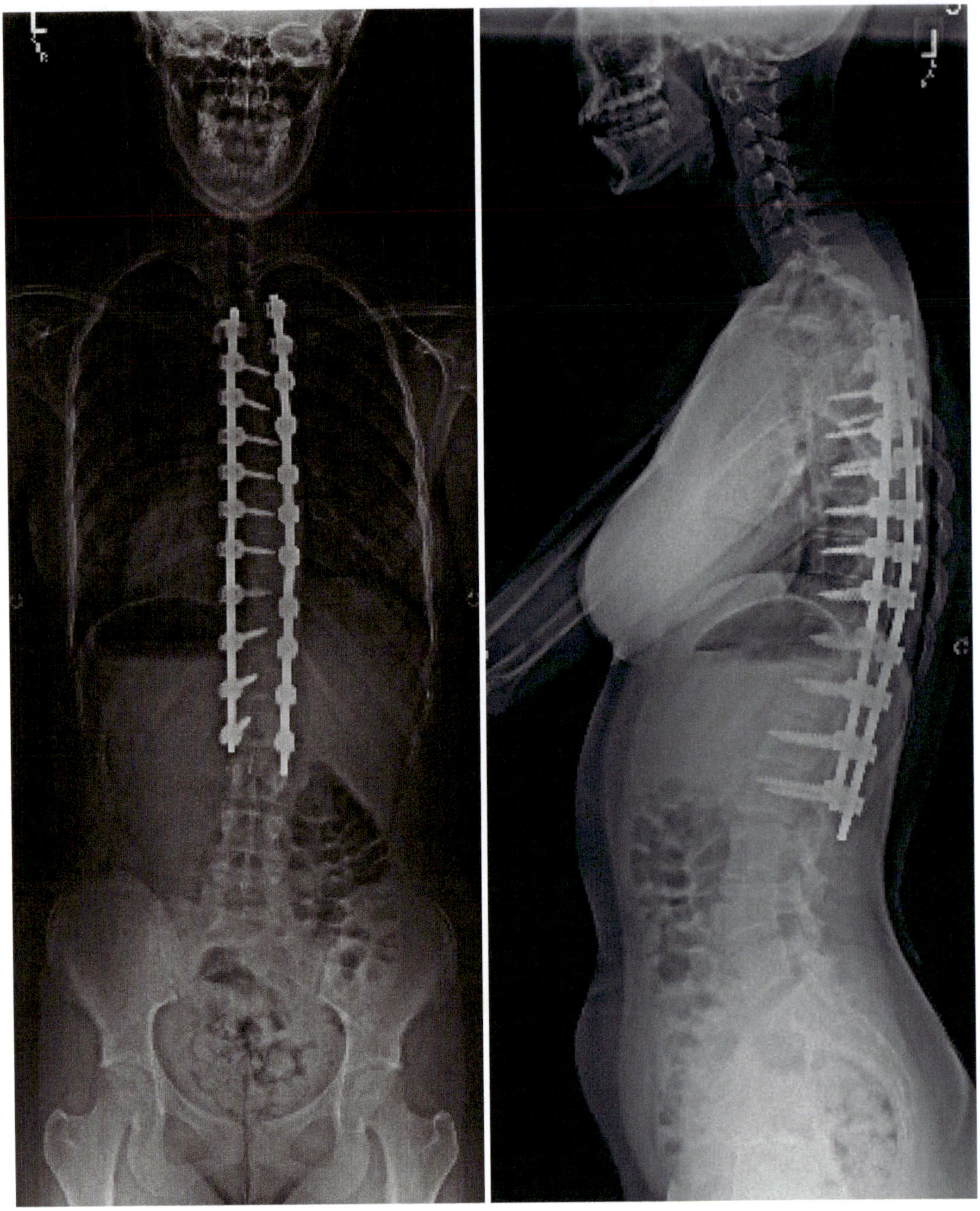

Fig. 17.1 Radiographs at 3-year follow-up after acute SSI and subsequent irrigation and debridement with implant retention

As mentioned above, late developing infections are thought to arise from a new, hematogenous seeding event or, more likely, an exacerbation of low-virulent bacteria at the time of initial surgery potentiated by local inflammation and irritation of surrounding tissue secondary to instrumentation. The most common organism responsible for these late developing infections is *P. Acnes*. *P. Acnes* is an anaerobic, aerotolerant Gram-positive bacteria common among the normal human skin flora, which typically requires >14 days to produce positive cultures. The results of Hahn et al.'s review of 7 cases of late presenting infections in adolescent spine surgery

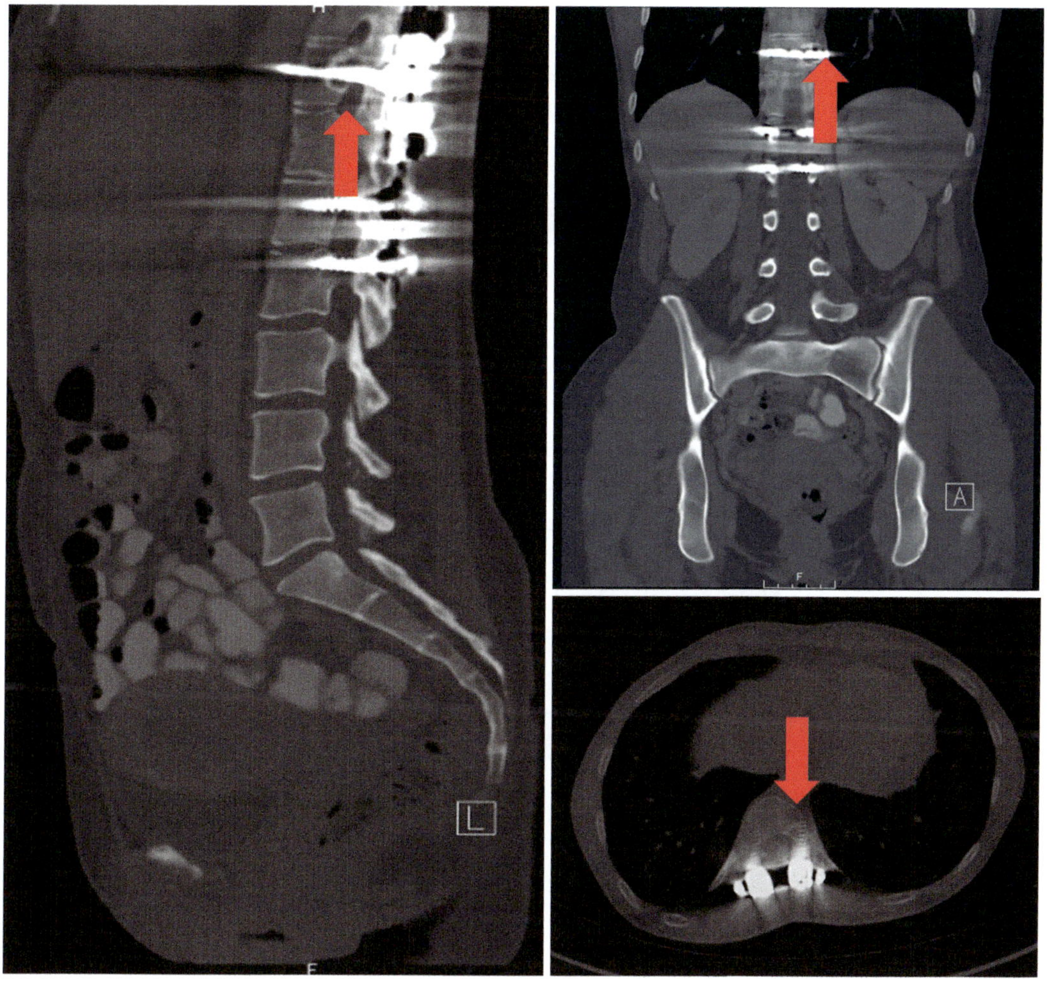

Fig. 17.2 The bold arrows in each image identify cystic changes with a sclerotic border within the pedicle and vertebral body around the pedicle screw, a common finding of loose instrumentation, indicative of potential infection

revealed that all had culture-positive *P. Acnes* infections [16]. These results were further echoed by LaGreca et al., who found the most common causative organism of a late infection, in a review of 42 patients, was *P. Acnes* [17]. The delayed culture results for these bacteria highlight the importance of following cultures for an extended period of time with these late-onset or chronic infections.

Neuromuscular Etiologies (See Box 17.3 for Case Example of Neuromuscular Etiology)

When studying the bacteria involved in neuromuscular patients, a number of patient factors must be considered. Sponseller et al. found the degree of cognitive impairment to be a significant risk factor for deep SSI in cerebral palsy and myelodysplasia patients [15]. In that same study, 52% of SSIs were polymicrobial with the most common organisms (60%) being coagulase-negative *Staphylococcus*, *Enterobacter*, *Enterococcus*, and *Escherichia coli*. These rates are similar to those reported by Mackenzie et al., evaluating a similar but unique patient population. Due to the increased incidence of enteric pathogens, it is likely many of these infections are secondary to contamination of wounds with feces or urine. In Warner et al.'s survey of all pediatric spinal SSIs, 46% were found to be polymicrobial, of which 83% of patients had a diagnosis of

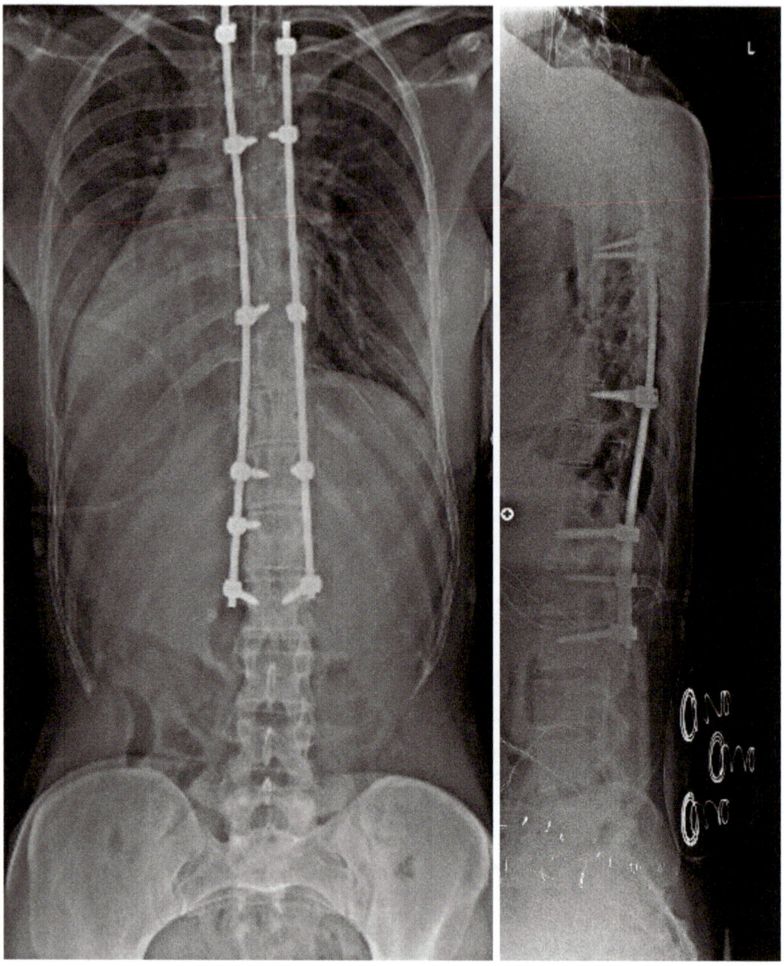

Fig. 17.3 AP/Lateral radiographs of revision instrumentation after clearance of chronic, deep infection

neuromuscular scoliosis, confirming the more diverse nature of bacterial infections in the neuromuscular population [8].

Box 17.3: Case 3: Postoperative Infection in a Neuromuscular Patient

Clinical Scenario: A 15-year-old male with ***myotonic dystrophy*** underwent T2-pelvis posterior spinal fusion. At the 5-week follow-up appointment, the patient had ***reported fevers*** and difficulty with oxygenation.

- Diagnostic Work-up
  - Laboratory tests: ***CRP 34.5, ESR 62***, WBC 11.9
  - CT scan with contrast (Fig. 17.4): Large paraspinal soft tissue fluid collection demonstrated along the lower thoracic spine
  - **Image-guided fluid aspiration performed: +** ***Gram-negative rods***
- Surgical Decision-Making
  - ***Acute surgical site infection (<6 weeks)***
  - Irrigation and debridement performed with preservation of implants
  - ***Negative pressure wound therapy applied***
  - Return to the operating room for ***two repeat debridements*** and reapplica-

tion of wound vac therapy, which remained in place for 6 weeks with bedside changes every 2–3 days.

- Medical Treatment
  - Infectious disease consultants recommended PICC line and ***IV ceftriaxone for 6 weeks*** due to ***Escherichia coli*** growth on initial intraoperative cultures.
  - Due to extensive pulmonary history, the patient's postoperative course was co-managed with the pediatric ***ICU team and pulmonary specialists***.
- Overall Outcome
  - Patient required a 2-month hospital stay due to continued respiratory issues, including a prolonged PICU stay. However, his incision healed without further infection, and once the patient's respiratory status improved, he was discharged home.

Non-idiopathic Etiologies

Similar to the neuromuscular population, patients with syndromic cases of scoliosis requiring surgical intervention have higher rates of SSI with more variability in causative organisms than idiopathic cases. Maesani et al. reviewed 30 cases of SSI in non-idiopathic patients, while *S. Aureus* remained the most common pathogen isolated, and typically as a single pathogen, Gram-negative bacteria were the second most frequent pathogens. Of these bacteria, *Pseudomonas aeruginosa* was most frequently causative and was often found in polymicrobial cultures with a high incidence of third-generation cephalosporin resistance [18]. Understanding this variability and the wide range of potential causative organisms in this patient population, surgeons and infectious disease specialists may then prescribe empiric antibiotic treatment regimens with broader-coverage spectrums until a specific bacterial profile is identified.

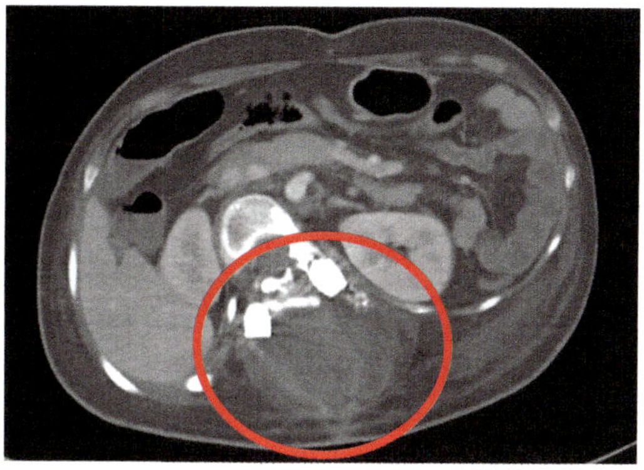

Fig. 17.4 Axial CT scan demonstrating a postoperative paraspinal fluid collection with rim enhancement which is commonly seen in abscess formation

Clinical Presentation and Examination

Not all SSIs will present with a similar constellation of symptoms. While one's suspicion should be increased when patients are febrile or have wound drainage, sometimes the presentation is not as clear and obvious. Typically patients with acute SSIs will have a more classic presentation of infection. Commonly there are superficial skin findings such as peri-incisional erythema, dehiscence, and drainage which may be seropurulent. Superficial fluctuance may also be evident upon further palpation and evaluation. In addition, if more virulent organisms such as MRSA are involved, patients may have more severe systemic findings such as fever, chills, and malaise.

Pain can also be a sign of underlying infection; however, the degree of pain may be variable, and some studies have reported a low incidence of pain as a presenting symptom. Many times in the setting of an acute SSI, the superficial and wound-related signs are more prominent at presentation and a more reliable indicator of underlying infection. However, it should be noted that, with delayed infections, pain after a symptom-free period should clue surgeons in on the potential of an underlying infection.

In review of presenting signs and symptoms for infection after spinal fusion for AIS, Rihn et al. found that back pain was the most common presenting symptom, followed by fullness along the posterior incision [19]. No patients in Rihn et al.'s series presented with fever, and only one patient reported intermittent fevers prior to presentation, demonstrating that delayed SSI may have a more indolent presentation without a robust systemic response.

Investigations and Clinical Work-up

After a thorough physical examination, several initial diagnostic steps should be performed including laboratory work-up to include complete blood count (CBC) to evaluate for an increased white-blood cell count (WBC), basic metabolic panel (BMP) for any electrolyte abnormalities, C-reactive protein (CRP), and erythrocyte-sedimentation rate (ESR) to assess for an inflammatory response which may be indicative of infection.

The interpretation of these studies can be clouded during the initial postoperative period as surgery itself will cause increases in the inflammatory markers. ESR may not peak until 5 days postoperatively and can potentially remain elevated up to 6 weeks. In comparison, CRP will peak closer to 3 days and normalize within 1–2 weeks, making it a more reliable indicator of acute infection in the immediate postoperative period. These values may be increased more so after instrumented surgery but should overall normalize at the same rate. Currently, there are no studies that provide validated expected CRP/ESR levels at specific postoperative timepoints after pediatric spine surgery. When treating neuromuscular or syndromic/non-idiopathic patients with multiple comorbidities, one should always consider additional sources of infection as potential causes of increased inflammatory markers. Pneumonia, urinary tract infections, and gastrointestinal infections may cause increases in inflammatory markers and are common in the immediate postoperative period. Newer biomarkers are currently being studied, such as procalcitonin, absolute neutrophil count, and serum-amyloid-a; however, there is limited evidence to substantiate their standardized use in diagnosis of pediatric spine SSI.

After confirmatory laboratory studies, basic and advanced imaging studies should be ordered to evaluate for any implant, bone, or soft tissue involvement. Beginning with plain radiographs, providers may progress to ordering advanced imaging, including ultrasound, CT scans, and MRIs.

Plain Radiographs

In the acute period after surgery, plain radiographs may not provide any diagnostic suggestion of an SSI. However, in a more delayed presentation, there are several clues that may indicate an underlying infection. In deformity surgery, any loss of correction or signs of instrumentation failure should raise suspicions of an SSI. Furthermore, peri-implant lucencies which may be indicative of loosening due to infection, as well as signs of nonunion and pseudoarthrosis may suggest a delayed infection as a potential cause. While typically the first line of imaging in the diagnostic work-up of SSI, plain radiographs are almost always followed by advanced imaging modalities to better investigate the potential infection or other causes of patients' symptoms.

CT Scan (See Imaging Include in Box 17.2 for Examples of Expected CT Findings)

Advanced imaging may involve CT scans with or without contrast which allow a better assessment of soft tissues compared to plain radiographs; a developing abscess within the paraspinal musculature or an epidural abscess is a finding associated with SSIs of the spine. The addition of contrast agents allows for improved specificity and sensitivity when identifying potential abscesses and fluid collections that may be present in an SSI. Further signs of SSI on CT include cystic bony changes, gas within the disc spaces, endplate osteolysis, and paravertebral soft tissue swelling. While CT myelograms have become less commonplace, there are certain scenarios in which they are a useful tool in the evaluation of an underlying infection. Patients with instrumentation that is not MRI-compatible or who have pacemakers, defibrillators, cochlear implants, or other contraindicated devices may need a myelogram to truly assess intraspinal infections [20].

More importantly than soft tissue evaluation, which would be more reliable with an MRI, CT allows for a detailed assessment of the underlying bone and fusion mass. If evaluating for pseudoarthrosis or nonunion, CT offers more distinct detail than plain radiographs. As will be discussed later, CT scans are essential in the decision-making of delayed SSIs when determining the need for implant removal. Evaluation of the fusion mass must be considered before removing implants in order to ensure the patient will be left with a stable spine if implants are not retained.

MRI (See Box 17.4 for Case Example of MRI Imaging in Spine SSI)

MRI remains the gold standard for evaluation of postoperative spinal SSIs despite the interference of compatible implants. The sensitivity and specificity are further enhanced with the addition of gadolinium contrast with reported values of 93% and 96% respectively [20]. MRI offers improved soft tissue contrast and higher accuracy in differentiating infection from other potential differential diagnoses, such as degeneration and neoplastic conditions. The most common findings include abscesses within the paraspinal muscles (93%) and subcutaneous fat (62.8%) as well as within laminectomy sites if performed (67.4%). The addition of contrast leads to peripheral or diffuse enhancement of abscesses and may also highlight the "pedicle screw fluid sign" in which fluid is seen outside the head of a pedicle screw on axial images.

Box 17.4: Case 4: Intradural Abscess after Lumbar Discectomy

Clinical Scenario: An 18-year-old male with L4–5 disc herniation and left-sided radicular leg pain who failed all conservative therapies was indicated for L4–5 bilateral laminotomies and discectomy. At 2-week follow-up, the patient had a wound dehiscence and continued drainage; he underwent serial irrigation and debridements, in which a dural tear was noted and repaired. After initial improvement, the patient became febrile with an **increase in CRP.**

- Diagnostic Work-up
  - Laboratory work-up: ***CRP 17.4 (from 6.5)***, WBC 8.3
  - ***Full spine MRI obtained*** (Fig. 17.5)
    - Fluid collection within the epidural space identified with ***surrounding enhancement*** and compression of the conus medullaris and cauda equina. Also, note the irregular endplates and abnormal disc space concerning for additional osteomyelitis and discitis.
- Surgical Decision-Making
  - Return to the operating room for irrigation and debridement with bilateral laminectomies T12-L3 and intradural debridement.
  - Initial wound vac placement followed by delayed primary wound closure by ***plastic surgery team*** (Fig. 17.6).
- Medical Treatment
  - Intraoperative cultures: ***Enterobacter aerogenes, Candida albicans***
  - ***Infectious disease specialist consulted:*** PICC line initiated with 6 weeks of IV ***meropenem/fluconazole***
  - Serial CRP measurements were followed for assessment of response. Patient was discharged on antibiotics and seen weekly for continued lab and clinical assessment.
  - Repeat MRI imaging completed before discharge to ensure no continued abscess
- Overall Outcome
  - At 1-year follow-up, the wound had healed, with no radicular symptoms or paraspinal back pain with return to normal activities and no repeat infections or admissions/surgeries.

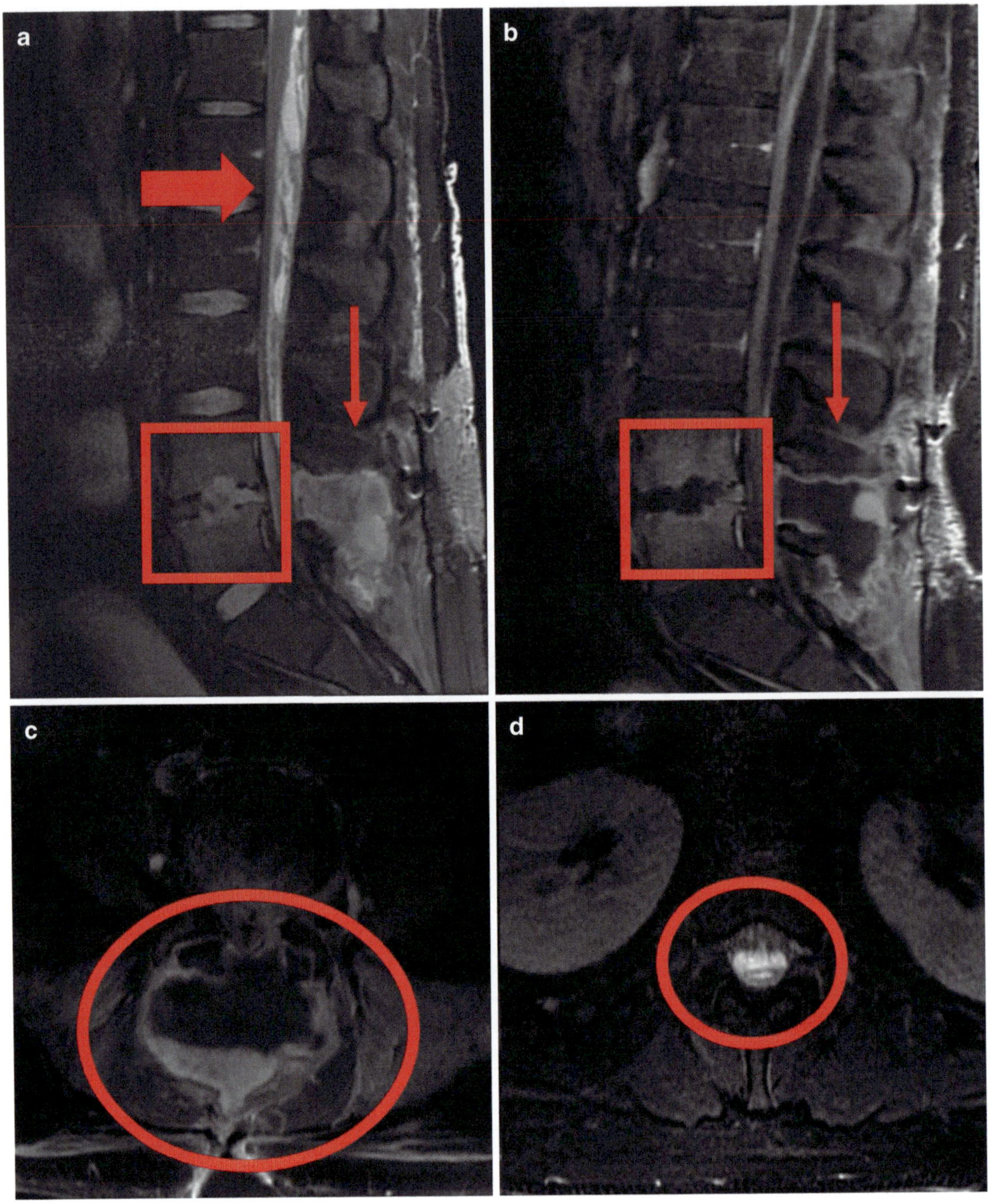

Fig. 17.5 Boxes seen in images (**a** and **b**) highlight endplate destruction seen in cases of discitis and vertebral osteomyelitis. The thick arrow in image (**a**) shows increased intradural signal and enhancement showing abscess formation. The thin arrows in image (**a** and **b**) correspond to the fluid collection outline in image (**c**) with rim enhancement within the paraspinal musculature. Image (**d**) highlights again the increase signal within the intradural abscess that can be clearly seen on axial imaging

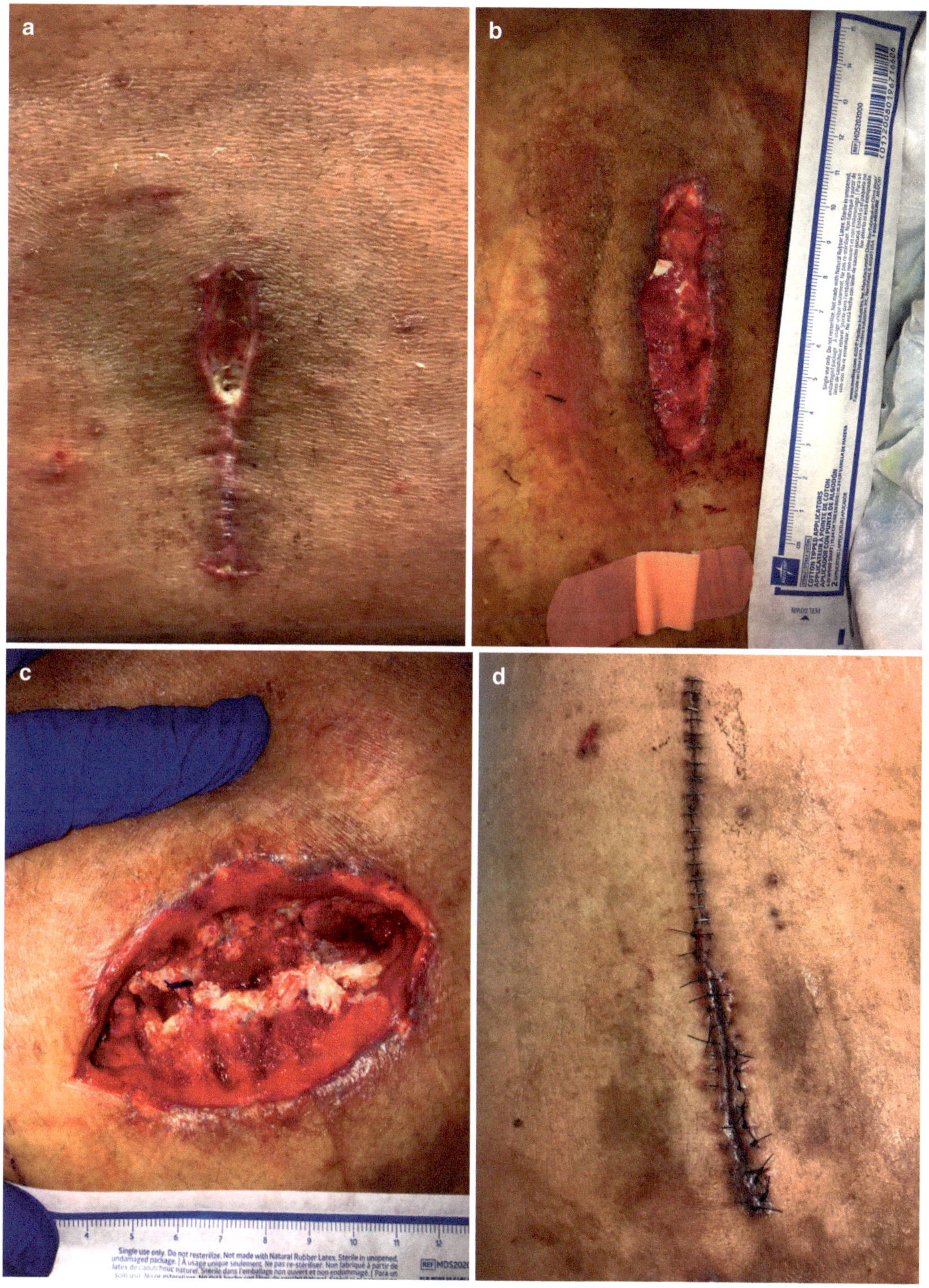

Fig. 17.6 (**a**) Initial presentation of acute wound dehiscence (**b** and **c**) Represent intraoperative images of initial serial debridements prior to intradural abscess (**d**) Final wound closure after last debridement and extensive decompression with the use of plastic surgery multilayered flap closure

Alternative Imaging Methods

While CT myelograms are one alternative to MRIs when contraindicated, newer technologies such as single-photon emission computed tomography (SPECT) may provide similar diagnostic accuracy to MRI [20].

Treatment Options

While we will outline recommendations for the treatment of diagnosed SSIs after pediatric spinal surgery, perhaps the most effective treatment is a thorough preventative strategy which identifies high-risk patients and provides evidenced based recommendations for the perioperative optimization of patients undergoing spine surgery. In addition to identifying risk factors for SSIs, this section will outline published consensus protocols, as well as the importance of a cohesive multidisciplinary team in efforts to decrease SSI rates.

Despite the means taken to limit SSIs in this population, it is inevitable that they will occur, and so we also discuss the appropriate use of antibiotic therapy as well as the indications for re-operation and decision-making on implant removal vs retention.

Identification of Risk Factors

Matsumoto et al. performed an extensive systematic review and meta-analysis of the available literature regarding SSIs in pediatric spine surgery, identifying potential risk factors, both modifiable and unmodifiable. [2] While their investigation spanned all etiologies, as mentioned earlier in this text, neuromuscular patients had a significantly higher risk of SSI than those with a non-neuromuscular etiology (relative risk, 2.84 [1.67–4.81]).

In evaluating preoperative patient characteristics associated with increased SSI risk, multiple studies demonstrated that non-ambulatory patients and those with gastrostomy tubes had significantly higher risk of developing an SSI. While these patients mostly had non-idiopathic scoliosis etiologies, when attempting to identify modifiable preoperative risks for patients with idiopathic scoliosis, the effect of obesity and/or BMI has been studied. In Matsumoto et al.'s review of the literature, patients classified as "overweight to obese" had a 2.5 times increased risk of developing an SSI compared to those considered "normal weight" [2]. Evaluating the other side of this equation, there was no increased risk of "underweight" patients when compared to those of normal weight. These findings are also corroborated by the reported results of Newton et al., who found BMI to be the only preoperative risk factor associated with postoperative SSI, with Lenke class and curve magnitude not demonstrating any significance [21].

In addition to preoperative factors, several intra-operative factors have been studied. Although not necessarily modifiable, patients undergoing fusion involving the pelvis have significantly higher SSI rates. When assessing the factors that may be influenced intra-operatively, blood loss was found to have an association with SSI, as those developing an SSI have on average 158 mL more blood loss [22]. Ho et al. also identified increased SSI risk with increasing operative time [22].

Along with surgical time, Ho et al. found patients with comorbid conditions, such as sickle cell trait, hypothyroidism, or severe acne were at an increased risk for SSI. Intra-operatively, increased drain output and cell saver amount returned were all associated with an increased risk. In addition, receiving a blood transfusion had a 3× increased risk for delayed infection, which was more significant the greater units of blood used in the transfusion.

Implementation of Best Practice Guidelines

In high-risk groups, such as neuromuscular, syndromic, and early-onset scoliosis patients, considerable work has been done to establish evidence-based guidelines in the perioperative management of these patients to decrease the risk of potential SSI. Recently, Glotzbecker et al. have outlined "Best Practice Guidelines" for the prevention of SSIs in Early Onset Scoliosis, including patients of all etiologies covering preoperative, intraoperative, and postoperative aspects [13].

Preoperative elements within the consensus statement include use of chlorhexidine skin wash the night prior to a lengthening or insertion procedure, as well as pulmonary and nutritional assessments prior to surgery. For patients with myelodysplasia, urine cultures should be obtained and, if positive, treated prior to surgery.

Intraoperatively, operating room access should be limited. Surgical prep should include a chlorhexidine-based solution, and the prep area should include access to all previous implants and be wide enough to allow a chest tube to be placed. When not contraindicated for allergy, intravenous cefazolin should be used as perioperative antibiotic coverage, with the addition of gram-negative coverage for patients with neuromuscular disease (including myelodysplasia).

Postoperatively, dressings should be impervious and changes minimized in the immediate postoperative period. Antibiotics started prior to incision should continue for 24 hours, but no longer, regardless of diagnosis. In total, consensus agreement was reached on 22 statements and principles which have been incorporated into the final recommendations of this group.

In the surgical treatment of AIS, many "Best Practice Guidelines" have been published with regard to decreasing intraoperative blood loss and postoperative hospital stays; however, no consensus has been published specifically addressing prevention of SSIs in this population. However, there is extensive evidence investigating a multitude of perioperative strategies to decrease SSIs. For example, the *Safety in Spine Project* has been established to bring together the stakeholders in spine surgery across multiple healthcare platforms to help identify ways to enhance the safety of spine surgery.

As mentioned earlier, increasing trends of MRSA have led to an increase in SSIs leading many within orthopedic surgery to engage in preoperative screening of *S. aureus* nasal colonization with subsequent decontamination prior to surgery. Mallet et al. applied these principles to AIS patients and found significantly decreased SSI rates (5.1–1.3%) with these practices [23]. In their study, nasal and cutaneous decontamination was done, respectively, by application of mupirocin (Bactroban ointment) twice a day into both anterior nostrils and by using Hibiscrub 4% during showers for 5 days before surgery. If methicillin-resistant *S. aureus* (MRSA) was isolated, one injection of vancomycin (15 mg/kg) 30 min before incision replaced usual antibiotic prophylaxis. All patients underwent preoperative skin preparation with two integral showers using povidone-iodine scrub. These results were corroborated through a meta-analysis by Ning et al., who demonstrated the importance of identifying MRSA carriers and proceeding with decontamination prior to surgery [24].

There is less objective data available on the use of preoperative skin cleansing prior to pediatric spinal deformity surgery; however, in a review of North American pediatric institutions, it is a near universal component of the implemented care bundles to decrease SSI. Most protocols include a chlorhexidine-based solution or a similar, antibacterial solution. These skin washes may be done the night prior to surgery or for several days leading up to surgery.

Intraoperatively, there has been more controversy regarding certain practices. While the use of vancomycin powder has been deemed safe to use in pediatric spine surgery, its overall influence on SSI rates is less conclusive. Garg et al. studied all pediatric patients undergoing posterior spinal fusion and found that, while the group receiving vancomycin powder had a lower infection rate (2% vs 3%), this was not significant [25]. Specifically reviewing a high-risk patient cohort undergoing growth-friendly surgeries, Thompson et al. demonstrated a benefit to use of vancomycin powder, regardless if it employed in the initial or one of the subsequent lengthening procedures [26]. Despite this evidence, a recent critical analysis review by Mistovich et al. concluded there is insufficient evidence to support the use of topical vancomycin in pediatric spinal deformity surgery [27].

The use of closed-suction wound drains postoperatively remains a point of contention among pediatric spine surgeons. While the use of a drain theoretically minimizes hematoma or edema from the cutaneous incision, it may also serve as a potential source of contaminant. Diab et al. found no increased risk of complications with the use of a postoperative drain; however, more patients with drains required transfusions. Conflicting data has been reported on the efficacy of drains in the prevention of SSIs, with Ho et al. demonstrating decreased SSI rates, while Blank et al. found no significant difference in SSI rates. Mistovich et al.'s critical analysis deemed no change in SSI risk with the use of postoperative drains [27].

High-Performance Teams

In today's healthcare system, it is essential to approach the management of complex disorders such as scoliosis with a cohesive, multidisciplinary team. While much of the focus in preventing SSIs occurs between incision and closure, the greatest potential for decreasing risk may lie in the preoperative and postoperative periods. Mackenzie et al. nicely outlines the important components of the multidisciplinary team in coherence with the "Comprehensive Unit-based Safety Program" [28].

In creating an overarching scoliosis protocol, orthopedic spine surgeons must enlist the help of a multitude of other specialties in determining the best evidence-based recommendations. Through multidisciplinary conferences, attended by the multitude of providers involved in the care of scoliosis patients, all aspects of the perioperative period from preoperative optimization to postoperative regimens are reviewed at these conferences.

For example, nutritional assessments are performed by gastroenterologists who may determine the need for potential preoperative gastric tube placement in order to optimize nutrition levels. Additionally, dermatology consults are utilized for excessive acne at incision sites, and anesthesiologists evaluate patients ahead of time to determine the need for any additional cardiopulmonary evaluation and treatments that may be required prior to surgery.

Within the operating room, the surgical team consists of a small pool of experienced nurses and technicians who are trained specifically in pediatric spine procedures and gain critical experience before becoming more active members of the team. Other surgical teams may be involved in the actual procedure, such as plastic surgery for wound closure. Many studies have supported the use of plastic surgery performing multilayered, tension-free flap closures in adult spinal deformity with more recent studies validating this in pediatric populations, especially neuromuscular patients at high risk of SSI and compromised soft tissues. Incorporation of the plastic surgery team is nicely demonstrated in the management of the patient presented in Box 17.4. The use of a multilayered flap closure decreases the amount of available dead space while creating a water-tight closure and well-vascularized muscle flap [29]. Most of the benefit in these closures has been found in the higher risk patient populations.

Acute Surgical Site Infection Treatment (See Box 17.1 (Idiopathic) and 17.3 (Neuromuscular) for Case Examples of the Management of Acute SSI)

When a surgical wound presents with active drainage in the acute postoperative period, aggressive debridement and irrigation should be performed in the operating room. Currently, there remains sparse data regarding a nonoperative approach to spine SSIs, i.e., relying on antibiotic therapy alone. Antibiotic suppression alone should be attempted only in cases where the patient may not be a good surgical candidate and the risk of surgery is high, or if the clinical exam demonstrates a superficial seroma or non-infectious process as illustrated in Box 17.5.

Box 17.5: Case 5: Acute Seroma after Discectomy

Clinical Scenario: An 18-year-old male with an L5/S1 disc extrusion and left posterior thigh and leg pain which had failed conservative treatments and was indicated for an L5-S1 discectomy. He returned in 1 week with localized swelling and drainage reported on his bandage.

- Diagnostic Work-up
  - ***Physical exam:*** Revealed superficial area of fluctuance with minimal ***serous drainage*** (Fig. 17.7). Patient had no neurological symptoms or deficits. No fevers.
  - Laboratory work-up: ***CRP 0.9 (expected value at 1-week post-surgery)***
- Surgical Decision-Making
  - Low CRP value and exam consistent with ***superficial seroma***
- Medical Treatment
  - The patient was prescribed ***10 days of oral antibiotics*** and close follow-up. Within 1 week, ***the seroma had resolved,*** and the wound healed.
- Overall Outcome
  - Patient was further managed with the usual postoperative regimen and returned to normal activities by 4 weeks without any additional wound healing issues or concern for infection.

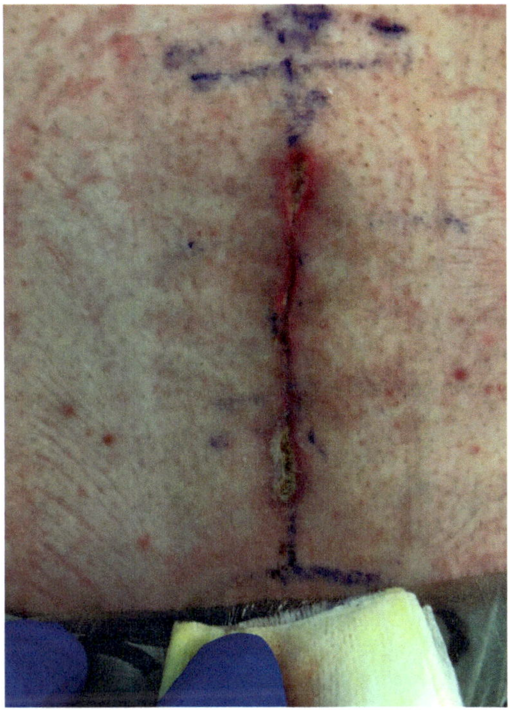

Fig. 17.7 Clinical image of postoperative seroma with serous drainage and soft tissue fullness appreciated around the operative incision

At this acute timepoint postoperatively, all implants should be retained given the immaturity of the fusion mass and the low concern for implant biofilm so soon after the index procedure. During the time of irrigation and debridement, tissue cultures should be obtained for aerobic, anaerobic, fungal, and mycobacterial species.

While the necessity of antibiotic therapy in the treatment of pediatric spine SSIs is well established, the more difficult decision points include selection of specific antibiotic agents and the duration of treatment, as well as incisional wound management. Many protocols may exist, but for the most part, patients are treated with a minimum of 4–6 weeks of parenteral antibiotics and, depending on the causative bacteria and extent of infection, may receive subsequent oral antibiotic treatment for several months afterwards. All antibiotic agent choices should be driven by culture results obtained at the time of debridement. In the same nature of the comprehensive care teams described earlier, infectious disease specialists should be consulted and involved in the decision-making process that follows proper antibiotic therapy guidelines.

After initial debridement and obtaining culture specimens, it is critical for surgeons to plan for potential repeat debridements and returns to the operative room, which has been reported to be required in up to 50% of cases. In order to better predict the need for multiple debridements, DiPaola et al. developed a scoring system based on multiple risk factors [30]. In their study, patients with positive MRSA cultures and presence of bacteremia were more likely to require serial debridements. In addition, the presence of instrumentation, posterior lumbar surgical location, and the use of non-autograft bone graft material led to multiple returns to the operating room, while diabetic patients were also considered high risk. While certain risk factors can be identified, the decision on serial debridements many times is based on the surgeon's clinical assessment and experience with the treatment of SSIs.

After thorough debridement is performed and antibiotics have been started, the last facet in the management of acute SSIs includes wound management. Canavese et al. first introduced the idea of vacuum-assisted closure for deep infection after scoliosis surgery, citing the facts that the subatmospheric pressure applied by the vacuum therapy induces the formation of granulation tissue, assists in debridement of necrotic tissue, and acts as a sterile barrier for the wound [31]. In the initial study, Canavese demonstrated resolution of acute, deep SSI in 14 patients with up to 6 years of follow-up. These results were mirrored by Van Rhee et al. who successfully treated six patients with an acute SSI using vacuum therapy and antibiotics after surgical debridement [32]. Since that time, extensive work has been done in studying the use of vacuum-assisted closure, as well as advancements in technology to include continuous irrigation suction systems. While these systems have shown efficacy, there appears to be no benefit when compared to a VAC system without irrigation as shown by Yuan et al. [33]

Delayed Surgical Site Infection Treatment (See Box 17.2 for Case Example of Chronic Infection Management)

Similar to the treatment of acute SSIs, irrigation and debridement remains the mainstay of treatment; however, the fate of implants may differ. There is ongoing controversy and debate regarding the need to remove implants at the time of surgery for a delayed SSI. One factor that must be investigated is the competency of the fusion mass, which should be thoroughly evaluated using plain radiographs, or advanced imaging such as CT scan. If there is any concern for an incomplete fusion, implants should be retained at least until fusion is obtained, with continued antibiotics during that time. Using a similar protocol, Collins et al. found that 60% of patients had continued colonization of bacteria when implants were eventually removed after confirmation of fusion [34].

The importance of spinal stability and maturity of the fusion mass must be balanced with the potential for biofilm formation in the case of a delayed, deep SSI. As with most orthopedic implants, bacteria are capable of forming a glycocalyx membrane which further allows the adherence of bacteria to the instrumentation while providing resistance and protection to the host's immune system response and antibiotic penetration. Once the biofilm has formed, there is little chance of infection resolution without removal of the implants. Hedequist et al. explain that, without implant removal, areas underneath the rods and pedicle screws or hooks are not completely debrided and may allow for continued infected tissue and potential for recolonization [35].

It is important, however, to understand that most underlying deep infections are soft tissue in nature and not chronic osteomyelitis. As has been shown by Richards et al., there was no sequestrum identified with a viable fusion mass [36]. Further studies investigating the retention of implants in these more chronic cases have demonstrated poor results with high rates of recurrent infection and the need for subsequent debridements until ultimately the implants were removed.

Removing implants after deformity surgery is not without its own risks. There is the potential for previous or residual deformity to progress further, leading to a possible revision surgery to correct new-onset deformity. Rathjen et al. reported a 7% rate of coronal curve progression of >10 degrees after implant removal in spine deformity patients, while Potter et al. reported an average 9 degree progression when implants were removed specifically for infection, with 6/21 patients requiring revision surgery within 16 months of implant removal [37, 38]. These values were corroborated by a more recent study by Hedequist et al., who cited an average of 12 degrees of coronal progression after implant removal [35].

Regardless of the patient characteristics or cause of the infection, the literature is conclusive that early recognition and thorough treatment protocols are effective in the treatment of SSIs. When following a protocoled management plan including organism identification, thorough surgical debridement, proper wound management, and antibiotic agents and duration, there are high rates of treatment success of delayed, deep SSI. In review of an institutional protocol for pediatric spine SSI, Moyano et al. reported just 1 reinfection (3.4% of their cohort) of pediatric posterior spinal fusion patients [39].

Complications

Significant complications are associated with SSIs in pediatric patients undergoing spinal surgery. As mentioned in the introduction, SSIs lead to prolonged hospital stays, increased rates of readmission, and higher reoperation rates. [40] The financial burden to the healthcare system may also be significant, and any management delays or errors can lead to increasing costs. Hedequist et al. found that the average hospital charge for a delayed, deep SSI was $81,828, which increased to $674,292 if the implants were not removed after 4 or more procedures [35].

Considering the patient's health status, repeat surgeries lead to increased risks of neurological injury secondary to the surgery itself or worsening infection. Additionally, while infections may present with mild burden to the patient, a lack of prompt recognition and treatment may lead to systemic sepsis and shock, with possible multiorgan failure. While the infection itself can produce numerous complications, as can its treatment. Prolonged antibiotic therapy may lead to *Clostridium difficile colitis*, as well as multiple-drug resistance for subsequent infections requiring antibiotics.

Summary

The incidence of spinal SSI in the pediatric population is variable, and all patient- and surgical-related factors must be considered when counseling patients and families on the potential risk of such complications during surgery. It is critical for surgeons to optimize all possible risk-factors and have a multidisciplinary team-based approach to the overall treatment of pediatric patients undergoing spine surgery.

When faced with a potential SSI after spine surgery, an organized and detailed clinical, laboratory, and imaging work-up is required to ensure a correct diagnosis is reached. Once identified, unless contraindicated secondary to underlying medical conditions, surgical intervention is the preferred treatment option, with thorough irrigation and debridement and obtaining tissue cultures for organism speciation.

The decision-making of implant retention or removal must be evidence-based and patient-specific. A full evaluation with imaging and intra-operative investigation should be performed to assess for an intact fusion mass in the case of deformity surgery. If adequate fusion has been achieved and maintained, surgeons will typically proceed with implant removal to decrease the risk of further infection due to an underlying biofilm formation, which is resistance to further treatment of antibiotics. The addition of adjunctive therapies such as negative pressure wound therapy, vancomycin powder, and surgical site drains have been debated in the literature; however, most data is supportive, and surgeons must use their clinical acumen and judgement on the utilization of these therapies.

It must also be highlighted that treatment is not surgical alone. Medical treatment with the involvement of infectious disease specialists to provide recommendations for antibiotic agents and duration based on culture-driven data should be included in the management of these SSIs. The use of imaging and serial laboratory values, such as CRP, is used to evaluate the efficacy of treatment and the eventual clearing of infection from the surgical site.

Overall, SSIs after pediatric spine surgery represent a significant burden to the healthcare system, but more importantly to patients and families. Having a protocoled and evidence-based approach to not only the treatment but, more importantly, the prevention of these complications will lead to improved outcomes for all parties involved.

References

1. Glotzbecker MP, Vitale MG, Shea KG, Flynn JM. Surgeon practices regarding infection prevention for pediatric spinal surgery. J Pediatr Orthop. 2013;33(7):694–9.
2. Matsumoto H, Simhon ME, Campbell ML, Vitale MG, Larson EL. Risk factors associated with surgical site infection in pediatric patients undergoing spinal deformity surgery: a systematic review and meta-analysis. JBJS Rev. 2020;8(3):e0163.
3. McLeod L, Flynn J, Erickson M, Miller N, Keren R, Dormans J. Variation in 60-day readmission for surgical-site infections (SSIs) and reoperation following spinal fusion operations for neuromuscular scoliosis. J Pediatr Orthop. 2016;36(6):634–9.
4. https://www.cdc.gov/nhsn/PDFs/pscManual/9pscSSIcurrent.pdf.
5. Smith JS, Shaffrey CI, Sansur CA, Berven SH, Fu KM, Broadstone PA, Choma TJ, Goytan MJ, Noordeen HH, Knapp DR Jr, Hart RA. Rates of infection after spine surgery based on 108,419 procedures: a report from the Scoliosis Research Society Morbidity and Mortality Committee. Spine. 2011;36(7):556–63.
6. Glotzbecker MP, Riedel MD, Vitale MG, Matsumoto H, Roye DP, Erickson M, Flynn JM, Saiman L. What's the evidence? Systematic literature review of risk factors and preventive strategies for surgical site infection following pediatric spine surgery. J Pediatr Orthop. 2013;33(5):479–87.
7. Sullivan BT, Abousamra O, Puvanesarajah V, Jain A, Hadad MJ, Milstone AM, Sponseller PD. Deep infections after pediatric spinal arthrodesis: differences exist with idiopathic, neuromuscular, or genetic and syndromic cause of deformity. JBJS. 2019;101(24):2219–25.
8. Warner SJ, Uppstrom TJ, Miller AO, O'Brien ST, Salvatore CM, Widmann RF, Perlman SL. Epidemiology of deep surgical site infections after pediatric spinal fusion surgery. Spine. 2017;42(3):E163–8.
9. Grossfeld S, Winter RB, Lonstein JE, Denis F, Leonard A, Johnson L. Complications of anterior spinal surgery in children. J Pediatr Orthop. 1997;17(1):89–95.
10. Janik JS, Burrington JD, Janik JE, Wayne ER, Chang JHT, Rothenberg SS. Anterior exposure of spinal deformities and tumors: a 20-year experience. J Pediatr Surg. 1997;32:852–9.
11. Hwang HS, Macagno A, Gupta MC, O'Brien MF. Complications in surgery for spinal deformity. In: Newton PO, O'Brien MF, Shufflebarger HL, Betz RR, Dickson RA, Harms J, editors. Idiopathic scoliosis. 1st ed. New York: Thieme Medical Publishers; 2010. p. 284–322.
12. Mackenzie WS, Matsumoto H, Williams BA, Corona J, Lee C, Cody SR, Covington L, Saiman L, Flynn JM, Skaggs DL, Roye DP Jr. Surgical site infection following spinal instrumentation for scoliosis: a multicenter analysis of rates, risk factors, and pathogens. JBJS. 2013;95(9):800–6.
13. Glotzbecker MP, St Hilaire TA, Pawelek JB, Thompson GH, Vitale MG. Best practice guidelines for surgical site infection prevention with surgical treatment of early onset scoliosis. J Pediatr Orthop. 2019;39(8):e602–7.
14. Kabirian N, Akbarnia BA, Pawelek JB, Alam M, Mundis GM Jr, Acacio R, Thompson GH, Marks DS, Gardner A, Sponseller PD, Skaggs DL. Deep surgical site infection following 2344 growing-rod procedures for early-onset scoliosis: risk factors and clinical consequences. JBJS. 2014;96(15):e128.
15. Sponseller PD, LaPorte DM, Hungerford MW, Eck K, Bridwell KH, Lenke LG. Deep wound infections after neuromuscular scoliosis surgery: a multicenter study of risk factors and treatment outcomes. Spine. 2000;25(19):2461–6.
16. Hahn F, Zbinden R, Min K. Late implant infections caused by Propionibacterium acnes in scoliosis surgery. Eur Spine J. 2005;14(8):783–8.
17. LaGreca J, Hotchkiss M, Carry P, Messacar K, Nyquist AC, Erickson M, Garg S. Bacteriology and risk factors for development of late (greater than one year) deep infection following spinal fusion with instrumentation. Spine Deformity. 2014;2(3):186–90.
18. Maesani M, Doit C, Lorrot M, Vitoux C, Hilly J, Michelet D, Vidal C, Julien-Marsollier F, Ilharreborde B, Mazda K, Bonacorsi S. Surgical site infections in pediatric spine surgery: comparative microbiology of patients with idiopathic and nonidiopathic etiologies of spine deformity. Pediatr Infect Dis J. 2016;35(1):66–70.
19. Rihn JA, Lee JY, Ward WT. Infection after the surgical treatment of adolescent idiopathic scoliosis: evaluation of the diagnosis, treatment, and impact on clinical outcomes. Spine. 2008;33(3):289–94.
20. Divi SN, Kepler CK, Segar AH, Russo GS, Bronson WH, Boody BS, Galetta MS, Goyal DK, Fang T, Schroeder GD, Vaccaro AR. Role of imaging, tissue

sampling, and biomarkers for diagnosis of SSI in spine surgery. Clin Spine Surg. 2020;33(5):E199–205.
21. Newton PO, Bastrom TP, Yaszay B. Patient-specific risk adjustment improves comparison of infection rates following posterior fusion for adolescent idiopathic scoliosis. JBJS. 2017;99(21):1846–50.
22. Ho C, Skaggs DL, Weiss JM, Tolo VT. Management of infection after instrumented posterior spine fusion in pediatric scoliosis. Spine. 2007;32(24):2739–44.
23. Mallet C, Caseris M, Doit C, Simon AL, Michelet D, Madre C, Mazda K, Bonacorsi S, Ilharreborde B. Does Staphylococcus aureus nasal decontamination affect the rate of early surgical site infection in adolescent idiopathic scoliosis surgery? Eur Spine J. 2018;27(10):2543–9.
24. Ning J, Wang J, Zhang S, Sha X. Nasal colonization of Staphylococcus aureus and the risk of surgical site infection after spine surgery: a meta-analysis. Spine J. 2020;20(3):448–56.
25. Garg S, Bloch N, Potter M, Quick H, Palmer C, Michael N, O'Donnell C, Erickson M. Topical vancomycin in pediatric spine surgery does not reduce surgical site infection: a retrospective cohort study. Spine Deformity. 2018;6(5):523–8.
26. Thompson GH, Poe-Kochert C, Hardesty CK, Son-Hing J, Mistovich RJ. Does vancomycin powder decrease surgical site infections in growing spine surgery?: a preliminary study. JBJS. 2018;100(6):466–71.
27. Mistovich RJ, Jacobs LJ, Campbell RM, Spiegel DA, Flynn JM, Baldwin KD. Infection control in pediatric spinal deformity surgery: a systematic and critical analysis review. JBJS Rev. 2017;5(5):e3.
28. Mackenzie WS, McLeod L, Wang K, Crotty J, Hope JE, Imahiyerobo TA, Ko RR, Anderson RC, Saiman L, Vitale MG. Team approach: preventing surgical site infections in pediatric scoliosis surgery. JBJS Rev. 2018;6(2):e2.
29. Garg S, Khechoyan D, Kim EB, French B. Multilayered and flap closure technique for pediatric spinal deformity surgery. J Am Acad Orthop Surg. 2020;28(3):e92–9.
30. DiPaola CP, Saravanja DD, Boriani L, Zhang H, Boyd MC, Kwon BK, Paquette SJ, Dvorak MF, Fisher CG, Street JT. Postoperative infection treatment score for the spine (PITSS): construction and validation of a predictive model to define need for single versus multiple irrigation and debridement for spinal surgical site infection. Spine J. 2012;12(3):218–30.
31. Canavese F, Gupta S, Krajbich JI, Emara KM. Vacuum-assisted closure for deep infection after spinal instrumentation for scoliosis. J Bone Joint Surg. 2008;90(3):377–81.
32. van Rhee MA, de Klerk LW, Verhaar JA. Vacuum-assisted wound closure of deep infections after instrumented spinal fusion in six children with neuromuscular scoliosis. Spine J. 2007;7(5):596–600.
33. Yuan W, Liu X, Zhou X, Pei L, Zhu Y. Management of early deep wound infection after Thoracolumbar Instrumentation: continuous irrigation suction system: versus: vacuum-assisted closure system. Spine. 2018;43(18):E1089–95.
34. Collins I, Wilson-MacDonald J, Chami G, Burgoyne W, Vineyakam P, Berendt T, Fairbank J. The diagnosis and management of infection following instrumented spinal fusion. Eur Spine J. 2008;17(3):445–50.
35. Hedequist D, Haugen A, Hresko T, Emans J. Failure of attempted implant retention in spinal deformity delayed surgical site infections. Spine. 2009;34(1):60–4.
36. Richards BS, Hasley BP, Casey VF. Repeat surgical interventions following "definitive" instrumentation and fusion for idiopathic scoliosis. Spine. 2006;31(26):3018–26.
37. Rathjen K, Wood M, McClung A, Vest Z. Clinical and radiographic results after implant removal in idiopathic scoliosis. Spine. 2007;32(20):2184–8.
38. Potter BK, Kirk KL, Shah SA, Kuklo TR. Loss of coronal correction following instrumentation removal in adolescent idiopathic scoliosis. Spine. 2006;31(1):67–72.
39. Moyano, Carlos A, et al. Infection recurrence in instrumented spinal fusion in children. Global Spine J. 2021;11(7):1040–5.
40. Basu S, Solanki AM, Srivastava A, Shetty AP, Rajasekaran S, Jayaswal A. Unplanned return to operation room (OR) following growing spinal constructs (GSCs) in early onset scoliosis (EOS)-a multi-centric study. Eur Spine J. 2020;29(8):2075–83.

18 Infections Related to External Fixators

James Widnall and Selvadurai Nayagam

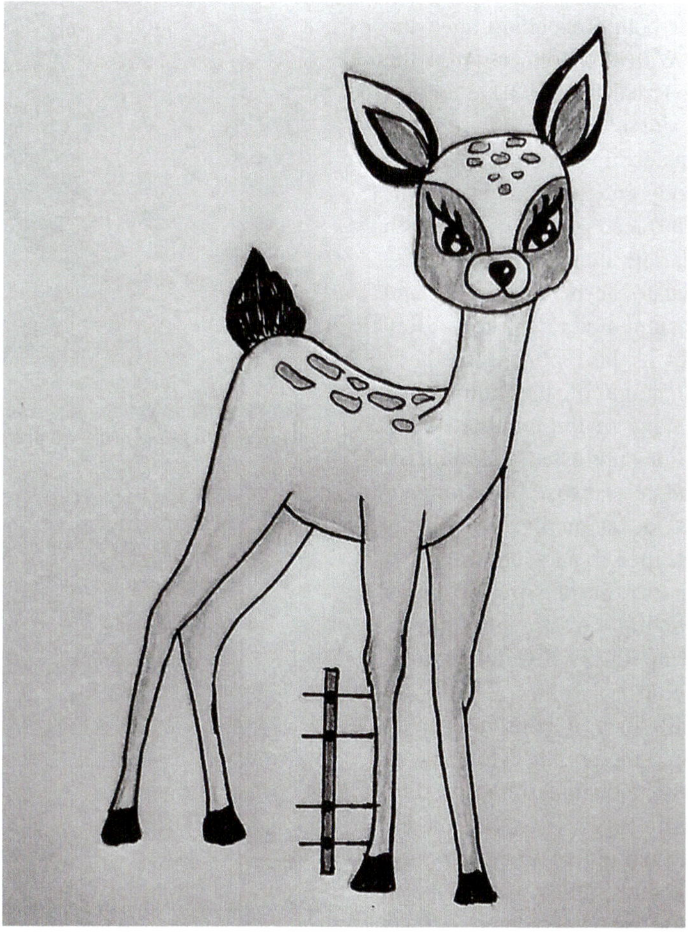

J. Widnall
Alder Hey Children's Hospital, Liverpool, UK
e-mail: james.widnall@alderhey.nhs.uk

S. Nayagam (✉)
Alder Hey Children's Hospital, Liverpool, UK

Royal Liverpool University and Broadgreen
University Hospitals, Liverpool, UK

© Springer Nature Switzerland AG 2022
M. V. Belthur et al. (eds.), *Pediatric Musculoskeletal Infections*,
https://doi.org/10.1007/978-3-030-95794-0_18

Infections Associated with External Fixation

The Problem

Extent of the Problem

External fixation as utilized in trauma and limb reconstruction vary in complexity from simple uniplanar devices to elaborate multiplanar circular ones. Both types anchor to the bone using half-pins or wires or both, depending upon the configuration used. With this connection to the bony skeleton, all external fixators have a common problem of pin site infection.

Pin site infections occur from skin penetration by a foreign body and subsequent colonization of the interface, most often with *Staphylococcus* [1]. The incidence of pin site infection is reported to be between 11% and 100% [2–4]. The documented rates vary widely owing to differences in the reporting methods used, from a percentage of the number of patients to a percentage of the number of pin sites. Pin site infections are usually skin infections which respond to increased cleaning or antibiotics or both. Occasionally, a cellulitis develops and may deepen to an acute osteomyelitis which can lead to pin or wire loosening prompting a potential treatment failure. (Figs. 18.1 and 18.2) Rarely, life-threatening infections may develop.

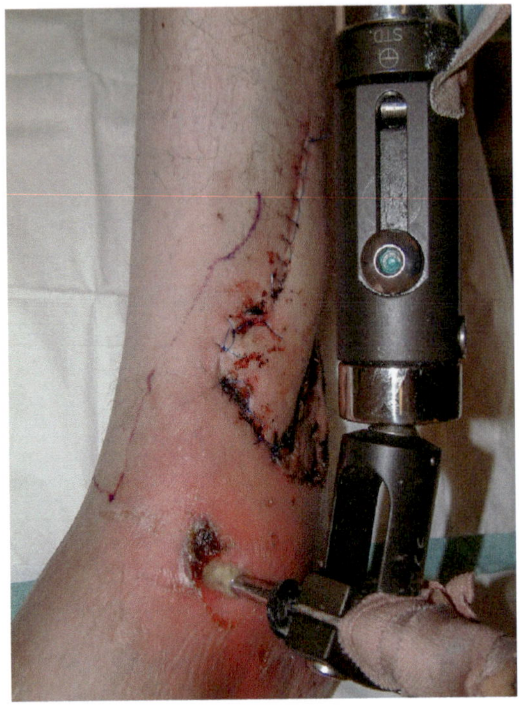

Fig. 18.1 Pin site infections can develop into an osteomyelitis with cellulitis if untreated promptly

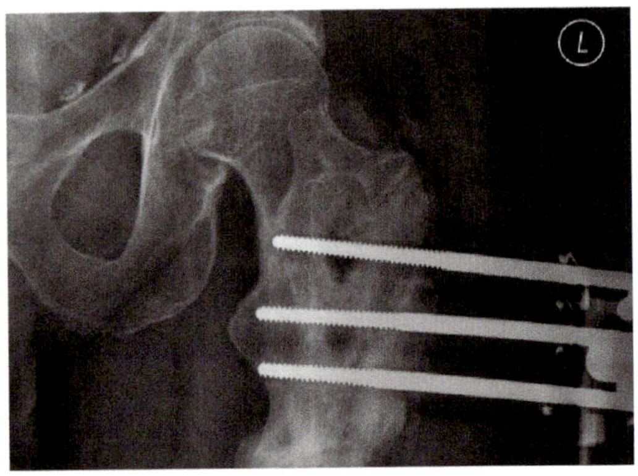

Fig. 18.2 Tell-tale signs of loosening from infection – there is lucency around the proximal half-pin

The likelihood of such a complication is dependent on multiple factors: the virulence of the infecting organism, techniques employed by the surgeon during half-pin or wire insertion, the aftercare provided to the pin site, and the presence of patient comorbidities. In diabetes mellitus, perioperative hyperglycaemia affects white cell function and can predispose to infection which, in turn, increases complications in patients undergoing fixator applications for foot and ankle conditions [5, 6]. As a parallel, those with acquired immune deficiency syndrome (AIDS) from HIV infection have high rates (42–72%) of infection using internal fixation for open tibial fractures [7, 8]. External fixation methods are thus the preferred treatment for this group. While the pin site infection rate does not appear to be significantly different between HIV-positive and HIV-negative patients, the HIV-positive status increases the likelihood for pharmaceutical or surgical intervention for pin site infections. Interestingly, no correlation has been shown between CD4 count and severity of pin site infection [3, 9].

Pin site infections are not unique to the human population. Canine and feline animals have showcased a similar rate of pin site infection following external fixation for trauma [10, 11].

Impact of the Problem

The clinical impact of a pin site infection and the potential for treatment failure underpin the need for clinicians to be aware of the problem, both to reduce the incidence and manage associated complications. Rarely, it may result osteomyelitis and life-threatening infections.

Potential Risk of Osteomyelitis

The majority of pin site infections (up to 94%) are superficial and settle quickly with a course of antibiotics [12]. Deep infections can be diagnosed if the pin site does not settle following an appropriate course of oral antibiotics, necessitating either intravenous administration or pin removal [13]. These often depict the development of an acute osteomyelitis around the pin in contrast to a localised skin infection. Intravenous followed by extended oral treatment with antibiotics may solve the problem – akin to treating osteomyelitis – but recurrence is common. Pin removal under continued antibiotic cover may then be needed and should be done in the operating room under general anaesthesia to a) allow thorough debridement and lavage of the pin track and b) permit alternative pin placement. Persisting with a half-pin or wire causing an acute osteomyelitis using antibiotic suppression is more likely to lead to a chronic problem and the possibility of ring sequestra.

Lethal Scenarios

Serious complications such as necrotising fasciitis (NF) and toxic shock syndrome have been described originating from pin site infections [14]. Necrotising fasciitis is a life-threatening polymicrobial soft tissue infection with horizontal spread along tissue planes needing urgent and radical surgical debridement. In a retrospective review from a tertiary centre, four patients over a 15-year period developed NF from treatment associated with an external fixator. All recovered with urgent recognition and treatment. Toxic shock syndrome is a T-cell-mediated response to endotoxins produced from *staphylococcal* or *streptococcal* organisms. Treatment is supportive. Frame removal in toxic shock syndrome is appropriate if frame treatment is near complete or if there is a clear causal pin site [14].

Conversion Scenarios

Increasingly, converting from external to internal fixation is common. The external fixation is either a temporizing stabiliser in long bone trauma or used for the correcting phases in limb reconstruction techniques. Pin site infections have potentially larger consequences when there is indwelling metalwork in proximity. The risks differ when plates or intramedullary nails are used.

Extraperiosteal Devices (Plates)

Initial treatment with spanning external fixation before definitive internal fixation is a recognised treatment pathway for high energy limb injuries. Concerns exist over the potential for deep infection because of pin site proximity to the internal fixation constructs (e.g., plates or screws). Studies into both tibial plateau and pilon injuries have produced conflicting advice on this risk [15–17]. There is agreement that initial temporary external fixation be placed in optimal configurations to gain fracture stability – thus achieving the objective of damage control – and for the time interval between external and internal fixation to be kept as short as possible [18].

Intramedullary Devices (Nails)

In limb lengthening, attempts are made to decrease the incumbency of external fixation. Strategies which combine the external fixator – which serves as the "mechanical motor" that drives the lengthening – with intramedullary nails, which hold and stabilise the lengthened bone until consolidation is complete, have evolved. These nails are inserted at the time of external fixation (lengthening over nail – LON – technique) or just before removal of the fixator (lengthening then nail – LTN – technique). Both techniques expose the intramedullary nail to a wire or half-pin site that is a portal to the exterior. Experiments have suggested that the medullary canal becomes contaminated early in such settings [19, 20].

Deep pin site sepsis thus heightens the risk of developing an intramedullary osteomyelitis. In a series of LON in the femur, Song et al. reported over 90% (20 out of 22 patients) pin site infection rate with 7 being deep infections [21]. Three of the 7 patients with deep pin site sepsis, all of whom had a history of osteomyelitis prior to the index procedure as well, went onto established intramedullary osteomyelitis requiring surgical treatment. In a series of similar tibial lengthenings by Kim et al., 19 infections were reported in 118 segments lengthened of which 6 were deep infections requiring nail removal [22].

In trauma, conversion from temporary external fixation to intramedullary nailing for open tibial fractures may risk osteomyelitis. Yokoyama et al. reported seven deep infections in 42 patients after conversion, with the deep infections occurring in Gustilo-Anderson type III injuries [23]. Using univariate analysis, the higher Gustilo-Anderson and AO fracture types, presence of a pin site infection, and a longer interval between external fixation and conversion to intramedullary nailing led to a higher risk of deep infection. With multivariate analysis, time to definitive skin closure exceeding 1 week was the principal influential variable; this parameter was emphasised again recently [24].

Factors which Make a Difference to Pin Site Infections

Factors which influence pin site sepsis have been the subject of much research. The results point to several broad areas:

1. Material properties of the pins and wires
2. Method of pin insertion
3. Location of the pin site
4. Function of the fixator and tenure of external fixation
5. Aftercare to the pin site

Material Properties of the Pins and Wires

Titanium

Pieske and colleagues proposed that titanium pins have a benefit over stainless steel due to a lower Young's modulus that improves osseointegration and decreases susceptibility to bacterial adhesion. In their RCT of external fixator pins used around the wrist, there were trends of increased pin-related complications, both loosening and infection, in the stainless steel group, but this did not reach statistical significance [25].

Silver

Silver has antibacterial properties due to decreased bacterial adhesion. Silver-coated screws in sheep iliac bones decreased *S. aureus* colony-forming units and screw loosening when compared to uncoated screws [1]. However, two RCTs found no differences when silver-coated pins were compared to stainless steel bacteriologically and clinically in patients with tibial fractures [26, 27].

Hydroxyapatite (HA) Coating

Piza et al. compared HA-coated pins against stainless steel pins in patients undergoing limb lengthening and found a significant difference in extraction torque required [28]. Using 150 N mm as a definition for loosening, they quoted an 80% rate of loosening in stainless steel pins compared to 4% in HA-coated pins, but no difference in pin site infection was found. Pommer et al. also found increased torque extraction requirements and a decrease in radiographic signs of loosening when comparing HA-coated stainless steel pins to uncoated titanium pins on a series of patients undergoing distraction osteogenesis [29]. Thirteen percent of the uncoated titanium pins had associated infection, while none occurred in the HA group. A systemic review was not able to confirm clinical benefit gained in terms of pin site infection from use of HA-coated pins but upheld the higher extraction torque requirements, inferring greater osseointegration [30].

Antiseptic and Antibiotic Coatings

HA coatings on pins have been combined with antiseptics to augment the benefits of osseointegration. DeJong et al. used a lipid-stabilised coating of HA with chlorhexidine on external fixation pins and compared these to uncoated pins in a contaminated goat model [31]. Significant improvements were noted in culture results, in clinical evaluations for infection and torque extraction data. An extension of this concept was to introduce local antibiotic delivery around the pin. Antibiotic-impregnated external fixation pin sleeves which elute antibiotics over time were studied by Marotta and colleagues [32, 33]. Using gentamicin, they found bactericidal activity was maintained in vitro for 20 weeks highlighting potential prophylaxis against the typical pathogens of pin site infections (e.g., *S. aureus*, *S. epidermidis*, *Pseudomonas*, and *E. coli*). The concentration locally was far higher than what would have been possible via systemic delivery. More recent in vivo studies, carried out on rabbit models, have confirmed persistent elution from antimicrobial pin coatings (in this case Triclosan) for up to 8 weeks resulting in a significant reduction in pin site infections with no overt detriment to the soft tissues adjacent to the pin [34].

Method of Pin Insertion

Several studies have suggested the mechanical qualities of pin anchorage are closely related to subsequent bacterial colonisation of the pin and potential infection [28, 29, 35, 36]. While this can depend on pin design and coatings, the surgeon can influence this interface too. One method is to maximise insertion torque, without risking microfracture, through pre-drilling with an appropriate and recommended drill size [37–39].

Due to the heterogeneous structure of bone and its poor thermal conductivity, thermal damage from drilling can produce bone death if local temperatures exceed 47 °C for 1 minute [40, 41]. Osteonecrosis secondary to thermal damage is a progressive process; osteocyte depletion with blood flow reduction and secondary osteoclastic bone resorption decrease pin anchorage.

Drill tip designs that increase cutting efficiency and bone swarf clearance reduce heat generation. External irrigation reduces bone chip clogging and temperature rises, as does intermittent drilling [40, 42]. Increases in drill spindle speed and applied axial load (feed rate) both add to a rise in temperature but also decrease the time of drilling. There are conflicting conclusions for optimising drill speed and feed rate as studies suggest that the linear relationship between spindle speed and temperature exists below 10,000 rpm, whereas this is inverse above 10,000 rpm [43, 44]. Modern orthopaedic battery-powered drills can deliver spindle speeds of 0–18,000 rpm thereby leaving firm recommendations on speed selection for reducing thermal necrosis difficult. Similarly, high feed rates increase the thrust force and torque between the drill margin and bone but shorten drilling duration, creating a similar paradox as with spindle speeds over heat generation. In general, unless using brand new drill bits for every operation, a stop-start method of drilling (peck-drilling) and external irrigation can limit heat generation and promote both heat dissipation and clearance of bone chip clogs especially when creating deep holes [42, 44, 45].

Location of the Pin Site

Impaled soft tissue bulk and excessive soft tissue movement around the pin site have been shown to increase the risk of pin site infection [46, 47]. Proximal tibial wire sites are more prone to infection than those more distal. Half-pins in periarticular regions are at increased risk too. The decreased rate of infection seen with diaphyseal half-pins in the tibia is due to the lack of transfixed soft tissues on the subcutaneous surface [48]. Despite this difference, the need to achieve bone segment purchase optimally through attention to safe corridors is paramount; hence transfixation of soft tissues or proximity to gliding structures cannot be avoided in some cases. Dressing techniques can be employed for these sites to reduce movement around wires and pins [49, 50].

Function of the Fixator and Tenure of External Fixation

The function (whether the fixator is a static device or used to effect a correction) and total time spent in the fixator influence the risk of pin site infection [46, 47, 51]. Fixators used for limb reconstruction procedures such as deformity correction or distraction osteogenesis produce greater stresses and trauma at the pin-bone interface [38]. Spanning external fixators applied for longer than 28 days before conversion to internal fixation are associated with an increased risk of deep infection [23, 52].

Aftercare to the Pin Site

Is There a Need to Manage Pin Sites?

A 'nihilistic' approach suggested by Gordon et al. reported a 4% rate of pin site infection (this proportion was measured through the number of pins observed infected over the number of observations made throughout the patients' follow-up). If the proportion is expressed using a more usual fraction i.e., the number of infected pin sites over the total number of pin sites, this changes the 4% to nearly 84% [46]. A randomised control trial by Camathias et al. of routine pin site care or none in half-pin external fixation suggested no difference in the outcome. The trial is notable for randomising the half-pins in the same patient thereby achieving intrasubject and intragroup randomisation [53]. This is a well-designed study methodologically, but the sample does not extrapolate well to the greater population of external fixation patients. The sample comprised trauma patients who had simple unilateral and uniplanar fixators applied and who remained as inpatients throughout treatment. The fixator constructs used were similar to those used for temporary spanning mode in trauma elsewhere and preclude sufficient stability to encourage eventual full weight-bearing in recovery. This may have been related to the setting in which the study was conducted (Solomon Islands) and, as such, important differences may limit extrapolation of the findings. The trial design has high internal validity but limited external validity.

Pin Site Care Regimes

Published studies give conflicting conclusions as to the pin site care regime that would lead to a reduction in infection. The issues which lead to these divergent recommendations may be with use of classifications of pin site infections that have yet to be validated, the inability to distinguish between one infection at a pin site and a recurrence at the same site soon after treatment as the one or two separate infections (analysis of recurrent events), and the omission of time in external fixation as an important variable in the calculations. Davies et al. attempted to address the issues above in their cohort-based observational study by avoiding an unvalidated classification system of pin site infection or the counting of the number of infections, whether of patients or of pin sites. Instead, they adopted the same methodology as used for studies of infections in joint prosthetic surgery [13]. By defining a clinically relevant pin site problem clearly (and including those subclinical infections which are painful pin sites that are negative to swab cultures but respond completely with anti-staphylococcal antibiotics) and performing time-to-event analysis of the data, they were able to overcome problems of counting repeat infections at the same pin site during the course of external fixation, different periods of external fixation in different patients, or a need to classify pin site infections [13]. A survival plot of data becomes a visual representation of the behaviour of the regimes compared e.g., Kaplan-Meier survival analysis was used to evaluate time to the first problematic pin site in two groups: one which had used a daily cleaning regime with normal saline, crust removal, and either non-adherent dressings or left uncovered and the second group using a protocol of pin site care adopted from the Russian Ilizarov Scientific Centre in Kurgan. In the latter, a combination of antiseptic usage, occlusive dressings, and pressure bandaging to minimise skin movement around the wire or half-pin was utilised. (Fig. 18.3) The survival time showed a 50% chance of a pin site infection after 24 days in the first protocol compared to the same risk after 92 days using the Russian protocol. This highlights the suitability of time-to-event analysis for pin site infection studies – by using the first pin site infection as an end point and omitting that case from the data pool at that point onwards. This form of data analysis will accommodate the increased risk of infection with increased time in frame, something that is overlooked when studies report on just infection rates through follow-up.

A table of randomised controlled trials of the last 15 years on pin site care regimens is presented with comments (Table 18.1). The risk of type 2 errors is raised for some studies with non-significant results as are concerns over details in randomisation in some other studies with significant results [51, 53–58]. In particular, in those studies where randomisation is detailed, none describe use stratified randomisation or the tech-

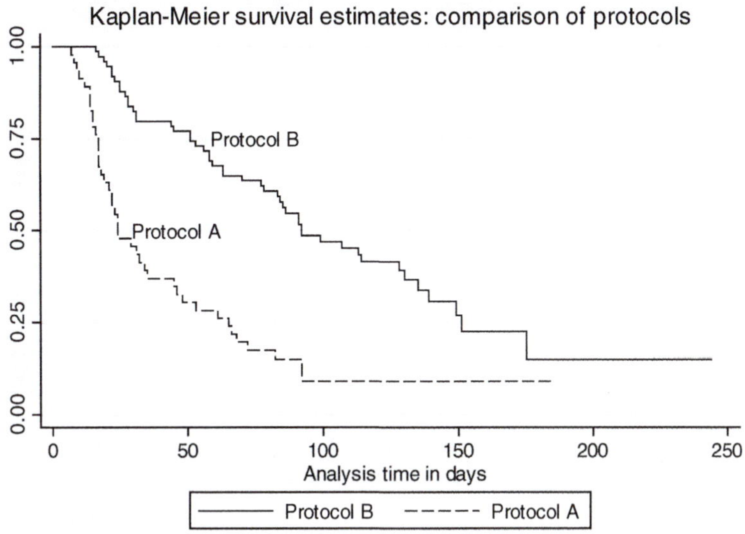

Fig. 18.3 Kaplan Meier analysis provides a clear visual depiction of the differences between the two regimes compared

nique of minimisation to ensure the groups are balanced in terms of patient characteristics. It would be important that the key influential characteristics (for pin site infections) in patients in each group were balanced e.g., fixators used in static mode or for correction. The lack of confidence interval reporting is notable.

All six studies have similar issues with the 'counting' of infected pin sites:

1. Those that use classification systems have categories which overlap (e.g., erythema and drainage) and that the systems have yet to be validated [54, 57]
2. Others have designed their own method of counting that prevent comparisons across other studies [46, 58]
3. The issue of a recurrent infection at the same pin site within a short period of treatment (whether through a change in cleaning frequency or a course of antibiotics) is not described whether counted as one (and the same) infection or a new second infection. This is an issue that may need recurrent event data analysis.
4. Patients have fixators on for different periods of time and as such are exposed to different risks of developing a pin site infection. As the process of randomisation is not clearly specified in some trials, it is uncertain if the patient characteristics in the samples are comparable.

As most pin site infections are skin infections producing pain, inflammation, discharge, and with only a small number progressing to an acute osteomyelitis or worse, and patients who have external fixators applied have them for varying reasons, a pragmatic approach to the design of such trials is required. This conclusion of a lack of strong evidence to recommend one regime over another, despite the availability of some randomised controlled trials, is repeated in the Cochrane Database of Systematic Reviews [59].

Microbiology of Pin Site Infections

The commonest organism causing a sero-purulent discharge from a pin site is *Staphylococcus aureus*. However, if positive cultures from swabs taken from pin sites are used to create a frequency table, then *Staphylococcus epidermidis* is top, with *S. aureus* and *E. coli* following [4, 60]. It suggests that skin commensals have a significant role in contributing to infections and local control measures (through cleaning or use of topical antiseptics) may have a place. This is supported in some reported studies [49, 51, 56, 57]. Conversely, some organisms have a tenacity to be persistent despite use of oral antibiotics, and this may reflect local bioavailability; this is the case with

Table 18.1 Summary and comments on several randomised controlled trials on pin site care regimes in the last 15 years

Authors	Year	Comparisons	Result	A priori power calculation	Confidence Intervals	Comments
Sáenz-Jalón et al.	2020	2% Alcoholic chlorhexidine v. 10% povidone-Iodine	No difference	No	Not reported	Method of randomisation not declared. At risk of type 2 error
Subramanyam et al.	2020	1. None v. povidone-iodine v. silver sulfadiazine v. chlorhexidine 2. Daily v. weekly dressings	No difference	Yes	Not reported but calculable from data in tables	Block randomisation method. This would have ensured a balance of numbers but not a balance of characteristics with patients in the four arms of the trial Novel method of counting infections at pin sites. Infections expressed as pin site infection days rate: $\frac{(\text{number of infected pin sites}) * (\text{days infected})}{(\text{number of pin sites observed}) * (\text{days observed})}$ Wide confidence intervals calculated from mean, number of pins and SD suggest the study to be underpowered. The authors, whilst having worked out a sample size of 561 pin sites in each arm for a power of 95% at a significance level of 0.05 then divided each arm into two groups with one having daily pin site care and the other weekly, thereby halving the sample sizes.
Ogbemudia et al.	2015	Daily with methylated spirit and dry sterile gauze v. Weekly with 1% silver sulphadiazine impregnated gauze	Significant difference	Yes	Not reported	Method of randomisation not declared. Prolonged in-patient stay (5 weeks) for most patients. Classification system used for pin site problems but actual data not reported.
Lee et al.	2012	Dry sterile gauze dressing v. polyhexamethylene biguanide impregnated gauze	Significant difference	Yes	Reported	Method of randomisation not declared. Relative risks with confidence intervals were reported as were the relative risk reductions.

Camathias et al.	2012	Daily pin site care using povidone-iodine dressings v. no pin site care	No difference	Yes	Only graphically as a boxplot for torsional stability of pins at extraction	Simple randomisation. Checks to ensure balance of characteristics across groups not described. Limited reporting of confidence intervals of results. Sample (type of fixator construct applied, treatment as inpatients for entire duration) may make extrapolation of results to external fixation in general trauma or limb reconstruction population limited.
Egol et al.	2006	Weekly dry dressing changes v. half-strength hydrogen peroxide daily pin site care v. weekly changes of chlorhexidine-impregnated discs (dressings)	No difference	Yes	Not reported	Simple randomisation. Checks to ensure balance of characteristics across groups not described. A covariate imbalance identified. Authors used a meaningful but as yet unvalidated classification system for degree of pin site complication. Overlap of the descriptors in the classification system would be expected. Absence of confidence intervals would make the non-significant result difficult to assess as these intervals may contain values that are meaningful.

MRSA and some gram-negative (*Pseudomonas Aeruginosa*) pin site infections [61]. Fortunately, the incidence of these problems is low.

Treating Pin Site Infections

While it is customary to try to grade pin site infections to tailor treatment, there is sufficient ambiguity and unreliability in the classifications so far proposed that to recommend a treatment protocol based on that will add to uncertainty. Most clinicians will take a pragmatic approach to the problem. The first symptom of a problem is pain and, while it is possible to have an 'innocent'-looking pin site and pain, some degree of erythema is usual. A swab for microbiological assay is a sensible step. While it is preferable to await the results before starting oral antibiotic therapy, the urgency for commencing treatment will depend on the impact of the problem. Pin sites discharging pus or the presence of areas of cellulitis warrant starting antimicrobial therapy promptly. In the absence of the results of swab cultures, an anti-staphylococcal with good bone and tissue bioavailability is recommended. Examples include cephalexin, ampicillin, clindamycin and erythromycin for good bioavailability and ciprofloxacin, doxycycline, rifampicin, and linezolid with excellent bioavailability. As always, it is preferable to consult a microbiologist even before prescribing empirical treatment.

Some pin site infections require more than oral therapy. These include those that do not or partially respond to oral antibiotics. The cause for the incomplete response should be sought before changing treatment. This may lie with the chosen antibiotic, the dose or dosing regimen, or one of the pin site where the problem is due to a biofilm becoming established and preventing antibiotic penetration, or that the infection has progressed to an established acute osteomyelitis. (Fig. 18.1) Signs of an osteomyelitis include radiolucency around the wire or half-pin on x-ray or the presence of a discharge and inflammation at both ends of a tensioned wire. (Fig. 18.2) For established biofilms and acute osteomyelitis complicating a pin site, a change of wire or half-pin is needed supplemented with continued targeted antibiotic use.

Occasionally, pin site problems persist even after extraction of the half-pin or wire. The ongoing problem is often the result of an osteomyelitis that has become chronic over a ring sequestrum. This problem originates at the time of drilling; the local track necrosis becomes a nidus which is overtaken by a local skin infection that ventures deep. Treatment will require debridement of this sequestrum by over-drilling the track and evacuating the swarf, followed with both systemic and local antibiotic delivery (Figs. 18.4, 18.5, and 18.6). The authors have used antibiotic impregnated calcium sulphate or bioactive glass for this purpose [62] Table 18.2.

Authors' Preference

A single winning formula for reducing pin site-related problems remains elusive. Continued efforts to separate the influential factors from those that matter less are needed. There is sufficient evidence that the following variables do matter (Boxes 18.1 and 18.2):

1. Material properties of the pins and wires
2. Method of pin insertion
3. Locations of the pin sites
4. Function of the fixator and tenure of external fixation
5. Aftercare regime to the pin site

The authors' unit has used two pin site care regimes in the last 24 years. Both were the subject of an observational study that revealed significant differences [13]. The better regime, adopted from the Ilizarov Institute in Russia, consisted of attention to most of the factors listed above. The dramatic reduction in superficial and deep pin site sepsis gave the unit confidence to engage in conversion surgery; switching from

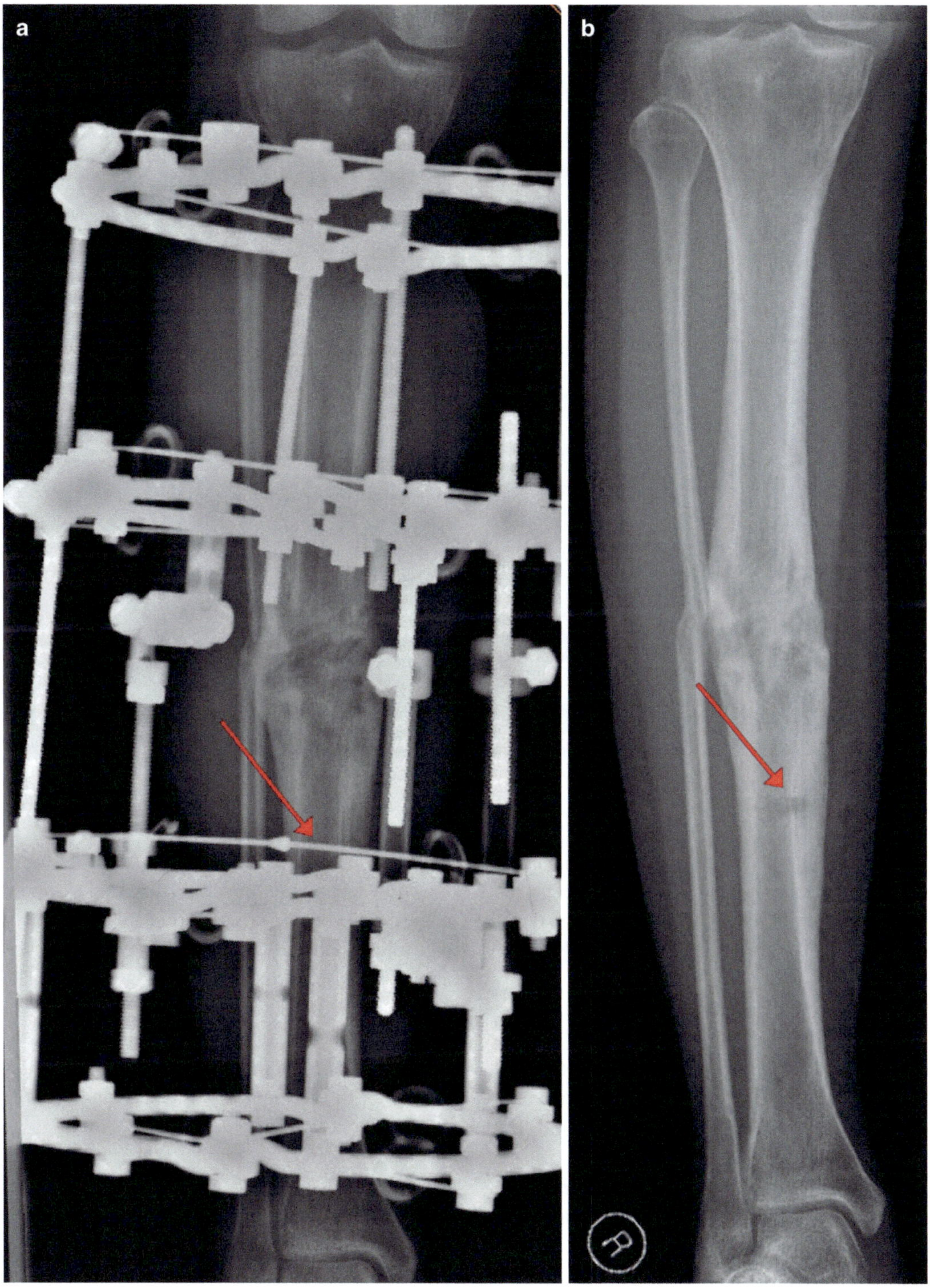

Figs. 18.4 (**a–d**) A wire inserted in this fixator (arrowed) became the focus of a chronic osteomyelitis. This is confirmed from the plain x-ray and PET-CT images

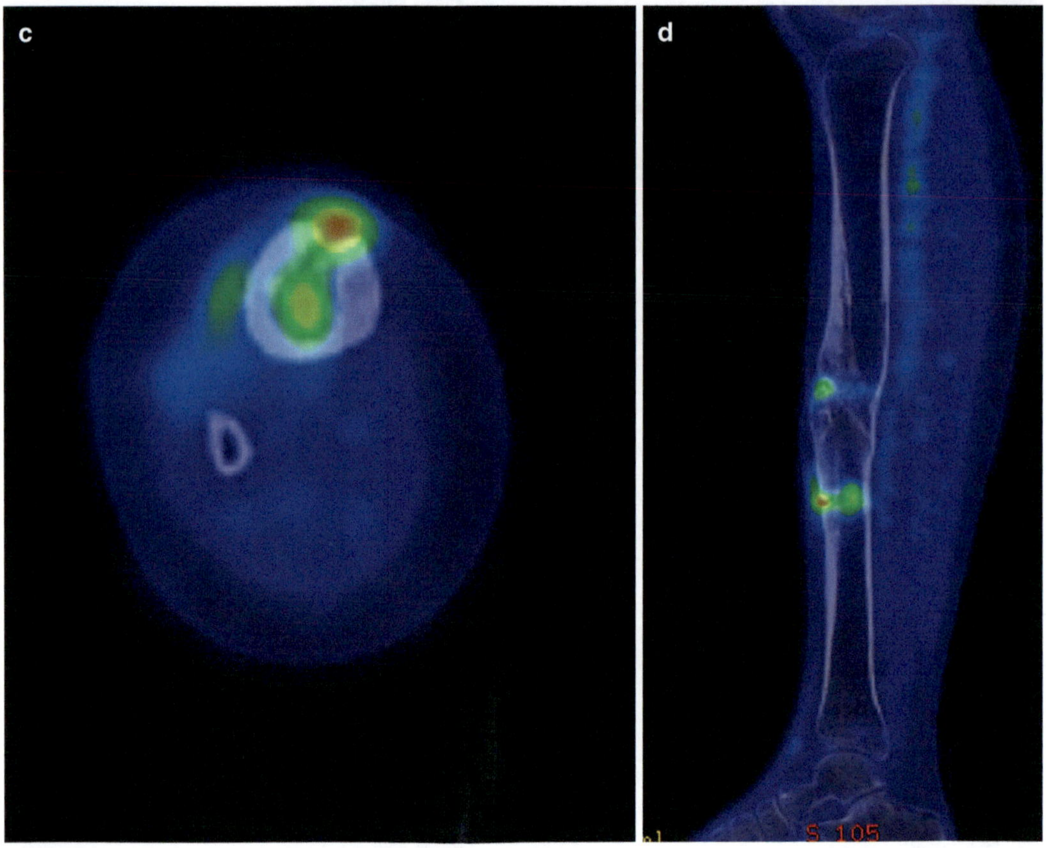

Fig. 18.4 (continued)

external to internal fixation in limb reconstruction surgery knowing that the risk of deep sepsis transfer was minimised. A pictorial of the pin site care regime is shown in Figs. 18.7, 18.8, 18.9, and 18.10.

Future work is needed to determine the optimum way to create and manage pin sites. An accurate localisation of pins and wires for purposes of data analysis, as recommended in the MUDEF system, should be considered [63]. Randomised controlled trials should have a priori sample size calculations based on size effects determined by previous published work. Clear descriptions of the manner of randomisation are important and stratified randomisation or minimisation techniques considered. Checks should be performed to ensure the groups compared are equivalent about the influential variables listed above other than the factor that is trialled. The samples will need to reflect the population for which the conclusions reached apply. A pragmatic approach to counting problematic pin sites has much to offer until a validated and reliable system of classification is produced. And, finally, the data should be subject to time-to-event analysis methods as this will account for different tenures of external fixation influencing the risk of pin site sepsis.

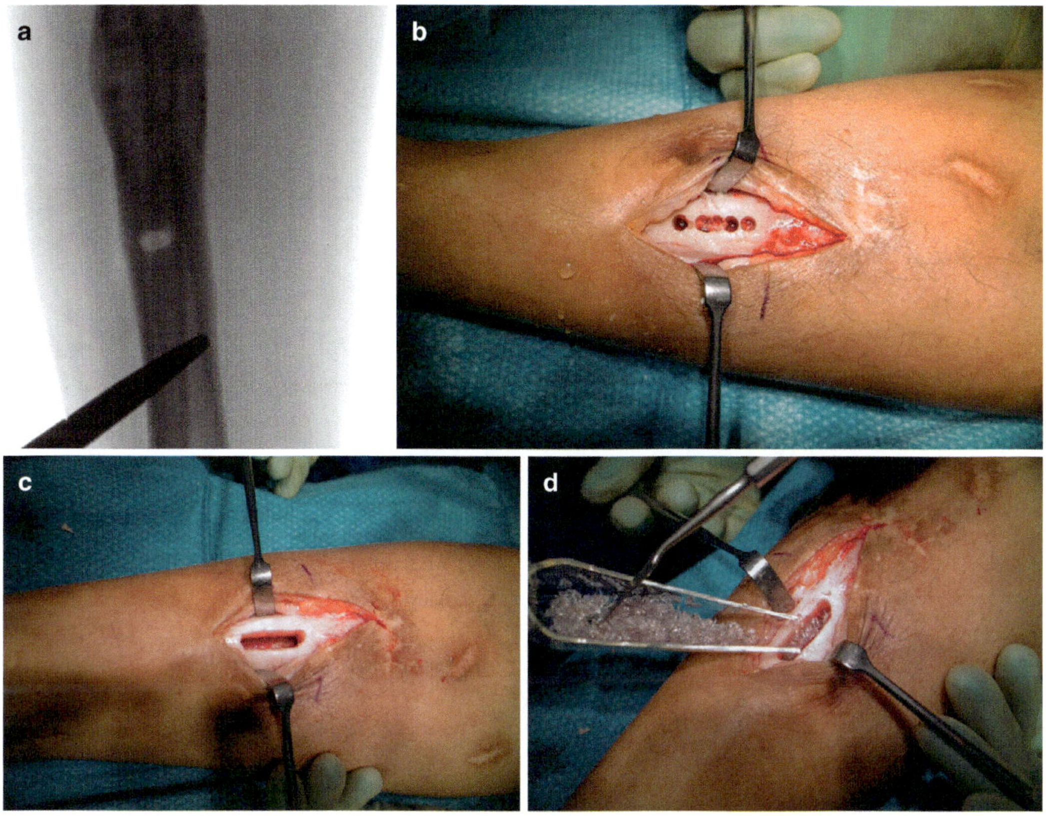

Fig. 18.5 (**a–d**) The previous track is over-drilled and enlarged to allow access to the medullary cavity. All swarf is removed, and the cavity lavaged before the cavity is filled with bioactive glass

Conclusion

Pin site infections remain a ubiquitous problem associated with external fixation. While an annoyance usually, these problems can evolve to a more serious infection that alters the course of treatment or, rarely, produce a limb- or life-threatening event. Evidence for managing pin sites is available but unfortunately point in different directions. The authors have considered the problem, its impact, and the most likely variables that influence the risk of pin site sepsis. Attention to all these variables is likely to reduce the extent of the problem until evidence emerges that points conclusively to one method of pin site care.

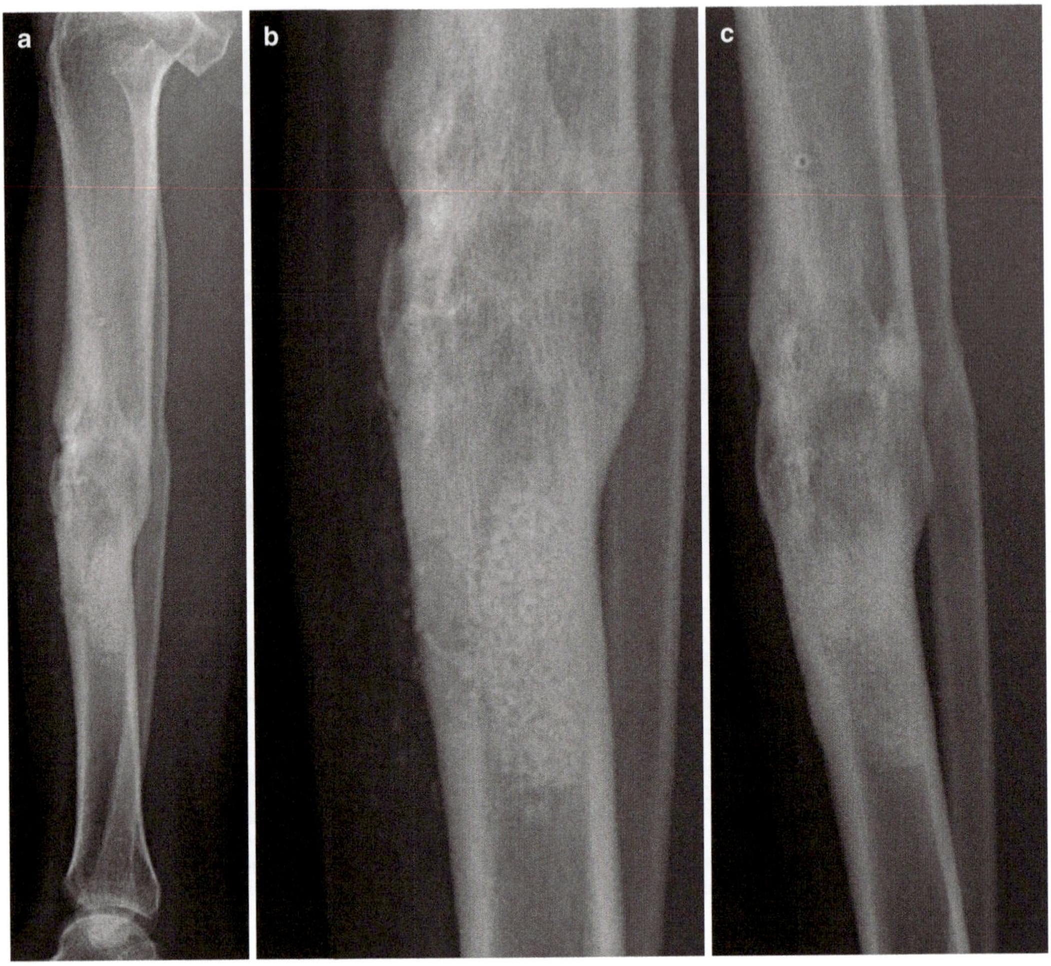

Fig. 18.6 (**a**–**c**) The lateral x-ray of the tibia shows the granular appearance of glass within the cavity. (**b**) is the close-up after surgery, and (**c**), at 5 years after surgery, confirms resolution of the problem and incorporation of the bioactive glass (less granular appearance)

Table 18.2 A suggested plan of action and treatment based on the presenting symptoms and signs of problem pin sites

Symptoms and signs	Action	Treatment
Pain without localised inflammation	Swab pin site and observe more frequently	Cleaning frequency may be increased
Pain with localised inflammation	Swab pin site and review with results	Cleaning frequency may be increased Oral antibiotic therapy based on results of swab culture and sensitivity report
Pain, localised inflammation, with seropurulent discharge	Swab pin site and review with results Consider x-ray for signs of lucency around pin or wire	Cleaning frequency may be increased Oral antibiotic therapy based on results of swab culture and sensitivity report Consider empirical antibiotic treatment after discussion with Microbiologist
Pain, localised inflammation, seropurulent discharge, with or without cellulitis Lucency on x-ray Discharge around both ends of wire	Swab pin site	Consider empirical antibiotic treatment after discussion with Microbiologist with change to appropriate antibiotics after swab results returned Consider wire or half-pin removal
Continued pain, inflammation and discharge after extraction of pin and wire	Swab pin site Consider CT scan of area	If chronic osteomyelitis around a ring sequestrum confirmed, consider track over-drilling and local and systemic antibiotic therapy

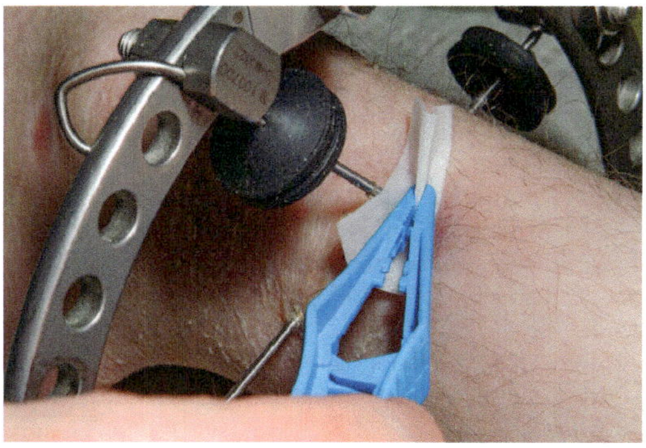

Fig. 18.7 The skin-pin interface and the wire are cleaned with alcohol

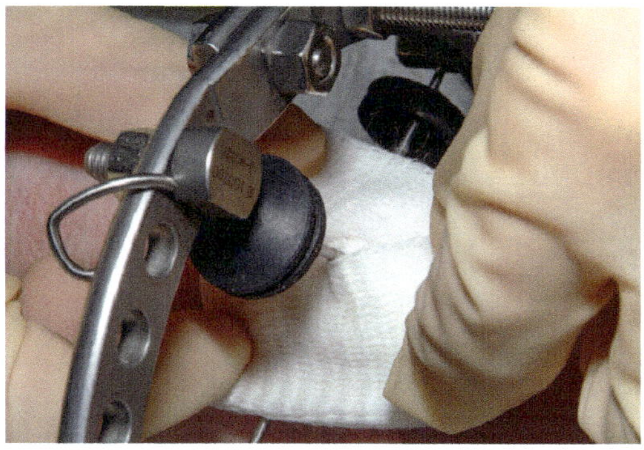

Fig. 18.8 A sterile dressing lightly dampened with alcoholic chlorhexidine is used to cover the pin or wire site

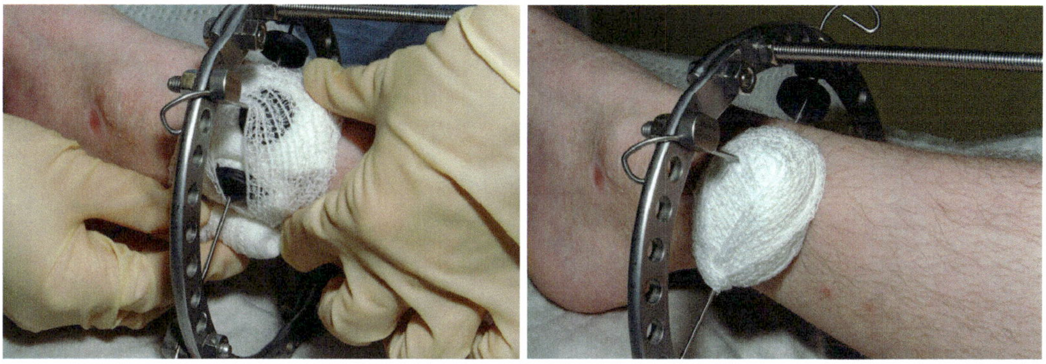

Figs. 18.9 and 18.10 A figure-of-8 bandage is wrapped over 2–3 pin sites to create an effective compression bandage that reduces skin movement around the wire or pin

Box 18.1: Key Learning Points

- Preventing pin site infections is a multi-step effort that includes the following:
  - Attention over the selection of types of pins and wires
  - Care during pin or wire insertion
  - An after-care regime to the pin site which aims to keep the local environment clean and stable
- Early diagnosis and treatment of pin site infections can prevent progression to an osteomyelitis.

Box 18.2: Pitfalls to Avoid

- Do not assume an after-care protocol alone will reduce the incidence of pin site problems.
- Have a system by which pin sites are reviewed regularly – whether by clinical staff or patients – as early intervention can prevent what is often a local skin infection from progressing into a localised acute osteomyelitis.
- Pin site infections that do not respond to appropriate oral antibiotics suggest the following with each requiring a different treatment response:
  - Incomplete cover by the chosen antibiotic or resistance by the microorganism

- Established biofilm problem with the affected half-pin or wire.
- Progression to an acute osteomyelitis
- Established chronic osteomyelitis with possible ring sequestra

References

1. Collinge CA, Goll G, Seligson D, Easley KJ. Pin tract infections: silver vs uncoated pins. Orthopedics. 1994;17(5):445–8.
2. Bibbo C, Patel DV, Gehrmann RM, Lin SS. Chlorhexidine provides superior skin decontamination in foot and ankle surgery: a prospective randomized study. Clin Orthop Relat Res. 2005;438:204–8.
3. Ferreira N, Marais LC. The effect of HIV infection on the incidence and severity of circular external fixator pin track sepsis: a retrospective comparative study of 229 patients. Strateg Trauma Limb Reconstr. 2014;9(2):111–5.
4. Parameswaran AD, Roberts CS, Seligson D, Voor M. Pin tract infection with contemporary external fixation: how much of a problem? J Orthop Trauma. 2003;17(7):503–7.
5. Rogers LC, Bevilacqua NJ, Frykberg RG, Armstrong DG. Predictors of postoperative complications of Ilizarov external ring fixators in the foot and ankle. J Foot Ankle Surg. 2007;46(5):372–5.
6. Turina M, Miller FN, Tucker CF, Polk HC. Short-term hyperglycemia in surgical patients and a study of related cellular mechanisms. Ann Surg. 2006;243(6):845–51; discussion 51–3.
7. Jellis JE. Orthopaedic surgery and HIV disease in Africa. Int Orthop. 1996;20(4):253–6.
8. Harrison WJ, Lewis CP, Lavy CB. Wound healing after implant surgery in HIV-positive patients. J Bone Joint Surg Br. 2002;84(6):802–6.
9. Norrish AR, Lewis CP, Harrison WJ. Pin-track infection in HIV-positive and HIV-negative patients with open fractures treated by external fixation: a prospective, blinded, case-controlled study. J Bone Joint Surg Br. 2007;89(6):790–3.
10. Beever L, Giles K, Meeson R. Postoperative complications associated with external skeletal fixators in cats. J Feline Med Surg. 2017;19(7):727–36.
11. Beever LJ, Giles K, Meeson RL. Postoperative complications associated with external skeletal fixators in dogs. Vet Comp Orthop Traumatol. 2018;31(2):137–43.
12. Schalamon J, Petnehazy T, Ainoedhofer H, Zwick EB, Singer G, Hoellwarth ME. Pin tract infection with external fixation of pediatric fractures. J Pediatr Surg. 2007;42(9):1584–7.
13. Davies R, Holt N, Nayagam S. The care of pin sites with external fixation. J Bone Joint Surg Br. 2005;87-B(5):716–9.
14. Jauregui JJ, Bor N, Thakral R, Standard SC, Paley D, Herzenberg JE. Life- and limb-threatening infections following the use of an external fixator. Bone Joint J. 2015;97-b(9):1296–300.
15. Laible C, Earl-Royal E, Davidovitch R, Walsh M, Egol KA. Infection after spanning external fixation for high-energy tibial plateau fractures: is pin site-plate overlap a problem? J Orthop Trauma. 2012;26(2):92–7.
16. Potter JM, van der Vliet QMJ, Esposito JG, McTague MF, Weaver M, Heng M. Is the proximity of external fixator pins to eventual definitive fixation implants related to the risk of deep infection in the staged management of tibial pilon fractures? Injury. 2019;50(11):2103–7.
17. Shah CM, Babb PE, McAndrew CM, Brimmo O, Badarudeen S, Tornetta P 3rd, et al. Definitive plates overlapping provisional external fixator pin sites: is the infection risk increased? J Orthop Trauma. 2014;28(9):518–22.
18. Eccles S, Handley B, Khan U, McFadyen I, Nanchahal J, Nayagam S. Skeletal stabilisation. In: Standards for the management of open fractures. Oxford, UK: Oxford University Press; 2020.
19. Clasper JC, Parker SJ, Simpson AH, Watkins PE. Contamination of the medullary canal following pin-tract infection. J Orthop Res. 1999;17(6):947–52.
20. Clasper JC, Stapley SA, Bowley DM, Kenward CE, Taylor V, Watkins PE. Spread of infection, in an animal model, after intramedullary nailing of an infected external fixator pin track. J Orthop Res. 2001;19(1):155–9.
21. Song HR, Oh CW, Mattoo R, Park BC, Kim SJ, Park IH, et al. Femoral lengthening over an intramedullary nail using the external fixator: risk of infection and knee problems in 22 patients with a follow-up of 2 years or more. Acta Orthop. 2005;76(2):245–52.
22. Kim SJ, Cielo Balce G, Huh YJ, Song SY, Song HR, Kim SJ. Deep intramedullary infection in tibial lengthening over an intramedullary nail. Acta Orthop Belg. 2011;77(4):506–15.
23. Yokoyama K, Uchino M, Nakamura K, Ohtsuka H, Suzuki T, Boku T, et al. Risk factors for deep infection in secondary intramedullary nailing after external fixation for open tibial fractures. Injury. 2006;37(6):554–60.
24. Eccles S, Handley B, Khan U, McFadyen I, Nanchahal J, Nayagam S. Timing of Soft Tissue Reconstruction. In: Standards for the Management of Open Fractures. Oxford, UK: Oxford University Press; 2020.
25. Pieske O, Geleng P, Zaspel J, Piltz S. Titanium alloy pins versus stainless steel pins in external fixation at

the wrist: a randomized prospective study. J Trauma. 2008;64(5):1275–80.
26. Coester LM, Nepola JV, Allen J, Marsh JL. The effects of silver coated external fixation pins. Iowa Orthop J. 2006;26:48–53.
27. Massè A, Bruno A, Bosetti M, Biasibetti A, Cannas M, Gallinaro P. Prevention of pin track infection in external fixation with silver coated pins: clinical and microbiological results. J Biomed Mater Res. 2000;53(5):600–4.
28. Piza G, Caja VL, Gonzalez-Viejo MA, Navarro A. Hydroxyapatite-coated external-fixation pins. The effect on pin loosening and pin-track infection in leg lengthening for short stature. J Bone Joint Surg Br Vol. 2004;86(6):892–7.
29. Pommer A, Muhr G, Dávid A. Hydroxyapatite-coated schanz pins in external fixators used for distraction osteogenesis : a randomized, controlled trial. J Bone Joint Surg Am. 2002;84(7):1162–6.
30. Saithna A. The influence of hydroxyapatite coating of external fixator pins on pin loosening and pin track infection: a systematic review. Injury. 2010;41(2):128–32.
31. DeJong ES, DeBerardino TM, Brooks DE, Nelson BJ, Campbell AA, Bottoni CR, et al. Antimicrobial efficacy of external fixator pins coated with a lipid stabilized hydroxyapatite/chlorhexidine complex to prevent pin tract infection in a goat model. J Trauma. 2001;50(6):1008–14.
32. Forster H, Marotta JS, Heseltine K, Milner R, Jani S. Bactericidal activity of antimicrobial coated polyurethane sleeves for external fixation pins. J Orthop Res. 2004;22(3):671–7.
33. Marotta JS, Coupe KJ, Milner R, Heseltine KE. Long-term bactericidal properties of a gentamicin-coated antimicrobial external fixation pin sleeve. J Bone Joint Surg Am. 2003;85-A Suppl 4:129–31.
34. Qu H, Knabe C, Radin S, Garino J, Ducheyne P. Percutaneous external fixator pins with bactericidal micron-thin sol-gel films for the prevention of pin tract infection. Biomaterials. 2015;62:95–105.
35. Moroni A, Vannini F, Mosca M, Giannini S. State of the art review: techniques to avoid pin loosening and infection in external fixation. J Orthop Trauma. 2002;16(3):189–95.
36. Pieske O, Kaltenhauser F, Pichlmaier L, Schramm N, Trentzsch H, Loffler T, et al. Clinical benefit of hydroxyapatite-coated pins compared with stainless steel pins in external fixation at the wrist: a randomised prospective study. Injury. 2010;41:1031–36.
37. Hyldahl C, Pearson S, Tepic S, Perren SM. Induction and prevention of pin loosening in external fixation: an in vivo study on sheep tibiae. J Orthop Trauma. 1991;5(4):485–92.
38. Pettine KA, Chao EYS, Kelly PJ. Analysis of the external fixator pin-bone Interface. Clin Orthop Related Res. 1993;293:18–27.
39. Walker JT, Rochat MC, Snider TA, Payton ME. The relevance of threaded external skeletal fixation pin insertion speed in canine bone with and without predrilling. Vet Comp Orthop Traumatol. 2014;27(4):249–56.
40. Lee J, Chavez CL, Park J. Parameters affecting mechanical and thermal responses in bone drilling: a review. J Biomech. 2018;71:4–21.
41. Eriksson A, Albrektsson T, Grane B, McQueen D. Thermal injury to bone. A vital-microscopic description of heat effects. Int J Oral Surg. 1982;11(2):115–21.
42. Kondo S, Okada Y, Iseki H, Hori T, Takakura K, Kobayashi A, et al. Thermological study of drilling bone tissue with a high-speed drill. Neurosurgery. 2000;46(5):1162–8.
43. Abouzgia MB, Symington JM. Effect of drill speed on bone temperature. Int J Oral Maxillofac Surg. 1996;25(5):394–9.
44. Lee J, Rabin Y, Ozdoganlar OB. A new thermal model for bone drilling with applications to orthopaedic surgery. Med Eng Phys. 2011;33(10):1234–44.
45. Basiaga M, Paszenda Z, Szewczenko J, Kaczmarek M. Influence of surgical drills wear on thermal process generated in bones. Acta Bioeng Biomech. 2013;15(4):19–23.
46. Gordon JE, Kelly-Hahn J, Carpenter CJ, Schoenecker PL. Pin site care during external fixation in children: results of a nihilistic approach. J Pediatr Orthop. 2000;20(2):163–5.
47. Sims M, Saleh M. External fixation – the incidence of pin site infection: a prospective audit. J Orthop Nurs. 2000;4(2):59–63.
48. Hutson JJ Jr, Zych GA. Infections in periarticular fractures of the lower extremity treated with tensioned wire hybrid fixators. J Orthop Trauma. 1998;12(3):214–8.
49. Davies R, Holt N, Nayagam S. The care of pin sites with external fixation. J Bone Joint Surg Br. 2005;87(5):716–9.
50. Nayagam S. Safe corridors in external fixation: the lower leg (tibia, fibula, hindfoot and forefoot). Strateg Trauma Limb Reconstr. 2007;2(2–3):105–10.
51. Sáenz-Jalón M, Sarabia-Cobo CM, Roscales Bartolome E, Santiago Fernández M, Vélez B, Escudero M, et al. A randomized clinical trial on the use of antiseptic solutions for the pin-site care of external fixators: chlorhexidine-alcohol versus povidone-iodine. J Trauma Nurs. 2020;27(3):146–50.
52. Bhandari M, Zlowodzki M, Tornetta PI, Schmidt A, Templeman DC. Intramedullary nailing following external fixation in femoral and tibial shaft fractures. J Orthop Trauma. 2005;19(2):140–4.
53. Camathias C, Valderrabano V, Oberli H. Routine pin tract care in external fixation is unnecessary: a randomised, prospective, blinded controlled study. Injury. 2012;43(11):1969–73.

54. Egol KA, Paksima N, Puopolo S, Klugman J, Hiebert R, Koval KJ. Treatment of external fixation pins about the wrist: a prospective, randomized trial. J Bone Joint Surg Am. 2006;88(2):349–54.
55. Nayagam S, Davies R, Holt N. Treatment of external fixation pins about the wrist. J Bone Joint Surg Am. 2006;88(11):2534–5; author reply 5
56. Lee CK, Chua YP, Saw A. Antimicrobial gauze as a dressing reduces pin site infection: a randomized controlled trial. Clin Orthop Relat Res. 2012;470(2):610–5.
57. Ogbemudia AO, Bafor A, Ogbemudia EJ, Edomwonyi E. Efficacy of 1% silver sulphadiazine dressings in preventing infection of external fixation pin-tracks: a randomized study. Strateg Trauma Limb Reconstr. 2015;10(2):95–9.
58. Subramanyam KN, Mundargi AV, Potarlanka R, Khanchandani P. No role for antiseptics in routine pin site care in Ilizarov fixators: a randomised prospective single blinded control study. Injury. 2019;50(3):770–6.
59. Lethaby A, Temple J, Santy-Tomlinson J. Pin site care for preventing infections associated with external bone fixators and pins. Cochrane Database Syst Rev. 2013;12:Cd004551.
60. Mahan J, Seligson D, Henry SL, Hynes P, Dobbins J. Factors in pin tract infections. Orthopedics. 1991;14(3):305–8.
61. Hamahashi K, Uchiyama Y, Kobayashi Y, Watanabe M. Delayed methicillin-resistant Staphylococcus aureus-induced osteomyelitis of the tibia after pin tract infection: two case reports. J Med Case Rep. 2017;11(1):23.
62. Lindfors N, Geurts J, Drago L, Arts JJ, Juutilainen V, Hyvonen P, et al. Antibacterial bioactive glass, S53P4, for chronic bone infections - a multinational study. Adv Exp Med Biol. 2017: 81–92.
63. Solomin L. Method of unified designation of external fixation (MUDEF). In: Solomin L, editor. The basic principles of external skeletal fixation using the Ilizarov and other devices. Springer-Verlag Mailand; 2012. p. 53–62.

Part III

Chronic Musculoskeletal Infections and Their Sequelae

19 Chronic Hematogenous Osteomyelitis

Deepika Pinto and Alaric Aroojis

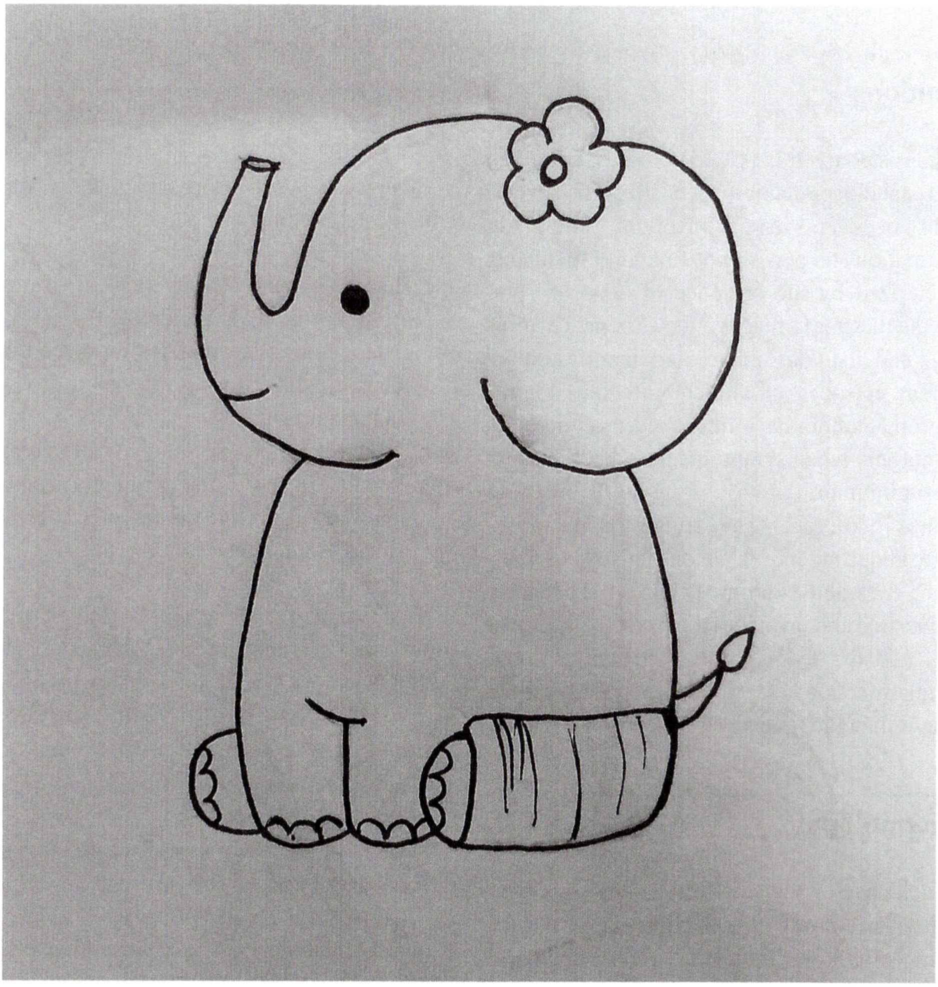

Both authors contributed to the study conception and design. Material preparation, data collection and analysis were performed by Deepika Pinto and Alaric Aroojis. The first draft of the manuscript was written by Deepika Pinto and both authors commented on previous versions of the manuscript. Both authors read and approved the final manuscript.

D. Pinto · A. Aroojis (✉)
Department of Paediatric Orthopaedics, Bai Jerbai Wadia Hospital for Children, Mumbai, India

© Springer Nature Switzerland AG 2022
M. V. Belthur et al. (eds.), *Pediatric Musculoskeletal Infections*,
https://doi.org/10.1007/978-3-030-95794-0_19

Introduction

Osteomyelitis is an ancient disease and has been known since time immemorial. The term "osteomyelitis" was introduced by Nelaton in 1844 [1]. It derives from "osteon" meaning bone, "myelo" meaning marrow, and "itis" meaning inflammation and thus describes the condition in which the bone and its marrow are inflamed, due to infection by microorganisms [2].

Definition

Chronic osteomyelitis (COM) broadly describes a long-standing infection (persisting for several months or even years), involving low-grade inflammation and persistence of microorganisms, characterized by the presence of dead necrotic bone (sequestrae), reactive new bone (involucrum), and fistulous tracts, and manifested by recurrent episodes of clinical infection [3, 4]. Numerous authors have described osteomyelitis to be chronic when symptoms have been present for a minimum duration ranging from 1 to 6 months [5, 6]; others have suggested that osteomyelitis requiring more than one episode of treatment be considered chronic [7]. It is the presence of sequestrae and involucra that is the hallmark of COM, and the radiographic evidence of long-standing infection is far more important for diagnosing it than the time since onset of symptoms.

Epidemiology

The incidence of acute as well as chronic osteomyelitis has considerably declined in most parts of the western world due to improvements in hygiene, nutrition, and the overall standards of living [1, 8, 9]. The same cannot be said for developing nations, where it is estimated that approximately 60 million children suffer from musculoskeletal impairment due to infection, a significant proportion of which will be COM [8]. Although the mortality from osteomyelitis has considerably declined with the advent of modern anti-microbial agents, the morbidity of COM is still considerably high.

The most commonly affected bone in COM is the tibia. The relatively poor vascularity of the tibia, coupled with the extensive periosteal stripping that occurs in severe acute hematogenous osteomyelitis (AHO), predisposes to progression to COM in the tibia [10]. The next most commonly affected bone is the femur followed by the humerus [11]. As in most other forms of musculoskeletal infection, *Staphylococcus aureus* continues to remain the most common causative organism in COM [12–14].

Etiology

Waldvogel in 1970 propounded three ways in which osteomyelitis can occur [15]:

(a) Hematogenous osteomyelitis – the form seen most commonly in children
(b) Osteomyelitis secondary to a contiguous focus of infection – occurring following trauma and surgery
(c) Osteomyelitis associated with peripheral vascular disease – predominantly seen in diabetics as foot soft-tissue infections which spread to the bone

In the pediatric age group, COM is most commonly the consequence of inadequately treated AHO, the so-called chronic hematogenous osteomyelitis (CHOM) [11]. Less commonly, COM in children may be seen following trauma or as a complication of bony surgeries [4].

Pathogenesis

Acute hematogenous osteomyelitis typically begins in the metaphysis of long bones in children. As the infection is established in the metaphysis, the bacteria multiply, an exudate is produced due to the host immune response, and ultimately pus is formed. The pus collects under pressure and can exit the metaphysis in one of three ways – into the diaphysis; across the physis into the epiphysis; or through the metaphyseal cortex into the sub-periosteal space [16]. In most instances, the pus breaks through the thin metaphyseal cortex and produces a sub-periosteal abscess. When left untreated, the pus eventually breaks through the periosteum and spreads into the soft tissues. It may eventually rupture through the skin producing a draining sinus.

The periosteum in a child is very thick and does not get ruptured until late. The periosteum, however, is loosely adherent to the underlying cortex and is easily raised, interrupting the periosteal blood supply to the bone. As the infection progresses unchecked, increased intramedullary pressure and thrombosis of medullary blood vessel cuts off the endosteal blood supply to the cortex as well. In this manner, affected parts of the cortex become avascular and necrotic. This avascular bone is called a *sequestrum*. In small children, large parts of bone, even the entire diaphysis, may become sequestered in this manner. The elevated periosteum retains its own blood supply from the overlying muscles and thus starts producing new bone. This newly formed reactive bone, which is produced in an effort to wall off the infection and maintain bony stability, is called the *involucrum*. The quality of the involucrum depends on the extent of damage to the periosteum. The breach in the cortex through which spontaneous drainage of pus occurs is termed as the *cloaca* [4].

Clinical Presentation

Most children with CHOM present with the diagnosis evident, with a history of prior AHO and its medical and surgical management. The typical history is of one of chronic pain along with a discharging wound. The disease may have been present for many months or even years, with episodes of recurrence interspersed between long quiescent periods. Fever, if present, is usually low grade. There may be a history of cyclical pain, which gradually increases in severity, associated with fever at its peak, which subsides on its own once pus breaks out through a sinus tract [17].

On examination, the affected limb is swollen due to both soft-tissue edema and bony overgrowth, and there is deep bony tenderness. Abnormal mobility may be found in case of a coexistent pathological fracture. The skin overlying the infected bone displays scars of previous surgery and typically one or more sinus tract openings. Adherence of the skin to the underlying bone is a characteristic feature of osteomyelitis [4]. Occasionally, a part of the bone may lie exposed (Fig. 19.1a,b). Some degree of shortening is often present in long standing cases, which may be due to bone loss, physeal injury, or both. Adjacent joints are stiff, most often due to scarring of muscles to the underlying infected bone, which limits their excursion. A reactive effusion may be present during acute exacerbations of disease.

Classification

Numerous classification systems have been proposed for COM. The Cierny and Mader osteomyelitis staging system (Table 19.1) was first published in 1984 and has since been widely used [18, 19]. This system combines the anatomic type of bone infection (Types I–IV) with the physiological class of the host (Classes I–III) to define 12 clinical stages of osteomyelitis. This system was developed primarily for use in adult osteomyelitis, particularly in cases of traumatic or iatrogenic osteomyelitis [8]. Childhood COM typically falls under Stage 4B – diffuse bone involvement in a host that is compromised either systemically or locally. This classification system has limited usefulness in the management of COM in children [8].

The Beit Cure classification system was developed by Jones et al. specifically for use in chronic hematogenous osteomyelitis in children, with the intention of having a system that would help decide surgical management as well as provide prognostic information [8, 20]. It is based on plain radiographic findings, which make it particularly useful in resource-poor settings, where the majority of cases of CHOM are seen. The first step is to identify whether or not a sequestrum is present [20]. Accordingly, one of the main types in this classification is the sequestrum/involucrum type (Type B). The other two types, where sequestrae are absent, are the Brodie type (Type A), characterized by metaphyseal abscesses, and the sclerotic type (Type C), where the bone is diffusely sclerotic.

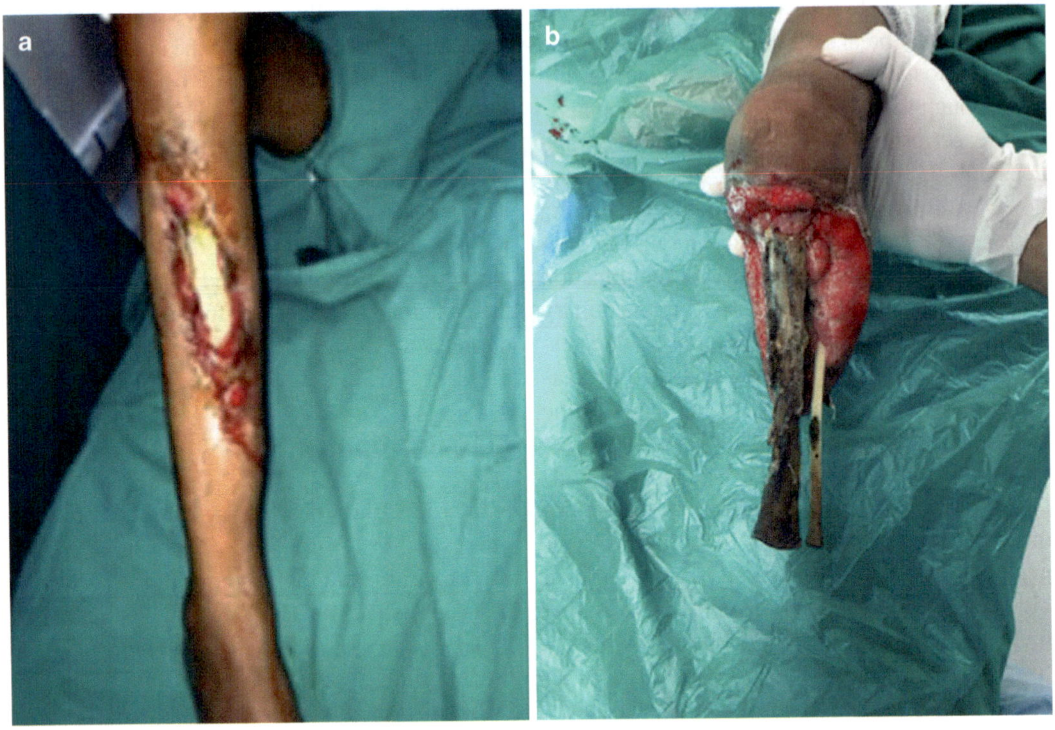

Fig. 19.1 Clinical presentations of CHOM. (**a**) A case of tibial osteomyelitis with exposed bone surrounded by scarred and unhealthy soft tissues. (**b**) An extreme case of neglected CHOM with sequestration and necrosis of the entire tibia and fibula. It eventually necessitated a below knee amputation

Table 19.1 Cierny and Mader osteomyelitis staging system

Anatomic type	
Stage 1	Medullary osteomyelitis
Stage 2	Superficial osteomyelitis
Stage 3	Localized osteomyelitis
Stage 4	Diffuse osteomyelitis
Physiological class	
A host	Normal host
B host	Systemically compromised host (Bs) or Locally compromised host (Bl) or Systemically and locally compromised host (Bls)
C host	Treatment worse than the disease (not a surgical candidate, requires suppressive or no treatment)
Clinical Stage = Anatomic type + Physiological class	

Type B is further subdivided into four types depending upon the size of the sequestrum in relation to the rest of the bone and the quality of the involucrum. In Type B1 (localized cortical sequestrum), only a peripheral strip of cortical bone is involved. In this type, removal of the sequestrum will not compromise the structural integrity of the bone. In the remaining three types, the entire circumference of the bone is affected. In these cases, the quality of the involucrum will determine whether some form of limb stabilization will be required after sequestrectomy. Where structural involucrum is present, and the consistency of the involucrum is relatively normal, it is designated Type B2 (sequestrum with normal involucrum). In addition, where structural involucrum is present, but it is of sclerotic consistency, it is designated Type B3 (sequestrum with sclerotic involucrum). Where there is no structural involucrum, it is designated as Type B4 (sequestrum without structural involucrum). Finally, where there is extensive metaphyseal involvement that is likely to damage the physis resulting in shortening or angular deformities, the suffix "P" (proximal) or "D" (distal) is added to denote the respective physis that is affected.

Investigations

The gold standard for establishing the diagnosis of CHOM is a positive culture from bone biopsy along with histopathology consistent with necrosis [21]. Blood investigations and imaging studies cannot conclusively prove or disprove the existence of an infectious process. They can only aid in diagnosis and help in planning surgical treatment.

Laboratory Investigations

Laboratory investigations generally lack any specificity for CHOM. The erythrocyte sedimentation rate (ESR) and C-reactive protein (CRP) are frequently elevated; however, the white blood cell (WBC) count is very often normal [22]. These investigations play an adjunctive role in management; they should be obtained at the outset so as to establish a baseline and thereafter to monitor the response to treatment [17].

Imaging Studies

Plain Radiographs

High-quality plain radiographs are usually the initial study obtained. Typical findings on plain radiographs include sequestrae, cortical destruction, periosteal new bone formation, loss of corticomedullary differentiation, osteopenia, sclerosis, cysts, and soft tissue changes. Assessment of the presence and size of sequestrae and the quality of the involucrum allow classification as per the Beit Cure system, which helps in surgical planning and prognostication [20].

Computerized Tomography (CT) Scan

CT provides better visualization of cortical bone destruction, periosteal reaction, and involucrum. It helps identify sequestrae and cloacae not seen on plain radiographs. On CT scanning, a sequestrum appears as a sclerotic lesion with a radiolucent rim [23]. Intramedullary gas is another ancillary sign of osteomyelitis, which is best seen on CT [23]. CT is also useful for evaluating bone defects and the extent of sclerosis. Finally, CT is also useful in guiding percutaneous aspirations and needle biopsies when the diagnosis is in doubt [24].

Magnetic Resonance Imaging (MRI)

MRI has emerged as the investigation of choice in osteomyelitis because of its excellent anatomical detail, superior assessment of soft tissues, and lack of ionizing radiation [23]. The main disadvantages of MRI are the high cost and the need for sedation in small children. The sequences most useful in the evaluation of osteomyelitis include fluid sensitive sequences (T2-weighted, fat-suppressed (FS), and short T1 recovery (STIR) sequences), for visualizing inflammatory changes and fluid collections, and gadolinium-enhanced fat-suppressed T1-weighted images, for assessing abscesses, sinus tracts, and differentiating from tumors.

Nuclear Medicine Imaging

Nuclear medicine studies are very sensitive for the detection of CHOM [23]. The newer targeted radionuclides and hybrid techniques such as single photon emission computed tomography-CT (SPECT-CT) provide greater specificity and more anatomical information respectively as compared to the conventional techniques [23]. The most commonly used nuclear medicine imaging studies in the diagnosis of osteomyelitis include the triple-phase bone scans, gallium scans, and white cell scans. Fluorodeoxyglucose positron emission tomography (FDG-PET) is a relatively newer technique. A systematic review and meta-analysis of the diagnostic accuracy of various imaging modalities for chronic osteomyelitis found that FDG-PET was the most sensitive technique for detecting COM and that its specificity was greater than that of white cell scans, triple-phase scans, and even MRI [25].

Tissue Sampling

There is no doubt that cultures from the infected tissue are essential not only for the diagnosis but also for guiding medical management of CHOM. The most representative cultures are usually those that are grown from deep samples obtained at the time of debridement. During surgery, it is important that every isolated pocket of pus and granulation tissue be sampled and cultured separately. Polymicrobial infection is known to occur in cases of chronic osteomyelitis, and hence, samples should be obtained from multiple sites so as to identify as many infecting organisms as possible [26]. This includes obviously purulent material, soft tissue, bone obtained from curettage, scrapings from the bed of the involved bone, and even material from the sinus tract [26]. Cultures must be repeated at every subsequent debridement procedure as well [19]. Samples obtained at the initial debridement must be sent for a complete microbiological panel, which includes Gram and acid-fast staining, aerobic and anaerobic cultures and sensitivity, fungal and mycobacterial cultures, and histopathology.

Salient features of COM
Characterized by hallmarks of dead necrotic bone (sequestrum) surrounded by reactive new bone (involucrum)
Most often the consequence of improperly treated AHO
Most commonly involved is tibia, followed by femur and humerus, respectively
Most common causative organism is *Staphylococcus aureus*
Clinically presents as recurrent or intermittent disease
Classification systems: Most useful in adults ➔ Cierny Mader classification Most useful in children ➔ Jones (Beit Cure) classification
Gold standard for diagnosis is biopsy from infected bone with histopathological and microbiological evaluation
Main differential diagnosis – malignant tumor (osteogenic sarcoma/Ewing's sarcoma)
Best way to prevent CHOM is to aggressively treat AHO

Treatment

The aims of treatment in CHOM are eradication of infection and restoration of limb function. In addition to the skeletal disease, these children have often previously undergone multiple surgeries and have compromised skin and soft tissue structures; besides having overall poor health due to chronic illness. The management of such children must be individualized and requires a multidisciplinary team effort, involving orthopedic surgeons, plastic surgeons, infectious disease (ID) specialists, physiotherapists, etc.

Optimization of the Host

Malnutrition and presence of coexistent infectious diseases are important systemic factors that influence the response to treatment. Simple measures to be considered at the start of treatment include nutritional supplementation with a high protein diet, correction of anemia with iron and folate supplements, multivitamin and mineral supplementation, de-worming agents, and improvement of hygiene.

Antimicrobial Therapy

Systemic Antibiotic Therapy

The antibiotic course must be tailored to the reports of culture-sensitivity testing, and this is best done in consultation with ID specialists. Antibiotics commonly used in childhood CHOM are listed in Table 19.2. The addition of oral rifampicin as a supplement to first-line anti-staphylococcal drugs has long been shown to improve cure rates [27]. When prolonged courses of intravenous antibiotics are considered necessary, outpatient parenteral antimicrobial therapy (OPAT) has been employed in order to reduce duration of hospital stay; however, it is not without complications [28]. Some authors have reported cure of CHOM with antibiotic therapy alone, in carefully selected cases (with absence

Table 19.2 Commonly used antimicrobials in childhood chronic osteomyelitis

Organism	Antibiotic
Methacillin-sensitive *Staphylococcus aureus* (MSSA)	First-generation cephalosporin (Cefazolin/ Cephalothin) Clindamycin
Methacillin-resistant *Staphylococcus aureus* (MRSA)	Vancomycin Clindamycin Linezolid Daptomycin
Streptococcus pyogenes	Penicillin G (intravenous) First-generation cephalosporin (Cephazolin/Cephalothin) Clindamycin
Streptococcus pneumoniae	Penicillin G (intravenous) First-generation cephalosporin (Cefazolin/ Cephalothin)
Gram-negative bacilli	Gentamycin Cefotaxime Ceftriaxone

of necrosis, abscesses, and joint involvement) [13]; however, this is unlikely to be successful in the majority of cases.

There is no consensus on the appropriate duration of antibiotic therapy. Traditionally, antibiotic regimens for CHOM have consisted of parenteral antibiotics for 4–6 weeks, followed by oral therapy for 2–5 months [29]. However, there is no evidence that prolonged parenteral antibiotics will be able to penetrate the necrotic bone [30]. Some authors suggest that, with the radical debridement procedures and effective muscle flaps that are used today, early revascularization of the diseased bone occurs, which implies that the duration of antibiotic therapy can be shortened accordingly [30]. In fact, some observational studies have shown that shorter antibiotic regimens have success rates comparable to those of longer regimens [29, 30].

Local Antibiotic Delivery Systems

These include the following:

(a) Antibiotic-impregnated polymethyl methacrylate (PMMA) beads and spacers
(b) Biodegradable antibiotic delivery systems
(c) Closed suction antibiotic irrigation systems

(a) *Antibiotic-Impregnated Polymethyl Methacrylate (PMMA) Beads and Spacers*

Antibiotic-loaded PMMA has been used for the prevention and treatment of skeletal infection for many years and has several advantages over systemic antibiotic therapy. Antibiotic from the PMMA is leeched into the wound hematoma and secretions, producing local antibiotic concentrations many times in excess of the minimal inhibitory concentrations (MIC), while at the same time maintaining low systemic levels and thus minimizing systemic toxicity. It is also considerably less expensive than prolonged systemic antibiotic therapy.

In children, antibiotic-loaded PMMA is typically used in the form of either beads or spacers. The mechanism of antibiotic elution is by leakage of the antibiotic through minute cracks in the cement; and as such, the size and shape of the PMMA significantly affects the concentrations of antibiotics released [31]. Antibiotic beads provide a much higher surface area for antibiotic release as compared to solid spacers. "Mini-beads" (3–5 mm) have been shown to release up to 93% of their antibiotic content as compared to 24% released by standard-sized (7 mm) beads [32]. Spacers are more useful for preserving local anatomy and reducing soft tissue ingrowth in large defects. Bar-on et al. recently described the successful use of antibiotic-impregnated cement rods inserted into the medullary canal and the rods being fashioned over Kirschner wires using chest tubes as molds [33].

The type of antibiotic is also an important consideration – clindamycin has been found to have the best elution profile, with the highest seroma, granulation tissue, and bone concentrations; vancomycin produces excellent bone concentrations, whereas tobramycin produces high serum and granulation tissue concentrations [31]. Cephalosporins, tetracycline, and rifampicin are not very suitable for use with PMMA [31, 32]. Mixing more than one antibiotic into the PMMA has been shown to have a synergistic effect; not only does the combination widen the antimicrobial spectrum but also improves the elution rates as well [31]. This is seen in combinations like vancomycin + tobramycin, gentamicin + vancomycin, and gentamicin + clindamycin [31, 32].

(b) *Biodegradable Antibiotic Delivery Systems*

The purported advantages of these alternatives to PMMA for the depot delivery of antibiotics include avoidance of second surgery for removal, delivery of the entire quantity of added antibiotic (whereas PMMA releases less than half of the total antibiotic added to it), and participation in the bone healing process, hence decreasing the need for secondary reconstructive procedures [31] (Fig. 19.2a–g).

The biodegradable substances belong to three categories [34]:

(i) Proteins: Collagen, gelatin, thrombin, fibrinogen, albumin, and autologous blood clot
(ii) Bone graft substitutes: Calcium sulfate, morselized cancellous bone, tricalcium phosphate, hydroxyapatite, and bioactive glass
(iii) Synthetic polymers: Polyanhydride, polylactide, polyglycolide, polyhydroxyalkanoate, etc.

Use of these biodegradable substances is still largely in experimental stages. Thus, if used, it is wise to limit the quantity of antibiotic added; the total quantity of antibiotic added should not exceed the dose that would be safe were it to be injected intravenously over 24 hours [34].

(c) *Closed Suction Antibiotic Irrigation Systems*

This technique, originally devised by Weber and Lautenbach, consists of the placement of a double lumen tube into the medullary canal after reaming, through which an antibiotic solution can be delivered into the canal and the effluent drained [35]. The advantages of this technique are that the antibiotic can be easily modified once culture reports become available and that culture of the effluent fluid can help ascertain if the infection is under control. Hung applied a similar technique of multiple cortical bone fenestrations and continuous antibiotic irrigation in 276 cases of tibial hematogenous osteomyelitis in children and found it to be safe and effective [36].

Surgery

The goals of surgery in CHOM are to evacuate all infected tissues so as to reduce the bacterial load

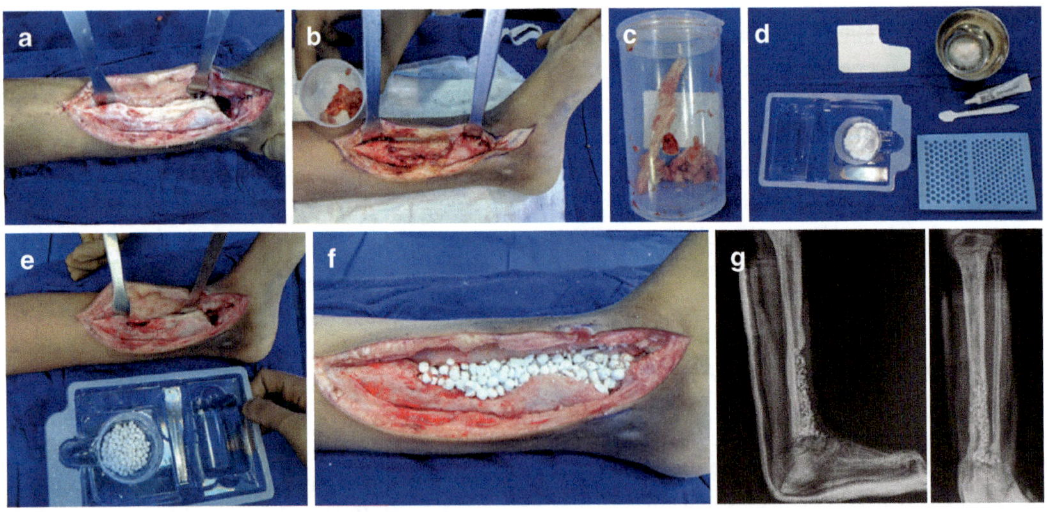

Fig. 19.2 Technique for preparation of biodegradable hydroxyapatite antibiotic beads. (**a**) CHOM of tibia with slough and sequestrum. (**b**) Radical debridement performed. (**c**) Excised sequestrum and slough. (**d**) Kit for preparation of hydroxyapatite antibiotic beads. (**e**) Beads prepared. (**f**) Beads inserted in gap. (**g**) Postoperative radiographs

and to improve local vascularity thus allowing better penetration of circulating antibiotics into the infected tissues. This typically requires multiple surgeries. The large prospective study by Cierny and Mader found an average of 3.8 procedures being required per adult patient [19], whereas a retrospective study in children by Yeargan et al. found the number of surgeries required to be 3.2 procedures per child [12].

Debridement

A good debridement is the cornerstone of treatment for CHOM. The debridement must be performed in a manner akin to musculoskeletal tumor surgery [19, 37]. The most common mistake is the tendency to perform an inadequate debridement, which is likely the most important cause for the high rate of recurrence in CHOM [38]. Table 19.3 provides an outline of the important steps during debridement surgery in CHOM.

There is some controversy regarding the appropriate time to perform a sequestrectomy. Many authors recommend early sequestrectomy as the sequestrum causes persistence of infection (Fig. 19.3a–d). Others advise delaying sequestrectomy until the involucrum has prop-

Table 19.3 Debridement and curettage in chronic osteomyelitis

Preoperatively
Careful preoperative planning – analyze imaging studies to determine extent of infection, number and location of sequestrae, site(s) of cloacae
Reserve blood – considerable blood loss can occur
Inject sinus tracts with methylene blue/fluorescein dye 24hours prior – makes them easier to locate and excise
Intraoperatively
Place incisions in between myo-cutaneous territories, so that future flap creation is not hampered.
Avoid incisions over the subcutaneous surfaces of bones
Center the incision over the sinuses wherever possible, and excise all sinus tracts completely
Incise the periosteum and elevate it adequately all around the infected bone
If a cloaca exists, widen it and perform the debridement through it.
Else, create a window in the weakest part of the involucrum
Using a drill, outline an oval cortical window – long axis of the window parallel to long axis of the bone (to avoid excessive focal weakening of the bone)
Connect the drill holes using an osteotome and de-roof the infected lesion
Excise any overhanging edges of bone to allow free drainage (saucerize the defect)
Remove all sequestrae, pus, granulation tissue, and scarred, non-viable tissue (both bone and soft-tissue)
Aggressively excise all necrotic bone, but leave intact the viable involucrum
Instruments useful for debridement include the following: Scalpels Rongeurs, osteotomes, curettes Straight stem and angled dental mirrors Pneumatic bone scalpel/dental burr
Often the lesion is surrounded by dense sclerotic bone. Use a rongeur or burr to excise this ischemic bone gradually until healthy bone is reached – as demonstrated by punctate bleeding bone (paprika sign)
Debride in a centrifugal pattern, until you reach a rim of healthy bone and soft tissue
Open the medullary cavity on both sides using a drill. This allows blood vessels to grow into the lesion
Give copious lavage with normal saline
Check stability of the bone: If >70% of cortical volume has been retained, the limb may simply be protected in a cast. If bone loss is greater, consider applying an external fixator
Wound closure
If the dead space is very small ⇒ Close it over a drain In case of a large defect:
If second surgery is not likely to be necessary ⇒ fill the defect with calcium sulfate granules/beads mixed with antibiotics
If repeat debridement/reconstruction will be necessary ⇒ place antibiotic-impregnated beads or spacer in the defect If soft tissue closure is not possible or it is only possible with excess tension ⇒ leave the wound open and plan definitive closure at the time of repeat debridement.
Postoperatively
Keep limb splinted to avoid pathological fracture during healing

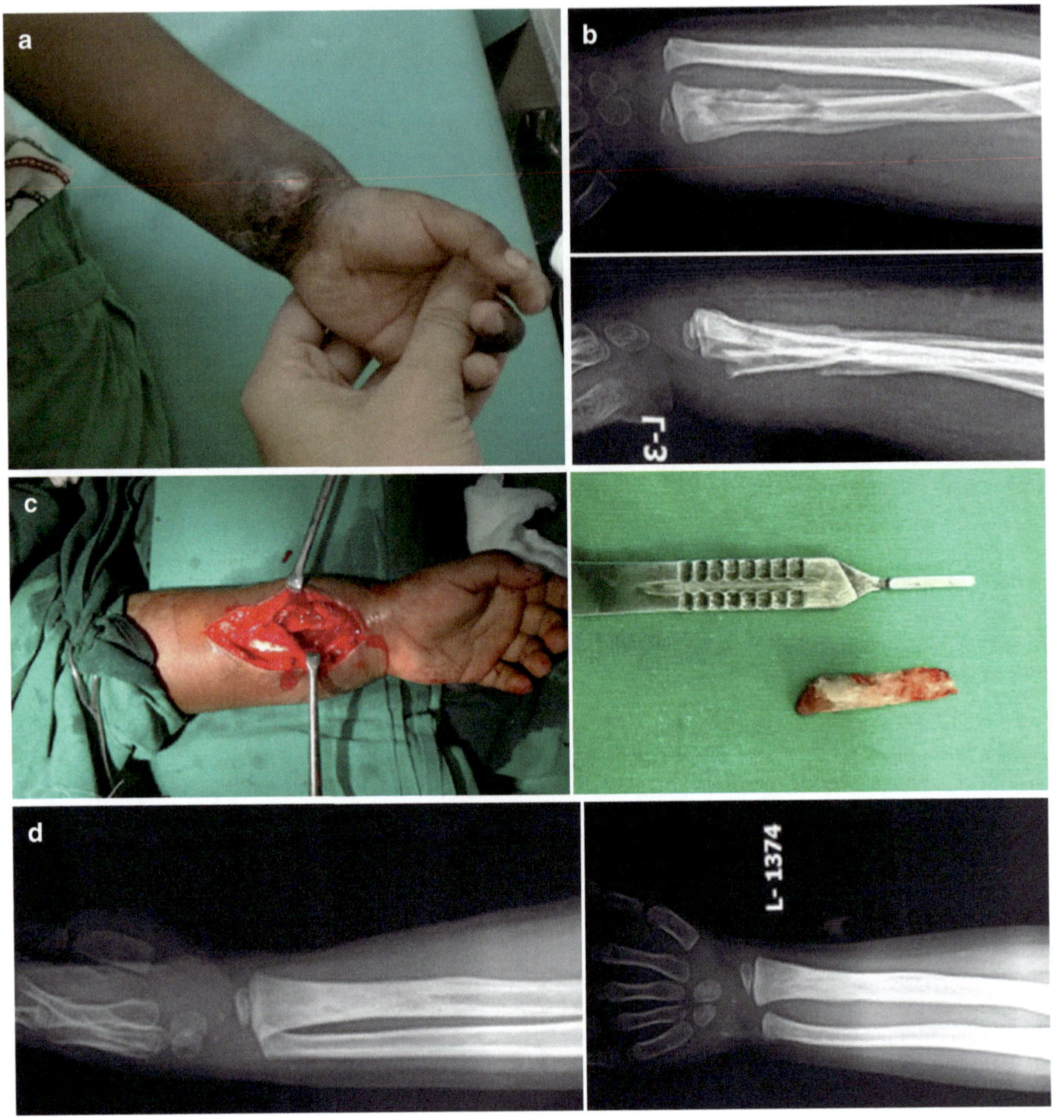

Fig. 19.3 Clinical and radiological findings in a case of chronic osteomyelitis of the radius. (**a**) Discharging sinus over the distal volar aspect of the forearm in a 5-year-old boy. (**b**) Anteroposterior and lateral radiographs of the forearm showing sequestration of the distal radial shaft, along with abundant periosteal reaction. Note that the involucrum bridges the proximal and distal radial segments, thus imparting structural stability. Also, the consistency of the involucrum is similar to that of normal bone. This is a Type B2 CHOM (sequestrum with normal involucrum) as per the Beit CURE classification system. (**c**) Intraoperative photographs demonstrating debridement up to healthy bleeding bone and the excised sequestrum. (**d**) Anteroposterior and lateral radiographs of the forearm one year after surgery. Note the restoration of normal anatomy of the radius and complete recovery

erly developed and attribute the occurrence of osseous defects to premature sequestrectomy [39]. Doaud et al. pointed out that it is the condition of the periosteum that determines the quality of the involucrum and that osseous defects probably occur due to the destruction of the periosteum during the acute stages of infection, due to both microbial activity and compression of periosteal vessels by a large sub-periosteal abscess [10]. In other words, the development of the involucrum depends on the activity and integrity of the periosteum, not on the presence of a sequestrum. In fact, the involucrum is more likely to develop better when the infection is controlled by sequestrectomy and antibiotic therapy [10].

Dead Space Management/ Reconstruction

Focal Bone Loss

Small defects, for example, an isolated metaphyseal abscess in sub-acute osteomyelitis, do not significantly diminish bony stability. Such defects may be simply closed over a drain and the limb kept protected in a cast or by application of an external fixator, until the bone regenerates. Young children have a remarkable capacity to form new bone; such defects and in some cases even areas of diaphyseal bone loss regenerate spontaneously after debridement, as long as the periosteal sleeve is intact [10]. Alternatively, the dead space may be filled with a bone substitute mixed with antibiotics [40].

Where there is focal bone loss in association with inadequate soft tissue cover, particularly in subcutaneous bones like the tibia, the Papineau technique (open bone grafting) is an appropriate strategy [41]. A modification of the Papineau technique implements a vacuum-assisted closure device in place of the wet to dry dressing changes [42]. The Papineau technique is an excellent option in places where microsurgical facilities for providing flap closure are unavailable [43].

Segmental Bone Defects

Extensive debridement, inadequate involucrum, and presence of pathological fractures with bone resorption can produce large bone defects, with or without associated shortening and angular deformities. Such defects invariably disrupt structural integrity and require some form of fixation as well. Options for the reconstruction of such bone defects include the following:

(a) Conventional bone grafting
(b) Vascularized bone graft
(c) Bone transport
(d) Bypass grafting

(a) *Conventional Bone Grafting*

As mentioned earlier, bone grafting is best done as a secondary procedure, once the infection is under control. Autologous bone graft is the first choice, and the fibula is an excellent source for reconstructing defects in long bones [44, 45] (Fig. 19.4a–e). Fibula grafts in weight-bearing extremities in children have been shown to undergo considerable hypertrophy and, after 2–3 years, function as native bone [46]. When care is taken to preserve the periosteal sleeve, the donor fibula also regenerates fully in most cases.

In the context of bone grafting, the Masquelet's induced membrane technique (IMT) requires special mention (Fig. 19.5a–e). In the first stage of this two-stage technique, the bone and soft tissues are debrided, followed by insertion of an antibiotic impregnated cement spacer, along with skeletal stabilization and soft tissue reconstruction as required. The presence of the spacer results in a foreign-body inflammatory reaction, leading to the formation of an organized pseudosynovial membrane that is rich in inductive molecules [47]. During the second stage (ideally 4 to 8 weeks later), the cement spacer is removed while preserving the membrane, the defect is filled with bone graft, and the membrane is closed over the graft without tension, along with definitive fixation of the bone if necessary. Corticalization of the reconstructed bone segment occurs within a few months of the second procedure and is independent of the initial size of the defect [48]. The gold standard for filling the defect is cancellous bone harvested from the iliac crest [48]. When the quantity of autograft is insufficient, it may be mixed with allograft or synthetic bone substitutes, but the ratio should be at least 70% autograft and 30% volume expander [47]. In a series of children with long bone COM treated by the IMT, Canavese et al. had satisfactory outcomes and in fact found that children appear to generate the periosteal membrane faster than adults [49].

(b) *Vascularized Bone Graft*

Vascularized bone grafting is indicated in cases with defects of >6cms in length, associated with poor soft tissue cover, and par-

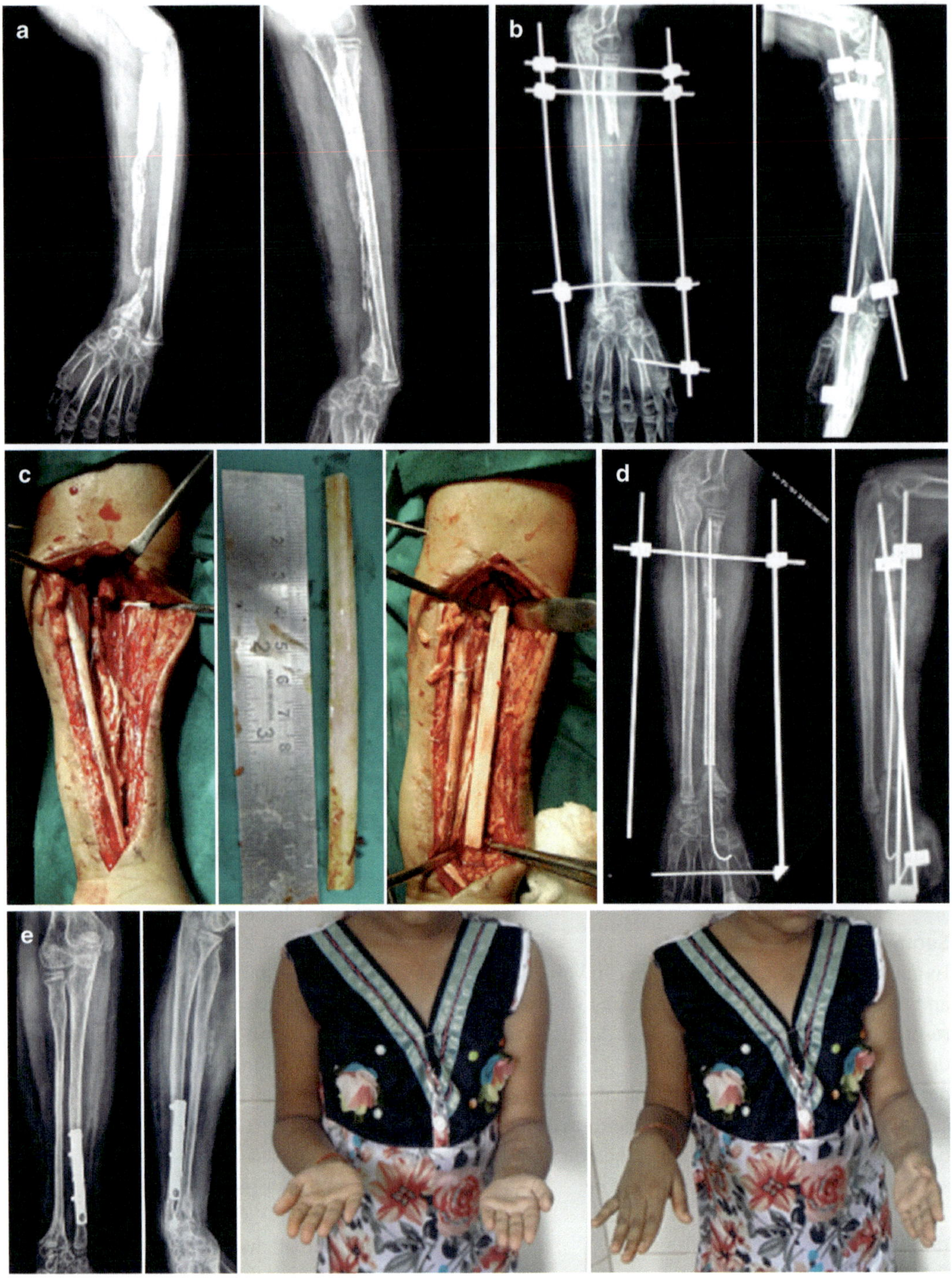

Fig. 19.4 Reconstruction of segmental bone defects with fibula strut graft in an 8-year-old girl. (**a**) Anteroposterior and lateral radiographs of the forearm showing osteomyelitis of the radius with a large diaphyseal sequestrum. (**b**) Anteroposterior and lateral radiographs of the forearm after the first stage involving radical debridement, sequestrectomy, and external fixator application. (**c**) Intraoperative photographs during the second stage showing repeat debridement with freshening of the bone ends, harvesting of fibula strut graft, and graft interposition in the radial defect. (**d**) Immediate postoperative radiographs showing the graft stabilized by an intramedullary Kirschner wire supplemented by the external fixator. (**e**) Anteroposterior and lateral radiographs and clinical photographs 2 years postoperatively showing excellent consolidation of the graft (an ulna shortening osteotomy was done to correct ulna-plus hand)

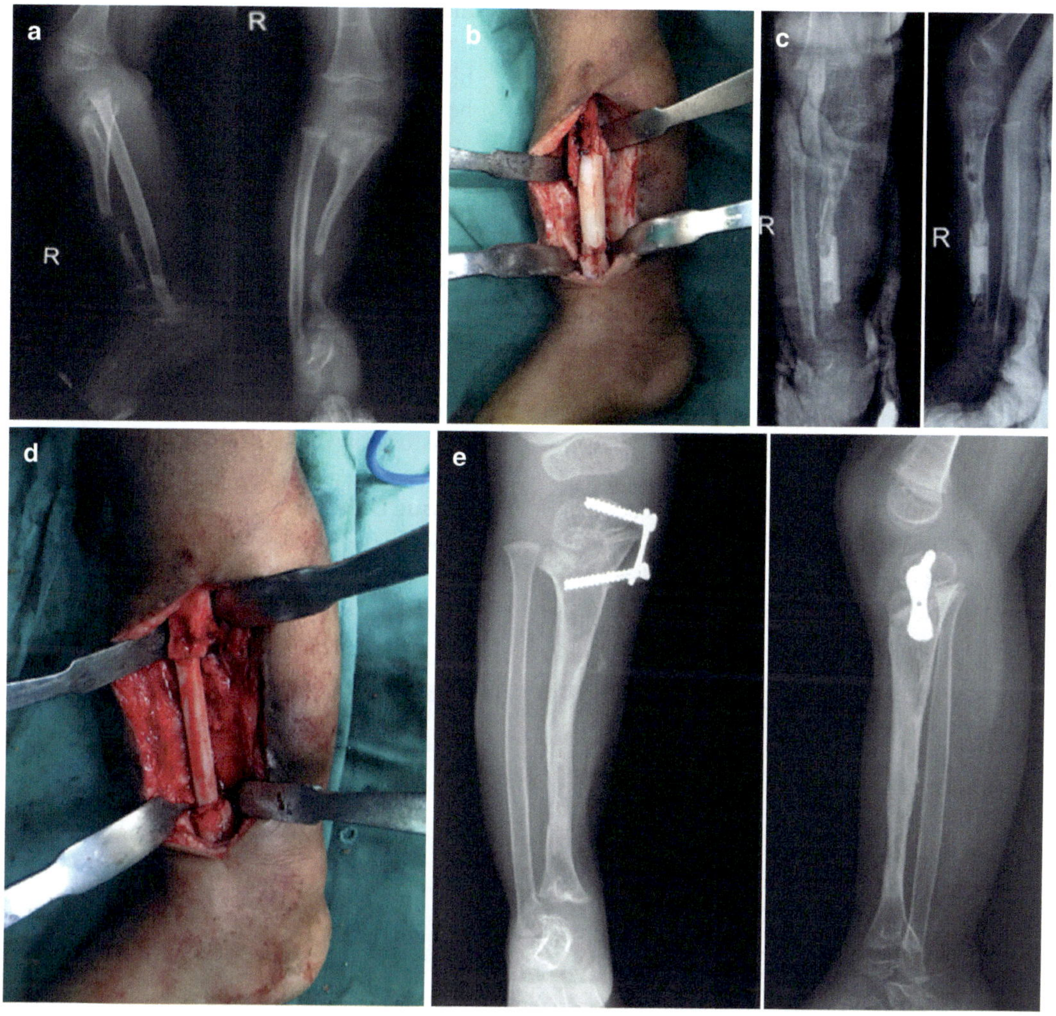

Fig. 19.5 Use of the Masquelet's induced membrane technique in the treatment of CHOM. (**a**) Anteroposterior and lateral radiographs of the right leg demonstrating tibial gap non-union secondary to chronic osteomyelitis in a 2-year-old boy. (**b**) Intraoperative photograph showing insertion of antibiotic impregnated cement spacer (Stage 1). (**c**) Anteroposterior and lateral radiographs of the right leg showing the cement spacer in situ. (**d**) Intraoperative photograph showing cement spacer removal and fibula grafting (Stage 2). (**e**) Anteroposterior and lateral radiographs of the right leg 12 months after the grafting procedure demonstrating healing of the non-union. Proximal medial tibial eight plates were used to correct a residual valgus deformity. Physeal damage of the proximal & distal tibia will necessitate lengthening later

ticularly when non-vascularized bone grafting has been attempted and failed [50]. The fibula is the most commonly used donor; others include ilium, scapula, and ribs [50]. The vascularized graft is useful in osteomyelitis because it brings in vascularity into a scarred and avascular bed, resists graft resorption, and is less likely to suffer stress fractures and reinfection than non-vascularized strut grafts.

(c) *Bone Transport*

In the Ilizarov method, a segment of healthy bone is transported longitudinally to fill a segmental defect. Proponents of this technique for the treatment of childhood COM with bone loss believe that this technique allows the surgeon to perform a more radical debridement [14]. Furthermore, the increased local blood flow secondary to distraction osteogenesis improves the effectiveness of antibiotic therapy. Another advantage is the ability to simultaneously correct angular deformities and limb length discrepancies. Kucukkaya et al. reported excellent results using the Ilizarov method in the treatment of chronic tibial osteomyelitis in children. They found that additional bone grafting at the docking site, frequently required in adults, was not necessary in children [14]. Complications with this technique include joint subluxation/stiffness, neurological and vascular injury, delayed consolidation at the distraction site, pin tract problems, and psychological intolerance.

(d) *Bypass Grafting*

When segmental bone loss affects either the tibia or one of the forearm bones, bypass grafting can serve as an alternative to the abovementioned reconstruction options. In the forearm, this entails creation of a single bone forearm (Fig. 19.6a, b). In case of the tibia, either posterolateral bone grafting can be done bone proximally and distally to create a cross union, or the fibula can be osteotomized at both levels and transferred into the tibial defect [4]. In either case, once union has occurred, and the fibula assumes load-bearing and usually hypertrophies in response to the increased loading. Bypass grafting is indicated in cases where a large portion of the diaphysis is lost, particularly when there is insufficient metaphysis available to allow distraction osteogenesis [4].

Soft Tissue Defects

In COM, the soft tissue envelope is very often compromised, and adequate debridement and sinus excision sometimes leave large soft-tissue

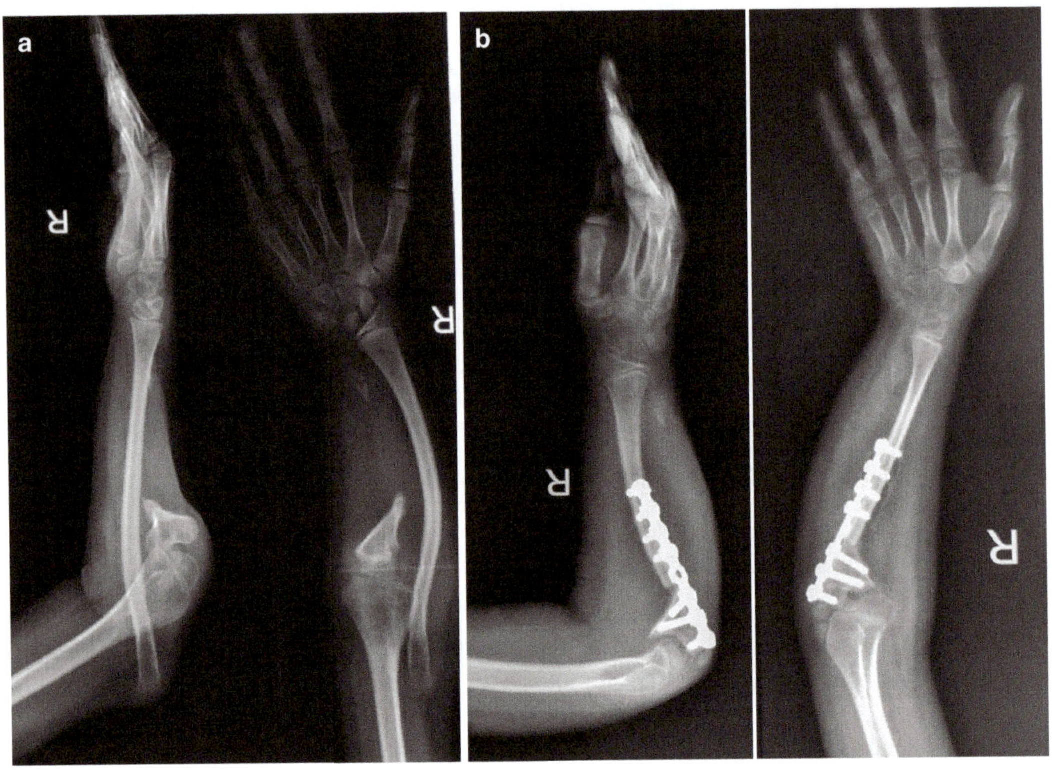

Fig. 19.6 Reconstruction of extensive bone loss by bypass grafting. (**a**) Anteroposterior and lateral radiographs of the right forearm showing complete destruction of the ulnar diaphysis secondary to chronic osteomyelitis in a 10-year-old girl. The resultant ulnar shortening has resulted in dislocation and proximal migration of the radial head. (**b**) Anteroposterior and lateral radiographs of the right forearm showing bypass reconstruction by creation of a single bone forearm

defects that cannot be closed primarily. It is not preferable to allow such defects to heal by secondary intention, as the resultant scar tissue is weak and often breaks down leading to recurrent drainage. The aim should be to replace the unhealthy scar tissue with durable, vascularized tissue, such as skin grafts, myocutaneous flaps, and even free flaps if necessary [19]. A recent study of adult tibial COM found that fasciocutaneous and perforator free flaps were as effective as muscular flaps in treating infection, while being more cosmetic and producing higher patient satisfaction [51]. A plastic surgeon experienced in such coverage techniques should be involved in treatment during the reconstructive phases.

Recent studies have shown negative pressure wound therapy (NPWT) to be beneficial in COM with soft-tissue problems [52]. In this procedure, after a thorough debridement of the tissues, a piece of foam is placed over the entire wound, a drain is placed over the foam, and a large piece of transparent, impervious tape is placed over the entire area, including the surrounding healthy tissue so as to secure the foam and drain over the wound. The tube is then connected to a vacuum source, which allows application of a negative pressure to the entire wound area, and the fluid drawn from the wound is collected in a disposable cannister. The device can be adjusted to provide varying degrees of negative pressure (between 20–60 kPa), either continuously or intermittently, and has an alarm that sounds if the pressure seal is broken or the cannister is full. The entire dressing is changed every 4–5 days, accompanied by debridement. NPWT can be discontinued once the wound is healthy enough to be closed surgically. NPWT acts by draining the wound of exudate and stimulating the growth of the surface tissues. The cited advantages in COM include better bacterial clearance, reduced frequency of dressing changes, fewer recurrences of infection, and decreased need for soft-tissue cover procedures [52].

Adjunctive Therapies

Of the several potential adjuncts that have been proposed in the treatment of refractory osteomyelitis, hyperbaric oxygen therapy (HBOT) is probably the foremost. HBOT involves intermittent inhalation of 100% oxygen at pressures of 2 to 2.5 atm absolute, each session lasting 90–120 minutes [53]. It is believed that, by raising the oxygen tension in the bone and soft tissues, HBOT enhances the bactericidal activity of leukocytes, enhances collagen synthesis and osteogenesis, induces angiogenesis, suppresses anaerobic organisms, and enhances antibiotic activity [53]. A number of other adjunctive therapies have been proposed (namely platelet-rich plasma, pulsed electromagnetic fields, ultrasound, and growth factor/gene therapy); however their role remains speculative at present [53].

Complications

The potential complications of COM include the following:

(i) *Recurrence of infection*: Relapse may occur even after several years [1, 54]. Factors affecting recurrence include adequacy of debridement, presence of comorbidities, and duration of the disease prior to treatment [38].

(ii) *Fractures:* Pathological fractures at the site of infection are common; these are more likely in the early stages of disease before the involucrum has properly formed [4]. Besides this, fractures in adjacent bones may also occur, due to disuse osteopenia in prolonged disease, particularly when these children start weight-bearing or have joint manipulation.

(iii) *Joint problems*: This can range from stiffness, which can be overcome with physiotherapy, to joint destruction with associated subluxation or dislocation due to spread of infection into the joint.

(iv) *Physeal damage*: Infection may directly damage the physis resulting in partial or complete arrest. This is manifested as progressive angular deformities or shortening as the child grows. Less commonly, physeal stimulation due to local hyperemia can result in overgrowth of the affected bone.

(v) *Non-union:* Fractures through infected bone are often complicated by non-union, with or without bone loss.

(vi) *Treatment-related complications:* This includes side effects from antibiotics, problems associated with external fixators, donor site morbidity from bone graft/flap harvest, etc.

Important steps in treatment		
Optimization of general health		
Antibiotic therapy	Based on tissue culture/sensitivity	
	Guided by ID specialists	
	Systemic vs local antibiotic delivery	
Surgery	Debridement	
	Osseous stabilization	
	Reconstruction of bone defects	Open bone grafting (Papineau)
		Segmental bone grafts (autografts, allografts)
		Vascularized bone grafts
		Induced membrane technique
		Bone transport
		Bypass grafting
	Soft tissue cover	Skin grafts/flaps
		Negative pressure wound therapy
Treatment adjuncts	Hyperbaric oxygen	

Conclusion

Chronic osteomyelitis continues to be a pernicious problem in poor countries with fragile healthcare systems and limited resources. Early referral to higher centers and a judicious management by a multidisciplinary medical team can mitigate the morbidity and complications associated with this chronic condition. The Beit CURE classification is useful in prognosticating the final outcome and in developing a rational treatment plan. The management of CHOM is primarily surgical and includes sequential phases of eradication of infection followed by reconstruction of soft-tissue and bone defects. Modern techniques of local antibiotic delivery systems, negative pressure wound therapy, and advanced methods of soft-tissue and bone reconstruction can help improve the outcomes of this difficult condition.

Declarations Funding support: This project has no funding support.

Consent to publish: The authors affirm that participants provided informed consent for publication of the images in Figs. 19.1, 19.2, 19.3, 19.4, 19.5, and 19.6.

Conflicts of Interest: The authors declare that they have no conflict of interest.

References

1. Klenerman L. A history of osteomyelitis from the Journal of Bone and Joint Surgery. J Bone Joint Surg Br. 2007;89-B:667–70.
2. Lazzarini L, Mader JT, Calhoun JH. Osteomyelitis in long bones. J Bone Joint Surg. 2004;86:2305–18.
3. Lew DP, Waldvogel FA. Osteomyelitis. Lancet. 2004;364:369–79.
4. Spiegel DA, Penny JN. Chronic osteomyelitis in children. Tech Orthop. 2005;20:142–52.
5. Dormans JP, Drummond DS. Pediatric hematogenous osteomyelitis: new trends in presentation, diagnosis, and treatment. J Am Acad Orthop Surg. 1994;2:333–41.
6. Weiland AJ, Moore JR, Daniel RK. The efficacy of free tissue transfer in the treatment of osteomyelitis. J Bone Joint Surg. 1984;66:181–93.
7. Schauwecker DS. Osteomyelitis: diagnosis with In-111-labeled leukocytes. Radiology. 1989;171:141–6.
8. Jones HW, Beckles VLL, Akinola B, Stevenson AJ, Harrison WJ. Chronic haematogenous osteomyelitis in children. J Bone Joint Surg Br. 2011;93-B:1005–10.
9. Craigen MA, Watters J, Hackett JS. The changing epidemiology of osteomyelitis in children. J Bone Joint Surg Br. 1992;74:541–5.
10. Daoud A, Saighi-Bouaouina A. Treatment of sequestra, pseudarthroses, and defects in the long bones of children who have chronic hematogenous osteomyelitis. J Bone Joint Surg Am. 1989;71:1448–68.
11. Beckles VLL, Jones HW, Harrison WJ. Chronic haematogenous osteomyelitis in children. J Bone Joint Surg Br. 2010;92-B:1138–43.
12. Yeargan SA, Nakasone CK, Shaieb MD, Montgomery WP, Reinker KA. Treatment of chronic osteomyelitis in children resistant to previous therapy. J Pediatr Orthop. 2004;24:109–22.
13. Reinehr T, Bürk G, Michel E, Andler W. Chronic osteomyelitis in childhood: is surgery always indicated? Infection. 2000;28:282–6.
14. Kucukkaya M, Kabukcuoglu Y, Tezer M, Kuzgun U. Management of childhood chronic tibial osteomyelitis with the ilizarov method. J Pediatr Orthop. 2002;22:632–7.

15. Waldvogel FA, Medoff G, Swartz MN. Osteomyelitis: a review of clinical features, therapeutic considerations and unusual aspects. N Engl J Med. 1970;282:316–22.
16. Green NE, Nania JJ. Bone and joint infections in children. In: Turek's Orthop. Princ. Their Appl. 6th ed. Lippincott Williams & Wilkins; 2005. p. 124–49.
17. Panteli M, Giannoudis PV. Chronic osteomyelitis: what the surgeon needs to know. EFORT Open Rev. 2016;1:128–35.
18. Mader JT, Shirtliff M, Calhoun JH. Staging and staging application in osteomyelitis. Clin Infect Dis. 1997;25:1303–9.
19. Cierny G, Mader JT, Penninck JJ. The classic: a clinical staging system for adult osteomyelitis. Clin Orthop Relat Res. 2003;414:7–24.
20. Jones HW, Harrison JW, Bates J, Evans GA, Lubega N. Radiologic classification of chronic hematogenous osteomyelitis in children. J Pediatr Orthop. 2009;29:822–7.
21. Hatzenbuehler J, Pulling TJ. Diagnosis and management of osteomyelitis. Am Fam Physician. 2011;84:1027–33.
22. Dabov GD. Osteomyelitis. In: Campbell's operative orthopaedics, vol. I. 12th ed. Elsevier; 2012. p. 725–48.
23. Lee YJ, Sadigh S, Mankad K, Kapse N, Rajeswaran G. The imaging of osteomyelitis. Quant Imaging Med Surg. 2016;6:184–98.
24. Pineda C, Espinosa R, Pena A. Radiographic imaging in osteomyelitis: the role of plain radiography, computed tomography, ultrasonography, magnetic resonance imaging, and scintigraphy. Semin Plast Surg. 2009;23:080–9.
25. Termaat MF, Raijmakers PGHM, Scholten HJ, Bakker FC, Patka P, Haarman HJTM. The accuracy of diagnostic imaging for the assessment of chronic osteomyelitis: a systematic review and meta-analysis. J Bone Joint Surg Am. 2005;87:2464–71.
26. Patzakis MJ, Wilkins J, Kumar J, Holtom P, Greenbaum B, Ressler R. Comparison of the results of bacterial cultures from multiple sites in chronic osteomyelitis of long bones. A prospective study. J Bone Joint Surg. 1994;76:664–6.
27. Norden CW, Fierer J, Bryant RE. Chronic staphylococcal osteomyelitis: treatment with regimens containing rifampin. Clin Infect Dis. 1983;5:S495–501.
28. Maraqa NF, Gomez MM, Rathore MH. Outpatient parenteral antimicrobial therapy in osteoarticular infections in children. J Pediatr Orthop. 2002;22:506–10.
29. Howard-Jones AR, Isaacs D. Systematic review of systemic antibiotic treatment for children with chronic and sub-acute pyogenic osteomyelitis. J Paediatr Child Health. 2010;46:736–41.
30. Haidar R, Der BA, Atiyeh B. Duration of post-surgical antibiotics in chronic osteomyelitis: empiric or evidence-based? Int J Infect Dis. 2010;14:e752–8.
31. Gogia J, Meehan J, Di Cesare P, Jamali A. Local antibiotic therapy in osteomyelitis. Semin Plast Surg. 2009;23:100–7.
32. van Vugt TAG, Arts JJ, Geurts JAP. Antibiotic-loaded Polymethylmethacrylate beads and spacers in treatment of orthopedic infections and the role of biofilm formation. Front Microbiol. 2019;10:1–11.
33. Bar-On E, Weigl DM, Bor N, Becker T, Katz K, Mercado E, Livni G. Chronic osteomyelitis in children: treatment by intramedullary reaming and antibiotic-impregnated cement rods. J Pediatr Orthop. 2010;30:508–13.
34. McLaren AC. Alternative materials to acrylic bone cement for delivery of depot antibiotics in orthopaedic infections. Clin Orthop Relat Res. 2004;427:101–6.
35. Hashmi MA, Norman P, Saleh M. The management of chronic osteomyelitis using the Lautenbach method. J Bone Joint Surg Br. 2004;86-B:269–75.
36. Hung NN. Cortical bone fenestrations with continuous antibiotic irrigation to mediate hematogenous tibial osteomyelitis in children. J Pediatr Orthop B. 2010;19:497–506.
37. Eckardt JJ, Wirganowicz PZ, Mar T. An aggressive surgical approach to the management of chronic osteomyelitis. Clin Orthop Relat Res. 1994;298:229–39.
38. Simpson AHRW, Deakin M, Latham JM. Chronic osteomyelitis. J Bone Joint Surg. 2001;83:403–7.
39. Fowles JV, Lehoux J, Zlitni M, Kassab MT, Nolan B. Tibial defect due to acute haematogenous osteomyelitis: treatment and results in twenty-one children. J Bone Joint Surg Br. 1979;61:77–81.
40. Andreacchio A, Alberghina F, Paonessa M, Cravino M, De Rosa V, Canavese F. Tobramycin-impregnated calcium sulfate pellets for the treatment of chronic osteomyelitis in children and adolescents. J Pediatr Orthop B. 2019;28:189–95.
41. Asomugha EU, Alexander IJ. Papineau open cancellous bone grafting for chronic osteomyelitis and infected nonunions of the distal lower extremity. Tech Foot Ankle Surg. 2014;13:108–17.
42. Archdeacon MT, Messerschmitt P. Modern papineau technique with vacuum-assisted closure. J Orthop Trauma. 2006;20:134–7.
43. Gunawan B, Wijaya MT, Pohan MAS. Reconstruction of tibial bone defect in new age using the old age Papineau technique: a case series. Ann Med Surg. 2019;48:109–14.
44. Steinlechner CWB, Mkandawire NC. Non-vascularised fibular transfer in the management of defects of long bones after sequestrectomy in children. J Bone Joint Surg Br. 2005;87-B:1259–63.
45. Patwardhan S, Shyam AK, Mody RA, Sancheti PK, Mehta R, Agrawat H. Reconstruction of bone defects after osteomyelitis with nonvascularized fibular graft. J Bone Joint Surg. 2013;95:e56.
46. Krieg AH, Hefti F. Reconstruction with non-vascularised fibular grafts after resection of bone tumours. J Bone Joint Surg Br. 2007;89-B:215–21.
47. Masquelet A, Kanakaris NK, Obert L, Stafford P, Giannoudis PV. Bone Repair Using the Masquelet Technique. J Bone Joint Surg Am. 2019;101:1024–36.
48. Masquelet AC. Induced membrane technique. J Orthop Trauma. 2017;31:S36–8.

49. Canavese F, Corradin M, Khan A, Mansour M, Rousset M, Samba A. Successful treatment of chronic osteomyelitis in children with debridement, antibiotic-laden cement spacer and bone graft substitute. Eur J Orthop Surg Traumatol. 2017;27:221–8.
50. Dinh P, Hutchinson B, Zalavras C, Stevanovic M. Reconstruction of osteomyelitis defects. Semin Plast Surg. 2009;23:108–18.
51. Buono P, Castus P, Dubois-Ferrière V, Rüegg EM, Uçkay I, Assal M, Pittet-Cuénod B, Modarressi A. Muscular versus non-muscular free flaps for soft tissue coverage of chronic Tibial osteomyelitis. World J Plast Surg. 2018;7:294–300.
52. Tan Y, Wang X, Li H, Zheng Q, Li J, Feng G, Pan Z. The clinical efficacy of the vacuum-assisted closure therapy in the management of adult osteomyelitis. Arch Orthop Trauma Surg. 2011;131:255–9.
53. Fang R, Galiano R. Adjunctive therapies in the treatment of osteomyelitis. Semin Plast Surg. 2009;23:141–7.
54. Ciampolini J. Pathophysiology of chronic bacterial osteomyelitis. Why do antibiotics fail so often? Postgrad Med J. 2000;76:479–83.

Chronic Post-traumatic Osteomyelitis

20

Ian Singleton, Premal Naik, Levent Eralp, and Mohan V. Belthur

Introduction

Chronic posttraumatic osteomyelitis is a source of significant healthcare burden and disability, particularly in the developing world [1–4]. Modern, evidence-based management is required to prevent the development of chronic osteomyelitis following pediatric injuries.

Definition

Chronic posttraumatic osteomyelitis is osteomyelitis that arises following trauma, commonly from open fractures of long bones (Fig. 20.6a, b) [1–3]. Similar to other types of chronic osteomyelitis, chronic posttraumatic osteomyelitis is a persistent destructive inflammatory process caused by infecting pathogens [1]. Chronic posttraumatic osteomyelitis arises from pathogens introduced via traumatic wounds and direct bacterial invasion from surrounding issues [1]. In addition, chronic posttraumatic osteomyelitis can be caused not only by traumatic injury but also as a postoperative complication of surgeries, especially orthopedic trauma procedures with retained implants (Figs. 20.2a–d and 20.5a–d) [1]. Patients with any etiology of chronic osteomyelitis can be in chronically poor health with considerable pain and significant disability.

Chronic osteomyelitis is typically delineated from acute osteomyelitis by persisting to 6 or more weeks after the initial bony infection and is characterized by the presence of bone destruction and formation of sequestra [5]. The pathologic definition of a bony sequestrum is a piece of devitalized bone that has become separated

Author Contributions: All the authors contributed to the study conception and design. Material preparation, data collection, and analysis were performed by Ian Singleton, Dr. Premal Naik, and Dr. Mohan Belthur. The first draft of the manuscript was written by Ian Singleton, and all the authors commented on subsequent versions of the manuscript. All the authors read and approved the final manuscript.

I. Singleton
University of Arizona College of Medicine – Phoenix, Phoenix, AZ, USA
e-mail: iansingleton@email.arizona.edu

P. Naik
NHL Municipal Medical College, Rainbow Super-speciality Hospital & Children's Orthopaedic Centre, Ahmedabad, Gujarat, India

L. Eralp
Istanbul Medical School, University of Istanbul, Istanbul, Turkey

M. V. Belthur (✉)
Department of Child Health & Orthopedics, University of Arizona College of Medicine, Phoenix, AZ, USA

Department of Orthopedics, Phoenix Children's Hospital, Phoenix, AZ, USA
e-mail: mbelthur@phoenixchildrens.com

© Springer Nature Switzerland AG 2022
M. V. Belthur et al. (eds.), *Pediatric Musculoskeletal Infections*,
https://doi.org/10.1007/978-3-030-95794-0_20

from the surrounding bone during the process of necrosis [6]. The necrotic bone of the sequestrum is separated from living bone by granulation tissue [7].

Epidemiology

Unlike the incidence of acute hematogenous osteomyelitis, which is largely a pediatric disease and has been steadily decreasing in developed nations, the incidence of chronic posttraumatic osteomyelitis has increased or remained steady in developed nations over the past 50 years [8–10]. In addition, the increased survival following traumatic injury has been accompanied by an increased occurrence of posttraumatic osteomyelitis [8, 11, 12].

In one study of pediatric osteomyelitis in the United States, approximately half (48%) of cases were hematogenous infections, 38% were trauma-related contiguous infections, and 14% were iatrogenic or diabetes-related infections. The overall incidence of osteomyelitis in children has remained relatively stable over time (eight to ten cases per 100,000 person-years), as well as the incidence by etiology [8]. Posttraumatic chronic osteomyelitis accounts for about 20–30% of all chronic osteomyelitis cases [2, 3, 13].

In the developing world, chronic osteomyelitis is encountered much more frequently. For example, in Gambia, osteomyelitis accounts for approximately 20% of pediatric surgical admissions and 15.4% of inpatient days [3]. This is due to insufficient medical care, poor access, food supply, and hygiene, especially in rural areas [3].

Etiology

Chronic osteomyelitis is one of the most serious posttraumatic complications in the treatment of long bone fractures. In adults, chronic osteomyelitis is a reported complication of open fractures of long bones in approximately 21–25%; however, children have an increased ability to heal bone, and infection rates in pediatric patients following open fractures are lower than that of adults [14–20]. The incidence of infection rises with the severity of the fracture [15]. In a series of 554 open fractures in pediatric patients, the authors reported a 3% overall infection rate, with rates of 2% (5/302) for type I fractures, 2% (3/154) for type II fractures, and 8% (8/98) for type III fractures [21]. In addition, Hutchins et al. reported five cases of osteomyelitis in children in association with 10 type III open femoral fractures, but no infections in association with 34 type I or II open femoral fractures [22]. Chronic posttraumatic osteomyelitis is also reported to occur in 5.3–27% of gunshot fractures and in 7.6–13.2% of cases after open reduction of closed fractures [13, 14]. *Staphylococcus aureus* is cultured in approximately 36% of monomicrobial infections [23].

Pathogenesis

The pathologic process in chronic posttraumatic osteomyelitis is associated with impaired circulation in the injured bone, with additional necrosis in the soft tissues that are directly involved in the injured area. As regional blood circulation and microcirculation in the tissues deteriorates due to the purulent and necrotic process, this causes local tissue ischemia and an increase in the volume of necrotic lesion [14]. Ischemia causes immunosuppression, slows and distorts reparative osteogenesis, and allows the maintenance of the infectious process. These pathologic processes ultimately lead to the formation of a sequestrum. The involucrum is a layer of reactive new bone which attempts to wall off the sequestrum, prevent the infection from reaching the bloodstream, and provide mechanical stability [7, 24, 25]. Perforation of tracks through the involucrum is termed cloaca, and those that reach the skin are known as sinuses [7]. A significant factor in the development of chronic osteomyelitis is the formation of biofilms by the invading bacteria [14]. Biofilms are organized communities of microorganisms enveloped in an extracellular matrix attached to a surface [25]. Biofilm can prevent antibiotics and phagocytes from reaching the surface bound bacteria, and biofilm formation substantially increases the difficulty of eradicating the pathogen and contributes to the persistence of infection [26].

Clinical Presentation

Acute osteomyelitis can be recognized by the four classical signs of infection: calor, dolor, rubor, and tumor. However, chronic posttraumatic osteomyelitis can present with a closed wound and no apparent signs of acute infection. Fever is typically absent in chronic osteomyelitis, and symptoms such as pain, erythema, swelling, and disability of the affected limb can mimic other common complications of fractures such as non-infected nonunion, posttraumatic arthrosis or symptomatic hardware [27, 28]. Because the infection may be clinically silent, a high index of suspicion is warranted. More obvious signs of chronic posttraumatic osteomyelitis are the development of draining sinuses or ulcers [29, 30]. Draining sinus tracts are particularly prevalent in the setting of posttraumatic osteomyelitis (Figs. 20.2e–g and 20.7a, b) [29]. Ulcers may result in exposed bone or bone encountered while probing the ulcer with a sterile instrument. While probing to bone is highly suggestive of osteomyelitis, the inability to probe to bone does not rule out osteomyelitis [29, 30]. Chronic infection after an open fracture may also present as persistent, incomplete wound healing or fracture nonunion [29].

Classification

There are two major classifications schemes for osteomyelitis. In 1970, Lew and Waldvogel proposed a system based on etiology. They described three pathophysiologic mechanism of osteomyelitis: (1) hematogenous osteomyelitis; (2) contiguous focus osteomyelitis from trauma, surgery, prosthetic material, or soft tissue spread; and (3) vascular insufficiency osteomyelitis as is often seen in diabetes mellitus. Additionally, any of these categories may be acute or chronic. This classification system does not take into account the severity of each type of infection or offer guidance as to treatment implications [24, 29].

In 1985, Cierny and Mader developed a classification of chronic osteomyelitis that combined four anatomic types with three host physiologic classes. The four anatomic types are (1) medullary, (2) superficial (cortical bone), (3) localized (medullary cavity and cortex), and (4) diffuse (entire thickness of the bone with loss of stability). The three physiologic classes are (A) normal host, (B) systemic or local compromise, and (C) treatment worse than disease [24, 29, 31]. Type B can be written as Bs for systemic compromise, Bl for local compromise, and Bls for both systemic and local compromise. Systemic compromise includes malnutrition, renal failure, hepatic failure, alcohol abuse, immune deficiency, diabetes mellitus, chronic hypoxia, malignancy, extremes of age, peripheral neuropathy, steroid therapy, and tobacco abuse. Local compromise includes chronic lymphedema, venous stasis, major vessel vascular disease, small vessel vascular disease, arteritis, extensive scarring, radiation fibrosis, and loss of sensation [29, 31, 32]. The Cierny-Mader classification system also offers guidance on treatment. However, it was primarily developed for use in adult patients and has limitations in pediatric patients [32]. Pediatric patients have an increased ability to resorb dead bone and remove the devitalized surfaces where bacteria can persist in a biofilm. In addition, it does not take into account the length of time the infection has been present [31, 33].

Another commonly used classification system, the Beit CURE, was developed by Jones et al. to be used in childhood chronic hematogenous osteomyelitis. This system does not apply to posttraumatic osteomyelitis [34].

Investigations

Laboratory Investigations

Serum inflammatory markers, such as leukocyte count, C-reactive protein, and erythrocyte sedimentation rate, are commonly used, but have limited diagnostic value for chronic posttraumatic osteomyelitis [28]. A single center study demonstrated white blood cells to be elevated in 13.41% of chronic osteomyelitis cases, while erythrocyte sedimentation rate was elevated in 56.87%, C-reactive protein in 44.54%, procalcitonin in 35.33%, interluekin-6 in 73.81%, and tumor necrosis factor alpha in 65.82% [23].

Imaging Studies

The imaging of chronic posttraumatic osteomyelitis presents special challenges when compared to the imaging of other forms of osteomyelitis [28]. The persistent tissue disruption from the original trauma and following surgical correction can make it difficult to differentiate a potential infection. In addition, the orthopedic implants used in the surgical fixation of fractures are typically retained and can obscure imaging. Currently, there is no consensus on the best imaging modality for chronic posttraumatic osteomyelitis [28, 35–37].

Plain Radiographs

Plain radiography is easily accessible and typically serves as the primary study [37]. Plain radiography can be used to assess the healing of the fracture and examine other possible explanations for the patient's symptoms. It can assess the position of metal implants, fracture stability, and bone healing (Figs. 20.1a, b, 20.3c, d, 20.4a–c,

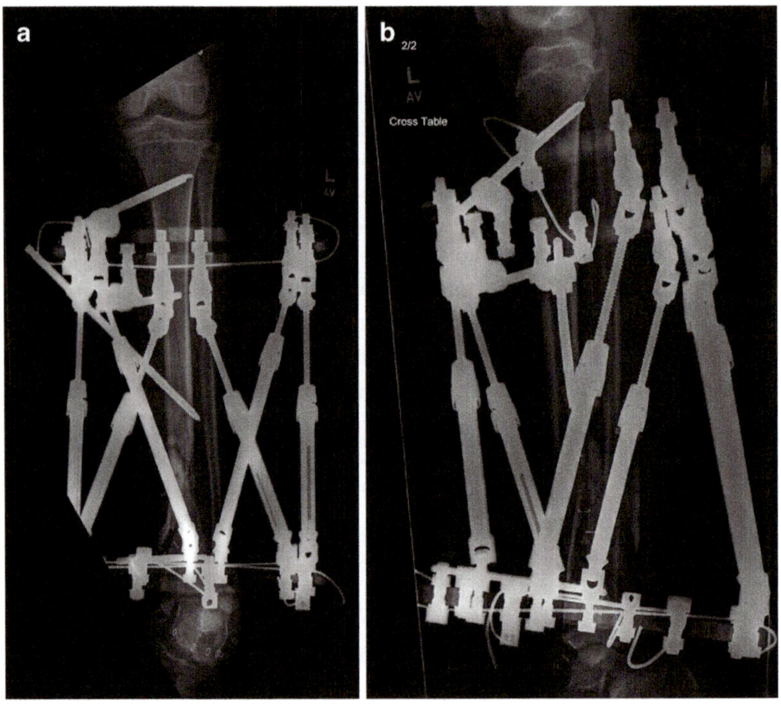

Fig. 20.1 (**a**, **b**) Radiographs of the left tibia in a 13-year-old girl, who sustained a grade 3A comminuted left distal tibia fracture which was treated at an outside facility with closed reduction and application of a circular external fixator with closure of the soft tissue wound. She developed posttraumatic osteomyelitis of the tibia with a discharging sinus over the anteromedial aspect of the leg with poor soft tissue envelop. (Courtesy of Dr. William Wood). (**c**, **d**) Radiographs of the left tibia 12 weeks from injury following debridement of soft tissue and bone with intramedullary nailing (IM) of the tibia, dead space management using an antibiotic spacer, and soft tissue reconstruction using a latissimus dorsi free flap was performed. (**e**, **f**) Radiographs of the left tibia 18 weeks from injury after subsequent reconstruction of the bone defect of 5 cm using the induced membrane technique with iliac crest autograft. This was done after the infection was controlled with antibiotic treatment. (**g**, **h**) Radiographs of the left tibia 9 months from injury showing a healed left distal tibia fracture with retained IM nail

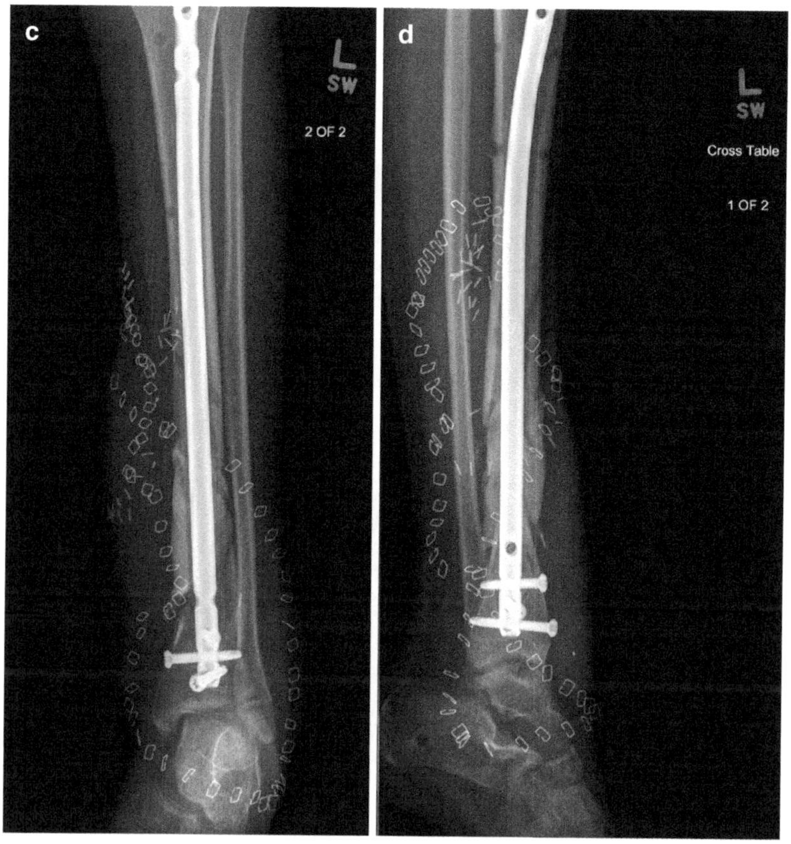

Fig. 20.1 (continued)

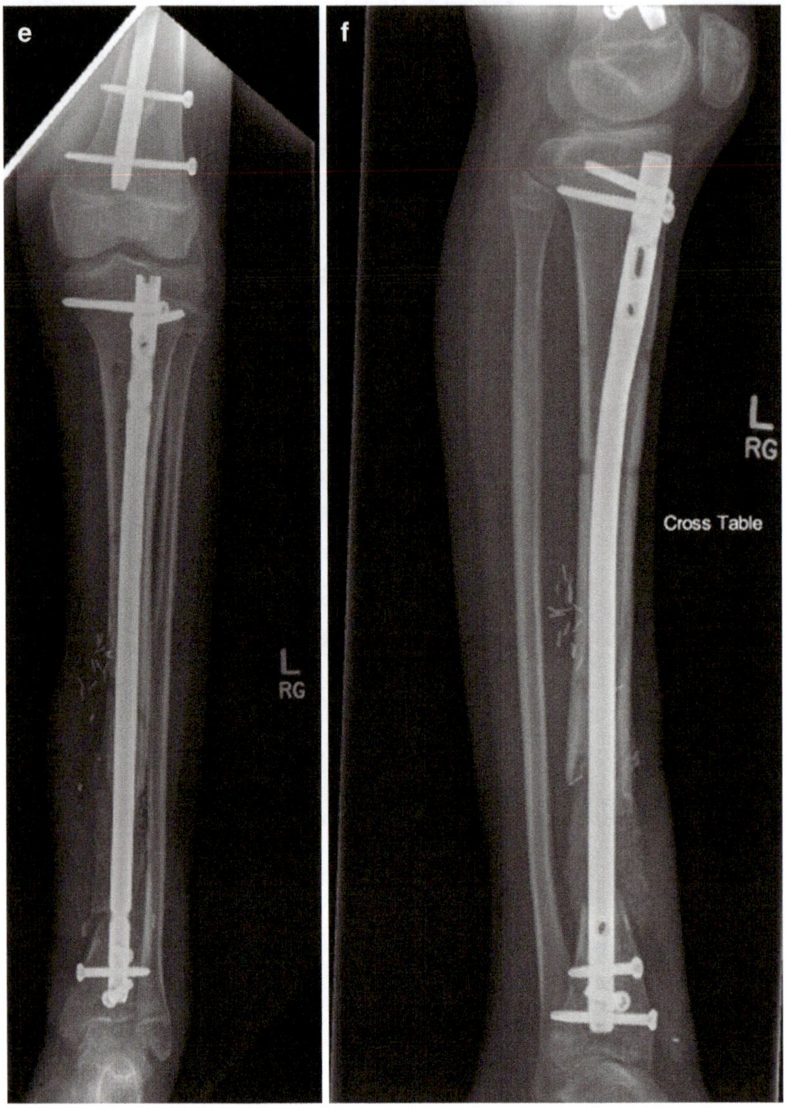

Fig. 20.1 (continued)

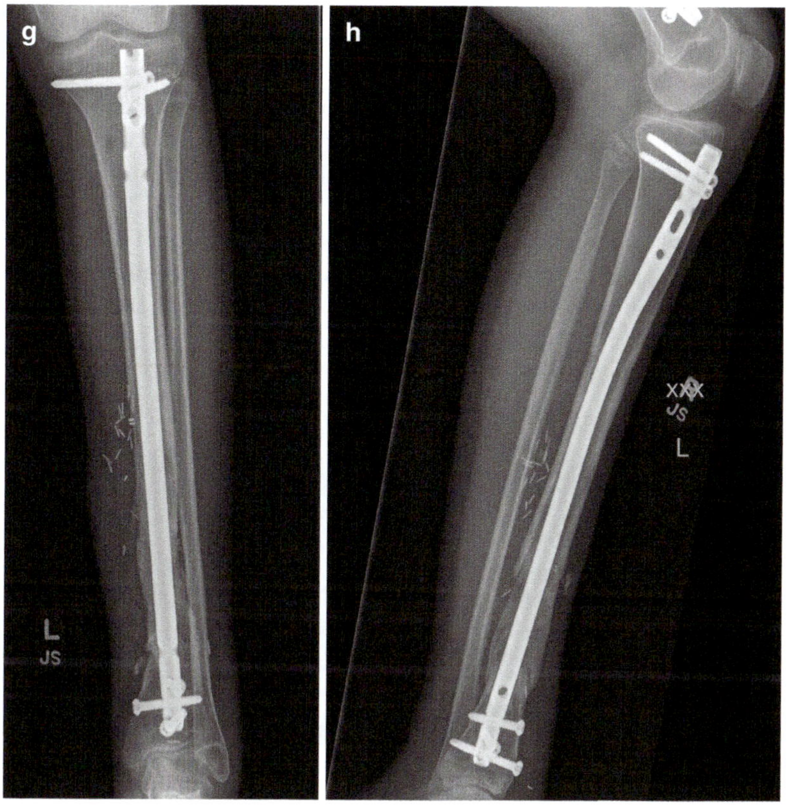

Fig. 20.1 (continued)

and 20.7b) [28]. Comparing serial radiographs is more valuable than interpreting a single image. Osteomyelitis can sometimes be detected by newly developed linear periosteal reaction, osteolysis, cavities, and cortical irregularities such as a "fuzzy" appearance of the cortex. Overall, the sensitivity and specificity are low (values of 14% and 70%, respectively), and radiologically detectable changes typically appear much later than the onset of the infection [28, 37]. In advanced disease, ulcer tracts may be seen as a lucent soft tissue defect at the skin surface with a foci of gas extending to the underlying bone. Bony destruction, bony sequestrum, and soft tissue or intraosseous gas may also be present [24].

Computerized Tomography (CT) Scan

Although in the past CT was complicated by artifact due to metal implants, improvements in imaging technology have made it possible to image bone with retained implants as well as the surrounding soft tissue [30, 35, 38]. Many newer scanners are equipped with metal artifact reduction algorithms that utilize iterative reconstruction to limit beam hardening artifacts [38]. Signs of posttraumatic osteomyelitis are similar to those seen in conventional radiography. However, high spatial resolution CT better demonstrates the details of cortical bone and the presence of sequestra. In addition, subtle changes such as cortical erosion or destruction, periosteal and endosteal reaction, and intraosseous fistulas are better visualized by CT. However, CT has limited soft tissue resolution. In cases of known infection, CT is often used for preoperative planning as it provides the best detail of bone structure (Fig. 20.5e–g) [27, 35].

Magnetic Resonance Imaging (MRI)

Like CT, only recently has it become possible to use MRI in the evaluation of osteomyelitis next to orthopedic hardware. Although MRI can typically be used in the presence of metal orthopedic implants, it has traditionally suffered from in-plane and through-plane data misregulation due to the magnetic susceptibility of implanted materials [30, 39]. Special sequences have been developed such as slice encoding for metal artifact correction (SEMAC) and multi-acquisition with variable-resonance image combination (MAVRIC) that allow for the optimization MR images with metallic implants. These are specific and advanced sequences that are not widely available at most hospitals [37]. In addition, the postoperative changes and reparative fibrovascular scar tissue may create signal intensities similar to those of infection for up to 1 year after surgery. This leads to false-positive results, although gadolinium enhancement may allow for discrimination of active infection from fibrovascular scarring (Figs. 20.2h–j and 20.3e, f) [27].

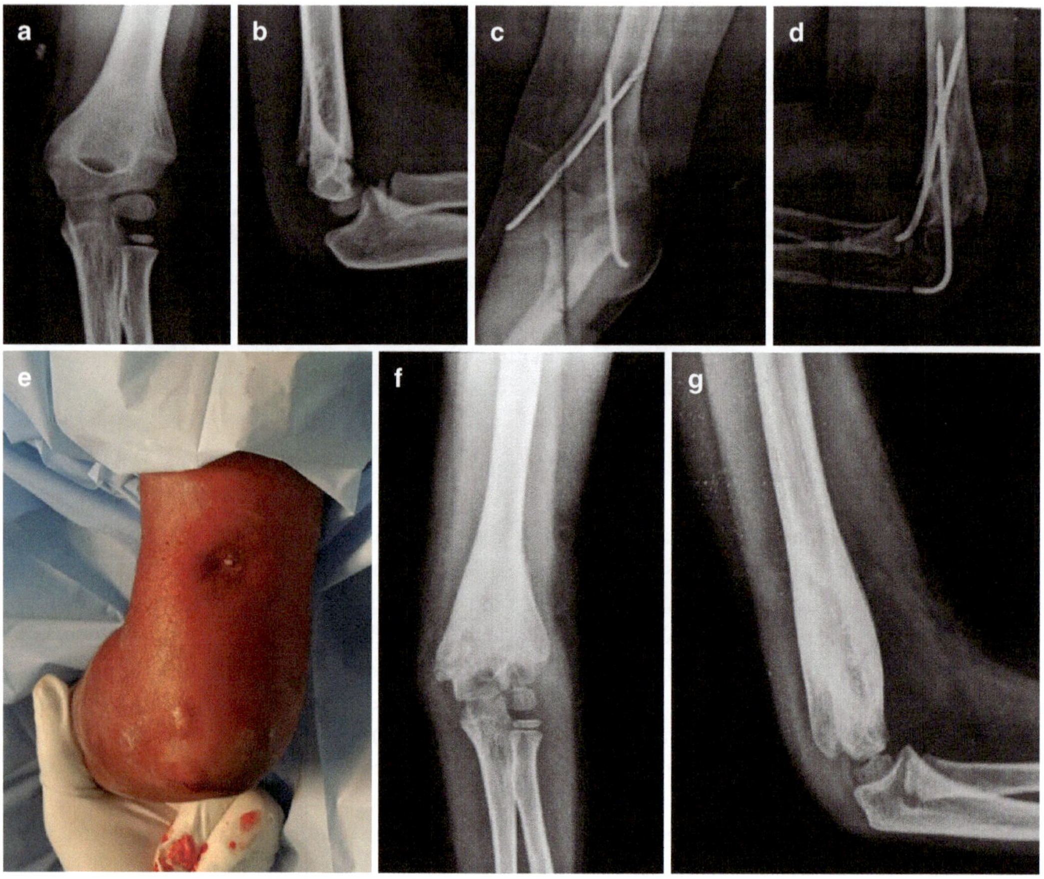

Fig. 20.2 (**a–d**) A 7-year-old male with a grade 2 supracondylar fracture of the left distal humerus treated with percutaneous pinning, who developed an infection around the lateral pin. (**e–g**) The boy presented with a chronic draining sinus 5 months after the initial surgery with changes of chronic osteomyelitis in the left distal humerus. (**h–j**) MRI of the left distal humerus shows intraosseous and extraosseous fluid collection and septic arthritis of left elbow. (**k–m**) Clinical photograph and radiographs of the left distal humerus showing treatment with debridement and antibiotic impregnated calcium sulfate beads. (**n, o**) Clinical photographs and radiographs of the left distal humerus showing complete resolution of osteomyelitis with absorption of calcium sulfate beads, successful healing of sinus and improvement in elbow movements at 2 months follow-up

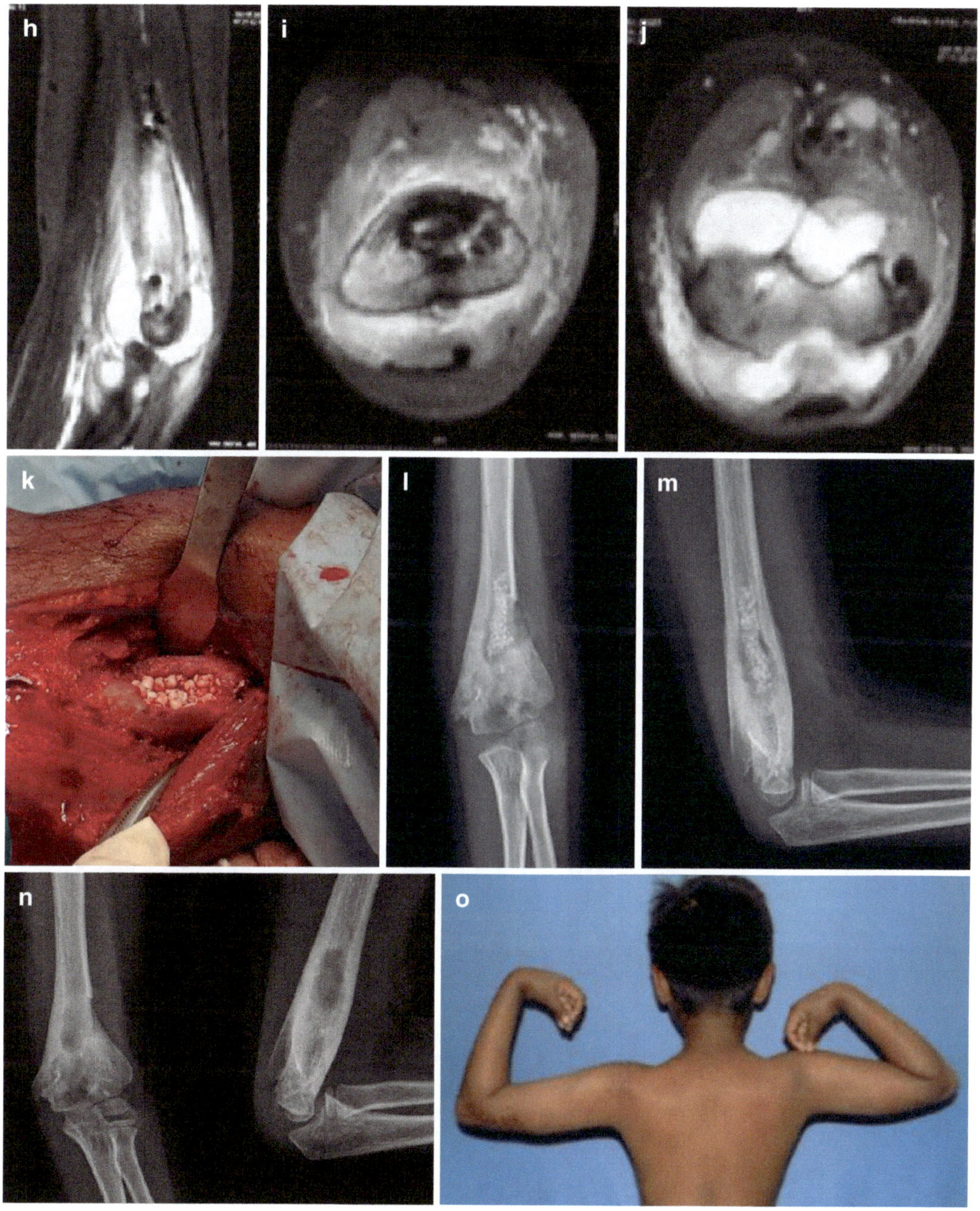

Fig. 20.2 (continued)

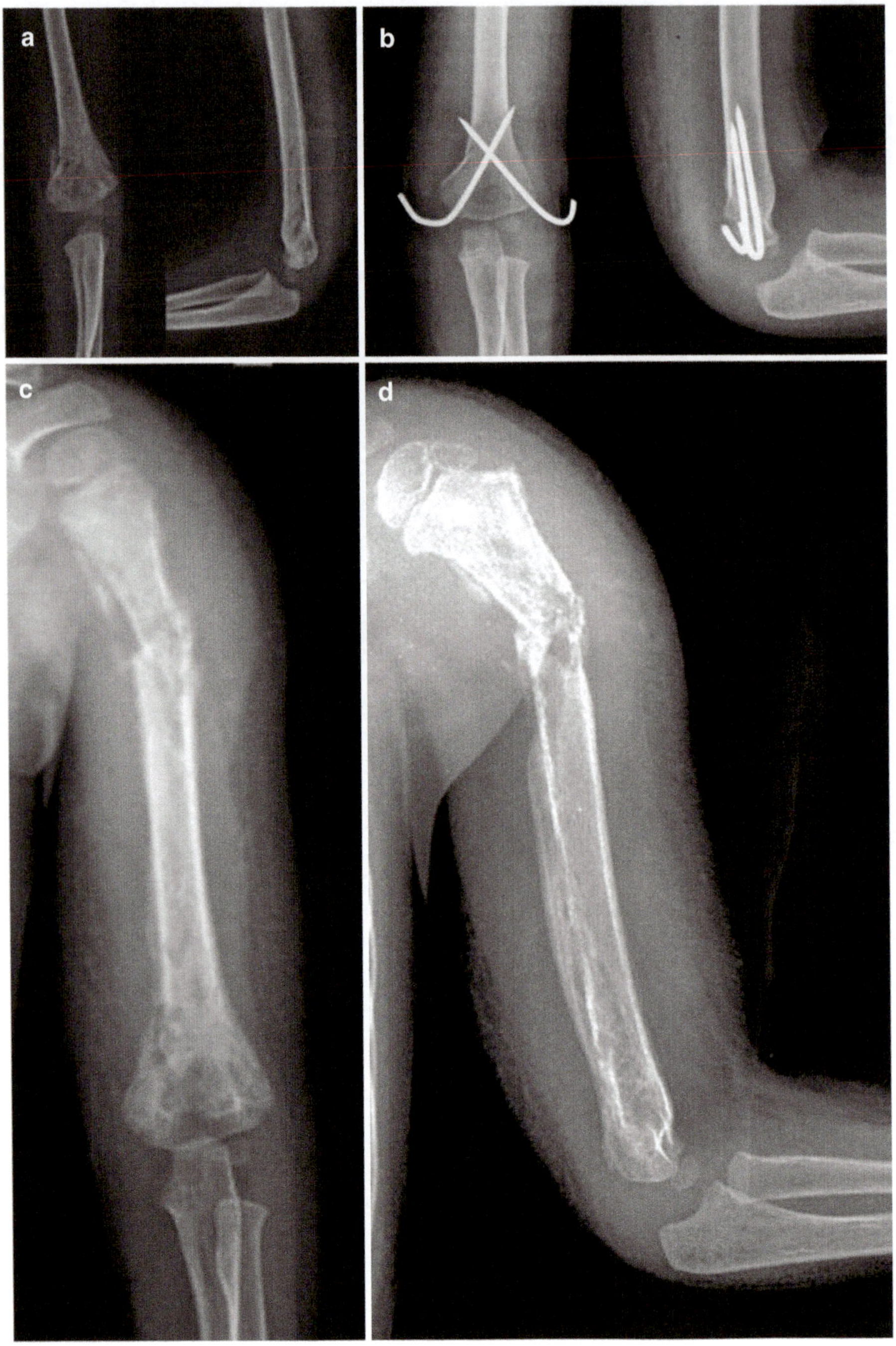

Fig. 20.3 (**a**, **b**) Radiographs of a 3-year-old male child with a left grade 2 extension supracondylar fracture treated with percutaneous pinning. He developed pain and swelling in the distal arm with discharge from pins after 2 weeks. The implants were removed, and child was put on oral antibiotics. (**c**, **d**) Child fell again and presented with severe pain, swelling, and fever 6 weeks after pinning; radiographs of the left arm showed panhumeral chronic osteomyelitis with a pathological fracture proximal third humerus shaft fracture. (**e**, **f**) An MRI of the left humerus confirmed pan-humeral osteomyelitis with a subperiosteal abscess around the pathological fracture. (**g**, **h**) Child was treated with antibiotics, drainage of the subperiosteal abscess, and stabilization of the left humerus pathologic fracture with a mini external fixator. (**i**, **j**) Radiographs of the left humerus at 2- and 6-month follow-up show complete resolution of osteomyelitis with excellent union of pathological fracture

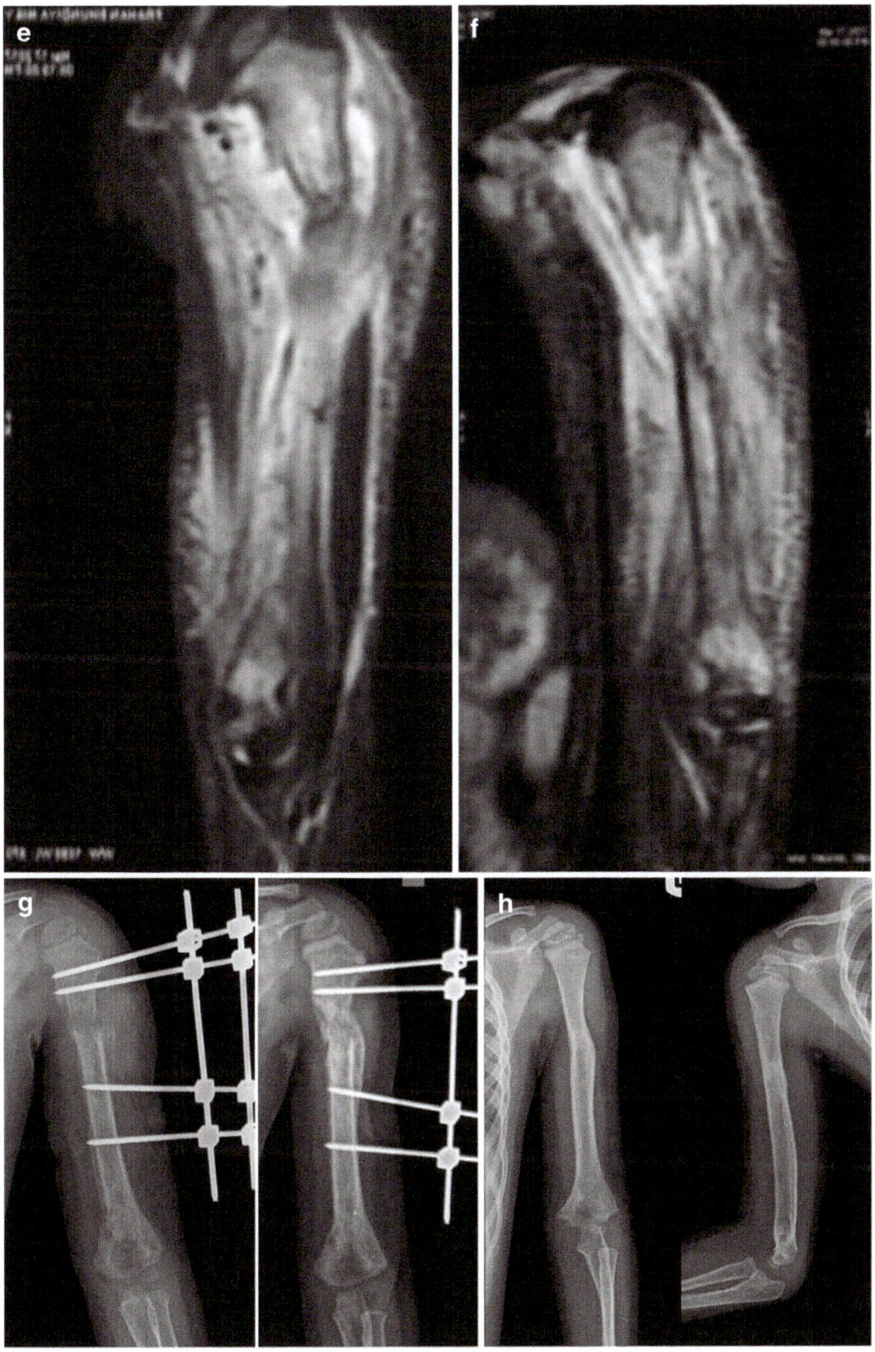

Fig. 20.3 (continued)

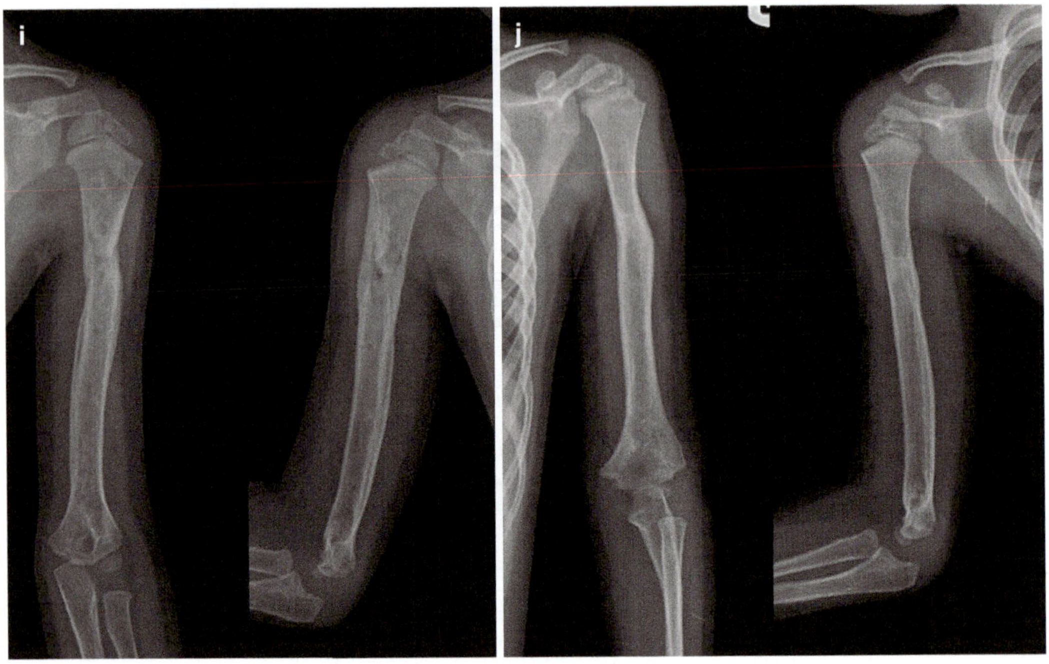

Fig. 20.3 (continued)

Nuclear Medicine Imaging

The three most commonly used nuclear medicine techniques to diagnose chronic posttraumatic osteomyelitis are the three-phase bone scan (with SPECT-CT), white blood cell scintigraphy (also called leukocyte scan) with SPECT-CT, and ^{18}F-fluorodeoxyglucose (FDG)-PET/CT [40]. While a normal three-phase bone scintigraphy scan rules out almost completely an existing bone infection due to the high sensitivity, it is not recommended for use within at least the first 1–2 years following the traumatic event as any recent alteration to the bone will result in a positive outcome [28, 40]. For example, it is known that a bone scan may be positive for at least 2 years after total hip arthroplasty and 5 years after total knee arthroplasty due to postoperative physiological bone remodeling [28, 40]. There is a lack of studies focusing on white blood cell scintigraphy for specifically diagnosing chronic posttraumatic osteomyelitis. However, it is the only existing imaging modality that is a specific indicator of an infection. One author reviewed WBC scintigraphy ± SPECT/CT in 114 patients with suspected PTO at their hospital and calculated a sensitivity, specificity, positive predictive value, and negative predictive value were 89, 95, 86, and 97%, respectively. Although rigorous studies do not yet exist for white blood cell scintigraphy in chronic posttraumatic osteomyelitis, current evidence suggests it can contribute important diagnostic information [28, 40]. PET/CT with ^{18}F-fluorodeoxyglucose (FDG) shares similar diagnostic complications as three-phase bone scintigraphy. It accumulates in healing tissues, in areas of inflammation, and in areas of infection, which makes its use limited following a traumatic event and subsequent fixation. Furthermore, no interpretation criteria presently exist as to when to declare an FDG-PET positive or negative for infection. It may have use in diagnosing chronic posttraumatic osteomyelitis that arises many years after the initial causative event, although this remains to be studied [28, 40].

Tissue Sampling

Microbiologic cultures obtained from the initial debridement are unreliable and only return positive for known causative pathogens of osteomyelitis in 25% of cases. Therefore, a microbiologic diagnosis does not occur during the initial debridement, but rather at subsequent debridements for a suspected infection. Causative organisms can originate from normal skin flora, soil contamination of the trauma, or nosocomial pathogens acquired during medical interventions. The most commonly isolated pathogens include *S. aureus*, coagulase-negative staphylococci, and aerobic gram-negative bacilli. Other causative microbes include enterococci, anaerobes, fungi, and mycobacteria [29].

Important features of chronic posttraumatic osteomyelitis

It accounts for about 20–30% of all chronic osteomyelitis cases.

Incidence is much less in children than adults as children resist infection and typically many pediatric fractures are managed by K-wires and nails. Large plates and the tissue dissection to apply them are not common in children, with adolescents being the exception.

Typically, it is a posttraumatic complication of long bone fractures.

It can also occur as a postoperative complication of surgeries, especially orthopedic trauma procedures with retained implants.

Antibiotic resistance can occur due to biofilm formation on the necrotic, devascularized bone and retained orthopedic implants.

Classification system: Cierny-Mader.

Serum inflammatory markers have limited diagnostic value in late presenting cases.

No consensus on the best imaging modality; new algorithms have shown significant improvement in masking metallic artifacts and improving the specificity of CT and MRI.

Microbiologic diagnosis occurs at subsequent debridement for a suspected infection.

Treatment and Management

Stage One: Debridement, Skeletal Stabilization, and Antibiotic Therapy

The treatment of chronic posttraumatic osteomyelitis requires a combination of medical and surgical management to restore function free of pain and infection. Communication and coordination between orthopedic surgeons, plastic surgeons, and infectious diseases specialists are essential for successful management [29, 41]. Surgical debridement is a cornerstone of therapy as antibiotics poorly penetrate dead or injured bone and infected fluid collections. Adequate surgical debridement decreases the bacterial load, removes necrotic tissue, and increases the chance that the host immune system and antibiotics will arrest infection [14, 29, 31]. Debridement also allows cultures to be obtained from deep tissues in order to target antibiotic therapy. Orthopedic hardware creates an avascular surface for microbial colonization and biofilm formation; its removal enhances the possibility of eliminating the infection. After the removal of infected dead tissue and hardware, nonunion of bone can be addressed when present. Placement of antibiotic-containing beads or cement spacers made of polymethylmethacrylate or calcium sulfate provides concentrated, targeted local antibiotic delivery (Figs. 20.1c, d and 20.7c, d) [42]. Finally, dead space can be exposed for flap coverage. Once surgical control of the affected area has been accomplished, effective antibiotic therapy can be administered [29].

Surgical Debridement

The first step of surgical treatment is a radical debridement of all nonviable and infected tissue, including skin, soft tissue, and bone [43]. It is imperative that multiple intraoperative specimens are sent for culture including sinus tract material, purulent fluid, soft tissue, curetted bone, and the bed of the involved bone [27]. Five samples should be taken if possible [1]. Debridement proceeds until well-perfused, noninfected tissue that actively bleeds is encountered at the margins of the resection [1, 27, 41]. Viable bone can be detected by punctuate bleeding ("paprika sign"), and bone bleeding can still be seen with an inflated tourniquet [1, 27]. In addition, abnormal bone splinters as it is cut, whereas healthy bone curls up like wood shavings [1]. Nonviable or infected tissue missed during debridement is sheltered from the microcirculation and will allow the infection to persist and prevent the subsequent antibiotic therapy from clearing the infection [11, 19, 23]. Thus, debridement should be radical and not limited by concerns about creating osseous or soft tissue defects; only the vascular and nerve supply should be preserved (Figs. 20.4d–h and 20.7c) [27, 41]. If the marrow is infected, it should be reamed out and irrigated [27, 41]. All foreign bodies such be removed,

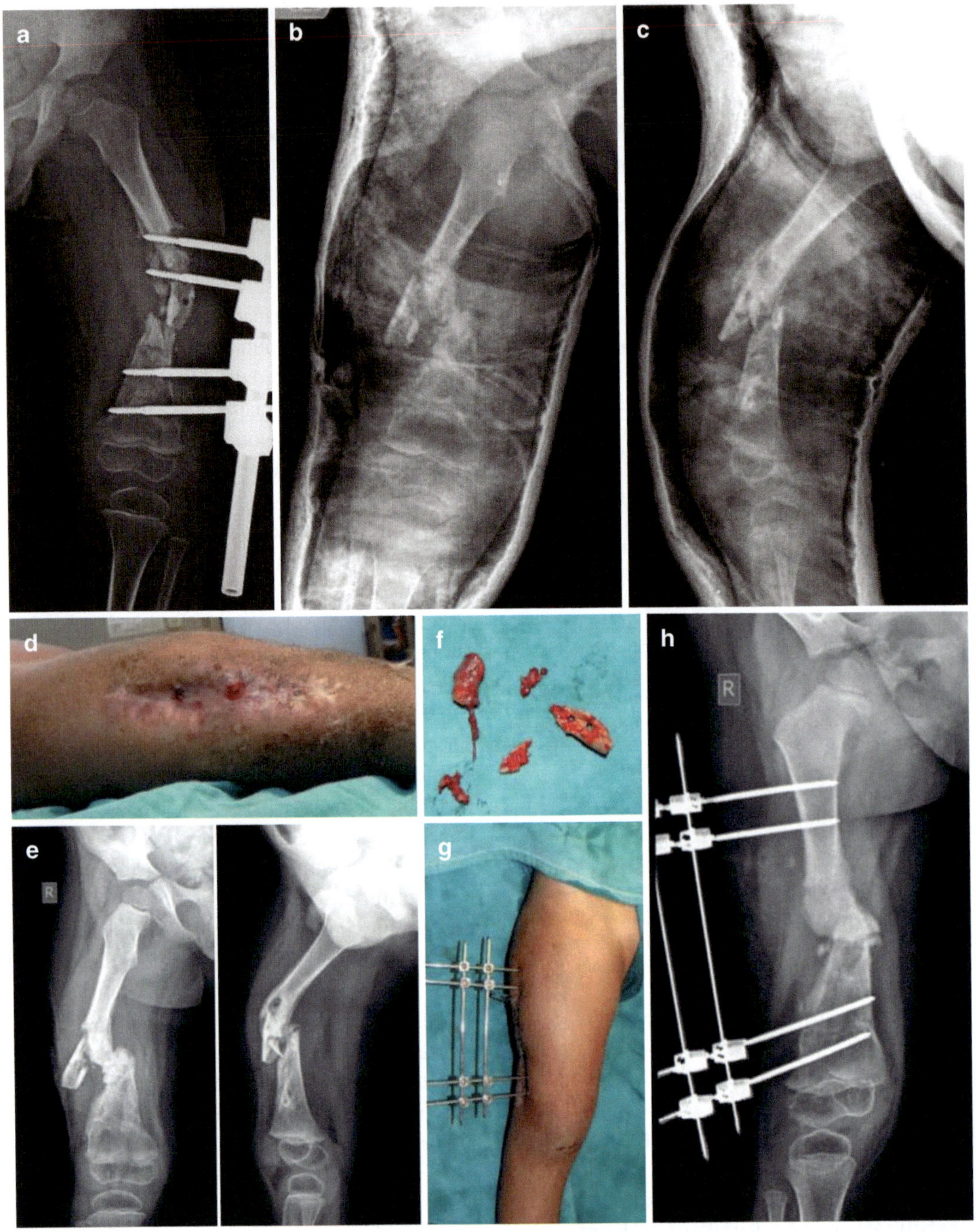

Fig. 20.4 (**a**–**c**) A 6-year-old male had a left fracture shaft femur treated with ORIF and plating. Subsequently developed sepsis, the plate was removed, and fracture was stabilized with an external fixator; child presented to us with a loose fixator and discharging sinus. Treatment included removal of the loose external fixator, spica cast, and antibiotics. (**d**–**h**) 3 weeks after the previous operation, the child was operated for a left femur sequestrectomy, debridement, and stabilization with a mini external fixator. (**i**–**l**) 6 months follow-up clinical photographs and radiographs show excellent union of the fracture with healing of the sinus and a mild procurvatum deformity of the left femur

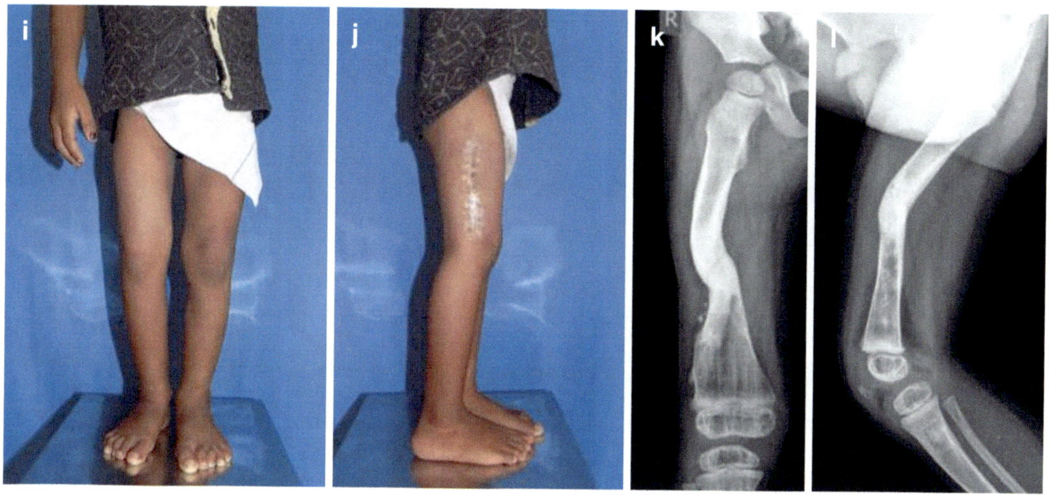

Fig. 20.4 (continued)

including orthopedic implants (Fig. 20.3a, b) [41, 44]. The wound is then irrigated with a large amount of saline, and antibiotics may be added to the irrigation fluid [27, 41, 44].

Skeletal Stabilization

Skeletal stabilization of ununited fractures is necessary for controlling the infection, and an assessment of the bone's stability is made intraoperatively following excision [1, 27]. Skeletal stabilization of the lower extremity allows postoperative weight bearing which is important to minimize worsening osteopenia, muscle wasting, and joint contracture, as well as promote bone healing [1]. Chronic osteomyelitis of bone with nonunion or bone defects is traditionally treated by a two-stage procedure involving initial debridement, antibiotic delivery, and external fixation, with definitive internal fixation following at a later date (Figs. 20.3g–h, 20.6c–f, and 20.7d) [31]. Splinting can also be considered in place of external fixation in certain cases where the osseous defect is not extensive and the bone is extremely osteopenic and/or for the upper extremities [44, 45].

Local Antibiotic Therapy

Polymethylmethacrylate (PMMA) impregnated with antibiotics is used to sterilize and temporarily fill the dead space created by the radical debridement. The osteoconductive carriers promote bone healing, while the carrier element gradually dissolves and releases a very high local concentration of the antibiotics with a low systemic level. The levels released are orders of magnitude higher than the concentrations achieved by parenteral antibiotics, but with a reduced risk of systemic side effects [1, 27, 31, 44].

PMMA can take the form of beads or a cement spacer [27, 29]. The cement spacer has several advantages over the beads. Cement spacers provide mechanical support to the bone which is important when a bony defect is created from debridement (Fig. 20.1c, d). Beads offer no mechanical support to the bone and are suitable when only part of the bone is removed with one or more cortices preserved. In addition, if an orthopedic implant must be retained, beads can be used to provide a high concentration of antibiotics in the area around the implant (Figs. 20.5h–j and 20.7c). Beads can also be difficult to remove as they are enveloped within the healing fibrous tissue. Furthermore, it can be challenging to prepare oval-ended beads that are small enough to feed on steel wire for removal in the short window before the cement hardens. Lastly, the cement spacer induces periosteal membrane formation that aids in bone healing, a technique first pioneered in 1986 by Masquelet.

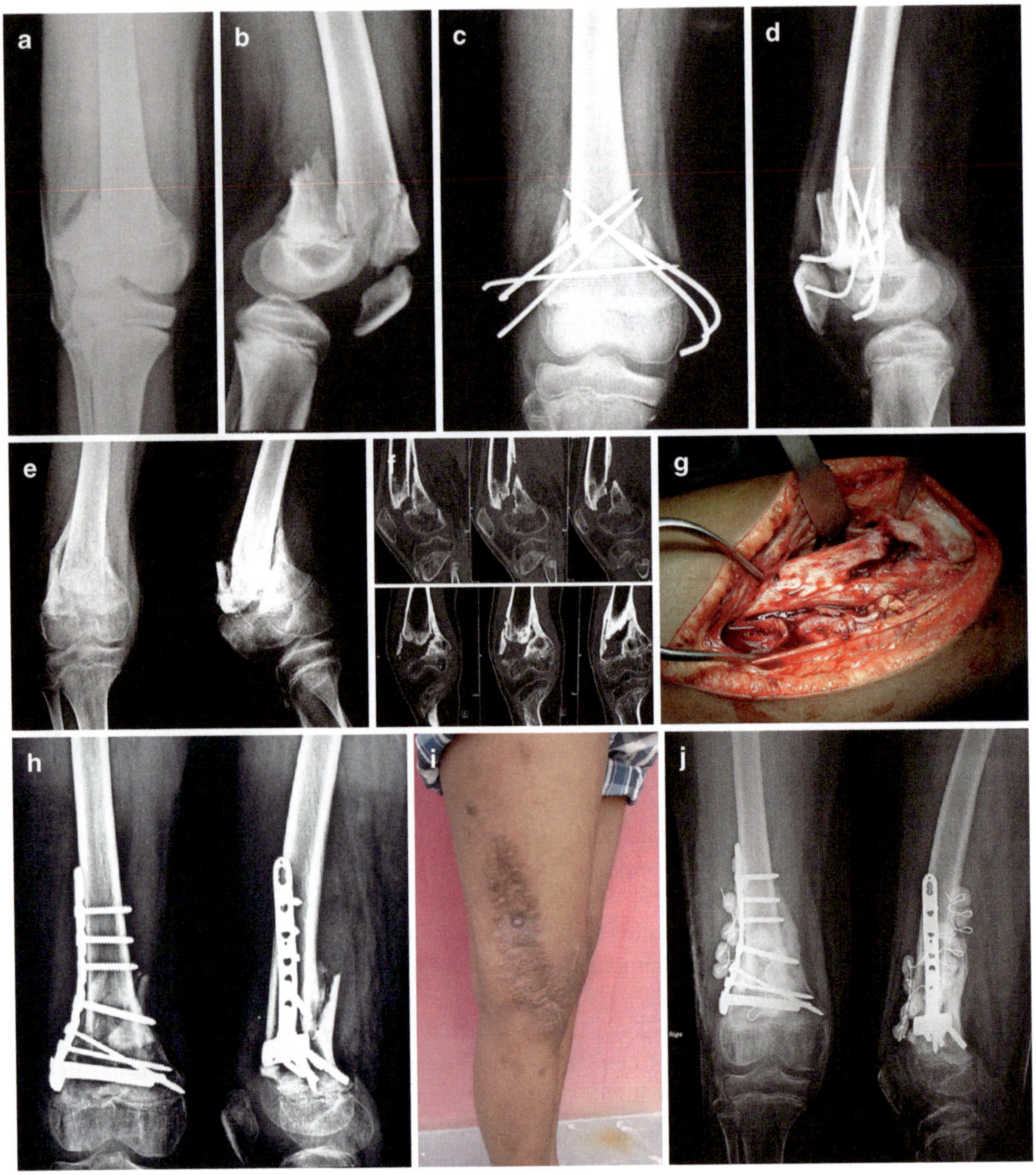

Fig. 20.5 (**a–d**) A 12-year-old male with a grade 2 open right distal femur fracture managed with closed reduction and percutaneous pinning. (**e–g**) Child presented 2 months after initial surgery with a swollen right knee with restricted movements. CT scan showed nonunion; thorough debridement with stabilization was done, and he was started on antibiotics. (**h–j**) The right femur nonunion was stabilized with plate fixation but presented with a discharging sinus after 2 months; successful union was achieved after repeat debridement, stabilization, and placement of antibiotic impregnated cement beads. (**k–n**) One and half years after the surgical treatment, the child presented with a discharging sinus, good distal femur union, and 5 cm of shortening; he was treated with removal of implants and contralateral epiphysiodesis for LLD and ended with 1 inch of shortening

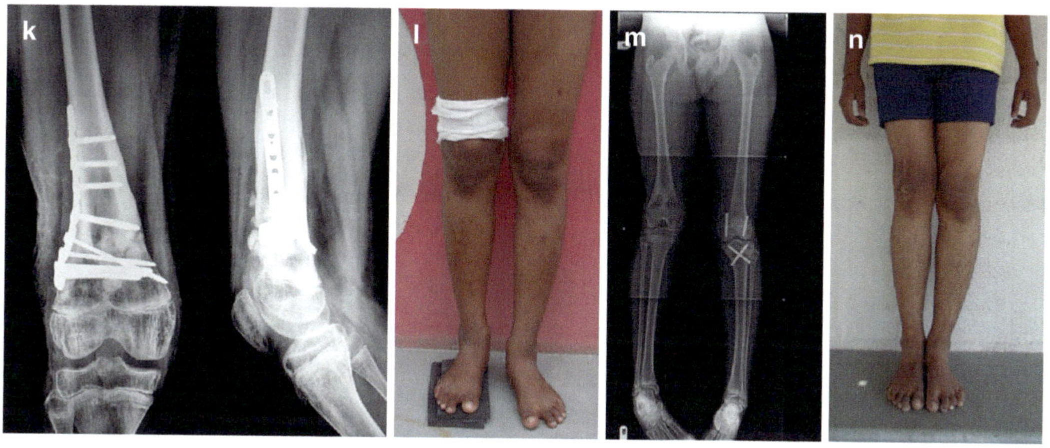

Fig. 20.5 (continued)

This is especially noticeable in pediatric patients as children may be able to regenerate a periosteal membrane faster than adults [19, 33, 44, 46]. The local antibiotics are left in the wound until the second surgical stage. Canavese et al. report timing the second stage based on the normalization of infectious markers, particularly WBC and CRP, with good results. This occurred between 3 weeks to 1 month after the implantation of PMMA [19, 33, 44].

In addition, bioabsorbable bone graft substitutes, such as α-hemihydrate calcium sulfate impregnated with antibiotics, are an option that allows for single-stage surgeries as they dissolve and do not need to be removed later. This is a newer technique and not as well studied as PMMA cement; however, the literature is promising (Fig. 20.2k–o) [20, 47].

Systemic Antibiotic Therapy

Initial systemic antibiotic therapy should provide coverage against the most common pathogens. The antibiotic regimen is then tailored to the specific organism once culture and sensitivity results are available. No consensus exists for antibiotic duration, although intravenous administration is generally given for 4–6 weeks and can be completed on an outpatient basis. Bone requires 3–4 weeks to revascularize after debridement surgery, and the paradigm is to protect the bone with antibiotics during this time [31, 41]. Canavese et al. report success with 3–4 weeks of intravenous antibiotics followed by 1.5–6 months of oral antibiotics [44].

Stage Two: Wound Management

If after debridement the remaining soft tissue envelope is adequate, delayed or primary closure may be possible. If the soft tissue is compromised, coverage should be achieved by a local or free tissue flap 3–7 days after the original procedure. Staged coverage has the benefit of allowing targeted antibiotics based on deep tissue cultures time to work as well as allowing a repeat debridement before soft tissue coverage. Muscle flaps have the advantage of providing durable coverage and improving vascularity at the recipient site which in turn enhances antibiotic delivery, host defense mechanisms, and healing [1, 27, 31]. In study of 925 cases of long bone osteomyelitis in adults, direct closure was possible 76%, while local flaps were required in 5% and free tissue transfer in 19% [1].

Stage Three: Management of Bone Defects

After the infection has been controlled, the soft tissue envelope has healed, and the muscle flap placed and viable, the PMMA can then be removed, and bone defects managed. If a flap was necessary, this typically occurs 6–8 weeks after the muscle transfer [27]. Otherwise, it can occur sooner based on the time required to eradicate the infection [44].

Bone Defects <6 cm

Children have a greater healing potential than adults and may be able to regenerate defects that adults cannot. Thicker and more active periosteum provides faster healing and greater fracture stability and provides significant potential to regenerate bone, even in the setting of considerable bone loss, and bone grafting is seldom required. However, for older children those healing potential approaches that of an adult, surgical correction of the bone defect may be necessary [15–17, 48, 49]. Typically, for defects up to 6 cm, autogenous iliac crest bone grafting or bone graft substitutes such as β-tricalcium phosphate are used (Fig. 20.1e, f) [27, 44]. The bone graft or substitute can again be impregnated with antibiotics [50]. Additionally, internal fixation or external fixation can be used to augment stability during this time if needed [44].

Acute shortening and compression can be used to safely reconstruct bone defects of up to 3–5 cm in the long bones [51, 52]. It is a simple and fast treatment for segmental bone loss that allows for early primary closure without soft tissue tension [52]. Compression of the bone edges promotes osteosynthesis, while shortening the length of the wound may prevent the need for a complex soft tissue procedure. An angular deformity can be introduced with the wound at the concavity of the deformity to facilitate wound closure in large or asymmetric defects [53]. However, challenges can occur due to noncompliance of soft tissues leading to bunching of soft tissues, difficulty with skin closure, and the potential for kinking of neurovascular structures. As a proportion of limb length, children tend to tolerate acute shortening better than adults, but care must be taken when greater than 4 cm is acutely shortened in pediatric patients [51, 54, 55].

Bone Defects >6 cm

For bone defects greater than 6 cm, specialized reconstructive procedures such as nonvascularized or vascularized bone grafts, distraction osteogenesis, or induced membrane technique may be required.

Non-vascularized or pedicled fibular graft is an excellent choice to reconstruct bone defects of the long bones [56–58]. The non-vascularized fibular graft is reported to have equivalent union rates to the free vascularized fibular grafts in pediatric patients, possibly due to the increased number of stromal cells in children [57]. Pedicle grafts have the advantage of maintaining the original blood supply as well as avoiding disrupting the contralateral normal limb, both of which occur in a free vascularized fibular graft [58]. In addition, a long microsurgical procedure is not needed [59].

The free vascularized fibular graft is a free tissue transfer that, in addition to bone, can also include the skin, fascia, and muscle (Fig. 20.7b–d). In addition to repairing large, combined bone, and soft tissue defects, it can also be used in patients who have had multiple previous operations and have a scarred soft tissue envelop and are opposed to external fixation [27]. However, this requires a long microsurgical procedure [59].

Distraction osteogenesis has a few advantages over vascularized bone grafts. In vascular bone grafting, refracture and issues with host-graft junction healing can occur. Distraction osteogenesis has the benefit of increasing the blood flow in the extremity by three to ten times in the extremity, which both promote healing and increase the impact of systemic antibiotics [48, 60]. Please refer to Chaps. 25 and 26 for a more detailed description of the rationale, principles, and description of these reconstructive techniques.

The induced membrane technique can be used to treat bone defects regardless of magnitude or etiology. It can correct segmental bone defects of 20–25 cm in length [19, 44]. A cement spacer is placed in the bony defect to induce a bioactive periosteal membrane, which is considered mature at 4–6 weeks after spacer placement [44]. The spacer is then removed and is replaced with graft from the posterior iliac crest. Graft expansion can be done by adding allograft chips that are mixed with the autograft and blood harvested during iliac crest graft extraction. The allograft thus takes on the same aspect as the autograft, and the blood impregnates the donor bone [19]. This technique is particularly viable in skeletally immature patients, who form a periosteal membrane quicker than in adults [44]. Please refer to Chap. 38 for a more detailed explanation of the rationale, principles, and description of the induced membrane technique.

Prevention

The most effective means to prevent the occurrence of chronic posttraumatic osteomyelitis is a careful and thorough treatment of the original injury. Preventing the development of an acute infection is the best measure against the development of a chronic infection [41]. Antibiotics administered within 2 hours of an open fracture substantially reduces the risk of an acute infection [61]. Performing the initial irrigation and debridement of an open fracture within 24 hours decreases the incidence of infection [49, 62]. Thorough surgical debridement, wound irrigation, and placing muscle flap or vascularized tissue grafts aid in the prevention of infection after trauma through removing dead tissue, decreasing the bacterial load, and filling the dead space with adequately vascularized tissue (Fig. 20.6a–h) [17, 18, 31].

Adequate sterile technique aids in the prevention of posttraumatic osteomyelitis following elective orthopedic cases. The typical rate of infection following elective orthopedic surgery is 1–2%; this rate has remained stable over time, and a small percentage of cases will invariable become infected despite following rigorous sterile technique [41].

Outcomes and Complications

Generally, infection control and union are achievable outcomes [3, 4, 13, 48, 63–67]. In a study by Yeargan et al. of 30 children with chronic osteomyelitis resistant to previous therapy, all of the patients who completed the study were able to achieve infection control (Figs. 20.1g, h, 20.3i, j, 20.4i–l, 20.5k–n, 20.6g, h, and 20.7f–h). Eighty percent were free of pain and had a leg length discrepancy of less than 2.5 cm, while 13% were able to activities of daily living without pain and had a leg length discrepancy of less than 3.5 cm. The hospital stay averaged 4.7 months and 3.2 procedures per patient, although the longest stay was 18 months [13].

In a study of 27 pediatric patients in developing countries by Wirbel et al., the recurrence rate after the assumed eradication of the infection was 11% within 3 months of discharge. In the same study, 22% of the children had a leg length discrepancy of greater than 2 cm, and 14.8% developed restrictions in the range of motion of an affected joint [3]. Ultimately, osteomyelitis in children may cause growth disturbances and deformities. These complications typically result from growth plate injury or substantial bone loss during debridement [48]. In addition, amputation may rarely be indicated, although the parents of pediatric patients are typically unwilling or very hesitant to give permission [27, 68, 69].

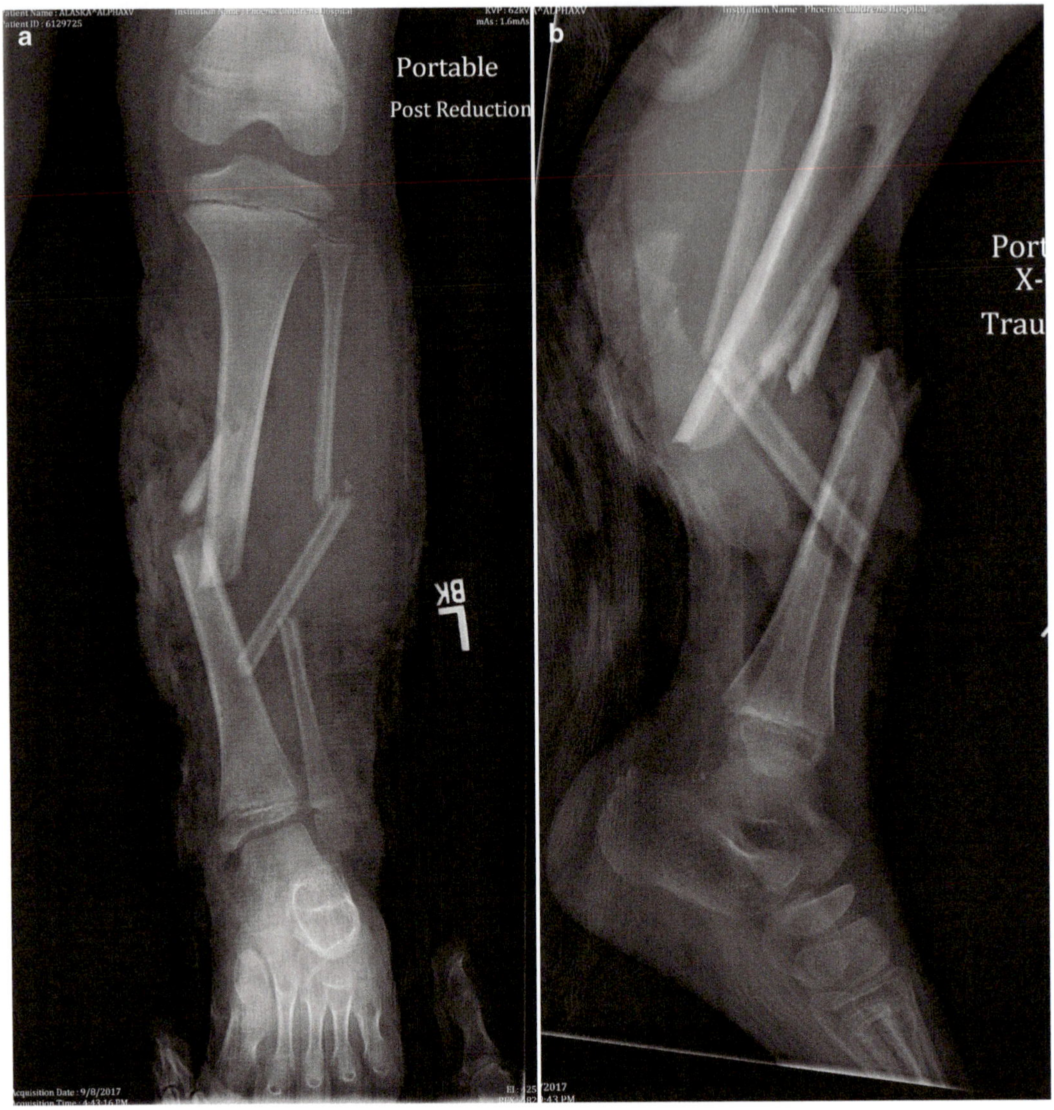

Fig. 20.6 (**a**, **b**) Radiographs of the left tibia in a 9-year-olds who presented with a grade 3B open comminuted tibial shaft and segmental fibular shaft fractures. (**c**, **d**) Radiographs showing reconstruction of the left tibia with open reduction and internal fixation using a 3.5 mm locking plate following a radical soft tissue debridement. The soft tissue defect was managed with a wound VAC initially followed by a gracilis free flap reconstruction and split thickness skin grafting within 72 hours. (**e**, **f**) Radiographs of the left tibia 3 months after surgical reconstruction showing healed and well-aligned tibia and fibula fractures with retained hardware. (**g**, **h**) Radiographs of the left tibia 3 years after treatment showing well-aligned tibia and fibula with excellent alignment following removal of hardware

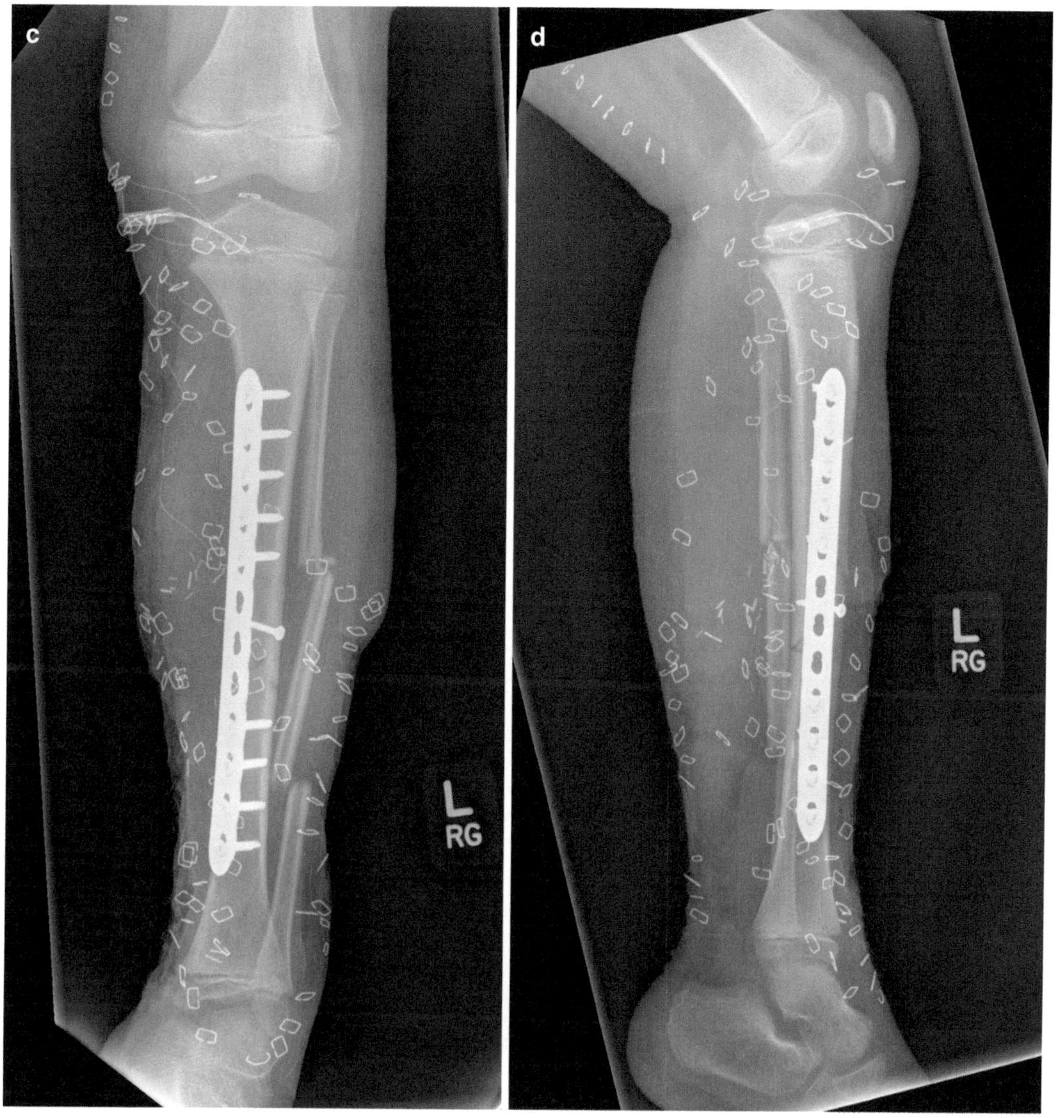

Fig. 20.6 (continued)

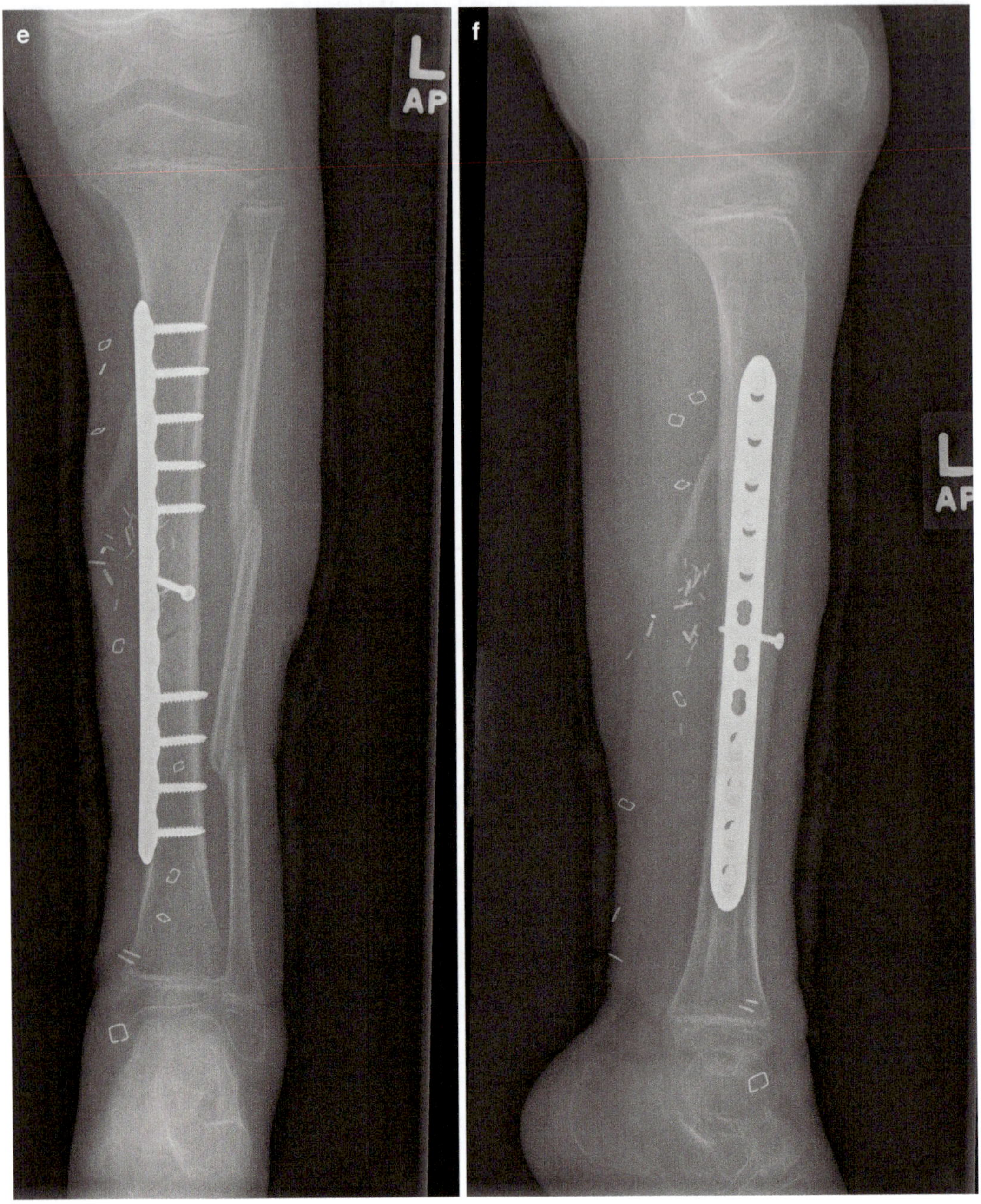

Fig. 20.6 (continued)

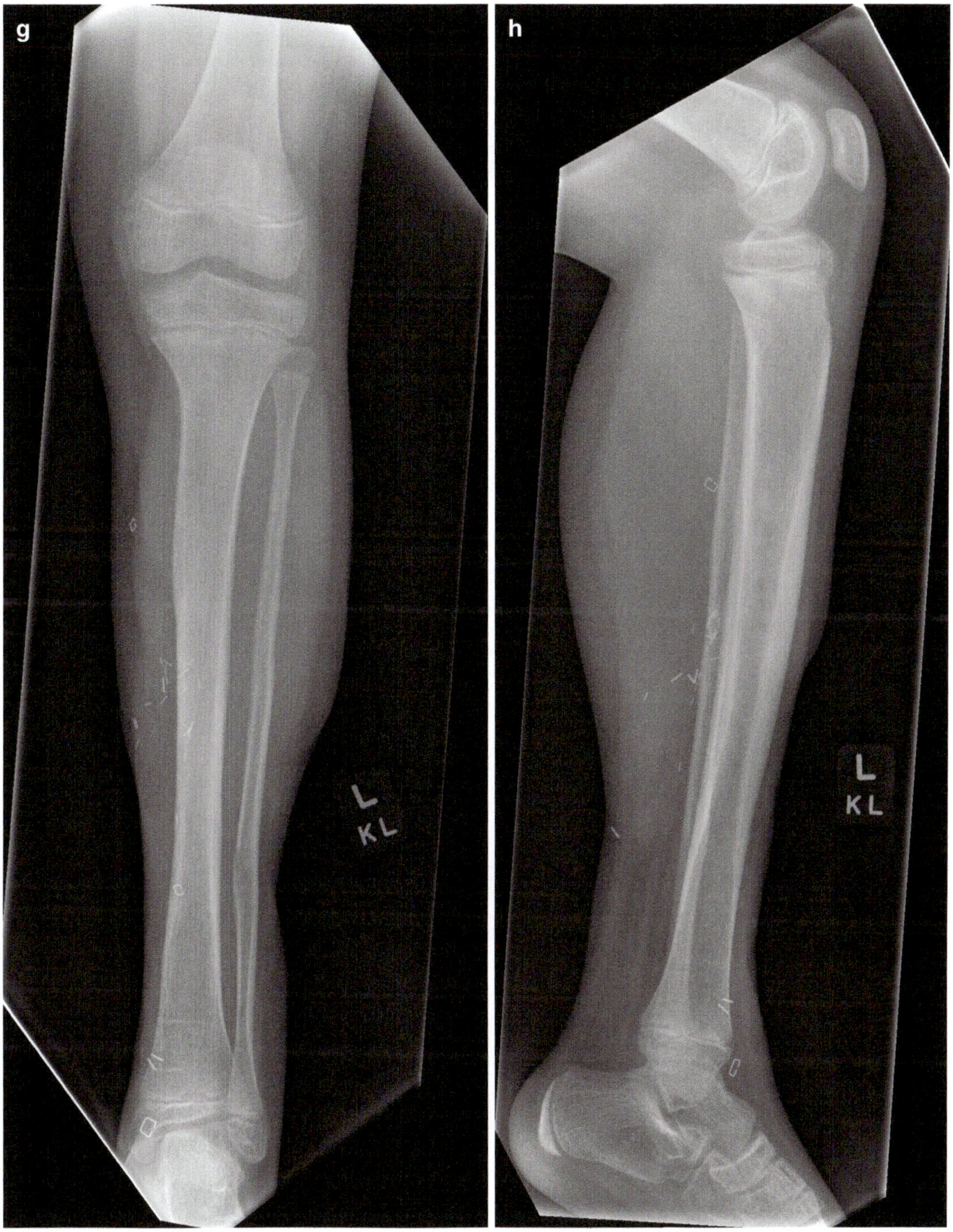

Fig. 20.6 (continued)

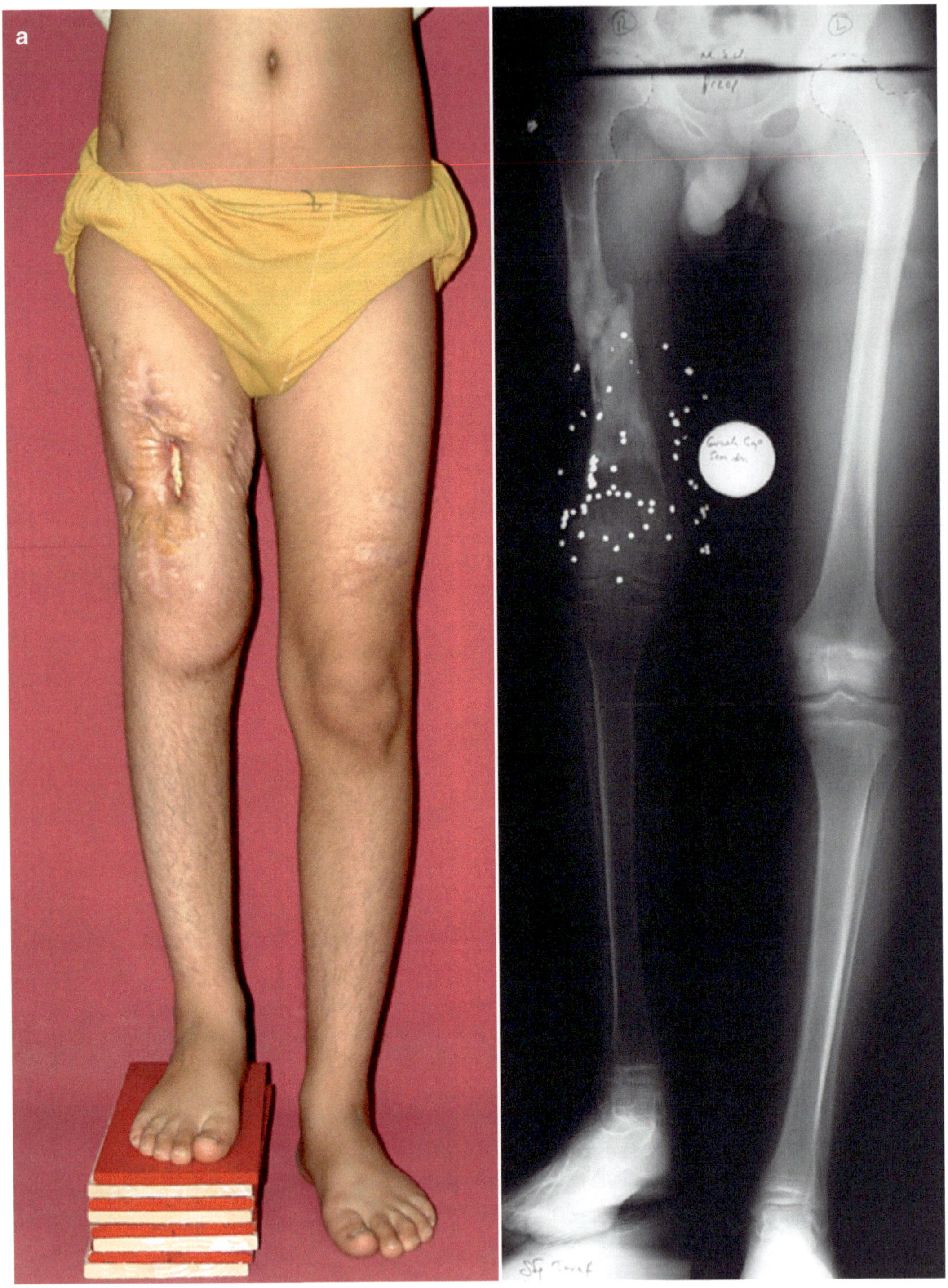

Fig. 20.7 (**a**, **b**) Show a 15-year-old male, sequela of gunshot wound, right femoral nonunion with 8 cm shortening. (**c**, **d**) Show the first Step: debridement + antibiotic loaded PMMA beads + soft tissue distraction to achieve equal femoral length (very stiff soft tissue around NU site). (**e**) This was followed by the second Step: free vascularized fibula graft (osteomyocutaneous) + IM nail. (**f**) Shows the final result, at 9 months (time to union + hypertrophy)

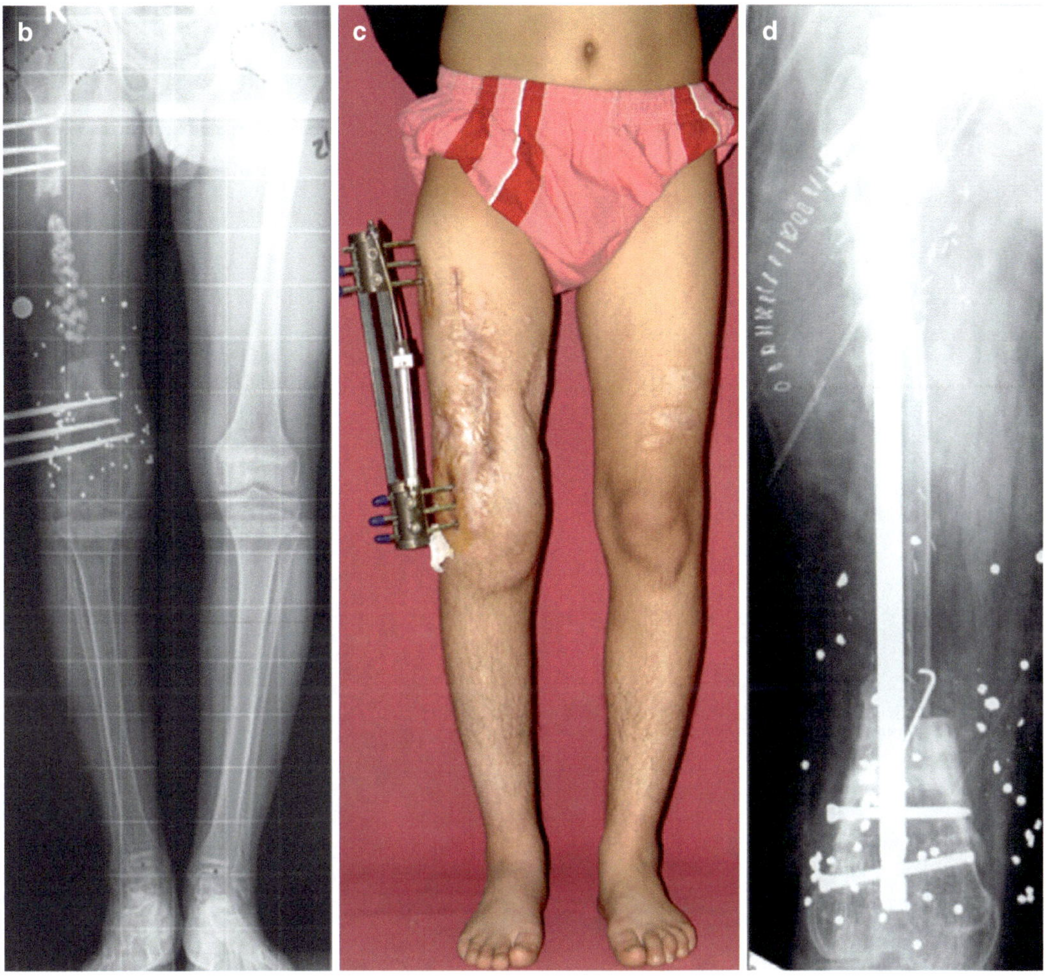

Fig. 20.7 (continued)

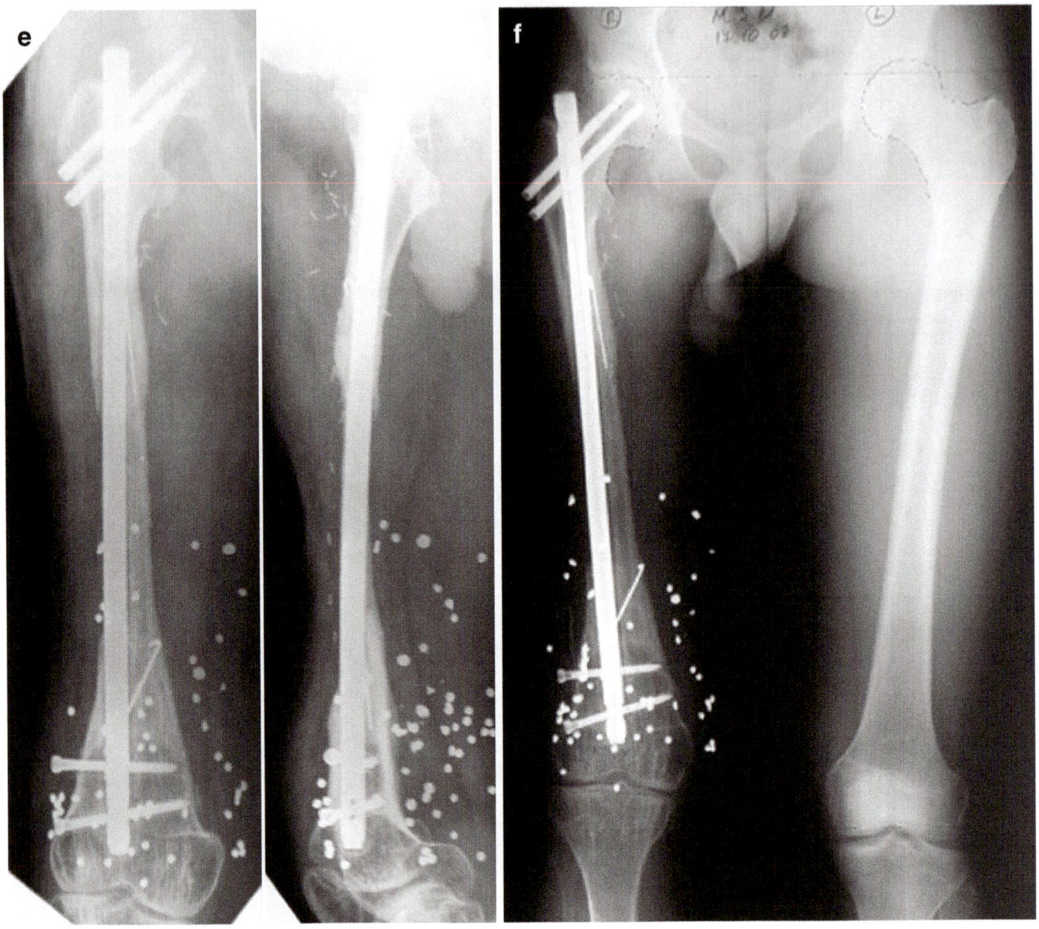

Fig. 20.7 (continued)

Conclusions

Chronic posttraumatic osteomyelitis is a significant complication of trauma or surgeries. It can be a devastating development with substantial long-term consequences for the patient. Preventing the development of an acute infection is the best measure against the development of a chronic infection. If a chronic infection does occur, a multistage surgery is typically required to eradicate the infection. The standard surgical treatment includes radical debridement, skeletal stabilization, temporary placement of local antibiotics for dead space management, soft tissue coverage, and management of the bony defect. This complex course of treatment requires a multidisciplinary collaborative team approach involving orthopedic and plastic surgeons, infectious disease specialists, and pediatricians to optimize care and patient safety.

Important steps in treatment
Early detection with high clinical suspicion and timely investigations
A radical debridement of all nonviable and infected tissue, including skin, soft tissue, and bone, is required.
Multiple intraoperative specimens are sent for culture to guide antibiotic management; at least five samples should be taken if possible, including bone and soft tissue.
Skeletal stabilization of ununited fractures is necessary for controlling the infection.
Polymethylmethacrylate or calcium sulfate impregnated with antibiotics can be used to sterilize and temporarily maintain the dead space created by the radical debridement.
If the soft tissue is compromised, coverage should be achieved by a local, regional, or free tissue flap within 3–7 days after the original procedure.
Children have a greater healing potential than adults and may be able to regenerate defects that adults cannot; bone defects less than 6 cm may not require specialized reconstructive techniques. For bone defects greater than 6 cm, specialized reconstructive procedures such as vascularized bone grafts, distraction osteogenesis, or induced membrane technique may be required. In resourced constrained centers, distraction osteogenesis is preferred over vascularized bone transfers.
Younger children should be followed long enough to diagnose and manage growth plate involvement related complications.

Box 20.1 Pearls to Stay Out of Trouble

Surgeries with retained implants

- Use standard aseptic precautions for any surgery with a retained implant in children, even if the implant is a K-wire.
- Postoperative fever, pain, swelling, and painful joint movements will be the first clinical clue of an infection. Patients/parents must be instructed to report them at the earliest sign.
- Do not delay investigating any child suspected of having a postoperative infection.

Open fractures

- Radical initial debridement is the most important intervention and decides the future course of events.
- As the final wound management may need a plastic surgeon, it is recommended to have a plastic surgeon during the first debridement.
  - The plastic surgeon may offer valuable inputs in debridement and may help in primary wound coverage, obviating need for further procedures.
- All dead and contaminated tissues except neurovascular structures must be removed.
- If primary stabilization is done with an external fixator, utmost care of pin tracts is mandatory.
- Early dead space and soft tissue defect management is essential.
- Early conversion to definitive stabilization is important.

Box 20.2 Tips and Tricks for Successful Outcome

- Check previous treatment details, investigations, radiographs, and other imaging before ordering new investigations.
- Collaborative multidisciplinary care with a team approach is important.
- In patients with large implants in situ, confirm compatibility of MRI, CT, or any other advance imaging to negate metallic artifacts with specialized algorithm.
- In established chronic osteomyelitis, thorough debridement with multiple sample collections to identify organism (preferably up to five samples) is a recommended practice.
- Remove all dead bone in primary debridement until punctuate bleeding ("paprika sign") is seen with the tourniquet inflated. Do not leave behind any dead bone for the fear of creating a bone defect.

- In patients with infected nonunions with retained implants, implant removal to eradicate biofilm may be necessary.
- Be ready with multiple strategies to reconstruct bone/soft tissue defects.
- After successful control of the infection and bone union, follow-up to skeletal maturity to diagnose any growth-related problems is **key.**

Box 20.3 Key Learning Points

- Chronic posttraumatic osteomyelitis, though uncommon in children, is a well-established entity and commonly seen after open fractures.
- Collaborative multidisciplinary care with a team approach is key.
- Advance imaging like CT, MRI, and PETCT with algorithm may be used to reduce metallic artifact.
- Debride thoroughly, collect multiple intraoperative tissue samples, and plan alternative fixation strategies beforehand.
- Use local antibiotic delivery systems wisely to manage the dead space.
- Wound coverage and bone defect management are integral part of treatment, involving expert consultation early on.
- Good outcomes can be expected, and follow-up to skeletal maturity is recommended.
- An ounce of prevention is better than a pound of cure.

Acknowledgments We would like to thank Dr. William Wood, MD, Pediatric Orthopedic Surgeon, Phoenix Children's Hospital, Phoenix, Arizona, USA, for contributing Fig. 20.1a–h.

Declarations

Funding Support: This project has no funding support.

Consent to Publish: The authors affirm that participants provided informed consent for publication of the images in Figs. 20.1, 20.2, 20.3, 20.4, 20.5, and 20.6.

Conflicts of Interest: The authors declare that they have no conflict of interest.

References

1. Chan JKK, Ferguson JY, Scarborough M, McNally MA, Ramsden AJ. Management of post-traumatic osteomyelitis in the lower limb: current state of the art. Indian J Plast Surg. 2019;52(1):62–72. https://doi.org/10.1055/s-0039-1687920.
2. Biruk WL, Wubshet K. Chronic osteomyelitis at Tikur Anbessa hospital, Addis Ababa University, Ethiopia. East Cent African J Surg. 2007;12(1):33–41.
3. Wirbel R, Hermans K. Surgical treatment of chronic osteomyelitis in children admitted from developing countries. African J Paediatr Surg. 2014;11(4):297–303. https://doi.org/10.4103/0189-6725.143133.
4. Mantero E, Carbone M, Calevo MG, Boero S. Diagnosis and treatment of pediatric chronic osteomyelitis in developing countries: prospective study of 96 patients treated in Kenya. Musculoskelet Surg. 2011;95(1):13–8. https://doi.org/10.1007/s12306-011-0104-0.
5. Panteli M, Giannoudis PV. Chronic osteomyelitis: what the surgeon needs to know. EFORT Open Rev. 2017;1(5):128–35. https://doi.org/10.1302/2058-5241.1.000017.
6. Jennin F, Bousson V, Parlier C, Jomaah N, Khanine V, Laredo J-D. Bony sequestrum: a radiologic review. Skelet Radiol. 2011;40(8):963–75. https://doi.org/10.1007/s00256-010-0975-4.
7. Pineda C, Espinosa R, Pena A. Radiographic imaging in osteomyelitis: the role of plain radiography, computed tomography, ultrasonography, magnetic resonance imaging, and scintigraphy. Semin Plast Surg. 2009;23(2):80–9. https://doi.org/10.1055/s-0029-1214160.
8. Kremers HM, Nwojo ME, Ransom JE, Wood-Wentz CM, Melton LJ III, Huddleston PM III. Trends in the epidemiology of osteomyelitis: a population-based study, 1969 to 2009. JBJS. 2015;97(10):837–45.
9. Klenerman L. A history of osteomyelitis from the Journal of Bone and Joint Surgery. J Bone Joint Surg Br. 2007;89-B(5):667–70. https://doi.org/10.1302/0301-620X.89B5.19170.
10. Peng J, Ren Y, He W, et al. Epidemiological, clinical and microbiological characteristics of patients with post-traumatic osteomyelitis of limb fractures in Southwest China: a hospital-based study. J Bone Jt Infect. 2017;2(3):149–53. https://doi.org/10.7150/jbji.20002.
11. Cierny G 3rd. Infected tibial nonunions (1981-1995). The evolution of change. Clin Orthop Relat Res. 1999;(360):97–105. https://doi.org/10.1097/00003086-199903000-00012.
12. Mader JT, Cripps MW, Calhoun JH. Adult posttraumatic osteomyelitis of the tibia. Clin Orthop Relat Res. 1999;360:14–21. https://doi.org/10.1097/00003086-199903000-00004.

13. Yeargan SA, Nakasone CK, Shaieb MD, Montgomery WP, Reinker KA. Treatment of chronic osteomyelitis in children resistant to previous therapy. J Pediatr Orthop. 2004;24(1):109–22. https://doi.org/10.1097/01241398-200401000-00021.
14. Mironov SP, Tsiskarashvili AV, Gorbatiuk DS. Chronic post-traumatic osteomyelitis as a problem of contemporary traumatology and orthopedics (literature review). Genij Ortopedii. 2019;25(4):610–21. https://doi.org/10.18019/1028-4427-2019-25-4-610-621.
15. Stewart DG Jr, Kay RMSD. Open fractures in children. Principles of evaluation and management. J Bone Joint Surg Am. 2005;87(12):2784–98.
16. Venkatadass K, Grandhi TSP, Rajasekaran S. Use of Ganga Hospital Open Injury Severity Scoring for determination of salvage versus amputation in open type IIIB injuries of lower limbs in children—an analysis of 52 type IIIB open fractures. Injury. 2017;48(11):2509–14. https://doi.org/10.1016/j.injury.2017.09.010.
17. Nandra RS, Wu F, Gaffey ABC. The management of open tibial fractures in children: a retrospective case series of eight years' experience of 61 cases at a paediatric specialist center. Bone Joint J. 2017;99-B(4):544–53. https://doi.org/10.1302/0301-620X.99B4.37855.
18. Ramseier LE, Bhaskar AR, Cole WG, Howard AW. Treatment of open femur fractures in children: comparison between external fixator and intramedullary nailing. J Pediatr Orthop. 2007;27(7):748–50. https://doi.org/10.1097/BPO.0b013e3181558b00.
19. Gouron R. Surgical technique and indications of the induced membrane procedure in children. Orthop Traumatol Surg Res. 2016;102(1, Supplement):S133–9. https://doi.org/10.1016/j.otsr.2015.06.027.
20. Andreacchio A, Alberghina F, Paonessa M, Cravino M, De Rosa V, Canavese F. Tobramycin-impregnated calcium sulfate pellets for the treatment of chronic osteomyelitis in children and adolescents. J Pediatr Orthop B. 2019;28(3):189–95.
21. Skaggs DL, Friend L, Alman B, et al. The effect of surgical delay on acute infection following 554 open fractures in children. J Bone Joint Surg Am. 2005;87(1):8–12. https://doi.org/10.2106/JBJS.C.01561.
22. Hutchins CM, Sponseller PD, Sturm P, Mosquero R. Open femur fractures in children: treatment, complications, and results. J Pediatr Orthop. 2000;20(2):183–8.
23. Jiang N, Ma Y-F, Jiang Y, et al. Clinical characteristics and treatment of extremity chronic osteomyelitis in southern China: a retrospective analysis of 394 consecutive patients. Medicine (Baltimore). 2015;94(42):–e1874. https://doi.org/10.1097/MD.0000000000001874.
24. Mandell JC, Khurana B, Smith JT, Czuczman GJ, Ghazikhanian V, Smith SE. Osteomyelitis of the lower extremity: pathophysiology, imaging, and classification, with an emphasis on diabetic foot infection. Emerg Radiol. 2018;25(2):175–88. https://doi.org/10.1007/s10140-017-1564-9.
25. Kavanagh N, Ryan EJ, Widaa A, et al. Staphylococcal osteomyelitis: disease progression, treatment challenges, and future directions. Clin Microbiol Rev. 2018;31(2):e00084–17. https://doi.org/10.1128/CMR.00084-17.
26. Tsukayama DT. Pathophysiology of posttraumatic osteomyelitis. Clin Orthop Relat Res. 1999;360:22–9.
27. Patzakis MJ, Zalavras CG. Chronic posttraumatic osteomyelitis and infected nonunion of the tibia: current management concepts. J Am Acad Orthop Surg. 2005;13(6):417–27.
28. Govaert GAM, Glaudemans AWJM, Ploegmakers JJW, Viddeleer AR, Wendt KW, Reininga IHF. Diagnostic strategies for posttraumatic osteomyelitis: a survey amongst Dutch medical specialists demonstrates the need for a consensus protocol. Eur J Trauma Emerg Surg. 2018;44(3):417–26. https://doi.org/10.1007/s00068-017-0783-9.
29. Schmitt SK. Osteomyelitis. Infect Dis Clin N Am. 2017;31(2):325–38. https://doi.org/10.1016/j.idc.2017.01.010.
30. Fritz JM, McDonald JR. Osteomyelitis: approach to diagnosis and treatment. Phys Sportsmed. 2008;36(1):nihpa116823. https://doi.org/10.3810/psm.2008.12.11.
31. Calhoun JH, Manring MM, Shirtliff M. Osteomyelitis of the long bones. Semin Plast Surg. 2009;23(2):59–72. https://doi.org/10.1055/s-0029-1214158.
32. Cierny G 3rd, Mader JT, Penninck JJ. A clinical staging system for adult osteomyelitis. Clin Orthop Relat Res. 2003;414:7–24.
33. Canavese F, Khan A. Chronic osteomyelitis in children treated with antibiotic-laden cement: a preliminary report. J Orthop Spine Trauma. 2016;2(2):e5283.
34. Stevenson AJ, Jones HW, Chokotho LC, Beckles VLL, Harrison WJ. The Beit CURE classification of childhood chronic haematogenous osteomyelitis--a guide to treatment. J Orthop Surg Res. 2015;10:144. https://doi.org/10.1186/s13018-015-0282-9.
35. Cyteval C, Bourdon A. Imaging orthopedic implant infections. Diagn Interv Imaging. 2012;93(6):547–57. https://doi.org/10.1016/j.diii.2012.03.004.
36. Govaert GA, IJpma FF, McNally M, McNally E, Reininga IH, Glaudemans AW. Accuracy of diagnostic imaging modalities for peripheral post-traumatic osteomyelitis – a systematic review of the recent literature. Eur J Nucl Med Mol Imaging. 2017;44(8):1393–407. https://doi.org/10.1007/s00259-017-3683-7.
37. Park BN, Hong SJ, Yoon MA, Oh JK. MRI diagnosis for post-traumatic osteomyelitis of extremities using conventional metal-artifact reducing protocols: revisited. Acad Radiol. 2019;26(11):e317–23. https://doi.org/10.1016/j.acra.2019.01.001.
38. Triche BL, Nelson JT, McGill NS, et al. Recognizing and minimizing artifacts at CT, MRI, US, and molecular imaging. Radiographics. 2019;39(4):1017–8. https://doi.org/10.1148/rg.2019180022.

39. Koff MF, Burge AJ, Koch KM, Potter HG. Imaging near orthopedic hardware. J Magn Reson Imaging. 2017;46(1):24–39. https://doi.org/10.1002/jmri.25577.
40. Govaert GAM, Glaudemans AWJM. Nuclear medicine imaging of posttraumatic osteomyelitis. Eur J Trauma Emerg Surg. 2016;42(4):397–410. https://doi.org/10.1007/s00068-016-0647-8.
41. Walter G, Kemmerer M, Kappler C, Hoffmann R. Treatment algorithms for chronic osteomyelitis. Dtsch Arztebl Int. 2012;109(14):257–64. https://doi.org/10.3238/arztebl.2012.0257.
42. Abosala A, Ali M. The use of calcium sulphate beads in periprosthetic joint infection, a systematic review. J Bone Jt Infect. 2020;5(1):43–9. https://doi.org/10.7150/jbji.41743.
43. Anderson RL Jr, Argamaso R. Management of extensive open fractures in children and teen-age patients. J Natl Med Assoc. 1976;68(1):20–45.
44. Canavese F, Corradin M, Khan A, Mansour M, Rousset M, Samba A. Successful treatment of chronic osteomyelitis in children with debridement, antibiotic-laden cement spacer and bone graft substitute. Eur J Orthop Surg Traumatol. 2017;27(2):221–8. https://doi.org/10.1007/s00590-016-1859-7.
45. Haidar LA, Sliwinski L, Warth RJ, Mansour AIII. Placement of provisional external fixation of pediatric femoral shaft fractures using radiopaque markers in the setting of severe polytrauma: a technical report. Tech Orthop. 2021;36(1):82–6.
46. Masquelet AC, Fitoussi F, Begue T, Muller GP. [Reconstruction of the long bones by the induced membrane and spongy autograft]. Ann Chir Plast Esthet. 2000;45(3):346–53.
47. Ferguson J, Diefenbeck M, McNally M. Ceramic biocomposites as biodegradable antibiotic carriers in the treatment of bone infections. J Bone Jt Infect. 2017;2(1):38–51. https://doi.org/10.7150/jbji.17234.
48. Kucukkaya M, Kabukcuoglu Y, Tezer M, Kuzgun U. Management of childhood chronic tibial osteomyelitis with the Ilizarov method. J Pediatr Orthop. 2002;22(5):632–7. https://doi.org/10.1097/01241398-200209000-00012.
49. Sharma A, Gupta V, Shashikant K. Optimizing management of open fractures in children. Indian J Orthop. 2018;52(5):470–80. https://doi.org/10.4103/ortho.IJOrtho_319_17.
50. Birt MC, Anderson DW, Bruce Toby E, Wang J. Osteomyelitis: recent advances in pathophysiology and therapeutic strategies. J Orthop. 2016;14(1):45–52. https://doi.org/10.1016/j.jor.2016.10.004.
51. El-Rosasy MA. Acute shortening and re-lengthening in the management of bone and soft-tissue loss in complicated fractures of the tibia. J Bone Joint Surg Br. 2007;89-B(1):80–8. https://doi.org/10.1302/0301-620X.89B1.17595.
52. Adamczyk A, Meulenkamp B, Wilken G, Papp S. Managing bone loss in open fractures. OTA Int. 2020;3(1):e059.
53. Pierrie SN, Hsu JR. Shortening and angulation strategies to address composite bone and soft tissue defects. J Orthop Trauma. 2017;31(Suppl 5):S32–5.
54. Pikkel YY, Wilson JJ, Kassis S, Lerner A. Acute shortening and angulation for limb salvage in a paediatric patient with a high-energy blast injury. BMJ Case Rep. 2014;2014:bcr2013203431. https://doi.org/10.1136/bcr-2013-203431.
55. Curran AR, Kuo KN, Lubicky JP. Simultaneous ipsilateral femoral and tibial lengthening with the Ilizarov method. J Pediatr Orthop. 1999;19(3):386–90.
56. Chacha PB. Salvage of severe open fractures of the tibia that might have required amputation. Injury. 1974;6(2):154–72. https://doi.org/10.1016/0020-1383(74)90009-6.
57. Patwardhan S, Shyam AK, Mody RA, Sancheti PK, Mehta R, Agrawat H. Reconstruction of bone defects after osteomyelitis with nonvascularized fibular graft: a retrospective study in twenty-six children. J Bone Joint Surg Am. 2013;95(9):e56, S1.
58. Gupta SP, Garg G. The Huntington procedure: still a reasonable option for large tibial defects in paediatric patients. J Child Orthop. 2014;8(5):413–21. https://doi.org/10.1007/s11832-014-0618-8.
59. Gerwin M, Weiland AJ. Vascularized bone grafts to the upper extremity: indications and technique. Hand Clin. 1992;8(3):509–23.
60. Parsons B, Strauss E. Surgical management of chronic osteomyelitis. Am J Surg. 2004;188(1A Suppl):57–66. https://doi.org/10.1016/S0002-9610(03)00292-7.
61. Penn-Barwell JG, Murray CK, Wenke JC. Early antibiotics and debridement independently reduce infection in an open fracture model. J Bone Joint Surg Br. 2012;94(1):107–12. https://doi.org/10.1302/0301-620X.94B1.27026.
62. Srour M, Inaba K, Okoye O, et al. Prospective evaluation of treatment of open fractures: effect of time to irrigation and debridement. JAMA Surg. 2015;150(4):332–6. https://doi.org/10.1001/jamasurg.2014.2022.
63. Leff W, Lohse F. Posttraumatische Osteomyelitiden im Kindesalter. Teil I: Pathogenese und Klinik [Post-traumatic osteomyelitis in childhood. I: Pathogenesis and clinical aspects]. Zentralbl Chir. 1983;108(13):777–89.
64. Hosny GA, Ahmed ASAA. Paediatric infected femoral nonunion; mid-term results of a rare problem with a single-stage treatment and up to eleven and half years follow-up. Int Orthop. 2020;44(3):503–9. https://doi.org/10.1007/s00264-019-04464-1.
65. Hosny GA, Ahmed ASAA. Infected tibial nonunion in children: is radical debridement mandatory? Injury. 2019;50(2):590–7. https://doi.org/10.1016/j.injury.2018.10.043.
66. Rousset M, Walle M, Cambou L, et al. Chronic infection and infected non-union of the long bones in paediatric patients: preliminary results of bone versus beta-tricalcium phosphate grafting after induced membrane formation. Int Orthop. 2018;42(2):385–93. https://doi.org/10.1007/s00264-017-3693-x.

67. Agarwal A, Yogendra Raj R, Shanker M. Clinicoradiological outcomes following single-stage treatment using external fixator, copious bone grafting and high dose antibiotics for infected post-osteomyelitic nonunion of femoral shaft. J Pediatr Orthop B. 2021;30(1):85–92.
68. Khan MAA, Javed AA, Rao DJ, Corner JA, Rosenfield P. Pediatric traumatic limb amputation: the principles of management and optimal residual limb lengths. World J Plast Surg. 2016;5(1):7–14.
69. Handayani YF, Hia B, Telaumbanua V, Widyadharma IPE. Chronic osteomyelitis after seven years neglected bone exposed in 12-year-old boy: a case report. Open Access Maced J Med Sci. 2019;7(4):610–3. https://doi.org/10.3889/oamjms.2019.100.

Chronic Recurrent Multifocal Osteomyelitis (Chronic Non-infective Osteitis)

21

Grainne M. Murray, Ethan S. Sen, and Athimalaipet V. Ramanan

Introduction and Epidemiology

Chronic non-infectious osteitis (CNO) is an autoinflammatory bone disorder characterised by inflammatory bone lesions that can cause pain and swelling [1, 2]. It shows significant variation in presentation, with a proportion of patients having monofocal disease, while others exhibit multifocal, frequently symmetrical bone involvement [3]. Nomenclature in the literature has frequently been confusing, where the term chronic recurrent multifocal osteomyelitis (CRMO) has been used. However, given that the disease is not uniformly multifocal and is an inflammation of bone without an infectious agent, CNO is generally preferred.

G. M. Murray
Department of Paediatric Rheumatology, University Hospitals Bristol NHS Foundation Trust, Bristol, UK
e-mail: murraygm@tcd.ie

E. S. Sen
Department of Paediatric Rheumatology, Great North Children's Hospital, Newcastle upon Tyne, UK

Faculty of Medical Sciences, Newcastle University, Newcastle upon Tyne, UK
e-mail: ethan.sen@nhs.net

A. V. Ramanan (✉)
Department of Paediatric Rheumatology, University Hospitals Bristol NHS Foundation Trust, Bristol, UK

Translational Health Sciences, Bristol Medical School, University of Bristol, Bristol, UK

The peak age of onset is 7–12 years, with females affected more than males (approximately 2:1). Detailed demographics on presentation features are shown in Table 21.1. While CNO mostly affects children and young adults, it shares similarities with SAPHO syndrome (synovitis, acne, pustulosis, hyperostosis and osteitis) that is predominantly seen in adults [4–6]. Autoinflammatory disorders are characterised by recurrent systemic inflammation in the absence of auto-antibodies, pathogens or antigen-specific T cells [7].

The incidence is questionable, as some studies have stated 1 per million though it is likely that this is a significant underestimation. A nationwide, prospective incidence survey in Germany from 2006 to 2008 estimated the annual incidence at 0.4 per 100,000 children [8]. A recent study has reported the institutional incidence to be almost equal to that of bacterial osteomyelitis [9]. A prospective incidence study is currently being undertaken by the British Paediatric Surveillance Unit in the UK to include all new diagnoses of CNO over a 13-month period [10]. Due to its rarity, it is a diagnosis which is frequently delayed or missed, with many studies reporting 12–18 months from onset of symptoms until definitive diagnosis [1, 11–13]. There are many unintended harms which can occur due to incorrect or delayed diagnosis, including pain and disability for the patient, prolonged hospital admissions for intravenous antibiotics, and

© Springer Nature Switzerland AG 2022
M. V. Belthur et al. (eds.), *Pediatric Musculoskeletal Infections*,
https://doi.org/10.1007/978-3-030-95794-0_21

Table 21.1 Clinical characteristics of CNO from large published studies (>80 patients)

	Jansson et al. [40]	Wipff et al. [13]	Schwarz et al. [51]	Girschick et al. [12]	Bhat et al. [19]	All (mean)
Year of publication	2007	2015	2015	2018	2018	–
Years of recruitment	1977–2005	1995 onwards	Not stated	2004–2016	2001–2016	–
Number of patients	89	178	93	486	131	–
Gender F:M (%)	65:35	69: 31	58:42	64:36	72:28	66:34
Age at disease onset (years)	10	9.8	10.9	9.9	9.5	10
Time to diagnosis (months)	21	17	11	12	12	14.6
Monofocal: Multifocal (%)	19:81	7:93	16:84	29:71	15:85	17:83
Associated arthritis (%)	6	11	25	29	7	16
Associated skin lesions (%)	24	12	10	19	11	15
Associated IBD[a] (%)	7	3	7.5	8	1	5.5
Bone biopsy completed (%)	58	67	86	58	56	65
Treatment (all %)						
NSAIDs	87	97	94	74	81	87
Steroids	15	8	20	23	10	15
Bisphosphonates	4	10	8	13	68	20
TNF blockers	2	7	4	7	15	7
Methotrexate	7[b]	8	0	12	14	8

[a]*IBD* inflammatory bowel disease
[b]7% received either methotrexate or azathioprine

unnecessary radiation exposure from repeated radiological investigations [1]. However, increasing awareness of this condition among local specialists has been shown to decrease time to diagnosis [1].

Pathology and Microbiology

Autoinflammatory disorders are characterized by an activation of the innate immune system in the absence of high-titre autoantibodies and (at least initially) no involvement of autoreactive lymphocytes. Several genetically inherited monogenic autoinflammatory conditions include early-onset noninfectious osteomyelitis, namely, Majeed syndrome, deficiency of interleukin-1 receptor antagonist (DIRA), and pyogenic arthritis, pyoderma gangrenosum, and acne syndrome (PAPA) [14]. The type I interferonopathies are another group of autoinflammatory disorders which can exhibit bone involvement [15].

The pathophysiology of CNO is not fully understood but is thought to represent an imbalance between pro- and anti-inflammatory cytokines and dysregulated inflammasome activation. An infectious agent was initially suspected to play a causative role, but this theory now seems unlikely given that no organism is reliably identified on bone biopsy, nor do these patients respond to antibiotics [16, 17].

A genetic component may play a role, particularly in PTSPIP1/2 gene. Studies with knockout mice have revealed similar patterns of disease, but, as yet, this has not translated into a diagnostic test for humans [18].

Clinical Presentation and Examination

The clinical presentation can vary substantially, from mild pain affecting a single bone to widespread osteitis with bony destruction, most often involving the metaphyses of long bones. Vertebral fractures are also seen. Patients may report pain which is usually insidious in onset, bony swelling, malaise, or low-grade fevers. A multicentre study, including 131 patients with CNO, reported that bone pain was the predominant symptom in 91% and swelling in 49% [19]. The pain may be worse at night [20]. The duration of symptoms is variable and can be difficult to pinpoint due to their vague nature [17].

These patients present to a variety of specialists, with one recent study showing that 51% were initially referred to an orthopaedic surgeon and 21% to a general paediatrician [1]. This emphasises the importance of awareness of this condition among all who assess children with bone pain.

A subset of patients (up to 20%, see Table 21.1) will have features of overlapping diseases such as inflammatory bowel disease, psoriasis, or palmoplantar pustulosis [9]. In adults, SAPHO syndrome includes synovitis, acne, pustulosis (palms and soles), hyperostosis, and osteitis. Therefore, the history in these patients should always include careful questioning about rashes and abdominal pain, diarrhoea, or passing blood per rectum. The family history may be significant for CNO, psoriasis, inflammatory bowel disease, or inflammatory arthritis, with up to 30% having an affected relative [13].

On examination, there may be evidence of bony or soft tissue swelling, warmth, and/or redness at the site of pain, and there may be arthritis affecting adjacent joints. Rashes may be evident. However, in some cases the examination findings are quite subtle, particularly during quiescent periods of disease.

Differential Diagnoses

There is a wide variety of differentials to be considered in a child presenting with features of CNO [21]. Some of the most important conditions to rule out include malignancy and bacterial osteomyelitis.

Malignancies such as leukaemia, lymphoma, neuroblastoma, or primary bone tumours may present with similar symptoms. Bacterial osteomyelitis, including unusual organisms such as *Kingella kingae*, brucellosis, typhoid fever, or tuberculosis, should also be considered [22]. Bacterial osteomyelitis may be classified as acute (less than 2 weeks), subacute (2 weeks to 3 months), and chronic (more than 3 months), with subacute or chronic more likely to be confused with CNO (see Boxes 21.1 and 21.2). Benign bone lesions such as osteoid osteoma are also a possibility. Less commonly, metabolic bone disorders, osteonecrosis, osteopetrosis, or vitamin C deficiency (scurvy) may present with features similar to CNO [20, 23].

Box 21.1 Tips to Differentiate CNO from Infectious Osteomyelitis

- Symmetrical and multifocal disease
- Lack of abscess, fistula, sequestra
- Lack of response to antibiotics
- History of inflammatory disorders: psoriasis, palmoplantar pustulosis, inflammatory bowel disease

In a young child, particularly one who is generally unwell (failing to thrive, organomegaly), monogenic autoinflammatory disorders, such as Majeed syndrome or DIRA, are an important consideration.

Box 21.2 Bacterial Osteomyelitis and CNO

- If a patient with presumed bacterial osteomyelitis is not responding to treatment as you would expect, consider CNO.
- Arranging an MRI or discussion with paediatric rheumatologist may be invaluable.

Blood tests may reveal mildly elevated CRP, ESR, and/or white cell count. These elevations tend to be lower than one would expect in bacterial osteomyelitis but cannot be relied upon [9]. Other investigations such as ANA, ANCA, and HLA-B27 are not particularly helpful in making a diagnosis, unless there are signs suggestive of JIA. There are, as yet, no specific biomarkers for CNO, though research is ongoing in this area [22, 27]. One study, which measured urinary N-terminal telopeptide, a biomarker of bone turnover, found no significant difference in levels between children with CNO and healthy controls, or between children with active versus inactive CNO [28]. Another study suggested that serum CCL 11/eotaxin and serum interleukin-6 are potential biomarkers to distinguish children with CNO from healthy controls and those with alternative diagnoses [29]. Further validation in larger cohorts is required to confirm these initial findings.

Therefore, in the initial phases, several subspecialists may be involved in the investigation of these patients. In a study comparing rates of bacterial osteomyelitis with CNO, the significant differences included those with bacterial osteomyelitis more often presenting with local inflammatory signs (68 vs 47% $p = 0.04$), fever (38 vs 12% $p = 0.003$), and abscesses (39 vs 0% $p < 0.001$) [9]. In patient surveys in Germany, 36% of patients report being initially diagnosed with a malignant tumour and 30% with bacterial osteomyelitis [11]. Sixty-nine percent of patients reported they consulted 2–5 doctors before receiving the final diagnosis [11].

Investigations/Work-Up

Investigations are aimed at firstly clarifying the diagnosis and secondly delineating the extent of the disease. In the absence of prospectively tested and widely accepted diagnostic criteria, CNO remains a diagnosis of exclusion. The main differential diagnoses include infectious (bacterial) osteomyelitis and malignancies, such as primary bone tumours or leukaemia/lymphoma. Several sets of criteria have been suggested and can be used as guidance during the diagnostic workup [1, 24]. Though slightly variable in details, all criteria proposed include the presence of typical clinical and radiological features, without significant evidence of systemic infection or inflammation [20]. An example of the proposed criteria is detailed in Fig. 21.1.

In the first instance, a plain X-ray of the affected bone is usually performed, which is useful to rule out commoner causes of limb pain, such as fractures. While it may be normal in the early phases of disease, features such as osteolysis, sclerosis, or new bone formation may be seen, as illustrated in Fig. 21.2 [25]. In the early phases, there may be no obvious signs to differentiate infectious osteomyelitis from CNO. In

Fig. 21.1 Bristol criteria for diagnosis of CNO [1]

- **The presence of typical clinical findings**
    - Bone pain +/- localised swelling without significant local or systemic features of inflammation or infection
- **AND**
- **The presence of typical radiological findings**
    - Plain X-ray showing combination of lytic areas, sclerosis, new bone formation or preferably STIR MRI showing bone marrow oedema +/- bone expansion, lytic areas, and periosteal reaction.
- **AND EITHER**
- **Criterion 1:** more than one bone, or clavicle alone, without significantly raised CRP (CRP < 30g/L)
- **OR**
- **Criterion 2:** if unifocal disease (other than clavicle) or CRP >30g/L, with bone biopsy showing inflammatory changes (plasma cells, osteoclasts, fibrosis, or sclerosis) with no bacterial growth whilst not on antibiotic therapy

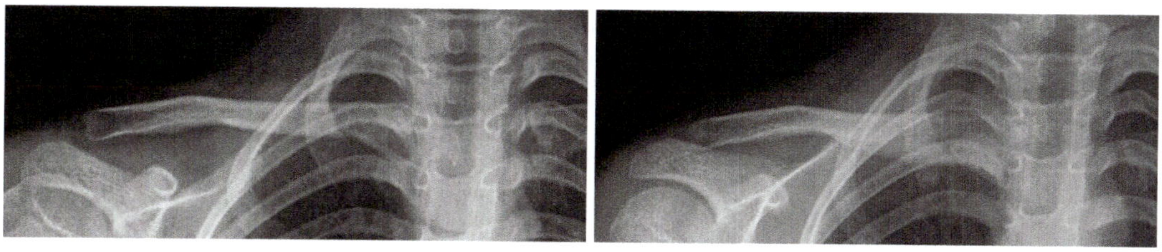

Fig. 21.2 AP radiographs of the normal medial right clavicle (on the left) and 4 months later (on the right), the marked hyperostosis and expansion

European cohorts, approx. 30–40% of patients are treated with antibiotics initially, but rates have declined over time, possibly as awareness of CNO has increased [12, 26].

Distribution of Lesions and Choice of Imaging

A whole body (WB) MRI is useful to identify mild or asymptomatic bony lesions. Arnoldi et al. reported that more active lesions were found on WB MRI than on clinical examination in almost 50% of patients [30]. Short tau inversion recovery (STIR) sequencing allows identification of bone marrow oedema, which appears as hyperintensity [25].

Several groups have recommended performing a WB MRI at time of diagnosis to identify asymptomatic lesions, particularly in the vertebral column [6, 17, 31, 32] (see Box 21.3). In the largest reported cases series of 486 patients, baseline MRI revealed a mean of 4.1 lesions per patient [12]. In addition, many children who have monofocal disease at onset will develop multifocal lesions at follow-up, with some studies reporting only 7–12% remaining monofocal [13, 26].

Box 21.3 Whole Body MRI Findings

In a child with a single symptomatic site, the presence of multiple lesions in typical sites on a WB MRI is highly suggestive of CNO.

Typical features include bone cortical thickening and lytic lesions with sclerosis and bone oedema on MRI [20]. An example of MRI findings in the clavicle is seen in Fig. 21.3. The importance of standardisation of WB MRI protocol and the interpretation of the MRI by an experienced radiologist are emphasised, given the key role that MRI can play in diagnosis and monitoring of treatment response [3, 33]. Scoring systems such as the radiological index for nonbacterial osteitis (RINBO) and the chronic nonbacterial osteomyelitis magnetic resonance imaging scoring (CROMRIS) which aim to standardise interpretation and reporting are in development [30, 34]. Pitfalls in the analysis of MRIs include high signal in the metatarsals, tarsals, and carpal bones, which is often a normal variant, as well as bilateral, symmetric metaphyseal high signal bands after a patient has been treated with bisphosphonates [33].

Analysis of typical lesion distribution patterns on WB MRI has revealed patterns of disease as demonstrated in Fig. 21.4:

(a) Tibio-appendicular multi-focal pattern: with tibial but no clavicular involvement
(b) Claviculo-spinal pauci-focal pattern: clavicular lesions, no tibial involvement, spinal lesions, and overall fewer lesions
(c) Tibio-clavicular crossover pattern: synchronous involvement of both, with relatively few other lesions [3]

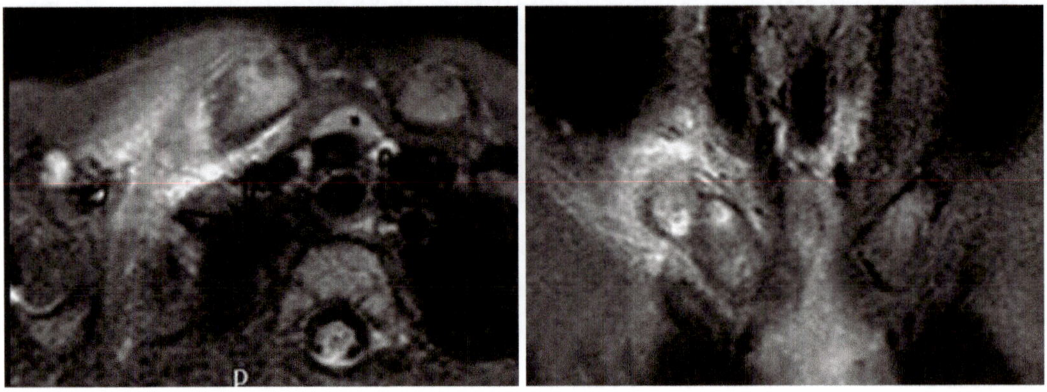

Fig. 21.3 Axial and coronal STIR imaging illustrating the enlarged right clavicle with increased intramedullary and juxtacortical signal, from the same patient as Fig. 21.1 *above*

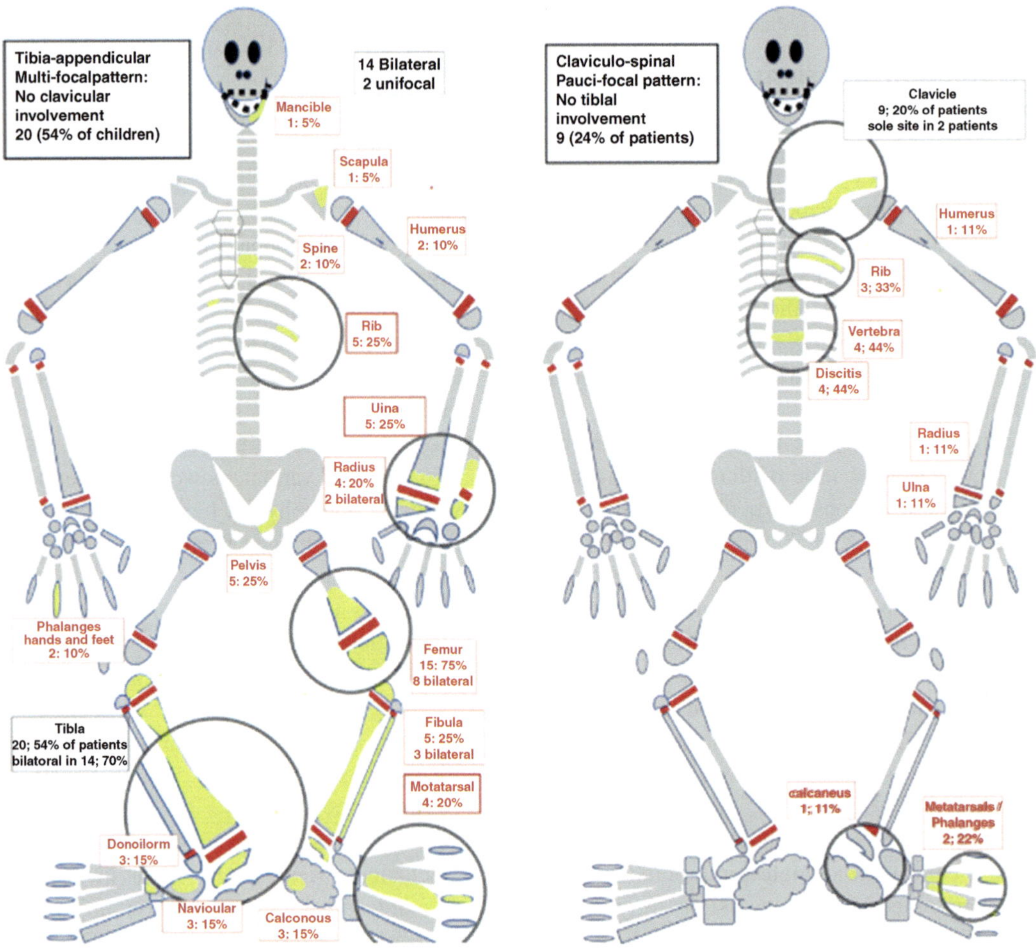

Fig. 21.4 Typical lesion distribution pattern in chronic noninfectious osteitis. (Reprinted from Andronikou et al. [3], with permission from Elsevier)

Clavicular lesions are strongly suggestive of CNO, since infective osteomyelitis is quite rare in this site [3, 17]. It is for this reason that unifocal clavicular lesions are felt 'typical' enough to be positive in the Bristol criteria (detailed in Fig. 21.1), negating the need for a biopsy [1]. Lesions can occur in any portion of the clavicle, with one recent study showing an even distribution of medial, lateral, and central lesions; however it is most common to involve the medial third of the clavicle in all age groups [3, 35]. Clavicle disease typically manifests as a lytic medullary process with surrounding periosteal reaction, which may have an 'onion skin' appearance [17].

Bilateral and symmetrical disease is often seen in those with involvement of the fibula, tibia, and phalanges of the feet (80%, 68%, and 67% bilateral, respectively [3]).

Vertebral lesions are a classic and common site for CNO, most often seen in the thoracic spine, and present in 8–26% in various studies [1, 3, 17, 36, 37]. Examples of vertebral lesions are seen in Fig. 21.5. Vertebral lesions may be asymptomatic, even when they are significant, and can cause deformity later in the course [37]. Vertebral height loss is the most commonly seen pathological fracture [17], with risk reported as up to 17% in some studies [13]. It is particularly important to detect spinal involvement for this reason.

Bone scintigraphy can be used to detect lesions but is not so useful for characterising them and requires a small dose of radiation. CT scans are also used in some centres, particularly when the diagnosis is unclear. However, due to the radiation dose and the ability to screen the whole body, MRI is generally preferred.

Role of Bone Biopsy

A bone biopsy may be necessary, predominantly to rule out malignancy. The Bristol criteria, outlined in Fig. 21.1, provide some guidance as to when a biopsy is needed. A biopsy is more likely to be needed if there is a single lesion in an atypical bony location, or other concerning symptoms such as weight loss or anaemia. An MRI may be useful in planning the most appropriate biopsy

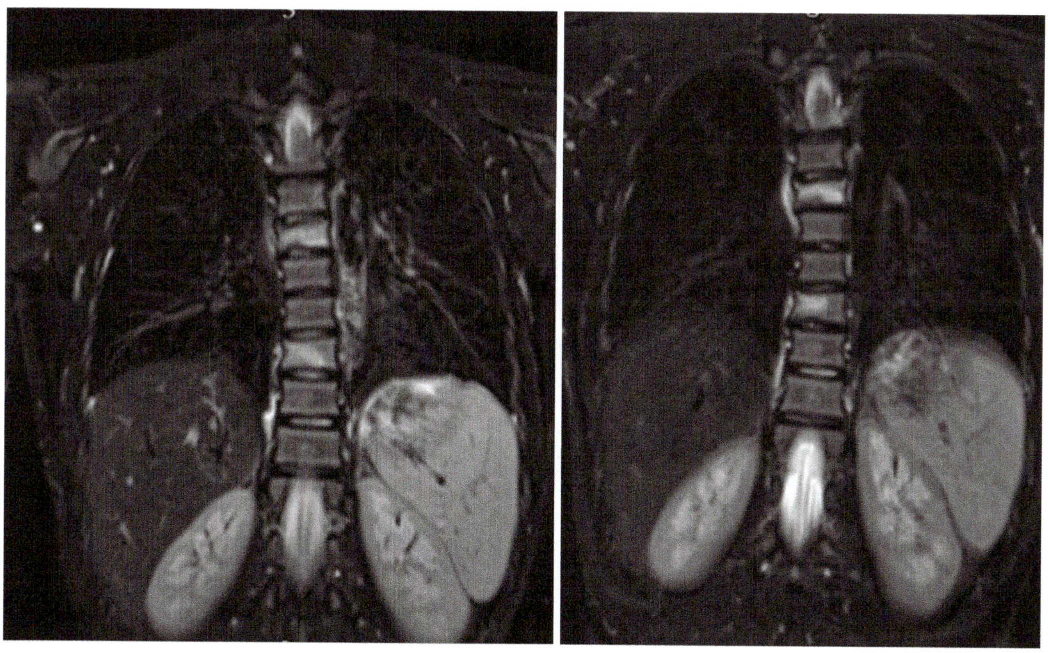

Fig. 21.5 Coronal STIR MR images demonstrating high signal of the T6 and T9 vertebral bodies, which themselves are of reduced height

site. The composition of the cellular infiltrates at a site of inflammation are related to the 'age' of the biopsied lesions, with neutrophils predominant early in disease, whereas lymphocytes, macrophages, and plasma cells detected later in the course of the illness [20, 38]. Osteoclastic bone resorption and necrosis may be present, with fibrosis becoming more prominent later in the disease, as well as signs of reactive new bone formation [38]. Biopsy cultures are expected to be negative.

Treatment Options

Treatment of CNO is empiric and, in the absence of clinical trials, based on small case series and expert opinion [2, 14, 26]. There are currently no reliable methods to differentiate the patients who will spontaneously resolve from those who will have persistent disease [25]. Therapeutic options include non-steroidal anti-inflammatory drugs (NSAIDs), (short-term) corticosteroids, bisphosphonates, and classical disease-modifying medications (DMARDs) such as methotrexate or biologic DMARDs, usually tumour necrosis factor alpha (TNF) inhibitors. Treatment pathways, physician preference, and access to these medications vary significantly between countries, as detailed in Table 21.1. The authors suggested treatment algorithm is detailed in Fig. 21.6.

Treatment aims at limiting and controlling inflammation to reduce pain, improve function, and maintain normal growth and development [39]. Based on published reports and an international consensus process, the Childhood Arthritis and Rheumatology Research Alliance (CARRA) recently released consensus treatment plans for CNO which is refractory to NSAIDs or includes active spinal lesions [32].

NSAIDs are useful for pain control and can also induce remission in a significant percentage of patients (43–83%) [36, 40]. A month of regular treatment is required to determine efficacy. It is thought that NSAIDs may (at least partially)

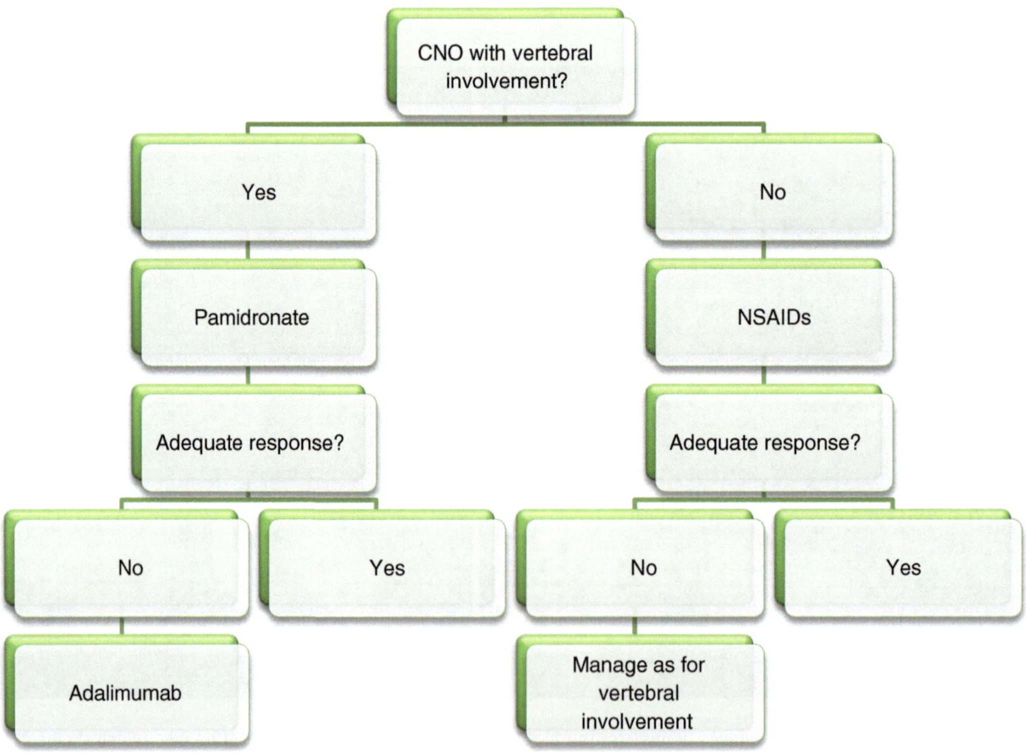

Fig. 21.6 Suggested treatment options for management of chronic noninfectious osteitis

correct increased osteoclast activity through the reduction of prostaglandin production [41]. A recent, long-term, retrospective study demonstrated that 50% of NSAID-treated CNO patients may develop flares, after a median of 29 months [26]. However, for a proportion of patients, particularly those with vertebral involvement or associated peripheral arthritis, NSAIDs are insufficient.

Corticosteroids may be used in the initial phases, particularly if there is widespread bony involvement. Owing to the risk of using high-dose systemic steroids in malignancy, a bone biopsy should strongly be considered before this course of treatment is undertaken.

DMARDS (disease-modifying antirheumatic agents) such as methotrexate and azathioprine are generally ineffective as a single agent, though methotrexate may have a role in combination with TNF inhibitors [40].

TNF α inhibitors, most often adalimumab, have been demonstrated to be effective [13, 40, 42]. They are also particularly beneficial for those with concomitant peripheral arthritis or inflammatory bowel disease [26]. In some centres, TNF inhibitors are used for active vertebral disease or persistent pain despite NSAID or other non-biologic DMARD [43].

Bisphosphonates, most often pamidronate, are safe and effective treatment for CNO [26, 39, 44–46]. They often provide rapid relief to pain, and additionally, radiological improvement of bone lesions is seen. They are particularly advocated for vertebral disease, as MRI has demonstrated improvement in vertebral modelling and height and in multifocal disease [13, 45]. Bisphosphonates are known to inhibit osteoclasts, and they also have an anti-inflammatory effect and have been used in rheumatoid arthritis and ankylosing spondylitis [47]. The most commonly used agent is pamidronate, which is administered intravenously for 3 consecutive days every 3 months. It is important to note that in follow-up MRI scans, bisphosphonates may produce linear hyperintense signal in the distal femurs particularly, which should not be mistaken for active disease [32, 34].

There are currently no head-to-head trials comparing the efficacy of bisphosphonates with TNF inhibitors; however such a study has been proposed with expert consensus opinion established prior to a Bayesian-design trial [48] .

Interleukin 1 antagonists Monogenic forms of CNO, such as Majeed syndrome and DIRA, respond well to interleukin-1 blockade with anakinra, and so this is an agent to be considered in refractory cases [15].

Monitoring Response to Treatment

Pain in patients with CNO may represent active disease, but may also represent mechanical problems, and therefore careful clinical examination and a low threshold for repeat MRI are often required prior to making decisions on escalating treatment [38]. Early aggressive treatment with a TNF inhibitor and methotrexate has been shown to significantly improve pain scores, patient, and physician global assessments, ESR, and CRP, without progression of skeletal damage when compared to NSAID monotherapy, albeit in a small group of patients ($n = 18$) [43].

A particular challenge in monitoring response to treatment is the issue of asymptomatic lesions. A difficulty can also arise as a high-sensitivity MRI may show signs of bone activity in children who are, in fact, in clinical remission. Therefore, the overall clinical picture, including the history of disease severity and bone involvement as well as the child's clinical condition and blood tests, should be considered. It is, therefore, important that MRIs are interpreted by a radiologist experienced with this condition to avoid over-treating based on MRI findings alone. In many centres, annual WB MRIs are a recommended part of care for patients requiring treatment with biologics or bisphosphonates.

Complications and Outcomes

There are many potential complications of CNO, which are exacerbated by delayed diagnosis and prolonged uncontrolled disease [13]. Poor prognostic factors include male sex, multifocal pattern at onset of disease, and a long time between onset of symptoms and diagnosis [13]. Although there are few studies detailing long-term outcomes, and those which are published are small, they suggest that the rates of physical or psychological sequalae are over 20% [26, 49].

Locally these include pain, which may become chronic, asymmetric bony growth leading to kyphosis or leg length discrepancy, and pathological fractures, particularly of vertebral bodies [32]. It has been reported that vertebral deformities can be seen in over 50% of those with spinal involvement, including 22% developing scoliosis or kyphosis requiring treatment [37]. Some of the reports of these were before biologics or bisphosphonates were routinely used for resistant symptoms [45]. Pathological vertebral fractures are seen in 11% in some studies [26]. CNO may evolve into spondyloarthropathy or the enthesitis-related arthritis (ERA) category of juvenile idiopathic arthritis, or patients may have ongoing symptomatology from co-existing conditions (inflammatory bowel disease, psoriasis).

More generally, children with CNO can struggle with psychosocial difficulties, sleep disruption, poor school attendance, and inability to participate in sport. A recent study comparing physical fitness with quality of life measures revealed that, though many patients were in remission or not on medication for their disease, their overall wellbeing (as measured on PedsQL3.0), as well as the CHAQ score (disability index), was significantly worse compared to healthy age-matched controls [50]. This was despite objective measurements of fitness which showed no differences from healthy controls. Silier et al. described that 79% of patients report a negative effect on school or work due to CNO [11] (Boxes 21.4 and 21.5).

Box 21.4 Key Learning Points

- CNO may present insidiously and frequently involves the clavicle, vertebral bodies, or metaphyses of long bones.
- Common differentials include infectious osteomyelitis and malignancy.
- Whole body MRI and/or bone biopsy are usually required to make a diagnosis.
- Treatment can include NSAIDs, bisphosphonates, and biologics.
- Delayed diagnosis may contribute to chronic pain, pathological fractures, and bony deformity.

Box 21.5 Pitfalls to Avoid

- CNO is rare in young children (<7 years of age).
- In a child with bone pain who is systemically unwell (with fevers, night sweats, weight loss, anaemia), CNO is less likely, and malignancy should be strongly considered.
- Initial plain films may be normal; repeat imaging (plain film or MRI) may be warranted.

Conclusion

CNO is an autoinflammatory condition which presents with bony pain, frequently involving the clavicle, vertebral bodies, or metaphyses of long bones. It may involve multiple bony sites, and the long-term prognosis is variable. Despite advances in the understanding of the pathophysiology in recent years, there are no specific biomarkers. Therefore, it remains a diagnosis of exclusion and requires close collaboration between paediatric orthopaedic surgeons, rheumatologists, and radiologists with experience in this condition. Treatments include non-steroidal anti-inflammatories, bisphosphonates, and biologics such as adalimumab.

Acknowledgements Many thanks to Dr. Mark Chopra for his assistance in preparing the figures used

References

1. Roderick MR, Shah R, Rogers V, Finn A, Ramanan AV. Chronic recurrent multifocal osteomyelitis (CRMO) - advancing the diagnosis. Pediatr Rheumatol Online J. 2016;14(1):47.
2. Hofmann SR, Schnabel A, Rösen-Wolff A, Morbach H, Girschick HJ, Hedrich CM. Chronic nonbacterial osteomyelitis: pathophysiological concepts and current treatment strategies. J Rheumatol. 2016;43(11):1956–64.
3. Andronikou S, Mendes da Costa T, Hussien M, Ramanan AV. Radiological diagnosis of chronic recurrent multifocal osteomyelitis using whole-body MRI-based lesion distribution patterns. Clin Radiol. 2019;74(9):737.e3–e15.
4. Guérin-Pfyffer S, Guillaume-Czitrom S, Tammam S, Koné-Paut I. Evaluation of chronic recurrent multifocal osteitis in children by whole-body magnetic resonance imaging. Joint Bone Spine. 2012;79(6):616–20.
5. Stern SM, Ferguson PJ. Autoinflammatory bone diseases. Rheum Dis Clin N Am. 2013;39(4):735–49.
6. Hedrich CM, Hofmann SR, Pablik J, Morbach H, Girschick HJ. Autoinflammatory bone disorders with special focus on chronic recurrent multifocal osteomyelitis (CRMO). Pediatr Rheumatol Online J. 2013;11(1):47.
7. Ferguson PJ, El-Shanti HI. Autoinflammatory bone disorders. Curr Opin Rheumatol. 2007;19(5):492–8.
8. Jansson AF, Grote V. Nonbacterial osteitis in children: data of a German Incidence Surveillance Study. Acta Paediatr. 2011;100(8):1150–7.
9. Schnabel A, Range U, Hahn G, Siepmann T, Berner R, Hedrich CM. Unexpectedly high incidences of chronic non-bacterial as compared to bacterial osteomyelitis in children. Rheumatol Int. 2016;36(12):1737–45.
10. Royal College Paediatrics and Child Health. BPSU study - Chronic recurrent multifocal osteomyelitis/chronic nonbacterial osteomyelitis (CRMO/CNO) 2020 [23/12/2020]. Available from: https://www.rcpch.ac.uk/work-we-do/bpsu/study-crmo.
11. Silier CCG, Greschik J, Gesell S, Grote V, Jansson AF. Chronic non-bacterial osteitis from the patient perspective: a health services research through data collected from patient conferences. BMJ Open. 2017;7(12):e017599.
12. Girschick H, Finetti M, Orlando F, Schalm S, Insalaco A, Ganser G, et al. The multifaceted presentation of chronic recurrent multifocal osteomyelitis: a series of 486 cases from the Eurofever international registry. Rheumatology (Oxford). 2018;57(7):1203–11.
13. Wipff J, Costantino F, Lemelle I, Pajot C, Duquesne A, Lorrot M, et al. A large national cohort of French patients with chronic recurrent multifocal osteitis. Arthritis Rheumatol. 2015;67(4):1128–37.
14. Hofmann SR, Kapplusch F, Girschick HJ, Morbach H, Pablik J, Ferguson PJ, et al. Chronic recurrent multifocal osteomyelitis (CRMO): presentation, pathogenesis, and treatment. Curr Osteoporos Rep. 2017;15(6):542–54.
15. Bader-Meunier B, Van Nieuwenhove E, Breton S, Wouters C. Bone involvement in monogenic autoinflammatory syndromes. Rheumatology (Oxford). 2018;57(4):606–18.
16. Buch K, Thuesen ACB, Brøns C, Schwarz P. Chronic non-bacterial osteomyelitis: a review. Calcif Tissue Int. 2019;104(5):544–53.
17. Khanna G, Sato TS, Ferguson P. Imaging of chronic recurrent multifocal osteomyelitis. Radiographics. 2009;29(4):1159–77.
18. Ferguson PJ, Bing X, Vasef MA, Ochoa LA, Mahgoub A, Waldschmidt TJ, et al. A missense mutation in pstpip2 is associated with the murine autoinflammatory disorder chronic multifocal osteomyelitis. Bone. 2006;38(1):41–7.
19. Bhat CS, Anderson C, Harbinson A, McCann LJ, Roderick M, Finn A, et al. Chronic non bacterial osteitis- a multicentre study. Pediatr Rheumatol Online J. 2018;16(1):74.
20. Taddio A, Ferrara G, Insalaco A, Pardeo M, Gregori M, Finetti M, et al. Dealing with chronic non-bacterial osteomyelitis: a practical approach. Pediatr Rheumatol Online J. 2017;15(1):87.
21. Menashe SJ, Aboughalia H, Zhao Y, Ngo AV, Otjen JP, Thapa MM, et al. The many faces of pediatric chronic recurrent multifocal osteomyelitis (CRMO): a practical location- and case-based approach to differentiate CRMO from its mimics. J Magn Reson Imaging. 2020;54(2):391–400.
22. Chen Z, Cheng L, Feng G. Bone inflammation and chronic recurrent multifocal osteomyelitis. Eur Rev Med Pharmacol Sci. 2018;22(5):1380–6.
23. Metz J, Holjar-Erlic I, Kelly A, Ramanan AV. Think about the 'C' (in custard and crackers). Arch Dis Child Educ Pract Ed. 2018;103(6):304–6.
24. Jansson AF, Müller TH, Gliera L, Ankerst DP, Wintergerst U, Belohradsky BH, et al. Clinical score for nonbacterial osteitis in children and adults. Arthritis Rheum. 2009;60(4):1152–9.
25. Roderick MR, Ramanan AV. Chronic recurrent multifocal osteomyelitis. Adv Exp Med Biol. 2013;764:99–107.
26. Schnabel A, Range U, Hahn G, Berner R, Hedrich CM. Treatment response and longterm outcomes in children with chronic nonbacterial osteomyelitis. J Rheumatol. 2017;44(7):1058–65.
27. Hofmann SR, Kubasch AS, Range U, Laass MW, Morbach H, Girschick HJ, et al. Serum biomarkers for the diagnosis and monitoring of chronic recurrent multifocal osteomyelitis (CRMO). Rheumatol Int. 2016;36(6):769–79.
28. Perkins A, Stevens AM, Ferguson PJ, Zhao Y. Urinary N-telopeptide as a biomarker of disease activity in patients with chronic nonbacterial osteomyelitis who

have not received bisphosphonates. J Rheumatol. 2020;47(12):1842–4.
29. Hofmann SR, Böttger F, Range U, Lück C, Morbach H, Girschick HJ, et al. Serum interleukin-6 and CCL11/eotaxin may be suitable biomarkers for the diagnosis of chronic nonbacterial osteomyelitis. Front Pediatr. 2017;5:256.
30. Arnoldi AP, Schlett CL, Douis H, Geyer LL, Voit AM, Bleisteiner F, et al. Whole-body MRI in patients with non-bacterial osteitis: radiological findings and correlation with clinical data. Eur Radiol. 2017;27(6):2391–9.
31. von Kalle T, Heim N, Hospach T, Langendorfer M, Winkler P, Stuber T. Typical patterns of bone involvement in whole-body MRI of patients with chronic recurrent multifocal osteomyelitis (CRMO). Rofo. 2013;185:655–61.
32. Zhao Y, Wu EY, Oliver MS, Cooper AM, Basiaga ML, Vora SS, et al. Consensus treatment plans for chronic nonbacterial osteomyelitis refractory to nonsteroidal antiinflammatory drugs and/or with active spinal lesions. Arthritis Care Res (Hoboken). 2018;70(8):1228–37.
33. Andronikou S, Kraft JK, Offiah AC, Jones J, Douis H, Thyagarajan M, et al. Whole-body MRI in the diagnosis of paediatric CNO/CRMO. Rheumatology (Oxford). 2020;59(10):2671–80.
34. Zhao Y, Sato TS, Nielsen SM, Beer M, Huang M, Iyer RS, et al. Development of a scoring tool for chronic nonbacterial osteomyelitis magnetic resonance imaging and evaluation of its interrater reliability. J Rheumatol. 2020;47(5):739–47.
35. Suresh S, Saifuddin A. Unveiling the 'unique bone': a study of the distribution of focal clavicular lesions. Skelet Radiol. 2008;37(8):749–56.
36. Beck C, Morbach H, Beer M, Stenzel M, Tappe D, Gattenlöhner S, et al. Chronic nonbacterial osteomyelitis in childhood: prospective follow-up during the first year of anti-inflammatory treatment. Arthritis Res Ther. 2010;12(2):R74.
37. Hospach T, Langendoerfer M, von Kalle T, Maier J, Dannecker GE. Spinal involvement in chronic recurrent multifocal osteomyelitis (CRMO) in childhood and effect of pamidronate. Eur J Pediatr. 2010;169(9):1105–11.
38. Roderick MR, Sen ES, Ramanan AV. Chronic recurrent multifocal osteomyelitis in children and adults: current understanding and areas for development. Rheumatology (Oxford). 2018;57(1):41–8.
39. Roderick M, Shah R, Finn A, Ramanan AV. Efficacy of pamidronate therapy in children with chronic non-bacterial osteitis: disease activity assessment by whole body magnetic resonance imaging. Rheumatology (Oxford). 2014;53(11):1973–6.
40. Jansson A, Renner ED, Ramser J, Mayer A, Haban M, Meindl A, et al. Classification of non-bacterial osteitis: retrospective study of clinical, immunological and genetic aspects in 89 patients. Rheumatology (Oxford). 2007;46(1):154–60.
41. Hedrich CM, Morbach H, Reiser C, Girschick HJ. New insights into adult and paediatric chronic non-bacterial osteomyelitis CNO. Curr Rheumatol Rep. 2020;22(9):52.
42. Eleftheriou D, Gerschman T, Sebire N, Woo P, Pilkington CA, Brogan PA. Biologic therapy in refractory chronic non-bacterial osteomyelitis of childhood. Rheumatology (Oxford). 2010;49(8):1505–12.
43. Zhao Y, Chauvin NA, Jaramillo D, Burnham JM. Aggressive therapy reduces disease activity without skeletal damage progression in chronic nonbacterial osteomyelitis. J Rheumatol. 2015;42(7):1245–51.
44. Kerrison C, Davidson JE, Cleary AG, Beresford MW. Pamidronate in the treatment of childhood SAPHO syndrome. Rheumatology (Oxford). 2004;43(10):1246–51.
45. Gleeson H, Wiltshire E, Briody J, Hall J, Chaitow J, Sillence D, et al. Childhood chronic recurrent multifocal osteomyelitis: pamidronate therapy decreases pain and improves vertebral shape. J Rheumatol. 2008;35(4):707–12.
46. Bhat CS, Roderick M, Sen ES, Finn A, Ramanan AV. Efficacy of pamidronate in children with chronic non-bacterial osteitis using whole body MRI as a marker of disease activity. Pediatr Rheumatol Online J. 2019;17(1):35.
47. Rogers MJ, Gordon S, Benford HL, Coxon FP, Luckman SP, Monkkonen J, et al. Cellular and molecular mechanisms of action of bisphosphonates. Cancer. 2000;88(12 Suppl):2961–78.
48. Ramanan AV, Hampson LV, Lythgoe H, Jones AP, Hardwick B, Hind H, et al. Defining consensus opinion to develop randomised controlled trials in rare diseases using Bayesian design: an example of a proposed trial of adalimumab versus pamidronate for children with CNO/CRMO. PLoS One. 2019;14(6):e0215739.
49. Catalano-Pons C, Comte A, Wipff J, Quartier P, Faye A, Gendrel D, et al. Clinical outcome in children with chronic recurrent multifocal osteomyelitis. Rheumatology (Oxford). 2008;47(9):1397–9.
50. Julia N, Katharina R, Hermann G, Annette HW, Henner M, Helge H, et al. Physical activity and health-related quality of life in chronic non-bacterial osteomyelitis. Pediatr Rheumatol Online J. 2019;17(1):45.
51. Schwarz T, Petzke S, Morbach H, Hofmann C, Beer M, Raab P, et al. Juvenile chronic non-bacterial osteomyelitis (CNO): long term course of disease and response to treatment in a large institutional cohort. Pediatr Rheumatol Online J. 2015;13(Suppl 1):P178–P.

22 Pathological Fractures with Osteomyelitis

Manoj Padman, Scott B. Rosenfeld, and Mohan V. Belthur

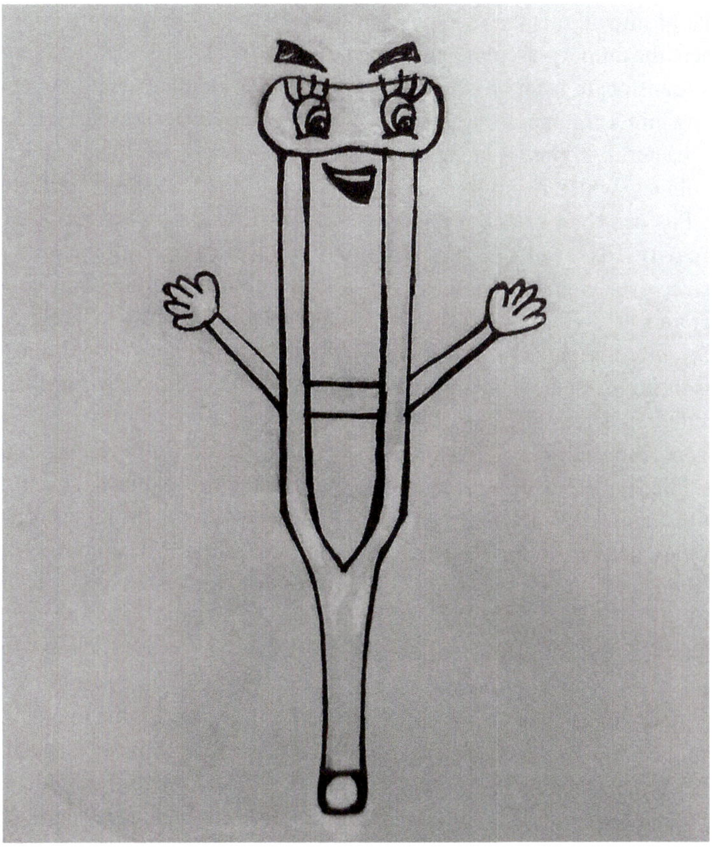

M. Padman (✉)
Centre for Paediatric Orthopaedics & Disabilities, Paediatric Orthopaedics, Rainbow Children's Hospital, Fortis Memorial Research Institute, Delhi NCR, New Delhi, India

S. B. Rosenfeld
Department of Orthopaedic Surgery, Texas Children's Hospital, Baylor College of Medicine, Houston, TX, USA
e-mail: sbrosenf@texaschildrens.org

M. V. Belthur
Department of Child Health & Orthopedics, University of Arizona College of Medicine, Phoenix, AZ, USA

Department of Orthopedics, Phoenix Children's Hospital, Phoenix, AZ, USA

© Springer Nature Switzerland AG 2022
M. V. Belthur et al. (eds.), *Pediatric Musculoskeletal Infections*,
https://doi.org/10.1007/978-3-030-95794-0_22

Introduction

Osteomyelitis, defined as inflammation of the bone and bone marrow due to a microbial pathogen, can occur by (a) local contiguous spread of infection from adjacent tissues or from a penetrating or infected wound, (b) hematogenous route, and (c) invasion of bone from an infected implant. Acute hematogenous osteomyelitis is by far the most common modality of infection in children and results from seeding of bones by bacteria circulating within the blood [1–5]. The most common site of infection is the metaphysis of long bones where the unique vascular anatomy allows bacteria to translocate from blood vessels into bone following minor trauma. Bone destruction is caused by bacterial toxins, ischemia, and inflammatory cytokines, which result in necrosis and suppuration. Pus can then extend along the intramedullary cavity as well as to the subperiosteal space, overlying soft tissues and into the adjacent joints [2, 5–7].

Staphylococcus aureus remains the most common organism isolated in acute hematogenous osteomyelitis in children across all ages [2–4, 8–12]. Other pathogens, especially Kingella kingae, are also being identified with increasing frequency in children under the age of 4 years, due to better diagnostic technology helping in the isolation of these fastidious organisms [3, 5, 6, 11].

The emergence of community-acquired methicillin-resistant *Staphylococcus aureus* (CA-MRSA) over the past two decades, as a major pathogen responsible for acute osteomyelitis especially in the USA, has been well documented. CA-MRSA has accounted for up to 30–50% of *Staphylococcus aureus* osteomyelitis in some series [8, 13–17]. Of late, there has been a shift in the epidemiology of invasive staphylococcal disease with a decline in the prevalence of MRSA and reciprocal increase in methicillin-sensitive *Staphylococcus aureus* (MSSA) [18–20].

The clinical course of CA-MRSA osteomyelitis has been shown to be protracted and severe in several studies with longer duration of hospital stay, increased number of surgeries, and higher incidence of complications [14, 15, 17, 21–25]. Higher inflammatory markers (ESR and CRP) at admission, prolonged fever with bacteremia, and multiple foci of infection should raise the suspicion of possible CA-MRSA infection [16, 21, 24, 26].

Staphylococcal infections have become increasingly problematic due to the resistance mechanisms developed by the bacteria to evade both the host immune system and antibiotic treatment [27]. The pathogenicity of *Staphylococcus aureus* is mediated through an array of toxins and virulence proteins which facilitate the formation of distinct biofilm on necrotic bone tissue and bone marrow as well as within the osteocyte canalicular networks of living bone [28].

Staphylococcus aureus carrying the genes encoding Panton-Valentine leukocidin (pvl^+ S aureus) has been shown to produce a more severe clinical course of infection compared to pvl^- strains [22, 23, 25, 29–32]. Panton-Valentine leukocidin (PVL) is a necrotizing exotoxin produced by *Staphylococcus aureus* and is thought to be responsible for producing severe infections in humans by its ability to cause death of polymorphonuclear leukocytes. Although PVL is more common in MRSA, it may be also present in MSSA resulting in similarly high severity of illness [32]. Pvl+ *Staphylococcus aureus* infections of the musculoskeletal system can present as multifocal osteomyelitis, contiguous septic arthritis, subperiosteal abscesses, and pyomyositis along with systemic sepsis, deep vein thrombosis, and septic embolism [16, 21–23, 25, 29–32].

Pathological fractures occur in bone which has been weakened due to alteration of its intrinsic mechanical and viscoelastic properties consequent to focal and/or systemic disease [33]. The risk of development of such a fracture is determined by the altered strength of bone and the amount of load applied to it. Normal biomechanical properties of the bone may be altered by intrinsic processes within the bone such as reduction of mineral density by the disease itself, as well as by extrinsic processes which create stress risers such as biopsy tracts, surgical debridement, and internal fixation [34, 35]. Quantitative CT-based evaluation of the mechanical properties of bone have been studied in order to help predict fracture risk, but these have been limited to the study of benign skeletal neoplasms [36, 37]. Pathological fractures typically happen following trivial trauma and in the case of osteomyelitis can occur at any stage of the disease: acute, subacute, or chronic.

Epidemiology and Risk Factors

Pathological fractures occurring as a complication of acute and chronic osteomyelitis have been reported both in adults and children, but have been relatively uncommon and limited to case reports or historical case series [38–47]. More recently, cases of pathological fractures in long bones following *Staphylococcus aureus* osteomyelitis have been reported both in children [22, 48] and in adults [49].

Chronic osteomyelitis has been shown to be the leading cause of pathological fractures in the long bones of Nigerian children, accounting for 74.5% of all pathological fractures, and such a high prevalence has been attributed to delay in diagnosis as well as inadequate treatment of acute hematogenous osteomyelitis [50]. Sickle cell disease has been shown to be a risk factor for osteomyelitis in these cases from Africa, and the predominant organism has been *Staphylococcus aureus*, both in children with and without sickle cell disease [51, 52].

Pathological fractures were reported in approximately 5% of cases of acute hematogenous *Staphylococcus aureus* osteomyelitis by Belthur et al. [53] and were shown to be associated with the USA300.0114 pulsotype of MRSA. They described 17 out of 364 children (mean age of 8.8 years) who developed a pathological long bone fracture after a mean of 72 days (range 20–150 days) from the onset of infection. Children who developed a pathological fracture showed a higher number of subperiosteal and intramuscular abscesses as well as larger circumference abscess surrounding the bone on initial MRI scans.

In a study of 286 cases of *Staphylococcus aureus* acute hematogenous osteoarticular infections reported by McNeil et al. [54], 27 patients (9.4%) developed musculoskeletal complications, of which pathological fractures (29.6%) were found to be the second most common complication after chronic osteomyelitis (51.8%). Infection with agr group III *S. aureus*, prolonged fever (>4 days after admission), and delayed source control were found to be independently associated with complications overall. Fracture risk increased substantially among patients who needed ≥3 surgical procedures, infection caused by pvl+ organisms, larger diameter bone abscesses, bacteremia, and prolonged fever.

In a selected series of 81 patients with acute severe staphylococcal osteomyelitis (both MSSA & MRSA) all of whom had undergone surgical drainage of extraosseous pus, Horn et al. [55] reported complications in 39 patients (48%) including pathological fractures in 19 patients (23%). The authors attributed such a high complication rate to a more severe disease group which included only those patients who were treated surgically and excluding patients who were managed only medically. A previous study from the same institution had reported a pathological fracture rate of 3.4% [56]. The dominant organism isolated was MSSA in 93% of patients, with MRSA accounting for only 2.4%. The authors did not identify any modifiable risk factors to predict the development of complications, though there was an association with significantly prolonged hospital stay and longer duration of antibiotic therapy. The extent of bone involvement on plain radiographs at 6 weeks from the onset of disease was found to correlate with the likelihood of developing complications, with the cut off being involvement of more than 45% of the shaft.

A poorly performed drainage of intraosseous abscess can also be a risk factor for developing a pathological fracture. A slot created in the cortex of the bone can act as a stress riser and precipitate a pathological fracture. Careful attention must be made to create a rectangular slot with a small width on the non-tension side of the bone to minimize reduction of the bone strength [57–59].

Clinical Presentation

Pathological fractures can present acutely in the presence of active infection or in a delayed fashion after source control has been achieved (Fig. 22.1). Sudden increase in pain in the infected long bone following trivial trauma, difficulty to weight bear, swelling, or angular deformity are the usual presenting features. Sometimes, they may present as a malunion (Fig. 22.2) or nonunion following delayed presentation or with inadequate follow-up after treatment of active infection. The mean time interval from onset of disease to diagnosis of pathological fracture has been reported to vary from 72.1 days [53] to 80.3 days [54].

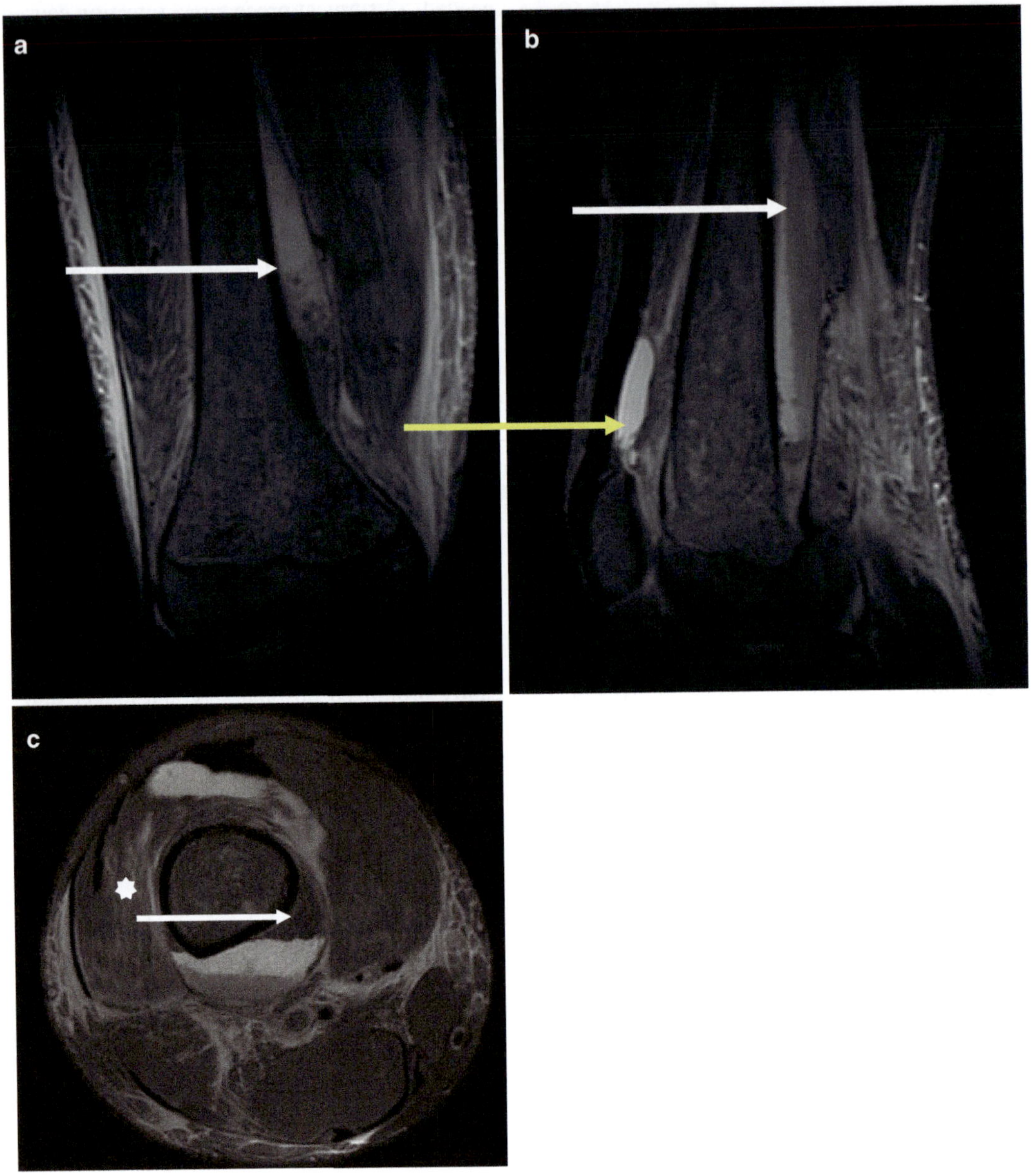

Fig. 22.1 (**a**–**g**) A 14-year-old male with right femoral MRSA osteomyelitis with associated deep vein thrombosis and bilateral pleural effusions. (**a**–**c**) MRI images (coronal STIR, sagittal STIR, and axial PD FS images) showing osteomyelitis of right distal femur with a very large subperiosteal abscess (white arrows), moderate to large knee effusion with marked synovial hyperemia most likely septic arthritis (yellow arrow), deep vein thrombosis of the popliteal vein, and regional cellulitis with myositis (white star), without myonecrosis. (**d**) Radiographs at presentation showing mild osteopenia. (**e**) Radiographs at 2 months showing permeative lucencies, sclerosis, and subperiosteal reaction. (**f**) Radiographs at 4 months showing extensive callus formation and periosteal reaction extending from the midshaft to distal metaphysis. Heterogenous area of sclerosis and lucency seen along distal half of the femoral shaft. (**g**) Radiographs at 5 months showing an angulated fracture of lower third of femoral shaft and features consistent with healing chronic osteomyelitis

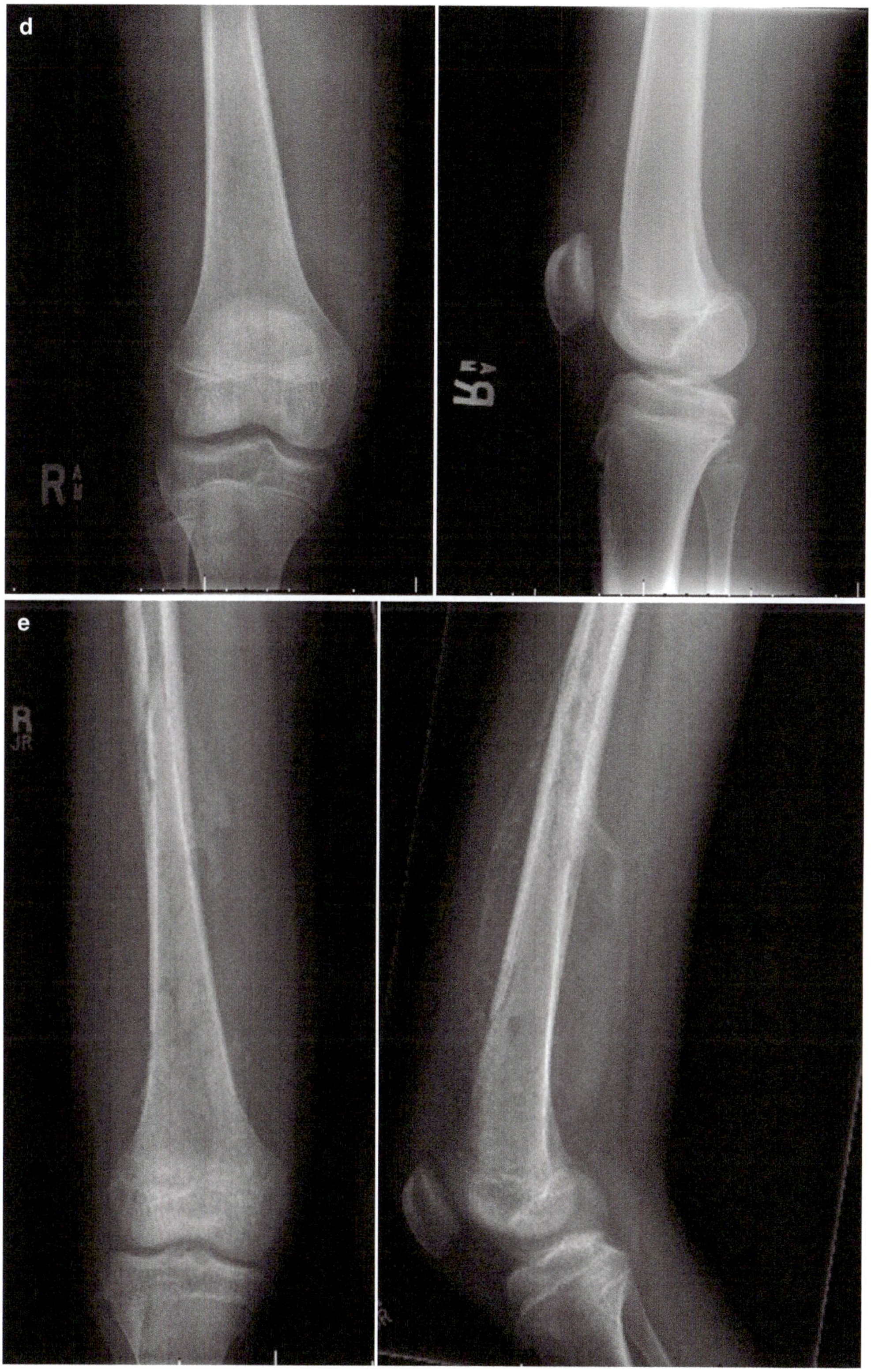

Fig. 22.1 (continued)

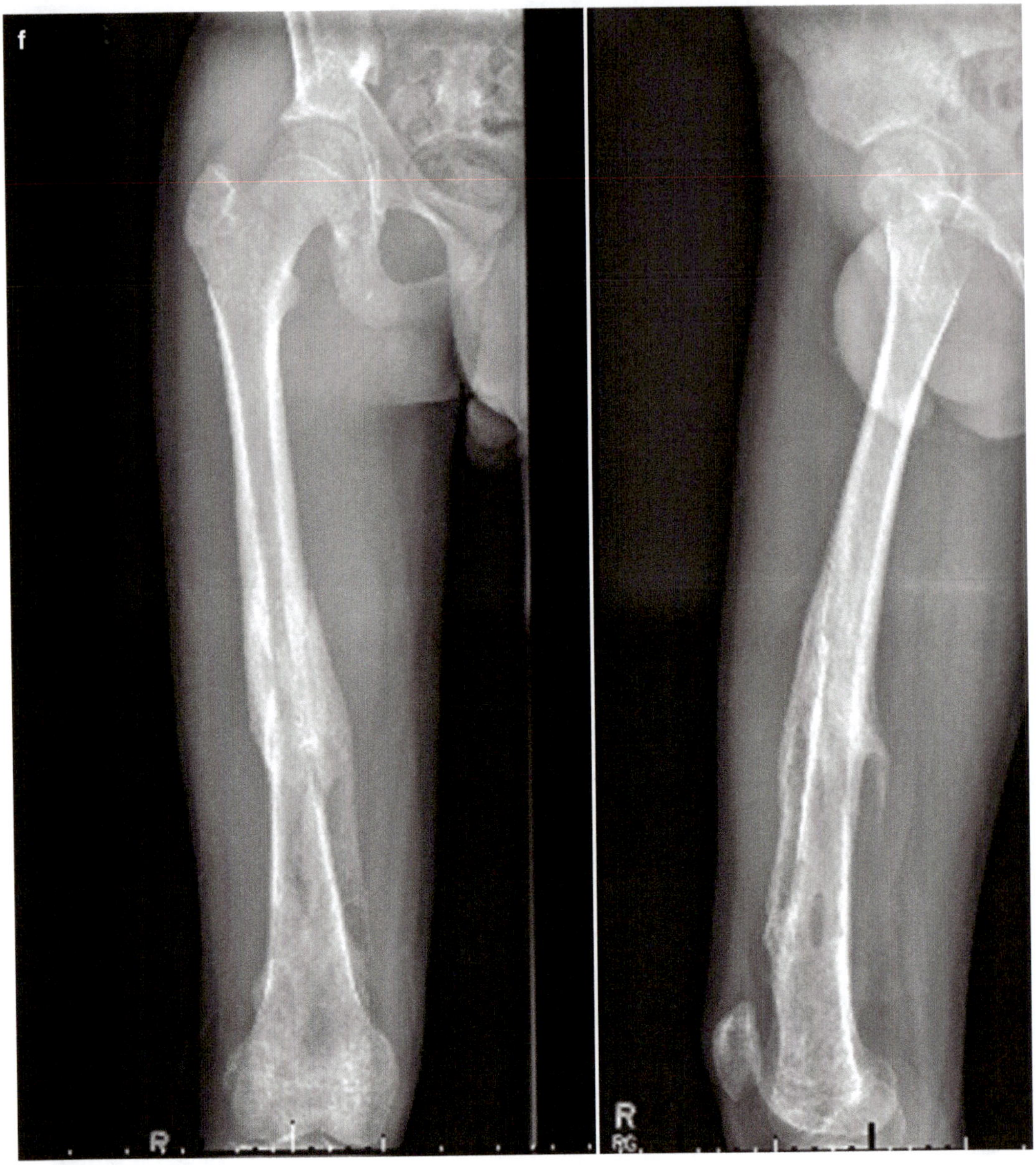

Fig. 22.1 (continued)

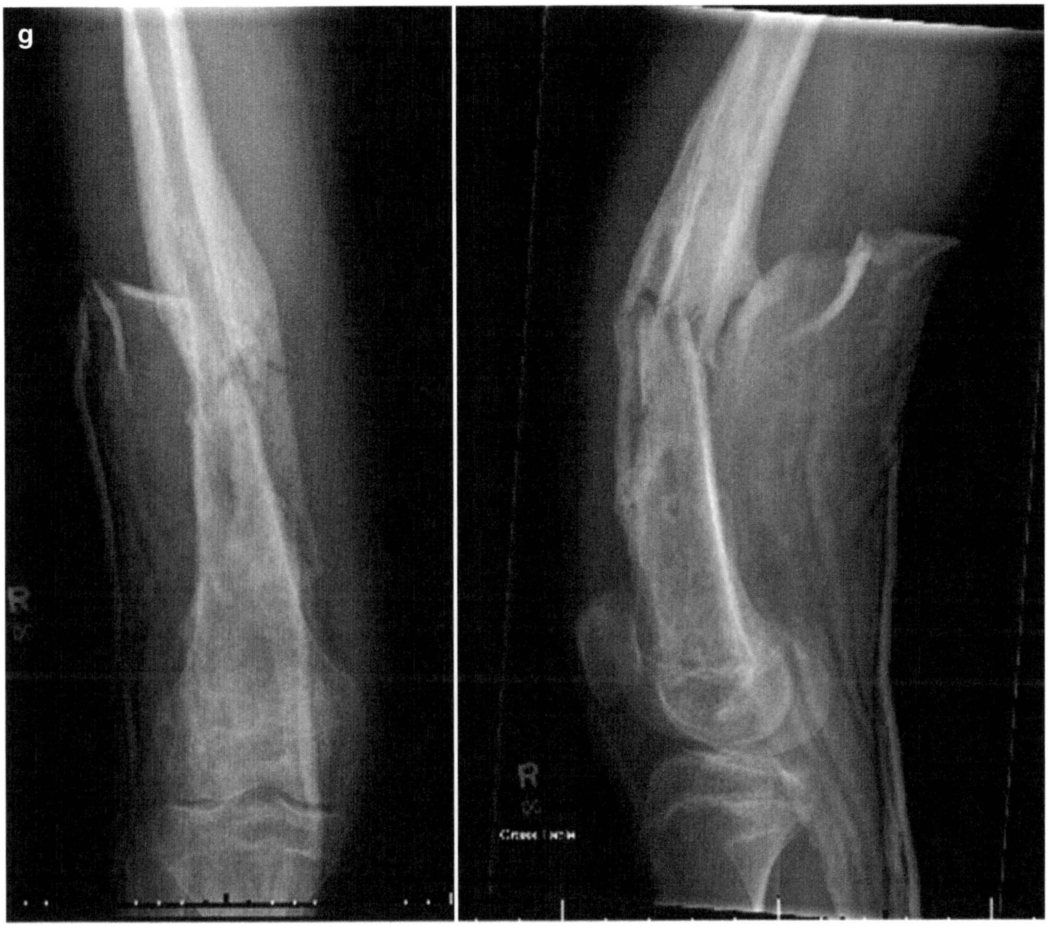

Fig. 22.1 (continued)

Investigations

Diagnostic evaluation of any clinically suspected musculoskeletal infection should be aimed towards confirmation of infection, localization of the source and extent of infection, and identification of the specific pathogen involved, with a view to planning targeted treatment [60]. Blood counts, measurement of inflammatory markers, and other acute phase reactants as well as microbiological analysis of tissue samples and blood have remained the key components of work up in a case of suspected musculoskeletal infection.

Though the initial radiographs may not show any changes indicative of infection, follow-up X-rays, especially in resource deprived environments, have been useful in identifying chronic infection [61, 62] as well as in determining the extent of bone involvement with a view to predicting the likelihood of developing sequelae [55, 63].

Magnetic resonance imaging (MRI) with and without contrast enhancement has become the preferred imaging modality for evaluation of any suspected case of osteomyelitis due to its high sensitivity in the identification of early marrow edema [64–66]. Additionally, MRI can help in detecting the true extent of infection within the involved bone as well as associated manifestations such as contiguous septic arthritis, subperiosteal abscess, pyomyositis, soft tissue collections, and deep vein thrombosis [11, 12, 16, 65, 67, 68] (Figs. 22.3 and 22.4). Belthur et al. [53] reported an increased incidence of

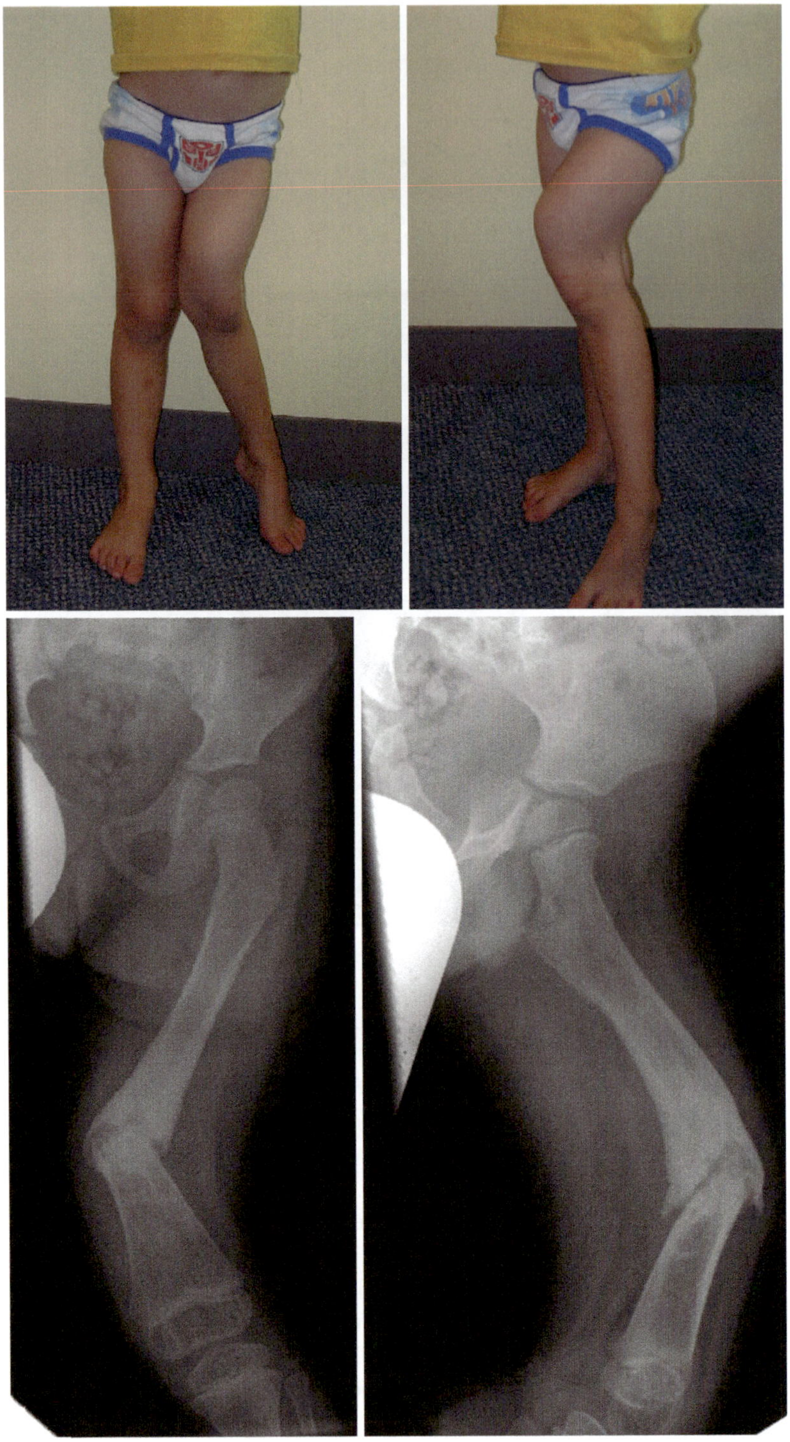

Fig. 22.2 An 8-year-old male presenting with malunion of left femur pathological fracture following acute hematogenous osteomyelitis

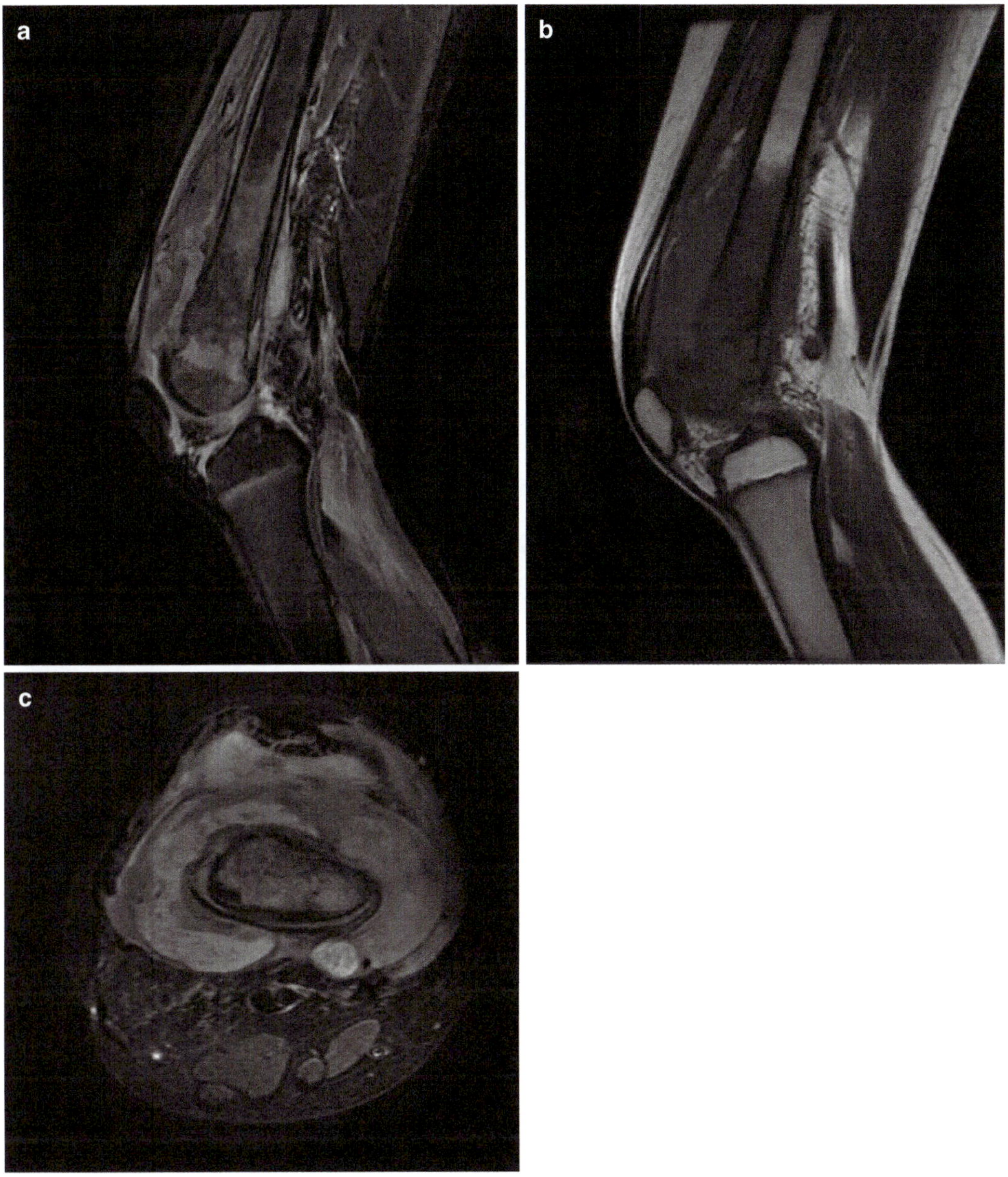

Fig. 22.3 (**a–e**) An 11-year-old male with right distal femoral osteomyelitis showing characteristic MRI findings. (**a**) Sagittal STIR (TR 6154 ms, TE 46 ms, TI 200 ms) showing diffuse hyperintense signal in the distal third of the right femur with extraosseous and subperiosteal abscess, anterior > posterior, and mild knee joint effusion. (**b**) Sagittal T1-weighted image (TR/TE 760 ms/16 ms) showing diffuse hypointense signal in the distal third of the right femur with blurring of the physis and extraosseous subperiosteal abscess, anterior > posterior. (**c**) Axial STIR (TR/TE/TI 5475 ms/44 ms/200 ms) image showing near circumferential subperiosteal abscess and diffuse intramedullary signal as well as cortical thickening. (**d**) Contrast-enhanced sagittal T1FS (TR/TE 453 ms/16 ms) image showing poorly defined enhancement in the distal third of the right femur extending to the subarticular bone, peripherally enhancing subperiosteal abscess and myofascial enhancement. (**e**) Contrast-enhanced axial T1 FS (TR/TE 453 ms/16 ms) image showing near circumferential peripherally enhancing subperiosteal abscess with absence of central enhancement. Poorly defined intramedullary enhancement in the femur corresponds to the area of infection. (Images courtesy Dr. Sriram Rajan, Consultant Radiologist, Mahajan Imaging, New Delhi)

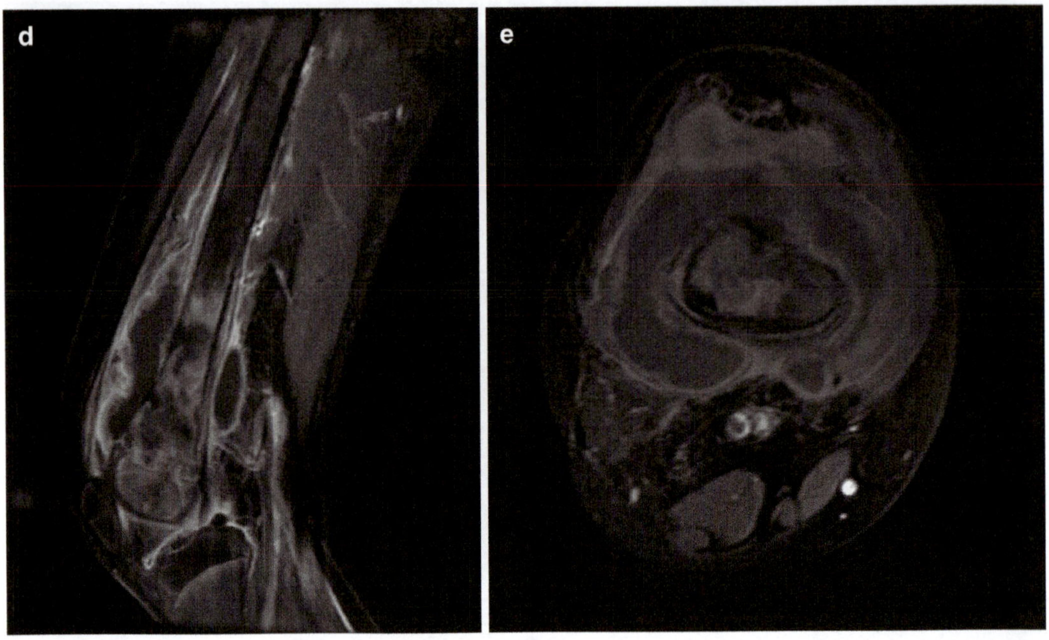

Fig. 22.3 (continued)

subsequent pathological fracture in patients with MRSA osteomyelitis, whose initial MRI images showed a sharp zone of decreased bone marrow enhancement or subperiosteal abscess extending to more than half the bone circumference.

Management

While there is fairly uniform consensus about the initial management of acute hematogenous osteomyelitis in terms of the primacy of appropriate and adequate antimicrobial therapy along with clearly specified and limited indications for operative intervention, there is paucity of guidance for the management of pathological fractures following osteomyelitis due to the relative infrequency of this complication. The following steps may be recommended based on our review of the literature:

1. Identifying children who are at high risk for developing complications (Table 22.1)
2. Adequate management (medical/surgical) of active infection if present
3. Realignment and stabilization of pathological fractures
4. Excision of sequestra, management of bone gap, and stimulation of the nonunion
5. Rehabilitation to optimize function
6. Long-term follow-up

An analysis of specific risk factors, clinical, microbiological, laboratory, and radiological, may help in identifying patients who are at risk of developing a pathological fracture [53–55]. Given the strong association between severity of the disease and development of various complications including pathological fractures, it is vital to identify those children who are likely to have a complicated course at an early stage of their illness. Using demographic, clinical, laboratory, and imaging parameters, from the time of presentation as well as within the first few days of hospitalization, risk assessment algorithms and scoring systems have been developed to identify children who may benefit from individualized and potentially aggressive management [69–71]. Specific to the context of risk of development of pathological fractures, those children who run the

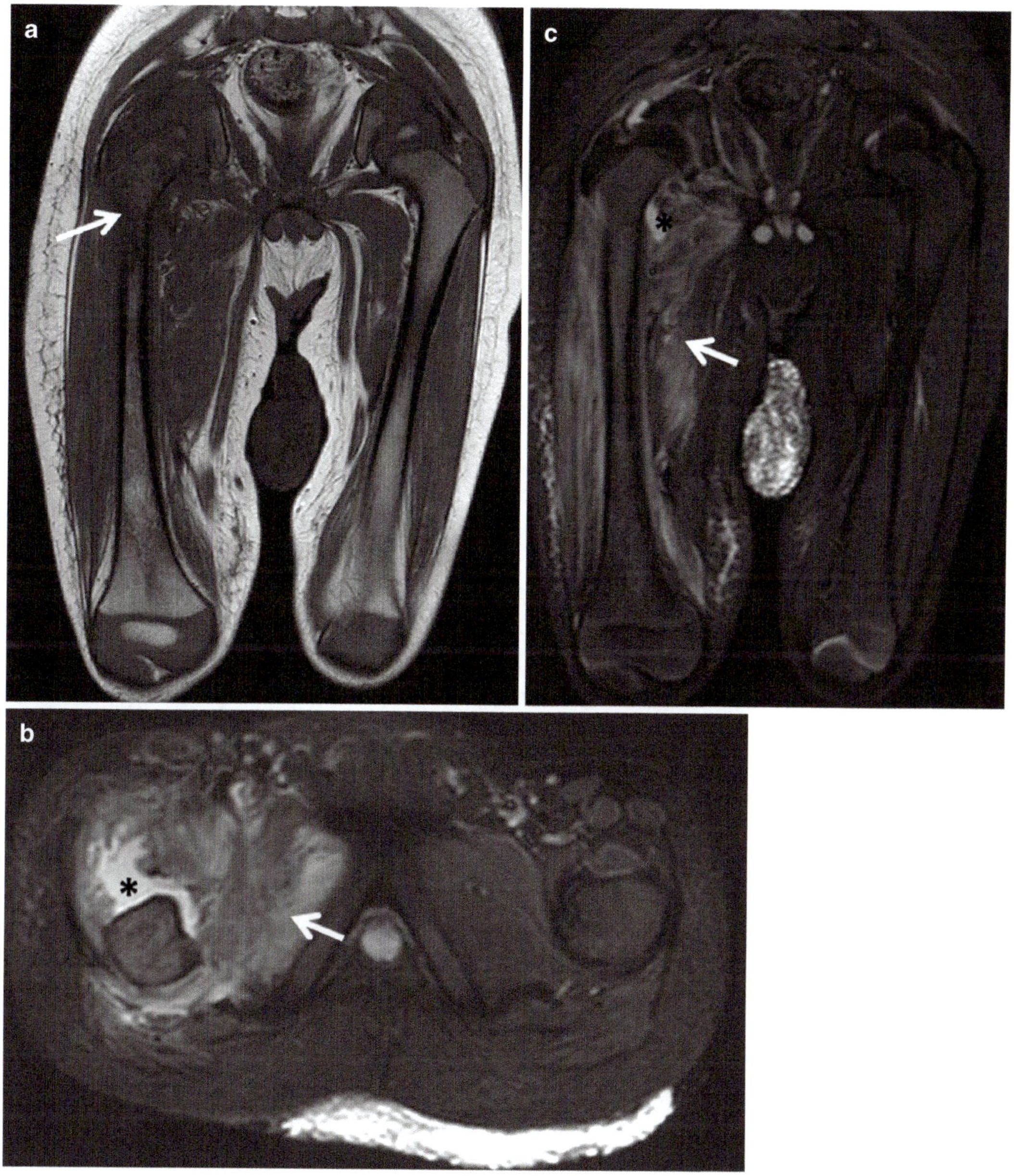

Fig. 22.4 (**a–e**) A 2½-year-old male with right proximal femoral osteomyelitis which resulted in a pathological fracture. (**a–c**) MRI images at presentation. (**a**) T1 coronal image showing large ill-defined area of hypointensity (white arrow) involving the proximal femur on right side. (**b**) MRI STIR (short tau inversion recovery) axial image showing diffuse edema in the muscles (white arrow) around the proximal femur on right side. Fluid collection (asterisk) is also seen anterior to the femur. (**c**) MRI STIR coronal image showing diffuse edema in the muscles of thigh (white arrow) with small fluid pockets (asterisk) around proximal femur on the right side. (MRI Images courtesy Dr. Amit Sahu, Consultant Radiologist, Max Healthcare, New Delhi). (**d**) Radiographs at presentation. (**e**) Radiographs at 6 months showing a pathological fracture of the proximal femur. (MRI Images courtesy Dr. Amit Sahu, Consultant Radiologist, Max Healthcare, New Delhi)

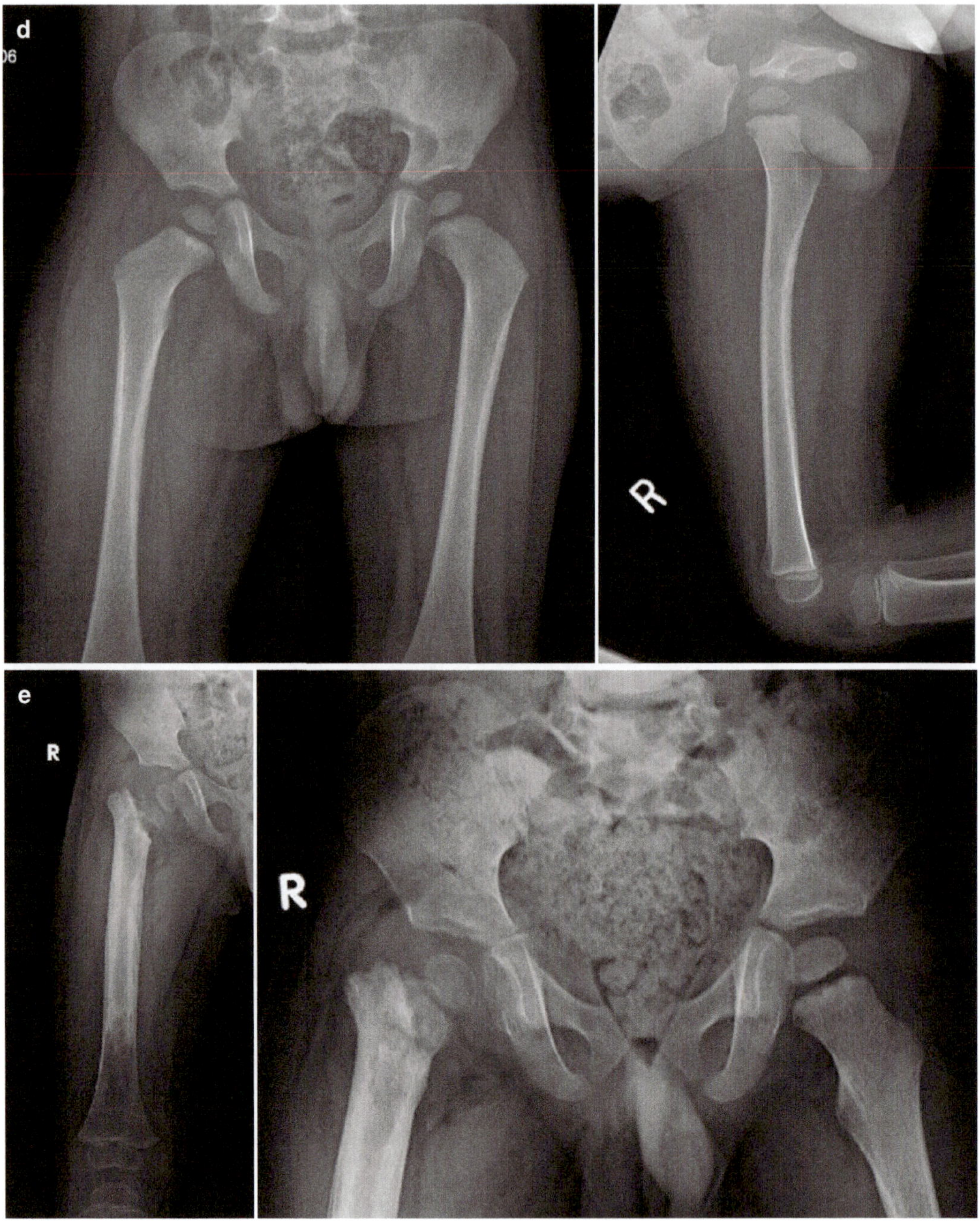

Fig. 22.4 (continued)

risk of developing a more severe infection may be candidates for lengthier duration of immobilization of their extremities, delayed weight-bearing, and activity restriction [53, 72].

Fracture stabilization can be achieved by several methods including immobilization of the extremity with plaster casts or braces and internal (intramedullary/extramedullary) (Fig. 22.5) or external fixation. The preference has been to avoid conventional internal fixation devices in the setting of infection for fear of these implants serving as nidus for bacterial biofilm. The objec-

Table 22.1 Risk factors for pathological fractures

Bacteriological	
	Infection with a virulent strain (pvl + Staph aureus)
	Agr group III Staphylococcus aureus
Clinical	
	Bacteremia
	Prolonged fever
	Delayed source control
	Number of surgical procedures ≥3
Imaging	
	Radiographs at 6 weeks – extent of bone involvement >45%
	Initial MRI
	Subperiosteal abscess of large circumferential size and involving >2/3rd length of bone
	Sharp transitional zone between diseased and normal marrow

tive of any management strategy would be to achieve bony union without evolving into chronic infection as well as to avoid the sequelae of angular deformity, length discrepancy, physeal growth arrest, or joint stiffness. Fracture nonunion is of utmost concern and may occur secondary to residual infection or the presence of necrotic bone at the fracture site.

In their series of 17 pathological fractures, Belthur et al. [53] reported the use of non-operative modalities for immobilization in 15 patients, namely casts for lower limb fractures and shoulder immobilizers for upper limb fractures and intramedullary nails in the remaining 2 patients. Though a high rate of osseous union was

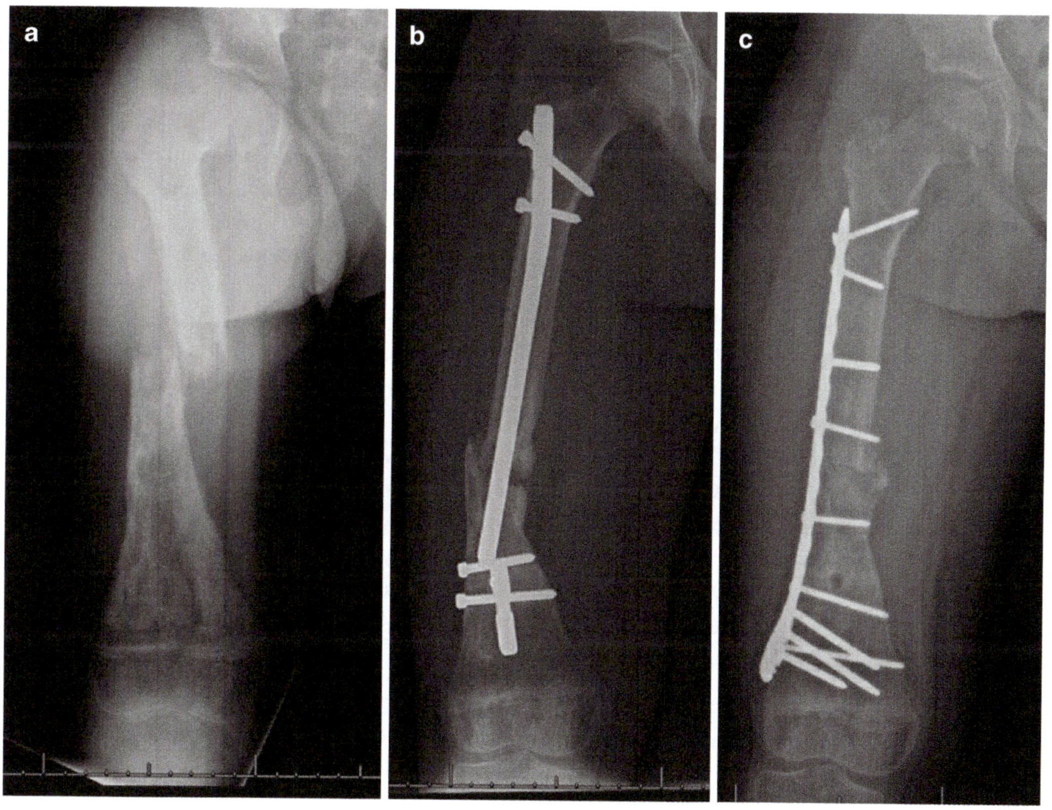

Fig. 22.5 (**a–c**) A 6-year-old female with history of multifocal MRSA infection including sepsis, endocarditis, septic pulmonary emboli, septic arthritis of the hip, and osteomyelitis of the right femur status post multiple debridements. (**a**) Pathological fracture of the right femoral diaphysis 3 months after initial presentation. (**b**) Persistent nonunion with implant failure after source control with intravenous and local antibiotics, local debridement, and intramedullary fixation. (**c**) Revision open reduction and internal fixation after debridement of devitalized bone

achieved (15 of 17 patients), angular deformities were seen in 41% of cases. Once the active infection is well controlled, immobilization of the extremity for an extended length of time may be adequate to achieve union in most cases (Fig. 22.6). Specific limitations of extended periods of immobilization are the prolonged duration of treatment with associated morbidities, stiffness of adjoining joints, and difficulty with plasters in the older, heavier child.

Stabilization of pathological fractures of long bones secondary to osteomyelitis must always be undertaken against the backdrop of optimum medical and surgical treatment of the infection itself, which usually involves adequate antibiotic therapy, drainage of abscesses, as well as debridement of nonviable and infected tissue. The challenges of management of pathological fractures of long bones during the early active phase of the infective process are different from those encountered during the late or chronic stage in which the infection is resolved, but other sequelae such as pseudoarthrosis or segmental bone loss are present.

Yildirim and colleagues [73] reported a 100% osseous union rate in 11 children and adolescents, with a mean age of 8.7 years who had pathologic fractures in the femur and tibia secondary to osteomyelitis, which were stabilized using internal, extramedullary fixation (a locking plate as an internal fixator). Cancellous bone graft harvested from the iliac crest was used as an adjunct to stimulate union after radical debridement, copious lavage, and stable fixation of bone ends with a locking plate. Though the authors have highlighted the benefits of placement of the locking plate a few millimeters away from the bone to reduce implant to bone contact surface ratio compared to intramedullary nails or conventional plate screw constructs thereby reducing potential infections, concerns remain about the routine use of internal fixation in the setting of osteomyelitis.

Belthur et al. [53] reported the use of intramedullary nails for stabilization of pathological fractures in 2 out of their 17 patients who were older and heavier (Fig. 22.7). Antibiotic cement nails and newer-generation antibiotic-coated intramedullary nails have been shown to be very successful in the treatment of intramedullary bone infection while providing stability to the affected bone, with most series showing success rates in the range of 80–100% [74–76]. The rationale behind the use of antibiotic nails conform to the principles of management of chronic osteomyelitis as outlined by Cierny and Mader, namely effective dead space management after debridement, stabilization of fracture or nonunion, and adequate local antibiotic levels [77, 78]. Delivery of antibiotics directly within the surgical field ensures adequate local concentrations which may not otherwise be possible with systemic administration when there is compromised vascularity at the infected fracture site, and polymethylmethacrylate (PMMA) has been used for a considerable length of time as an effective material for dead space management as well as a carrier for antibiotic delivery [79]. Despite several series showing highly successful outcomes with antibiotic nails in adults [74–76, 80, 81], their use has not been

Fig. 22.6 (**a–f**) A 5½-year-old female with left tibial *Staphylococcus aureus* osteomyelitis with subperiosteal and extraosseous abscesses. (**a–c**) MRI images at presentation. (**a**) T1 coronal image showing abnormal hypointense geographical areas within the marrow of proximal tibia on left side (white arrow). Similar smaller areas of abnormality are also seen in distal tibia (black arrow). (**b**) Contrast-enhanced MRI T1 fat saturated coronal image showing heterogeneous enhancement of marrow in proximal tibia (white arrow) representing osteomyelitis. Mild abnormal enhancement is also seen in distal tibia. There is a subperiosteal abscess around the proximal tibia showing peripheral enhancement (black arrow). (**c**) Contrast-enhanced MRI T1 fat saturated axial image showing multi-loculated extraosseous abscess in the subcutaneous plane as well as circumferential subperiosteal abscess (white arrows) around the proximal tibia. (MRI Images courtesy Dr. Amit Sahu, Consultant Radiologist, Max Healthcare, New Delhi). (**d**) Radiographs at 6 weeks showing extent of bone involvement. (**e**) Radiographs at 3 months showing pathological fracture of proximal tibia. (**f**) Radiographs at 9 months showing united fracture after non-operative management with extended period of immobilization in plaster. (MRI Images courtesy Dr. Amit Sahu, Consultant Radiologist, Max Healthcare, New Delhi)

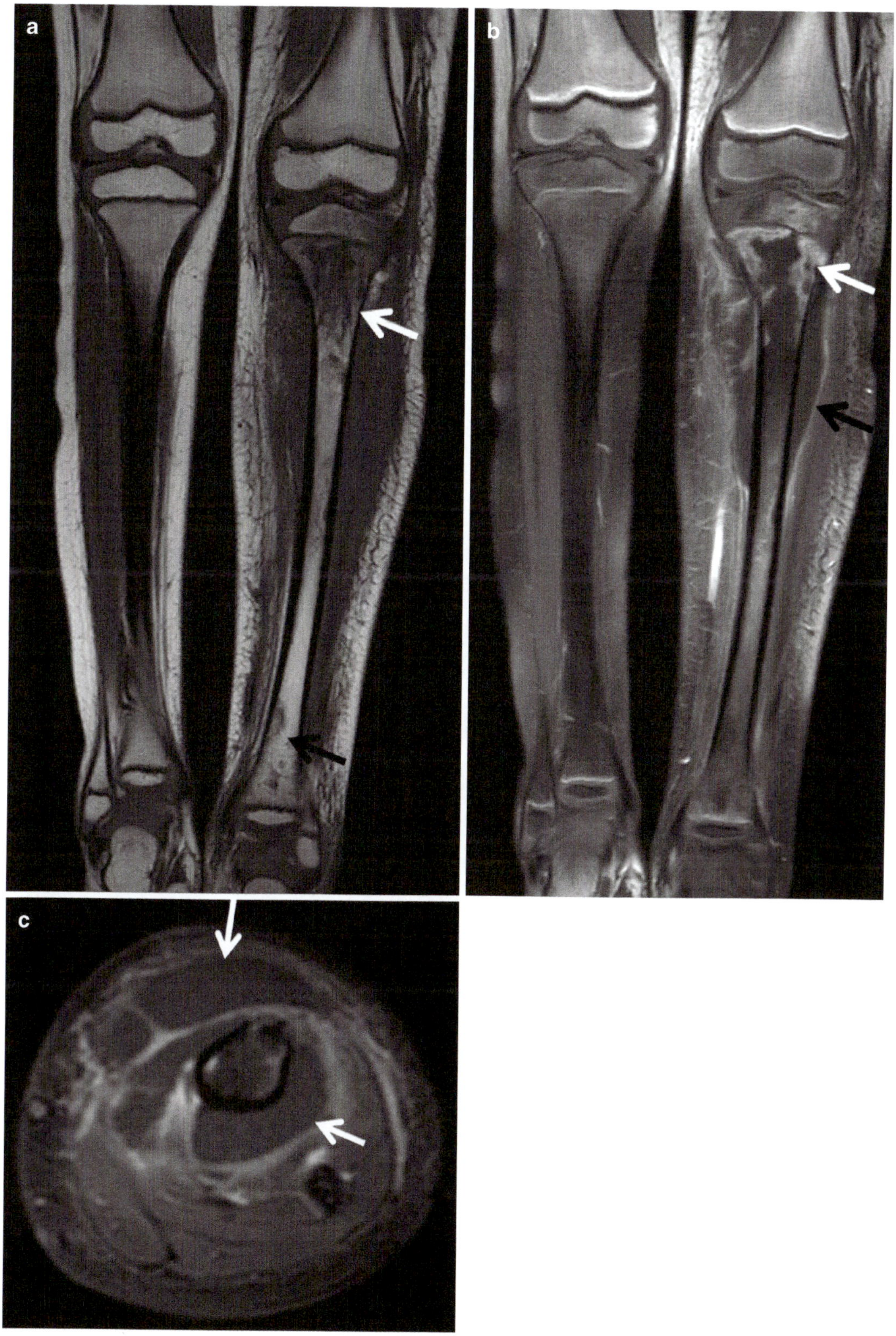
a
b
c

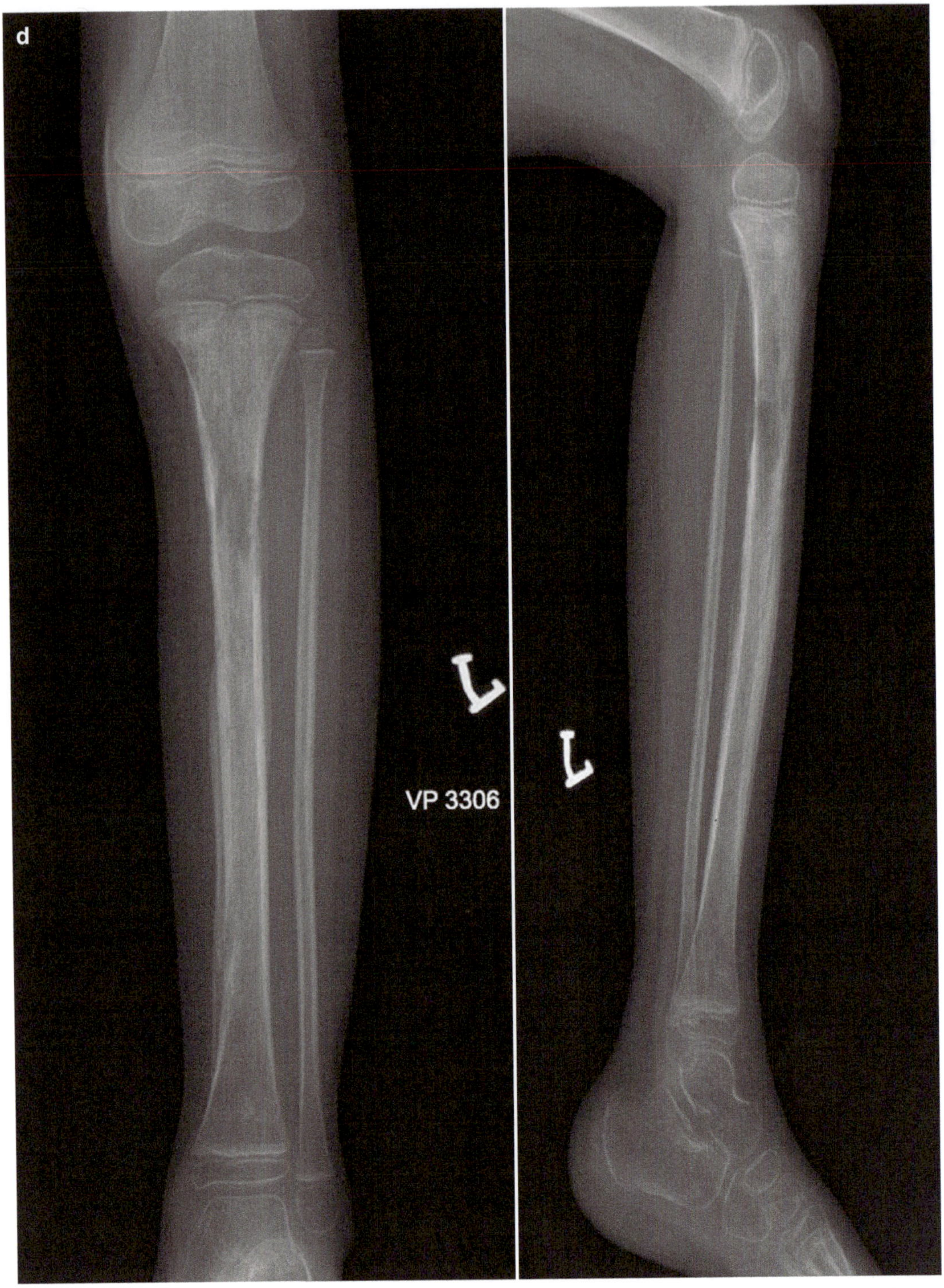

Fig. 22.6 (continued)

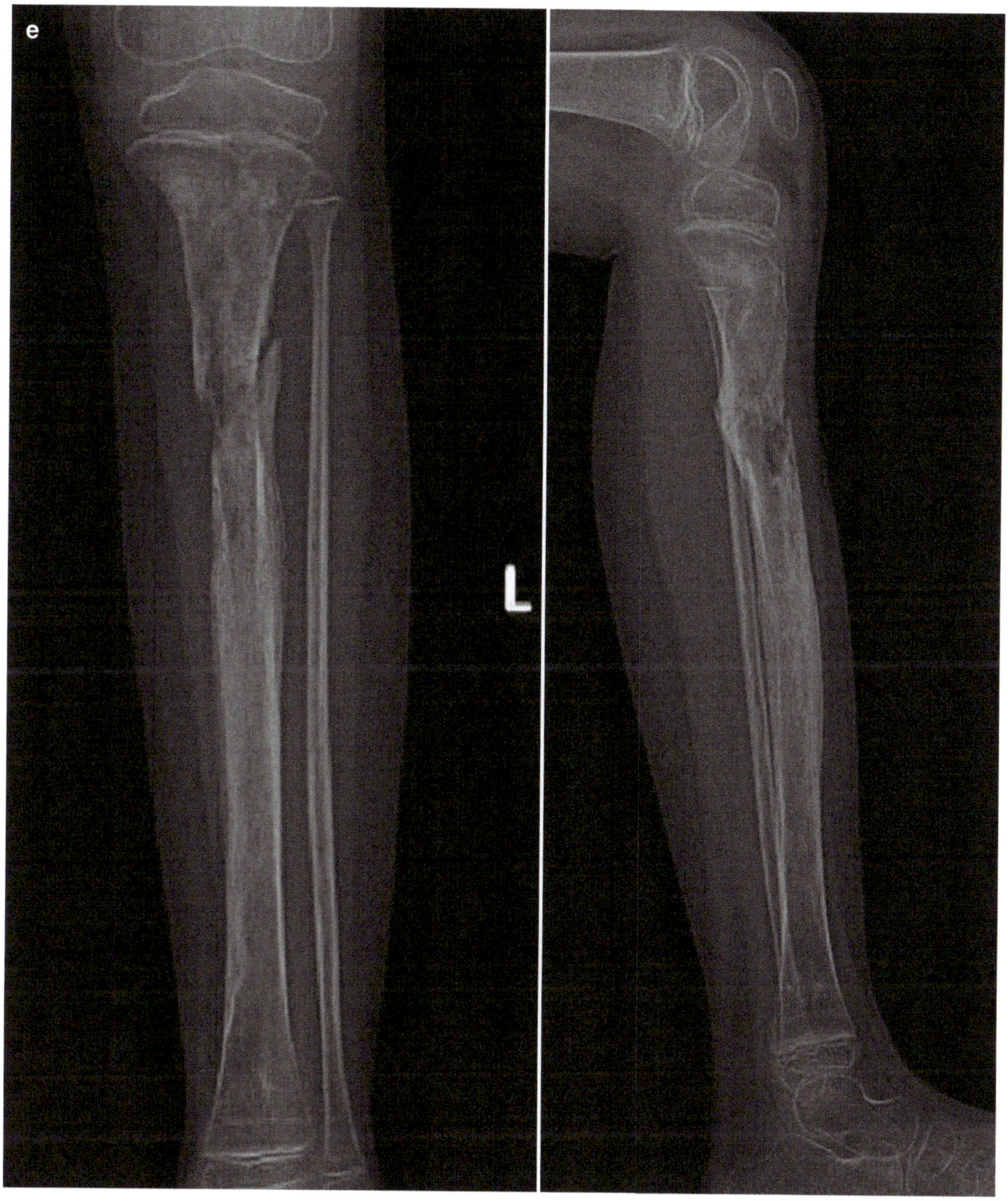

Fig. 22.6 (continued)

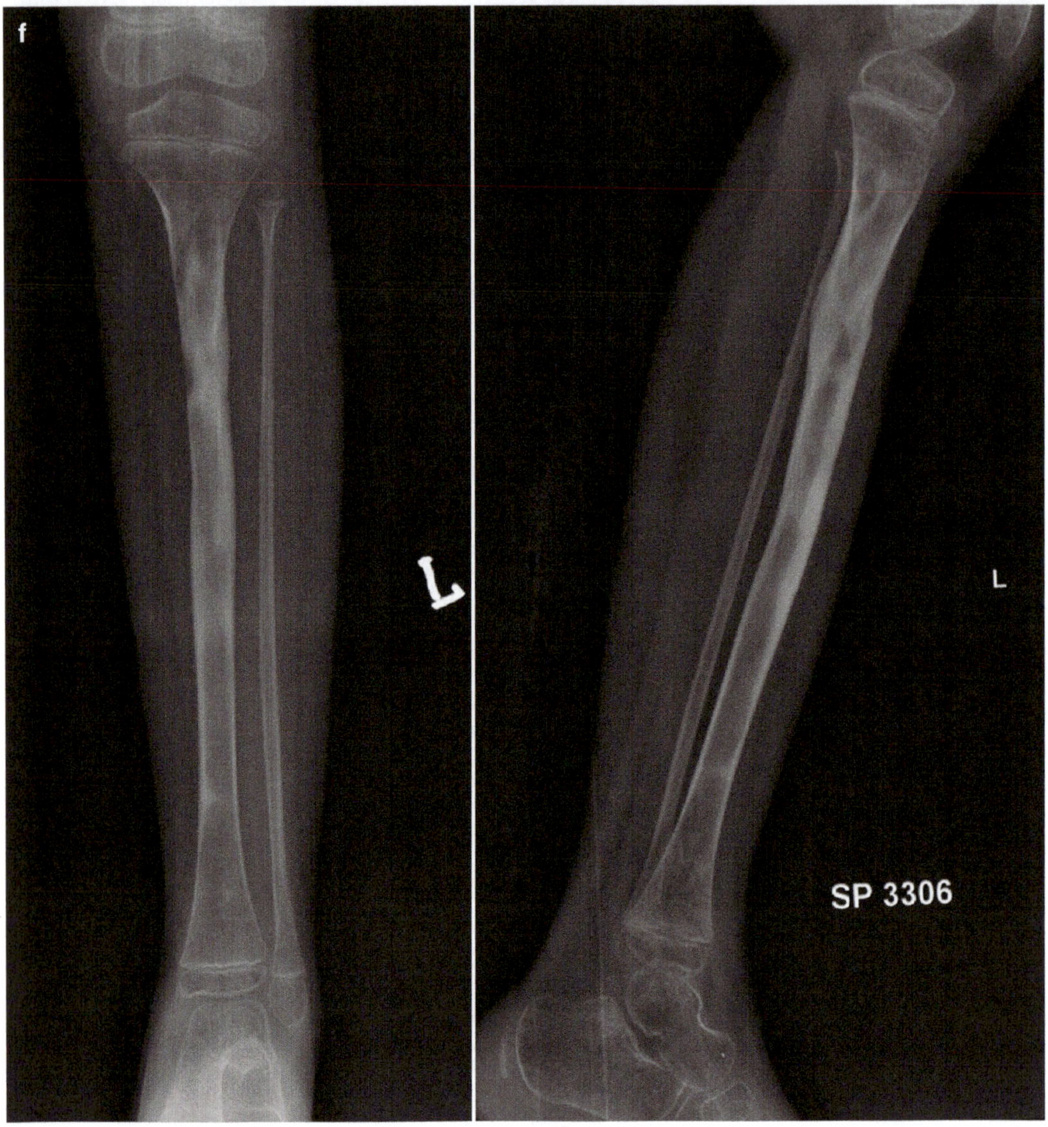

Fig. 22.6 (continued)

advocated in children under the age of 16 years due to the open physes limiting nail insertion and the need for extensive reaming of the medullary cavity as part of debridement [81]. In the only published series about antibiotic cement nails in children, Bar-on et al. [82] have reported the safe and effective usage of antibiotic impregnated cement rods in four children with chronic osteomyelitis who underwent debridement and lavage, reaming of the intramedullary canal, and insertion of gentamicin impregnated cement rods into the canal.

Extending the established principles of use of the Ilizarov circular external fixator in the management of posttraumatic osteomyelitis and infected nonunions of tibia [83], external fixators have been used to stabilize pathological fractures secondary to osteomyelitis using

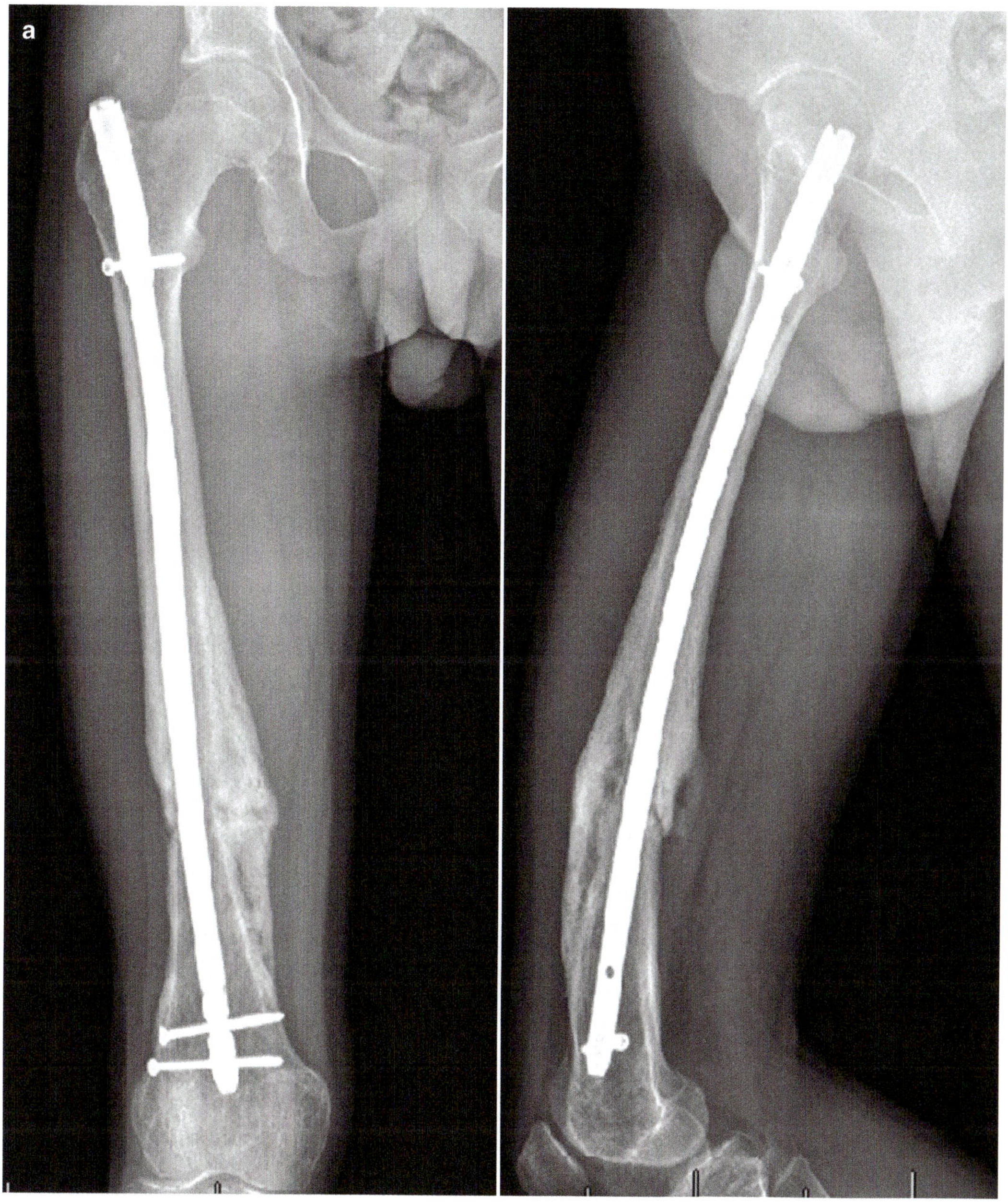

Fig. 22.7 (**a**, **b**) Same case as Fig. 22.1. (**a**) Radiographs after 6 months showing intramedullary nail fixation of right distal femoral fracture with evidence of healing. (**b**) Long leg radiographs after 2 years showing healed osteomyelitis and healed fracture with satisfactory limb alignment and no limb length discrepancy

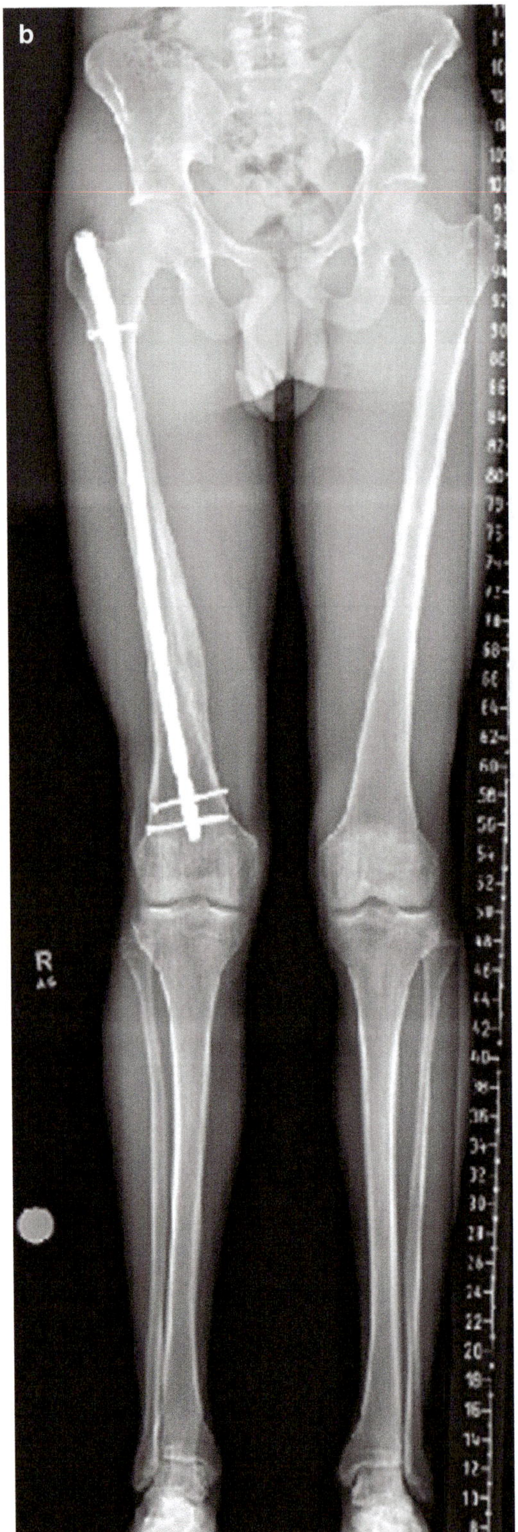

Fig. 22.7 (continued)

monolateral fixators in children [84] and circular ring fixators in adults [85]. Where there is structural instability of bone in the setting of chronic osteomyelitis (radiological evidence of sequestrum without adequate involucrum – Biet CURE Type B4 childhood chronic hematogenous osteomyelitis), sequestrectomy and removal of dead bone will result in creation of a bony defect which will then need to be addressed along with stabilization of bone either simultaneously or in a staged manner [62]. One of the advantages of stabilization with the Ilizarov circular external fixator is the ability to address any segmental defect which may develop following sequestrectomy by either bone transport or fibular grafting (Fig. 22.8). The major disadvantages of Ilizarov circular fixator are the difficult application especially in small and short bone segments, poor patient tolerance, and pin site infections.

Masquelet's induced membrane technique is well recognized as a strategy for management of bone defects from a variety of etiologies [86]. Since its original description in adults [87, 88], the use of this technique has been extended to biological reconstruction of long segment bone loss in children as well [89]. The technique has been shown to be effective in the staged management of pathological fractures with large bone defects secondary to chronic osteomyelitis and infected non-unions in children and adolescents [90–92].

Outcomes

Given that pathological fractures themselves are a complication of hematogenous osteomyelitis, outcomes of fracture management will inevitably be heavily influenced by the course of the underlying infective process. While nonunion and malunion resulting in angular or rotational deformity are clearly poor outcomes of fracture management, other adverse outcomes such as length discrepancy, joint stiffness, and persistent chronic osteomyelitis may also be due to concomitant physeal involvement, joint involvement, and a more virulent infection.

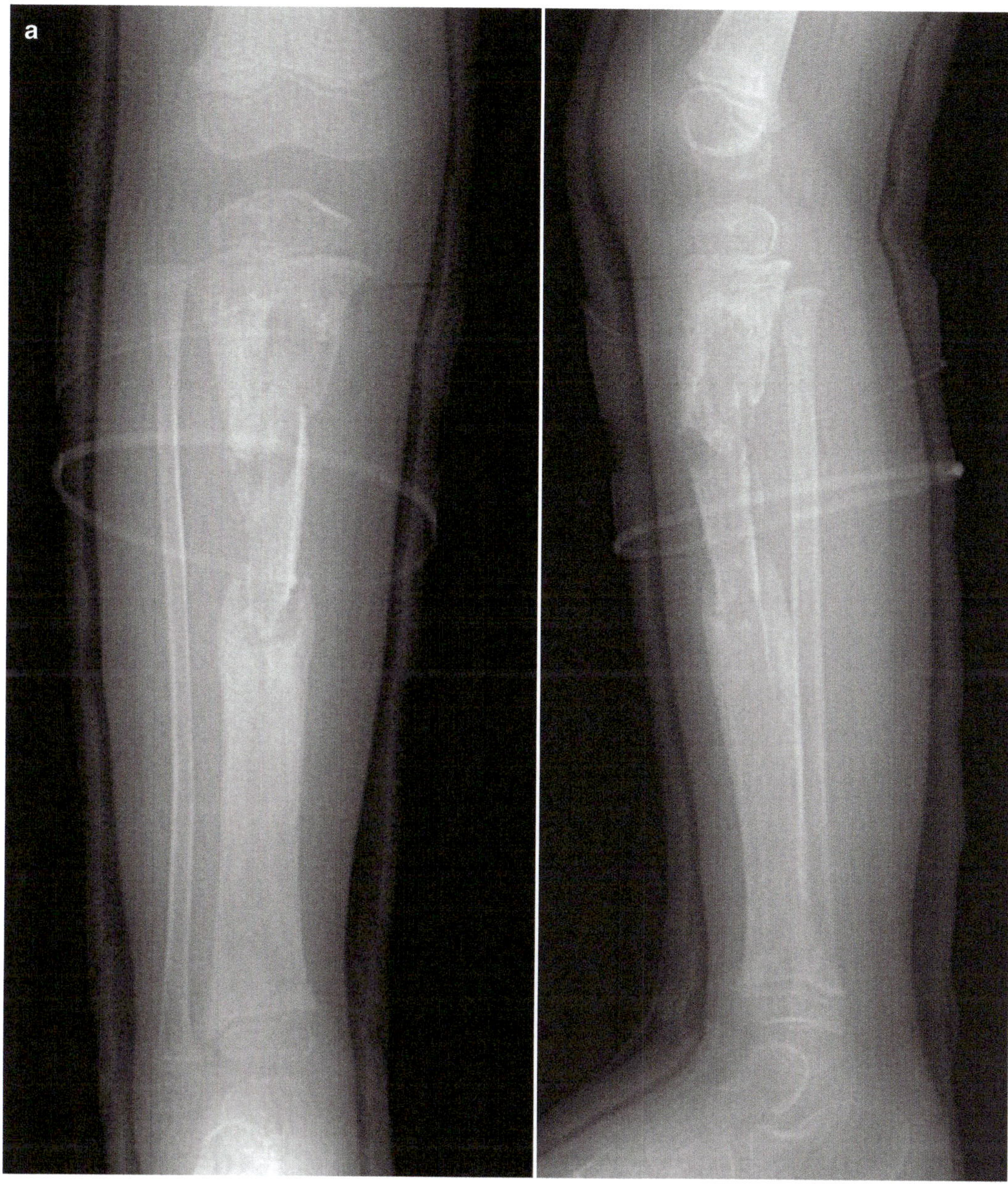

Fig. 22.8 (**a–d**) A 2½-year-old female with 3-month history of right tibial osteomyelitis – structural instability with large sequestrum and no involucrum (Biet CURE B4 type chronic osteomyelitis), with no active signs of infection, total count, and inflammatory markers normal. (**a**) Radiographs of tibia at presentation showing segmental pathological fracture with large sequestrum with no involucrum. (**b**) CT scan showing pathological fracture with extensive sequestrum and no involucrum. (**c**) Postoperative radiographs showing Ilizarov circular external fixator stabilizing the tibia after sequestrectomy and intercalary nonvascularized fibular strut grafting. (**d**) Radiographs 1 year after index surgery, showing healed fracture with complete integration of graft

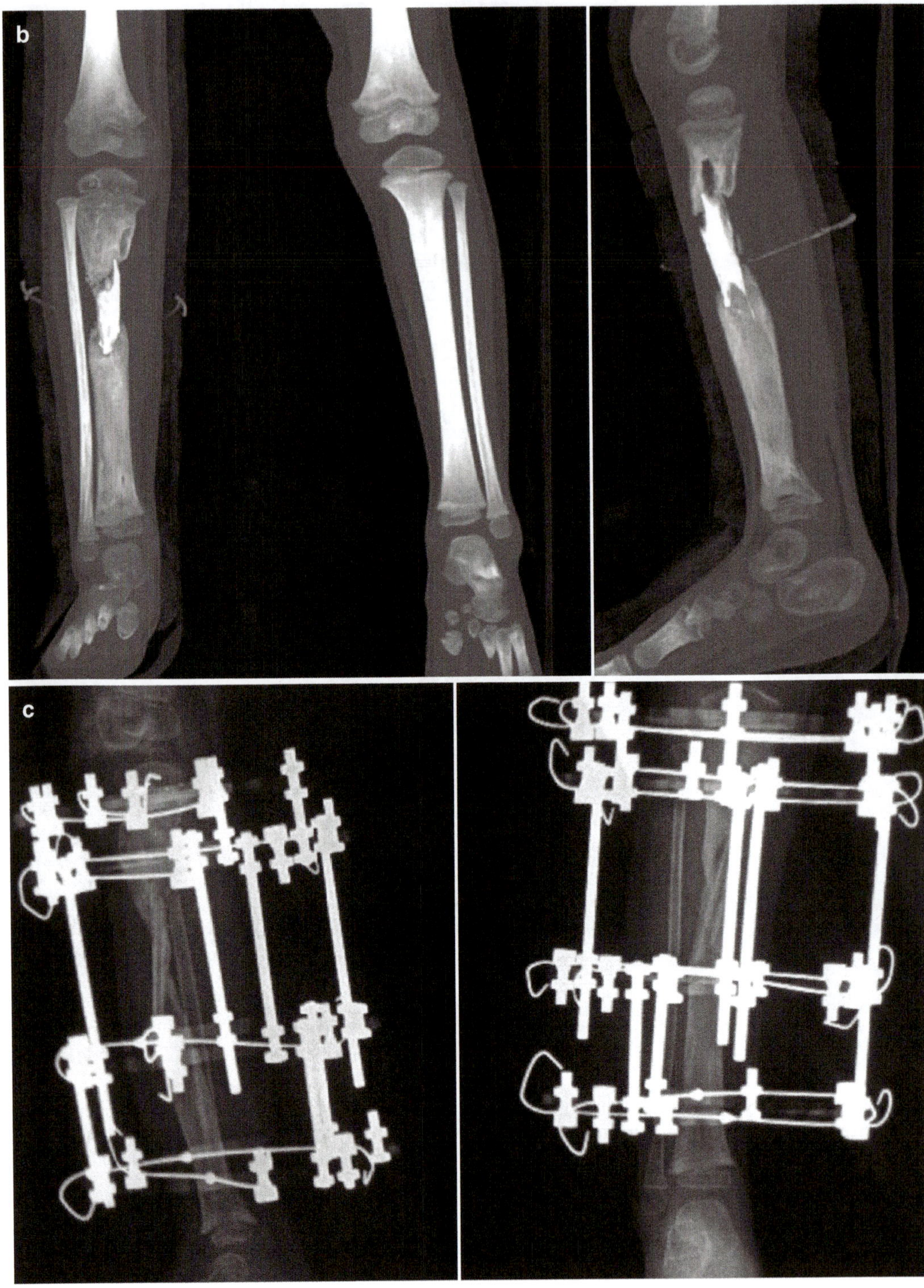

Fig. 22.8 (continued)

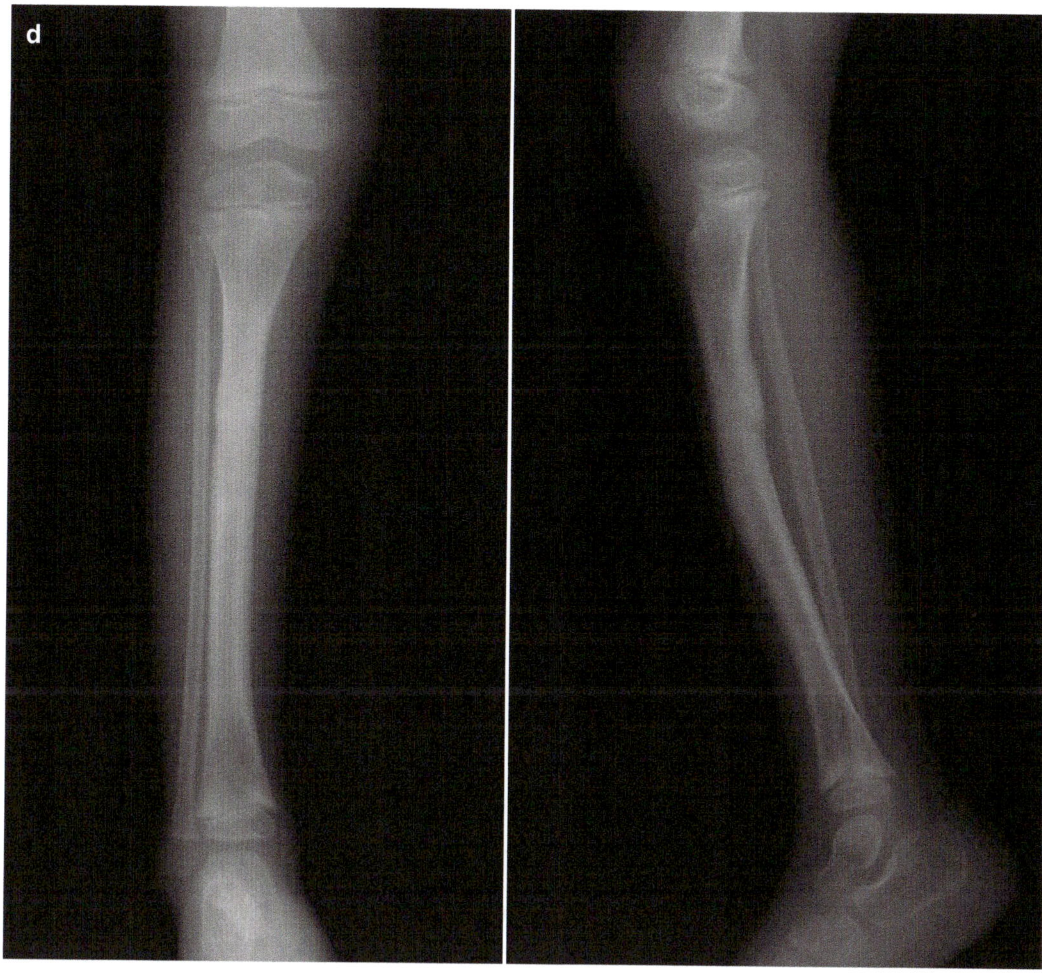

Fig. 22.8 (continued)

Belthur et al. [53] reported 88% osseous union in their series of 17 patients, with the 2 patients who had nonunion of their fractures needing supplementary bone grafting with internal fixation and bone transport with external fixation. However, the fracture healed with angular deformity in 41% of their cases which required either surgery or monitoring with possible surgery later. Yildirim et al. [73] reported a 100% healing of fractures in their series of 11 patients with no angular deformity or recurrence of infection, though 2 of their patients had shortening of 2–2.5 cm at a mean follow-up of 55.45 months (range 34–76 months).

Conclusion

The last two decades have shown an increase in the incidence and severity of musculoskeletal infections caused by CA-MRSA and more virulent strains such as pvl+ *Staphylococcus aureus*. Infections caused by these organisms are characterized by a more severe clinical course, multifocal infections, concomitant septic arthritis, and extra osseous abscesses. They are also more likely to result in sequelae such as progression to chronic osteomyelitis and pathological fractures. Demographic, clinical, laboratory, microbiological, and imaging characteristics at presentation as well as early in the course of disease have been used to predict the likelihood of developing complications. Those patients at risk of developing a complicated disease course may benefit from more aggressive, closely monitored, and individualized treatment, which may include delayed weight-bearing and activity restriction to prevent the development of pathological fractures. Once a pathological fracture occurs, resolution of the active infection is paramount, and the majority can be managed non-operatively. Internal or external fixation may be required for stabilization in weight-bearing bones or if the fracture alignment cannot be maintained otherwise.

Box 22.1 Key Messages

- Incidence of pathological fractures following hematogenous osteomyelitis is 3–5%.
- Severity of infection and virulence of organism is linked with risk of fracture.
- Extent of bone involvement, extent of subperiosteal abscess, increased number of surgical interventions – key risk factors
- Extended period of immobilization and delayed resumption of activities – useful strategy to prevent fractures
- Conservative management usually achieves union.
- Stable fixation with enhanced delivery of local antimicrobials is an alternative option to prevent malalignment and progression to chronic infection.

References

1. Lew DP, Waldvogel FA. Osteomyelitis. N Engl J Med. 1997;336(14):999–1007. https://doi.org/10.1056/nejm199704033361406.
2. Copley LAB, Herring JA. Infections of the musculoskeletal system. In: Herring JAMD, editor. Tachdjian's pediatric orthopaedics; 2014. p. 1024–76.e10.
3. Peltola H, Pääkkönen M. Acute osteomyelitis in children. N Engl J Med. 2014;370(4):352–60. https://doi.org/10.1056/NEJMra1213956.
4. Iliadis AD, Ramachandran M. Paediatric bone and joint infection. EFORT Open Rev. 2017;2(1):7–12. https://doi.org/10.1302/2058-5241.2.160027.
5. Le Saux N. Diagnosis and management of acute osteoarticular infections in children. Paediatr Child Health. 2018;23(5):336–43. https://doi.org/10.1093/pch/pxy049.
6. Funk SS, Copley LA. Acute hematogenous osteomyelitis in children: pathogenesis, diagnosis, and treatment. Orthop Clin North Am. 2017;48(2):199–208. https://doi.org/10.1016/j.ocl.2016.12.007.
7. Baker ADL, Macnicol MF. Haematogenous osteomyelitis in children: epidemiology, classification, aetiology and treatment. Paediatr Child Health. 2008;18(2):75–84. https://doi.org/10.1016/j.paed.2007.11.002.
8. Arnold SR, Elias D, Buckingham SC, Thomas ED, Novais E, Arkader A, et al. Changing patterns of acute hematogenous osteomyelitis and septic arthritis: emergence of community-associated methicillin-resistant Staphylococcus aureus. J Pediatr Orthop. 2006;26(6):703–8. https://doi.org/10.1097/01.bpo.0000242431.91489.b4.
9. Dodwell ER. Osteomyelitis and septic arthritis in children: current concepts. Curr Opin Pediatr. 2013;25(1):58–63. https://doi.org/10.1097/MOP.0b013e32835c2b42.
10. Pääkkönen MMDP, Peltola HMDP. Bone and joint infections. Pediatr Clin N Am. 2013;60(2):425–36. https://doi.org/10.1016/j.pcl.2012.12.006.
11. Saavedra-Lozano J, Falup-Pecurariu O, Faust SN, Girschick H, Hartwig N, Kaplan S, et al. Bone and joint infections. Pediatr Infect Dis J. 2017;36(8):788–99. https://doi.org/10.1097/inf.0000000000001635.
12. Gornitzky AL, Kim AE, O'Donnell JM, Swarup I. Diagnosis and management of osteomyelitis in children: a critical analysis review. JBJS Rev. 2020;8(6):e1900202. https://doi.org/10.2106/JBJS.RVW.19.00202.
13. Hensinger RN. Impending danger: community-acquired methicillin-resistant Staphylococcus aureus. J Pediatr Orthop. 2006;26(6):701–2. https://doi.org/10.1097/01.bpo.0000246917.16370.a3.
14. Saavedra-Lozano J, Mejías A, Ahmad N, Peromingo E, Ardura MI, Guillen S, et al. Changing trends in acute osteomyelitis in children: impact of methicillin-resistant Staphylococcus aureus infections. J Pediatr Orthop. 2008;28(5):569–75. https://doi.org/10.1097/BPO.0b013e31817bb816.
15. Kini AR, Shetty V, Kumar AM, Shetty SM, Shetty A. Community-associated, methicillin-susceptible, and methicillin-resistant Staphylococcus aureus bone and joint infections in children: experience from India. J Pediatr Orthop B. 2013;22(2):158–66. https://doi.org/10.1097/BPB.0b013e32835c530a.
16. Kaplan SL. Recent lessons for the management of bone and joint infections. J Infect. 2014;68:S51–S6. https://doi.org/10.1016/j.jinf.2013.09.014.
17. Sarkissian EJ, Gans I, Gunderson MA, Myers SH, Spiegel DA, Flynn JM. Community-acquired

methicillin-resistant Staphylococcus aureus musculoskeletal infections: emerging trends over the past decade. J Pediatr Orthop. 2016;36(3):323–7. https://doi.org/10.1097/bpo.0000000000000439.
18. Hultén KG, Mason EO, Lamberth LB, Forbes AR, Revell PA, Kaplan SL. Analysis of invasive community-acquired methicillin-susceptible Staphylococcus aureus infections during a period of declining community acquired methicillin-resistant Staphylococcus aureus infections at a large children's hospital. Pediatr Infect Dis J. 2018;37(3):235–41. https://doi.org/10.1097/inf.0000000000001753.
19. Crandall H, Kapusta A, Killpack J, Heyrend C, Nilsson K, Dickey M, et al. Clinical and molecular epidemiology of invasive Staphylococcus aureus infection in Utah children; continued dominance of MSSA over MRSA. PLoS One. 2020;15(9):e0238991. https://doi.org/10.1371/journal.pone.0238991.
20. Weiss L, Lansell A, Figueroa J, Suchdev P, Kirpalani A. Declining prevalence of methicillin-resistant Staphylococcus aureus septic arthritis and osteomyelitis in children: implications for treatment. Antibiotics (Basel). 2020;9:101. https://doi.org/10.3390/antibiotics9030101.
21. Martínez-Aguilar G, Avalos-Mishaan A, Hulten K, Hammerman W, Mason EO Jr, Kaplan SL. Community-acquired, methicillin-resistant and methicillin-susceptible Staphylococcus aureus musculoskeletal infections in children. Pediatr Infect Dis J. 2004;23(8):701–6. https://doi.org/10.1097/01.inf.0000133044.79130.2a.
22. Dohin B, Gillet Y, Kohler R, Lina G, Vandenesch F, Vanhems P, et al. Pediatric bone and joint infections caused by Panton-Valentine leukocidin-positive Staphylococcus aureus. Pediatr Infect Dis J. 2007;26(11):1042–8. https://doi.org/10.1097/INF.0b013e318133a85e.
23. Mitchell PD, Hunt DM, Lyall H, Nolan M, Tudor-Williams G. Panton-Valentine leukocidin-secreting Staphylococcus aureus causing severe musculoskeletal sepsis in children. A new threat. J Bone Joint Surg Br. 2007;89(9):1239–42. https://doi.org/10.1302/0301-620x.89b9.19485.
24. Hawkshead JJI, Patel NB, Steele RW, Heinrich SD. Comparative severity of pediatric osteomyelitis attributable to methicillin-resistant versus methicillin-sensitive Staphylococcus aureus. J Pediatr Orthop. 2009;29(1):85–90. https://doi.org/10.1097/BPO.0b013e3181901c3a.
25. Vander Have KL, Karmazyn B, Verma M, Caird MS, Hensinger RN, Farley FA, et al. Community-associated methicillin-resistant Staphylococcus aureus in acute musculoskeletal infection in children: a game changer. J Pediatr Orthop. 2009;29(8):927–31. https://doi.org/10.1097/BPO.0b013e3181bd1e0c.
26. Davis WT, Gilbert SR. Comparison of methicillin-resistant versus susceptible Staphylococcus aureus pediatric osteomyelitis. J Pediatr Orthop. 2018;38(5):e285–e91. https://doi.org/10.1097/bpo.0000000000001152.
27. Kavanagh N, Ryan EJ, Widaa A, Sexton G, Fennell J, O'Rourke S, et al. Staphylococcal osteomyelitis: disease progression, treatment challenges, and future directions. Clin Microbiol Rev. 2018;31(2):e00084–17. https://doi.org/10.1128/CMR.00084-17.
28. Muthukrishnan G, Masters EA, Daiss JL, Schwarz EM. Mechanisms of immune evasion and bone tissue colonization that make Staphylococcus aureus the primary pathogen in osteomyelitis. Curr Osteoporos Rep. 2019;17(6):395–404. https://doi.org/10.1007/s11914-019-00548-4.
29. Bocchini CE, Hulten KG, Mason EO, Gonzalez BE, Hammerman WA, Kaplan SL. Panton-Valentine Leukocidin genes are associated with enhanced inflammatory response and local disease in acute hematogenous *Staphylococcus aureus* osteomyelitis in children. Pediatrics. 2006;117(2):433–40. https://doi.org/10.1542/peds.2005-0566.
30. Crary SE, Buchanan GR, Drake CE, Journeycake JM. Venous thrombosis and thromboembolism in children with osteomyelitis. J Pediatr. 2006;149(4):537–41. https://doi.org/10.1016/j.jpeds.2006.06.067.
31. Gonzalez BE, Teruya J, Mahoney DH Jr, Hulten KG, Edwards R, Lamberth LB, et al. Venous thrombosis associated with staphylococcal osteomyelitis in children. Pediatrics. 2006;117(5):1673–9. https://doi.org/10.1542/peds.2005-2009.
32. Ritz N, Curtis N. The role of Panton-Valentine leukocidin in Staphylococcus aureus musculoskeletal infections in children. Pediatr Infect Dis J. 2012;31(5):514–8. https://doi.org/10.1097/INF.0b013e31824f18cb.
33. Canavese F, Samba A, Rousset M. Pathological fractures in children: diagnosis and treatment options. Orthop Traumatol Surg Res. 2016;102(1 Suppl):S149–59. https://doi.org/10.1016/j.otsr.2015.05.010.
34. Ortiz EJ, Isler MH, Navia JE, Canosa R. Pathologic fractures in children. Clin Orthop Relat Res. 2005;432:116–26. https://doi.org/10.1097/01.blo.0000155375.88317.6c.
35. De Mattos CB, Binitie O, Dormans JP. Pathological fractures in children. Bone Joint Res. 2012;1(10):272–80. https://doi.org/10.1302/2046-3758.110.2000120.
36. Snyder BD, Hauser-Kara DA, Hipp JA, Zurakowski D, Hecht AC, Gebhardt MC. Predicting fracture through benign skeletal lesions with quantitative computed tomography. JBJS. 2006;88(1):55–70. https://doi.org/10.2106/jbjs.D.02600.
37. Leong NL, Anderson ME, Gebhardt MC, Snyder BD. Computed tomography-based structural analysis for predicting fracture risk in children with benign skeletal neoplasms: comparison of specificity with that of plain radiographs. J Bone Joint Surg Am. 2010;92(9):1827–33. https://doi.org/10.2106/JBJS.I.00871.
38. Capener N, Pierce KC. Pathological fractures in osteomyelitis. JBJS. 1932;14(3):501–10.
39. Kuznetsov IB. [Pathological fractures in osteomyelitis]. Ortop Travmatol Protez. 1960;21:14–6.

40. Ismailova VN. Pathological fractures in children with hematogenous osteomyelitis. Vestn Khir Im I I Grek. 1965;94:93–5.
41. Kovalevich MD, Makletsov GP. [Pathological fractures in hematogenous osteomyelitis]. Khirurgiia (Mosk). 1966;42(2):100–4.
42. Lee CK, Hansen HT, Weiss AB. Pathological fracture in chronic osteomyelitis. Orthopedics. 1979;2(1):46–9. https://doi.org/10.3928/0147-7447-19790101-09.
43. Pick RY, Segal D. Case report. Pathological subtrochanteric fracture in an infant: an unusual disease complex and a successful result. J Pediatr Orthop. 1981;1(2):209–13. https://doi.org/10.1097/01241398-198110000-00013.
44. Walmsley BH. Pathological fracture in acute osteomyelitis in an adult. J R Soc Med. 1983;76(1):77–8.
45. Bassey LO. [Pathologic fractures as a complication of osteomyelitis. Report of experiences from the tropics of southeast Nigeria]. Unfallchirurg. 1987;90(8):394–8.
46. Barczyński A, Gaździk TS, Pasierbek M. Atypical course of hematogenous osteomyelitis of the hip: a case report and clinical considerations. Ortop Traumatol Rehabil. 2003;5(1):92–9.
47. Krebs NM, Krebs RC, Yaish AM. Femoral osteomyelitis presenting as a pathologic fracture in a 53 year old male: a rare case report. J Orthop Case Rep. 2017;7(6):85–8. https://doi.org/10.13107/jocr.2250-0685.962.
48. Taylor MN, Chaudhuri R, Davis J, Novelli V, Jaswon MS. Childhood osteomyelitis presenting as a pathological fracture. Clin Radiol. 2008;63(3):348–51. https://doi.org/10.1016/j.crad.2007.07.022.
49. Gelfand MS, Cleveland KO, Heck RK, Goswami R. Pathological fracture in acute osteomyelitis of long bones secondary to community-acquired methicillin-resistant Staphylococcus aureus: two cases and review of the literature. Am J Med Sci. 2006;332(6):357–60. https://doi.org/10.1097/00000441-200612000-00010.
50. Akinyoola AL, Orimolade EA, Yusuf MB. Pathologic fractures of long bones in Nigerian children. J Child Orthop. 2008;2(6):475–9. https://doi.org/10.1007/s11832-008-0141-x.
51. Oyemade GA, Dawodu AH, Olusanya AO. Osteomyelitis in Nigerian children (a review of 40 cases). J Trop Med Hyg. 1977;80(9):183–6.
52. Ebong WW. Pathological fracture complicating long bone osteomyelitis in patients with sickle cell disease. J Pediatr Orthop. 1986;6(2):177–81. https://doi.org/10.1097/01241398-198603000-00011.
53. Belthur MV, Birchansky SB, Verdugo AA, Mason EO Jr, Hulten KG, Kaplan SL, et al. Pathologic fractures in children with acute Staphylococcus aureus osteomyelitis. J Bone Joint Surg Am. 2012;94(1):34–42. https://doi.org/10.2106/jbjs.J.01915.
54. McNeil JC, Vallejo JG, Kok EY, Sommer LM, Hulten KG, Kaplan SL. Clinical and microbiologic variables predictive of orthopedic complications following Staphylococcus aureus acute hematogenous osteoarticular infections in children. Clin Infect Dis. 2019;69(11):1955–61. https://doi.org/10.1093/cid/ciz109.
55. Horn A, Wever S, Hoffman E. Complications following acute severe haematogenous osteomyelitis of the long bones in children. SA Orthop J. 2019;18:23–9.
56. Broodryk APSP, Hoffman EB. Fractures following acute haematogenous osteomyelitis in children. SA Bone Joint Surg. 1997;VII(4):20–2.
57. Clark CR, Morgan C, Sonstegard DA, Matthews LS. The effect of biopsy-hole shape and size on bone strength. J Bone Joint Surg Am. 1977;59(2):213–7.
58. Bickels J, Jelinek JS, Shmookler BM, Neff RS, Malawer MM. Biopsy of musculoskeletal tumors. Current concepts. Clin Orthop Relat Res. 1999;368:212–9.
59. Iwai T, Hoshi M, Oebisu N, Orita K, Shimatani A, Takada N, et al. Exploration of the optimal shape for bone tumour biopsy. Anticancer Res. 2019;39(8):4191–7. https://doi.org/10.21873/anticanres.13579.
60. Moore-Lotridge S, Gibson B, Duvernay M, Martus J, Thomsen I, Schoenecker J. Current concept review pediatric musculoskeletal infection - an update through the four pillars of clinical care and immunothrombotic similarities with COVID-19. 2020.
61. Jones HW, Harrison JW, Bates J, Evans GA, Lubega N. Radiologic classification of chronic hematogenous osteomyelitis in children. J Pediatr Orthop. 2009;29(7):822–7. https://doi.org/10.1097/BPO.0b013e3181b76933.
62. Stevenson AJ, Jones HW, Chokotho LC, Beckles VL, Harrison WJ. The Beit CURE classification of childhood chronic haematogenous osteomyelitis – a guide to treatment. J Orthop Surg Res. 2015;10:144. https://doi.org/10.1186/s13018-015-0282-9.
63. Roine I, Arguedas A, Faingezicht I, Rodriguez F. Early detection of sequela-prone osteomyelitis in children with use of simple clinical and laboratory criteria. Clin Infect Dis. 1997;24(5):849–53. https://doi.org/10.1093/clinids/24.5.849.
64. Browne LP, Mason EO, Kaplan SL, Cassady CI, Krishnamurthy R, Guillerman RP. Optimal imaging strategy for community-acquired Staphylococcus aureus musculoskeletal infections in children. Pediatr Radiol. 2008;38(8):841–7. https://doi.org/10.1007/s00247-008-0888-8.
65. Jaramillo D, Dormans JP, Delgado J, Laor T, St Geme JW 3rd. Hematogenous osteomyelitis in infants and children: imaging of a changing disease. Radiology. 2017;283(3):629–43. https://doi.org/10.1148/radiol.2017151929.
66. Manz N, Krieg AH, Heininger U, Ritz N. Evaluation of the current use of imaging modalities and pathogen detection in children with acute osteomyelitis and septic arthritis. Eur J Pediatr. 2018;177(7):1071–80. https://doi.org/10.1007/s00431-018-3157-3.
67. Pineda C, Vargas A, Rodríguez AV. Imaging of osteomyelitis: current concepts. Infect Dis Clin N Am. 2006;20(4):789–825. https://doi.org/10.1016/j.idc.2006.09.009.
68. Monsalve J, Kan JH, Schallert EK, Bisset GS, Zhang W, Rosenfeld SB. Septic arthritis in children: frequency of coexisting unsuspected osteomyelitis and implications on imaging work-up and management.

AJR Am J Roentgenol. 2015;204(6):1289–95. https://doi.org/10.2214/ajr.14.12891.
69. Copley LA, Barton T, Garcia C, Sun D, Gaviria-Agudelo C, Gheen WT, et al. A proposed scoring system for assessment of severity of illness in pediatric acute hematogenous osteomyelitis using objective clinical and laboratory findings. Pediatr Infect Dis J. 2014;33(1):35–41. https://doi.org/10.1097/inf.0000000000000002.
70. Martin AC, Anderson D, Lucey J, Guttinger R, Jacoby PA, Mok TJ, et al. Predictors of outcome in pediatric osteomyelitis: five years experience in a single tertiary center. Pediatr Infect Dis J. 2016;35(4):387–91. https://doi.org/10.1097/inf.0000000000001031.
71. Benvenuti MA, An TJ, Mignemi ME, Martus JE, Mencio GA, Lovejoy SA, et al. A clinical prediction algorithm to stratify pediatric musculoskeletal infection by severity. J Pediatr Orthop. 2019;39(3):153–7. https://doi.org/10.1097/bpo.0000000000000880.
72. Daoud A, Saighi-Bouaouina A. Treatment of sequestra, pseudarthroses, and defects in the long bones of children who have chronic hematogenous osteomyelitis. J Bone Joint Surg Am. 1989;71(10):1448–68.
73. Yildirim A, Kapukaya A, Atiç R, Mertsoy Y, Yiğit Ş, Çaçan MA, et al. The use of an "internal fixator technique" to stabilize pathologic fractures developing secondary to osteomyelitis. J Pediatr Orthop. 2017;37(3):222–6. https://doi.org/10.1097/bpo.0000000000000619.
74. Wasko MK, Kaminski R. Custom-made antibiotic cement nails in orthopaedic trauma: review of outcomes, new approaches, and perspectives. Biomed Res Int. 2015;2015:387186. https://doi.org/10.1155/2015/387186.
75. Barger J, Fragomen AT, Rozbruch SR. Antibiotic-coated interlocking intramedullary nail for the treatment of long-bone osteomyelitis. JBJS Rev. 2017;5(7):e5. https://doi.org/10.2106/jbjs.Rvw.16.00095.
76. Koury KL, Hwang JS, Sirkin M. The antibiotic nail in the treatment of long bone infection: technique and results. Orthop Clin North Am. 2017;48(2):155–65. https://doi.org/10.1016/j.ocl.2016.12.006.
77. Mader JT, Shirtliff M, Calhoun JH. Staging and staging application in osteomyelitis. Clin Infect Dis. 1997;25(6):1303–9. https://doi.org/10.1086/516149.
78. Cierny GI, Mader JT, Penninck JJ. The classic: a clinical staging system for adult osteomyelitis. Clin Orthop Relat Res. 2003;414:7–24. https://doi.org/10.1097/01.blo.0000088564.81746.62.
79. Metsemakers WJ, Fragomen AT, Moriarty TF, Morgenstern M, Egol KA, Zalavras C, et al. Evidence-based recommendations for local antimicrobial strategies and dead space management in fracture-related infection. J Orthop Trauma. 2020;34(1):18–29. https://doi.org/10.1097/bot.0000000000001615.
80. Thonse R, Conway J. Antibiotic cement-coated interlocking nail for the treatment of infected nonunions and segmental bone defects. J Orthop Trauma. 2007;21(4):258–68. https://doi.org/10.1097/BOT.0b013e31803ea9e6.
81. Kanakaris N, Gudipati S, Tosounidis T, Harwood P, Britten S, Giannoudis PV. The treatment of intramedullary osteomyelitis of the femur and tibia using the Reamer-Irrigator-Aspirator system and antibiotic cement rods. Bone Joint J. 2014;96-b(6):783–8. https://doi.org/10.1302/0301-620x.96b6.32244.
82. Bar-On E, Weigl DM, Bor N, Becker T, Katz K, Mercado E, et al. Chronic osteomyelitis in children: treatment by intramedullary reaming and antibiotic-impregnated cement rods. J Pediatr Orthop. 2010;30(5):508–13. https://doi.org/10.1097/BPO.0b013e3181e00e34.
83. Patzakis MJ, Zalavras CG. Chronic posttraumatic osteomyelitis and infected nonunion of the tibia: current management concepts. J Am Acad Orthop Surg. 2005;13(6):417–27. https://doi.org/10.5435/00124635-200510000-00006.
84. Saibaba BGN, Behera P, Santhanam SS. Prospective role of uniplanar compressible external fixation devices in the management of pathological diaphyseal fractures secondary to osteomyelitis in children. J Postgrad Med Edu Res. 2017;51(1):17–21.
85. Fenton P, Phillips J, Royston S. The use of Ilizarov frames in the treatment of pathological fracture of the femur secondary to osteomyelitis: a review of three cases. Injury. 2007;38(2):240–4. https://doi.org/10.1016/j.injury.2006.08.051.
86. Masquelet A, Kanakaris NK, Obert L, Stafford P, Giannoudis PV. Bone repair using the masquelet technique. JBJS. 2019;101(11):1024–36. https://doi.org/10.2106/jbjs.18.00842.
87. Masquelet AC, Fitoussi F, Begue T, Muller GP. [Reconstruction of the long bones by the induced membrane and spongy autograft]. Ann Chir Plast Esthet. 2000;45(3):346–53.
88. Masquelet AC, Begue T. The concept of induced membrane for reconstruction of long bone defects. Orthop Clin North Am. 2010;41(1):27–37; table of contents. https://doi.org/10.1016/j.ocl.2009.07.011.
89. Gouron R. Surgical technique and indications of the induced membrane procedure in children. Orthop Traumatol Surg Res. 2016;102(1, Supplement):S133–S9. https://doi.org/10.1016/j.otsr.2015.06.027.
90. Canavese F, Corradin M, Khan A, Mansour M, Rousset M, Samba A. Successful treatment of chronic osteomyelitis in children with debridement, antibiotic-laden cement spacer and bone graft substitute. Eur J Orthop Surg Traumatol. 2017;27(2):221–8. https://doi.org/10.1007/s00590-016-1859-7.
91. Mansour TM, Ghanem IB. Preliminary results of the induced membrane technique for the reconstruction of large bone defects. J Pediatr Orthop. 2017;37(1):e67–74. https://doi.org/10.1097/bpo.0000000000000663.
92. Rousset M, Walle M, Cambou L, Mansour M, Samba A, Pereira B, et al. Chronic infection and infected non-union of the long bones in paediatric patients: preliminary results of bone versus beta-tricalcium phosphate grafting after induced membrane formation. Int Orthop. 2018;42(2):385–93. https://doi.org/10.1007/s00264-017-3693-x.

Post Infective Deformities: Strategies for Limb Reconstruction

23

Mohan V. Belthur, Melissa Esparza,
James A. Fernandes, and Milind M. Chaudhary

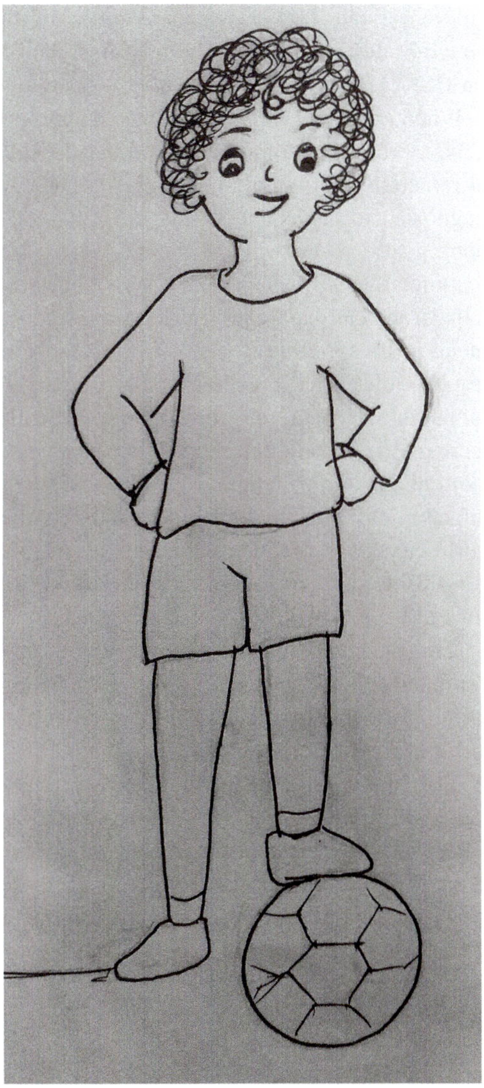

Author Contributions: All authors contributed to the study conception and design. Material preparation, data collection and analysis were performed by all authors. The first draft of the manuscript was written by Mohan Belthur and all the authors commented on previous versions of the manuscript. All the authors read and approved the final manuscript.

M. V. Belthur (✉)
Department of Child Health & Orthopedics, University of Arizona College of Medicine, Phoenix, AZ, USA

Department of Orthopedics, Phoenix Children's Hospital, Phoenix, AZ, USA
e-mail: mbelthur@phoenixchildrens.com

M. Esparza
Department of Child Health & Orthopedics, University of Arizona College of Medicine, Phoenix, AZ, USA

Department of Orthopedics, Phoenix Children's Hospital, Phoenix, AZ, USA
e-mail: mesparza@phoenixchildrens.com

J. A. Fernandes
Sheffield Children's Hospital NHS Foundation Trust, University of Sheffield, Sheffield, UK
e-mail: james.fernandes@nhs.net

M. M. Chaudhary
International Deformity & Lengthening Institute, Akola, Maharashtra, India
e-mail: milind@ilizarov.org

© Springer Nature Switzerland AG 2022
M. V. Belthur et al. (eds.), *Pediatric Musculoskeletal Infections*,
https://doi.org/10.1007/978-3-030-95794-0_23

Introduction

Pediatric musculoskeletal infections are common and constitute one of the top five conditions contributing to the burden of musculoskeletal disease in childhood [1]. With early diagnosis and appropriate treatment, the clinical course and outcomes of musculoskeletal infections are mostly benign [1, 7, 8]. However, poor outcomes, a wide spectrum of post-infective sequela, and significant functional impairment can occur, especially in the setting of delayed diagnosis, inadequate and inappropriate treatment, or infection caused by virulent organisms like Panton-Valentine leukocidin-producing strains of SA [8, 14, 15, 18, 29–37, 42]. This chapter provides an overview of the epidemiology, pathogenesis, spectrum of sequela, principles of management, and reconstructive options for post-infective sequela of the extremities. We discuss in detail the management options for growth plate arrest, deformity, and limb length discrepancy in this chapter. The subsequent chapters discuss management of bone defects of the upper and lower extremity, pathologic fractures, and sequelae of septic arthritis of the hip.

Epidemiology

Musculoskeletal infections (MSKI) are a significant source of pediatric morbidity worldwide [1]. The estimated incidence of pediatric osteoarticular infections in developed countries has been reported as 1 to 25 per 100,000, with osteomyelitis being more common than septic arthritis [2–8]. Approximately, 33% of these cases occur in children during their first 2 years of life [2–8]. The incidence of concurrent osteomyelitis and septic arthritis has been reported at a rate of 17–33% [2, 3, 9]. Other infectious conditions such as pyomyositis, discitis, and vertebral osteomyelitis also contribute to the global burden of MSKI [1].

The burden of disease of MSKI is even higher in low- and middle-income countries (LMIC), where more than 80% of the world's children live [1, 10, 11]. A higher incidence of disease is further exacerbated by limited access to care. A 2020 survey on the burden of pediatric musculoskeletal disease worldwide reports that more than one third of the world's population live in low-income countries but receive only 3.5% of the world's surgical care [1]. Within developed countries, there are also substantial health disparities in the incidence and outcomes of patients with MSKI [2, 3, 12]. Recent surveys from the nationwide Kids Inpatient Database report that children living in lower-income areas in the United States are more likely to be hospitalized for MSKI [2, 3].

When identified early and managed appropriately, morbidity and mortality of musculoskeletal infections can be minimized [6, 7]. Delay in diagnosis and inadequate or inappropriate treatment can result in sequelae [10, 11]. Postinfectious sequelae of the bones, joints, and soft tissues can have harmful long-term consequences for a child [8, 13–15]. Orthopedic sequelae of MSKI include chronic osteomyelitis, pathologic fracture, growth arrest, avascular necrosis, joint contracture, angular deformity, shortening, limb length discrepancy, bone defects, and early arthritis. Various studies worldwide have reported complication rates of 4.7–48% for orthopedic and medical complications of MSKI [8, 13–18].

Over the past 20 years, multiple studies have evaluated the changing epidemiology of MSKI, particularly the increase in MRSA infections and other antibiotic-resistant organisms. [7, 8, 19, 20]. Many of these studies have reported the rise in antibiotic resistance and virulence factors resulting in increased severity and invasiveness of musculoskeletal infections [19, 20] and, consequently, more long-term sequelae [14, 19, 20].

Impact

MSK infections represent a heavy burden on health systems and on the society at large as significant resources are needed for their diagnosis and management. MSK infections and their sequelae can cause functional impairment resulting in poor overall health, disability, social isolation, and restriction from school. The social burden of neglected infections affects not only the patients but also their families. It has been shown that prolonged hospital admission during childhood is associated with behavioral problems, delinquency, and even unstable job patterns in adulthood. Parents may have to spend extended periods away from work and may even lose their jobs because of the child's condition [1, 11].

Pathogenesis

The role of the acute-phase response (APR) in the pathogenesis of acute MSKI has been well described in recent studies [26–28]. While the acute-phase response plays an important role in the body's response to acute infection and trauma, including wound healing and pathogen clearance, it paradoxically can also result in long-term damage to the involved and neighboring tissues. Dysregulation of the coagulation and inflammatory response to an infectious insult, described as "hijacking the acute-phase response," can impair musculoskeletal regeneration and lead to long-term sequelae of the bones, joints, and soft tissues [27]. Different organisms have developed various mechanisms "for evading and hijacking the hemostatic, tissue regenerative, and antimicrobial properties of the acute-phase response."

Multiple studies have evaluated risk factors for developing complications and long-term sequelae of MSKI [29–37]. These risk factors align with the framework of the dysregulated acute-phase response described by the Vanderbilt group [26–28]. As the severity or duration of an infection increases, tissue damage progressively worsens due to overactive inflammatory and coagulation cascades. This dysregulation of inflammatory and coagulation responses can result in medical complications of septic DVT/PE, septic shock, and death in the most severe cases [28]. The same processes are responsible for some of the orthopedic sequelae due to the disrupted vascularity of developing bone in children. For example, disruption of vascularity to the femoral head may cause avascular necrosis and subsequent bone loss and joint destruction. Vascular disruption can affect any portion of the bone, which may lead to stiffness, joint contractures, weak bone and secondary pathologic fractures, angular deformity, and bone defects. Vascular disruption to the growth plate can result in partial or complete growth arrests.

Reported risk factors for developing sequelae of osteomyelitis include delayed source control, prolonged fever (100.4°) for >4 days, resistant infectious organisms, increased virulence of the infective organism (agr group III), increased magnitude and duration of CRP levels, immunocompromised state, and other comorbidities [13–15, 32–34].

Risk factors for developing sequelae of septic arthritis include delayed diagnosis >4 days, inadequate treatment, neonatal risk factors (prematurity, hypoxia, central venous catheterization), concurrent osteomyelitis, MRSA, PVL+ strains, and sickle cell disease [17, 25, 34, 36]. Late sequelae are more frequently seen after septic arthritis of the hip and shoulder than after septic arthritis of the of the other joints (knee, ankle, elbow, and wrist), because septic arthritis in these joints is more common, diagnosed later and is more frequently associated with concurrent osteomyelitis [21–25, 36].

Several studies have evaluated the efficacy of using total CRP to predict the risk of thrombotic events and found that increased peak CRP and the duration of its elevation are associated with infection severity and risk for thrombotic complications. Various institutions have evaluated some of these risk factors to propose predictive classification systems, severity of illness scores, and evidence-based guidelines [29, 38, 39]. These can help to risk stratify, utilize resources appropriately, guide management to optimize short- and long-term outcomes, and predict which patients are at risk for developing complications [38–40].

Risk factors for developing MSKI sequelae

Septic arthritis	Osteomyelitis
Delayed diagnosis >4 days	Delayed source control
Inadequate treatment	Prolonged fever (100.4°) for >4 days
Neonatal risk factors (prematurity, hypoxia, central venous catheterization)	Resistant infectious organisms
MRSA, PVL+ strains	Increased virulence (agr group III)
Sickle cell disease	Increased magnitude/ duration of CRP levels
Concurrent osteomyelitis	Immunocompromised state/other comorbidities

Spectrum of Disease

A diverse spectrum of post-infective sequelae can be seen depending on the site of infection, patient's age, infecting organism, host resistance, timing and adequacy of initial treatment, and severity/extent of damage to the affected bone (involvement of the physis/epiphysis) [8, 18, 21–24].

Complications of MSKI can occur during the acute infectious phase, subacutely, and as long-term sequelae. While this chapter focuses on musculoskeletal sequelae of acute and chronic infections, it is equally important to note the significant medical complications that are associated with MSKI. Pediatric patients with disseminated musculoskeletal infections can develop deep vein thromboses (DVT), pulmonary or other emboli (PE), pulmonary edema, pleural effusion, pericardial effusion, septic shock, multiorgan failure, and even death [33, 34, 37, 42].

Orthopedic complications often present subacutely, either following resolution of the infection or with inadequate clearance of the infection. Inadequate clearance of the infection following acute hematogenous osteomyelitis can result in the development of chronic osteomyelitis, sequestrum, and malignant transformation (rarely) [11, 18, 32]. Pathologic fractures may occur through the weakened bone following osteomyelitis and result in subsequent nonunion and malunion, with or without or segmental bone loss [18, 43–46]. Involvement of the physis in the affected area can cause physeal disturbance and growth arrest and secondary angular deformities of the long bones or limb length discrepancy [8, 18, 21, 47–49].

Septic arthritis may cause a spectrum of consequences for involved joints, ranging from joint stiffness in the short term to more permanent joint contractures and chondrolysis, ankylosis, or joint instability. Damage to the epiphysis and/or physis secondary to direct destruction by the infecting organism or secondary to avascular necrosis can result in post-infective articular and juxta-articular deformities [8, 21–25, 41, 48, 49].

Concurrent osteoarticular infections may cause any combination of the above, with both joint damage and bony deformity. These are more common around the shoulder and hip, as the metaphysis is intra-articular [8, 9, 36, 104].

Soft tissue infections such as pyomyositis, necrotizing fasciitis, and gas gangrene can also result in significant complications, morbidity, and mortality [50–52]. Complications reported include joint contractures, compartment syndrome, and concurrent osteomyelitis [117].

Classification

The ABCDS classification was proposed by Chaudhary et al. to facilitate creating a problem list and develop management strategies/solutions to treat sequelae of osteomyelitis. We propose a modification that can be used for all MSKI [53].

The ABCDs of MSKI sequelae

Arrest (partial or complete growth arrest)

Bone gap, pathologic fractures, sequestra

Contractures or instability (joint contractures, joint instability)

Deformity in all 3 planes (coronal, sagittal, transverse)

Shortening/lengthening (limb length discrepancy)

Other: relapse, avascular necrosis, malignant transformation

Presentation

The above sequelae can present early (infection is active) or late (infection has been controlled). Patients can present with pain, deformity, loss of function (difficulty to ambulate in the lower extremity or difficulty with reach/activities of daily living with upper extremity problems, respectively), limb length discrepancy, or joint instability (Figs. 23.1, 23.2, 23.3, 23.4, 23.5, 23.6, 23.7, 23.8, 23.9, and 23.10).

Evaluation

Proper evaluation, based on a thorough history, musculoskeletal examination, and imaging studies, allows the surgeon to create a problem list that identifies factors causing functional impairment, develop effective treatment solutions to address each problem, have the goal of optimizing the functional potential of the patient.

Management

Treatment of these post-infective sequelae can be challenging. However, timely, well-planned, and well-executed reconstructive options can ensure continued growth and development of the limb by restoring the mechanical axis of the limb, individual joint alignment, and stability, thus providing the best possible joint mechanics at skeletal maturity.

A: Growth Arrest/Growth Plate Disturbances

One of the most serious and challenging long-term complications of bone and joint infection in infants and children is growth disturbance.

Incidence The incidence of physeal arrest secondary to osteoarticular infections is not well established, but rates have been reported in several cohorts of patients [18, 41, 47, 54, 55]; in one series, the incidence of growth arrest was approximately 20% of 100 cases collected from 1943 to 1970 [54]. In another series of neonatal osteomyelitis, 71% had concurrent joint infection, and half of these patients developed a growth arrest. Tudisco et al. reported an incidence of 15% in a group of 26 patients with chronic osteomyelitis followed to skeletal maturity [47]. Ecklund et al. described MRI patterns of physeal arrest in 111 patients, of which 70.3% were posttraumatic, 7.2% secondary to infection, and the remainder from other causes [55]. Horn et al. reported on a cohort of 103 South African patients who were treated surgically for AHO in the long bones, with 39 patients

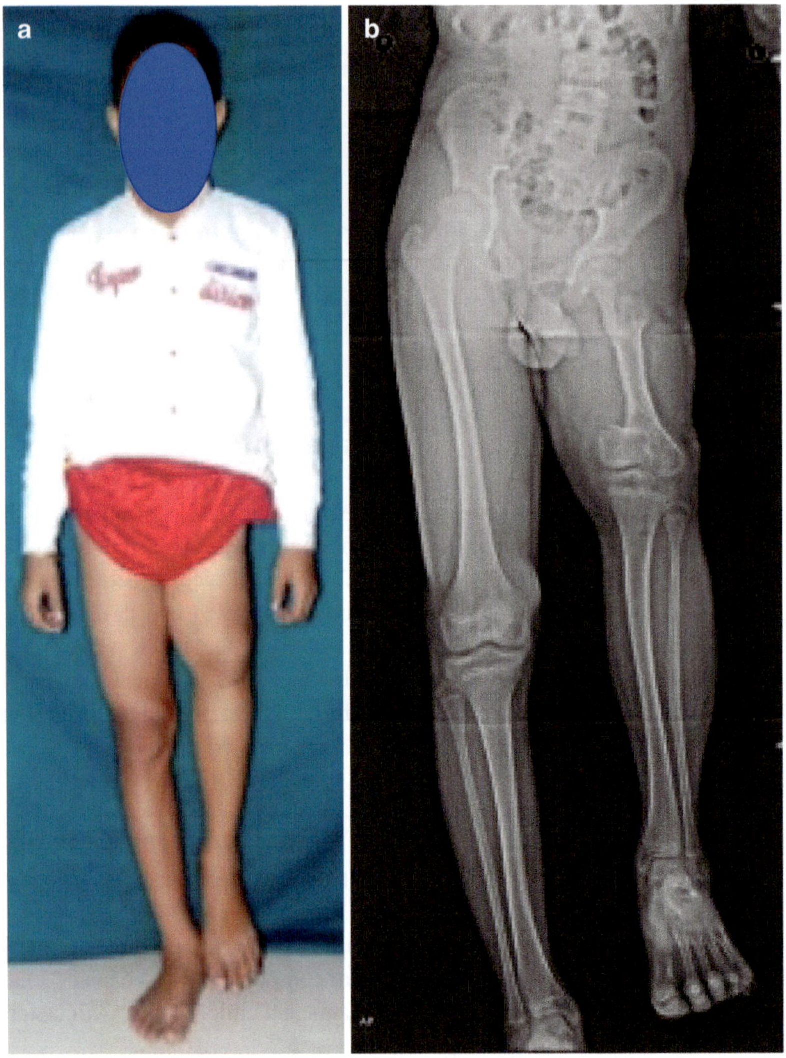

Fig. 23.1 Case 1: Shortening left femur. (Courtesy Dr. Milind Chaudhary). (**a**, **b**) A 10-year-old male with dramatic shortening of 14 cm and mild varus of the left femur secondary to complete growth arrest of the left distal femur growth plate s/p neonatal left knee septic arthritis with concurrent osteomyelitis. He also has mild valgus of the proximal tibia. His predicted LLD at maturity is 20 cm. (**c**, **d**) He had gradual lengthening of his left femur of 9 cm through a proximal femoral osteotomy using a monolateral limb reconstruction rail. (**e**, **f**) 1-year postop, showing a residual 5 cm LLD with mild distal femur varus. He will need a second lengthening with a contralateral epiphysiodesis to equalize his LLD at skeletal maturity. He will also need correction of his distal femur varus

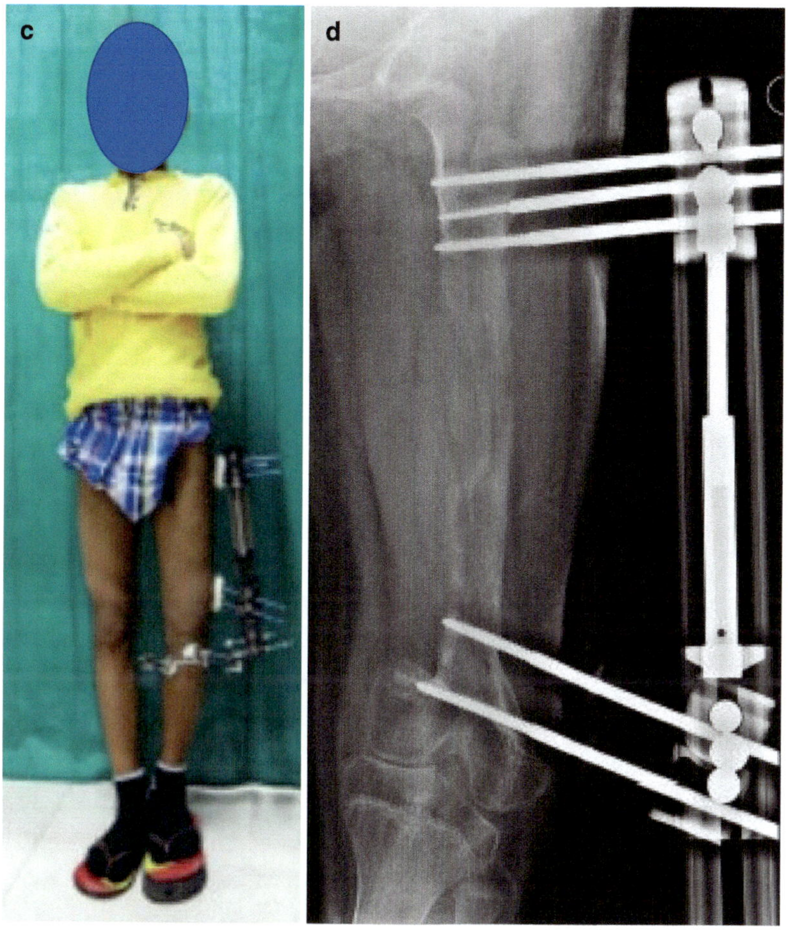

Fig. 23.1 (continued)

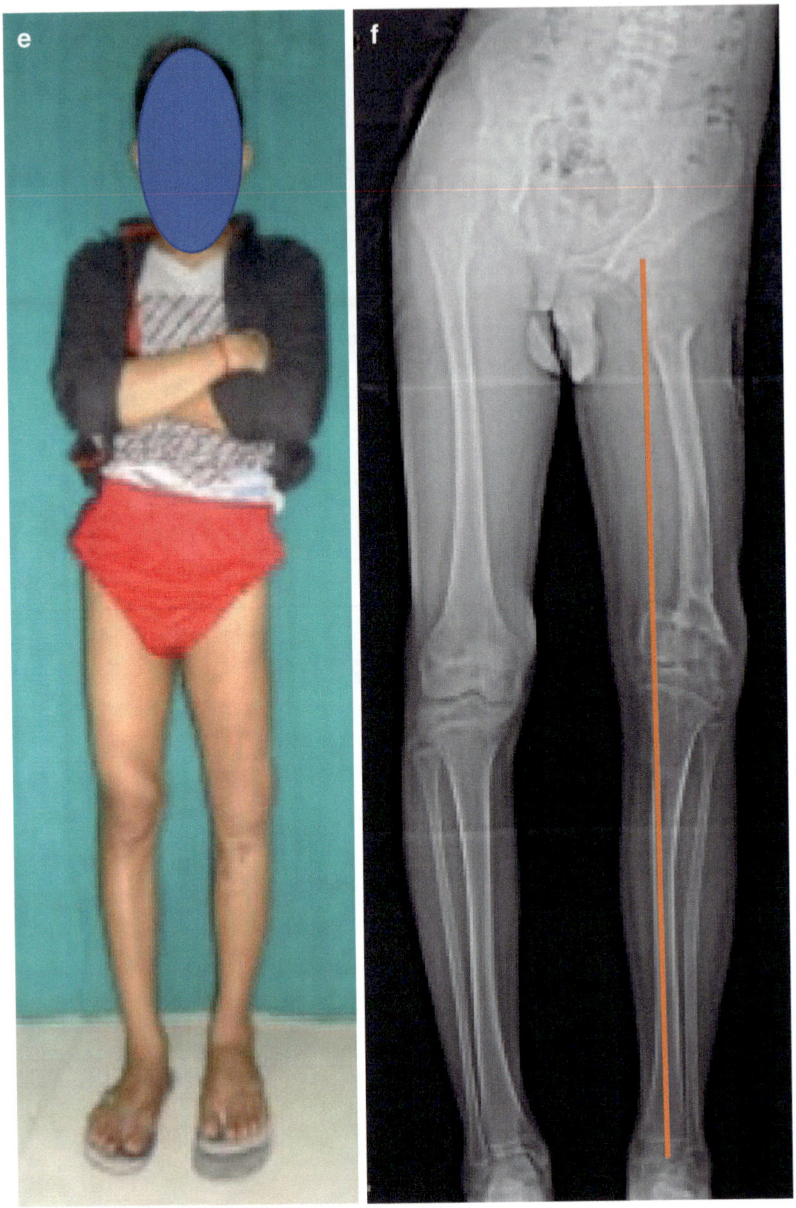

Fig. 23.1 (continued)

developing 67 complications. Growth arrest accounted for 9 of the 67 (13.4%) complications, with 3 of those 9 resulting in limb length discrepancies greater than 2 centimeters [18]. Peters et al. reported on long-term sequelae of a cohort of 6 patients with physeal injury secondary to neonatal septic arthritis and osteomyelitis treated from 1960 to 1989 [41]. The treatment protocol during the initial presentation of these patients included antibiotics and joint aspiration, with surgical incision and drainage (I&D) performed in only one patient. Sequelae included shortening, deformity, and dislocation. The authors stressed the importance of appropriate antibiotics and surgical drainage and the current standard of care in the modern era.

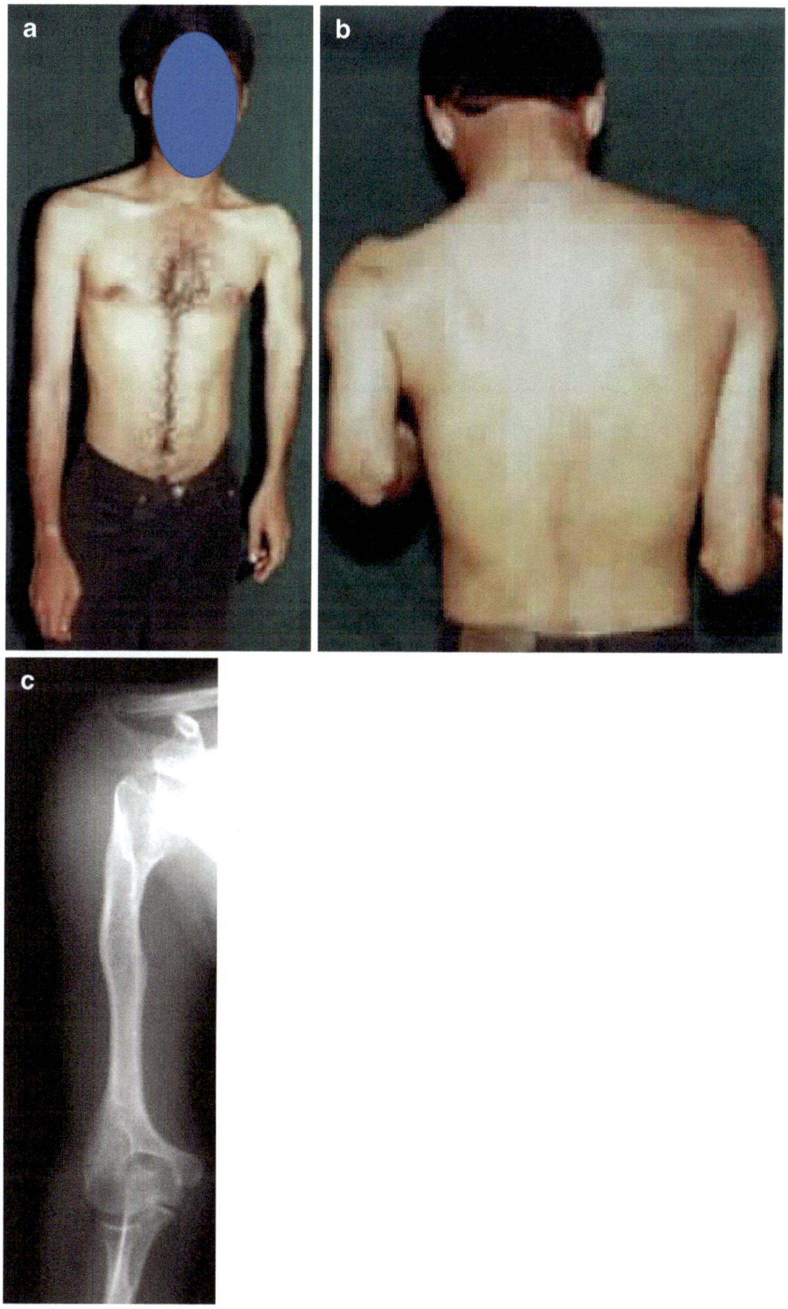

Fig. 23.2 Case 2: Shortening of Left Humerus. (Courtesy Dr. Milind Chaudhary). (**a**–**c**) An 18-year-old male with mild proximal humerus varus and shortening of 11 cm of left humerus, s/p concurrent neonatal osteomyelitis, and septic arthritis of the left shoulder with growth arrest of proximal humerus. (**d**–**g**) Gradual left humeral lengthening using a circular external fixator. (**h**–**k**) 1-year postop, with equalized limb lengths and good alignment. (**l**, **m**) Clinical photos showing excellent range of motion left elbow

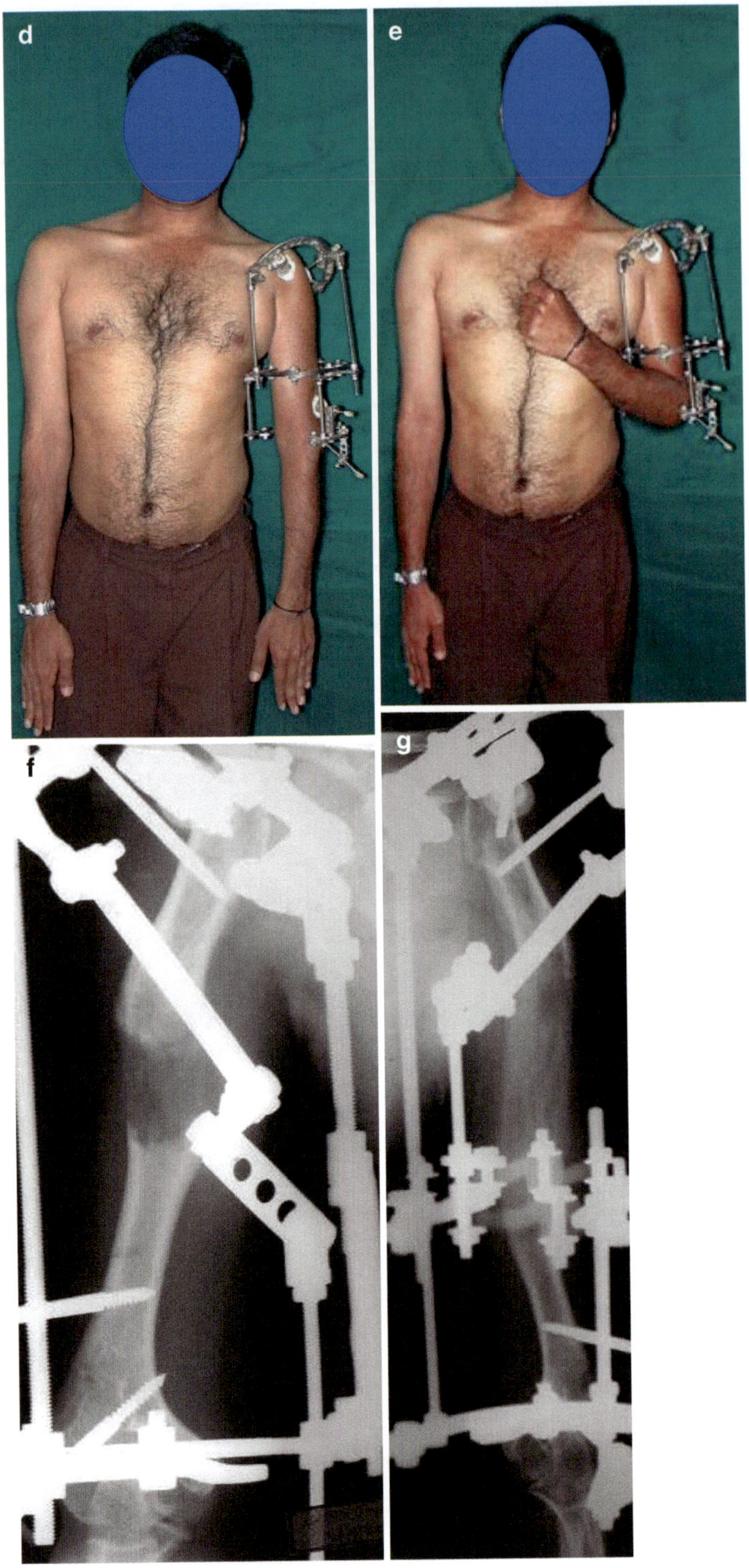

Fig. 23.2 (continued)

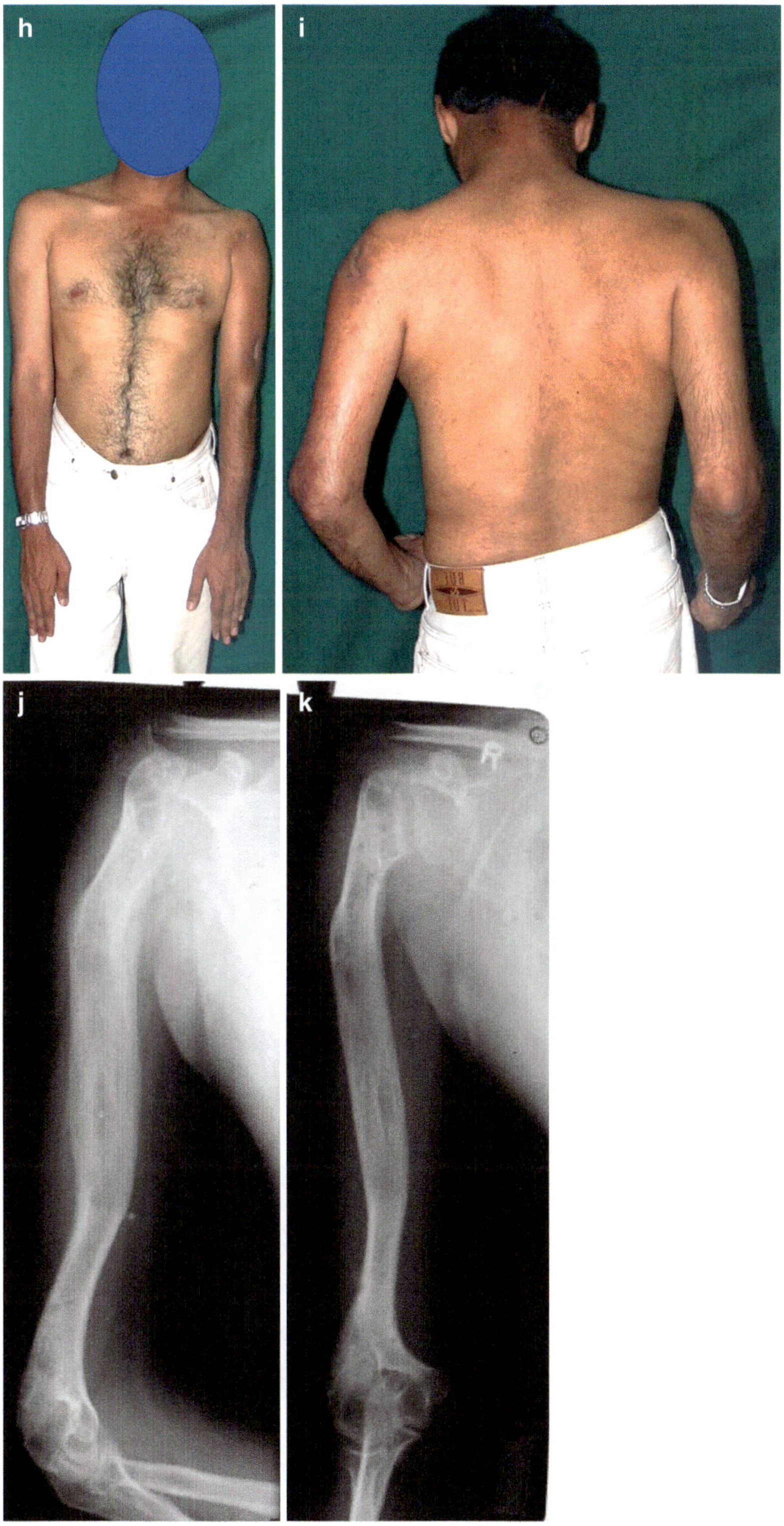

Fig. 23.2 (continued)

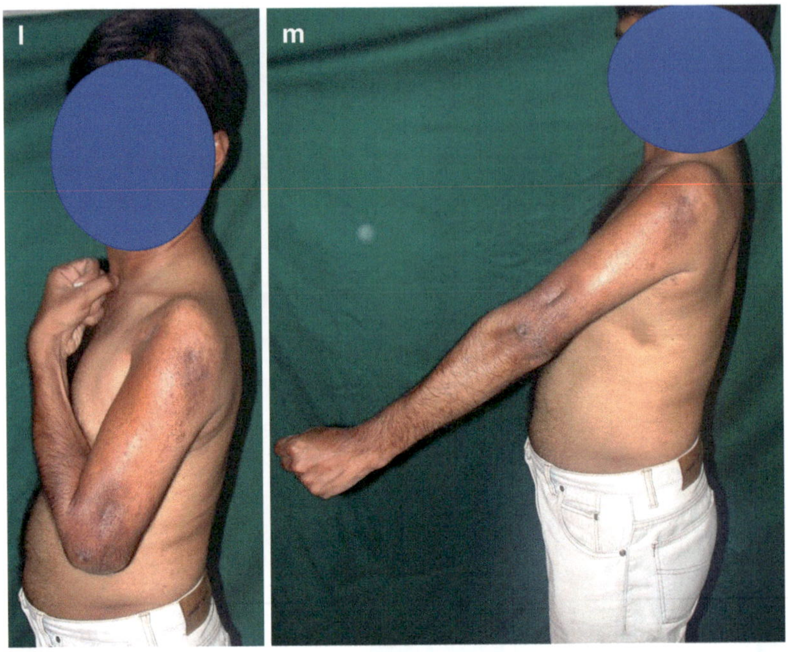

Fig. 23.2 (continued)

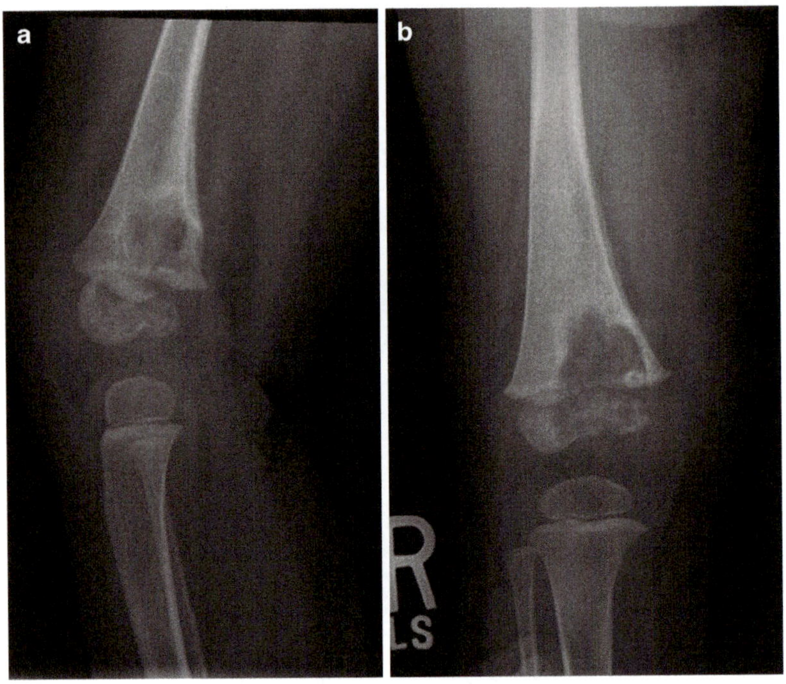

Fig. 23.3 Case 3: Growth arrest partial central. (Courtesy Dr. William Wood). (**a, b**) 1+ 3-year-old girl with AP/Lat radiographs of the right knee showing transphyseal osteomyelitis of the distal femur. (**c–d**) Radiographs of Rt knee s/p treatment of osteomyelitis. (**f–h**) Radiographs of Rt knee and LEs at age 3+3 years, showing a partial central growth arrest of Rt distal femur. Bar resection proposed but lost to follow-up. (**i, j**) Bone length radiographs at age 10+3 & 10+9 years, showing increasing LLD (6 cm) due to growth arrest of Rt distal femur. Predicted LLD 10 cm. (**k–m**) Age 11 years, 3 months postop radiographs s/p intramedullary lengthening with a precise nail, showing healing osteoplasty Rt femur with residual 1.4 cm LLD Rt < left femur. 4.5 cm of length achieved. Will need a further lengthening nearer to skeletal maturity

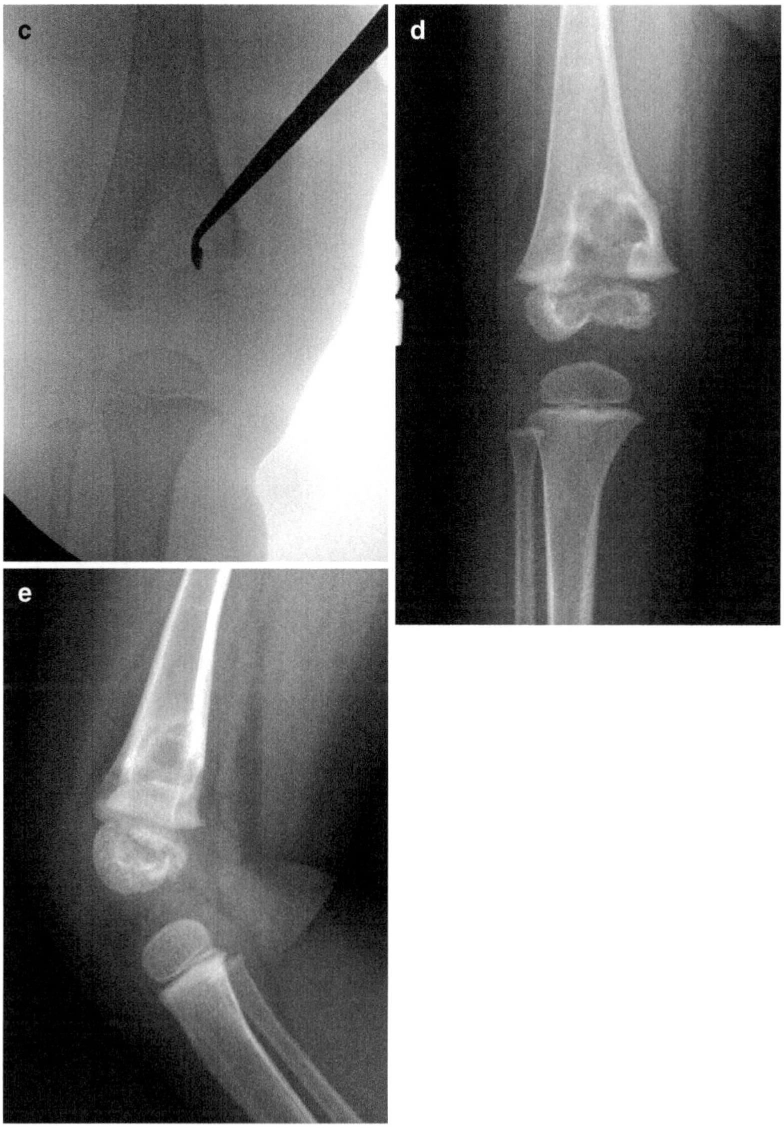

Fig. 23.3 (continued)

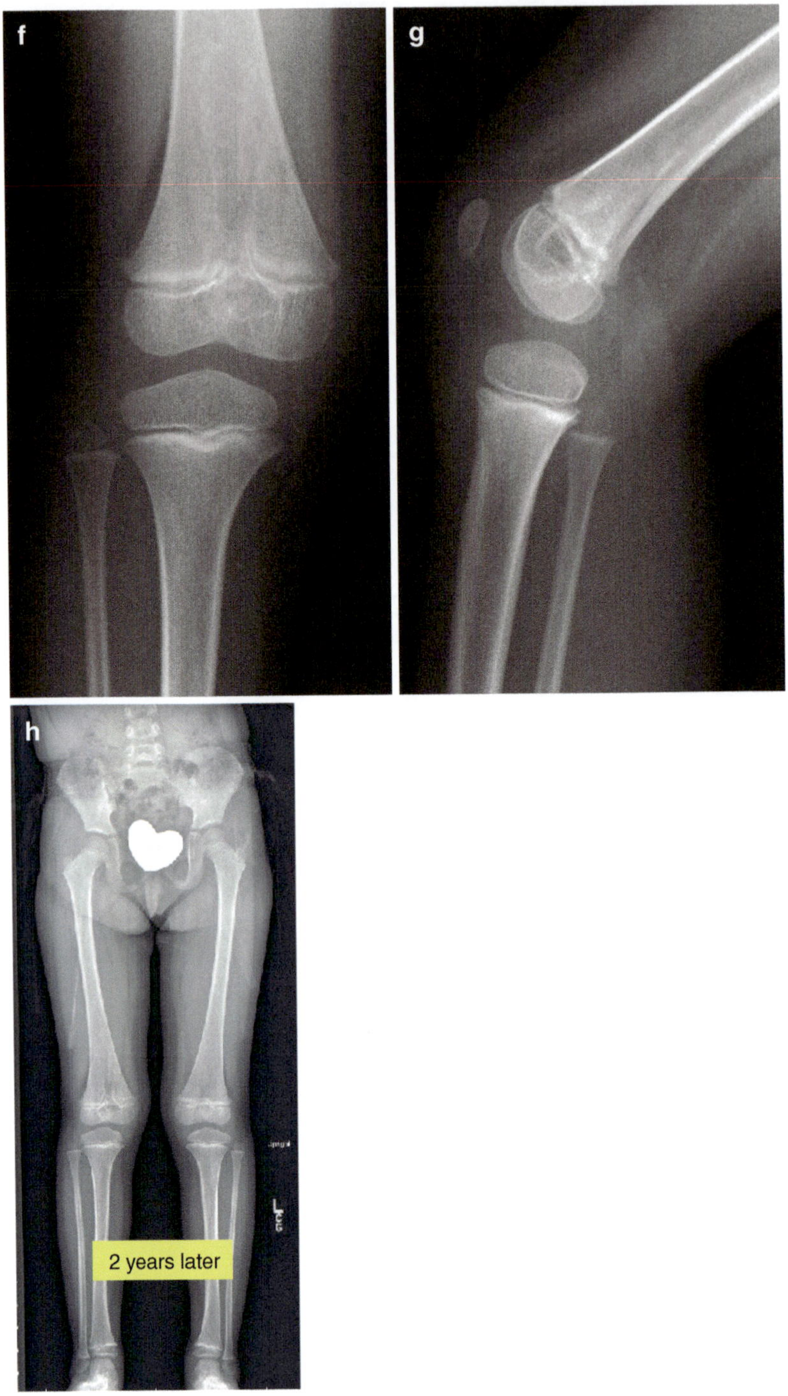

Fig. 23.3 (continued)

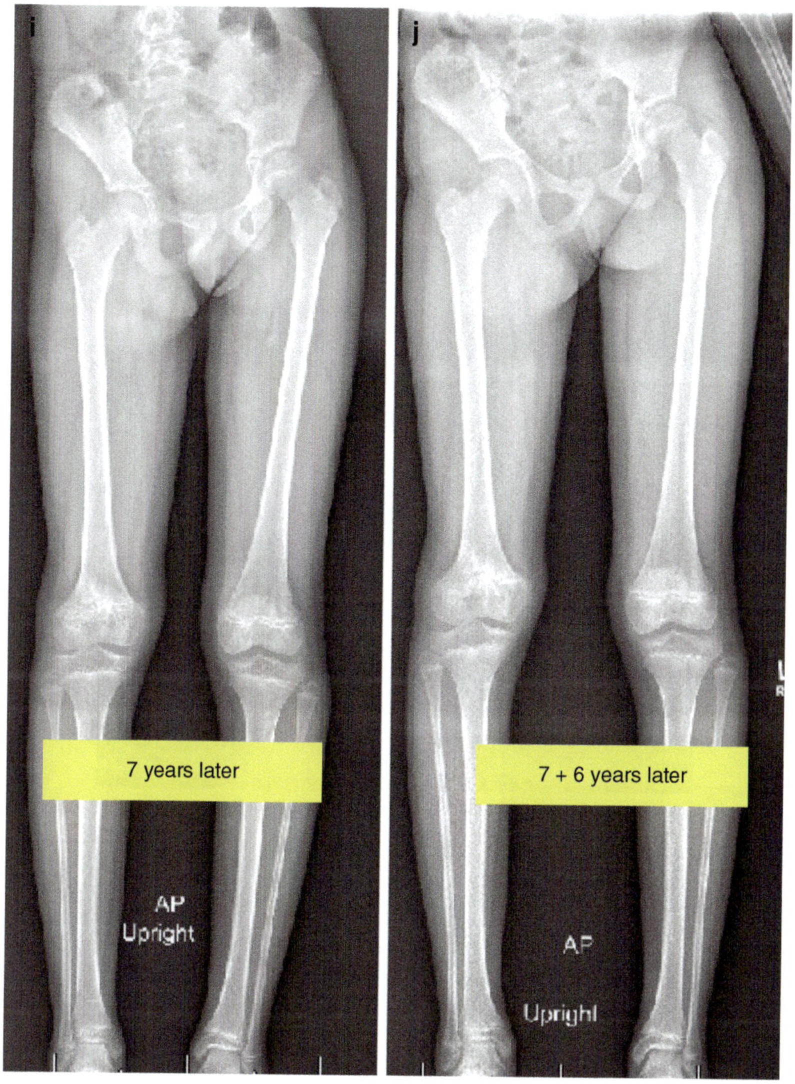

Fig. 23.3 (continued)

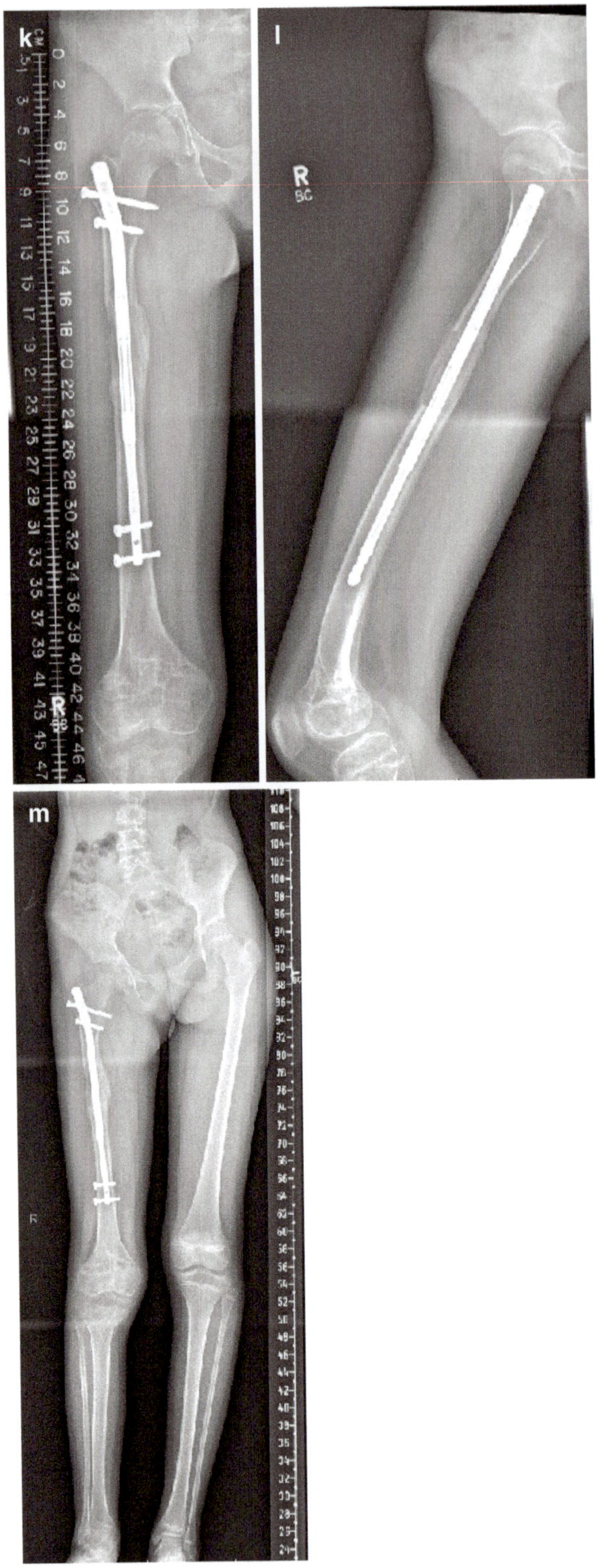

Fig. 23.3 (continued)

Location The distal and proximal femur are involved in 50% of cases, followed in frequency by the proximal and distal tibia, proximal humerus, distal radius, distal ulna, distal fibula, metacarpals, phalanges, and metatarsals. Multifocal growth arrest can occur and is usually secondary to multifocal septic arthritis and less commonly due to multifocal osteomyelitis [56].

Risk factors Infants with osteomyelitis have a greater propensity to develop growth arrest and resultant severe deformities than older children, as they have less immunity, transphyseal blood vessels, bony trabeculae that are weaker, a higher prevalence of concurrent osteomyelitis and adjacent joint septic arthritis, and chondrocytes that are more susceptible to damage. Delayed diagnosis and inadequate/inappropriate treatment increase the risk for developing growth arrests [8, 22–24, 56].

Pathogenesis Infection can cause physeal damage directly by spread of infection to the epiphysis through the transphyseal vessels, resulting in

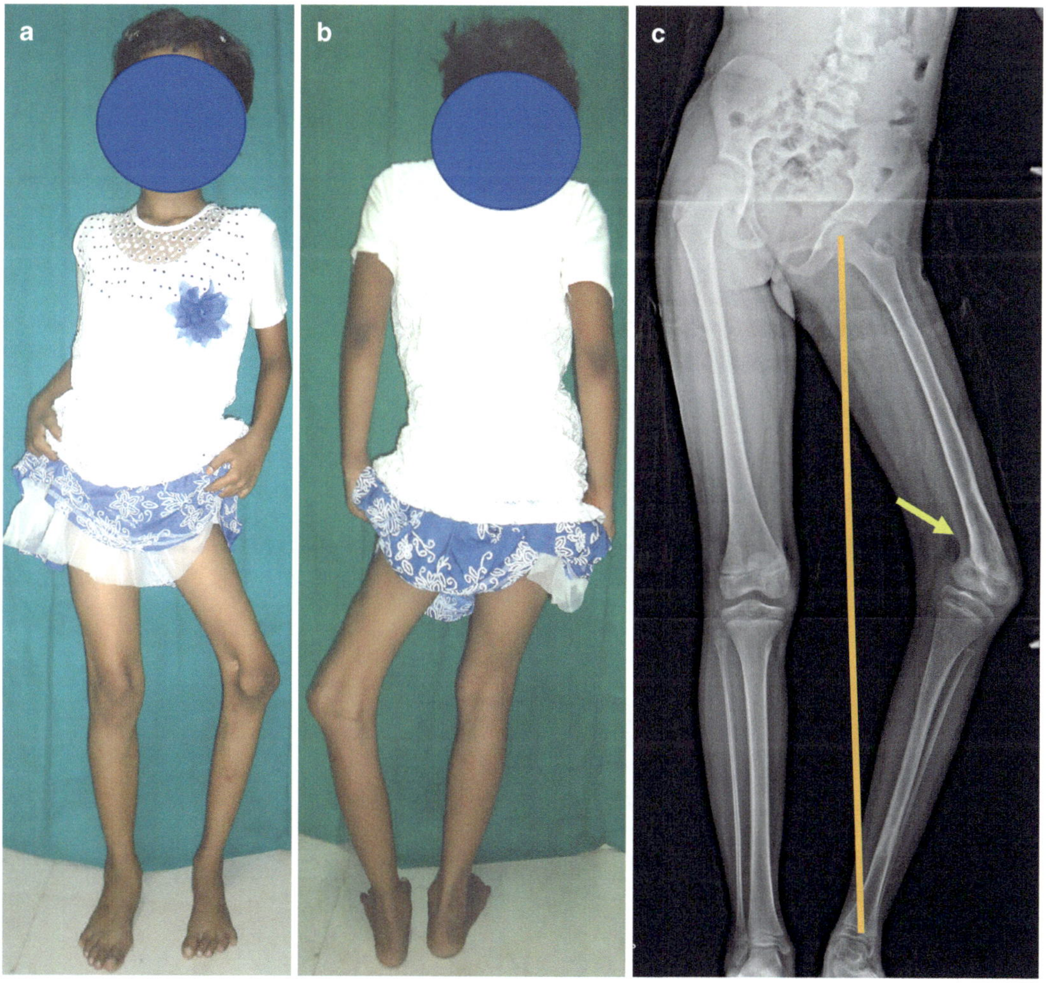

Fig. 23.4 Case 4: Growth arrest partial peripheral. (Courtesy Dr. Milind Chaudhary). (**a**–**c**) An 11-year-old girl with a left distal femur medial physeal bar with varus deformity and dramatic shortening. (**d**–**g**) Physeal bar excision through a laterally based triangular osteotomy and lengthening/deformity correction through the metaphyseal face of the triangular osteotomy. (**h**–**j**) 1-year postop, she is overlengthened and slightly overcorrected. A long-standing deformity like this is always overcompensated by the adjacent segment. Notice the valgus in the proximal tibia. The overlengthening will compensate the discrepancy for some more years

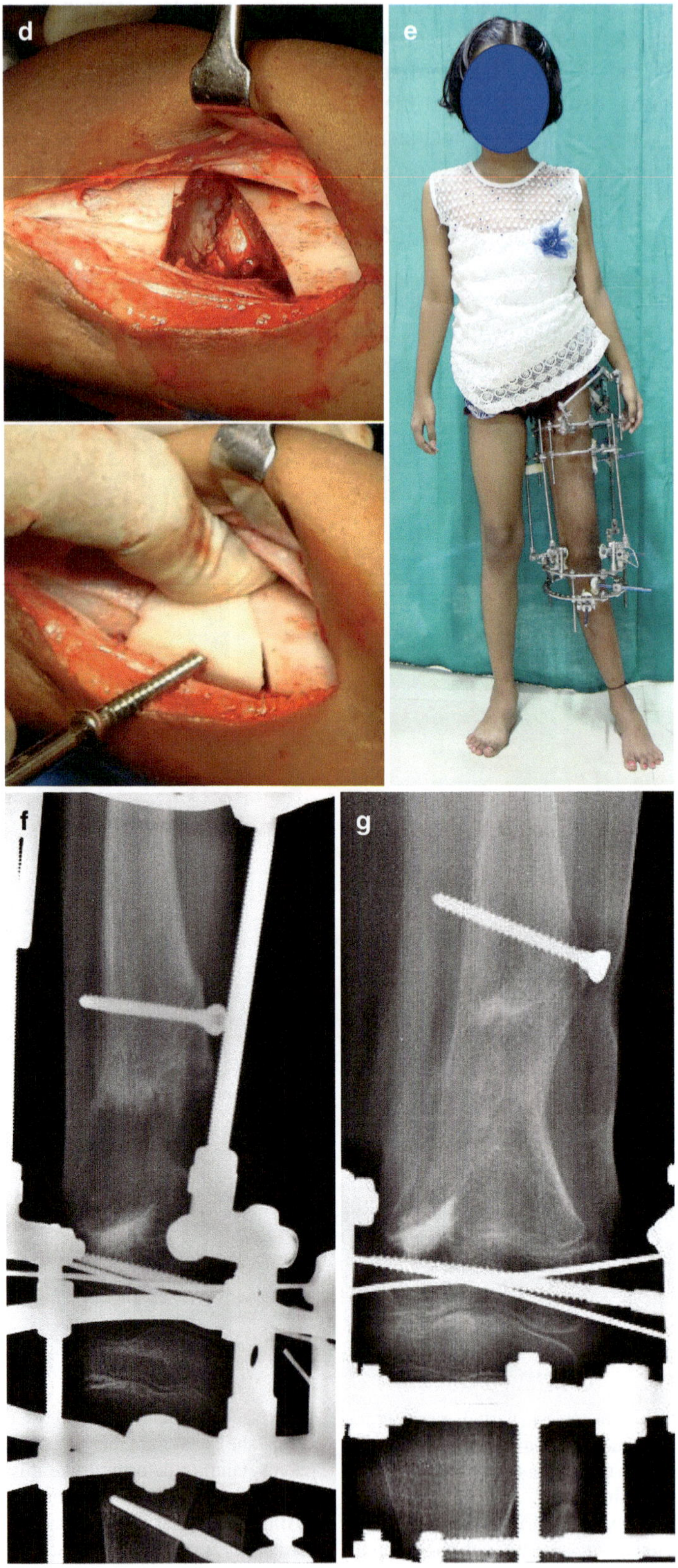

Fig. 23.4 (continued)

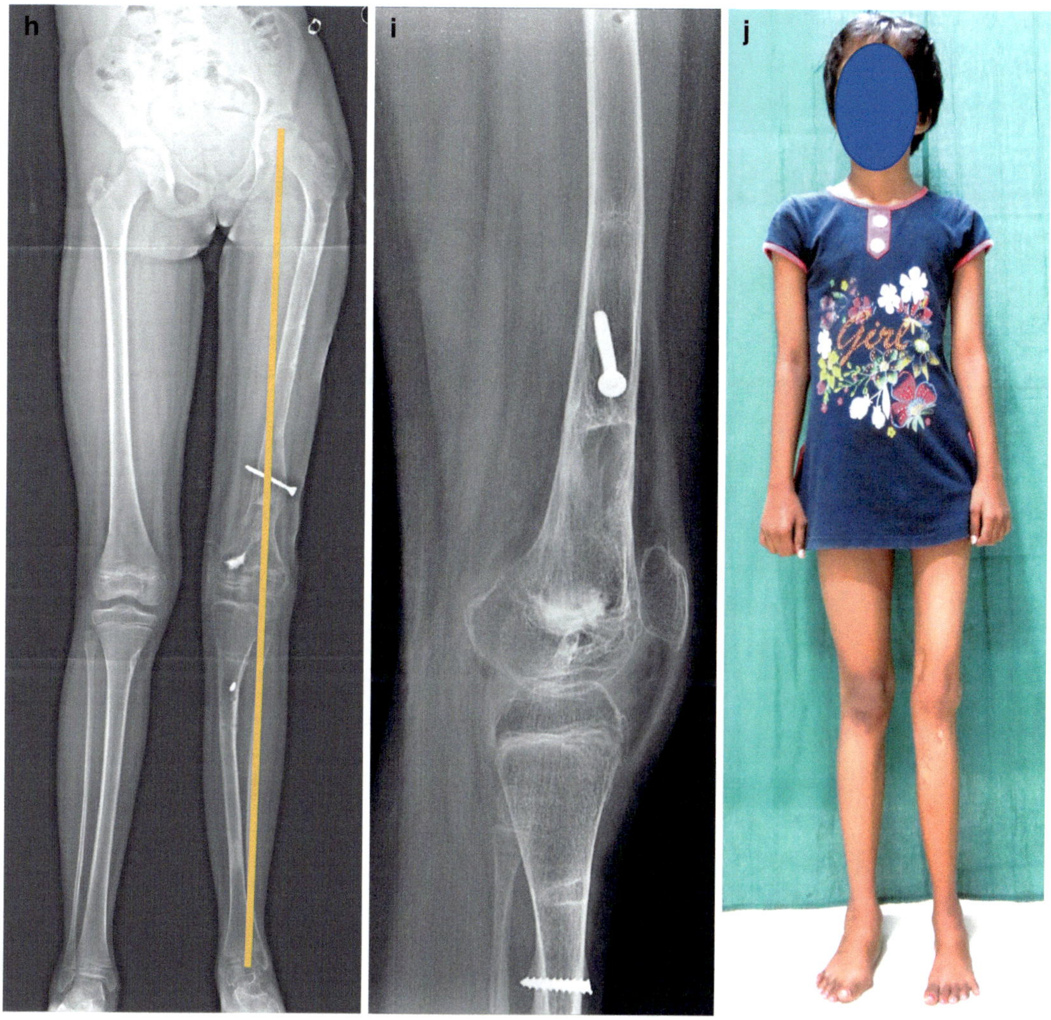

Fig. 23.4 (continued)

chondrolysis or indirectly by ischemia due to compression of the epiphyseal arcade of vessels by the septic process [56, 57]. In contrast to the classic belief that the avascular growth plate serves as a barrier to the transphyseal spread of infection, relatively recent data indicate that up to 81% of patients 2–16 years of age with pyogenic infection have MR imaging findings of transphyseal spread that has been postulated to represent direct injury of the underlying growth plate [58]. Physeal damage can result in the formation of a physeal bar, a variably sized bridge of bone from the metaphysis across the physis to the epiphysis, an entity also known as premature partial physeal arrest or closure. Physeal arrest can be complete or partial, with partial being more common. The osseous bar tethers the growth of the remaining normal physis, which results in deformities of the metaphysis, physis, and epiphysis, relative shortening of the involved bone, and angular deformity of the limb if the bar is eccentric [55–57].

Pathology In 1979, Ogden described the pathogenesis of physeal injury due to osteoarticular infection in neonates [57]. His conclusions were based on his findings of histologic evaluations of 55 foci of osteomyelitis and 11 septic joints in specimens from five affected patients. Differences in the pathophysiologic processes of osteomyeli-

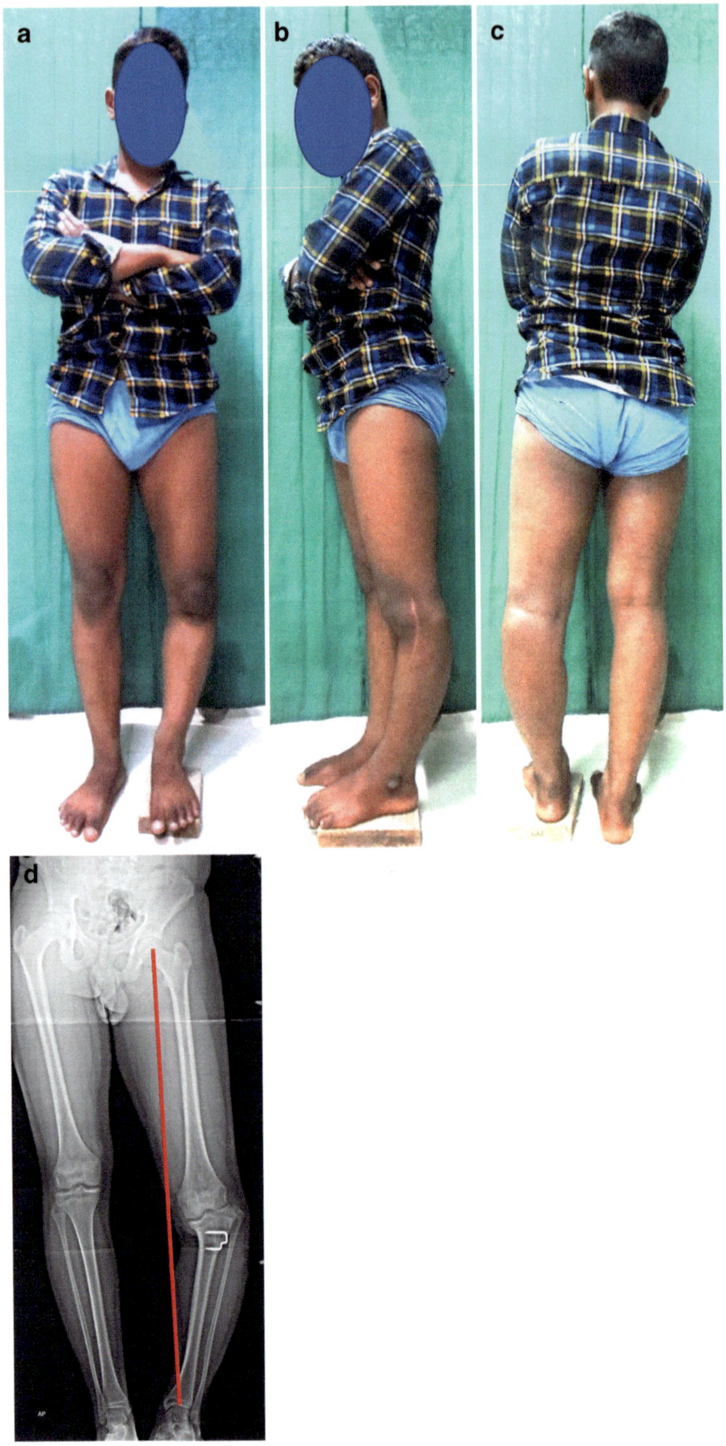

Fig. 23.5 Case 5: Growth arrest partial peripheral. (Courtesy Dr. Milind Chaudhary). (**a–d**) A 17-year-old male with a left 5 cm shortening and varus-recurvatum deformity of the proximal tibia following a partial growth arrest. (**e–h**) Gradual correction of left proximal tibia varus deformity with lengthening using a circular external fixator. (**i–m**) 1-year postop, both the deformity and LLD are well corrected

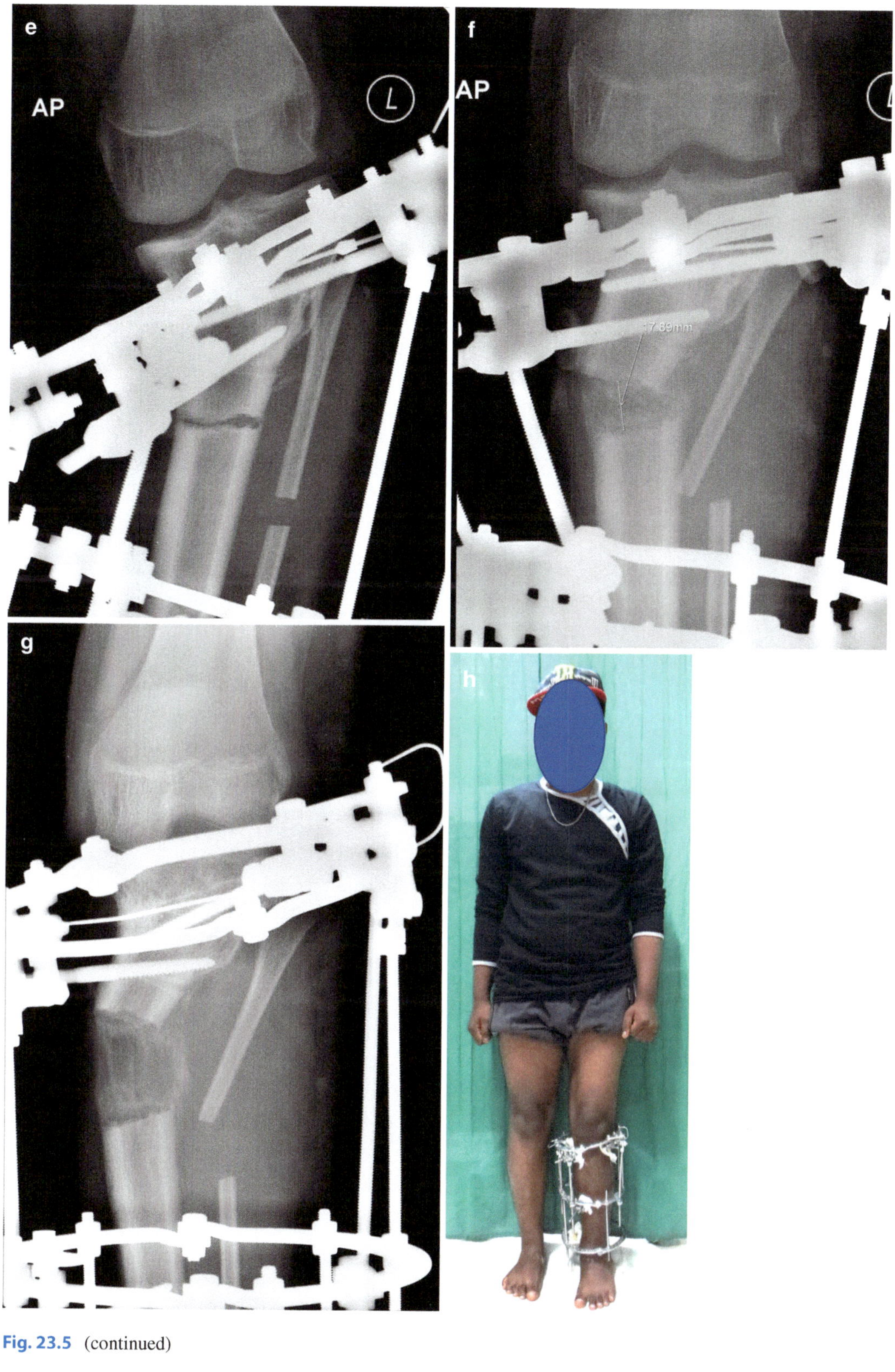

Fig. 23.5 (continued)

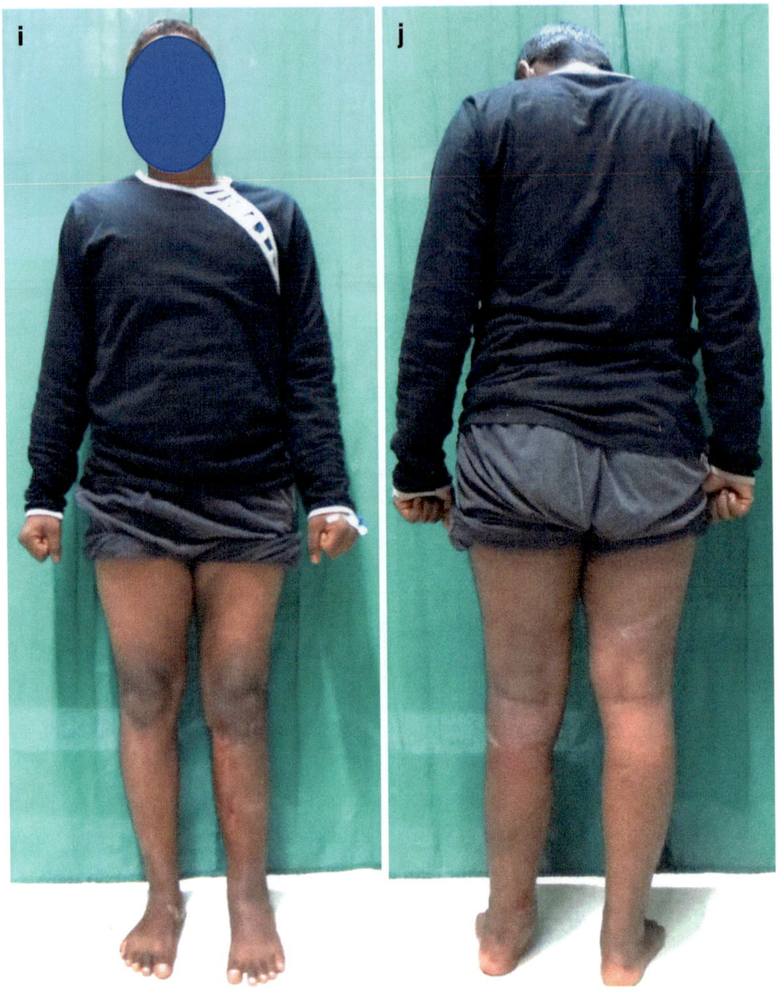

Fig. 23.5 (continued)

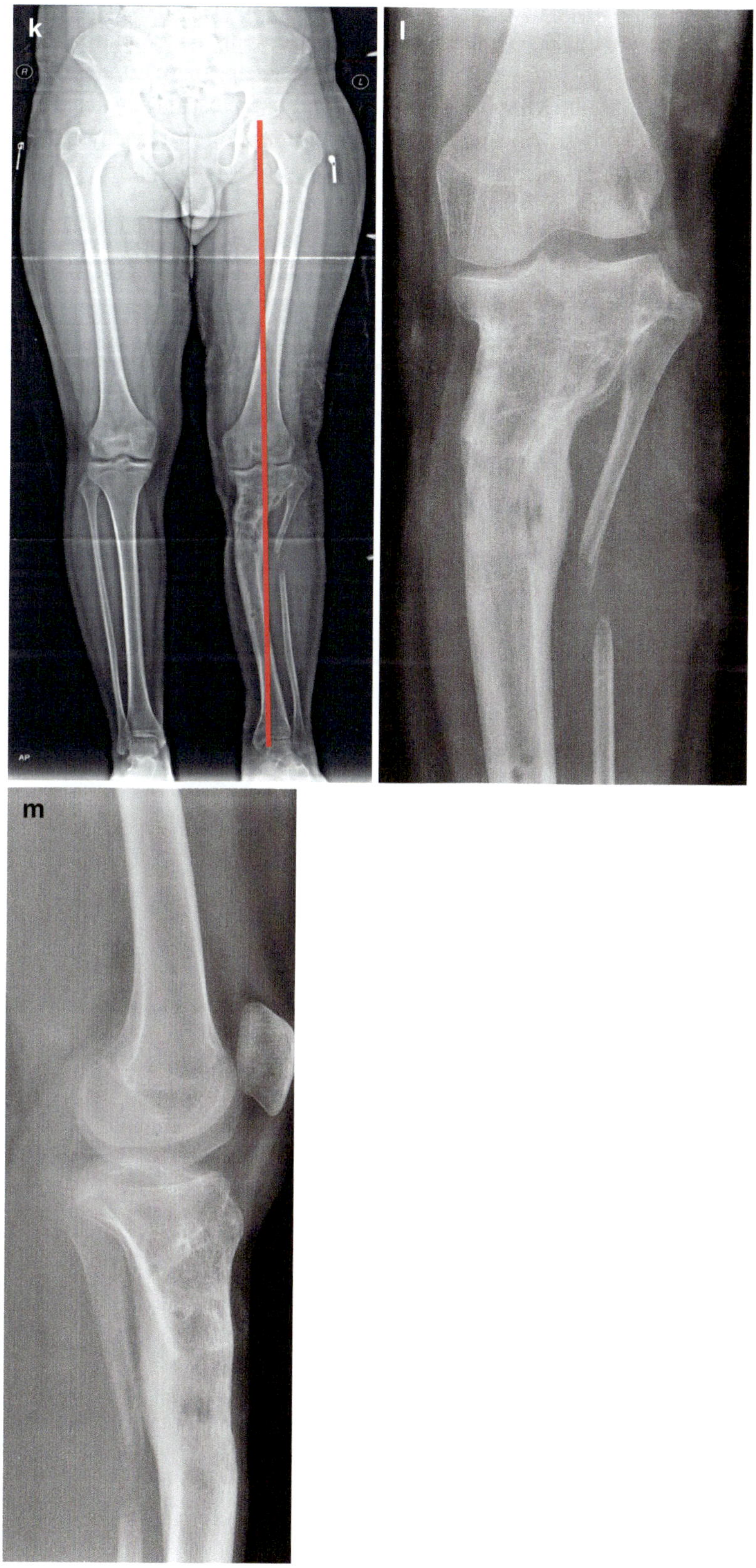

Fig. 23.5 (continued)

tis in different age groups of pediatric patients had previously been described, but Ogden was the first to provide histopathologic evidence to corroborate these theories. He lists the important findings as (a) multiple bone involvement; (b) multiple joint sepsis, always in association with, and seemingly secondary to an osteomyelitic focus; (c) highly varied destruction of the growth plate; (d) epiphyseal cartilage destruction; (e) variable occlusion of arteries, veins, and capillaries within the cartilage canal systems; and (f) an important role for transphyseal vessels in allowing spread of infection from the metaphysis into the epiphysis.

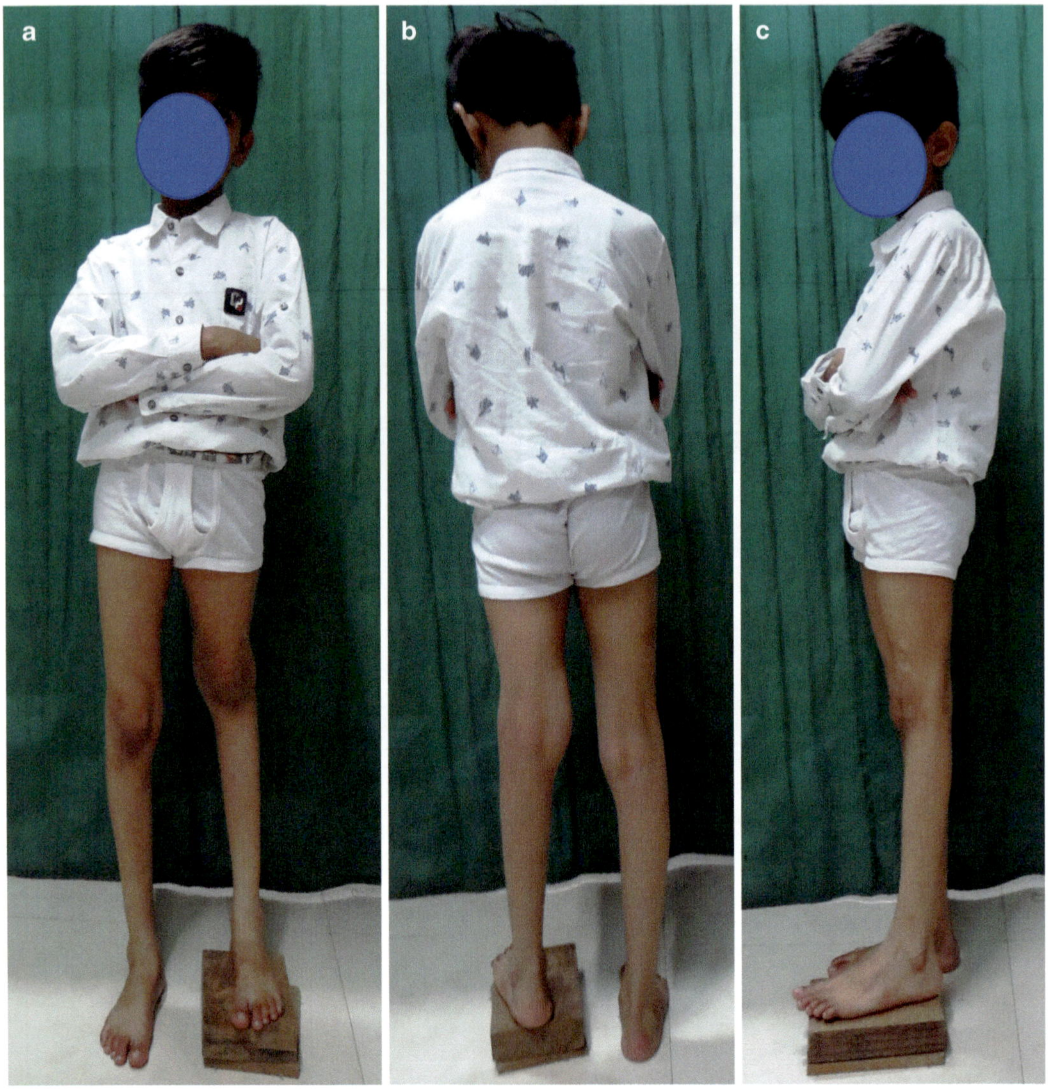

Fig. 23.6 Case 6: Growth arrest partial central. (Courtesy Dr. Milind Chaudhary). (**a–e**) This is an 8-year-old boy, with a left distal femur partial central growth arrest who had an attempt at physeal bar excision with bone cement. He presented with a 6 cm shortening and recurvatum deformity, 2 years of physeal bar excision. (**f–h**) Gradual left distal femur lengthening with correction of recurvatum was performed with a circular external fixator through a distal femoral osteotomy. (**i–l**) The recurvatum is well corrected. He will need another lengthening to equalize LLD closer to skeletal maturity with an intramedullary lengthening nail

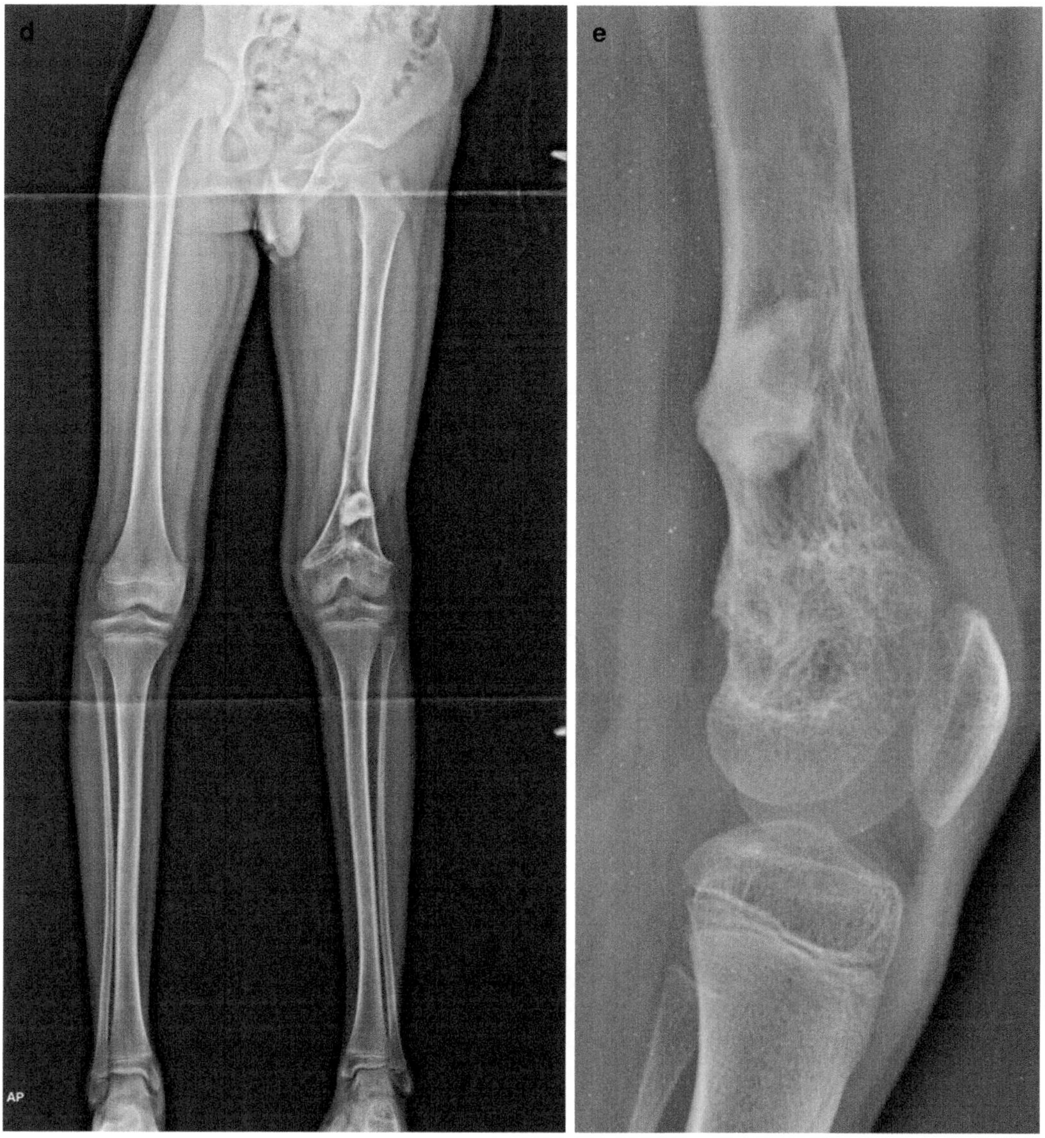

Fig. 23.6 (continued)

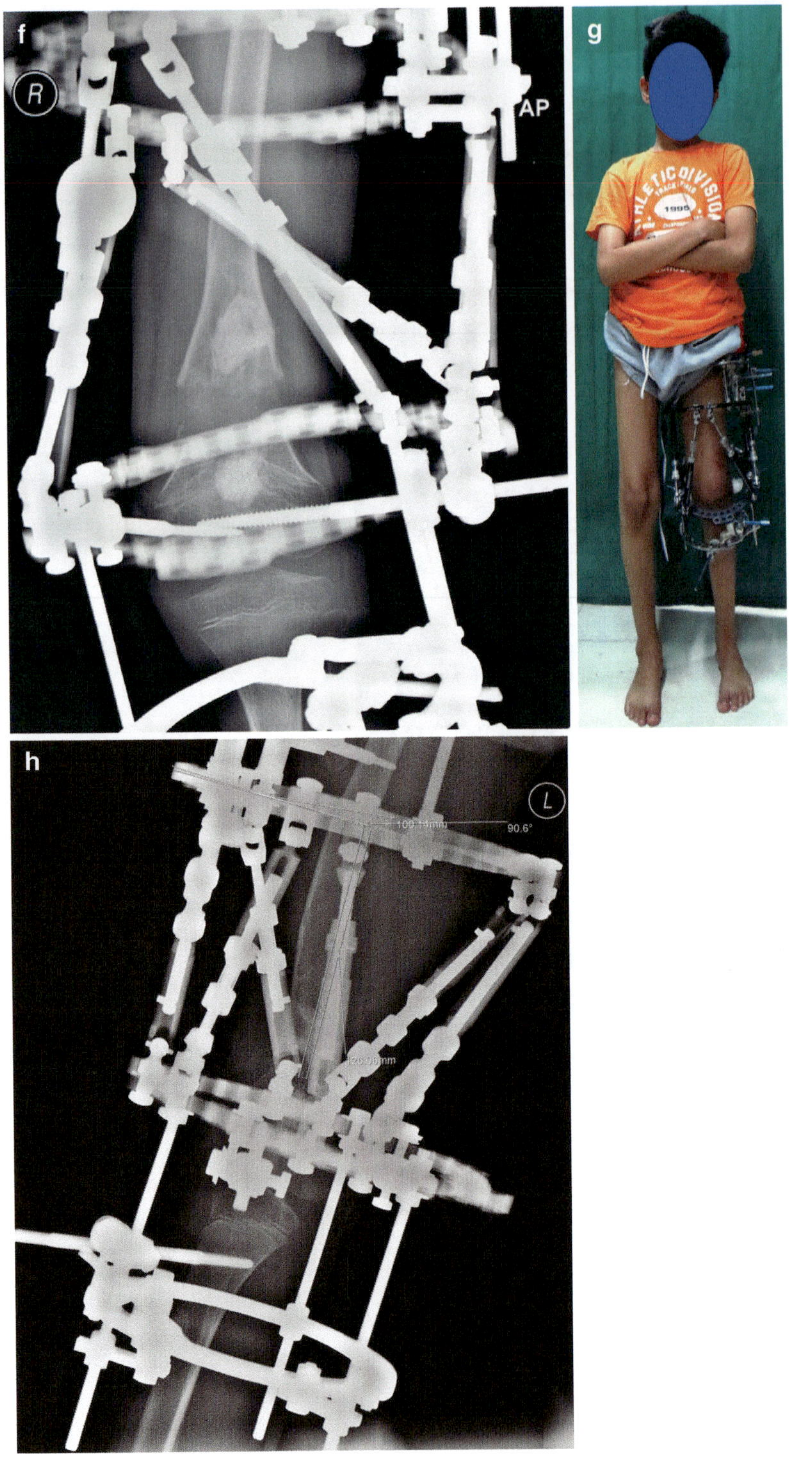

Fig. 23.6 (continued)

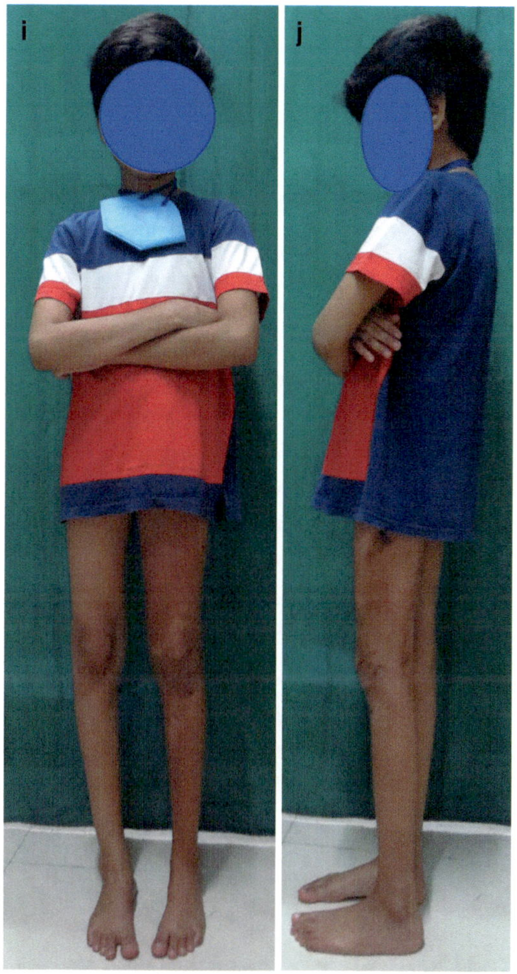

Fig. 23.6 (continued)

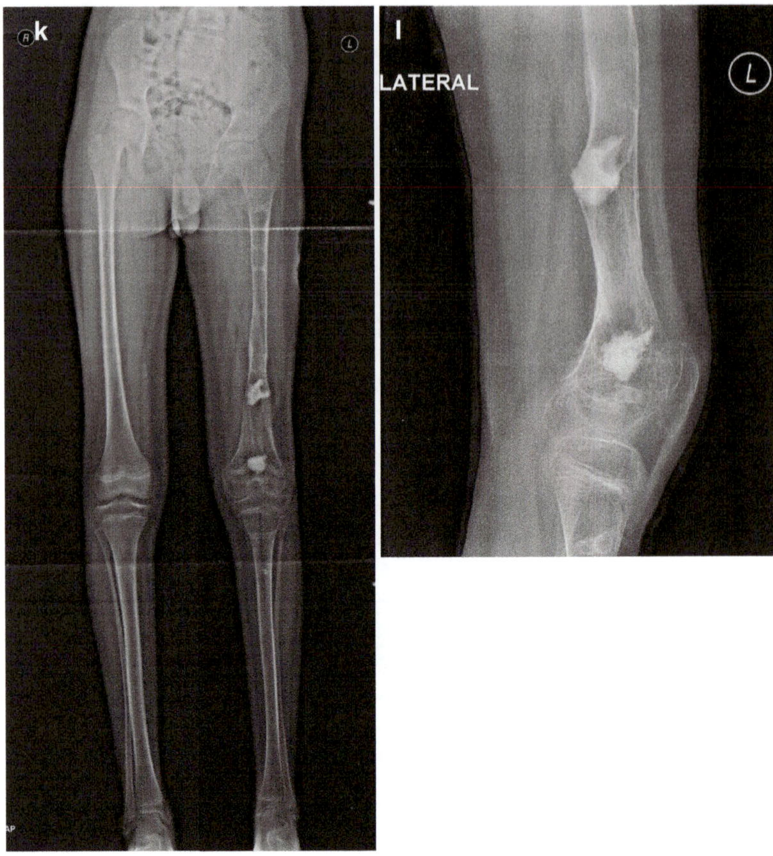

Fig. 23.6 (continued)

It was previously thought that the physis was a barrier to infectious spread from the metaphysis to the epiphysis. Ogden provided histologic evidence against this hypothesis, showing that in neonates, transphyseal vessels are a key component of this process. The transphyseal vessels typically disappear by 18 months of age, or with the appearance of the secondary ossification center. While physeal damage is most extensive in the neonatal period, it occurs in older children as well, which Ogden described as likely due to focal, direct bacterial and enzymatic destruction of small areas of the physis [56, 57].

Types of Growth Disturbances [48, 55, 56, 59–66]

A1. *Complete growth arrest:* Premature complete physeal closure is uncommon and may take months or years to develop. The subsequent relative bone shortening is dependent on the age of the child at the time of closure. The bones most commonly requiring treatment are those with the most growth: the femur, tibia/fibula, or humerus/radius [48, 56, 62, 63] (Figs. 23.1 and 23.2).

A1. *Partial growth arrest:* Premature partial physeal closure (a physeal bar) may occur at any age during growth and often cannot be predicted. The size and location of the bar determine the clinical deformity. Partial central physeal closure is relatively common following metaphyseal osteomyelitis and results in diminished longitudinal growth. If the partial physeal closure is eccentric, it will result in an angular deformity [48, 56, 62, 63] (Figs. 23.3 and 23.4).

A3. *Physeal bar equivalent (PBE):* Premature partial physeal arrest without the formation

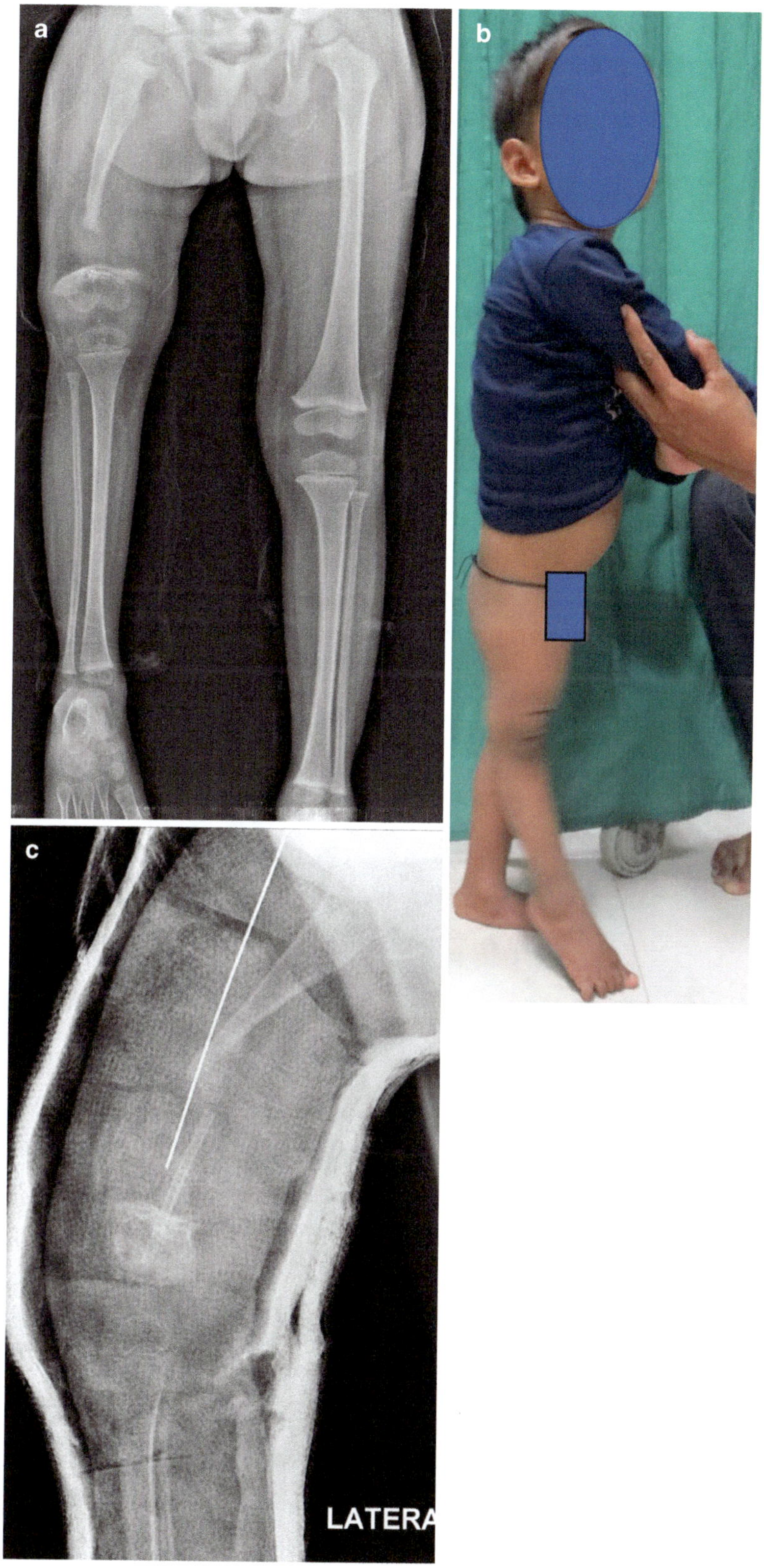

Fig. 23.7 Case 7: Bone gap with LLD. (Courtesy Dr. Milind Chaudhary). (**a**–**c**) A 2-year-old boy with a Rt distal femoral bone gap, with a completely destroyed, distal femoral physis as well as shortening. Reconstruction with a non-vascularized fibula graft with a K wire and a spica cast did not do the job, and we can see a loss of fixation within a few days of surgery. (**d**–**h**) The fixation was converted to an Ilizarov fixator and a proximal femoral corticotomy was added above. The Ilizarov fixator did a good job of holding the fibula in place, while the femur was lengthened by 6 cm proximally. (**i**–**l**) 9 months postop, a spica cast allowed him to walk after external fixator removal, and he went on to heal well. A minimal shortening remains which will of course need to be corrected in future

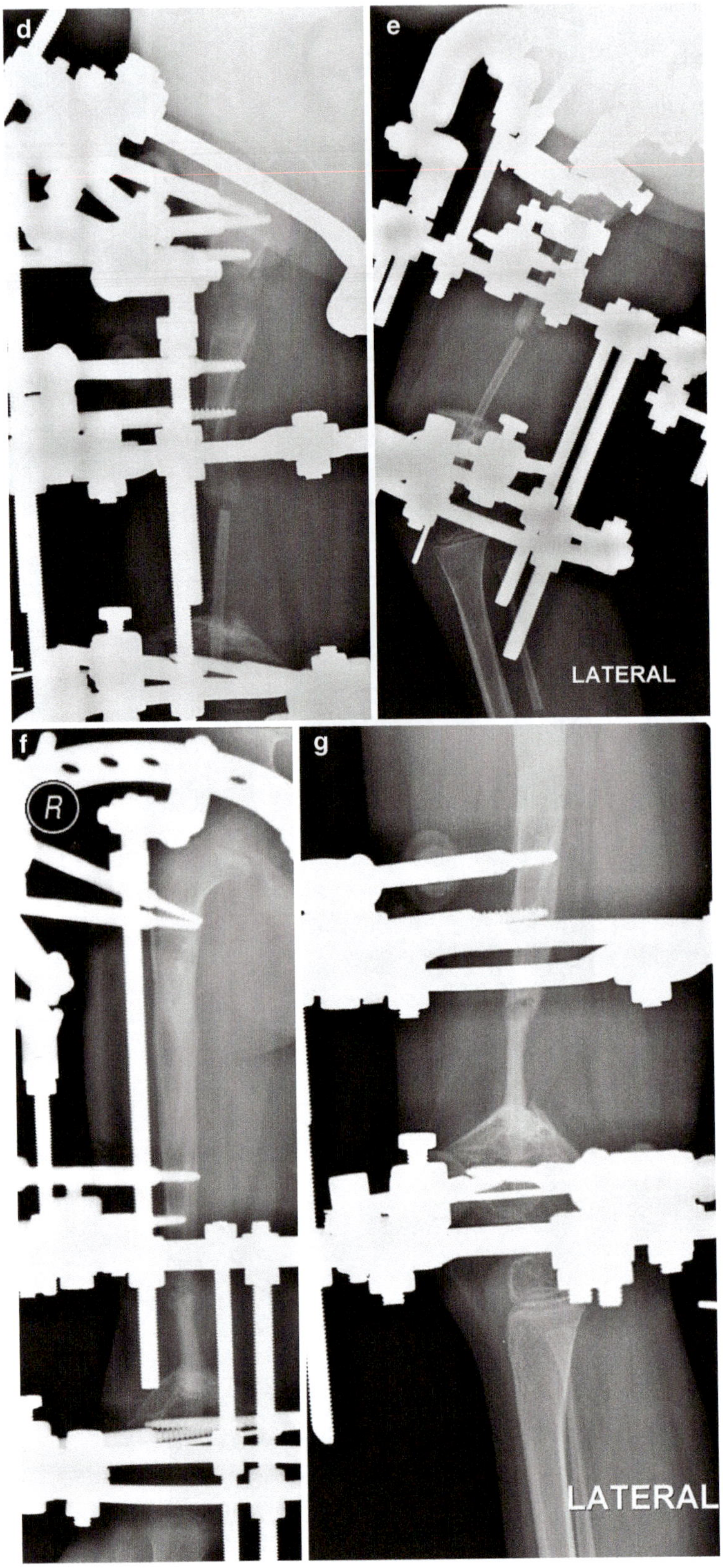

Fig. 23.7 (continued)

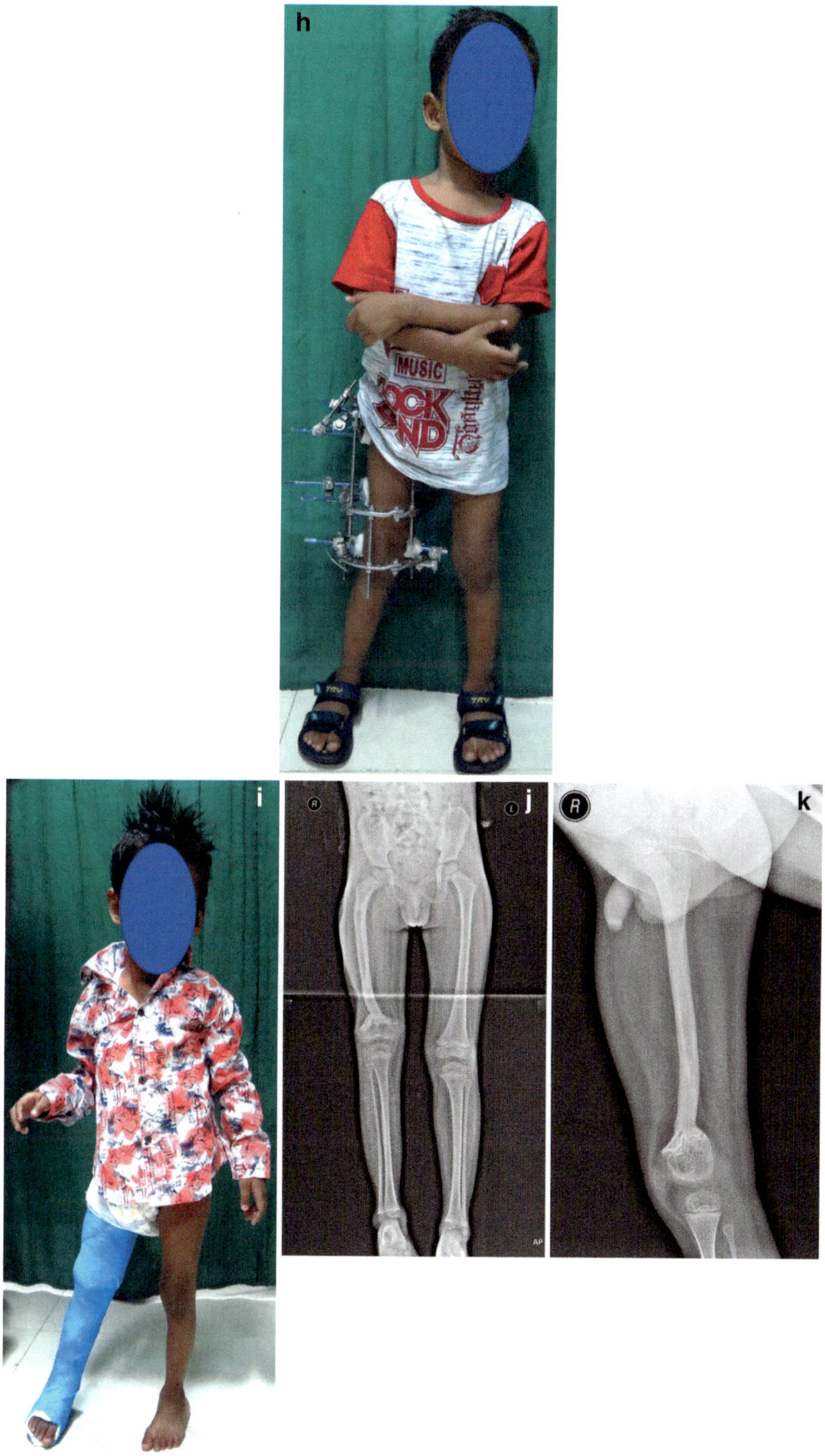

Fig. 23.7 (continued)

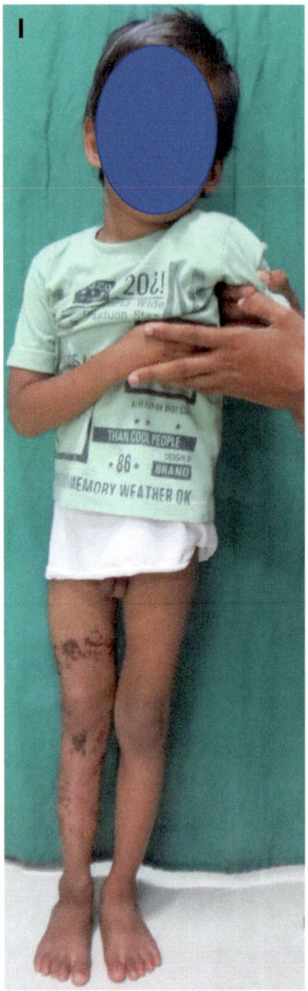

Fig. 23.7 (continued)

of an osseous bar may occur but is uncommon. It results from cell death in a portion of the physis and results in similar tethering deformities of the metaphysis, physis, and epiphysis, causing shortening and angular deformity of the bone. Early recognition and treatment of PBE is required to avoid severe limb-length inequality and angular deformity [56, 59].

A5. *Growth plate separation:* Displacement or complete separation of the epiphysis from the metaphysis is a rare complication of metaphyseal osteomyelitis and occurs primarily in the neonatal age group. The most common sites are the proximal and distal femur. Centrifugal extension of a metaphyseal abscess in the zone of trabecular calcification and the hypertrophic zone of the physis is associated with variable osteolysis, with or without cortical perforation and periosteal stripping. This promotes mechanical loosening of the epiphysis and predisposes to complete separation and slipping. These slipped epiphyses do not necessarily develop growth arrest because the germinal cell layer is spared. The potential for recovery appears to be excellent, provided an early diagnosis is made using imaging modalities and prompt treatment by anatomic reduction of the displaced epiphysis is instituted. The treatment of physeal separation includes decompression and debridement of the abscess, followed by reduction of the epiphysis. If reduction cannot be maintained with external immobilization, pins across the physis, despite the presence of infection, have been successful [56, 60, 61].

A5. *Epiphyseal disappearance and regeneration:* Epiphyseal disappearance followed by regeneration is an uncommon phenomenon that has been reported following septic arthritis, primary epiphyseal osteomyelitis, or with metaphyseal osteomyelitis with extension into the epiphysis. The proximal and distal femur epiphyses and the proximal tibia epiphysis are the most common sites, potentially leading to varus or valgus deformity. The largest series of disappearance and regeneration of the epiphysis is 15 cases. Despite the portentous early appearance of the epiphysis, many cases showed spontaneous re-ossification of the epiphysis with restoration of the femoral/tibial condyles and preservation of joint congruity. The valgus or varus deformity was treated satisfactorily with one or more osteotomies. The potential for regeneration of the epiphysis following infantile osteomyelitis suggests these cases should be treated expectantly regarding joint congruity [64–66].

Clinical Presentation Physeal arrest may occur at any time following infection but may not become clinically manifest for years. The average time from infection to manifest growth arrest is between 6 and 12 years [48, 56, 59] (Figs. 23.1, 23.2, 23.3, 23.4, 23.5, and 23.6).

Imaging Studies Plain radiographs may show a converging Park-Harris growth arrest line or a bony physeal bridge. CT traditionally has been used to estimate the size and location of a bridge. On CT images, an osseous bridge appears as a focal loss of normal growth plate hypoattenuation, with or without adjacent reactive sclerosis. With CT, fibrous bridges are missed, and this modality is less accurate when applied to multiplanar and tortuous growth plates. Currently, the imaging modality of choice is thin-section (< 1 mm) three-dimensional fat-saturated cartilage-sensitive MR sequences [55, 67, 68].

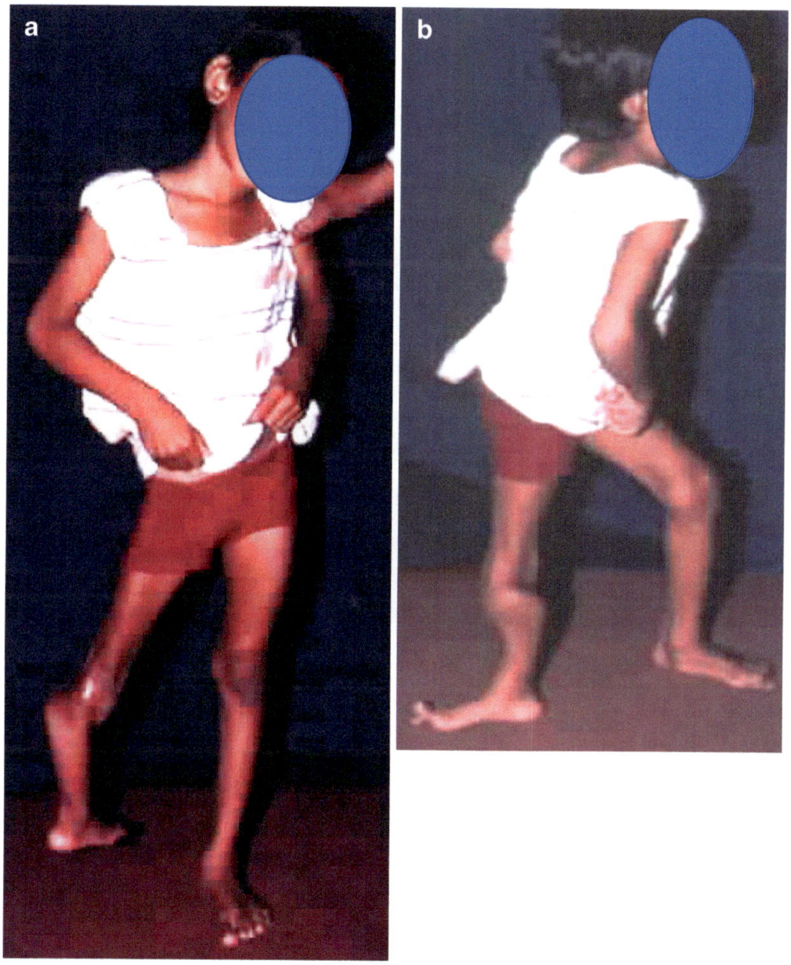

Fig. 23.8 Case 8: Bone gap with LLD and deformity. (Courtesy Dr. Milind Chaudhary). (**a–d**) A 4-year-old with a bone gap in the Rt proximal tibia with significant fibular overgrowth and severe internal rotation deformity and shortening. There was complete growth arrest of the upper tibial physis which led to this problem. (**e–g**) The Rt tibia was lengthened and de-rotated at the lower level and distracted apart at the upper level using a circular external fixator. In this space, the opposite non-vascularized fibula was inserted to fill and heal the bone gap. (**h–k**) 1-year postop, he has a straight Rt lower limb and realigned and healed bone gap with equalization of a 10 cm leg length discrepancy

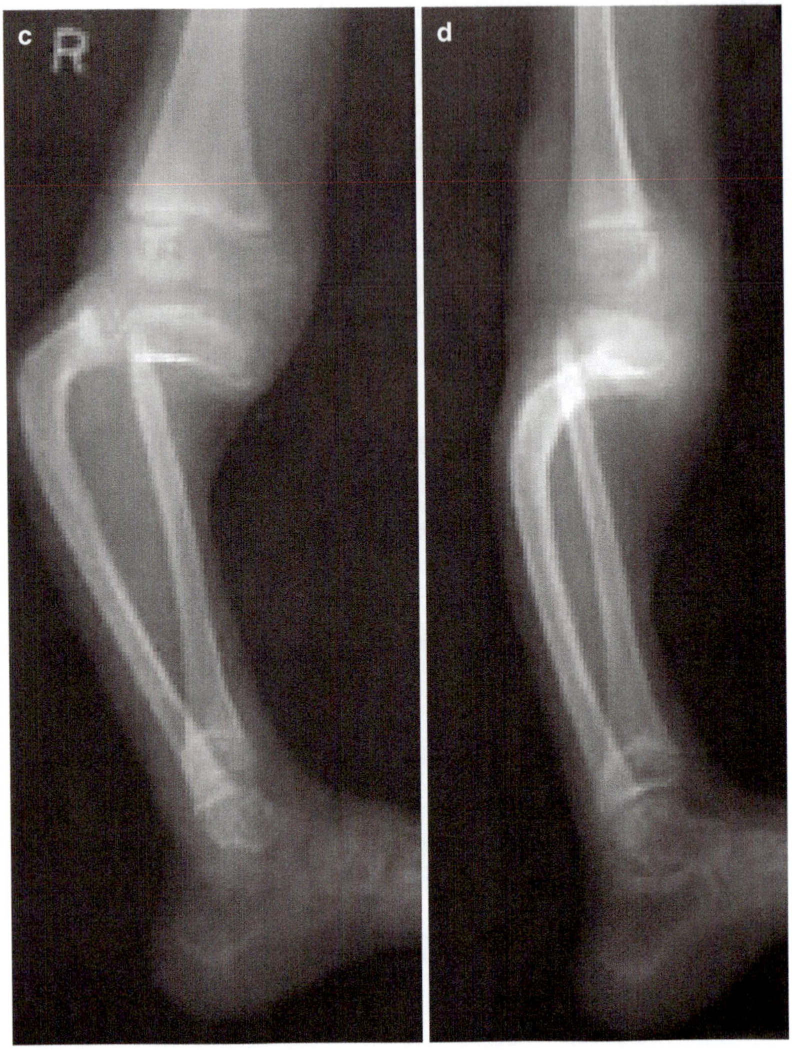

Fig. 23.8 (continued)

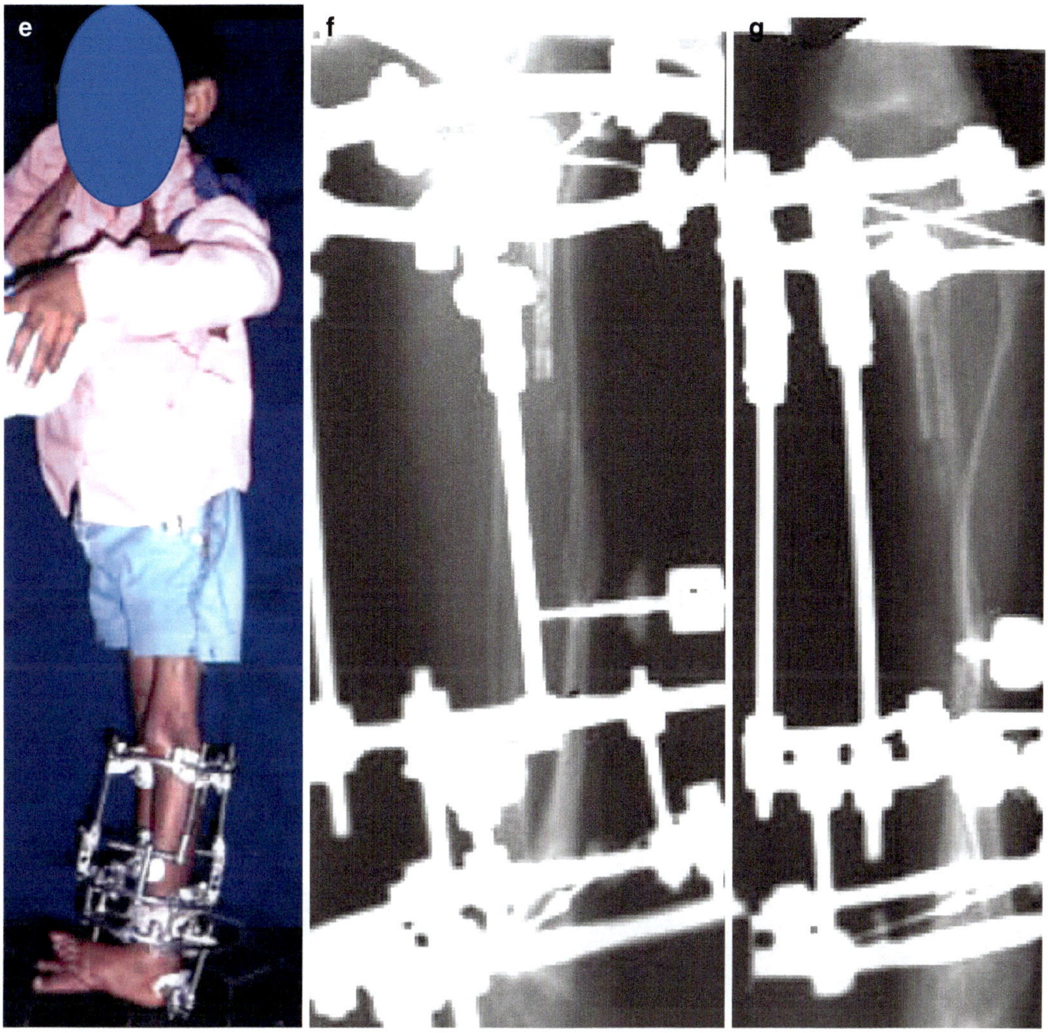

Fig. 23.8 (continued)

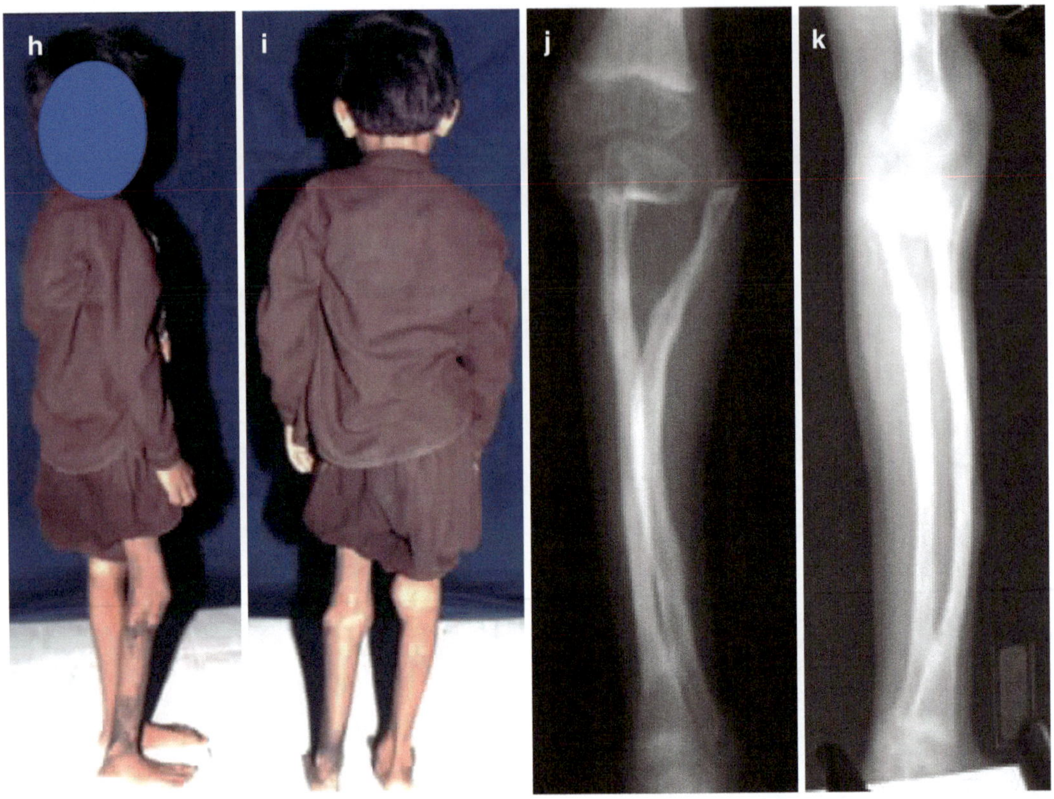

Fig. 23.8 (continued)

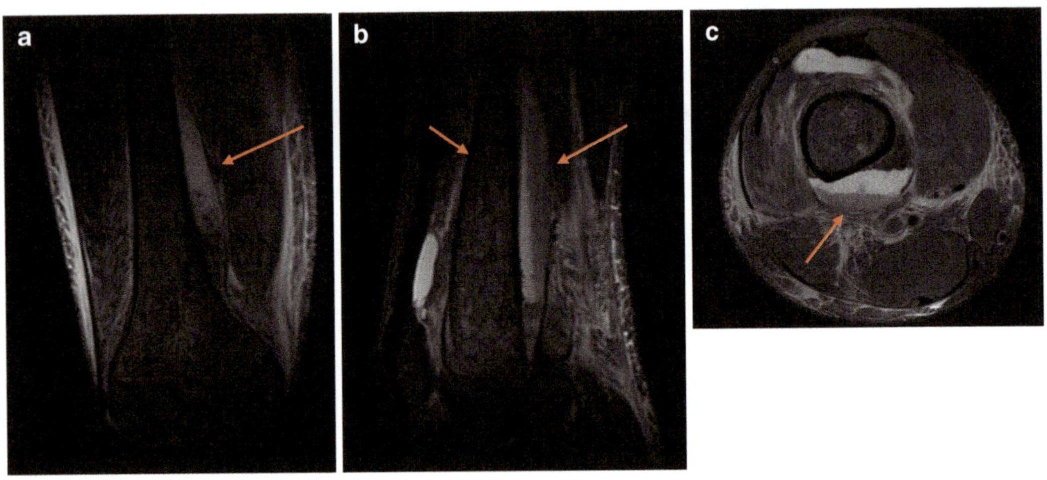

Fig. 23.9 Case 9: Pathologic fracture following OM Rt femur. (Courtesy Dr. Mohan V Belthur). (**a–e**) A 14-year-old male with Rt MRSA distal femur osteomyelitis, DVT, B/L pleural effusions. Index MRI and radiographs. (**f, g**) Radiographs at 4 months – There is extensive callus formation and periosteal reaction extending from the mid-shaft to the distal metaphysis of the femur. Heterogeneous area of sclerosis and lucency again seen along the distal half of the femoral shaft. (**h, i**) Radiographs at 5 months showing an acute angulated L/3 femur fracture with changes consistent with healing chronic osteomyelitis. (**j, k**) Radiographs at 6 months showing IM nail fixation of right distal femur fracture with healing. (**l**) Bone length radiograph at 2 years + 3 m showing healed osteomyelitis and healed fracture Rt distal femur with excellent alignment and no LLD

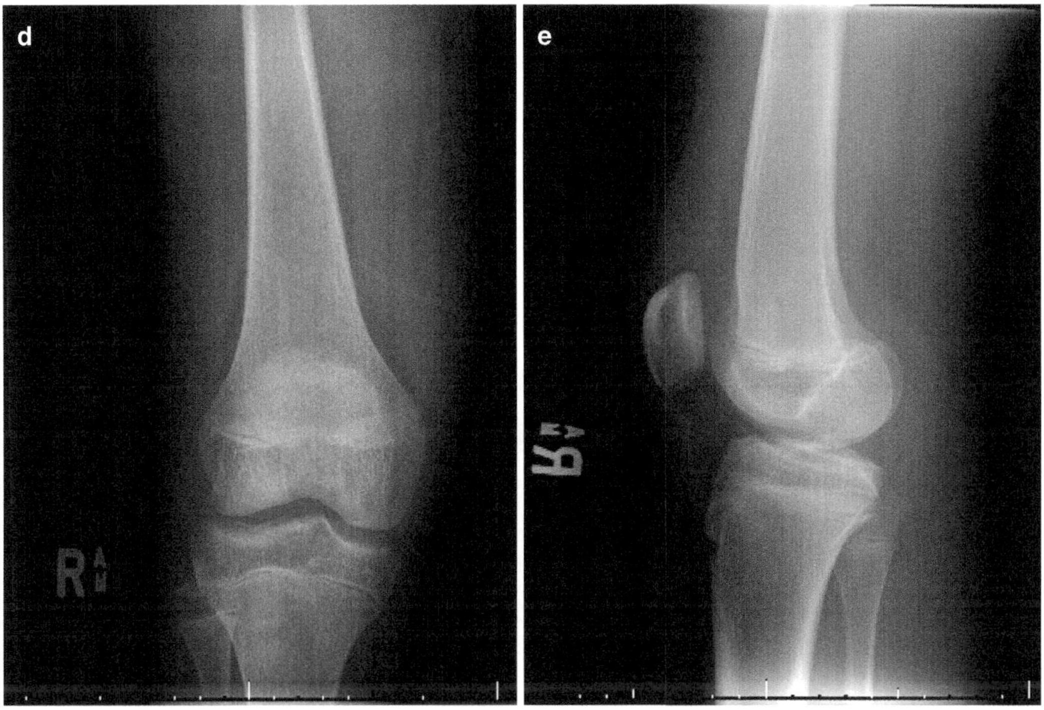

Fig. 23.9 (continued)

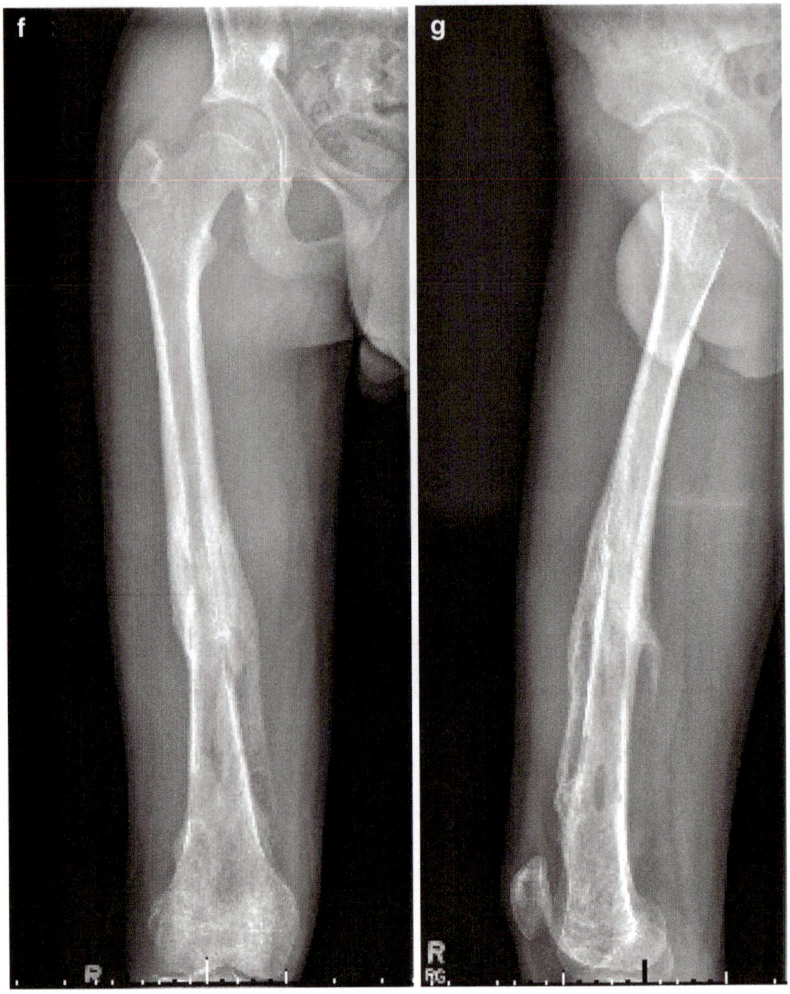

Fig. 23.9 (continued)

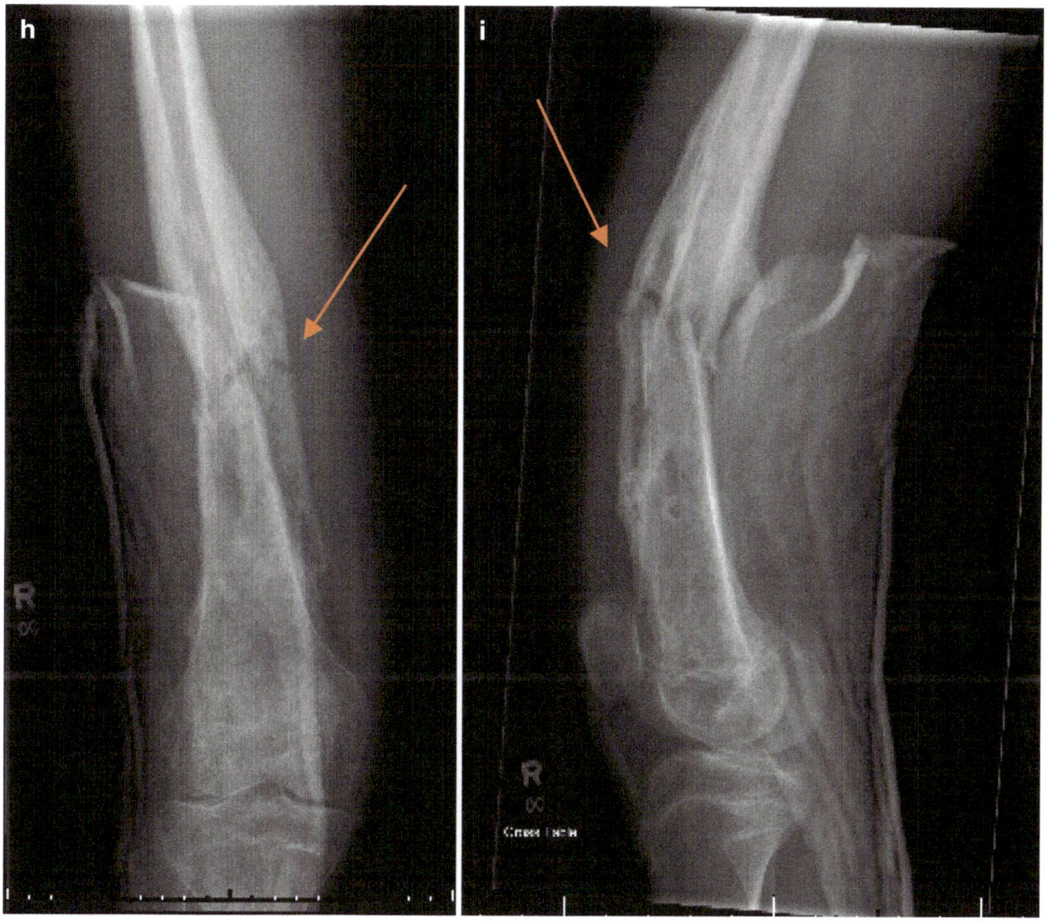

Fig. 23.9 (continued)

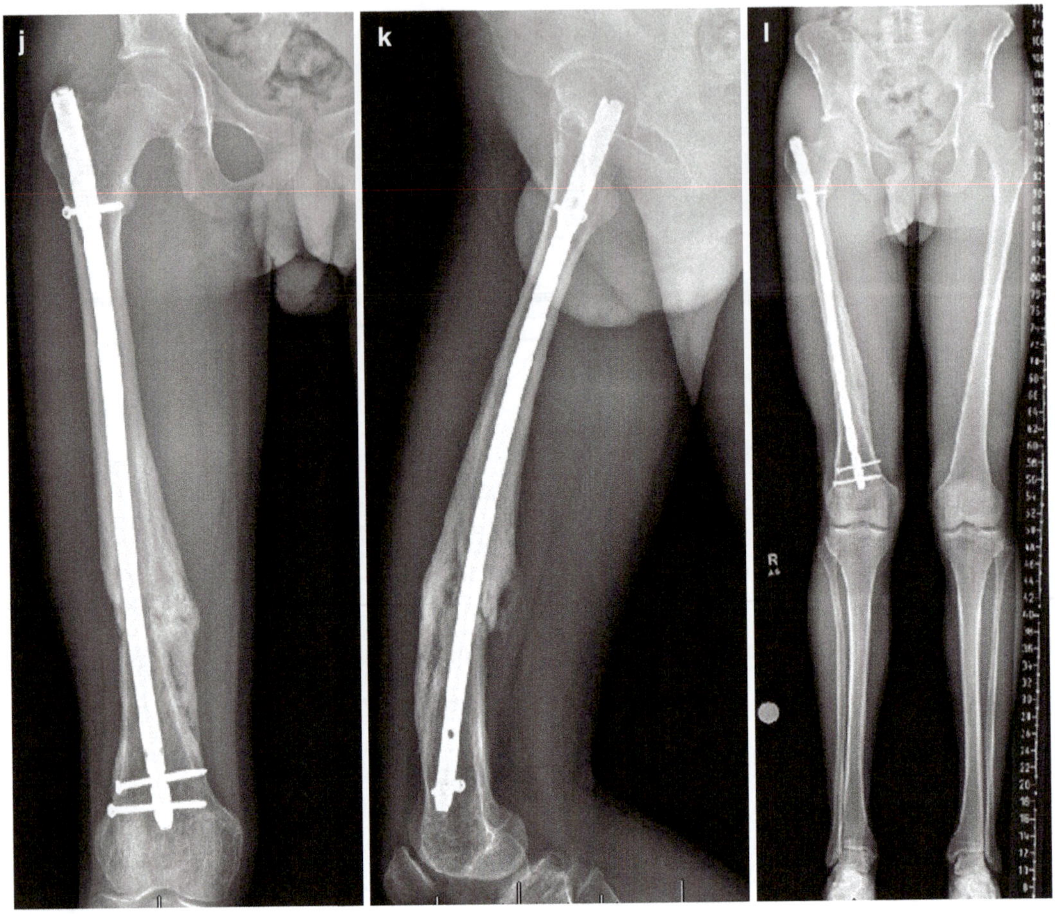

Fig. 23.9 (continued)

Treatment Principles Early diagnosis and appropriate management of bone and joint infections with antibiotics and surgery are necessary to prevent growth arrests. Delicate surgical technique is essential to avoid further damage to the physis during surgery to control infection. Early recognition and treatment of growth arrests is required to avoid severe limb-length inequality and angular deformity. Treatment options for physeal arrests are chosen based on the bone and physis involved, the amount of relative shortening, and the age of the patient, which determines the amount of growth remaining [48, 56, 59, 62, 63].

Treatment Options [48, 56, 59, 62, 63] Nonsurgical treatment is reserved for patients who are nearing skeletal maturation and have small bridges that involve less than 30% of the total growth plate area and affect the central portions of the growth plate.

Complete closure in the femur or humerus may be managed by options used for treating limb length discrepancies including a shoe lift, contralateral epiphysiodesis, shortening of the unaffected side, or lengthening of the affected bone (Figs. 23.7 and 23.8). When one of two paired bones (such as the tibia/fibula or radius/ulna) is involved, the result is relative overgrowth of the companion uninfected bone (Fig. 23.11). This usually requires secondary length equalization surgery.

A partial peripheral arrest of > 50% in an older child can be managed by a corrective osteotomy, combined with closure of the remaining physis and closure of the contralateral physis. In a

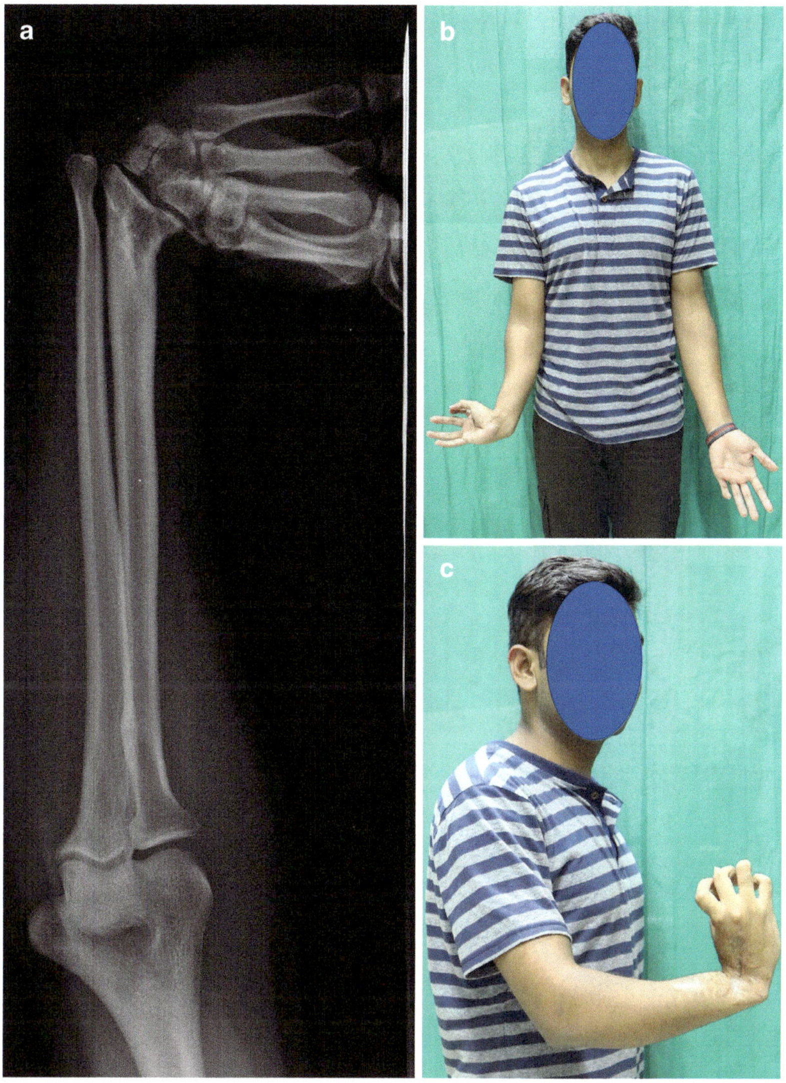

Fig. 23.10 Case 10: Contracture Rt wrist. (Courtesy Dr. Milind Chaudhary). (**a**–**c**) A 25-year-old male s/p Rt distal radial osteomyelitis has a severe valgus-dorsiflexion contracture of wrist with scars and a distal radial shortening and deformity. (**d**, **e**) A circular external fixator is applied to the Rt forearm and hand. In the first stage, the wrist contracture is gradually distracted. (**f**–**h**) In the 2nd stage, a Rt distal radial osteotomy is done, and the distal radius is lengthened, and the deformity is corrected. (**i**–**l**) 1-year postop, with a realigned Rt wrist and forearm

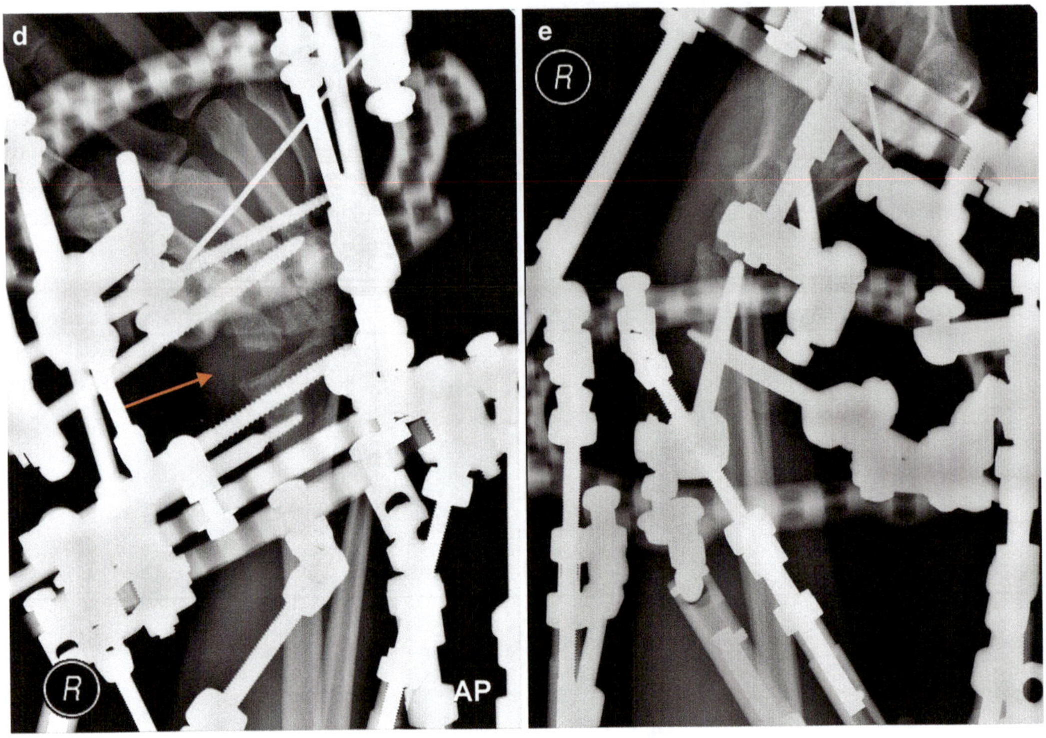

Fig. 23.10 (continued)

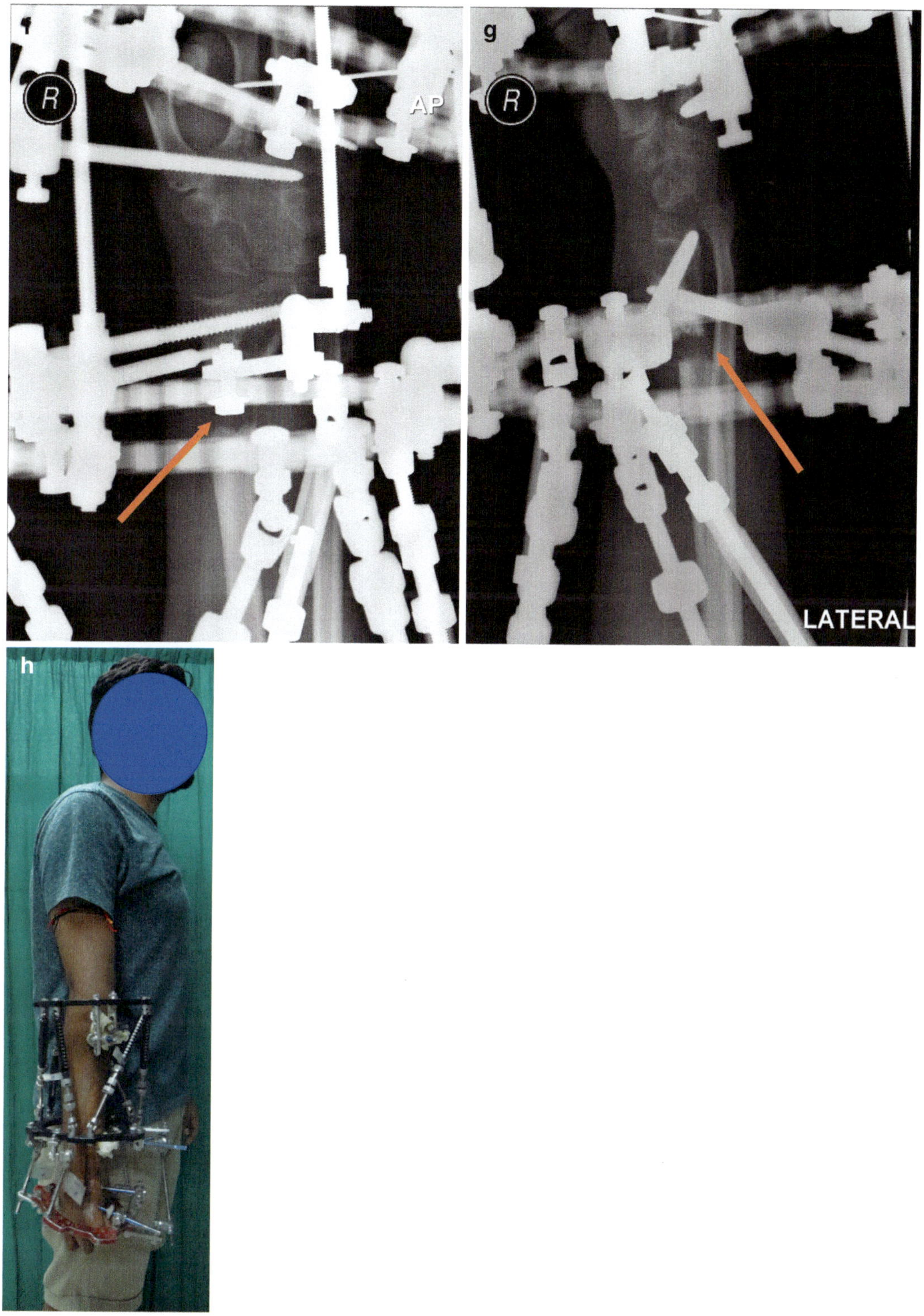

Fig. 23.10 (continued)

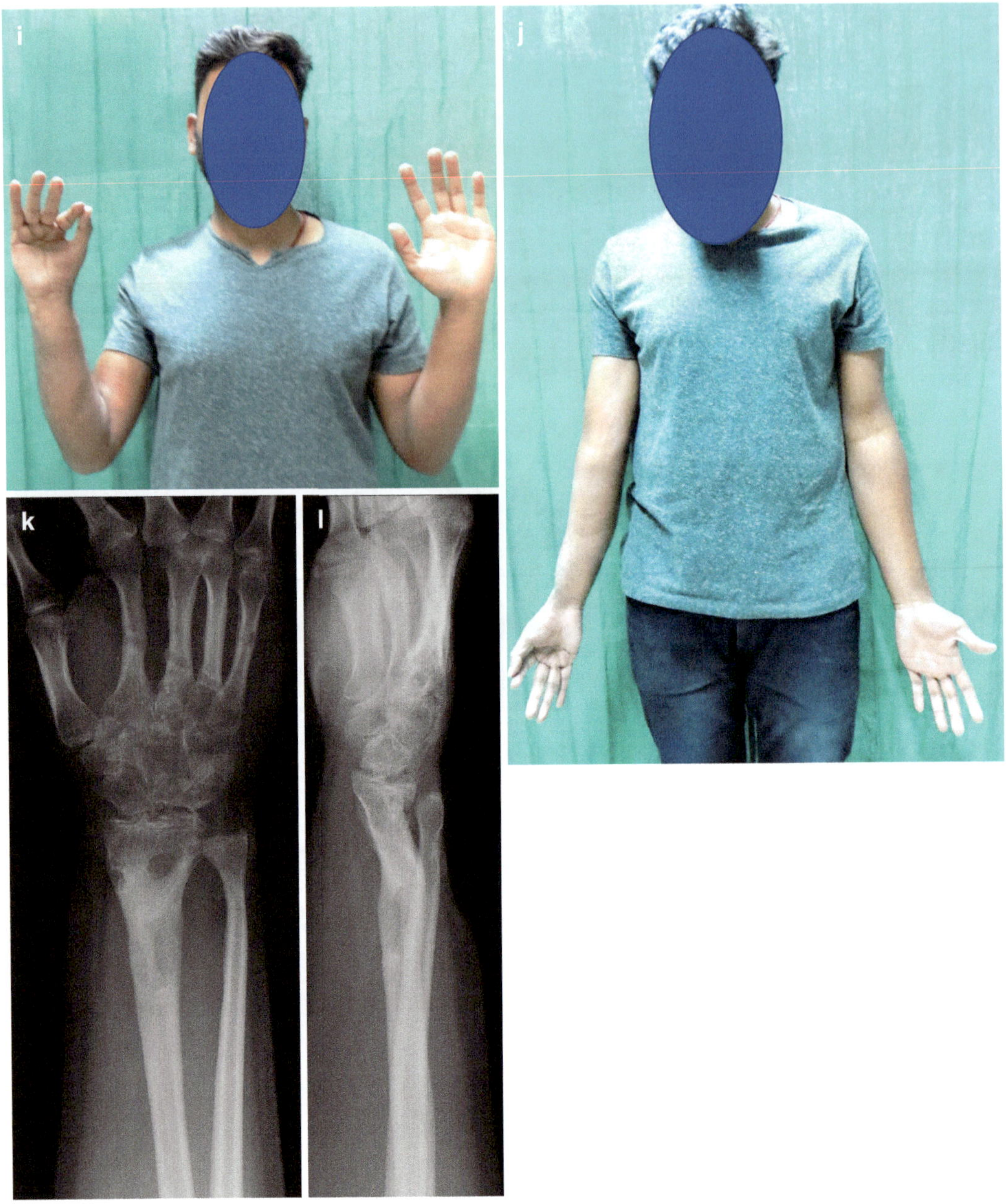

Fig. 23.10 (continued)

younger child, with a physeal bar involving < 50% of the growth plate, excision of the bar has the potential to reestablish growth and allow the angular deformity to correct. Osteotomy, if necessary, can be done concurrently if the deformity is greater than 20 degrees at the time of bar resection (Figs. 23.4 and 23.5).

A central partial closure results in relative shortening with little or no angular deformity. The object of treatment is to equalize the bone lengths and avoid cupping (Fishtail deformity) from becoming marked, resulting in joint line deformity and articular incongruity. This can be done by surgical arrest of the remaining physis

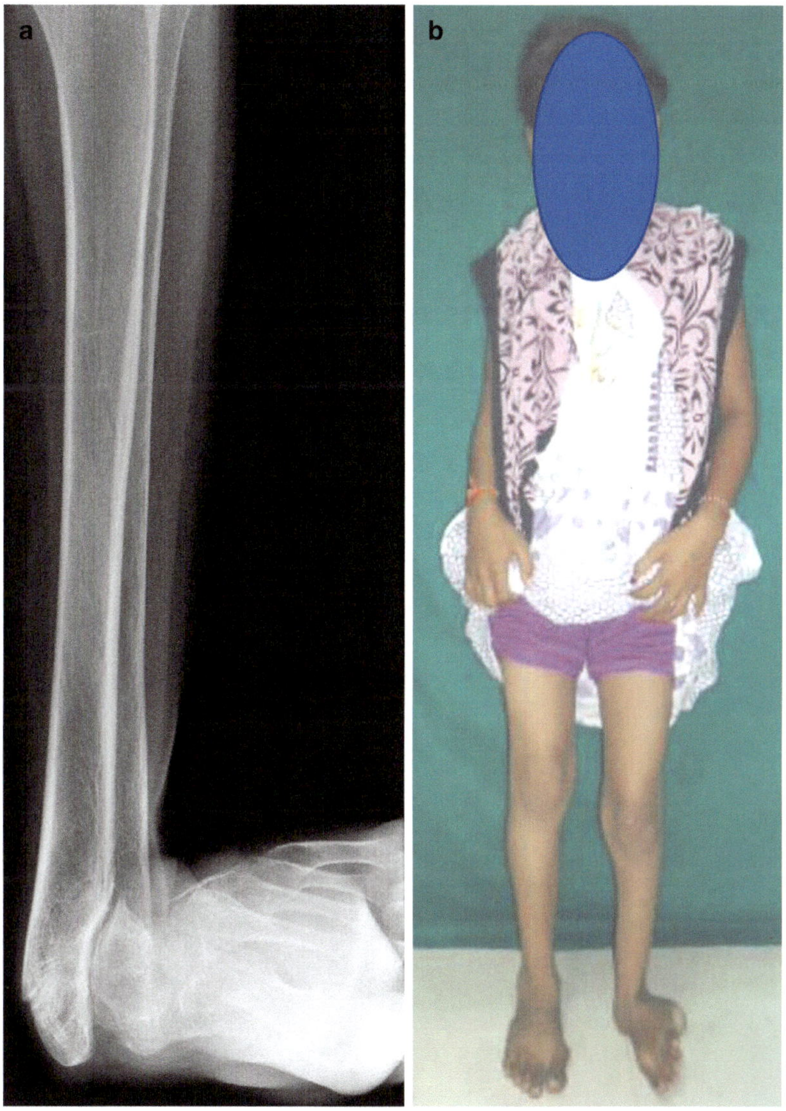

Fig. 23.11 Case 11: Deformity left ankle. (Courtesy Dr. Milind Chaudhary). (**a–d**) A 12-year-old girl s/p childhood osteomyelitis with a growth arrest of the left lateral distal tibial physis causing a severe left ankle juxta-articular valgus with shortening. (**e–g**) Left distal tibia and fibula osteotomy with realignment using a circular external fixator. (**h–j**) 1-year postop, she has a good correction and almost equal limb lengths and may need a second lengthening after few years

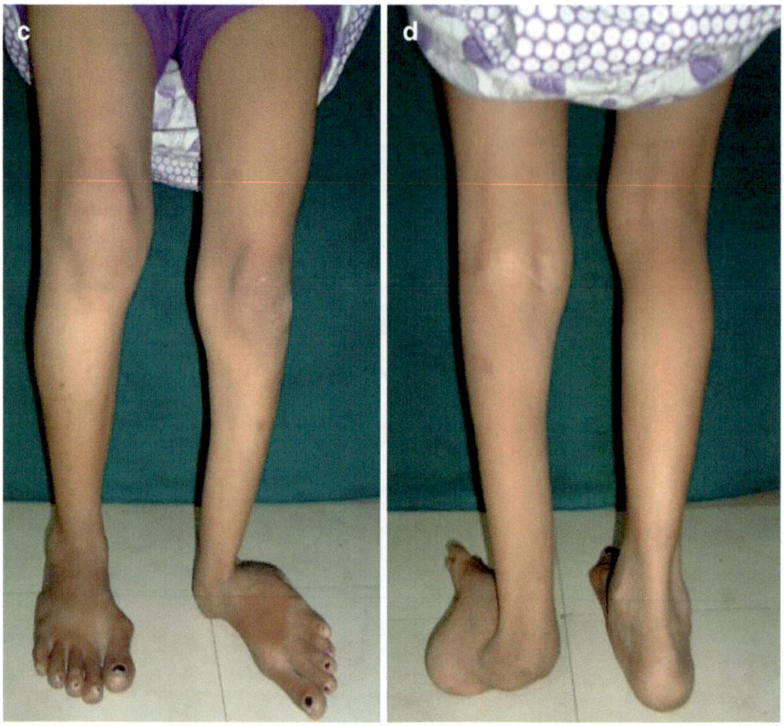

Fig. 23.11 (continued)

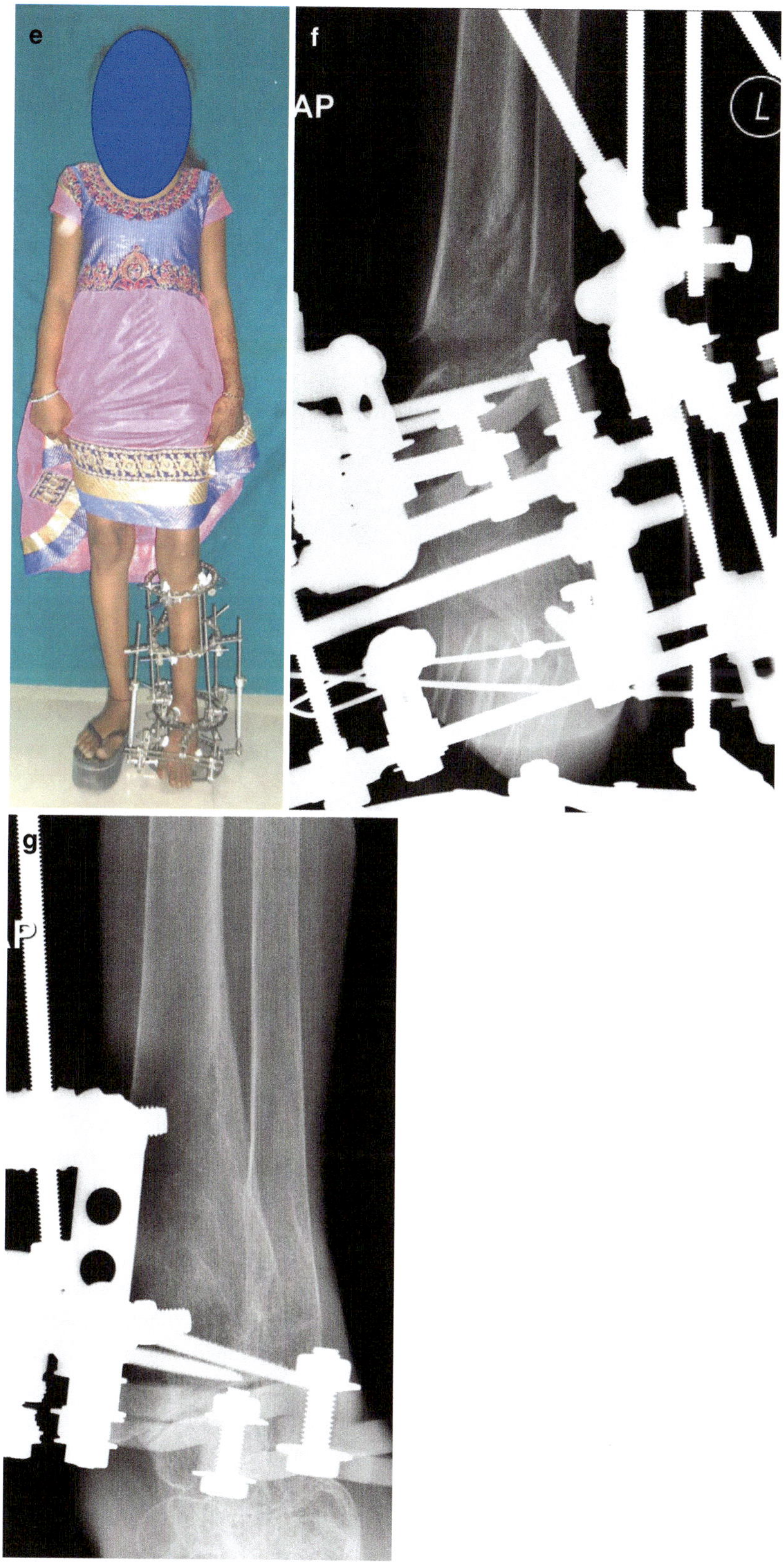

Fig. 23.11 (continued)

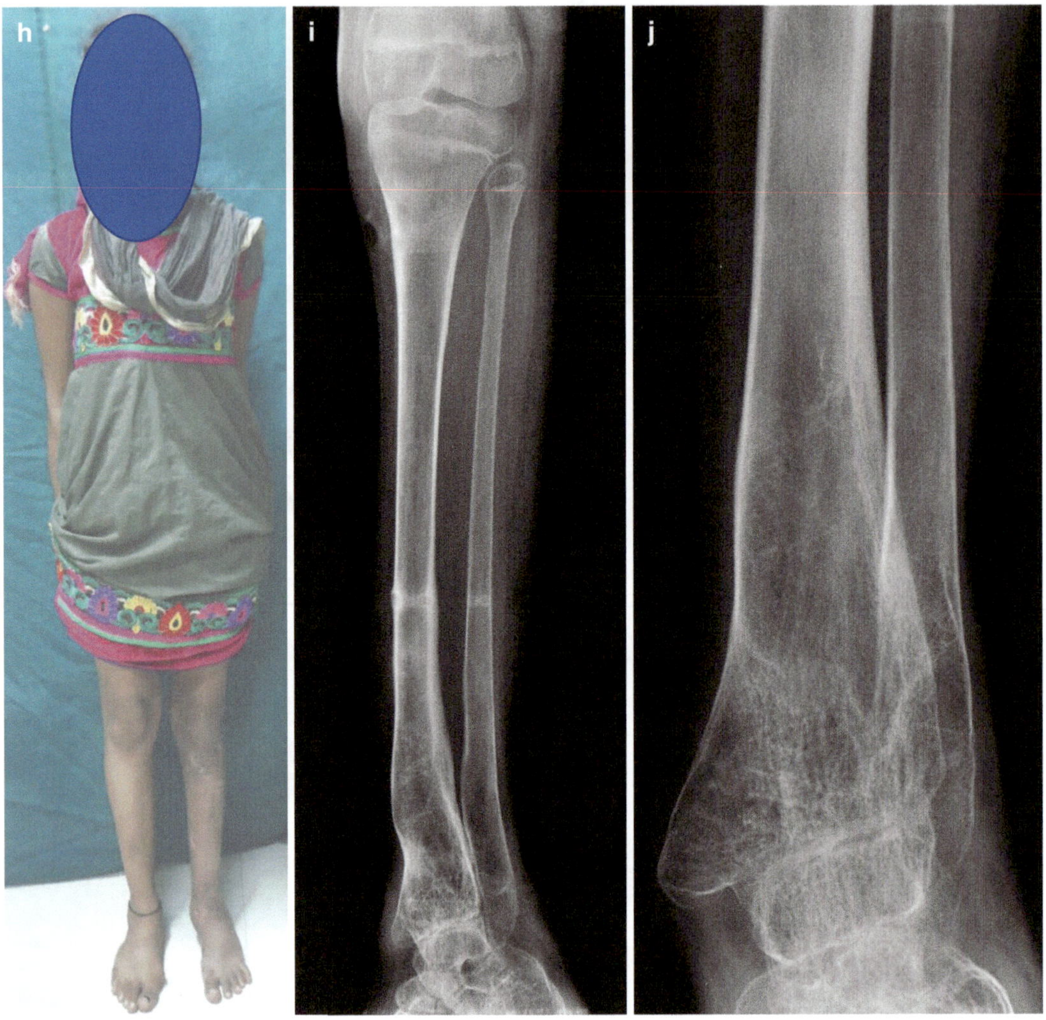

Fig. 23.11 (continued)

of the partially arrested physis combined with arrest and/or shortening of the contralateral normal bone, or by excision of the bar. Successful bar excision may be less predictable (Fig. 23.6).

Outcomes Successful physeal bar excision may be less predictable than in cases caused by fracture. Following infection, the bar found at surgery is sometimes larger than anticipated from the preoperative evaluation. An additional fear of bar excision is failure due to recurrent infection. Nevertheless, even though bar excision may be unpredictable, it has been successful following osteomyelitis, using both fat and cranioplast as interposition materials [48, 62, 63].

Petersen et al. reported on the long-term outcomes of physeal bar excision in 48 patients of mixed etiology followed to skeletal maturity. Fourteen patients (29%) had bar excision alone with no other accompanying or subsequent surgery. Thirty-four patients (71%) had an additional 1 to 4 accompanying procedures, including leg length discrepancy or angular correcting procedures. They concluded that physeal bar excision when applied to the appropriate patient is a useful procedure, reducing the number of surgical limb length equalizing procedures, but that careful follow-up until maturity is needed. Subsequent limb reconstruction procedures may be necessary to realign the limb or equalize leg length discrepancy [56, 62, 63].

B: Bone Issues

Bone-related sequelae (sequestra, pathologic fractures, and bone gap) are unusual complications of childhood osteomyelitis in healthcare systems that are advanced with good access to care but have been reported in up to 20 % of patients with chronic osteomyelitis in studies from LMICs [10, 11, 18, 44, 69]. The tibia is the commonest site of involvement. Most children present late with severe disease, requiring aggressive surgical intervention and prolonged hospitalization. The chronic form of the disease may lead to extensive necrosis of bone, pathological fractures, and formation of sequestra, with resulting segmental defects, cavities, discharging sinuses, and pseudarthroses. The next few chapters in this textbook, on pathologic fractures and bone gaps in the lower and upper extremity, will explore the relevant clinical features and the principles of management that are available for the successful treatment of bone-related sequelae following pediatric MSKIs (Figs. 23.7, 23.8, and 23.9).

C: Joint Contractures or Instability

C1: Joint Contractures

Inadequate and inappropriate treatment of musculoskeletal infections, especially septic arthritis, and soft tissue infections like pyomyositis can result in joint contractures [53, 70, 71].

Prevalence The most common joints involved include the knee, hip, shoulder, ankle, and elbow. The sagittal plane contractures are most disabling, but contractures could involve other planes of motion as well [70–72].

Pathogenesis Joint contractures can be caused by the following [53, 72–74]:

1. Cartilage destruction: This is caused by proteolytic enzymes released by the bacteria, synovium, and the white blood cells. In addition, the chondrocytes and polymorphonuclear leukocytes, which have both neutral and acid proteases, may be stimulated to release these either by bacterial lipopolysaccharides or by interleukin 1. Bacterial antigens and bacterial exotoxins stimulate T-lymphocyte proliferation, which can occur even though the bacteria have been killed. T lymphocytes then degrade the ground substance and destroy articular cartilage. This can start as early as 8 hours following infection, resulting in chondrolysis and arthrofibrosis.
2. Intraarticular deformity: This is caused by destruction of subchondral bone and collapse, avascular necrosis, or a central growth arrest resulting in a fishtail deformity (distal femur).
3. Juxta-articular deformity: This is caused by bone destruction resulting in a fracture with malunion or an incomplete growth arrest.
4. Soft tissue contracture: This is caused by either a capsular contracture or a muscle contracture due to pain, prolonged immobilization, and/or inflammation with fibrosis of the capsule and surrounding muscle.
5. Bony ankylosis: Bone and cartilage destruction can result in bony ankylosis in an unacceptable, nonfunctional position.

Evaluation

1. Careful clinical examination is necessary to evaluate the plane of the contracture, the remaining joint range of motion, compensation from adjacent joints, and the resulting functional deficit. Differentiation between soft tissue and bony causes of the contracture is also a critical part of the exam. A complete neurovascular examination is another essential component of the evaluation.
2. A detailed review of the plain radiographs is needed to identify intra- and extra-articular bony deformity, aiding in the differentiation between bone and soft tissue causes of joint deformity. Advanced preoperative evaluation may include ultrasonography, computed tomography (CT), magnetic resonance imaging (MRI), and MR angiography (MRA).

3. Detailed analysis and preoperative planning of the deformity, using principles of deformity correction and paying special attention to sagittal plane deformities, are the final steps before surgery.

Management

1. Treatment options for soft tissue contractures include physical therapy, serial stretch casting, and static or dynamic stretch orthoses for smaller degrees of contractures (< 20 degrees). For larger degrees of contractures, capsular/muscle releases in combination with serial casting or stretch orthoses can be used. For severe contractures, joint distraction and correction with external fixators may be indicated [75–83].
2. Treatment options for contractures caused by extra-articular deformities include careful preoperative planning followed by deformity correction of the extra-articular deformities [84–86] (Fig. 23.10).
3. Treatment options for contractures caused by intra-articular deformities include careful preoperative deformity evaluation and deformity correction by intra-articular osteotomies [87] (Fig. 23.12).
4. Treatment options for contractures caused by fibrous ankylosis include soft tissue releases, muscle/tendon lengthening, capsulotomy, arthrolysis, and joint distraction techniques using external fixation [77–85].
5. Treatment options for contractures caused by a bony ankylosis in an unacceptable position includes an osteotomy through the fusion mass and gradual realignment with or without lengthening to equalize any associated leg length discrepancies using circular external fixation [73, 84] (Fig. 23.13).

C2: Joint Instability

Septic arthritis remains an important infection and is associated with significant mortality and morbidity. It is well established that the prognosis of septic arthritis in children is associated with the site of infection, history of prematurity, age of the child, diagnosis and treatment delay, presence of concurrent osteomyelitis, and the organism responsible (staphylococcus being the most common and most virulent). The hip is known to be the most frequently involved site and has the poorest outcomes of all joints [8, 21, 103, 104].

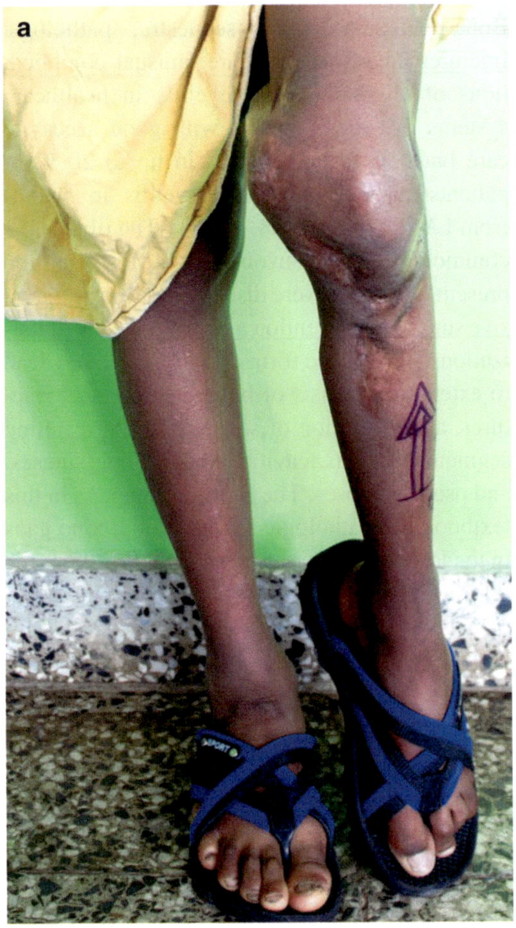

Fig. 23.12 Case 12: Contracture & shortening left knee. (Courtesy Dr. Tim Nunn). (**a–d**) An 11-year-old male with post-septic posterolateral left knee subluxation, flexion contracture of 90°, and distal femoral physeal arrest with femoral segment shortening and stuck down patella. Radiographs and sagittal CT reformat of left knee showing posterolateral left knee subluxation, flexion contracture, and a distal femoral physeal bar. (**e, f**) Transepiphyseal resection of left distal femur and tibia, common peroneal nerve release, partial acute correction, and gradual residual correction with a hexapod external fixator. (**g, h**) Fusion of left knee completed in extension fusion with attempted tibial growth plate preservation. Contralateral distal femur physeodesis was also performed for equalizing LLD.

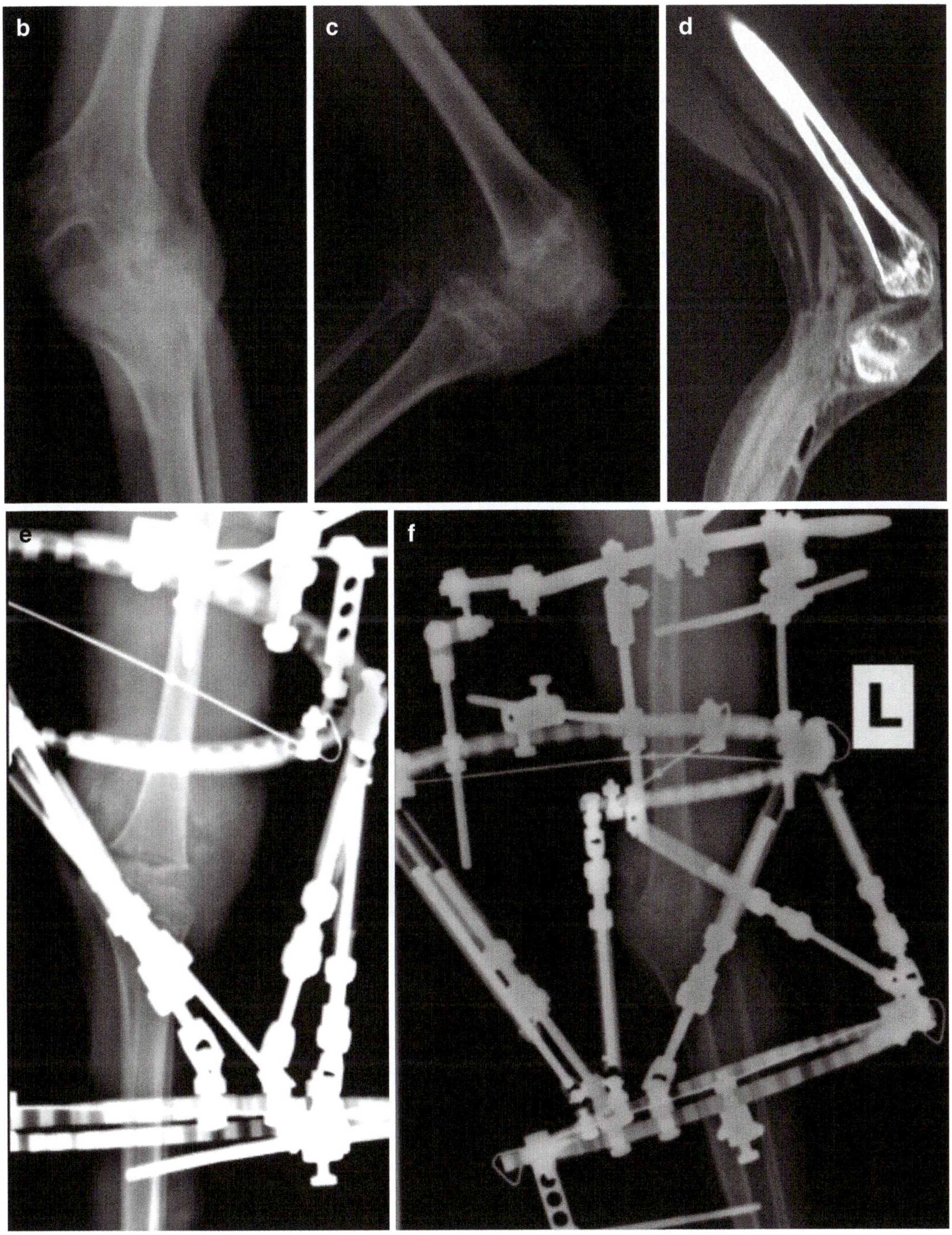

Fig. 23.12 (continued)

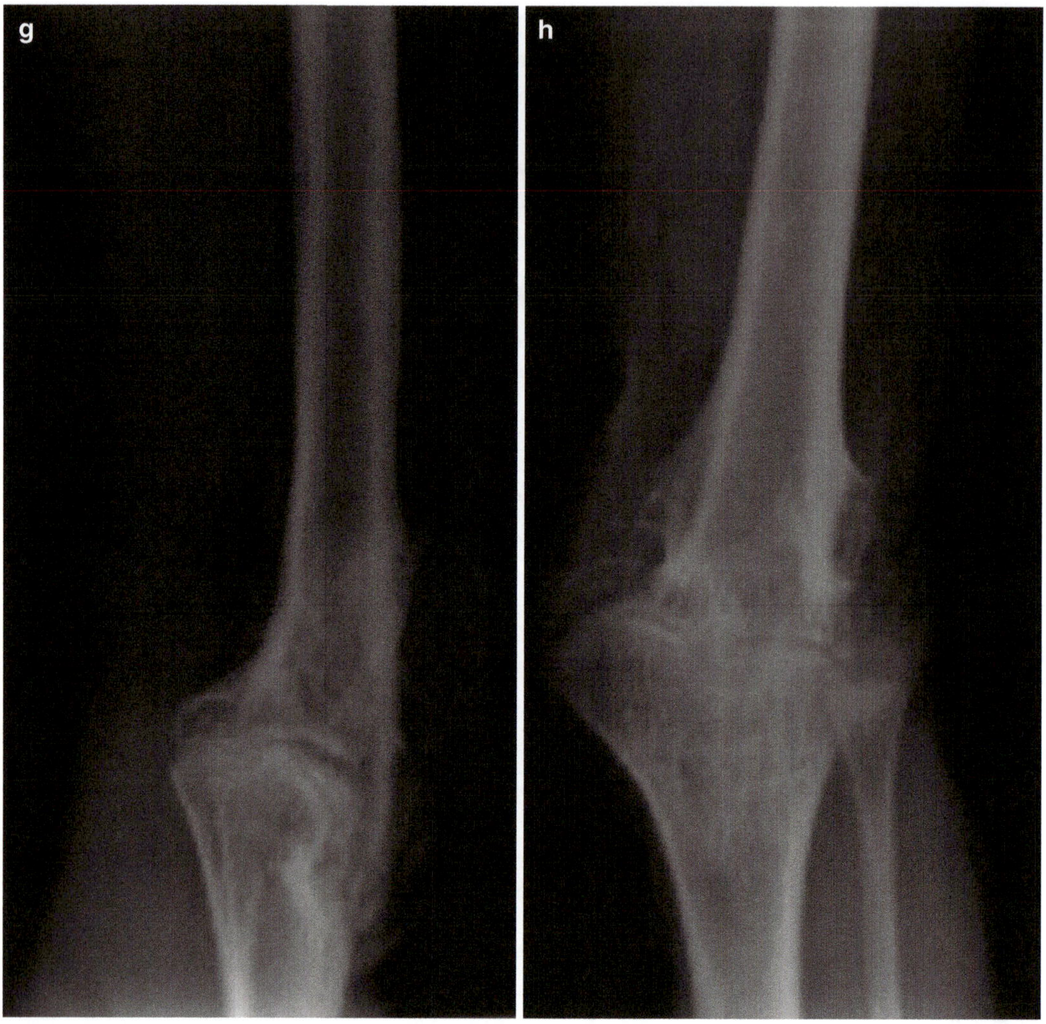

Fig. 23.12 (continued)

Joint instability following septic arthritis is a less recognized sequela which can present acutely as well as late. It is more frequently seen in LMICs due to delayed presentation. It is most commonly seen after septic arthritis of the hip joint but has also been described after MSKI of the shoulder, elbow, knee, and ankle [103–114] (Figs. 23.14 and 23.15).

Pathogenesis Instability can be caused acutely by stretching of the capsule by increased intra-articular hydrostatic pressure and destruction of ligaments by the septic process. Delayed instability can be caused by deformity of the bone caused by a growth plate arrest (e.g., a partial growth arrest of the proximal femur), dysplasia (e.g., acetabular dysplasia caused by growth arrest of the triradiate cartilage), or loss of static support (e.g., destruction or excision of the distal fibula) [103–114].

Evaluation A high index of suspicion and careful clinical evaluation with imaging studies are necessary to prevent delayed or missed diagnosis. It is important to obtain additional investigations in the form of MRI, ultrasound, or arthrogram. At the hip, MRI yields information about the condition of the capital femoral epiphysis (CFE), articular cartilage, acetabular labrum and capsule, and soft tissue interposing factors [108, 109].

Management At the hip, when joint instability is present acutely with septic arthritis, closed reduction and stabilization (e.g., hip spica cast application) may be successful. When the presentation is late, as a sequela of septic arthritis, the capital femoral epiphysis (CFE) may not be well visualized on radiographs because of the delayed ossification, and these hips may be mistakenly classified as dislocations with absence of the CFE. Differentiating between loss of the CFE and delayed ossification of the CFE is important for making appropriate management decisions [108, 109].

Examination under anesthesia with an arthrogram is indicated, followed by an attempt at closed reduction. Adductor tenotomy may be needed to achieve successful, congruent reduction; CR is successful in about 35% of cases. Surgical intervention is indicated in failed closed reduction cases and an age of more than 2 years. A combination of procedures may be required to obtain a congruous reduction, which may not always be achieved. Open reduction with femoral shortening ± varus derotation osteotomy ± acetabular osteotomy may be needed. Surgeries for septic hip dislocations are difficult because of adhesions, femoral head changes, acetabular changes, and cartilage changes. Risk factors for poor outcome include hip stiffness on exam, avascular necrosis of the CFE, premature fusion of the triradiate cartilage, and cartilage thinning on MRI identified preoperatively. On intraoperative evaluation, femoral head flattening and coxa magna, cartilage erosions, and marked fibrosis and adhesions were associated with poor out-

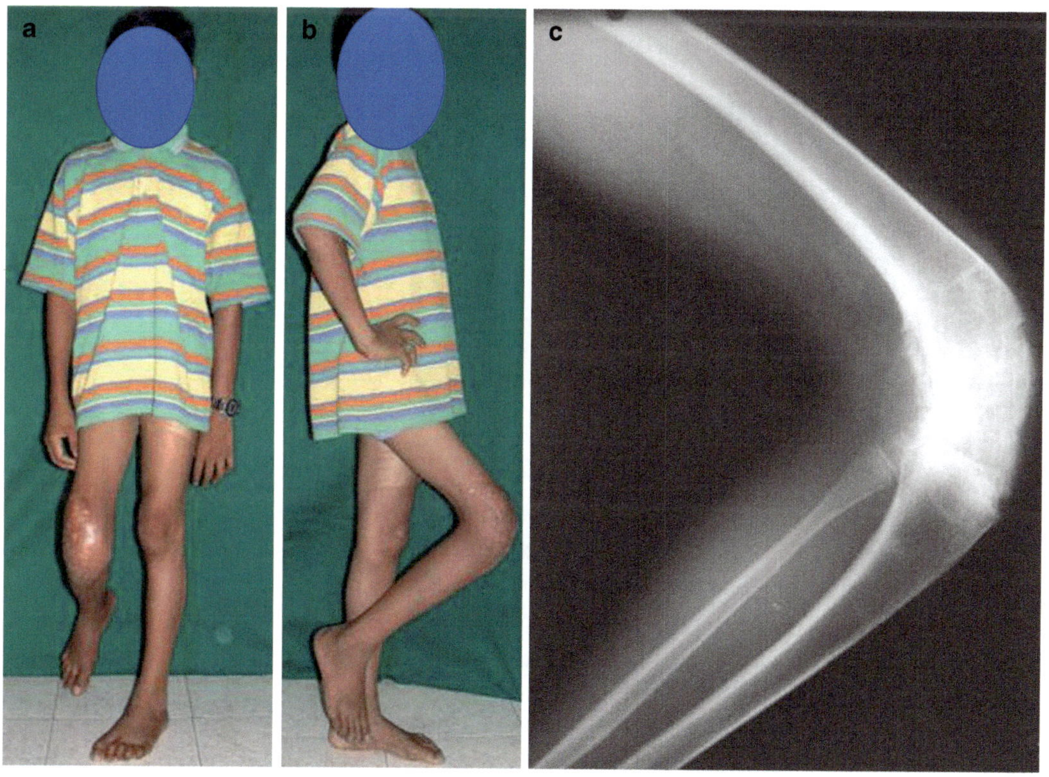

Fig. 23.13 Case 13: Contracture right knee. (Courtesy Dr. Milind Chaudhary). (**a**–**c**) A 10-year-old boy, with a right knee fusion (bony ankylosis) in 90 degrees flexion with paper thin skin because of osteomyelitis in childhood. (**d**–**g**) Gradual correction through a supracondylar osteotomy, away from bad skin using a circular external fixator and osteotomy Rule 3. (**h**–**k**) 1-year postop, he has a straight right knee. The mild residual anterior translation gives a simulation of a mild FFD which is needed for easy ambulation

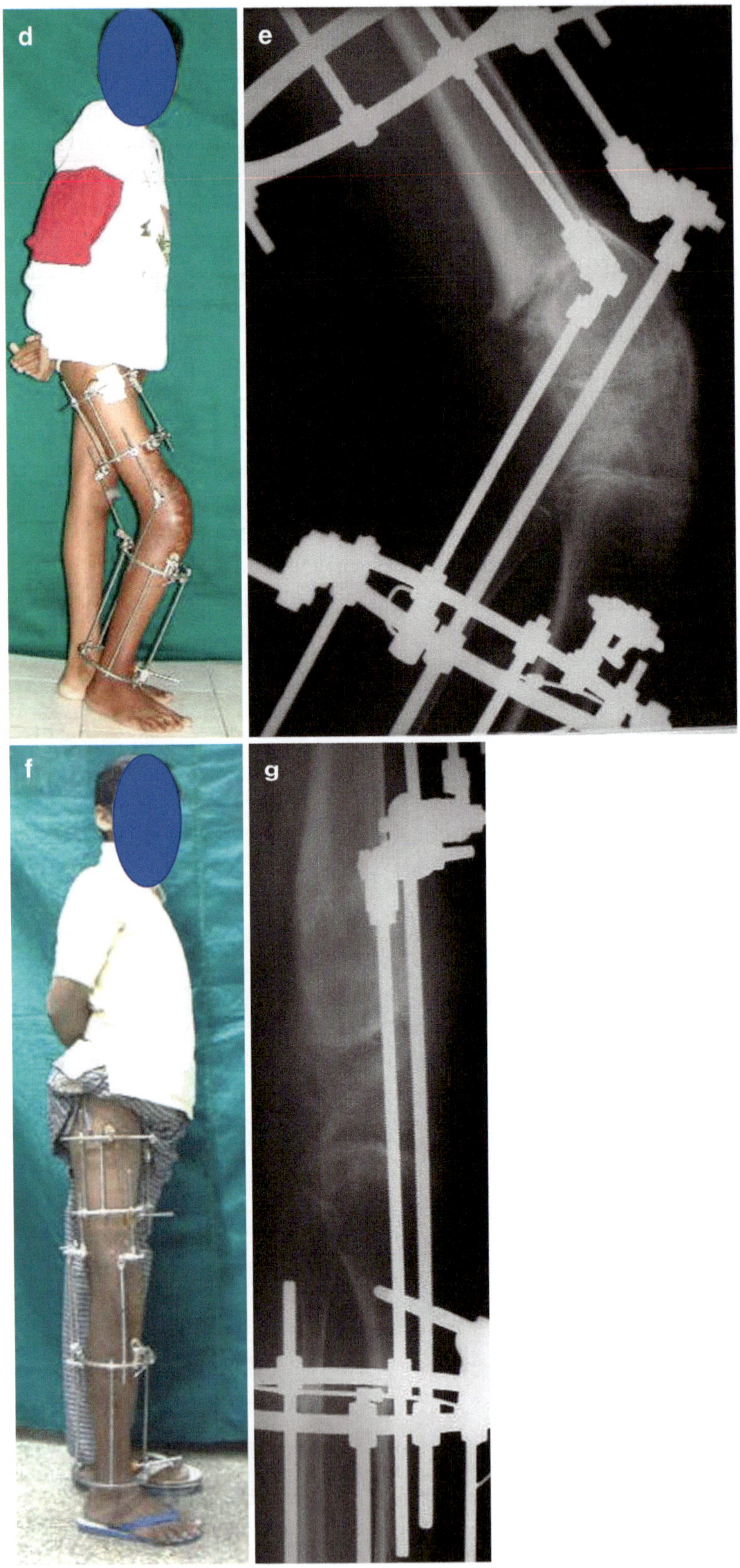

Fig. 23.13 (continued)

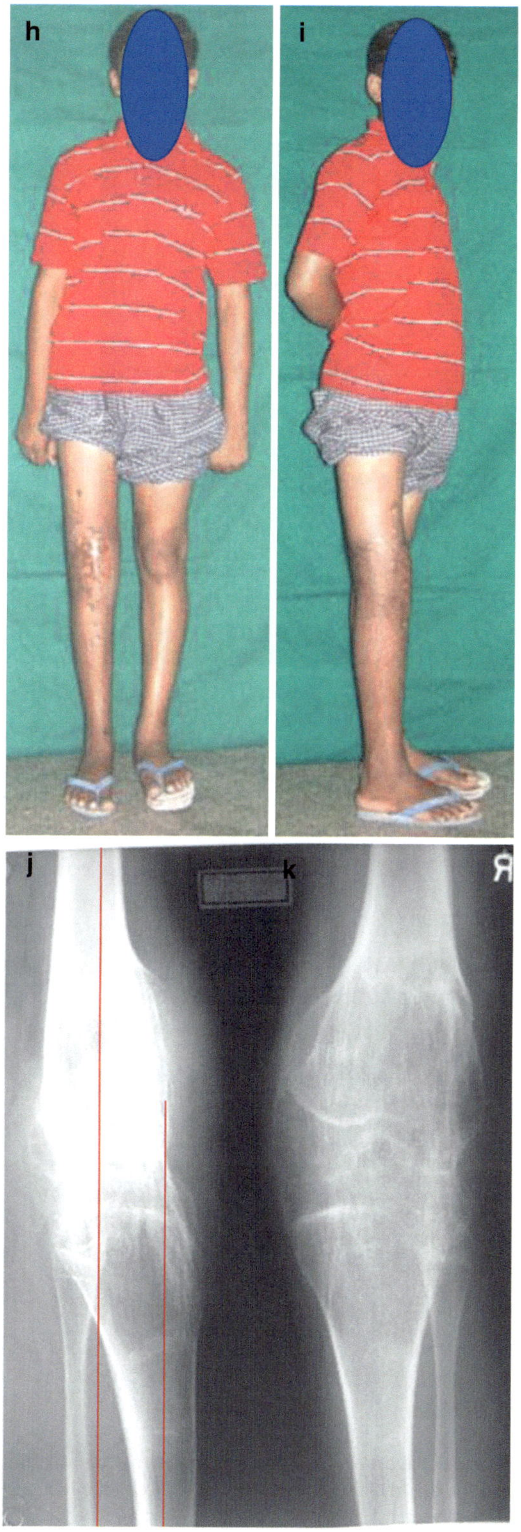

Fig. 23.13 (continued)

comes. Follow-up to skeletal maturity is needed to assess the long-term outcomes. Outcomes following open reduction for late presenting post-septic hip dislocations have been reported to be better than closed reduction. Open reduction potentially alters the natural history of post-septic sequelae of hips with dislocation and contributes to better hip mechanics and function [108, 109].

At other joints, delayed presentation of joint instability may require deformity correction or even salvage procedures like arthrodesis (e.g., at the ankle or knee) [73, 84] (Figs. 23.14 and 23.15).

D: Deformity

Post-infective deformities can be localized to the articular, juxta-articular, or metadiaphyseal areas. Articular and juxta-articular deformities are caused by septic arthritis with concurrent metaphyseal osteomyelitis resulting in growth plate damage, joint destruction and incongruity, impingement, accompanying ligamentous laxity, and joint instability [8, 21, 53]. The most serious sequelae are seen following musculoskeletal infections in the first 2 years of life [13]. Metadiaphyseal deformities usually result from malunion or nonunion of pathologic fractures following osteomyelitis. Soft tissue considerations, like scarring of the soft tissue envelope and neurologic issues, can contribute to the development and progression of the deformities [8, 21, 53] (Figs. 23.11, 23.16, 23.17, and 23.18).

Incidence Deformities are more frequently seen after septic arthritis of the hip and shoulder than after septic arthritis of the other joints (knee, ankle, elbow, and wrist) because septic arthritis in these joints is more common, is often diagnosed later, and is frequently associated with concurrent osteomyelitis [18, 21–25].

Evaluation Deformities can vary widely with respect to the site and plane of involvement, magnitude, integrity of the soft tissue envelope, and natural history. Hence, it is essential to have a comprehensive approach to evaluation of the deformity [8, 21, 53, 89]. This includes a detailed

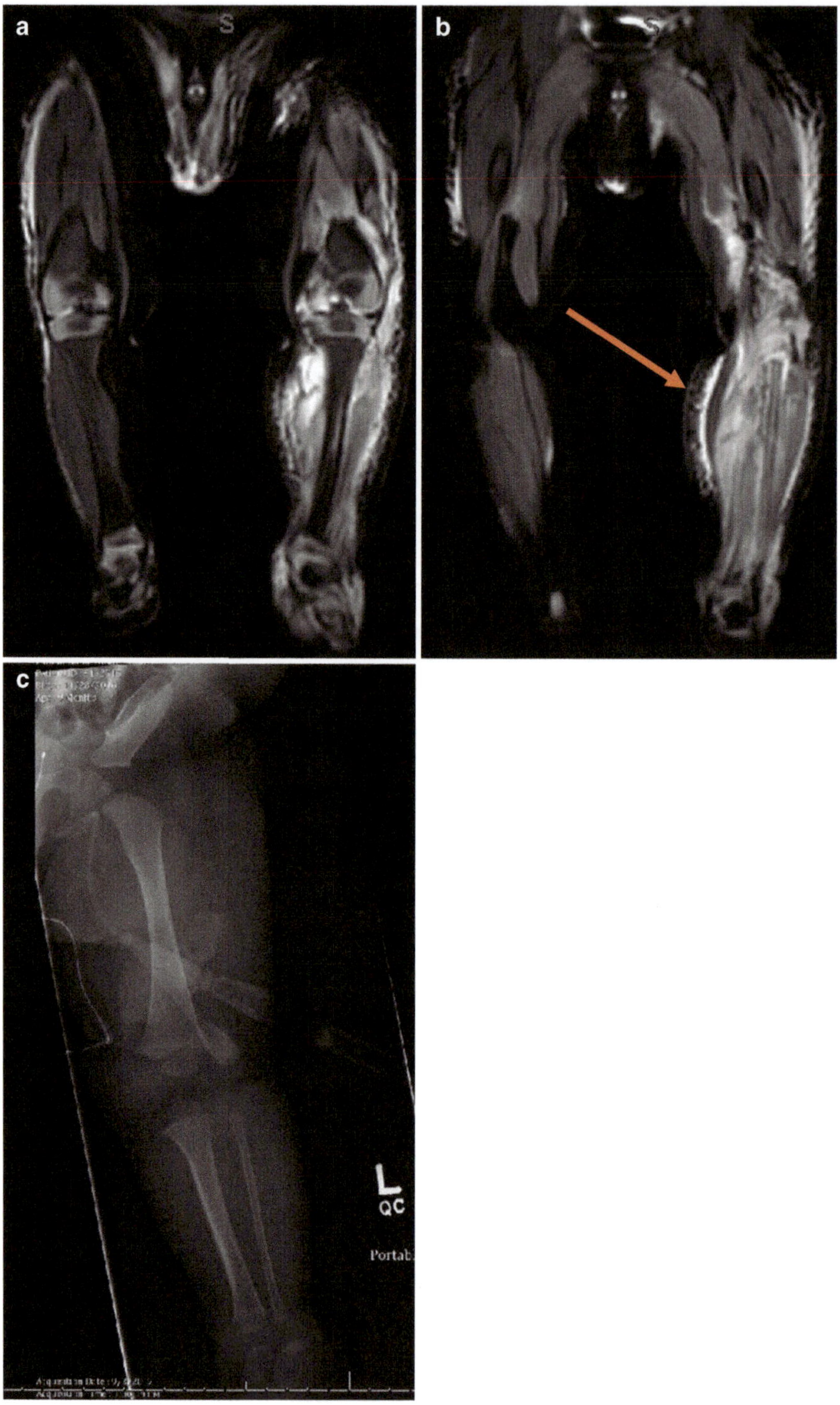

Fig. 23.14 Case 14: Left ankle subluxation following extensive fibular AHO. (Courtesy Dr. Mohan V Belthur). (**a–c**) T2 W MRI in a 9-month-old boy showing extensive myonecrosis involving left leg anterior, lateral, and deep posterior compartment musculature. Abnormal signal within left fibula with subperiosteal abscess. Radiograph shows soft tissue swelling left leg. (**d, e**) Radiographs of left leg at age 11 months show complete resection of fibula for pan fibular osteomyelitis. (**f–h**) Radiographs at age 2 + 6 years show superolateral subluxation of the left ankle with absence of fibula. (**i, j**) Radiographs at age 4 years, 9 months postop, show healed left ankle arthrodesis with good alignment

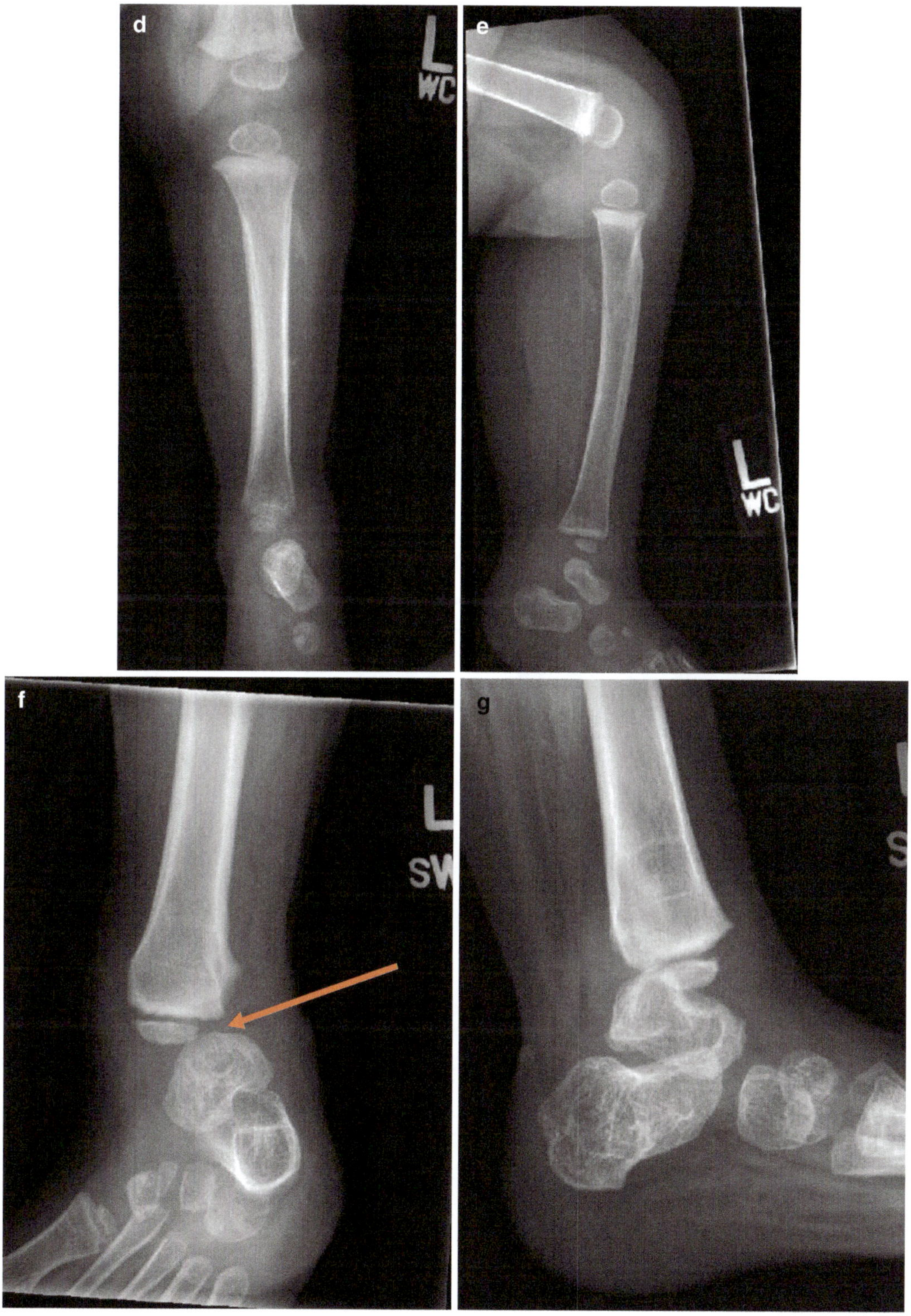

Fig. 23.14 (continued)

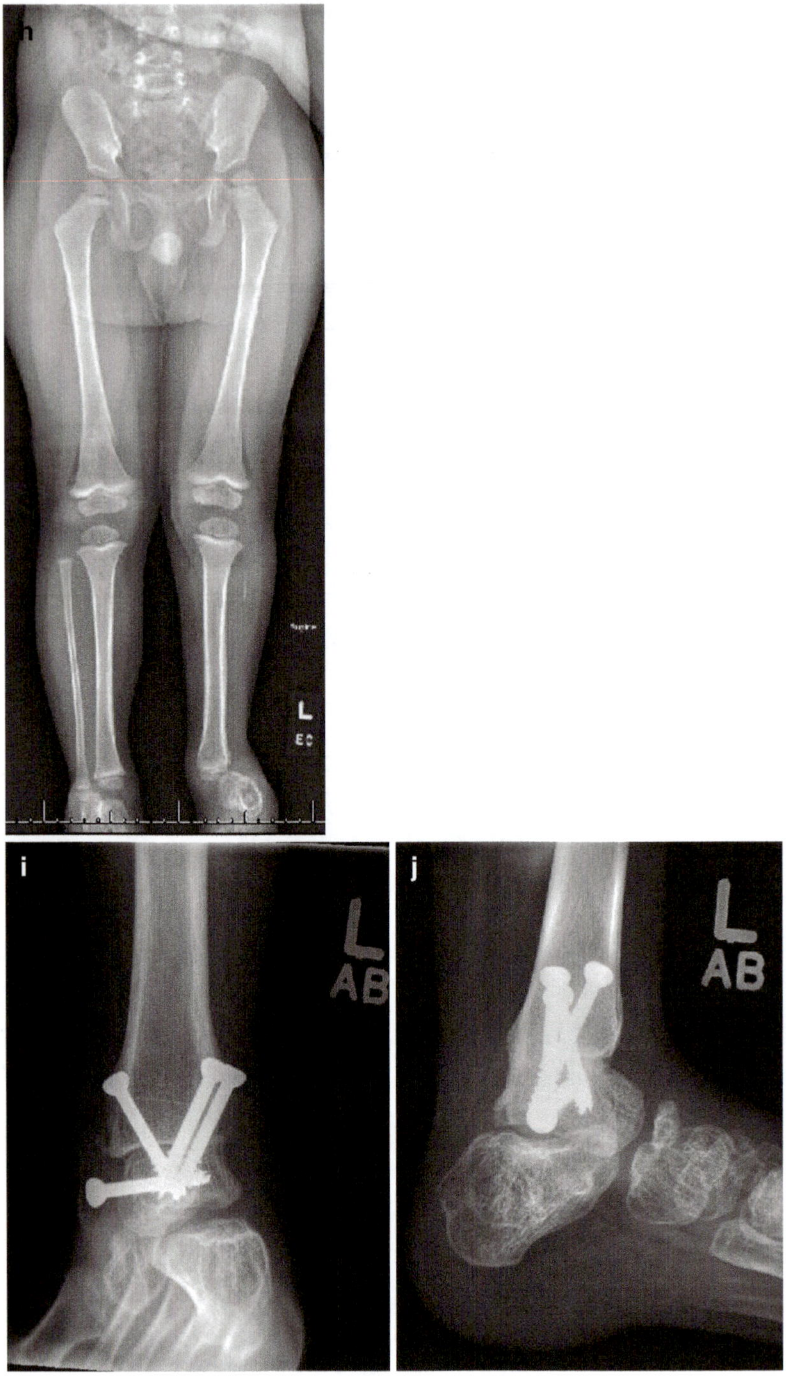

Fig. 23.14 (continued)

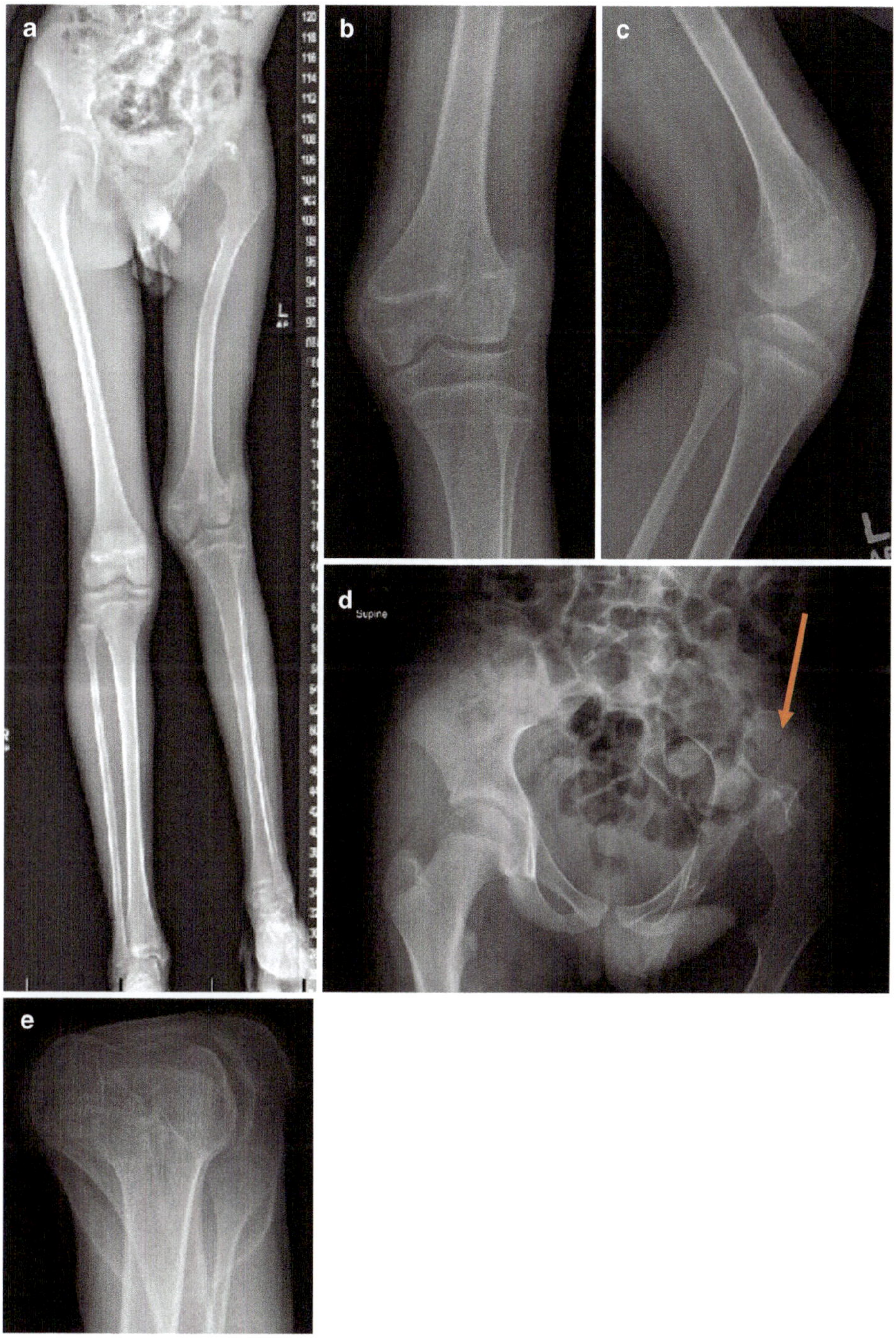

Fig. 23.15 Case 15: Postseptic left hip and PFJ dislocation with Left distal femur partial growth arrest. (Courtesy Dr. Mohan V Belthur). (**a–e**) In a 12-year-old male, radiographs show left hip dislocation with acetabular dysplasia, left distal femur valgus with a dislocated left patella, and LLD left < Rt 9.5 cm, s/p septic arthritis left hip and knee with concurrent osteomyelitis. (**f–h**) Coronal, sagittal, and axial MRI showing left distal femur lateral growth arrest with dislocation of patella. (**i–k**) 3 month postop radiographs, showing healed left distal femur osteotomy with corrected genu valgum, relocated patella with an LLD of 9.5 cm with a dislocated left hip, and Rt pan genu screw epiphysiodesis. (**l, m**) C arm pictures showing Rt femoral shortening osteotomy of 4.5 cm. (**n**) 15 + 6 yo skeletally mature with no functional LLD with realigned left LE and excellent function left knee/PFJ with a left hip high dislocation. He will need an Ilizarov hip reconstruction for his left hip and to equalize his residual LLD. (**o, p, q**) Plain radiographs of the knee showing well aligned left patellofemoral joint after realignment for Left chronic patellar lateral dislocation

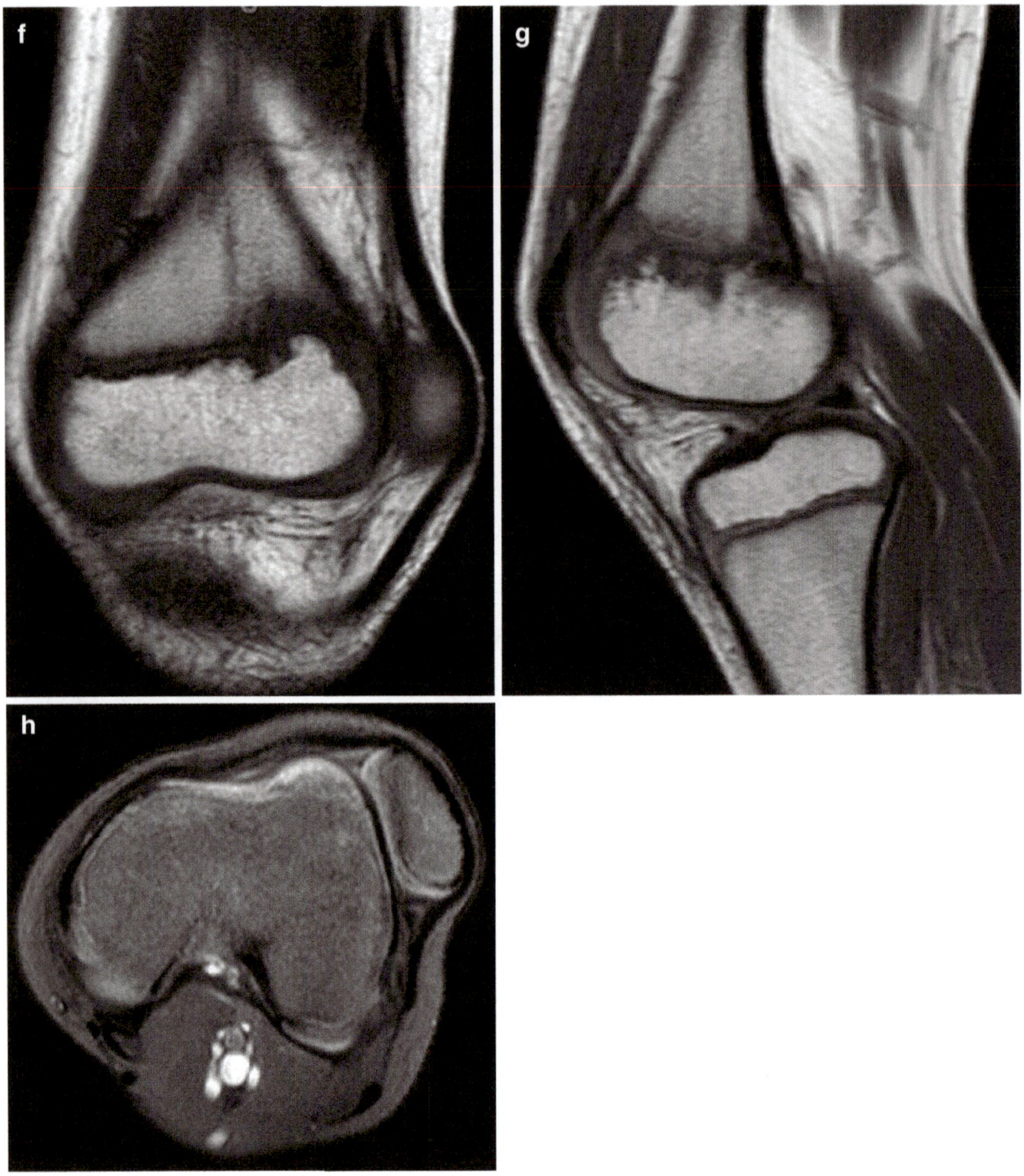

Fig. 23.15 (continued)

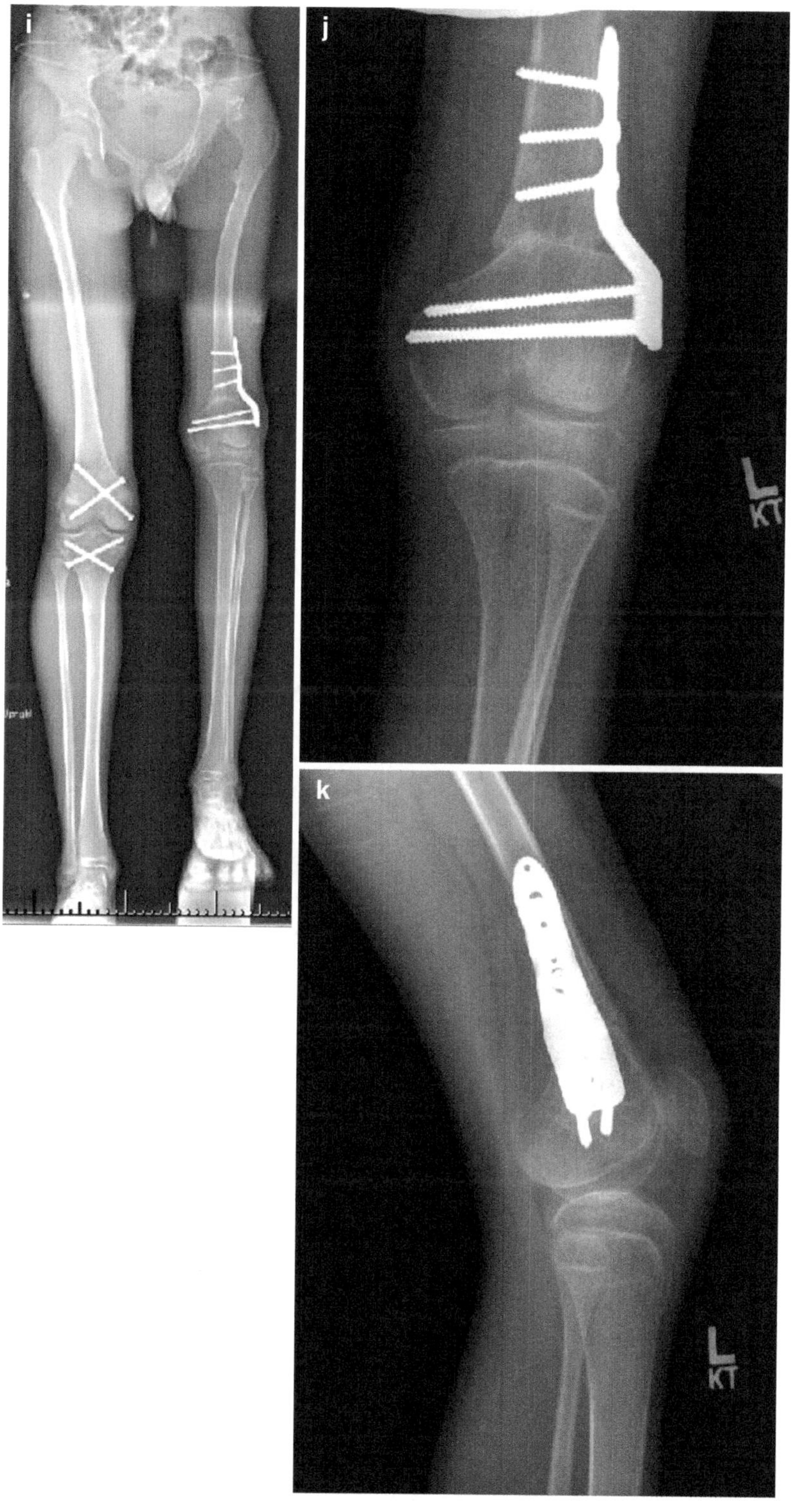

Fig. 23.15 (continued)

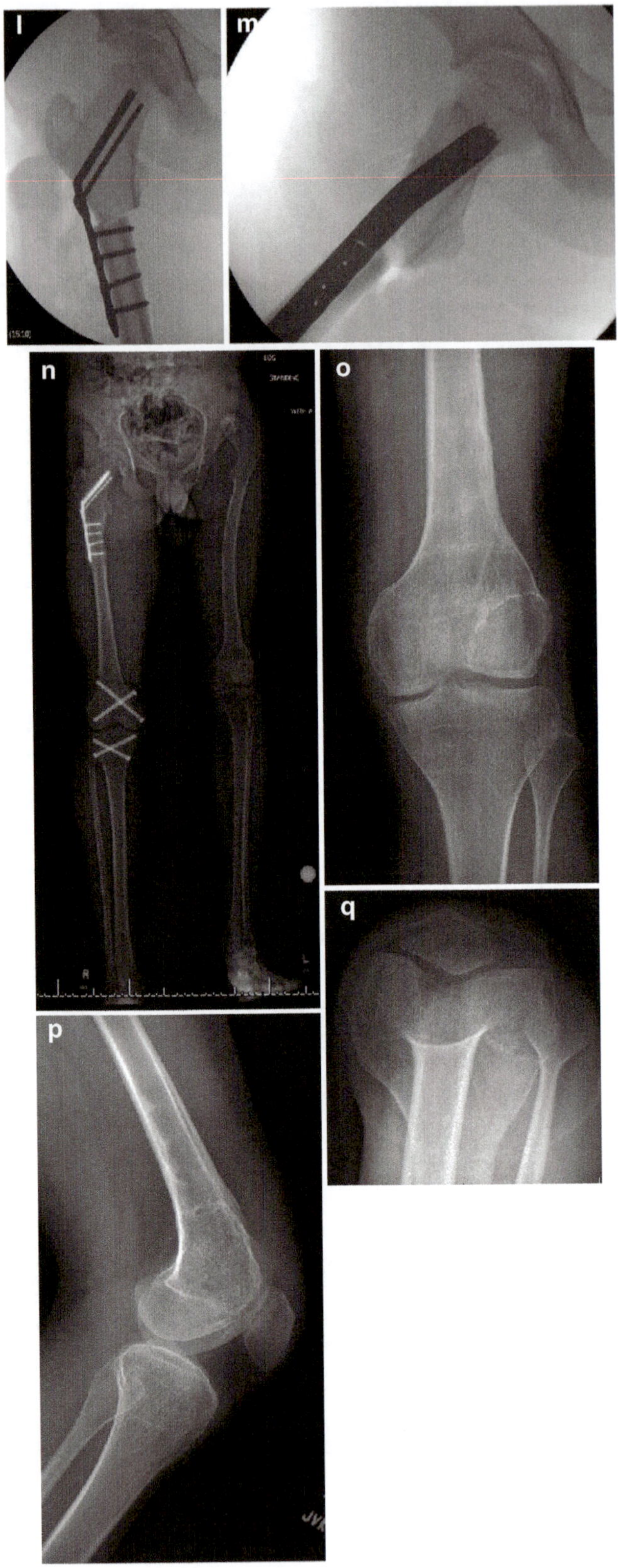

Fig. 23.15 (continued)

history, a systematic examination, and accurate imaging studies to develop a comprehensive problem list outlining the pathology associated with the involved limb.

When obtaining the history, a chronological account of the development of the deformity as well as current symptoms of pain, instability, neurologic changes, and functional limitations

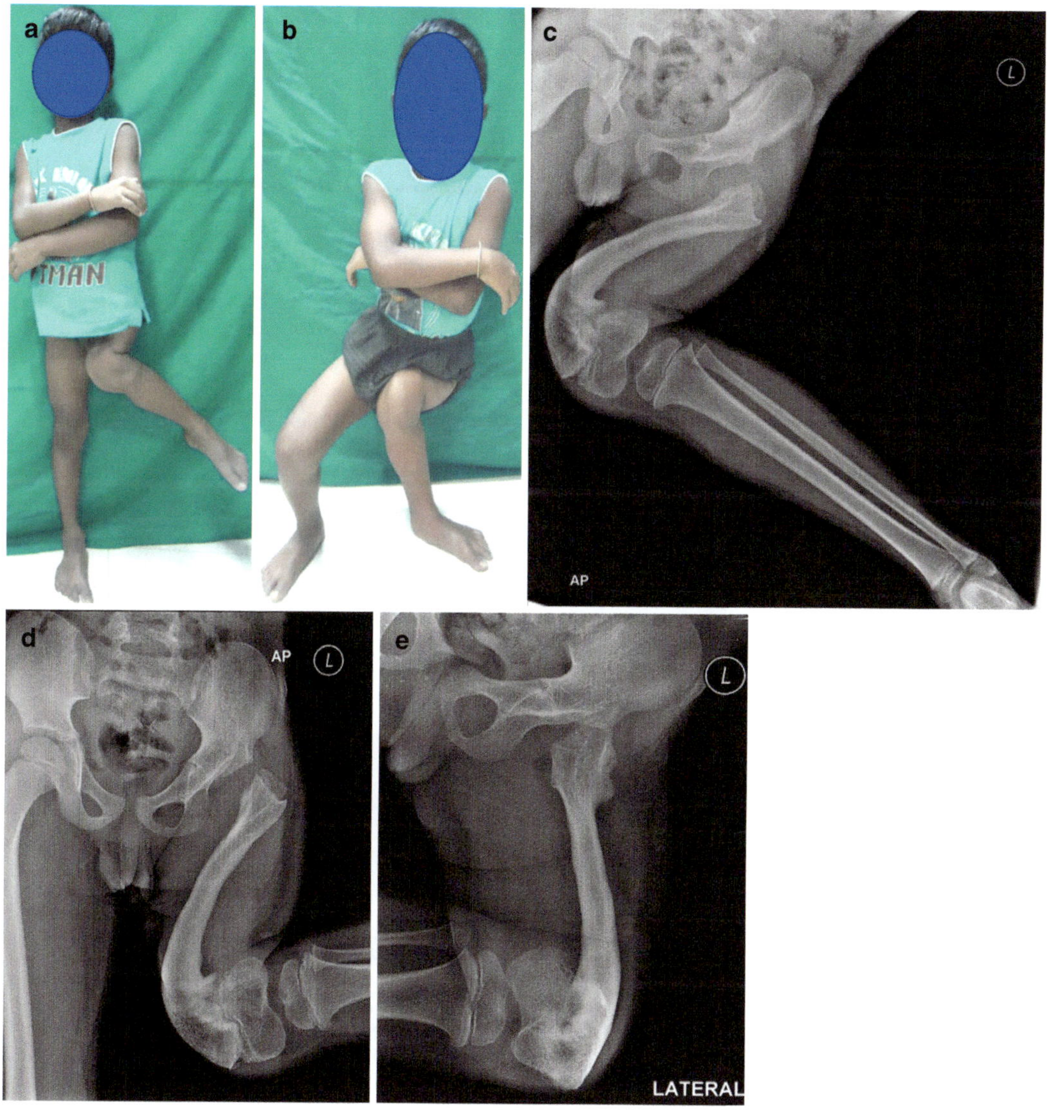

Fig. 23.16 Case 16: Deformity left distal femur and hip dislocation. (Courtesy Dr. Milind Chaudhary). (**a–e**) A 6-year-old boy with dislocation and destruction of the left femoral head as well as a multiplanar severe valgus, procurvatum, and external rotation deformity of the left distal femur with shortening due to a partial growth arrest, secondary to concurrent osteomyelitis and septic arthritis of the hip and knee. (**f–i**) Gradual correction of the left distal femur deformity was achieved using a circular external fixator. Fixation of distal femur was enhanced by spanning the knee. An outrigger allowed him to walk straight while the deformity corrected. (**j–n**) 1-year postop, with his left distal femur deformity corrected, we now plan on performing an Ilizarov hip reconstruction for his unstable left hip

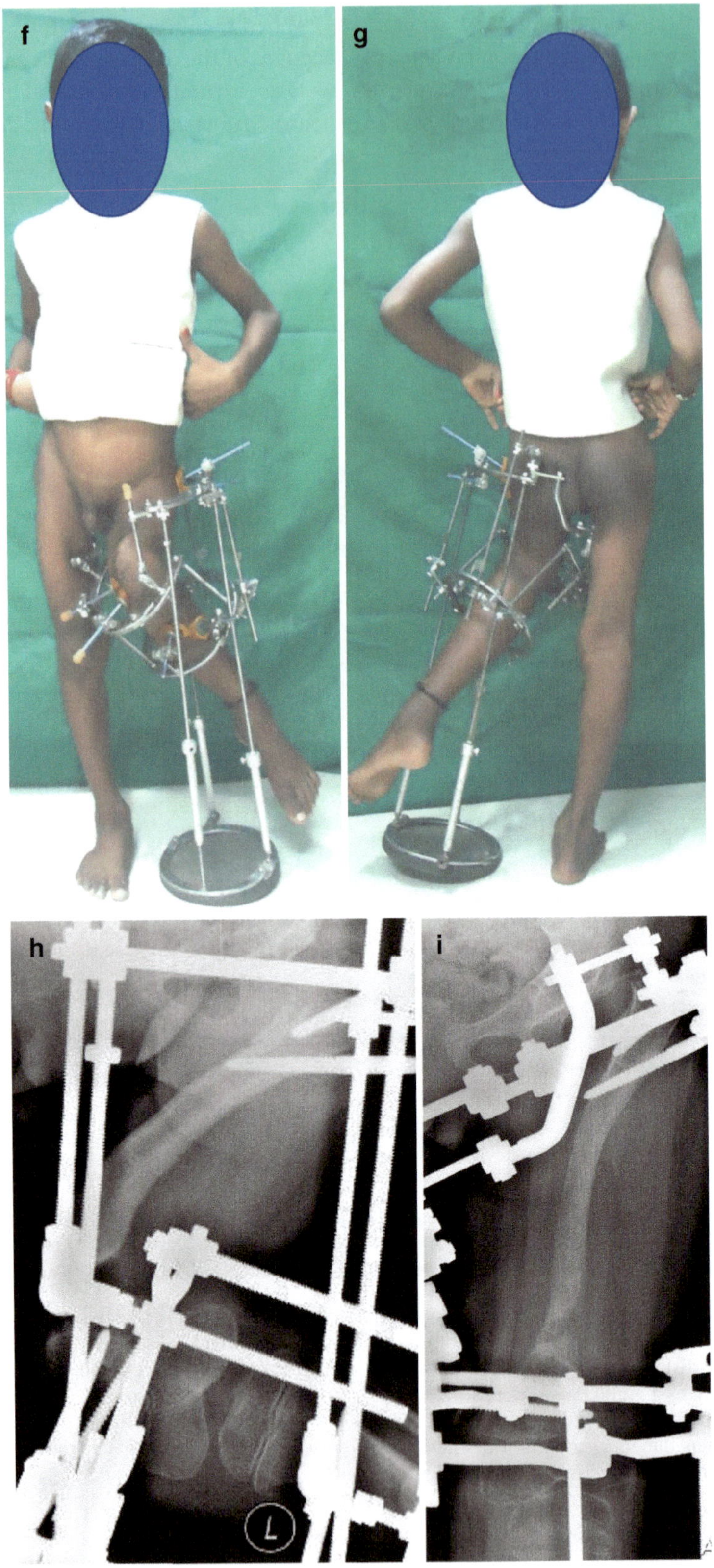

Fig. 23.16 (continued)

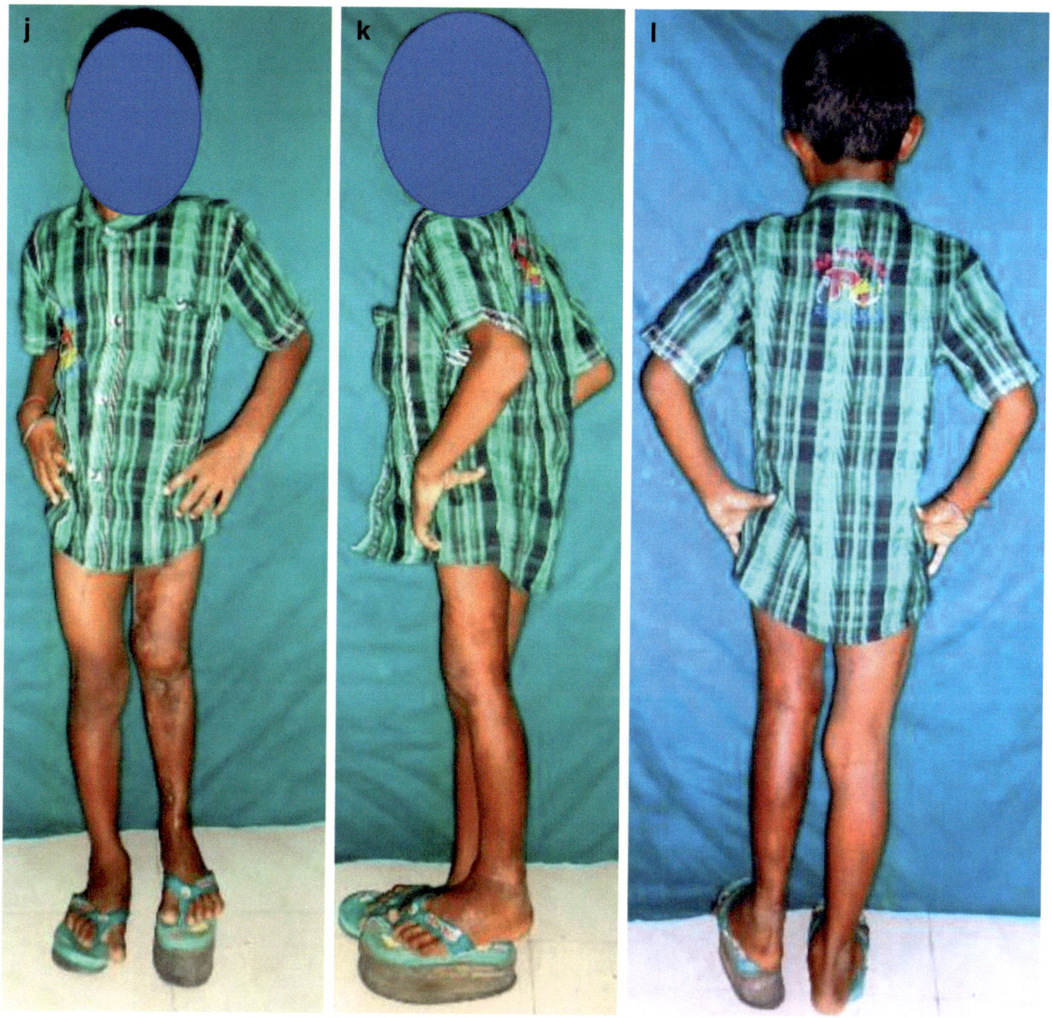

Fig. 23.16 (continued)

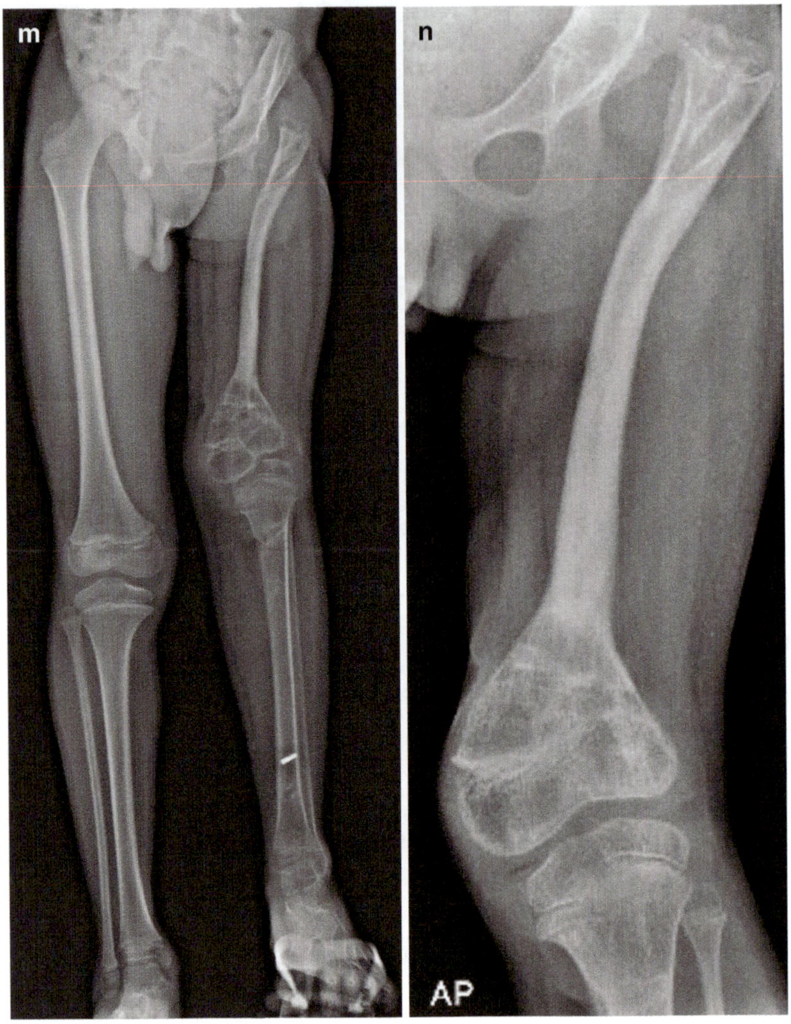

Fig. 23.16 (continued)

must be elicited. Past medical history including chronic medical conditions and previous treatment history can influence the decision-making.

Examination usually starts with evaluation of function (gait in the lower extremity and reach in the upper extremity) and should include assessment of range of motion and stability of all major joints. Coronal, sagittal, and transverse plane alignment of the upper and lower extremity must be evaluated. Patients with juxta-articular deformity may also have a compensatory fixed deformity at an adjacent bone and joint. Correction of this compensatory deformity must also be considered in the treatment plan to avoid malorientation of the joint, leading to altered biomechanics resulting in long-term disability.

Imaging Studies Meticulous analysis of the complex deformity of the limb by determining the location, magnitude, and direction of the deformity would be the first step in characterizing the deformity. Mechanical axis deviation, mechanical and anatomical alignment, and joint orientation should be accurately determined. In addition, limb length discrepancy (current and predicted at skeletal maturity), the presence of joint instability, and loss of mobility secondary to

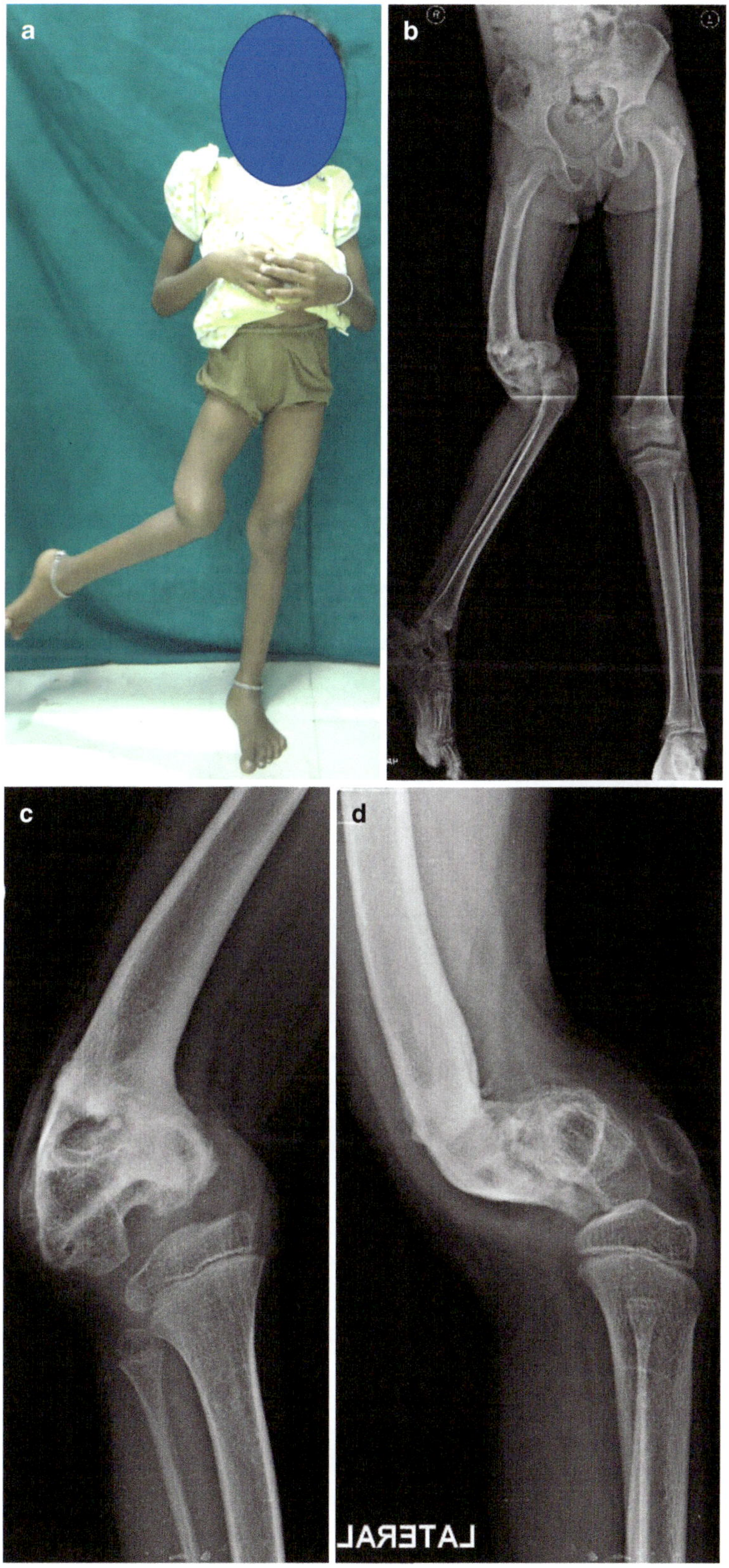

Fig. 23.17 Case 17: Deformity right distal femur. (Courtesy Dr. Milind Chaudhary). (**a**–**d**) A 12-year-old girl with a grotesque deformity of the right distal femur after osteomyelitis and growth arrest. Careful analysis reveals a varus, internal rotation and recurvatum in the distal femur. (**e**–**g**) A distal femur osteotomy allows us to recreate the physis, correct her deformities, and lengthen with hinges. Rate of lengthening in this deformity was reduced to allow the sclerotic bone to form a good regenerate. A proximal femoral corticotomy was done to add to the length gain. (**h**–**j**) 1-year postop, showing corrected deformity and equalized limb length discrepancy

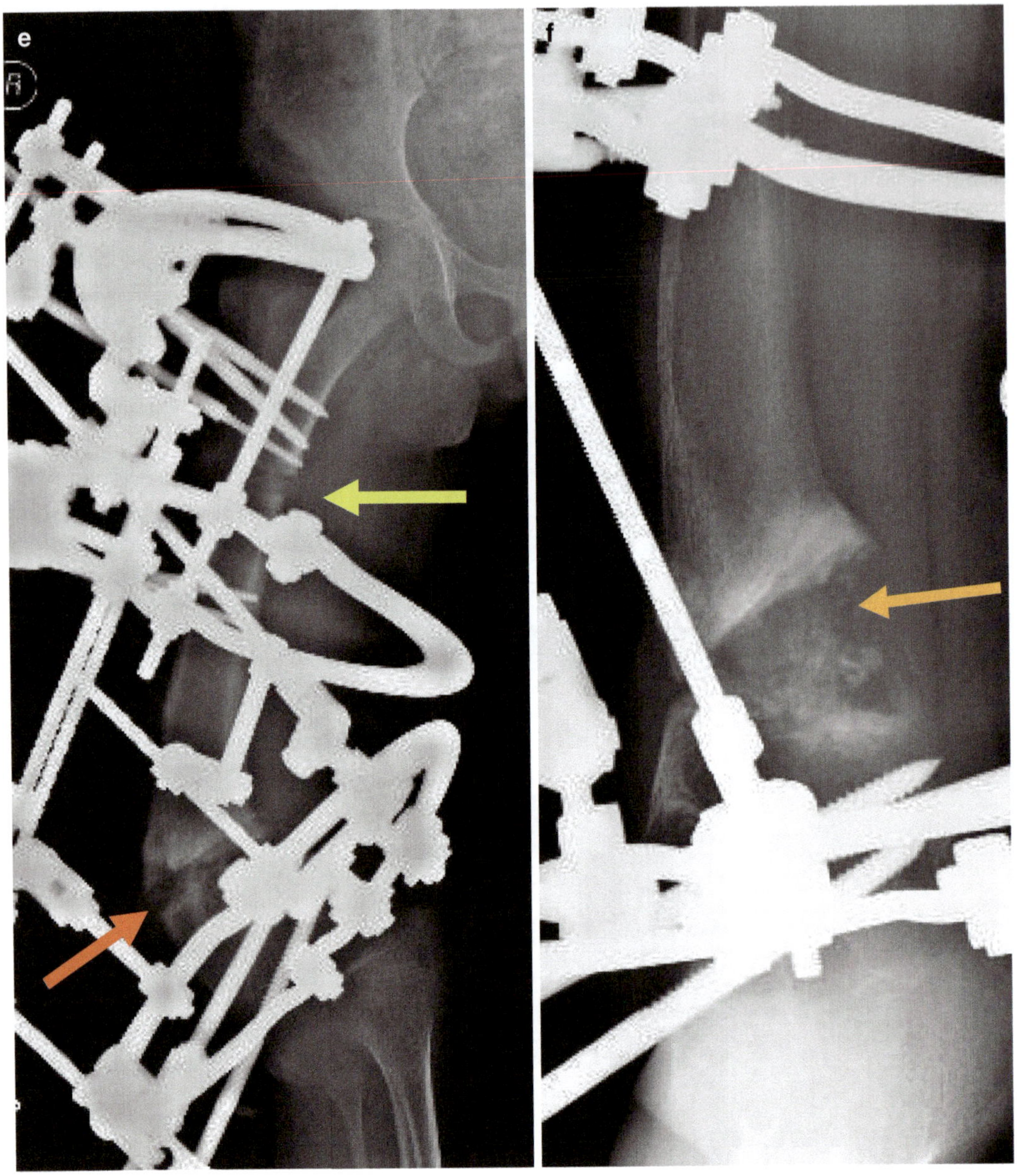

Fig. 23.17 (continued)

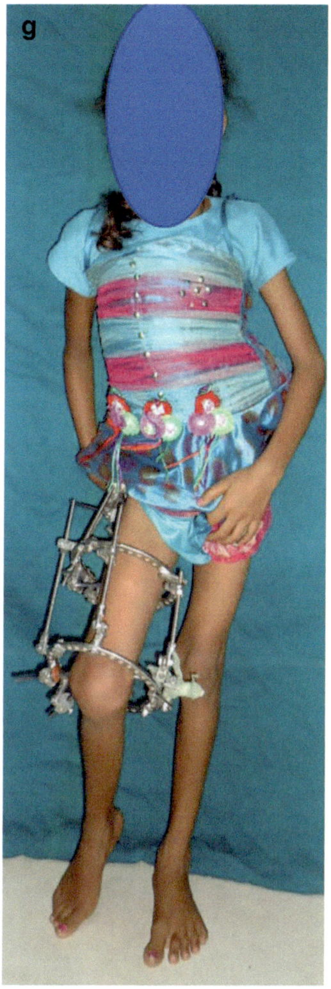

Fig. 23.17 (continued)

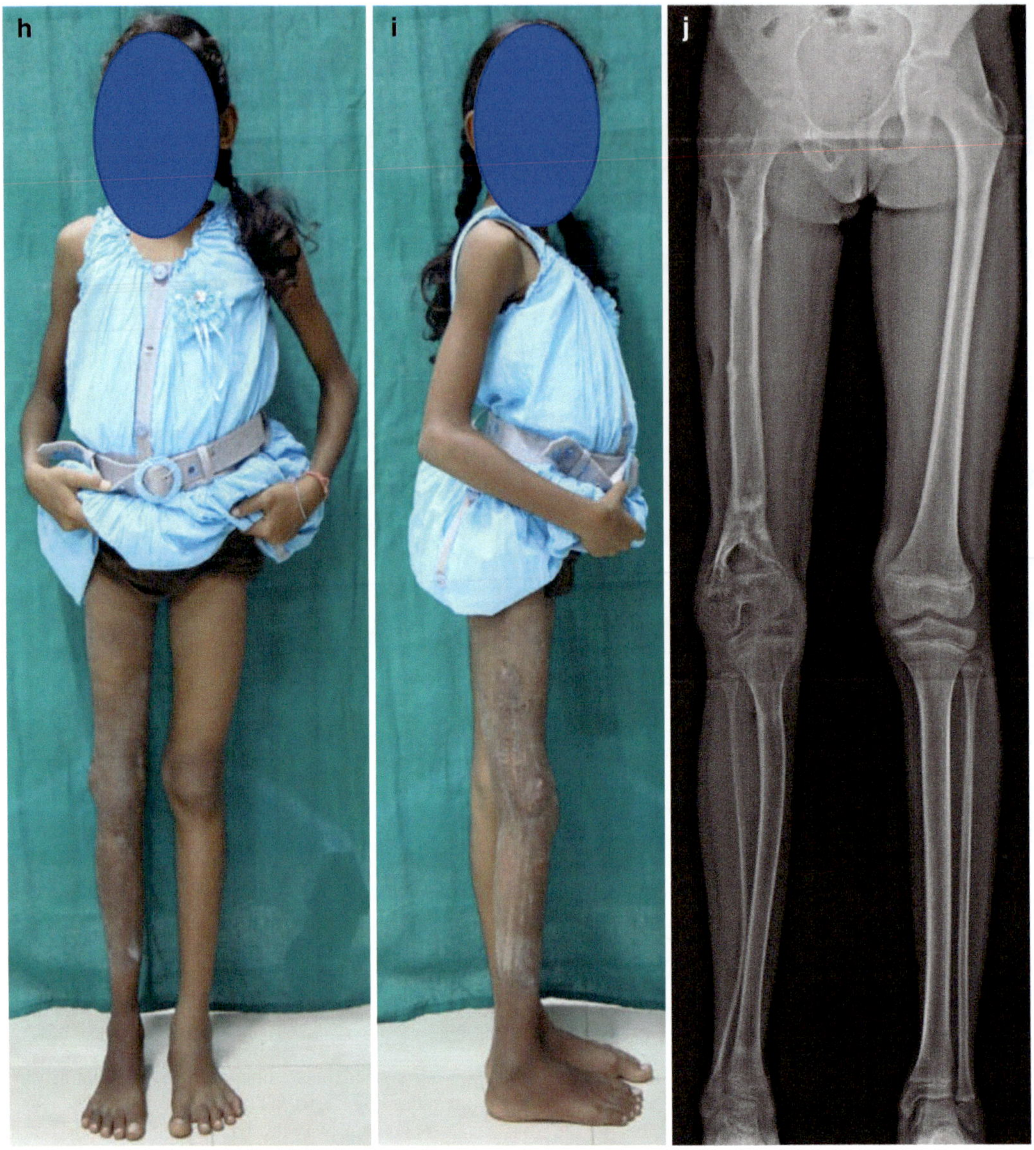

Fig. 23.17 (continued)

soft tissue contractures and/or juxta-articular skeletal deformity should be evaluated [21, 89].

Full length radiographs of the whole limb in the coronal and sagittal planes (standing in the lower limb) are helpful to evaluate mechanical axis of the limb, alignment of each individual limb segment, joint malorientation, joint instability, and limb length discrepancy. Full length radiographs of the extremity provide information about the static deformity in both the coronal and sagittal planes. Components of the deformity can include angulation, translation, length, and rotation. Of these, angulation, translation, and length can be ascertained from the radiographs. Rotation is often best ascertained by examining the patient, although specialized rotational studies like EOS (EOS Imaging, Paris, France), CT, and MRI can complement the physical examination in selected situations. Gait analysis can provide information about the dynamic contributions to the deformity in three planes in selected cases.

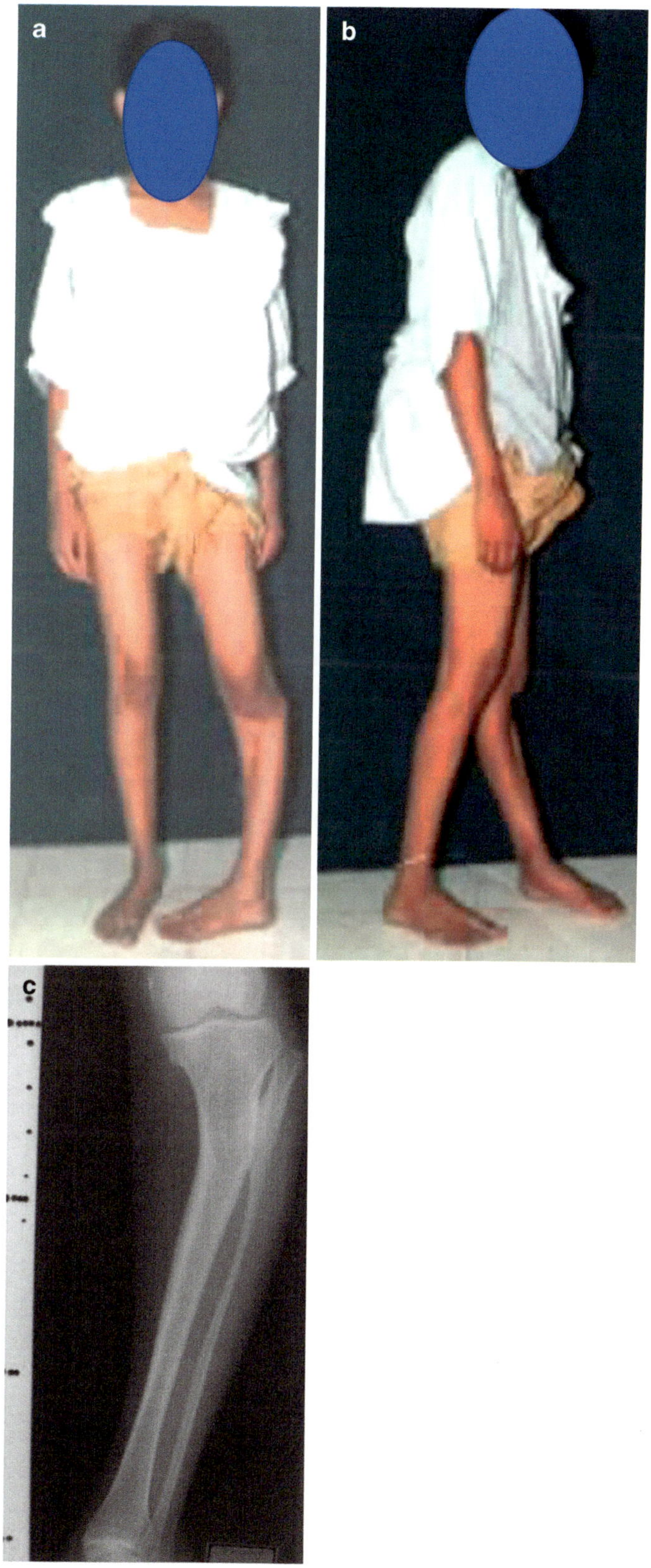

Fig. 23.18 Case 18: deformity right tibia. (Courtesy Dr. Milind Chaudhary). (**a–c**) A 20-year-old female with varus, internal rotation, recurvatum, and shortening of the left tibia s/p childhood osteomyelitis. (**d–h**) Left tibia and fibular osteotomy with gradual correction of deformity and shortening with a circular external fixator. (**i–k**) 1-year postop, with full correction of all left deformities of the left tibia and equal leg lengths

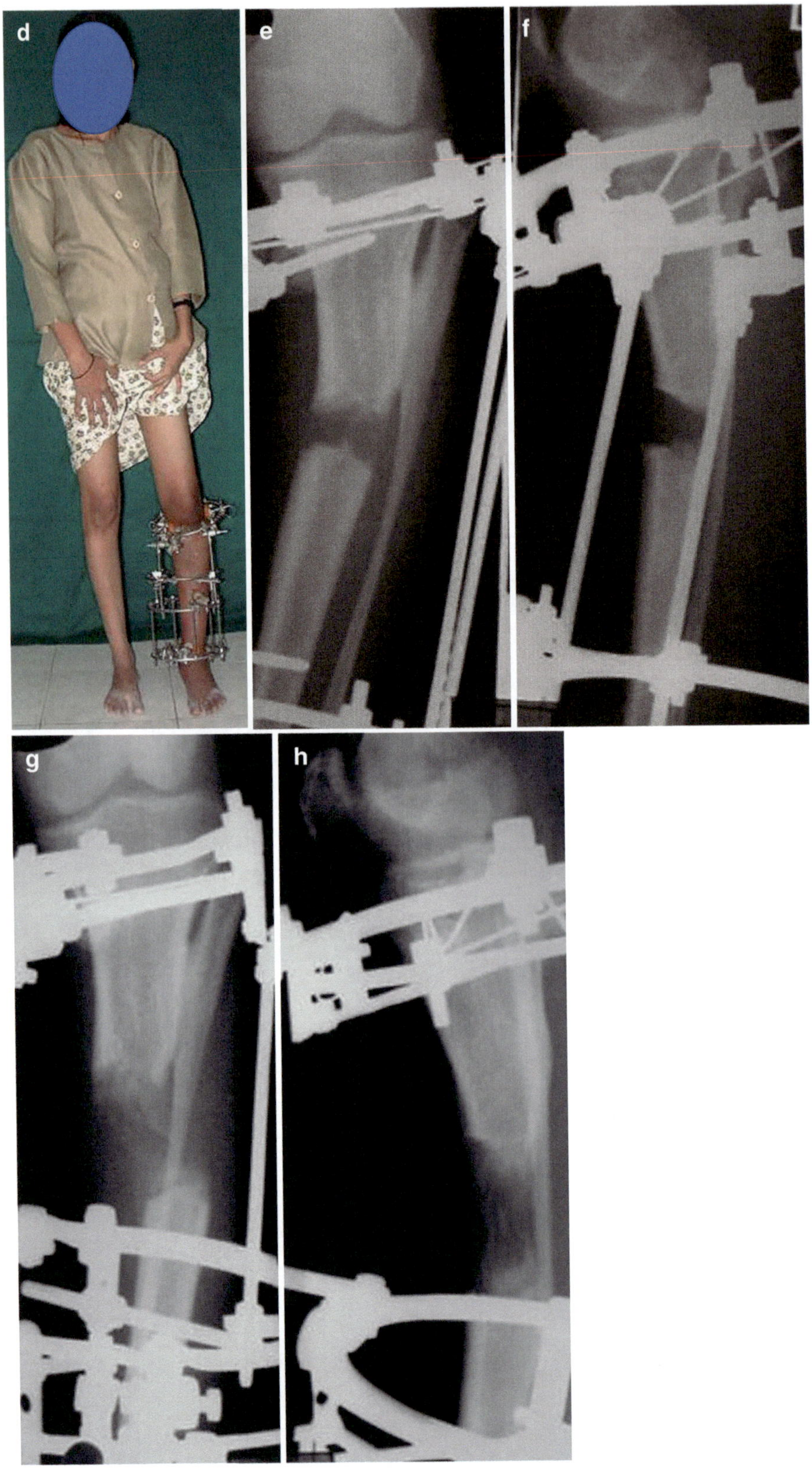

Fig. 23.18 (continued)

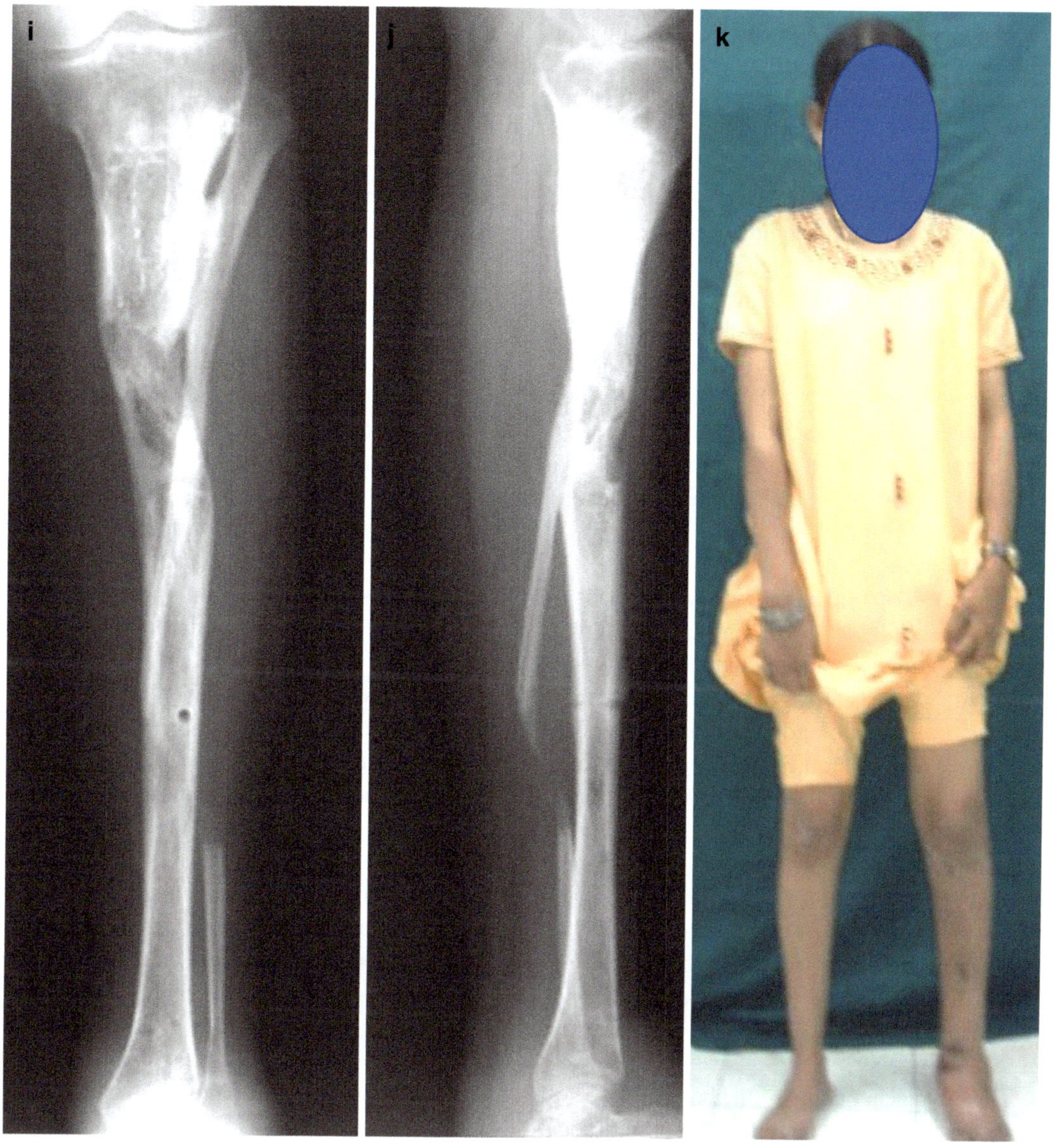

Fig. 23.18 (continued)

Advanced imaging modalities like MRI, 2D/3D CT with reconstruction, fluoroscopy, and/or arthrography may be needed to visualize the unossified cartilaginous structure of the epiphysis, to determine the osseocartilaginous geometry of the joint surface, and to understand the dynamic articular motion. 3D-printed models may be helpful for understanding the complex deformity, for preoperative planning, and for creating patient-specific solutions/implants [8, 21, 89].

One must also evaluate the social situation of the patient, as well as psychologic issues and family dynamics, when planning deformity correction. The ability of the patient and family to comply with the proposed treatment regimen must be evaluated. The surgeon's skills, system considerations, and availability of medical resources must also be considered when developing a treatment plan.

The history, physical examination, imaging studies, patient and family goals and preferences for treatment, and the dynamics of the situation must be brought together by the surgeon to formulate a problem list. After a problem list has been created, the anatomy and biology of the underlying deformity (including soft tissue and neurovascular considerations) should be considered before developing treatment strategies. The limb lengthening and reconstruction society AIM index is one such system of evaluation that reliably quantifies the severity of a deformity in seven domains [90]. Functional outcome scores such as PODCI (pediatric outcomes data collection instrument) and Peds QL (pediatric quality of life) questionnaires can be used to evaluate the patient's overall function before and after treatment [91].

Management Principles The management of post-infective deformities can be challenging. However, timely, well-planned, and well-executed reconstructive treatment strategies can ensure growth and development of the extremity with restoration of limb function. The goal of treating these deformities is to preserve joint function and prevent osteoarthritis from developing in the affected and adjacent joints by restoring the mechanical axis of the limb and normalizing the joint orientation, as both these factors contribute to abnormal loading of the affected joint, resulting in compartmental osteoarthritis of the affected joint [8, 21, 53, 85, 88, 89].

The biological quality of the bone and the soft tissue envelope is often reduced because of local changes and because of multiple surgeries. Consequently, wide areas of scar tissue and sclerotic bone may be present. The apex of the deformity is in most cases identical with the focus of the active or inactive infection. Detailed preoperative planning and experience with deformity correction using external and internal methods is essential when treating these deformities [89].

Management Options The decision to correct a given deformity and the treatment strategy must be patient-specific, and there are no absolute rules. The available reconstructive treatment options include physeal modulation or ablation, acute or gradual deformity correction, and soft tissue modification. These options can be used alone or in combination to provide solutions to the problem list developed after evaluation [8, 21, 53, 89] (Figs. 23.11, 23.16, 23.17, and 23.18).

Physeal modulation may include physeal bar excision or hemiepiphysiodesis with plates, screws, or staples, or by drilling. Physeal ablation involves a permanent epiphysiodesis to prevent progression or recurrence of deformity [8, 21, 53, 89].

Soft tissue surgery can be effective either as a solitary procedure or in conjunction with bony surgery [2, 8, 53, 89].

Acute deformity correction with an osteotomy using external or internal fixators or a combination is usually done for deformities of smaller magnitude, less complexity, and with minimal limb length discrepancies, without placing undue stress on the neurovascular structures [21, 53, 86–89].

Gradual deformity correction remains the workhorse of complex multiplanar deformities of larger magnitude with limb length discrepancies. This can be achieved using external or internal fixation or a combination of the two methods [84–89].

For correction of juxta-articular and metadiaphyseal deformities, realignment through an osteotomy as close to the apex of the deformity as possible is preferred if the biologic considerations permit, as this leads to a more anatomic reorientation without causing secondary translational deformities. Intra-articular deformities cause joint incongruity and may require well-planned and well-executed intra-articular osteotomies with stable internal fixation to restore joint congruity and preserve joint function [21, 87–89].

For juxta-articular deformities of the ankle and wrist, the relative lengths of the two bones (distal tibia/fibula in the ankle and radius/ulna in the wrist), physeal integrity of the two bones, orientation of the adjacent joint (ankle/wrist) in the coronal and sagittal planes, and compensatory deformity must be evaluated. A combination of physeal modulation and osteotomy is usually necessary to address these deformities [8, 21, 49, 84–89].

Sometimes, salvage procedures like arthrodesis, resection of a joint, or joint replacement arthroplasty may be necessary when the joint cannot be preserved or reconstructed. The decision to perform either a reconstructive or salvage procedure should be individualized depending on the type of residual deformity [8, 21, 92–94].

S: Limb Length Discrepancy (LLD)

S1: Shortening

Prevalence Wilson et al. reported an incidence of 21.8 % of shortening following AHO. The infection almost always involved the epiphyseal line and damaged the physis [95].

Pathogenesis This can be caused predominantly by a growth arrest (that is complete or partial but involves the central part of the growth plate). A pathologic fracture or a segmental bone defect with deformity may also contribute to shortening. The profile of postinfectious growth arrest is most often linear (Shapiro type I), making the prediction of the final discrepancy relatively reliable, but types IV (linear, then a plateau, and then delayed progression) can also be encountered, notably in the proximal femur [8, 21, 53, 95].

Evaluation Clinical evaluation combined with imaging studies is used to determine the cause, site, and severity of the limb length discrepancy as well as to predict the limb length discrepancy at skeletal maturity. Although several techniques have been described for measurement of limb length discrepancy, a standing teleroentgenogram offers the best combination of benefits (accurate, easily available, technically easily, low cost, good reproducibility) with few shortcomings (dose of irradiation). More recently, use of low-dose EOS stereoradiography has been particularly advantageous because it can quantify (in 3 dimensions) the discrepancy, even in the case of fixed sagittal deformities, and can minimize the dose of irradiation [89].

The prediction of limb length discrepancy in the lower extremities can be done using several methods. Three commonly used methods include the arithmetic or "rule of thumb" method of Menelaus, the multiplier method described by Paley et al., and Mosley's straight line graph. All these methods are based on the longitudinal data presented by Anderson et al. [89, 101]. Using more than one method of prediction and incorporating bone age data have been shown to improve the accuracy of the predictions [101].

In the upper extremity, prediction of limb length discrepancy can be done using several methods including the growth remaining method of Pritchett et al. and the multiplier method of Paley et al. [99, 100].

Treatment Principles Treatment principles involve making an early diagnosis of LLD due to growth plate arrest and making accurate predictions of future LLD at skeletal maturity. In the lower extremity, treatment is aimed at equalizing LLD greater than 2 cm before skeletal maturity to prevent low back pain and long leg hip arthritis [21, 89].

Treatment Options

Lower Limb Length Discrepancy: Treatment is guided by the child's age, the prognosis in terms of final height, and the predicted discrepancy at the end of growth. Treatment is recommended in cases in which the projected LLD at maturity is greater than 2 cm. In a skeletally immature child with a LLD between 2 and 5 cm, progressive shortening using epiphysiodesis of the unaffected distal femur/tibia/both remains the treatment of choice, though lengthening can be considered. The key component of the treatment remains the planning stage, which should be repeated and carried out rigorously to determine the site and correct timing of the contralateral epiphysiodesis. In a skeletally mature patient, extemporaneous shortening at the end of growth can be performed in the femur/tibia. In cases of greater discrepancy (> 5 cm) or at the end of growth, progressive lengthening of the affected limb can be performed, possibly associated with epiphysiodesis of the opposite side. The principle is based on lengthening of the osseous callus (callotasis), at a speed of 1 mm per day, while maintaining joint range of motion and monitoring the adjacent joints. This principle of "distraction histogenesis" was developed by Gavril A Ilizarov [92, 118, 119]. The traditional method of lengthening has been via an external fixator, circular, or monoplanar, but the recent trend is by serial lengthening of an intramedullary nail, a technique better accepted by patients and with limited scarring compared to external fixators. In the postinfectious context, a careful evaluation of the medullary cavity will be necessary, because modifications in its diameter can make nailing difficult. An assessment of the risk of reactivating infection and an evaluation of the mobility and stability of the adjacent joints are also necessary [8, 21, 53, 89, 102] (Figs. 23.1 and 23.3).

Upper Limb Length Discrepancy: Damage to the proximal humeral growth plate in the young child can result in major shortening (8–10 cm) of the upper limb. Shortening of the upper limb, up to 4 cm, is better tolerated than in the lower extremity. Lengthening with an external fixator, either monoplanar or circular, can be performed in cases of discrepancy greater than 4 cm, with a bone union speed slower than what has been observed for the lower limbs. The main complications reported are fractures, elbow stiffness, varus deviations, and paralysis of the radial nerve. Recently, intramedullary lengthening techniques have been developed as it is better accepted by patients and limits disfigurement from scarring (Fig. 23.2).

S2: Lengthening Due to Growth Plate Stimulation

Temporary stimulation of growth in a long bone may occur during and shortly after osteomyelitis [95–98]. This "overgrowth" is attributed to hyperemia of epiphyseal vessels because of local inflammation. Lengthening was reported in 21.8 % of patients by Wilson et al. following AHO [95]. The infections that resulted in lengthening always involved the diaphysis and did not damage the physis. Norrish et al. reported an incidence of lengthening following COM of 31% [97]. They speculate that this may be related to prolonged duration of symptoms due to late presentation and delay in diagnosis. In most cases, the lengthening did not result in a LLD > 2–3 cm. This type of limb length discrepancy usually follows a type 3 pattern of development (the discrepancy increases with time, and then a plateau is reached, and it will not change throughout the remaining growth) as described by Shapiro et al. [96]. This can be managed by a shoe lift or by epiphysiodesis of the unaffected lower extremity or shortening of the affected extremity after skeletal maturity to equalize LLD [21, 53, 89].

O: Other Serious Sequelae

O1: Avascular Necrosis

Avascular necrosis in infants and children is an uncommon but severe complication of septic arthritis of the hip and can lead to marked deformity of the femoral head, particularly in children aged 6 ± 16 years. It has an incidence of about 10%, with the most important risk factor being a delay in definitive treatment of about 5 or more days. It is caused by increased intra-articular hydrostatic pressure of the intra-articular pus that exceeds the arterial pressure of the retinacular vessels (approximately 40 mmHg), which supply the immature femoral head, or septic thrombosis of the epiphyseal vessels. Total head involvement was seen in 60 % of affected hips and partial head involvement (with better long-term outcomes) in 40% of cases [103, 105, 106].

Prevention It is crucial to avoid any increase of the intra-articular hydrostatic pressure by establishing an early diagnosis and starting definitive medical and surgical treatment, preferably within 4 days of the onset of the joint infection. Definitive surgical treatment should include immediate arthrotomy and drainage of the joint effusion combined with decompression of the proximal femoral metaphysis when there is a suspicion of osteomyelitis.

Treatment Principles of treatment are like those used for Perthes avascular necrosis disease of the hip, with the aim to achieve containment of the femoral head in the acetabulum while maintaining joint range of motion. Treatment options in the pre-collapse phase include nonoperative options like physical therapy, activity modification, and surgical treatment including soft tissue/capsular release, joint distraction, and core decompression. In the post-collapse phase, reconstructive options include osteotomies of the femur or pelvis to improve containment. Salvage options include arthrodiatasis, arthrodesis, and joint replacement surgery [103, 105, 106].

O2: Relapse of Infection

Osteomyelitis in childhood can relapse later in adulthood, especially in patients with multifocal osteomyelitis and inadequate care during the index episode. This is an uncommon complication in developed countries. Clerc et al., in a multicenter retrospective study, reported on 37 immune-competent, adult patients who relapsed their osteomyelitis at a median time of 26 years (13–45 years) from the index infection (AHO). Patients presented at an average age of 40 years (28–56 years) and were predominantly migrants and male (70%). Most patients had inadequate treatment of the index infection (65%). The most common clinical features were local inflammatory manifestations (92%), discharging sinus (46%), and fever (27%). The most common site of involvement was the distal femur. Most patients had elevated inflammatory markers and intramedullary gadolinium deposition (with or without abscess) on MRI. Most relapses were monomicrobial infections (82%). At relapse, *S. aureus* was the most common (82%) pathogenic organism detected, sometimes producing PVL or sometimes expressing the SCV phenotype. Surgical management (97%) and prolonged antimicrobial therapy (12 weeks at least) are required to cure the relapse. These patients are at risk for fracture when they resume walking (2 patients). All patients had a favorable outcome, no patient died, and no further relapse occurred. The authors highlight the importance of early diagnosis, multidisciplinary care with appropriate antibiotic therapy, and timely surgical intervention to increase the chance of successful outcome for these patients [46].

O3: Treatment-Related Complications

Street et al. reported that 124 (15.2%) patients with acute hematogenous osteomyelitis in a cohort of 883 patients, treated over a 10-year period, developed treatment-related complications. These included reactions to antibiotic therapy 95 patients (11.2%) such as neutropenia/urticaria, and in complications related to peripherally inserted catheters, 23 patients (2.8%) and 6 (0.7%) patients had both [4].

O4: Malignant Transformation

Marjolin ulcer refers to a malignant transformation arising in areas of chronic inflammation or injury of the skin, regardless of the origin of the lesion or the type of malignancy. Malignant transformation following chronic osteomyelitis is a relatively rare and late complication with a declining incidence in the modern world. The rate of malignant transformation is around 1.5–23%. The incidence is higher in LMICs due to delayed presentation and inadequate care. Most patients are middle-aged men, with malignant transformation presenting at a median time interval of 28 years (18–72 years) following the index bacterial infection. The diagnosis of malignant transformation in a chronic discharging sinus requires a high index of clinical suspicion. The common clinical features include increased pain, a foul smell, and changes in wound drainage. Early diagnosis is facilitated by wound biopsy. Squamous cell carcinoma is the most common presenting malignancy. Definitive treatment is amputation proximal to the tumor or wide local excision, combined with adjuvant chemotherapy and radiation therapy in selected patients. Early diagnosis may sometimes allow en bloc excision and limb salvage. However, the most effective treatment is prevention with early diagnosis, multidisciplinary care, and definitive medical and surgical treatment of the osteomyelitis, including adequate debridement and early reconstruction [45].

Conclusions

Although the clinical course of pediatric MSKI is mostly benign, functional impairment due to sequelae can still occur, resulting in significant socioeconomic impact and diminution of quality of life. Risk factors for developing sequelae include neonatal age at the time of infection, concurrent infections, multifocal involvement, delayed diagnosis, inappropriate and inadequate treatment, the presence of sickle cell disease, immunocompromised associated conditions, and infection caused by Panton-Valentine leukocidin-producing strains of *Staphylococcus aureus* (SA). Early diagnosis, multidisciplinary evaluation, and appropriate treatment are essential to treat MSKI and prevent development of complications. Comprehensive multidisciplinary evaluation, detailed preoperative planning, and experience with deformity correction principles using internal and external fixation are essential to optimize outcomes. Long-term follow-up to skeletal maturity is recommended.

Box 23.1 Key Learning Points

1. Pediatric MSK infections are the most common causes of MSK-related disease burden in children.
2. Delayed diagnosis and inadequate or inappropriate treatment can lead to sequelae.
3. Post-infective sequelae can be predicted based on risk factors.
4. Common risk factors are neonatal age, concurrent infections, virulent organisms, multilevel involvement, and increased levels of acute-phase reactants.
5. Significant morbidity, functional impairment, and disability are complications of pediatric MSK infections.
6. The best way to avoid serious complications is by early diagnosis and appropriate management.

Box 23.2 Tips and Tricks for Successful Management of Deformity

1. Before proceeding with surgical management of complications, perform a detailed history, physical examination, and evaluation of imaging studies.
2. Careful deformity analysis, preoperative planning, and knowledge of osteotomy rules will improve outcomes.
3. Create and prioritize a problem list with appropriate solutions prior to proceeding to the OR.
4. Counsel families regarding the possible need for multilevel treatment and repeat episodes of surgeries for growth arrest or shortening.
5. Understand the biomechanics of intra- and extramedullary devices to provide stable fixation, and alter the mechanical environment as needed to optimize healing when surgically managing deformity after MSK infections.
6. Familiarity with hardware and software considerations of different external fixators will facilitate safe and successful corrections of deformities.
7. Discuss the anesthesia protocol and postoperative pain management before surgery with the family and the multidisciplinary care team.
8. Knowledge of anatomy, the structures at risk, and safe zones for insertion of wires and half pins are essential for the surgeon.
9. Safe wire and pin insertion technique is mandatory to minimize surgical complications.
10. For difficult cases, use a 3D-printed bone model for patient education and surgical simulation, and consider creating patient-specific implants.
11. Use hybrid techniques for lengthening and deformity correction to reduce external fixator time and scarring.
12. Consider joint spanning to optimize stability of the fixation when deformity

correction or lengthening is done close to the joint, as in juxta-articular deformities.

13. Intra-articular osteotomies are needed at times in the presence of intra-articular deformities.
14. Rehabilitation, strict adherence to postoperative protocol, and pin site care are needed to prevent complications and optimize function.

Box 23.3 Pitfalls to Avoid

1. Inadequate planning preoperatively
2. Lack of knowledge of implant biomechanics
3. Underestimating the complexity of the problem
4. Poor understanding of the biology of distraction histogenesis, especially in bone that had been previously infected
5. Failing to adopt a multidisciplinary team approach to optimizing function
6. Poor judgement of the family dynamics and social situation
7. Inadequate discussion of expectations with the family regarding outcomes of reconstructive surgery

Declarations Funding support: This project has no funding support.

Consent to publish: The authors affirm that participants provided informed consent for publication of the images in Figs. 23.1, 23.2, 23.3, 23.4, 23.5, and 23.6.

Conflicts of Interest: The authors declare that they have no conflict of interest.

References

1. Schwend RM. The burden of pediatric musculoskeletal diseases worldwide. Orthop Clin North Am. 2020;51(2):207–17.
2. Okubo Y, Nochioka K, Testa M. Nationwide survey of pediatric acute osteomyelitis in the USA. J Pediatr Orthop B. 2017;26(6):501–6.
3. Okubo Y, Nochioka K, Marcia T. Nationwide survey of pediatric septic arthritis in the United States. J Orthop. 2017;14(3):342–6.
4. Street M, Puna R, Huang M, Crawford H. Acute pediatric hematogenous osteomyelitis. J Pediatr Orthop. 2015;35:634–9.
5. Swarup I, LaValva S, Shah R, Sankar WN. Septic arthritis of the hip in children: a critical analysis review. JBJS Rev. 2020;8(2):e0103.
6. Safdieh G, Silberman J, Nguyen J, Doyle SM, Blanco JS, Scher DM, Green DW, Widmann RF, Dodwell ER. Pediatric septic arthritis and osteomyelitis in the USA: a national KID database analysis. HSS J. 2019;15(2):159–66.
7. Iliadis AD, Ramachandran M. Pediatric bone and joint infections. EFORT Open Rev. 2017;2(1):7–12.
8. Ilharreborde B. Sequelae of pediatric osteoarticular infection. Orthop Traumatol Surg Res. 2015;101(1 Suppl):S129–37.
9. Montgomery CO, Siegel E, Blasier RD, Suva LJ. Concurrent septic arthritis and osteomyelitis in children. J Pediatr Orthop. 2013;33(4):464–7.
10. Beckles VLL, Jones HW, Harrison WJ. Chronic haematogenous osteomyelitis in children: a retrospective review of 167 patients in malawi. J Bone Joint Surg Br. 2010;92-B:1138–43.
11. Wynn Jones H, Beckles VLL, Akinola B, Stevenson AJ, Harrison WJ. Chronic haematogenous osteomyelitis in children. An unsolved problem. J Bone Joint Surg Br. 2011;93-B:1005–10.
12. Young JD, Dee EC, Levine A, Sturgeon DJ, Koehlmoos TP, Schoenfeld AJ. Does universal insurance and access to care influence disparities in outcomes for pediatric patients with osteomyelitis? Clin Orthop Relat Res. 2020;478(7):1432–9.
13. Bergdahl S, Ekengren K, Ericksson M. Neonatal hematogenous osteomyelitis: risk factors for long term sequelae. J Pediatr Orthop. 1995;5:564–8.
14. Martin AC, Anderson D, Lucey J, Guttinger R, Jacoby PA, Mok TJ, et al. Predictors of outcome in pediatric osteomyelitis: five years' experience in a single tertiary center. Pediatr Infect Dis J. 2016;35(4):387–91.
15. Alhinai Z, Elahi M, Park S, Foo B, Lee B, Chapin K, Koster M, Sánchez PJ, Michelow IC. Prediction of adverse outcomes in pediatric acute hematogenous osteomyelitis. Clin Infect Dis. 2020;71(9):e454–64.
16. Martin N, Ahmed H, Dix-Peek S, Hoffman E. Acute osteomyelitis in children: a 20 year study. Orthop Proc. 2005;87-B (Supp III):279
17. Ahmed H, Dix-Peek S, Martin N, Hoffman E. Septic arthritis in children: a 20 year study. Orthop Proc. 2005;87-B (Supp III):279
18. Horn A, Wever S, Hoffman EB. Complications following acute severe haematogenous osteomyelitis of the long bones in children. SA Orthop J. 2019;18(3):23–9.
19. Gafur OA, Copley LA, Hollmig ST, Browne RH, Thornton LA, Crawford SE. The impact of the current epidemiology of pediatric musculoskeletal infection on evaluation and treatment guidelines. J Pediatr Orthop. 2008;28(7):777–85.
20. Sarkissian EJ, Gans I, Gunderson MA, Myers SH, Spiegel DA, Flynn JM. Community-acquired

Methicillin-resistant Staphylococcus aureus musculoskeletal infections: emerging trends over the past decade. J Pediatr Orthop. 2016;36(3):323–7.
21. Choi IH. Postinfectious deformities of the lower limb. Chapter 31, pg 589-603. S Sabharwal (ed). Pediatric lower limb deformities. Springer International Publishing Cham 2016.
22. Samora JAAOS 2013 Septic arthritis of the neonatal hip- acute management and late reconstruction
23. Samora JB, Klingele K. Septic arthritis of the neonatal hip: acute management and late reconstruction. J Am Acad Orthop Surg. 2013;21(10):632–41. https://doi.org/10.5435/JAAOS-21-10-632. PMID: 24084437.
24. Strong M, Lejman T, Michno P, Hayman M. Sequelae from septic arthritis of the knee during the first two years of life. J Pediatr Orthop. 1994;14(6):745–51.
25. Frederiksen B, Christiansen P, Knudsen FU. Acute osteomyelitis and septic arthritis in the neonate, risk factors and outcome. Eur J Pediatr. 1993;152:577–80.
26. An TJ, Benvenuti MA, Mignemi ME, Thomsen IP, Schoenecker JG. Pediatric musculoskeletal infection: hijacking the acute-phase response. JBJS Rev. 2016;4(9):e4.
27. Benvenuti M, An T, Amaro E, Lovejoy S, Mencio G, Martus J, Mignemi M, Schoenecker JG. Double-Edged Sword: musculoskeletal infection provoked acute phase response in children. Orthop Clin North Am. 2017;48(2):181–97.
28. Amaro E, Marvi TK, Posey SL, Benvenuti MA, An TJ, Dale KM, Lovejoy SA, Martus JE, Johnson ME, Mencio GA, Moore-Lotridge SN, Thomsen IP, Schoenecker JG. C-reactive protein predicts risk of venous thromboembolism in pediatric musculoskeletal infection. J Pediatr Orthop. 2019;39(1):e62–7.
29. Athey AG, Mignemi ME, Gheen WT, Lindsay EA, Jo C, Copley LA. Validation and modification of a severity of illness score for children with acute hematogenous osteomyelitis. J Pediatr Orthop. 2019;39(2):90–7.
30. Paterson MP, Hoffman EB, Roux P. Severe disseminated Staphylococcal disease associated with osteitis and septic arthritis. J Bone Joint Surg Br. 1990;72B(1):94–7.
31. Benvenuti MA, An TJ, Mignemi ME, Martus JE, Mencio GA, Lovejoy SA, Schoenecker JG, Williams DJ. A clinical prediction algorithm to stratify pediatric musculoskeletal infection by severity. J Pediatr Orthop. 2019;39(3):153–7.
32. McNeil JC, Vallejo JG, Kok EY, Sommer LM, Hultén KG, Kaplan SL. Clinical and microbiologic variables predictive of orthopedic complications following Staphylococcus aureus acute hematogenous osteoarticular infections in children. Clin Infect Dis. 2019;69:1955–61.
33. Chiappini E, Krzysztofiak A, Bozzola E, Gabiano C, Esposito S, Lo Vecchio A, Govoni MR, Vallongo C, Dodi I, Castagnola E, Rossi N, Valentini P, Cardinale F, Salvini F, Bona G, Bossi G, Olivieri AN, Russo F, Fossali E, Bottone G, Dellepiane M, De Martino M, Villani A, Galli L. Risk factors associated with complications/sequelae of acute and subacute haematogenous osteomyelitis: an Italian multicenter study. Expert Rev Anti Infect Ther. 2018;16(4):351–8.
34. Hamdy RF, Dona D, Jacobs MB, Gerber JS. Risk factors for complications in children with Staphylococcus aureus Bacteremia. J Pediatr. 2019;208:214–220.e2.
35. Pierrie SN, Scannell BP, Brighton BK, Vanderhave KL. Characteristics of pyogenic musculoskeletal infections in older children and adolescents. Orthopedics. 2020;43(4):e291–8.
36. Jackson MA, Burry VF, Olson LC. Pyogenic arthritis associated with adjacent osteomyelitis: identification of the sequela-prone child. Pediatr Infect Dis J. 1992;11(1):9–13.
37. Mitchell PD, Hunt DM, Lyall H, Nolan M, Tudor-Williams G. Panton Valentine leukocidin-secreting Staphylococcus aureus causing severe musculoskeletal sepsis in children. A new threat. J Bone Joint Surg Br. 2007;89:1239–42.
38. Copley LA, Barton T, Garcia C, et al. A proposed scoring system for assessment of severity of illness in pediatric acute hematogenous osteomyelitis using objective clinical and laboratory findings. Pediatr Infect Dis J. 2014;33(1):35–41.
39. Mignemi ME, Benvenuti MA, An TJ, Martus JE, Mencio GA, Lovejoy SA, Copley LA, Williams DJ, Thomsen IP, Schoenecker JG. A novel classification system based on dissemination of musculoskeletal infection is predictive of hospital outcomes. J Pediatr Orthop. 2018;38(5):279–86.
40. Rosenfeld SB, Copley LA, Mignemi M, An T, Benvenuti M, Schoenecker J. Key concepts of musculoskeletal infection. Instr Course Lect. 2017;15(66):569–84.
41. Peters W, Irving J, Letts M. Long-term effects of neonatal bone and joint infection on adjacent growth plates. J Pediatr Orthop. 1992;12(6):806–10.
42. Vander Have KL, Karmazyn B, Verma M, Caird MS, Hensinger RN, Farley FA, Lubicky JP. Community-associated methicillin-resistant Staphylococcus aureus in acute musculoskeletal infection in children: a game changer. J Pediatr Orthop. 2009;29(8):927–31.
43. Stevenson AJ, Wynn Jones H, Chokotho LC, Beckles VLL, Harrison WJ. The Beit CURE Classification of Childhood Chronic Haematogenous Osteomyelitis—a guide to treatment. J Orthop Surg Res. 2015;10:144.
44. Rasool MN. The treatment of tibial defects following chronic pyogenic haematogenous osteomyelitis in children. SA Orthop J. 2008;7:34–42.
45. Panteli M, Puttaswamaiah R, Lowenberg DW, Giannoudis PV. Malignant transformation in chronic osteomyelitis: recognition and principles of management. J Am Acad Orthop Surg. 2014;22:586–94.

46. Clerc A, Zeller V, Marmor S, Senneville E, Marchou B, Laurent F, Lucht F, Desplaces N, Lustig S, Chidiac C, Ferry T. Hematogenous osteomyelitis in childhood can relapse many years later into adulthood: a retrospective multicentric cohort study in France. Medicine. 2020;99(20):e19617.
47. Tudisco C, Farsetti P, Gatti S, Ippolito E. Influence of chronic osteomyelitis on skeletal growth: analysis of 26 cases affected during childhood. J Pediatr Orthop. 1991;11:358–63.
48. Peterson HA. Partial growth plate arrest and its treatment. J Pediatr Orthop. 1984;4(2):246–58.
49. Gauger EM, Casnovsky LL, Gauger EJ, Bohn DC, Van Heest A. Acquired upper extremity growth arrest. Orthopedics. 2017;40(1):e95–e103.
50. Vij N, Ranade A, Kang P, Belthur MV. Primary bacterial pyomyositis in children: a systematic review. Submitted to JPO 2021.
51. Schröder A, Gerin A, Firth GB, et al. A systematic review of necrotising fasciitis in children from its first description in 1930 to 2018. BMC Infect Dis. 2019;19:317.
52. Burnham JP, Kollef MH. Treatment of severe skin and soft tissue infections: a review. Curr Opin Infect Dis. 2018;31(2):113–9.
53. Chaudhary MM. ABCD'S of reconstruction after childhood osteomyelitis. Personal Communication, 14th Oct 2018. https://ilizarov.org/pediatric-orthopedics/attachment/abcds-of-recosntruction-for-childhood-osteomyelitis. Accessed on 9/13/2020. Presented at the CME of 63rd Annual conference of Indian Orthopaedic Association, 2018, Coimbatore, India.
54. Morrey BF, Peterson HA. Hematogenous pyogenic osteomyelitis in children. Orthop Clin North Am. 1975;6(4):935–51.
55. Ecklund K, Jaramillo D. Patterns of premature physeal arrest: MR imaging of 111 children. AJR. 2002;178:967–72.
56. Peterson HA. Chapter 3. Physeal injury other than fracture. Heidelberg Dordrecht London New York: Springer; 2012. p. 65–109.
57. Ogden JA. Pediatric osteomyelitis and septic arthritis: the pathology of neonatal disease. Yale J Biol Med. 1979;52:423–48.
58. Gilbertson-Dahadal D, Wright JE, Krupinski E, McCurdy WE. Taljanovic transphyseal involvement of pyogenic osteomyelitis is considerably more common than classically taught. AJR. 2014;203:190–5.
59. Peterson HA, Shaughnessy WJ, Stans AA. Physeal bar equivalent. J Pediatr Orthop B. 2017;26:507–14.
60. Aroojis A, Johari AN. Epiphyseal separations after neonatal osteomyelitis and septic arthritis. J Pediatr Orthop. 2000;20(4):544–9.
61. Wyers MR, Samet JD, Mithal LB. Physeal separation in pediatric osteomyelitis. Pediatr Radiol. 2019;49:1229–33.
62. Yuan BJ, Stans AA, Larson DR, Peterson HA. Excision of physeal bars of the distal femur, proximal and distal tibia followed to maturity. J Pediatr Orthop. 2019;39(6):e422–9.
63. Kim HT, Lim KP, Jang JH, Ahn TY. Resection of a physeal bar with complete transverse osteotomy at the metaphysis and Ilizarov external fixation. Bone Joint J. 2015;97-B(12):1726–31.
64. Miller B. Regeneration of the lateral femoral condyle after osteomyelitis in infancy. A case report with 20-year follow-up. Clin Orthop. 1969;65:163–6.
65. Roberts PH. Disturbed epiphysial growth at the knee after osteomyelitis in infancy. J Bone Joint Surg. 1970;52B:692–703.
66. Song KS, Kim HKW. Regeneration of the proximal tibial epiphysis after infantile osteomyelitis. Report of three cases with an eight-to-22 year follow-up. J Bone Joint Surg. 2005;87B:979–83.
67. Nguyen JC, Markhardt BK, Merrow AC, Dwek JR. Imaging of pediatric growth plate disturbances. Radiographics. 2017;37:1791–812.
68. Jaramillo D, Dormans JP, Delgado J, et al. Hematogeneous osteomyelitis in infants and children: imaging of a changing disease. Radiology. 2017;283:629–43.
69. Stevenson AJ, Wynn Jones H, Chokotho LC, Beckles VLL, Harrison WJ. The Beit CURE Classification of Childhood Chronic Haematogenous Osteomyelitis—a guide to treatment. J Orthop Surg Res. 2015;10:144. Published online 2015 Sep 17
70. Howard JB, Highenboten CL, Nelson JD. Residual effects of septic arthritis in infancy and childhood. JAMA. 1976;236:932–5.
71. Hunka L, Said SE, MacKenzie DA, Rogala EJ, Cruess RL. Classification and surgical management of severe sequelae of septic hips in children. Clin Orthop. 1982;171:30–6.
72. Paley D. Sagittal plane knee considerations. In: Paley D, editor. Principles of deformity correction. 1st ed. Berlin/Heidelberg/New York: Springer; 2002.
73. Franceschi F, Okello J, Loro A. Simultaneous joint fusion and limb lengthening for knee deformities in children: a one-stage procedure The Kampala experience. SA Orthop J. 2009;48:47–52.
74. Langenskiold A. Growth disturbance after osteomyelitis of femoral condyles in infants. Acta Orthop Scand. 1984;55(1):1–13.
75. Westberry DE, Davids JR, Jacobs JM, Pugh LI, Tanner SL. Effectiveness of serial stretch casting for resistant or recurrent knee flexion contractures following hamstring lengthening in children with cerebral palsy. J Pediatr Orthop. 2006;26(1):109–14.
76. Bhave A, Shabtai L, Ong PH, Standard SC, Paley D, Herzenberg J. Custom knee device for knee contractures after internal femoral lengthening. Orthopedics. 2015;38:e567–72.
77. Ebraheim NA, Saddemi SR, De Troye RJ. Results of Judet quadricepsplasty. J Orthop Trauma. 1993;7:327–30.
78. Heydarian K, Akbarnia BA, Jabalameli M, Tabador K. Posterior capsulotomy for the treatment of severe

flexion contractures of the knee. J Pediatr Orthop. 1984;4:700–4.
79. Volkov MV, Oganesian OV. Restoration of function in the knee and elbow with a hinge-distractor apparatus. J Bone Joint Surg Am. 1975;57(5):591–600.
80. Devalia KL, Fernandes JA, Moras P, Pagdin J, Jones S, Bell MJ. Joint distraction and reconstruction in complex knee contractures. J Pediatr Orthop. 2007;27(4):402–7.
81. Aldegheri R, Trivella G, Saleh M. Articulated distraction of the hip. Conservative surgery for arthritis in young patients. Clin Orthop Relat Res. 1994;301:94–101.
82. Marijnissen AC, van Roermund PM, van Melkebeek J, Lafeber FP. Clinical benefit of joint distraction in the treatment of ankle osteoarthritis. Foot Ankle Clin. 2003;8(2):335–46.
83. Herzenberg JE, Davis JR, Paley D, et al. Mechanical distraction for treatment of severe knee flexion contractures. Clin Orthop. 1994;301:80–8.
84. Laurenteeva-Ilizarova SG. Correction of knee deformity with simultaneous lengthening in patients with sequelae of haematogenous osteomyelitis of the distal end of the femur. PhD thesis, Kurgan, 1987
85. Wang CT, Huang SC. The Ilizarov technique for treatment of sequelae of childhood-acquired bone and joint infection. J Formos Med Assoc. 1999;98(3):175–82.
86. Paley D. Part 1: corrective osteotomies for lower limb deformities. Curr Orthop. 1994;8(3):182–95.
87. Paley D. Intra-articular osteotomies of the hip, knee, and ankle. Oper Tech Orthop. 2011;21:184–19.
88. Suger G, Schmelz A, Kinzl L, Liener U. Deformity correction in osteomyelitis. Orthopade. 2000;29(1):9–17.
89. Paley D. Principles of deformity correction (ed Rev). Berlin: Springer-Verlag; 2005.
90. McCarthy JJ, Iobst CA, Rozbruch SR, Sabharwal S, Eisman EA. Limb Lengthening and Reconstruction Society AIM index reliably assesses lower limb deformity. Clin Orthop Relat Res. 2013;471(2):621–7.
91. Daltroy LH, Liang MH, Fossel AH, Goldberg MJ. The POSNA pediatric musculoskeletal functional health questionnaire: report on reliability, validity and sensitivity to change. J Pediatr Orthop. 1998;18(5):561–71.
92. Ilizarov GA, Samchukov ML. Ilizarov hip reconstructive surgery in the treatment of hip osteoarthritis. Orthop Travmatol Protez. 1988;6:124–9.
93. Rozbruch SR, Paley D, Bhave A, Herzenberg JE. Ilizarov hip reconstruction for the sequelae of infantile hip infection. JBJS Am. 2005;71:686–91.
94. Chen CE, Wang JW, Juhn RJ. Total hip arthroplasty for primary septic arthritis of the hip in adults. Int Orthop. 2008;32(5):573–80.
95. Wilson JC, McKeever FM. Bone growth disturbance following acute hematogenous osteomyelitis. JBJS. 1936;107(15):1188–93.
96. Shapiro F. Developmental patterns in lower-extremity length discrepancies. J Bone Joint Surg Am. 1982;64:639–51.
97. Norrish A, Bates J, Harrison WJ. Chronic long bone osteomyelitis and limb length discrepancy: a prospective series of 42 patients. Orthopaedic proceedings 2009;91-b(Supp_I).
98. Pulido PG, Hotchen A, Gojanur A, Corbett J, Stohr KK. Brodie's abscesses can stimulate the growth plate in children. J Bone Joint Infect. 2019;4(6):264–7.
99. Pritchett JW. Growth and predictions of growth in the upper extremity. JBJS Am. 1988;70(4):520–5.
100. Paley D, Gelman A, Shualy MB, Herzenberg JE. Multiplier method for limb-length prediction in the upper extremity. J Hand Surg Am. 2008;33(3):385–91.
101. Hubbard EW, Liu RW, Iobst CA. Understanding skeletal growth and predicting limb-length inequality in pediatric patients. J Am Acad Orthop Surg. 2019;27(9):312–9.
102. Green SA, Dahl MT. Intramedullary limb lengthening: principles and practice. 1st ed. Cham: Springer; 2018.
103. Choi IH, Pizzutillo PD, Bowen JR, Dragann R, Malhis T. Sequelae and reconstruction after septic arthritis of the hips in infants. J Bone Joint Surg Am. 1990;72:1150–65.
104. Belthur MV, Palazzi DL, Phillips WA, Weinberg J. A clinical analysis of shoulder and hip joint infections in children. J Pediatr Orthop. 2009;29(7):828–33.
105. Maguire KJ, Otsuka NY. Septic shoulder presenting as a shoulder dislocation in the pediatric patient: a case report. J Pediatr Orthop B. 2017;26(3):270–3.
106. Saisu T, Kawashima A, Kamegaya M, Mikasa M, Moriishi J, Moriya H. Humeral shortening and inferior subluxation as sequelae of septic arthritis of the shoulder in neonates and infants. J Bone Joint Surg Am. 2007;89(8):1784–93.
107. Bagheri F, Ebrahimzadeh MH, Sharifi SR, Ahmadzadeh-Chabok H, Khajah-Mozaffari J, Fattahi AS. Pathologic dislocation of the shoulder secondary to septic arthritis: a case report. Cases J. 2009;2:9131.
108. Johari AN, Dhawale AA, Johari RA. Management of post septic hip dislocations when the capital femoral epiphysis is present. J Pediatr Orthop B. 2011;20(6):413–21.
109. Rastogi P, Agarwal A. Management of post septic sequelae of hips with dislocation in children. Int Orthop. 2020;44(10):2139–46.
110. Walker JL, Rang M. Radial head dislocation following septic arthritis of the elbow. Orthopedics. 1993;16(3):313–5.
111. Bonnaig NS, Casstevens EC, Freiberg R. Posterior knee dislocation following septic arthritis of the knee. Geriatr Orthop Surg Rehabil. 2012 Mar;3(1):45–7.
112. Babhulkar SS, Pande KC, Babhulkar S. Ankle instability after fibular resection. JBJS Br. 1995;77B:258–61.
113. Forlin E, Milani C. Sequelae of septic arthritis of the hip in children. A new classification and a review of 41 hips. J Pediatr Orthop. 2008;5:524–8.

114. Mitchell GP. Management of acquired dislocation of hip in septic arthritis. Orthop Clin North Am. 1980;11:51–64.
115. Vidigal EC Jr, Vidigal EC, Fernandes JL. Avascular necrosis as a complication of septic arthritis of the hip in children. Int Orthop. 1998;21(6):389–92.
116. Munting TW, Hoffman EB, Hastings CJ. Avascular necrosis following septic arthritis of the hip in children. Orthopaedic proceedings. 2002;84-b(Supp_I).
117. Vij N, Ranade A, Kang P, Belthur MV. Primary pediatric bacterial pyomyositis: a systematic review. (Submitted to JPO 2021).
118. Ilizarov GA. The tension-stress effect on the genesis and growth of tissues. Part I. The influence of stability of fixation and soft-tissue preservation. Clin Orthop Relat Res 1989;(238):249–81.
119. Ilizarov GA. The tension-stress effect on the genesis and growth of tissues: part II. The influence of the rate and frequency of distraction. Clin Orthop Relat Res 1989 (239):263–85.

24 Sequelae of Septic Arthritis of the Hip and Late Reconstruction

In-Ho Choi and Hyung-Chul Cho

Introduction

The negative growth sequelae following septic arthritis of the hip in childhood are diverse depending on the time of diagnosis, the age of occurrence, infecting organism, host resistance, timing and effectiveness of the initial treatment, and the extent, location, and pattern of the damage [1–4]. The long-term sequelae are most profound when the infection occurs in neonates and young infancy in whom a major part of the proximal femur is composed of unossified hyaline cartilage. Thus, if untreated or treated improperly, unossified epiphysis and the growth plate can be destroyed extensively. Once the capital femoral epiphysis has developed, early proper treatment can result in a completely normal hip, or mild coxa magna due to increased vascularity [1, 3, 5]. Late sequelae are closely related to predominantly involved regions of the proximal femur. The extent and location of physeal and juxtaphyseal damage mostly determines the pattern of residual deformities of the proximal femur. Partial asymmetric damage and premature fusion of the physis will result in coxa vara or valga, and abnormal torsion of proximal femur, whereas complete damage can result in coxa breva with relative greater trochanteric overriding. When the osteomyelitis focus within the femoral neck spreads directly into the hip joint cavity and is controlled after the destruction of the femoral neck has occurred, the femoral head (FH) shape may become distorted with either malorientation of the epiphysis or a pseudarthrosis of the femoral neck [5, 6]. Compared to infantile septic arthritis of the hip, infection in older children in whom major part of the femoral epiphysis has already ossified, cartilage insult may be predominantly limited to the articular cartilage [5]. The decision to perform either reconstructive or salvage procedures must be made on an individual basis, after carefully evaluating the clinical findings and imaging studies. Admittedly, appropriate and timely reconstructive operations would benefit growth and development of the hip by providing the best possible hip joint mechanics at skeletal maturity. This will improve overall function of the lower limb.

I.-H. Choi (✉)
Department of Orthopedic Surgery, Chung-Ang University, Seoul, South Korea

Department of Orthopedic Surgery, Division of Pediatric Orthopaedics, Seoul National University, Seoul, South Korea

Division of Pediatric Orthopaedics, Seoul National University Children's Hospital, Seoul, Republic of Korea
e-mail: inhoc1@caumc.or.kr

H.-C. Cho
Department of Orthopedic Surgery, Chung-Ang University Hospital, Seoul, South Korea
e-mail: dhccho@caumc.or.kr

© Springer Nature Switzerland AG 2022
M. V. Belthur et al. (eds.), *Pediatric Musculoskeletal Infections*,
https://doi.org/10.1007/978-3-030-95794-0_24

Clinical Problems Related to Post-septic Hip Sequelae

The resulting pathomechanisms of late sequelae can lead to gait abnormalities due to stiffness, instability, femoro-acetabular impingement (FAI), lever arm dysfunction, and leg-length discrepancy (LLD). All these problems are the results of distorted femoral head shape, avascular necrosis, premature symmetric or asymmetric physeal closure, pseudarthrosis of the femoral neck, acetabular dysplasia, relative greater trochanteric overriding, subluxation/dislocation, and severe destruction of the femoral head and neck.

Radiographic Classifications of Post-septic Hip Sequelae

Several radiographic classifications exist on late sequelae of infantile septic arthritis of the hip. The treating surgeon should understand current radiographic classification systems, which may be helpful when selecting appropriate surgical options to improve hip function. In 1990, Choi et al. reported a classification of residual proximal femoral deformities based on the nature and extent of damage and radiographic appearance at the final follow-up or at skeletal maturity into four major types and each major type was further divided into two subtypes (Table 24.1, Fig. 24.1) [1]. Their classification incorporates discrete observations made over several decades including those of Hunka et al. (1982) [8]. In the literature, other authors, including Johari et al. (2002) [9, 10] and Forlin and Milani (2008) [11], also reported different radiographic classifications of post-septic hip sequelae. However, the radiographic classifications reported by other authors [8–11] do not have a subtype equivalent to the Choi type IIIA (slipping at the femoral neck, resulting in coxa vara or valga with severe anteversion or retroversion). We believe that any classification system should be devised with a prime principle, that is, the severity of involvement from best to worst in order: prognosis-related or oriented, treatment-related or oriented, intuitive, fast to understand to differentiate, easy to remember, and inclusive of all or most of the conditions. In this regard, Choi et al.'s classification system is worthy of acceptance. However, all existing radiographic classifications have a major drawback—they were devised mainly based on the changes noted on the plain radiographs. A new, comprehensive three-dimensional (3D) radiographic classification depicting both bony and cartilaginous structures of the hip is warranted considering the rapid advancement in the imaging technology [12].

Table 24.1 Classification of post-septic hip sequelae

Type	Pathoanatomy	Suggested pathomechanism
I	A. Slippage: No residual deformity	Transient ischemia
	B. Coxa magna	
II	A. Coxa breva with a deformed head due to symmetric, premature physeal closure	Epiphyseal, physeal, and metaphyseal involvement due to severe ischemic insult or limited direct destruction
	B. Progressive coxa vara or coxa Valga due to asymmetric, premature physeal closure	
III	A. Slipping at the femoral neck, resulting in coxa vara or Valga with severe anteversion or retroversion	Infection episode predominantly in the region of the neck; malorientation of the physis; disturbed biomechanics of the femoral head-neck-shaft; rapid progression of complex deformity
	B. Pseudarthrosis of the femoral neck	Persistent pseudarthrosis of the neck; stiff versus mobile nonunion
IV	A. Destruction of femoral head and neck, with a persistent small medial remnant of the neck	Massive dissolution of the chondroepiphysis of the proximal femur
	B. Complete loss of femoral head and neck and no vestige of articulation of the hip	

Source: Choi et al. [1]

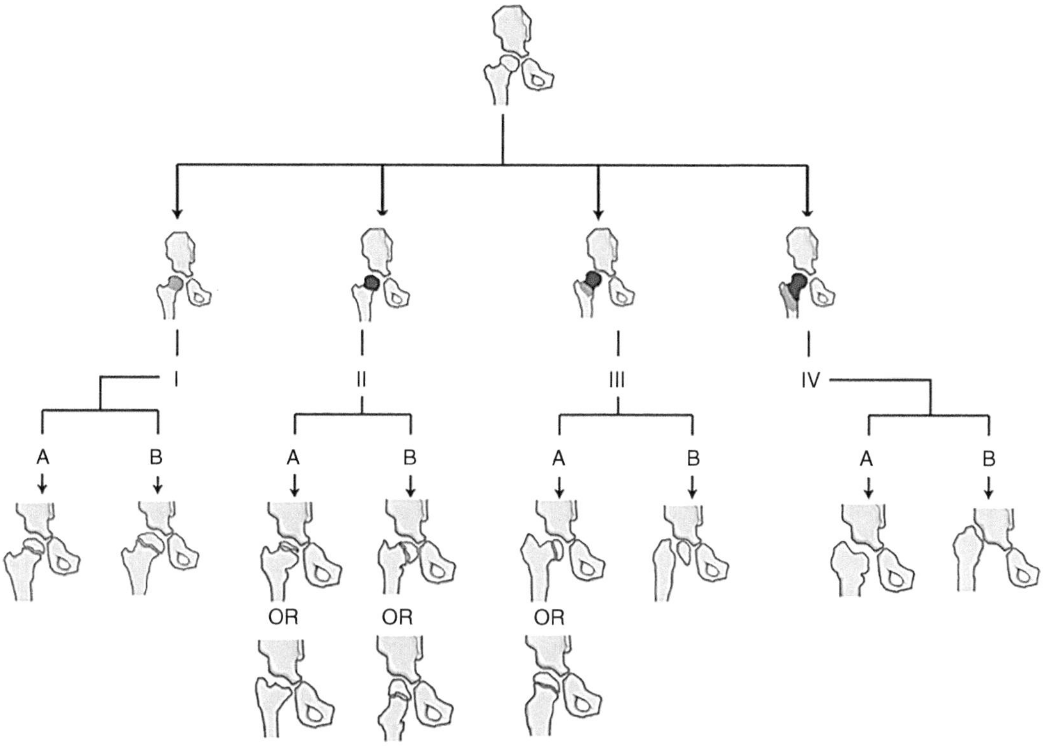

Fig. 24.1 Classification of sequelae of infantile septic arthritis of the hip

Treatment Approaches to Post-septic Hip Sequelae

The treatment approaches to late sequelae will vary profoundly depending on the severity and pattern of residual deformities. Accordingly, specific treatment plans should be individualized, based upon careful analysis of complex three-dimensional pathomorphologic features of the hip. The treating surgeon should identify the most efficacious, safe, and practical treatment strategies to accomplish the goals of treatment and optimize the outcome. Undoubtedly, they should have profound knowledge and surgical skills to deal with a variety of late sequelae.

Goals of Treatment

The aims of either a reconstructive or a salvage surgical procedure are to provide the best possible biomechanics of the hip and lower limb at skeletal maturity, thereby reducing the risk of development of early degenerative arthritis [1, 6, 8]. This can be accomplished by restoring hip stability, correcting deformities of proximal femur and acetabulum, improving hip joint congruity, retaining hip mobility, eliminating potential pain source such as FAI, and achieving level pelvis and lower-limb and length equalization without residual axial or rotational malalignment (Table 24.2). Figure 24.2 depicts the goals of treatment for FAI in older children with type II and III hips.

Considering Factors for Planning of Treatment

It is of paramount importance to carefully evaluate the status of the epiphysis, physis, femoral neck, acetabulum, and the greater trochanter (GT). Deformed unossified osseocartilaginous geometry of the proximal femur should be assessed in three

Table 24.2 Treatment options for reconstruction or salvage of the hips with post-septic hip sequelae

Condition (Indication)	Aim	Procedures
Subluxation or dislocation	Reduction/containment	Open reduction; soft-tissue release (adductor-iliopsoas tenotomy)
Joint incongruity	Optimization of congruity	Proximal femoral realignment osteotomy (varus or valgus osteotomy with a sagittal/rotational component); redirectional acetabular osteotomy (salter, Pemberton, and Dega osteotomies; triple innominate osteotomy; Ganz periacetabular osteotomy)
Abnormal femoral Neck-shaft angle	Normalization of the neck-shaft angle	Proximal femoral varus osteotomy or medial screw hemiepiphysiodesis; valgus osteotomy
Acetabular dysplasia	Normalization of the acetabular roof angle (lateral and anterior center edge [CE] angles)	Acetabuloplasties (e.g., Pemberton, Dega) or redirectional acetabular osteotomy (triple innominate osteotomy; Ganz periacetabular osteotomy)
Inadequate coverage	Normalization of femoro-acetabular coverage	Redirectional acetabular osteotomy; salvage acetabuloplasty (e.g., Chiari, shelf operation); femoral head reduction osteotomy
Anteverted or retroverted femur and acetabulum	Correction of abnormal version of the proximal femur and acetabulum	Proximal femoral rotational/derotational osteotomy; redirectional acetabular osteotomy (e.g., triple innominate osteotomy; Ganz periacetabular osteotomy)
Torn labrum or articular cartilage lesion	Management of intra-articular pathology of the cartilage or labrum	Labral debridement or refixation; articular cartilage repair using microfracture technique or osteochondral grafting or chondrocyte transplantation
Femoro-acetabular impingement	Elimination of cam or pincer lesion; restoration of head-neck offset	Osteochondroplasty via safe surgical hip dislocation or arthroscopy; excision of the femoral head and neck remnant (Choi type IVA or mobile nonunion type of IIIB)
Greater trochanteric overriding; short femoral neck	Correction of coxa brevis to improve abductor muscle function	Greater trochanteric advancement; true or relative femoral neck lengthening (Ganz, Wagner, or Morscher osteotomy)
Femoral neck nonunion	Repair of pseudarthrosis of the femoral neck	Bone grafting, often combined with proximal femoral valgus osteotomy
Destruction of the femoral head and neck	Reconstruction of the femoro-pelvic articulation	Greater trochanteric arthroplasty; pelvic support osteotomy; Ilizarov hip reconstruction (Choi type IVB or failed type IVA); L'Episcopo, Albee, or Harmon operation; Ilizarov femoral neck lengthening; femoral neck reconstruction using vascularized bone grafting (Choi type IVA)
Limb-length shortening	Equalization of the lower limb and length to obtain level pelvis	Lengthening by distraction osteogenesis; contralateral epiphysiodesis or shortening of the femur; Ilizarov hip reconstruction
Unstable hip with advanced osteoarthritis not amenable to the above-mentioned reconstructive procedures	Management of painful unstable hip as a last resort	Total hip replacement arthroplasty; arthrodesis; Ilizarov hip reconstruction after excision of the femoral head and neck remnant

dimensions using magnetic resonance imaging (MRI), ultrasonography, arthrography, and 2D/3D computed tomography (CT). The dynamics of articular motion between the deformed femoral head (FH) and acetabulum should be assessed. When open reduction is performed to restore stability of the hip, the status of articular cartilage of the femoral head and acetabulum should be carefully assessed pre- and intra-operatively. It is because restoring the stability at the expense of mobility is never an acceptable approach [5, 12]. Additionally, full-length standing radiograph visualizing the entire lower limbs is helpful not only to identify associated sequelae at other sites, if any, but also to determine axial malalignment, joint malorientation, and LLD [12].

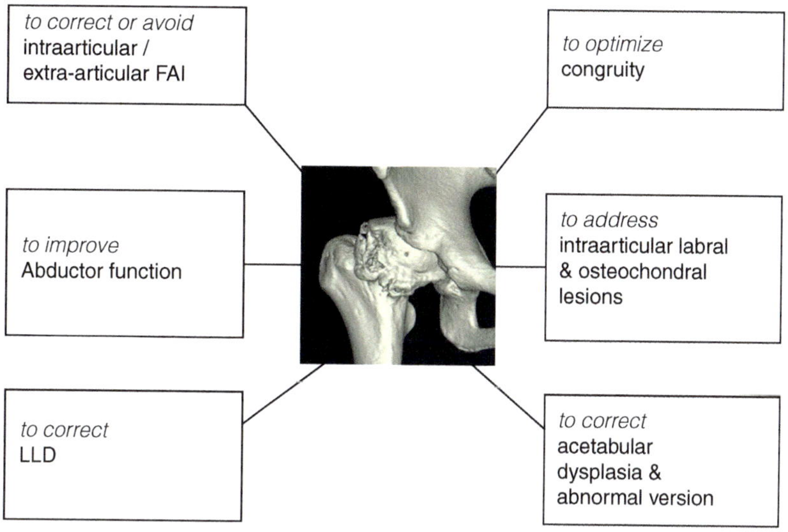

Fig. 24.2 Goals of treatment for FAI in older children with type II and III hips

Recommended Treatment Guidelines

The recommended primary and secondary surgical options are as varied as the types of deformities; therefore, treatment strategies should be individualized. However, an overall outline of treatment options for post-septic hip sequelae is summarized in Table 24.2. Definitive and adjunctive surgical treatment methods can be used alone or in combination. Tips and tricks for successful outcome and pitfalls to avoid are shown in Table 24.3. The principles that apply in the treatment of subluxation or dislocation associated with post-septic hip sequelae are generally the same as those used in the management of developmental dislocation of the hip, but with some modification because of special features of localized tissue destruction.

Specific Surgical Options

Choi Type I Deformity

Type 1 deformity appears to be the result of transient ischemia of the epiphysis. Thus, most Type I hips do not need reconstruction. Very rarely, a child with type I deformity may present with an unexceptionally enlarged femoral head with secondary acetabular dysplasia. In such case, the same reconstructive surgical interventions as those used in the management of developmental dislocation of the hip can be utilized not only to contain the femoral head but also to improve acetabular coverage (Fig. 24.3).

Choi Type II and III Deformities

Type II and III hips are fundamentally the result of an abnormally shaped, sized, or oriented femoral head and neck, altered head-neck offset, and acetabular dysplasia. Thus, remarkably diverse residual deformities can be seen on radiographs, ranging from deformities like those in Perthes disease with coxa vara/valga, coxa plana, coxa breva, coxa magna, coxa irregularis, relative greater trochanteric overriding, sagging rope sign [13], and acetabular dysplasia to the more deformed proximal femur visualized as beard, collared, staghorn, or rugby-ball-shaped FH [12, 14, 15]. Children with type II or III hips may remain asymptomatic in their younger age, but, in (pre)adolescence, these children often present with clinical problems such as pain, limp, joint instability or contracture, restriction of motion, LLD, spinal disorders, and even emotional disturbances. In children with type II and III hips, the surgeon should pay attention to see if the deformity is progressive and the sources of pain-

Table 24.3 Tips and tricks for successful outcome and pitfalls to avoid

Tips and tricks	Attentive identification of progressive deformity and the source of pain, e.g., femoro-acetabular impingement, is crucial. Secondary or concomitant deformities at other sites, if any, should be carefully evaluated to improve overall function of the affected lower limb. Specific treatment plan should be individualized after reviewing the clinical findings and imaging studies on the pathomorphologic features of the hip. It is important to set up realistic goals aiming at restoring hip stability, correcting deformities that may compromise hip function, retaining the hip mobility, eliminating the source of pain, and correcting the limb-shortening. Reconstructive surgical procedures should start on time to provide the best possible hip joint mechanics. When open reduction is performed to restore stability of the hip, the status of articular cartilage of the femoral head and acetabulum should be carefully assessed pre- and intra-operatively. In type IIIB hips, it is crucial to check the mobility between the chondro-osseous epiphysis and the acetabular floor. Ilizarov hip reconstruction is a highly effective treatment modality for the management of Choi type IVB and IVA hips in which the previous reconstructive surgery has failed, or there is late presentation with a severe abductor lurch and a considerable limb-length shortening, particularly in the adolescents and young adults in whom arthrodesis or hip arthroplasty is not suitable.
Pitfalls to avoid	Children with type II and type III hips may remain asymptomatic in younger age. Restoring stability at the expense of mobility is not an acceptable approach. Subcapital osteotomy for type IIIA sequelae may increase the risk of avascular necrosis of the femoral head. In type IIIB hips with no substantial mobility between the epiphysis and acetabular socket, aggressive open procedure to reconstruct the head and neck is not an acceptable approach because of high risk of avascular necrosis and potential postoperative stiffness, which can be quite disabling. In type IVA hips, any reconstructive procedure performed in ages older than 6 years seems to be relatively contraindicated due to limited remaining remodeling capacity. In type IVB hips, greater trochanteric arthroplasty for reconstruction of femoro-pelvic articulation is a technically demanding procedure with unpredictable outcomes, particularly when performed in older age. Ilizarov hip reconstruction should not be performed in younger age because of gradual straightening of the proximal femur at the site of valgus angulation, with a resultant loss of pelvic support.

ful limp compromise normal hip function (Table 24.2, Fig. 24.4). Treatment should start on time to correct subluxation, joint incongruity, abnormal neck-shaft angle, excessive femoral or acetabular version, acetabular dysplasia, inadequate femoro-acetabular coverage, and epiphyseal tilting or slipping due to asymmetrical premature fusion of the capital physis. It is noteworthy that a painful limp, followed by a limited range of motion, can be associated with FAI with or without chondro-labral damage. The conceptual recognition of FAI and safe surgical hip dislocation or arthroscopic management have revolutionized the diagnostic and therapeutic algorithms for joint-preserving surgery for type II and type III hips [12, 18]. Treating surgeons should have profound knowledge and skills to tackle various intra- and extra-articular FAI-related problems; they should be familiar with the surgical techniques including osteochondroplasty of the femoral head and neck, labral debridement or refixation, proximal femoral realignment osteotomy, triple innominate osteotomy (TIO), periacetabular osteotomy (PAO), relative or true femoral neck lengthening with distal advancement of the greater trochanter (GT), Chiari osteotomy or femoral head reduction osteotomy, and other hip reconstructive procedures [12, 16–24]. Additionally, attentive care should be given to correct marked shortening and deformity of the affected limb.

Certain limitations and difficulties of reconstruction for type III sequelae deserve mention. In young children with type IIIA hips with very severe coxa vara or coxa valga with epiphyseal slipping leading to severe torsional malalignment, one is left with the decision *where* to perform corrective osteotomy – whether near to the physis, that is, subcapital realignment, or away from the physis, that is, base of neck osteotomy

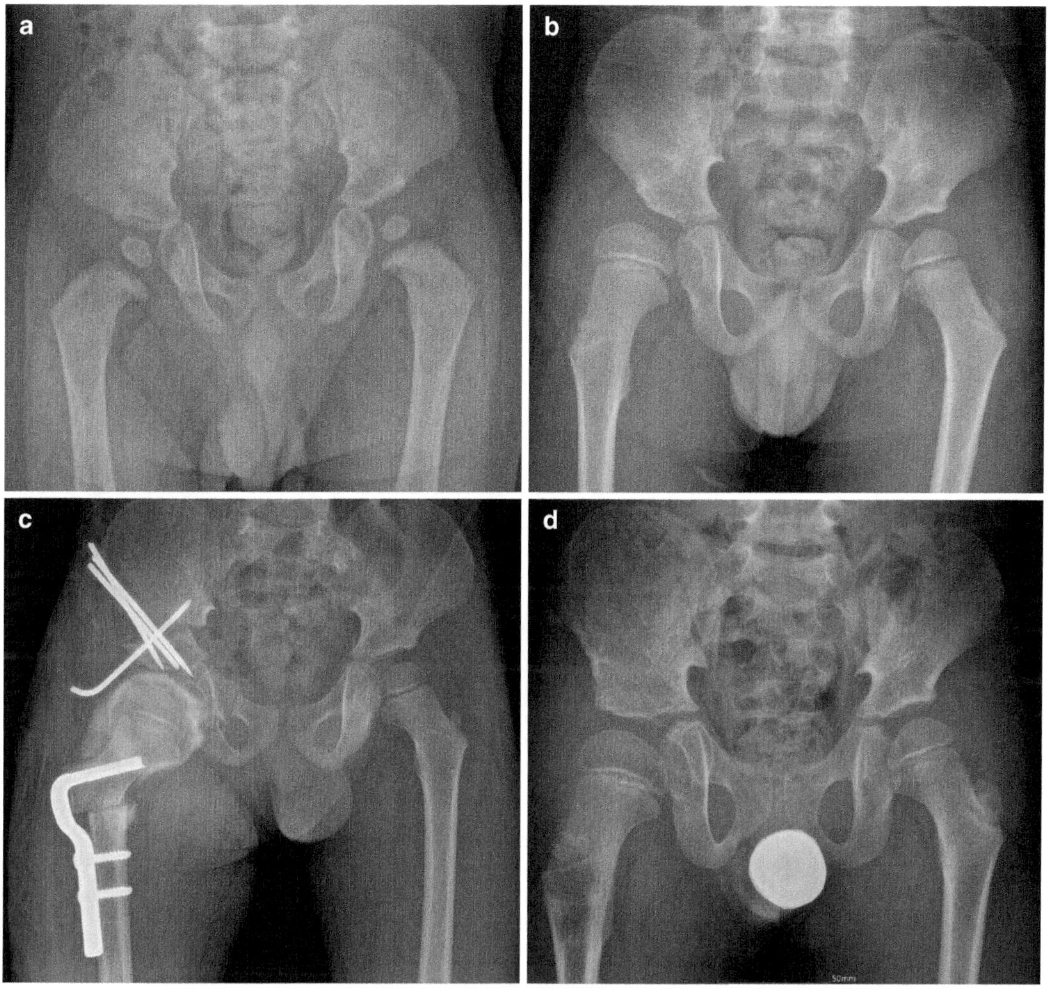

Fig. 24.3 A radiograph in a boy presented with type IB sequelae in the right hip showing unacceptably enlarged femoral head (coxa magna) and accompanying acetabular dysplasia due to infantile septic arthritis. He had a previous history of neonatal care in the intensive care unit (ICU) due to prematurity and low birth weight (820 g). (**a**) A pelvis anteroposterior (AP) radiograph taken at 11 months of age at other hospital. (**b**) A radiograph taken at 4 years of age at referral. (**c**) He underwent femoral varus and shortening osteotomy in conjunction with a triple pelvic osteotomy. (**d**) A radiograph taken at 6 years and 1 month of age showing improved containment, congruency, and coverage of the hip. Modified Harris hip score at the latest follow-up was 71

or inter- or sub-trochanteric osteotomy. This is an open question to be explored in the future. Anyhow, based upon deformity correction principles, subcapital realignment would be the best option because of the center of rotation of the angular deformity being located in the vicinity of the capital physis. However, the incidence of osteonecrosis is greatest with subcapital osteotomy and progressively decreases with more distal osteotomies owing to the unique characteristics of blood supply to the femoral head. The risk of FAI and degenerative arthritis can be avoided or decreased once the epiphysis can be reduced without developing osteonecrosis in type IIIA hips. However, we currently advocate corrective osteotomy at the base of neck or high intertrochanteric area instead of subcapital osteotomy for fear of potential avascular necrosis in young children. As opposed to type IIIA, type IIIB sequelae are more difficult to treat, particularly when associated with a mobile nonunion of the femoral neck. In type IIIB hips with no

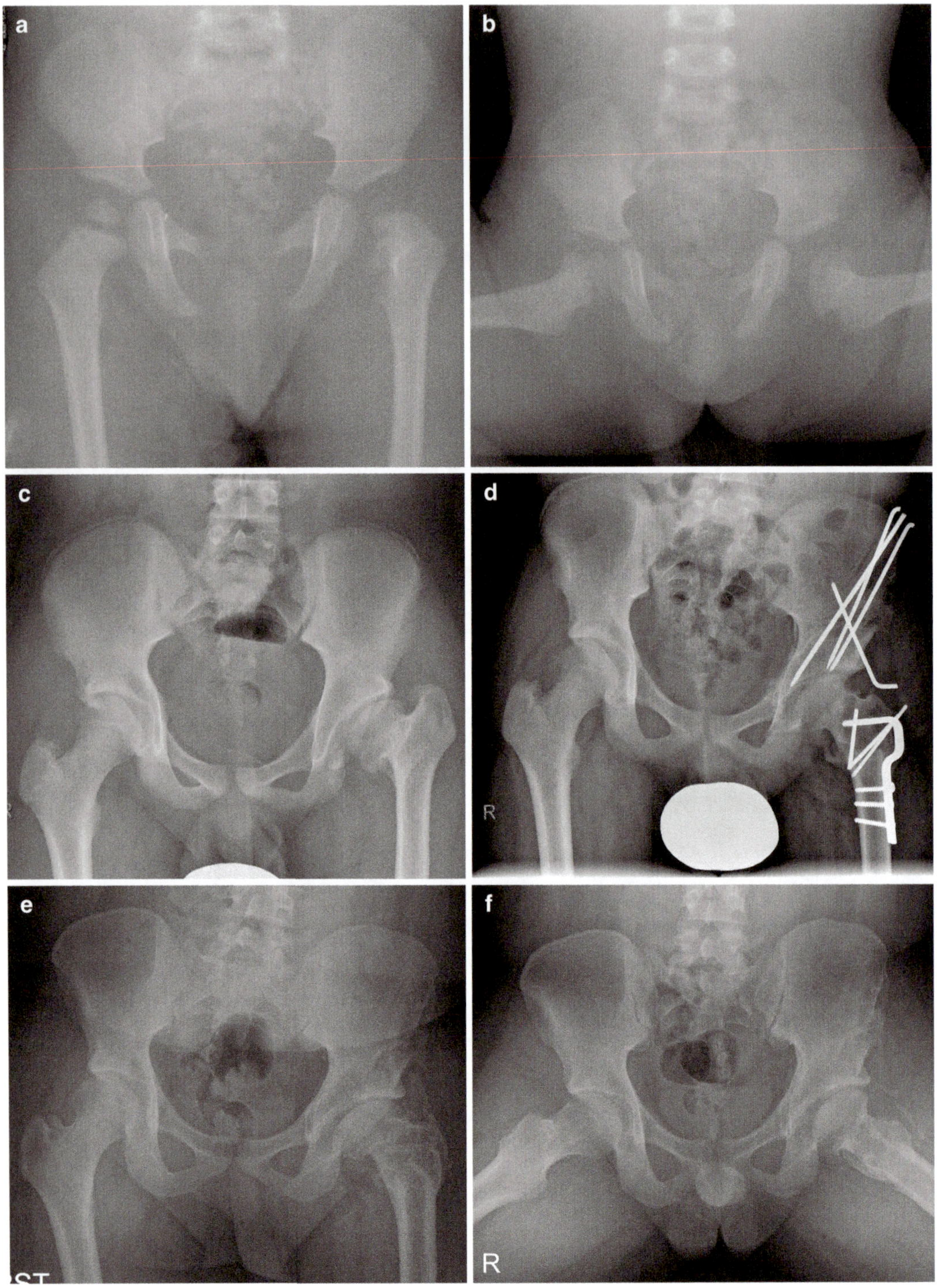

Fig. 24.4 An adolescent presented with type IIB sequelae in the left hip showing progressive coxa vara due to infantile septic arthritis. He had a previous history of greater trochanteric epi- and apo-physiodesis and 4 cm of femoral lengthening using a monolateral fixator at age 6 years and 7 months. (**a**, **b**) Radiographs taken at 16 months of age. (**c**) Radiographs taken at 14 years and 5 months of age at referral. (**d**) He underwent a combined procedure consisting of osteochondroplasty via safe surgical hip dislocation, femoral valgus osteotomy, and Ganz periacetabular osteotomy. (**e**, **f**) A radiograph taken at 19 years and 2 months of age showing improved containment, congruency, and coverage of the hip and the head-neck offset. Modified Harris hip score at the latest follow-up was 89

substantial mobility between the epiphysis and acetabular socket, aggressive open procedure to reconstruct the head and neck is not an acceptable approach because of high risk of avascular necrosis and potential postoperative stiffness, which can be quite disabling. Recently, Kumar et al. [25] reported satisfactory results in 15 of 16 patients with type IIIB hips; 14 patients were treated by closed reduction, fibular graft, and valgus osteotomy and 2 patients with short femoral neck along with pseudarthrosis were treated by Wagner double intertrochanteric osteotomy [24] with a fibular graft. However, they did not mention as to whether the hips treated had stiff or mobile nonunion in the femoral neck before operation.

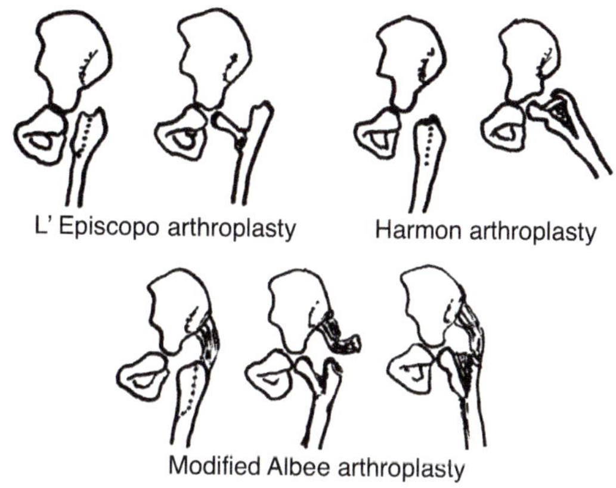

Fig. 24.5 Schematic drawings of L'Episcopo arthroplasty, Harmon arthroplasty, and modified Albee arthroplasty for reconstruction of type IVA hips

Choi Type IV Deformity

The management of severe deformities that occur because of fulminant septic arthritis of the hip is clinically challenging. Available reports include only small numbers of patients with severe sequelae, with relatively few long-term follow-up studies. When there is severe destruction of the femoral head and neck, with or without a small medial remnant of the neck, it is difficult to maintain a stable reduction. If instability and dislocation persist, the surgeon can either neglect the deformity or can attempt reconstruction to create a stable femoro-acetabular articulation [5, 12, 26]. However, the available surgical options for reconstruction of type IV hips are limited, and, in general, have not yielded satisfactory long-term results [1, 2, 5–9, 12, 21, 25–29]. In young children with type IVA sequelae with a reasonably sized unossified cartilaginous cap as a medial remnant, open reduction can be attempted. Femoral remnant can be fashioned to articulate with the acetabulum to create a stable femoro-acetabular articulation by utilizing the Albee [30], L'Episcopo [31], Harmon [32], or modified Albee procedures [33] (Fig. 24.5). In 1935, Dr. Albee [30] described an arthroplasty procedure providing a neck-lengthening effect by splitting a remnant of the femoral neck covered by unossified hyaline cartilage, beginning from above and proceeding downward into the shaft of femur in the sagittal plane, and by creating an incomplete greenstick fracture at the base of the medial portion of sectioned femur. One year later, Dr. L'Episcopo [31] reported another similar technique recommending the medial portion of the sectioned femur bent medially producing an angle of about 125° between the fragment and the shaft. In 1942, Harmon [32] also reported a similar technique by making an incomplete, spring opening wedge osteotomy at the base of the femoral remnant adjoining the greater trochanter. The resulting opening wedge gap can be filled with a block of corticocancellous bone graft or osteochondral graft taken from the iliac apophysis. These procedures produce a femoral neck-lengthening effect by repositioning the greater trochanter away from the acetabular margin. Dr. Li et al. [33] reported a modification of original technique of Albee or Harmon arthroplasty; any rough or uneven cartilage surfaces of the acetabulum can be trimmed with a small ball-shaped reamer, the greater trochanter is removed 0.5 cm below the physis, the width of the splitted medial fragment—serving as the new femoral head—is formed by approximately two-thirds of the diameter of the femoral segment, and the greater trochanter with attached gluteus medius and gluteus minimus are then sutured to the lateral fragment so that muscle tension is restored. They recommended creating a 135–145° angle between the

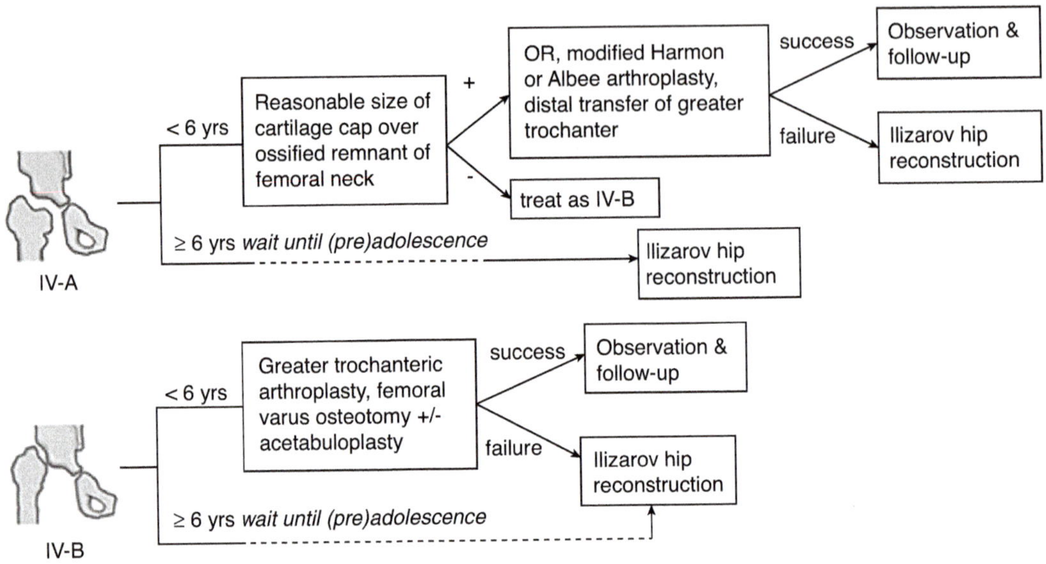

Fig. 24.6 Treatment approaches to type IV hips

"new" femoral head and the proximal part of the femoral shaft. Subsequent stability and fulcrum of the hip will depend on the amount of the osteochondral tissue assuming a femoral head and neck produced. We think that various surgical options for reconstruction of type IVA hips are applicable only when the acetabular cartilage is undamaged or altered to only a minor degree, preferably in younger ages around second and third years of life. Nonetheless, the results are not predictable in view of hip mobility and function when open reduction and reconstruction is performed in older children. Therefore, we think that, in children older than 6 years of age, type IVA hips should be treated in the same manner as type IVB hips (Fig. 24.6) [2, 12]. Admittedly, neglecting or postponing the treatment of type IVB hips will produce proximal iliac dislocation that may contribute to degenerative changes in the lumbosacral spine and hips [12, 26] with the passage of time. The patients may present with a marked abductor lurch, telescoping limp, and LLD, although they may remain asymptomatic for a number of years [5, 6, 12, 26].

In the literature, various treatment modalities for reconstructing a femoro-pelvic articulation in type IVB hips have been reported, including hip reconstruction with vascularized iliac crest grafting [34], arthrodesis, greater trochanteric arthroplasty (GTA) [12, 35–40] with adjunctive or secondary procedures, pelvic support osteotomy (PSO) [40–45], and Ilizarov hip reconstruction (IHR) [45–60]. Of these treatment modalities, GTA, PSO, and IHR are probably the most commonly performed procedures; an intra-articular femoro-acetabular articulation can be created with GTA, whereas extra-articular stability can be created with PSO or IHR [12]. Hip fusion is not recommended in young children in this era.

Greater Trochanteric Arthroplasty Versus Pelvic Support Osteotomy (Ilizarov Hip Reconstruction)

GTA is performed to place the greater trochanter into the acetabulum to function similarly to the femoral head, while the detached abductor muscles are transferred distally to provide hip stability and some degree of abductor function. GTA, basically and originally described by Colonna [35], has been popularized by Westin [36] and others [26, 27, 37, 38]. The underlying concept of GTA is based on the assumption that the trochanteric apophysis that is covered by hyaline cartilage will remodel into a globular shape similar to that of an FH [1, 2, 12, 17, 27, 29, 35–40, 45]. Subsequent progressive subluxation following the "stick femur" procedure in most patients necessitates additional procedures, such as femoral varus osteotomy to create the semblance of a "neck-shaft" angle, pelvic osteotomy including Chiari osteotomy, or shelf acetabuloplasty to improve FH coverage. However, GTA is a technically demanding procedure with highly unpredictable outcomes, despite some satisfactory reports [26, 27, 35, 36, 38–40]. Multiple problems can be ensued following GTA: development of avascular necrosis of the proximal segment, gradual straightening of the proximal femur, abductor weakness, stiffness, recurrent subluxation, degenerative arthritis, and difficulty during conversion to total hip arthroplasty in adulthood [1, 2, 12, 26, 27, 37, 38, 52]. According to our observation, the transferred GT can assume a globular shape with time, but with no or incomplete formation of head-neck offset with a resultant FAI (Fig. 24.7). We have experienced that the results of GTA are influenced by the patient's age at operation, preoperative hip range of motion, and abductor power [2, 12]. We found that satisfactory results can be obtained only in those children who underwent GTA under the age of 6 years—young enough to allow remodeling of the

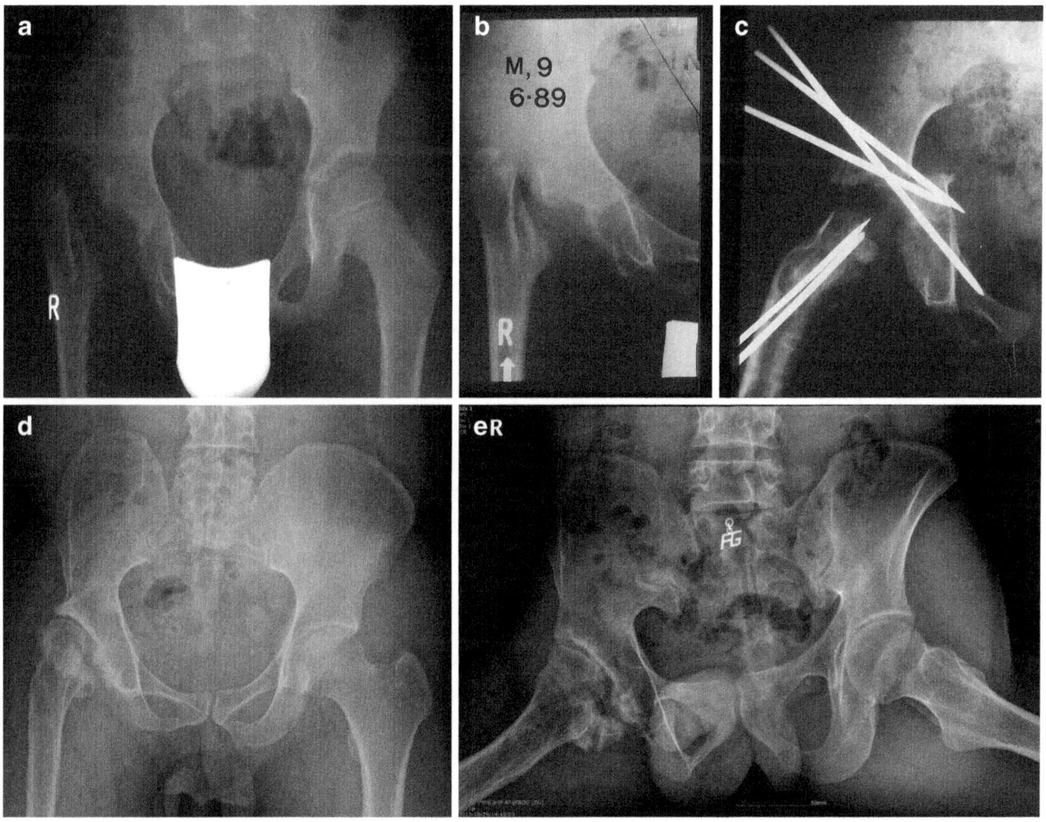

Fig. 24.7 A case of greater trochanteric arthroplasty for type IVB sequelae in the right hip after infantile septic arthritis. (**a**, **b**) A radiograph in a 9-year-old boy with Choi type IVB sequelae in the right hip. (**c**) He initially underwent greater trochanteric arthroplasty known as "stick femur" procedure, and subsequently femoral varus osteotomy was added in conjunction with Chiari osteotomy to prevent subluxation. (**d**, **e**) Radiographs taken at 38 years and 5 months of age showing advanced degenerative arthritis of the right hip joint, despite a well-remodeled greater trochanter that had assumed a globular shape like the femoral head. At the last follow-up, he presented with marked gluteal lurch. He alluded that his hip function has rapidly deteriorated for the past few years despite an acceptable range of hip motion. He is ready for a total hip replacement arthroplasty. Modified Harris hip score at the latest follow-up was 76

transferred GT. Unsatisfactory results are common virtually in all patients who underwent GTA over the age of 6 years [2, 12].

The "pelvic support osteotomy" (PSO) for creating extra-articular femoral-pelvic stability was developed in the 1910s and popularized by Milch and others [41–46]. The proximal femur is osteotomized around the level of the ischial tuberosity and the distal fragment is angulated laterally; the degree of valgus angulation is approximately 15° more than the range of passive adduction. As a result, the efficiency of abductor muscle improves in view of lever arm function with medially displaced center of gravity and ground reaction force [12, 45, 47]. However, the clinical application of traditional PSO is limited due to its indigenous drawbacks. The most difficult problem encountered in performing PSO is, to what extent the optimal valgus angulation is achieved. If the amount of angulation is too large, genu valgum, fixed pelvic obliquity, and impingement pain on adduction of the lower limb to neutral position may occur. On the other hand, if the angular correction is too small, the result would be an insufficient improvement in hip biomechanics. Most importantly, the issue of persisting LLD cannot be addressed with the PSO. Ilizarov developed and popularized a modified PSO technique called Ilizarov hip reconstruction (IHR), in which a second distal femoral varus osteotomy is performed to realign the knee joint and to correct the LLD in addition to proximal femoral valgus osteotomy for pelvic support [45–60]. Ilizarov emphasized the importance of extension of the proximal osteotomy to correct fixed hip flexion contracture, if any, and to permit locking of the hip joint [45–48, 50–59]. We have the same opinion with others that IHR is highly effective in eliminating or substantially reducing the Trendelenburg gait and in equalizing the lower limb length, so the stability and range of motion of the hip joint can be obtained at the same time [45, 48–60]. Hence, we believe that IHR is a viable option for type IVB and IVA hips in which the previous reconstructive surgery has failed, or there is late presentation with a severe abductor lurch and a considerable LLD, particularly in adolescents and young adults in whom arthrodesis or hip arthroplasty is not suitable [12, 45, 51]. Reported complications following IHR include knee stiffness, pin tract infection, delayed consolidation, refracture, obturator nerve entrapment, straightening of proximal valgus angulation, ischiofemoral impingement, and persistent Trendelenburg gait. Of note, an average of 30% (range, 0–62.5%) of patients have a persistent positive Trendelenburg sign after IHR, although it is reduced in severity in most of the patients [12, 45]. Recently, IHR with internal fixation devices otherwise named as "Pelvic Support Hip Reconstruction" has been reported with promising early results [61]. This technique avoids common complications associated with external fixators and facilitates faster rehabilitation. However, it is more technically demanding than gradual correction with external fixation.

IHR is not ideal for young children. It is because gradual straightening of the proximal femur tends to occur at the site of valgus angulation in accordance with Wolff's law with a resultant loss of pelvic support [12, 45, 47, 52, 53, 56, 57, 59, 60] (Fig. 24.8). Therefore, it is important to add empirically as much as 25–40° of overcorrection when performing IHR at an age before adolescence due to the possibility of straightening of the proximal femur after IHR [12, 45, 47, 52]. For this reason, some authors recommend performing the IHR at or near skeletal maturity. When there is marked shortening of affected limb in growing children, two options can be chosen. The first option is performing femoral lengthening without a PSO, inserting half pins into the pelvis to prevent proximal migration of the femur, at a younger age and subsequent IHR at or near skeletal maturity as a second procedure. The second option is to perform repeat IHR [12, 45, 56]. We prefer to perform IHR in preadolescents with type IVB hips with marked shortening despite a concern for repeat IHR. We believe that early stabilization of the hip with newly reconstructed fulcrum of femoral-pelvic articulation would help build up abductor muscle power, and, consequently, lead to an improved gait in emotionally sensitive adolescents.

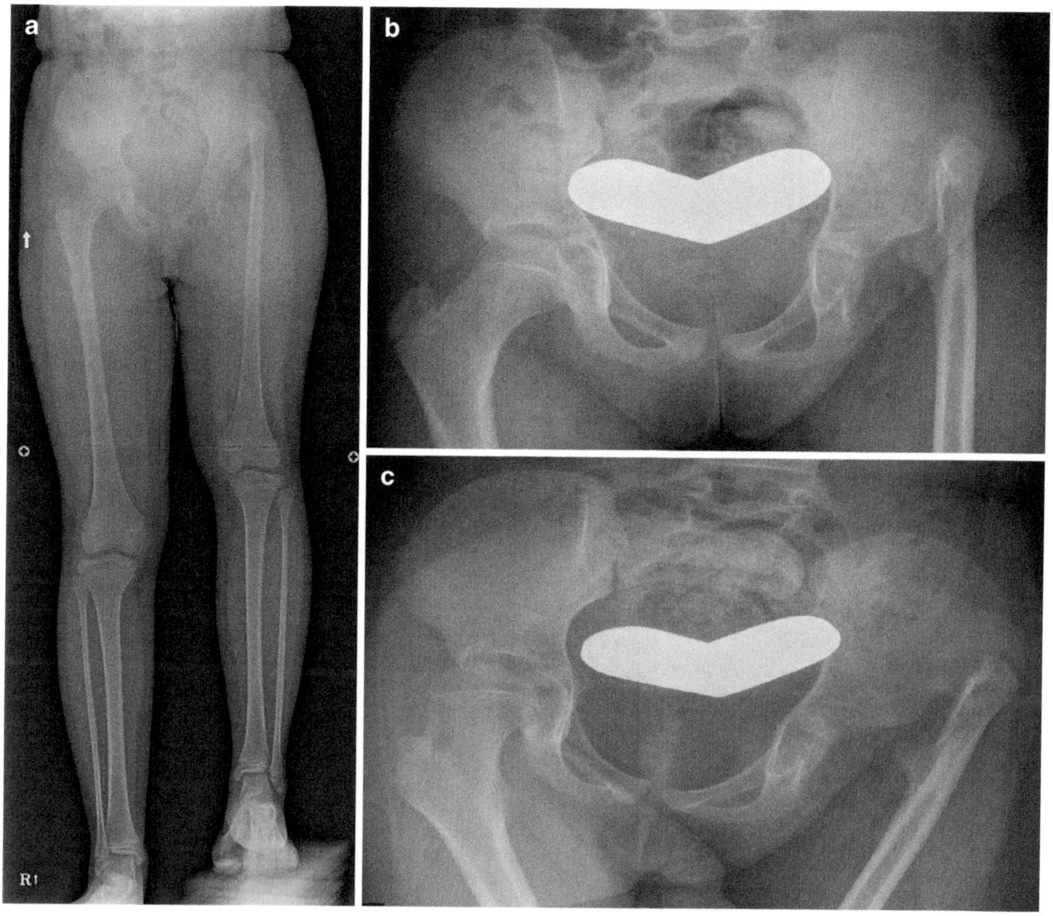

Fig. 24.8 A case of Ilizarov hip reconstruction for type IVB sequelae in the left hip after infantile septic arthritis. (**a–c**) Radiographs showing complete loss of femoral head and neck with marked proximal migration in a 10-year and 3-year-old girl. She presented with severe abductor lurch with occasional back pain. (**d**) She underwent Ilizarov hip reconstruction using a modification of a monolateral fixator (Dyna-ATC®, Seoul, Korea) with a 40° of proximal femoral valgus osteotomy for pelvic support and 8 cm of distal diaphyseal lengthening for leg length equalization. (**e**) On the teleradiograph taken at 23 years of age, it is noteworthy to observe remodeled, straightened proximal femur; however, the center of gravity and ground reaction force have been medially displaced, suggestive of improved efficiency of abductor muscle. (**f–h**) Overall function of the hip and affected lower limb was rated "satisfactory" except mild abductor lurch. She had no pain or discomfort around the hip. Modified Harris hip score at the latest follow-up was 88

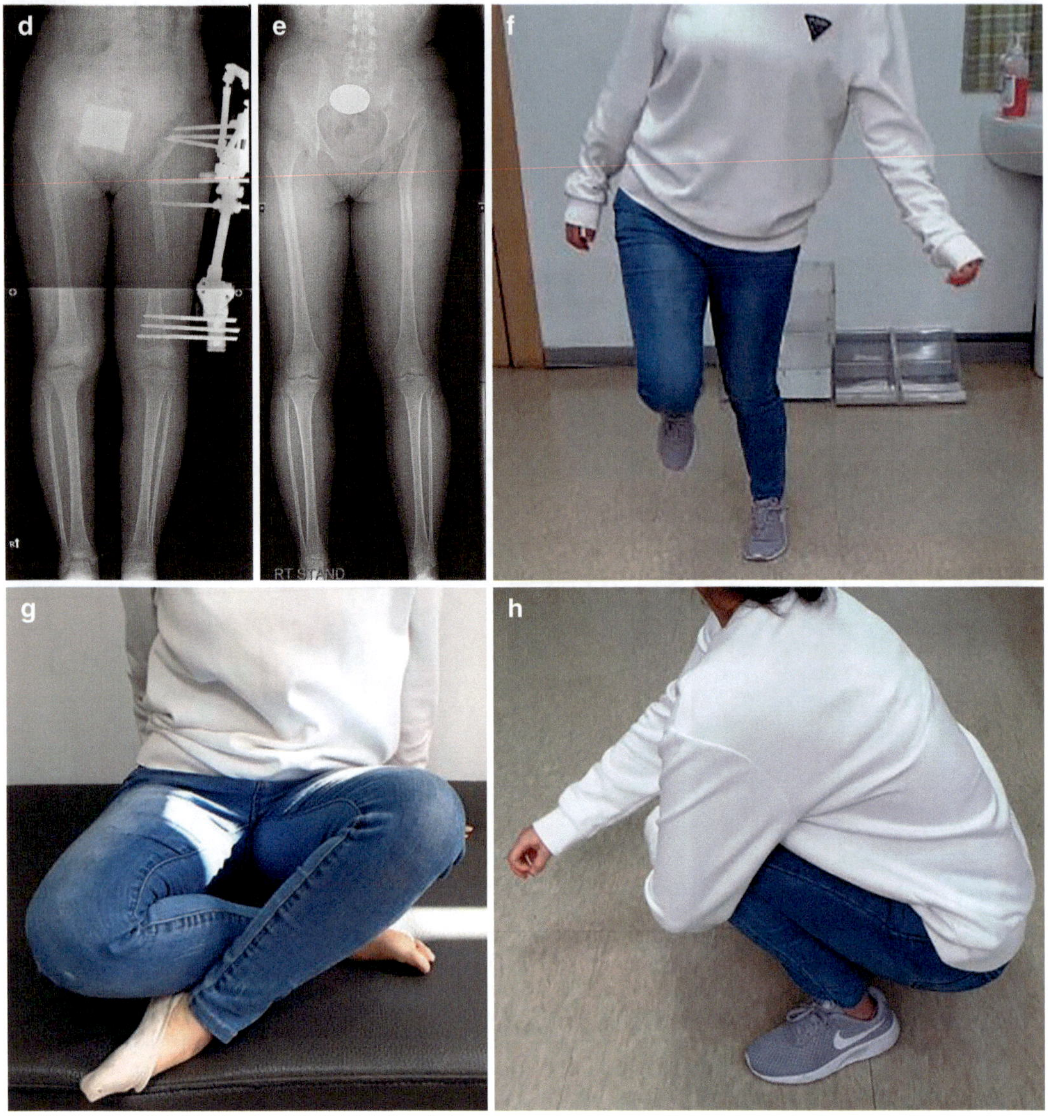

Fig. 24.8 (continued)

References

1. Choi IH, Pizzutillo PD, Bowen JR, Dragann R, Malhis T. Sequelae and reconstruction after septic arthritis of the hip in infants. J Bone Joint Surg Am. 1990;72:1150–65.
2. Choi IH, Yoo WJ, Cho TJ, Chung CY. Operative reconstruction for septic arthritis of the hip. Orthop Clin N Am. 2006;37:173–83.
3. Shapiro F. Pediatric orthopedic deformities. Basic science, diagnosis, and treatment. London: Academic Press; 2001. p. 897–909.
4. Agarwal A, Kumar KHV. Suppurative arthritis of hip in a walking child: effect of patient's age, delay in surgical drainage, and organism virulence. J Orthop Surg. 2020;28(1):1–8.
5. Joseph B. Post-infective hip dysplasia. In: Joseph B, Nayagam S, Loder R, Torode I, editors. Paediatric orthopaedics. A system of decision-making. 2nd ed. Boca Raton: CRS Press; 2005. p. 229–37.
6. Choi IH, Shin YW, Chung CY, Cho TJ, Yoo WJ, Lee DY. Surgical treatment of the severe sequelae of infantile septic arthritis of the hip. Clin Orthop. 2005;434:102–9.
7. Ilharreborde B. Sequelae of pediatric osteoarticular infection. Orthop Traumatol Surg Res. 2015;101:S129–37.
8. Hunka L, Said SE, MacKenzie DA, Rogala EJ, Cruess RL. Classification and surgical management

of the severe sequelae of septic hips in children. Clin Orthop. 1982;171:30–6.
9. Johari AN. Residual problems in septic arthritis of the hips in childhood. Thesis submitted for the MCh Ortho, University of Liverpool 1988. In: Varghese M, editor. Current concept: septic arthritis in childhood. Trends in paediatric orthopaedics. London: Macmillan (I) Ltd.; 2002. p. 25–32.
10. Johari AN, Dhawale AA, Johari RA. Management of post septic hip dislocations when the capital femoral epiphysis is present. J Pediatr Orthop B. 2011;20:413–21.
11. Forlin E, Milani C. Sequelae of septic arthritis of the hip in children: a new classification and a review of 41 hips. J Pediatr Orthop. 2008;28:524–8.
12. Choi IH. Postinfectious deformities of the lower limb. In: Sabharwal S, editor. Pediatric lower limb deformities. Principles and techniques of management. Cham: Springer; 2016. p. 589–603.
13. Kim HT, Eisenhauer E, Wenger DR. The "sagging rope sign" in avascular necrosis in children's hip disease – confirmation by 3D CT studies. Iowa Orthop J. 1995;15:101–11.
14. El-Tayeby HM. Osteochondroplasty of the femoral head in hip reconstruction for type II late sequelae of septic arthritis: a preliminary report. J Child Orthop. 2008;2:431–41.
15. Shin SJ, Choi IH, Cho TJ, Yoo WJ, Chung CY, Park MS. Unusual osteocartilaginous prominence or bump causing femoroacetabular impingement after septic arthritis of the hip: a report of 2 cases in preadolescence. J Pediatr Orthop. 2009;29:459–62.
16. Wenger DR, Pring ME. Triple innominate osteotomy. In: Flynn JM, Wiesel SW, editors. Operative techniques in pediatric orthopaedics. Philadelphia: Lippincott Williams and Wilkins; 2011. p. 515–26.
17. Ganz R, Klaue K, Vinh TS, Mast JW. A new periacetabular osteotomy for the treatment of hip dysplasias: technique and preliminary results. Clin Orthop. 2004;418:3–8.
18. Ganz R, Huff TW, Leunig M. Extended retinacular release soft-tissue flap for intra-articular hip surgery: surgical technique, indications, and results of application. Instr Course Lect. 2009;58:241–55.
19. Leunig M, Ganz R. Relative neck lengthening and intracapital osteotomy for severe Perthes and Perthes-like deformities. Bull NYU Hosp Jt Dis. 2011;69(suppl 1):S62–7.
20. Hasler CC, Morscher EW. Femoral neck lengthening osteotomy after growth disturbance of the proximal femur. J Pediatr Orthop B. 1999;8:271–5.
21. Standard SC. Treatment of coxa brevis. Orthop Clin N Am. 2011;42:373–87.
22. Wagner H. Femoral osteotomies for congenital hip dislocation. In: Weil UH, editor. Progress in orthopedic surgery, Acetabular dyplasia and skeletal dysplasia in childhood, vol. 2. New York: Springer-Verlag; 1978. p. 85.
23. Hefti F, Morsher E. The femoral neck lengthening osteotomy. Orthop Traumatol. 1993;2:144–51.
24. Paley D. The treatment of femoral head deformity and coxa magna by the Ganz femoral head reduction osteotomy. Orthop Clin N Am. 2011;42:389–99.
25. Kumar Knojia R, Gupta S, Kumar A, Reddy BK. Closed reduction, osteotomy, and fibular graft are effective in treating pediatric femoral neck pseudarthrosis after infection. Clin Orthop Relat Res. 2018;0:1–12. https://doi.org/10.1097/01.blo.0000533616.93007.46.
26. Dobbs MB, Sheridan JJ, Gordon JE, Corley CL, Szymanski DA, Schoenecker PL. Septic arthritis of the hip in infancy: long-term follow-up. J Pediatr Orthop. 2003;23:162–8.
27. Freeland AE, Sullivan DJ, Westin GW. Greater trochanteric hip arthroplasty in children with loss of the femoral head. J Bone Joint Surg Am. 1980;62:1351–61.
28. Agarwal A, Rastogi P. What factors contribute to Choi IV sequelae? A retrospective analysis of 15 septic hips. Clin Orthop Trauma. 2020;11(supplement 4):S645–9.
29. Wada A, Fujii T, Takamura K, Yanagida H, Urano N, Surijamorn P. Operative reconstruction of the severe sequelae of infantile septic arthritis of the hip. J Pediatr Orthop. 2007;27:910–4.
30. Albee FH. Arthroplasty of the hip and the preservation of its stability. Ann Surg. 1935;102:108–14.
31. L'Episcopo J. Stabilization of pathological dislocation of the hip in children. J Bone Joint Surg. 1936;18:737–42.
32. Harmon PH. Surgical treatment of the residual deformity from suppurative arthritis of the hip occurring in young children. J Bone Joint Surg. 1942;24:576–85.
33. Li XD, Chen B, Fan J, Zheng CY, Liu DX, Wang H, et al. Evaluation of the modified Albee arthroplasty for femoral head loss secondary to septic arthritis in young children. J Bone Joint Surg Am. 2010;92:1370–80.
34. Cheng JC, Aguilar J, Leung PC. Hip reconstruction for femoral head loss from septic arthritis in children. A preliminary report. Clin Orthop. 1995;314:214–24.
35. Colonna PC. A new type of reconstruction operation for old ununited fractures of the neck of the femur. J Bone Joint Surg. 1935;17:110–22.
36. Westin GW. The stick femur. In: Proceedings and reports of university colleges, councils and associations. J Bone Joint Surg Br. 1970;52:778–9.
37. Axer A, Alan A. A new technique for greater trochanteric hip arthroplasty. J Bone Joint Surg Br. 1984;66:331–3.
38. Weissman SL. Transplantation of the trochanteric epiphysis into the acetabulum after septic arthritis of the hip: report of a case. J Bone Joint Surg Am. 1967;49:1647–51.
39. Ferrari D, Libri R, Donzelli O. Trochanteroplasty to treat sequelae of septic arthritis of the hip in infancy. Case series and review of the literature. Hip Int. 2011;21:653–6.
40. Abrishami S, Karami M, Karimi A, Soufali AP, Aslani HR, Badizadeh K. Greater trochanteric preserving hip

arthroplasty in the treatment of infantile septic arthritis: long-term results. J Child Orthop. 2010;4:137–41.
41. Milch H. The pelvic support osteotomy. J Bone Joint Surg. 1941;23:581–95.
42. Milch H. The "pelvic support" osteotomy. Clin Orthop. 1989;249:4–11.
43. Peltier LF. The classic. The "pelvic support" osteotomy. Clin Orthop. 1989;249:4–11.
44. Schiltenwolf M, Carstens C, Bernd L, Lukoschek M. Late results after subtrochanteric angulation osteotomy in young patients. J Pediatr Orthop B. 1996;5:259–67.
45. Choi IH, Cho TJ, Yoo WJ, Shin CH. Recurrent dislocations and complete necrosis: the role of pelvic support osteotomy. J Pediatr Orthop. 2013;33(Suppl 1):S45–55.
46. Ilizarov GA. Treatment of disorders of the hip. In: Green SA, editor. Transosseous osteosynthesis. Berlin: Springer; 1992. p. 668–96.
47. Pafilas D, Nayagam S. The pelvic support osteotomy: indications and preoperative planning. Strategies Trauma Limb Reconstr. 2008;3:83–92.
48. Ilizarov GA, Samchukov ML, Kurtov VM. Ilizarov restorative reconstruction surgery in the treatment of hip osteoarthritis, congenital and pathological hip dislocation in children and adults. In: Materials of Second International Symposium. Experimental, theoretical, and clinical aspects of transosseous osteosynthesis developed in Kurgan Scientific Research Institute. Kurgan, USSR, 1986, pp. 100–102.
49. Ilizarov GA, Samchukov ML. Ilizarov reconstructive surgery in the treatment of hip osteoarthritis. Ortop Travmatol Protez. 1988;6:10–3.
50. Kadykalo OA, Kuftyev LM. Some biomechanical principles of the hip reconstruction with defect on head and neck of the femur by Ilizarov method. In: The value of general biological patterns in regeneration tissue opened by G. A. Ilizarov. Scientific works collection 13th Edition, The Ministry of Health, The RSFSR (The Russian Soviet Federative Socialist Republic) Kurgan All-union scientific center. Rehabilitation Traumatology Orthopedics, 1988, pp. 124–129.
51. Samchukov ML, Ivanova IV, Dolganov DV. Analysis of pelvo-trochanteric muscles and weight-bearing after Ilizarov femoral reconstruction in patients with hip osteoarthritis. In: The congress of scientific and technical advances of the young scientists of the Urals. USSR, 1986, pp. 86–87.
52. Paley D. Hip joint considerations. In: Paley D, editor. Principles of deformity correction. Berlin: Springer; 2002. p. 647–94.
53. Kocaoglu M, Eralp L, Sen C, Dincyurek H. The Ilizarov hip reconstruction osteotomy for hip dislocation. Outcome after 4-7 years in 14 young patients. Acta Orthop Scand. 2002;73:432–8.
54. Manzotti A, Rovetta L, Pullen C, Catagni MA. Treatment of the late septic arthritis of the hip. Clin Orthop. 2003;410:203–12.
55. Samchukov ML, Birch JG. Pelvic support femoral reconstruction using the method of Ilizarov: a case report. Bull Hosp Joint Dis. 1992;52:7–11.
56. Rozbruch SR, Paley D, Bhave A, Herzenberg J. Ilizarov hip reconstruction for the late sequelae of infantile hip infection. J Bone Joint Surg Am. 2005;87:1007–18.
57. El-Mowafi H. Outcome of pelvic support osteotomy with the Ilizarov method in the treatment of the unstable hip joint. Acta Orthop Belg. 2005;71:686–91.
58. Mahran MA, Elgebeily MA, Ghaly NA, Thakeb MF, Hefny HM. Pelvic support osteotomy by Ilizarov's concept: is it a valuable option in managing neglected hip problems in adolescents and young adults? Strategies Trauma Limb Reconstr. 2011;6:13–20.
59. Inan M, Bomar JD, Kucukkaya M, Harma A. A comparison between the use of a monolateral external fixator and the Ilizarov technique for pelvic support osteotomies. Acta Orthop Traumatol Turc. 2004;38:252–60.
60. El-Rosasy MA, Ayoub MA. Ilizarov hip reconstruction for late sequelae of childhood septic arthritis. Egypt Orthop J. 2018;53:1–7.
61. Metikala S, Kurian BT, Madan SS, Fernandes JA. Pelvic support hip reconstruction with internal devices: an alternative to Ilizarov hip reconstruction. Strategies Trauma Limb Reconstr. 2020;15(1):34–40.

25 Post Infective Bone Gap Management of the Upper Extremity

Milind M. Chaudhary, Ashish S. Ranade, and James A. Fernandes

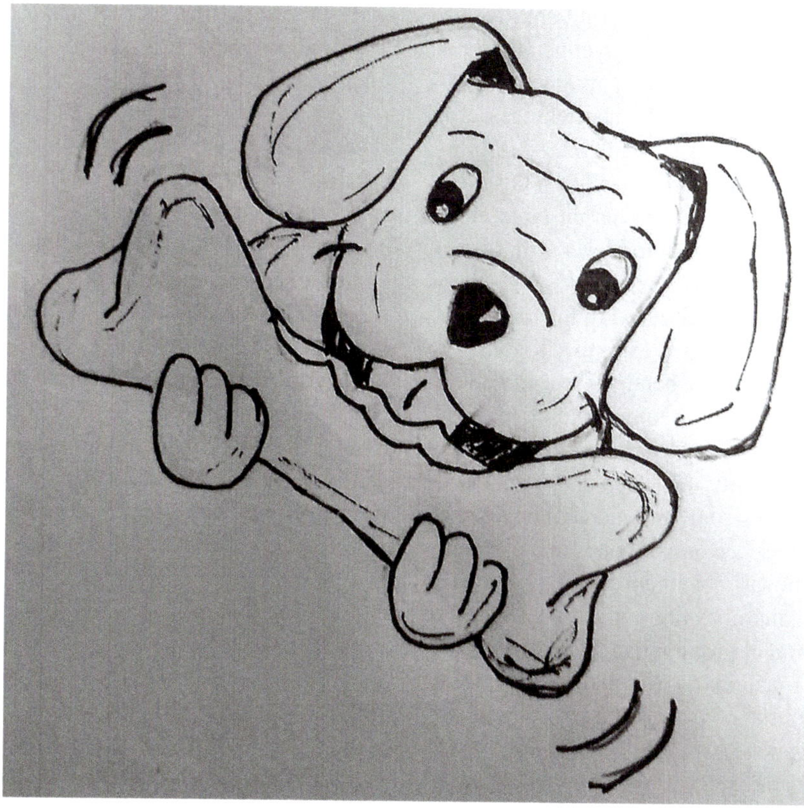

M. M. Chaudhary
International Deformity & Lengthening Institute, Akola, Maharashtra, India

A. S. Ranade (✉)
Blooming Buds Centre for Pediatric Orthopaedics, Deenanath Mangeshkar Hospital, Pune, Maharashtra, India
e-mail: ranadea2@gmail.com

J. A. Fernandes
Sheffield Children's Hospital NHS Foundation Trust, University of Sheffield, Sheffield, UK
e-mail: james.fernandes@nhs.net

© Springer Nature Switzerland AG 2022
M. V. Belthur et al. (eds.), *Pediatric Musculoskeletal Infections*,
https://doi.org/10.1007/978-3-030-95794-0_25

Introduction and Epidemiology

Bone and joint infections are common in children. Osteomyelitis does not commonly affect bones of the upper extremity [1]. The exact incidence of bone gap after upper extremity osteomyelitis remains unknown. In the Beit Cure classification, type B4 represents the bone gap following osteomyelitis [2]. In a study by Stevenson et al., Type B4 formed 20% of all childhood chronic osteomyelitis cases. Of those with B4 type osteomyelitis, only 10% had humeral involvement, and forearm bones formed a minority of cases [2]. Osteomyelitis and septic arthritis of the upper extremity may lead to loss of range of motion (ROM), shortening, deformity, persistent discharge, and joint instability. Humeral gap non-unions behave like a false joint close to the elbow and create an unstable elbow due to the loss of the structural lever arm. Loss of pronosupination of the forearm, loss of elbow ROM, and wrist deformity lead to functional loss as these affect the upper extremity's ability to reach and position the hand in space. Patients with bone gaps may need longer and more reconstructive procedures compared to other types of chronic osteomyelitis [2]. Gap management of the forearm poses some unique challenges considering the presence of two bones in the forearm and the rotational movement of the radius. The treatment entails not only gap management but also restoration of proximal and distal radioulnar joint (DRUJ) anatomy to restore forearm rotation. Sparse information about managing post-osteomyelitis bone gap of upper extremity exists because of its rarity.

In this chapter, we describe treatment principles of management of the bone gap in the upper extremity. Bone gap management lacks evidence-based recommendations, despite the many treatments described.

Pathology and Microbiology

Staphylococcus aureus is the commonest causative organism for hematogenous osteomyelitis. *Staphylococcus epidermidis* and *Pseudomonas* are other common pathogens [1]. Osteomyelitis of long bones commonly causes sequestra, pathological fractures, and bone gaps. A dead bone segment leads to chronic osteomyelitis with discharging sinuses. Surgical removal of the sequestrum, especially before formation of the involucrum, is the commonest cause of the bony gap. Deformed and short arms or forearms with discrepancy between the radius and ulna lead to functional limitations. A differential length difference between the radius and ulna leads to subluxation of the proximal and distal radioulnar joints in addition to shortening. Joint contractures, and shortening, lead to worsened function.

Clinical Presentation and Evaluation

Clinical examination forms an integral part of the treatment decision-making. The examination should also include assessing skin condition, and the position and range of motion of the shoulder, elbow, forearm, and wrist joint. Functional evaluation of the hand, including grip strength, should also be done. In the arm, a humeral bone defect may present as a shortened extremity. It may be associated with loss of ROM at the shoulder and the elbow. There might be a discharging sinus or sinuses. The bone defect in the forearm can present as an acquired radial or ulnar clubhand or as a shortening of the extremity [3, 4]. The examination should include distal radioulnar joint (DRUJ) examination as the ulnar head may be unstable or dislocated when the radial defect is large, and the DRUJ anatomy is disturbed. Compare lengths of both forearms placed together, with elbows resting on a table to assess the degree of shortening. Perform a detailed neurological examination besides assessing vascularity. Active infection is obvious even to cursory examination. Do not forget to evaluate the child's nutritional status as it affects the result.

Investigations and work up: Plain radiographs of the upper extremity bone segment including the joint above and below should be obtained. Radiographs should be assessed to determine the size of the defect; however, this may change depending on intraoperative findings of the bone viability. Examine physis on radiographs for irregular shape, and partial absence or presence of a physeal bar. Magnetic resonance imaging (MRI) with contrast helps identify the extent of the infection, and involvement of the physis and the soft tissues. Computed tomography (CT) angiography will reveal presence, location, and diameter of donor and recipient blood vessels for a vascularized bone graft. Laboratory investigations include complete blood count, C-reactive protein (CRP), and erythrocyte sedimentation rate (ESR). Obtain deep tissue samples from two locations during the surgery for culture to find the most useful antibiotics (Fig. 25.1).

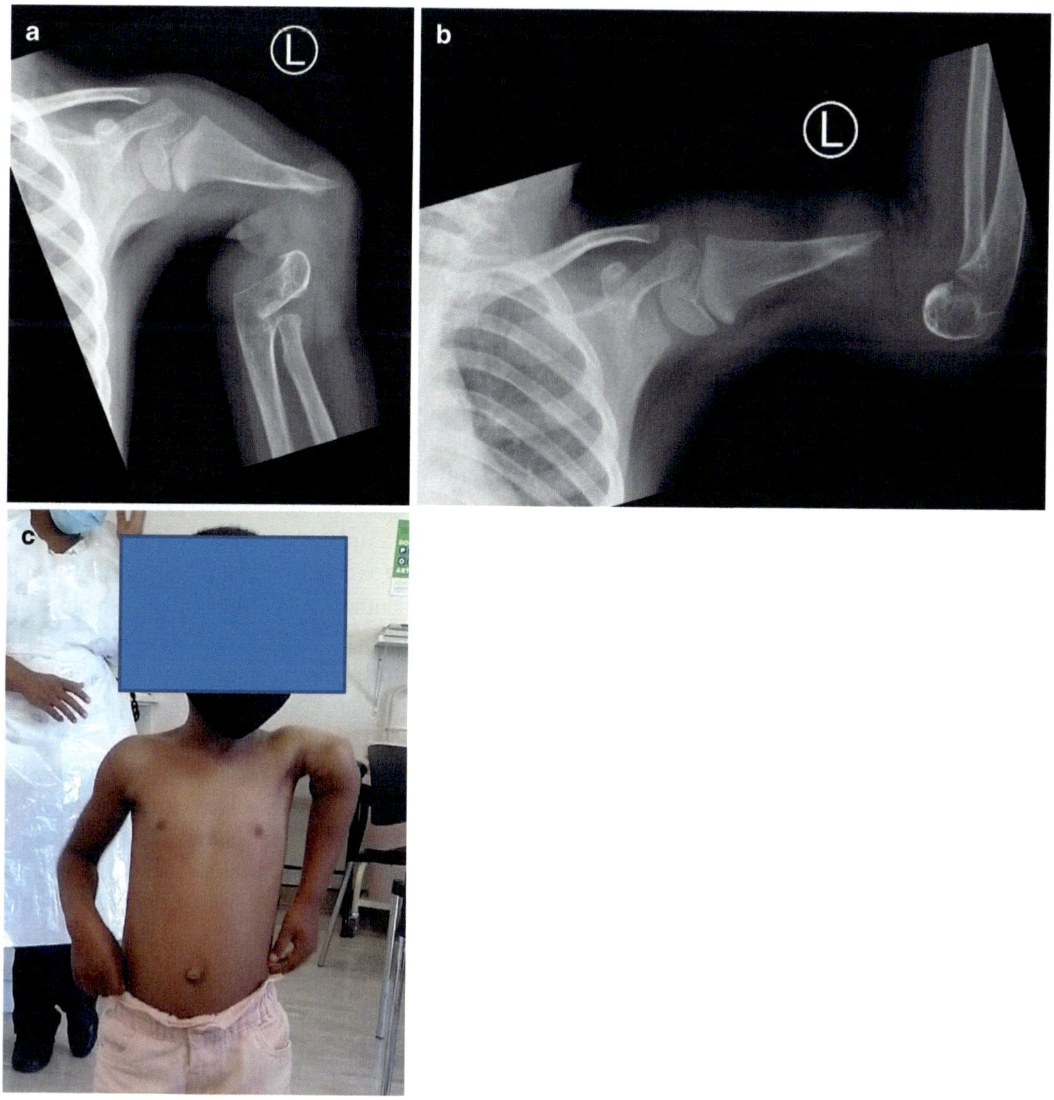

Fig. 25.1 (**a–c**) A left humerus gap in a 4-year-old girl as a sequela of methicillin-resistant *Staphylococcus aureus* (MRSA) osteomyelitis involving the left humerus at the age of 4 months. The bone defect has led to shortening, deformity, and instability of the arm; restricted motion at the elbow; and loss of function of the left upper extremity. (Images **a–c**, Case courtesy: Dr. Anria Horn, FCS Ortho [SA], MMed Orth [UCT], MBChB [Pret], Cape Town, South Africa)

Treatment Options

Restoration of bony anatomy, alignment, and length following chronic osteomyelitis of the upper extremity with defects is challenging. The treatment has a high rate of complications, including a significant risk of non-union. The treatment principles consist of three stages: (1) control infection by radical debridement and management of resulting dead space and by local antibiotic therapy, (2) reconstruct the bone defect and restore anatomy, alignment, and length, and (3) rehabilitate to restore function and use of upper extremity. Remove pus, granulation tissue, and all dead bone to eliminate infection. Stabilize bone with either casting, or internal or external fixation to prevent recurrence. Repeat these steps to get healthy and viable bone edges and a healthy and supple soft tissue cover. Choose antibiotics by culture sensitivity reports to eliminate infection. Reassess gap length and soft tissue status to formulate a definitive and comprehensive treatment plan. A bone defect of up to 6 cm can be treated with an autologous bone graft. Non-vascularized bone grafts can fill up smaller gaps, but those greater than 6 cm need vascularized grafts for union. This is the conventional thinking. However, this has been recently challenged. There is no clear evidence to justify the need for a vascularized bone graft for gaps of more than 6 cm [5]. Allsopp has proved otherwise [5]. The options could be reconstructive or salvage options [6, 7]. Treatment can aim for either reconstruction or salvage: [6,7]

1. Use of non-vascularized fibula and other autografts.
2. Use of vascularized fibula graft.
3. Bone transport with distraction osteogenesis using external fixator or internal lengthening devices.
4. Induced membrane technique.
5. Use of tissue-engineered bone graft substitutes and other new modalities.
6. Creation of single-bone forearm.
7. Bone shortening.
8. Amputation.

Use of Non-vascularized Bone Grafts

Cortico-cancellous iliac crest grafts do not provide structural support in filling bone gaps, but are in common use. Cancellous iliac crest grafts work well for smaller defects, and tricortical strut grafts may provide structural stability and osteogenic potential [8–10]. These are, however, unsuitable for larger defects and inadequate for reconstructing tubular defects [1]. Dugdale et al. successfully used tibial cortico-cancellous grafts for small mid-radial defects smaller than 3.5 cm [11].

Non-vascularized fibular graft (NVFG) provides an excellent alternative to bridge the gap in a tubular bone (Figs. 25.2 and 25.3), such as in the forearm and humerus in children [12–16]. Resect a segment of the fibula subperiosteally, insert in the gap, and stabilize either with intramedullary (IM) Kirschner (K)-wires or plates at proximal and distal junctions with host bone, or with an external fixator. A minimally invasive technique has been described using two or three small incisions for harvesting the fibula [17]. Swamy et al. used NVFG to fill large gaps averaging 8 cm in nine humeri, two in radius, and one in the ulna. Authors used cancellous bone grafting at the proximal and distal ends of the fibular graft. The authors recommend using stable fixation by using a plate at the ends of NVFG [12]. In various reports, the mean time for the union for NVFG was an average of 9 weeks (range, 7–15 weeks) [12, 14, 15].

After harvesting a fibular graft, donor-site morbidity remains a problem. Ankle instability, valgus deformity of the ankle due to proximal migration of the distal fibula, stress fracture of the fibular graft, and non-union are the possible complications [18]. One solution to the instability is to use a longitudinally lateral half of the fibula, leaving the medial end intact and in continuity. Ankle instability can be prevented by using one or two screws to fix the distal tibiofibular syndesmosis or create tibiofibular synostosis. The stress fracture occurs due to the graft not getting incorporated in the recipient bone. The risk is maximal in the initial few months [19]. Drill

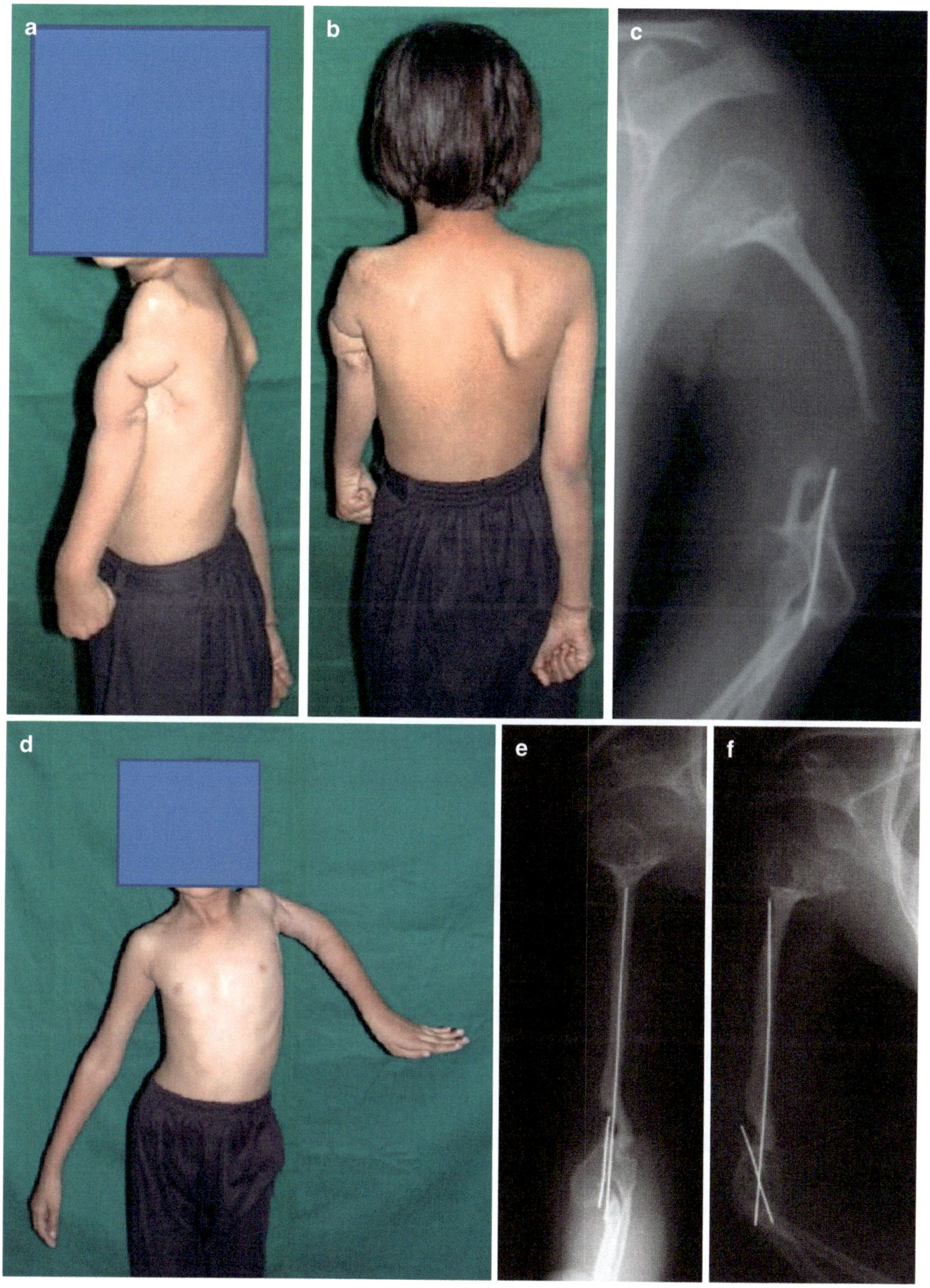

Fig. 25.2 (**a–c**) A 5-year-old child having a post-osteomyelitis sequela with a large gap in the mid-lower shaft of the humerus with a spontaneous fusion of the elbow joint. This has resulted from the infection as well as the debridement, which may damage the periosteum when done well before the formation of an involucrum, leading to a large bone gap. The proximal ends of the humerus are pencil thin, precluding a solution like bone transport. (**d–f**) Images showing treatment with a non-vascularized fibula with an intramedullary K-wire for stabilization along with shoulder spica immobilization

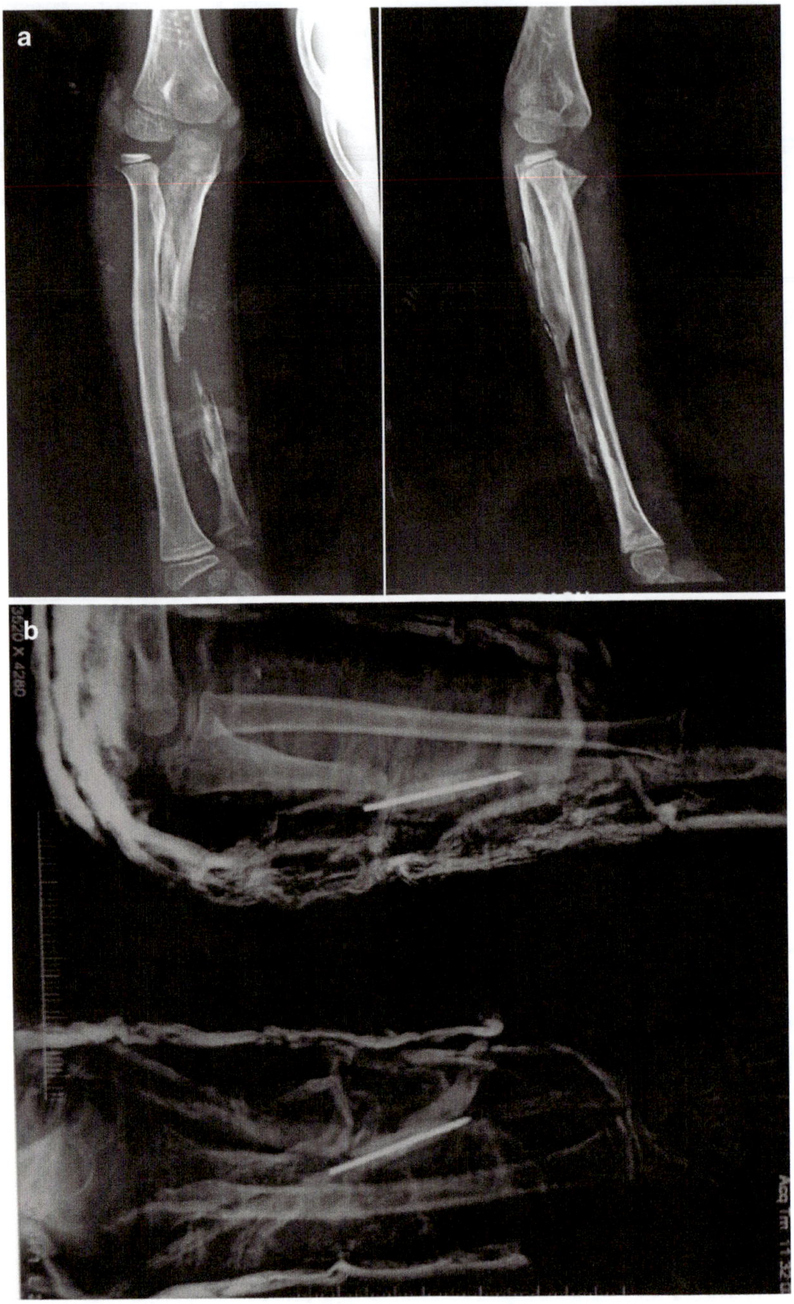

Fig. 25.3 (**a**) Anteroposterior (AP) and lateral radiographs of a 9-year-old boy with MRSA chronic osteomyelitis of the ulna with a bone defect and sequestrum. (**b**) Radiographs after debridement and the placement of vancomycin impregnated cement spacer. (**c**) Radiographs showing bridging the ulnar gap with the placement of an NVFG and an intramedullary K-wire. (**d**) The fibular donor site at 2-month follow-up. (**e**) Radiograph at 1-year follow-up. The K-wire has been removed. (**f–i**) The ranges of motion at the wrist and the elbow. There were no signs of infection at 2-year follow-up

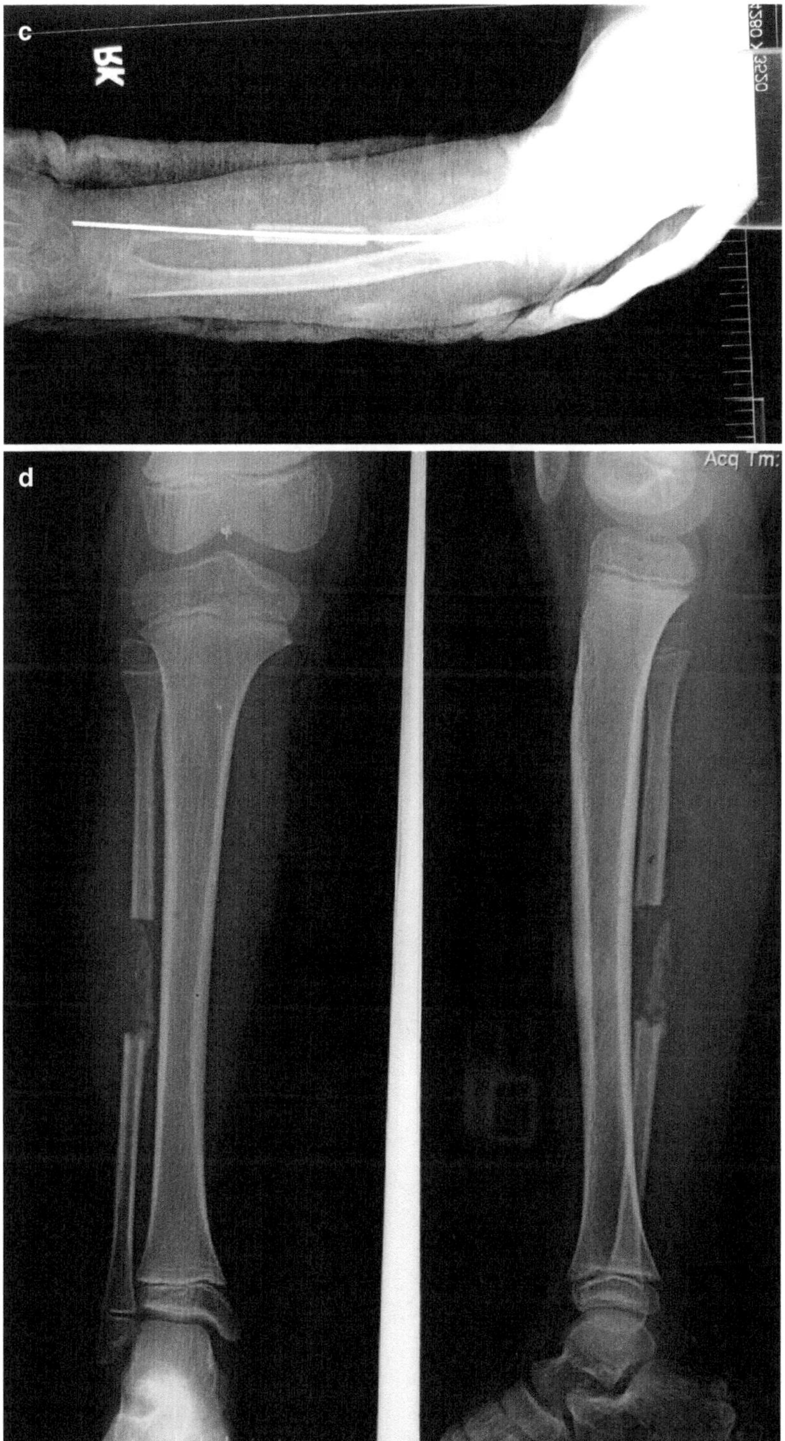

Fig. 25.3 (continued)

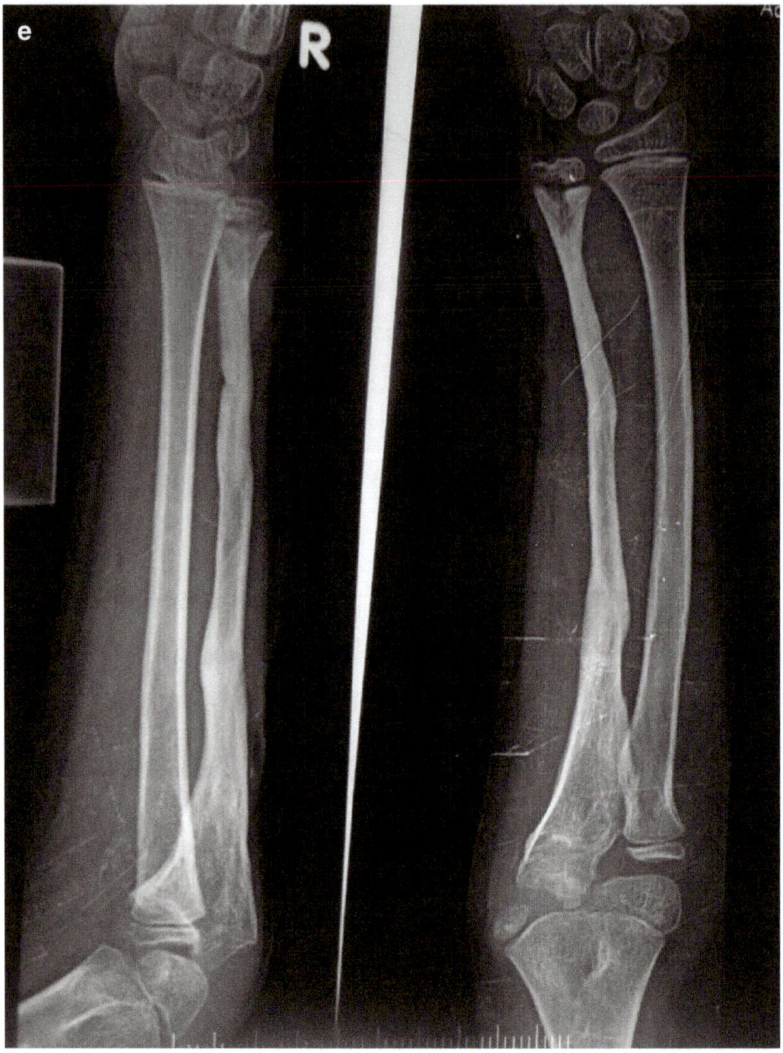

Fig. 25.3 (continued)

multiple holes in the fibular graft with saline cooling using 1 mm wires, for rapid healing and preventing stress fractures. Al-Zahrani et al. grafted the ends of NVFG strut with cancellous grafts to prevent non-union at its ends [19]. Recently, Agarwal and co-authors have described a fibular onlay graft technique on top of the fibular strut. They drove the ends of the fibular graft inside proximal and distal metaphyseal ends after filling an average gap of 5.8 cm. An intramedullary K-wire was used to stabilize the graft. The strut and junctional areas were covered with fibular matchstick grafts [14].

Long-term clinical and functional results using NVFG for bone gap treatment are unknown. Also, donor-site fibular regeneration and its consequences on the ankle are not known in the long run (Box 25.1).

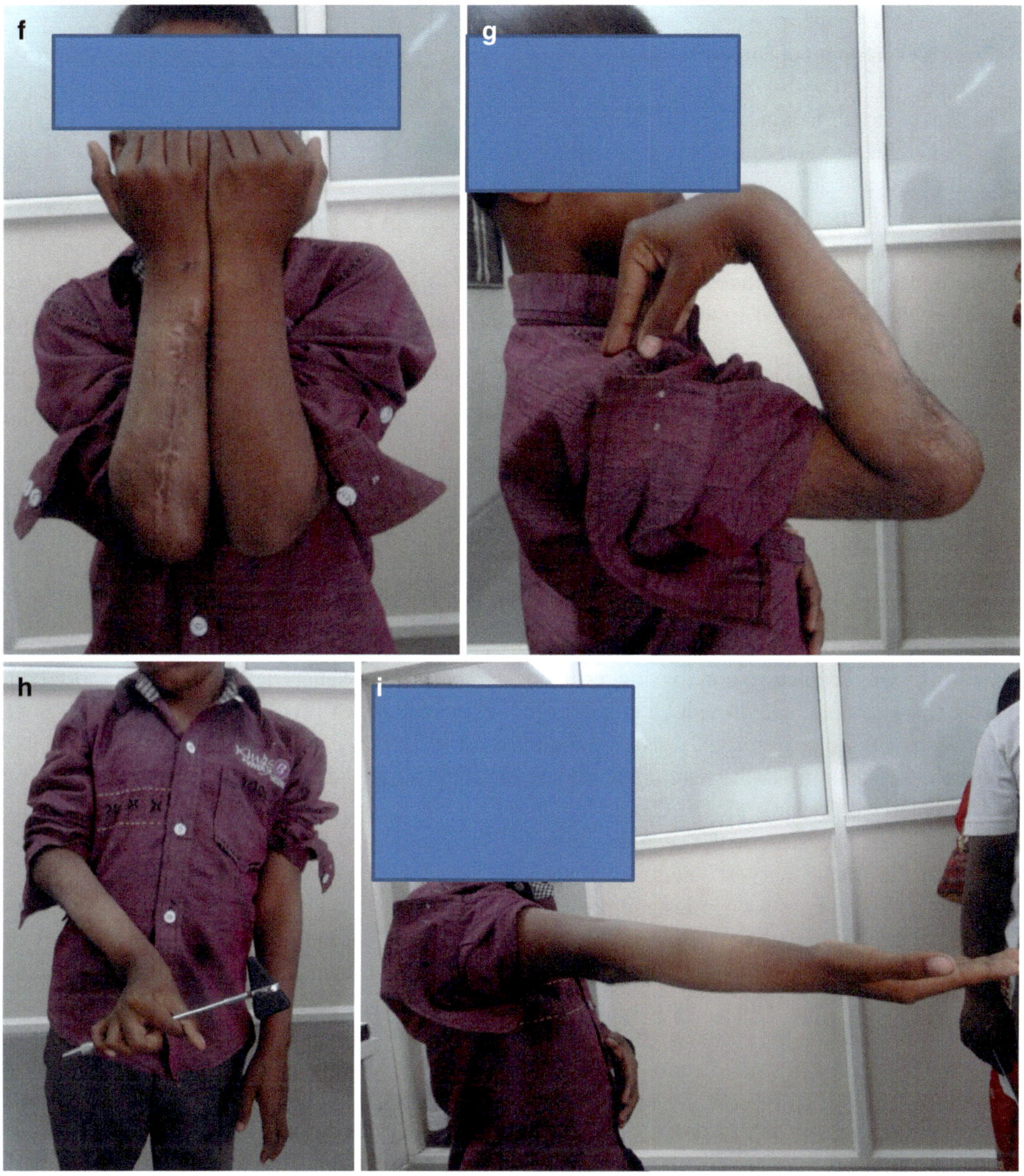

Fig. 25.3 (continued)

Box 25.1 Treatment of Forearm Bone Defects

- An external fixator may be used for simultaneous correction of joint contracture and to restore the length and normal relationship of the distal radioulnar joint.
- Fibular graft and induced membrane technique offer good options for treating the bone gap.
- Staged treatment may be necessary to bring back dislocated radial head.

Use of Vascularized Fibular Bone Graft (VFG)

The vascularized fibula is the commonest choice for filling bony defects 6 cm or longer. The tubular shape of the fibula provides a good fit for long bones of the extremity. It also provides biomechanical stability to the long tubular bone. The vascularized fibular graft (VFG) can hypertrophy to reach the size of the recipient bone. Approach the fibular harvest laterally between peroneus brevis and gastrocnemius and preserve its periosteum by marbelizing, that is, retaining some muscle fibers on the bone and periosteum. Osteotomize the fibula with a Gigli saw distally and locate and section the peroneal artery and tie it to the distal fibular end. Section the fibula proximally and rotate it internally to reach and harvest the peroneal artery near the trifurcation [20, 21]. Principles of treatment [22] are as follows:

- Debridement with the removal of non-vascularized and infected bone.
- Transverse osteotomy at the bone ends—use of plate and screws for stabilization.
- The cut end can be placed inside the medullary cavity if there is a mismatch in the diameter.
- Microvascular anastomosis to the deep humeral artery in the humerus and the radial artery or the anterior interosseous artery in the forearm.

In the forearm, the typical time for consolidation was 2–8 months, an average of 6 months [22, 23]. The advantages and disadvantages of the VFG are summarized in Table 25.1 (Fig. 25.4).

Use of an External Fixator

The external fixator can be used in various roles in treating the post-osteomyelitic upper extremity bone gap. The indications are as follows:

1. To distract soft tissues and to correct joint contractures [25].
2. To stabilize bone ends when the gap has been bridged by a bone graft or a cement spacer [15].
3. For bone lengthening through osteotomy [26, 27].
4. To do deformity correction and lengthening—radial clubhand, deformity, and shortening secondary to physeal growth arrest or bone loss [28, 29].
5. To reduce dislocated radioulnar joints by ulnar lengthening to bring down a proximally dislocated radial head and to bring ulnar head to station at distal radioulnar joint [30].

We can use either intramedullary devices or unilateral, circular, or hexapod external fixators for the task. [29, 31, 32]

The role of external fixators in treating post-osteomyelitic bone gaps in children has received scant attention in the literature. There is neither

Table 25.1 Advantages and disadvantages of using a vascularized fibular graft

Advantages	Disadvantages [24]
1. One-stage procedure 2. Probably quicker healing in longer bone defects 3. Resistance to infection 4. May provide skin cover	1. Needs technical expertise 2. Donor-site morbidity 3. Fracture of the graft—more common in the lower extremity 4. Failed anastomosis, and thrombosis of the feeding vessel 5. Infection 6. Wound-healing problems 7. Ankle instability, chronic pain, and sensory deficit

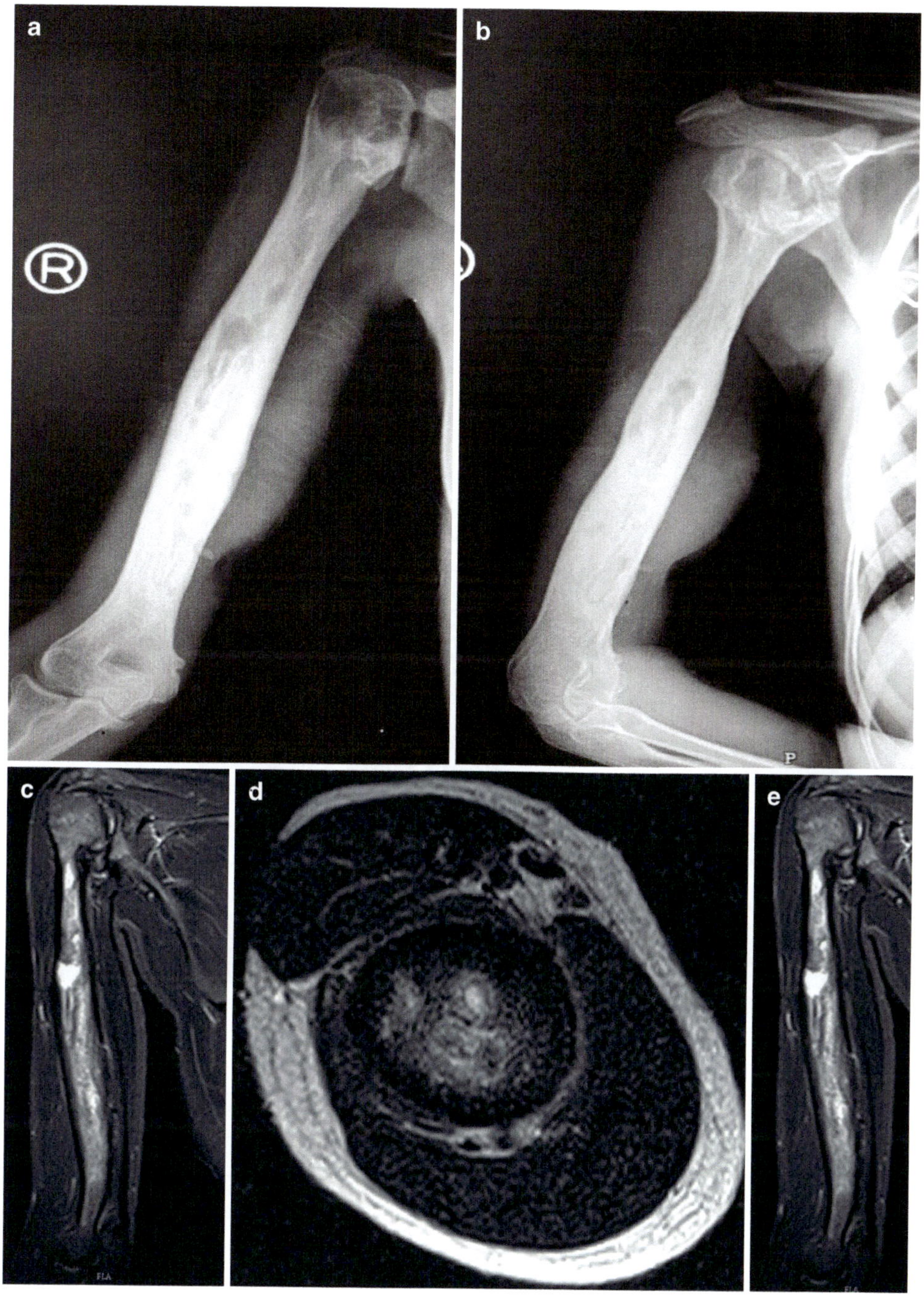

Fig. 25.4 (**a**, **b**) Radiographs showing chronic osteomyelitis of the right humerus in a 16-year-old. The patient had multiple surgeries in the past for the osteomyelitis and had a sinus on the medial side of the arm. (**c–e**) MRI showing segmental involvement of the humerus. Cor Stir, Cor T1 post-contrast, and axial T2 images through the humeral shaft show an intramedullary peripherally enhancing fluid collection with cortical thickening and periosteal reaction consistent with an intramedullary abscess. (**f**, **g**) Radiographs after segmental resection, placement of vancomycin loaded cement spacer, and external fixator placement. (**h**, **i**) Radiographs showing vascularized fibular graft placement after resection of the infected bone segment. (**j**, **k**) At 1-year follow-up, patient had developed re-infection. (**l**, **m**) Radiographs after implant removal and debridement. The VFG was viable and stable and hence was retained. (**n**, **o**) Radiographs at 2-year follow-up after the implant removal. The patient remains free of infection

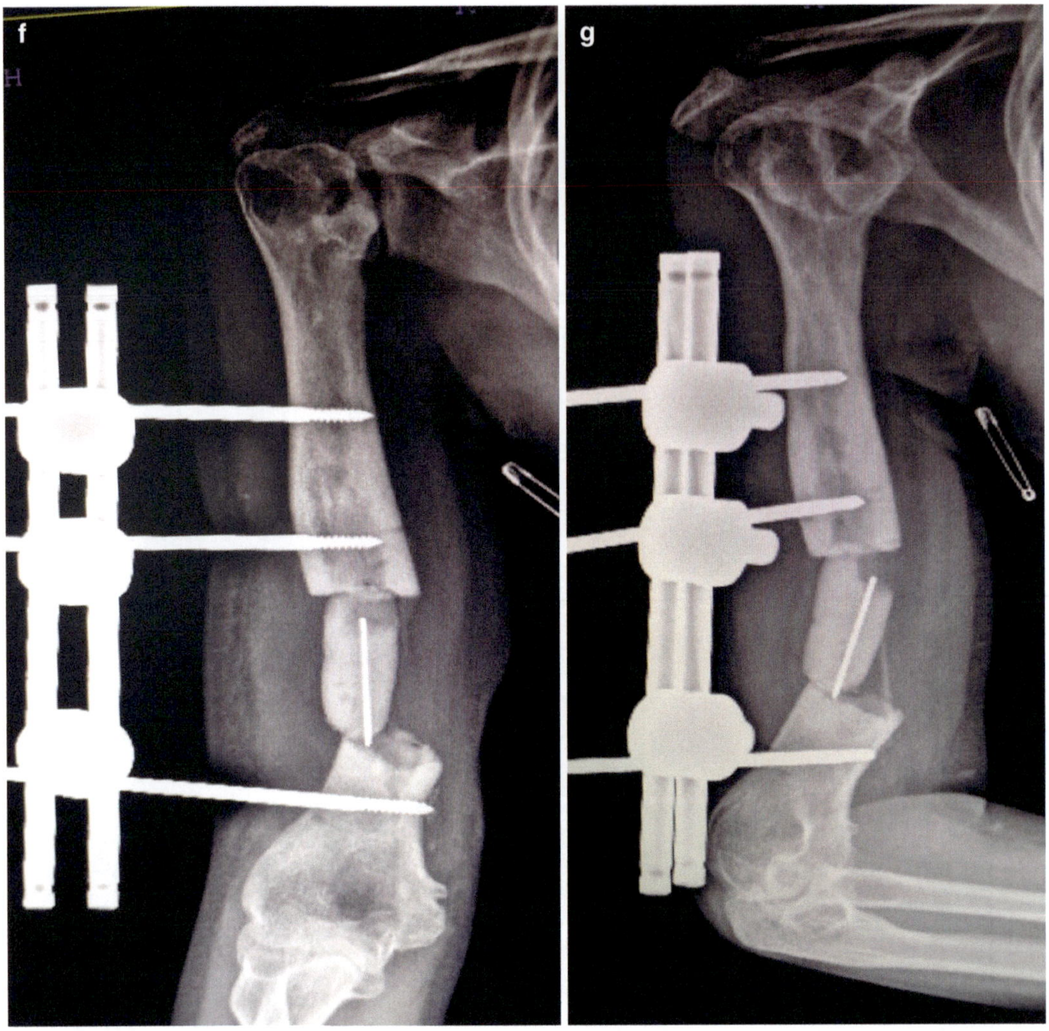

Fig. 25.4 (continued)

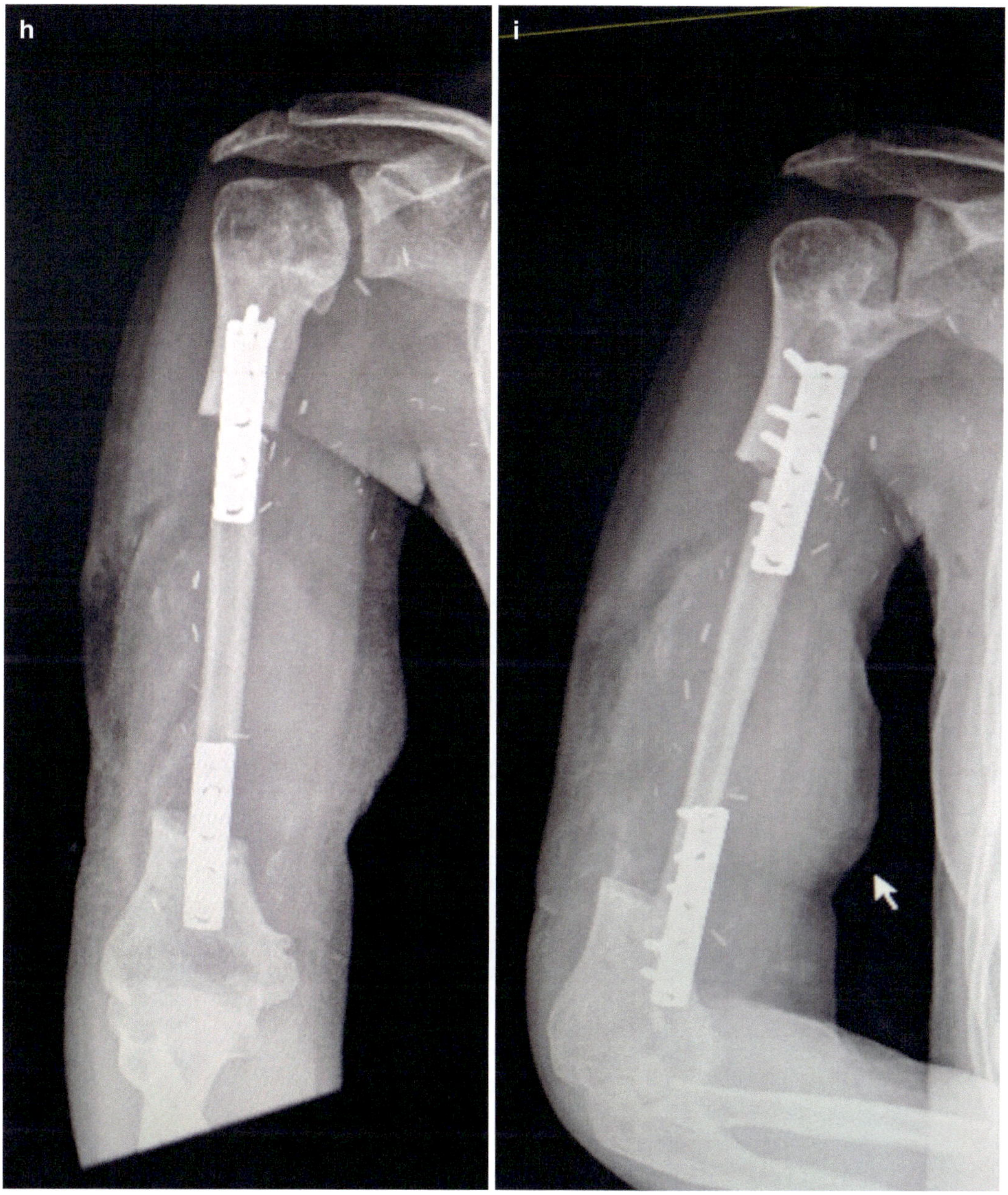

Fig. 25.4 (continued)

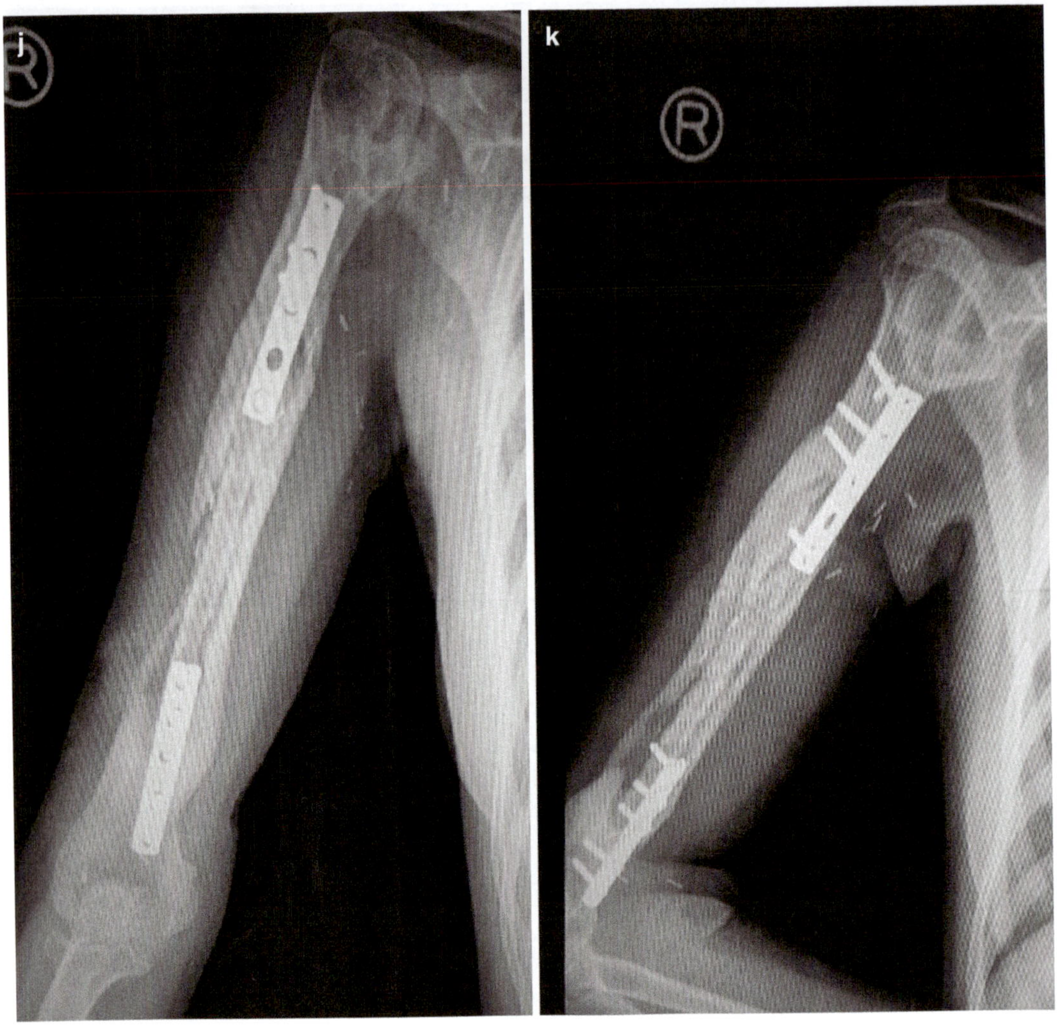

Fig. 25.4 (continued)

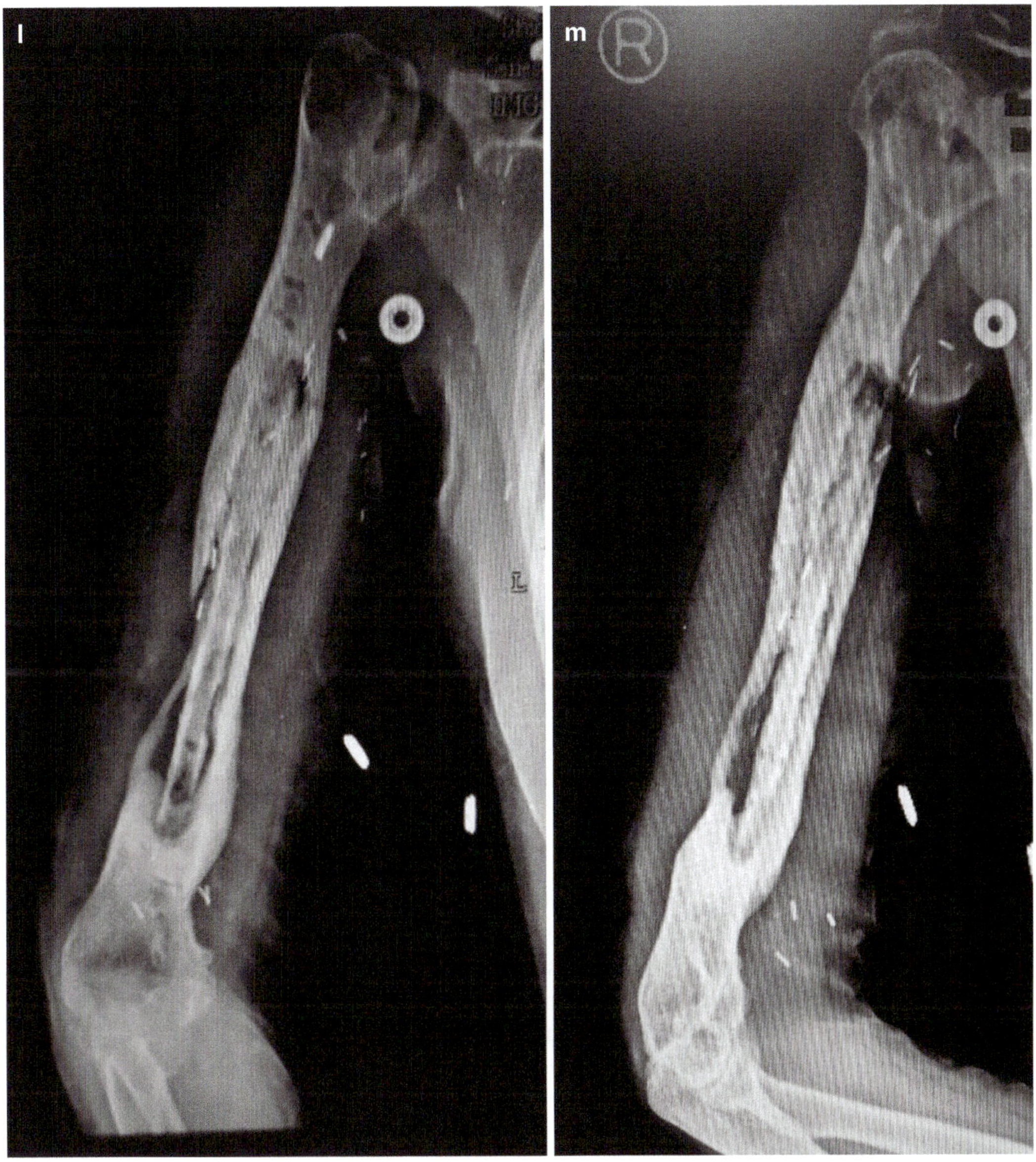

Fig. 25.4 (continued)

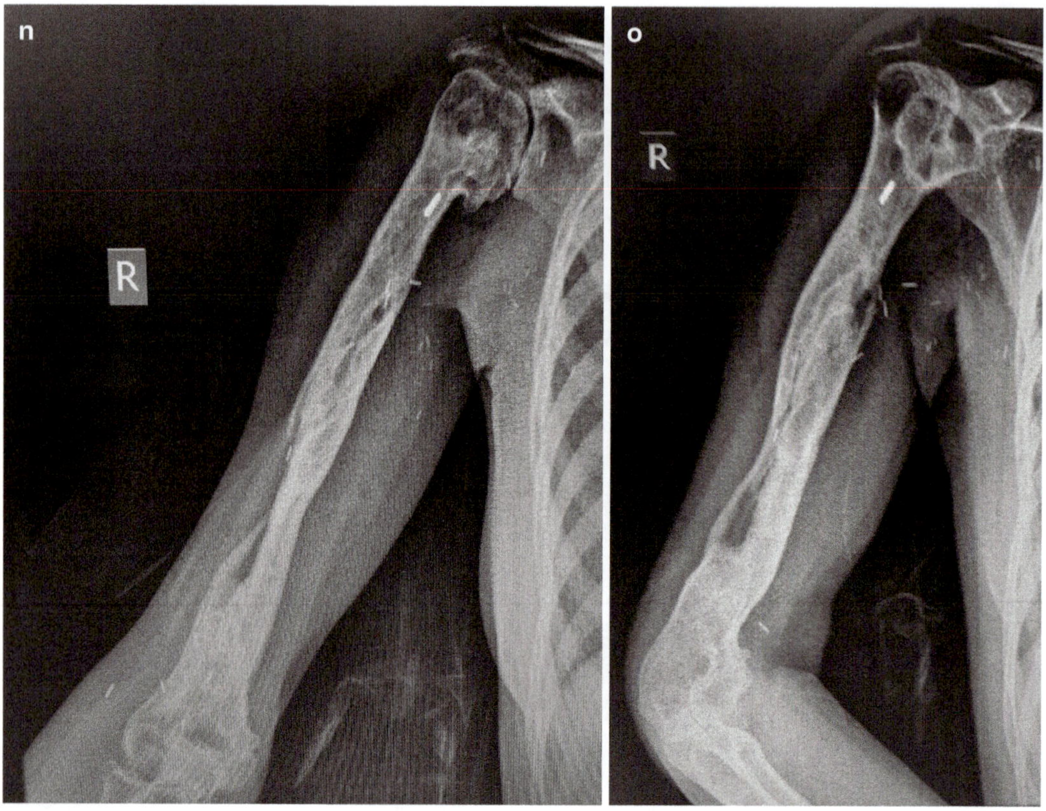

Fig. 25.4 (continued)

consensus on indications for surgery and which devices to use, nor are long-term outcomes reported. Recommended distraction rate is less than 1 mm/day for the radius and ulna, and 1 mm/day for the humerus. Upper extremity lengthenings have a high complication rate. They include pin-track infections, nerve injuries, non-unions, joint dislocation, regenerate fractures, and failures of fixation [33].

A unilateral external fixator is preferred while lengthening a single bone in the forearm or the humerus. Complex deformities or shortening with joint contractures are treated with circular frames or hexapod type six-axis correction devices. Liu used a unilateral external fixator for treating a post-osteomyelitic defect of the ulna, which they filled with distraction and brought down a dislocated radial head [30]. The average defect size was 5.4 cm, and the healing time was 31 weeks (46.5 days/cm) [27]. Hosny has described humeral lengthening in 11 patients using a ring fixator. The average bone healing index was 29.5 days/cm. He recommended bracing after frame removal as there was a high risk of regenerate fracture [29]. Delayed union or poor regenerate remains a problem with forearm lengthening. The use of intramedullary nails can shorten external fixator time. In a prospective study by Jager et al., a combination of elastic stable intramedullary nailing (ESIN) with the circular external fixator was used for an average lengthening of 4.5 cm. The healing index was 30% better when the combined technique was used (22 days/cm for the combined technique, and 32 days/cm for the external fixator without ESIN group) [34].

A monolateral external fixator has been described to treat manus valgus deformity associated with significant radial bone loss secondary to infection. A unilateral external fixator placed from the ulna to the second metacarpal was used to distract the contracture and achieve DRUJ alignment. This is followed by osteotomy of the ulna and translation of the proximal end of the ulna toward the distal radial remnant to achieve bony fusion. This technique creates a single-bone forearm after correcting the manus valgus deformity [25] (Boxes 25.2 and 25.3).

Box 25.2 Technical Pearls for the External Fixation of the Humerus

- Half pins are preferred over wires, especially in the proximal and middle 1/third of the humerus.
- Protect the axillary nerve, 5–6 cm below the acromion (depending on the humerus' length).
- Use a sharp-pointed drill bit to prevent "walking" and nerve entrapment.
- Palpate radial nerve in the lateral groove and drill a K-wire at least 1 cm away and then predrill with cannulated drill bit over it.
- Wires may be useful for small or osteoporotic distal fragments; typically, three wires are used.
- The first olive wire (lateral to medial) is passed just distal to the olecranon fossa.
- The second olive wire ascends (lateral to medial) above the olecranon fossa and exits medially.
- A third olive wire is passed from medial epicondyle, goes over the olecranon fossa, and exists at the lateral supracondylar ridge; these three wires subtend a triangle in the coronal plane, skirting the olecranon fossa.
- A 5/8th ring is used distally with an open anterior part to allow for elbow flexion; the first wire is attached directly to the ring, and the second and third ones are attached using three- or four-hole posts above and below the ring.

Box 25.3 Technical Pearls for the External Fixation of the Forearm

- Half pins are preferred over the wires to reduce the risk of neurovascular injury.
- Typically, the hand is fixed with a wire across the second, third, fourth, and fifth metacarpal bases; alternately, a thin tapering half pin can be passed radial to ulnar in the bottom of second or third metacarpals.
- Rings are preferred as they allow the insertion of half pins at various angles, and attached hinges allow angular, translatory, or rotational maneuvers.
- Proximally segment fixation is usually done with a 5/eighth ring with its anterior portion open to allow elbow flexion.
- Radius and ulna can be fixed separately.
- The use of different rings' sizes allows for separate connections and actions for the radius and ulna.

Humeral shortening due to osteomyelitis can be severe and is an obvious deformity. In a small minority of cases, there is a defect in the humerus. This can be treated with an NVFG and stabilized with either IM K-wires and a shoulder spica in a small child or an adjuvant external fixator. Recent developments allow simultaneous correction of deformities of the humerus with lengthening using the hexapod software-controlled external fixator. After correcting angular and rotational deformities, Kadhim and Herzenberg changed the hexapod to an Orthofix Limb Reconstruction System (LRS) fixator for easier rehabilitation. [35] Motorized IM lengthening nails ease humeral lengthening if resources and bony length and diameter allow (Figs. 25.5 and 25.6). [36]

Induced Membrane Technique and Newer Modalities

The Masquelet induced membrane technique is a relatively newer addition to the existing options to treat the bone defect following infection. It is a

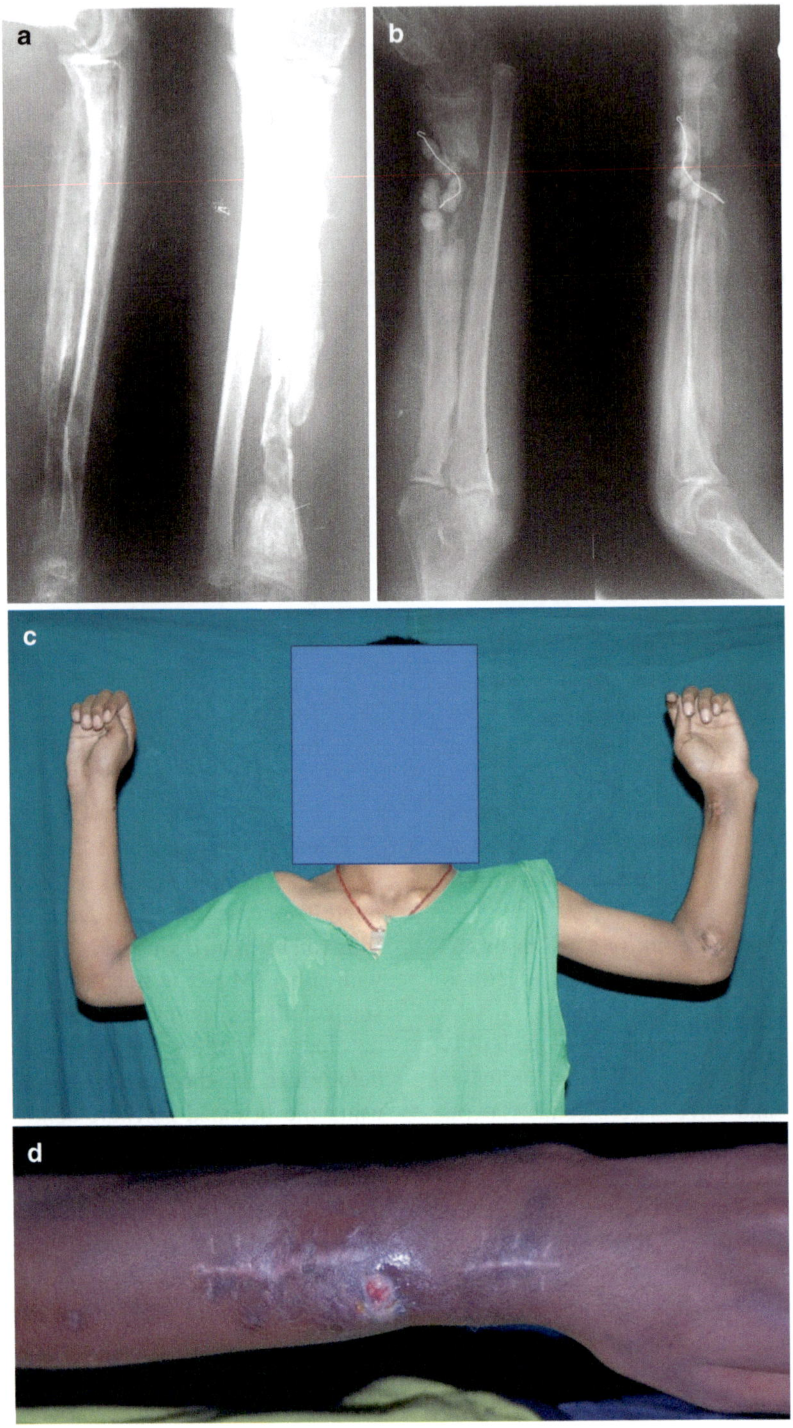

Fig. 25.5 (**a–d**) A 14-year-old comes with an actively draining infection in the lower third radius. Debridement is done and antibiotic loaded bone cement beads inserted, and antibiotics given to eradicate the infection. (**e, f**) In the next stage, the ring fixator pulls the distal radius out to length and fresh antibiotic beads help to address the dead space and completely eradicate the infection. (**g**) In the next stage, a vascularized fibular graft is performed with an intramedullary K-wire giving fixation in both the proximal and distal bone ends. The fixator is retained to provide stability. (**h–j**) The infection is completely eradicated, and the gap is filled. DRUJ is congruous and wrist movements are full

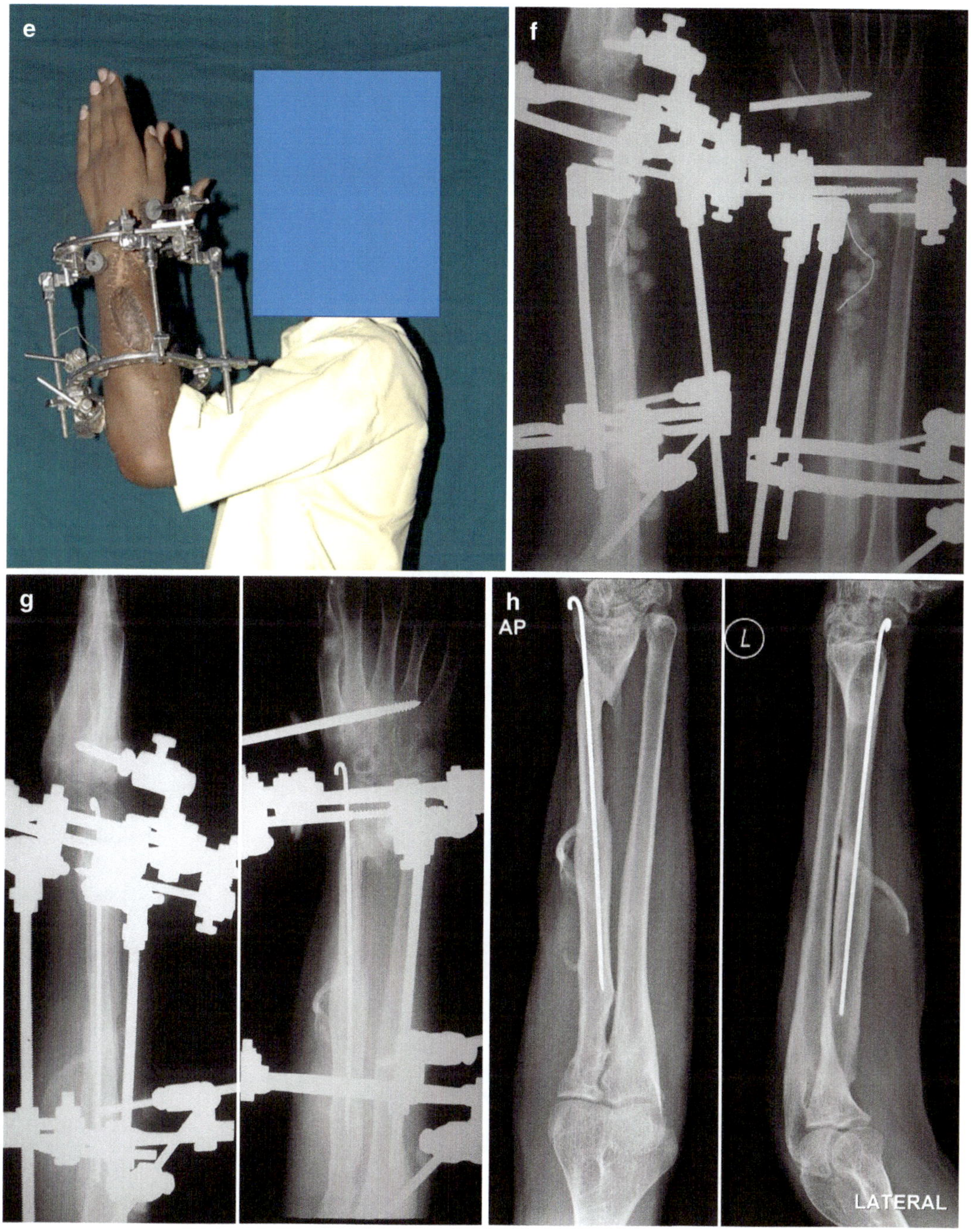

Fig. 25.5 (continued)

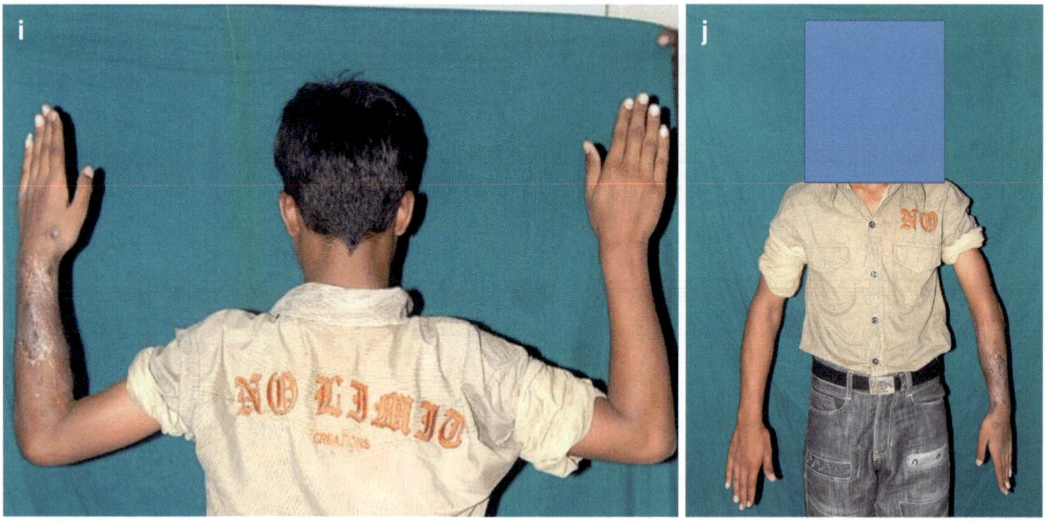

Fig. 25.5 (continued)

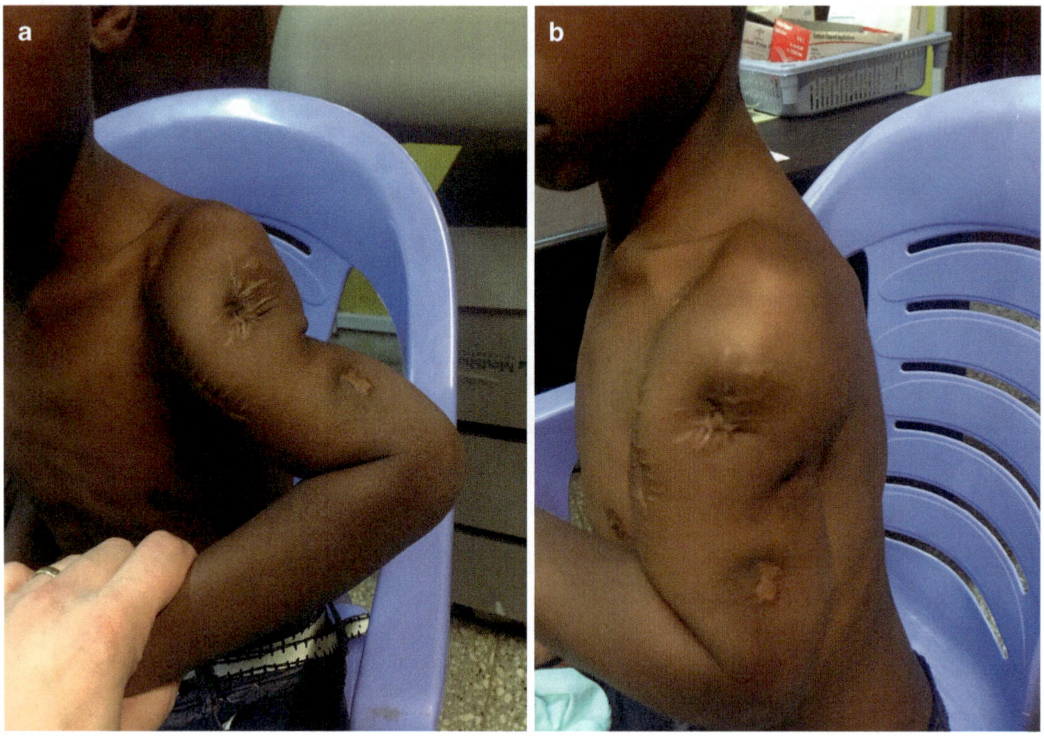

Fig. 25.6 (**a**, **b**) Left humerus bone defect secondary to chronic osteomyelitis with multiple surgeries in the past. (**c**, **d**) Images showing active and passive range of motion of the shoulder. (**e**) Radiograph with a bone defect in the left humerus. Implants from previous attempts of NVFG are seen. (**f**) Radiograph showing bony defect after removal of the implant and debridement. (**g**, **h**) Clinical photographs after placement of ring fixator to achieve compression and stabilization after NVFG with an intramedullary K-wire. (**i**, **j**) Radiograph after the surgery and the active range of motion of the left shoulder. (**k**) Radiographs after external fixator removal. (**l–n**) Clinical photographs showing good range of motion of the left shoulder and the elbow. (Images **a–n**: Case courtesy: Dr. Tim R. Nunn, FRCS [Tr & Orth], CURE Ethiopia Children's Hospital, Addis Ababa, Ethiopia)

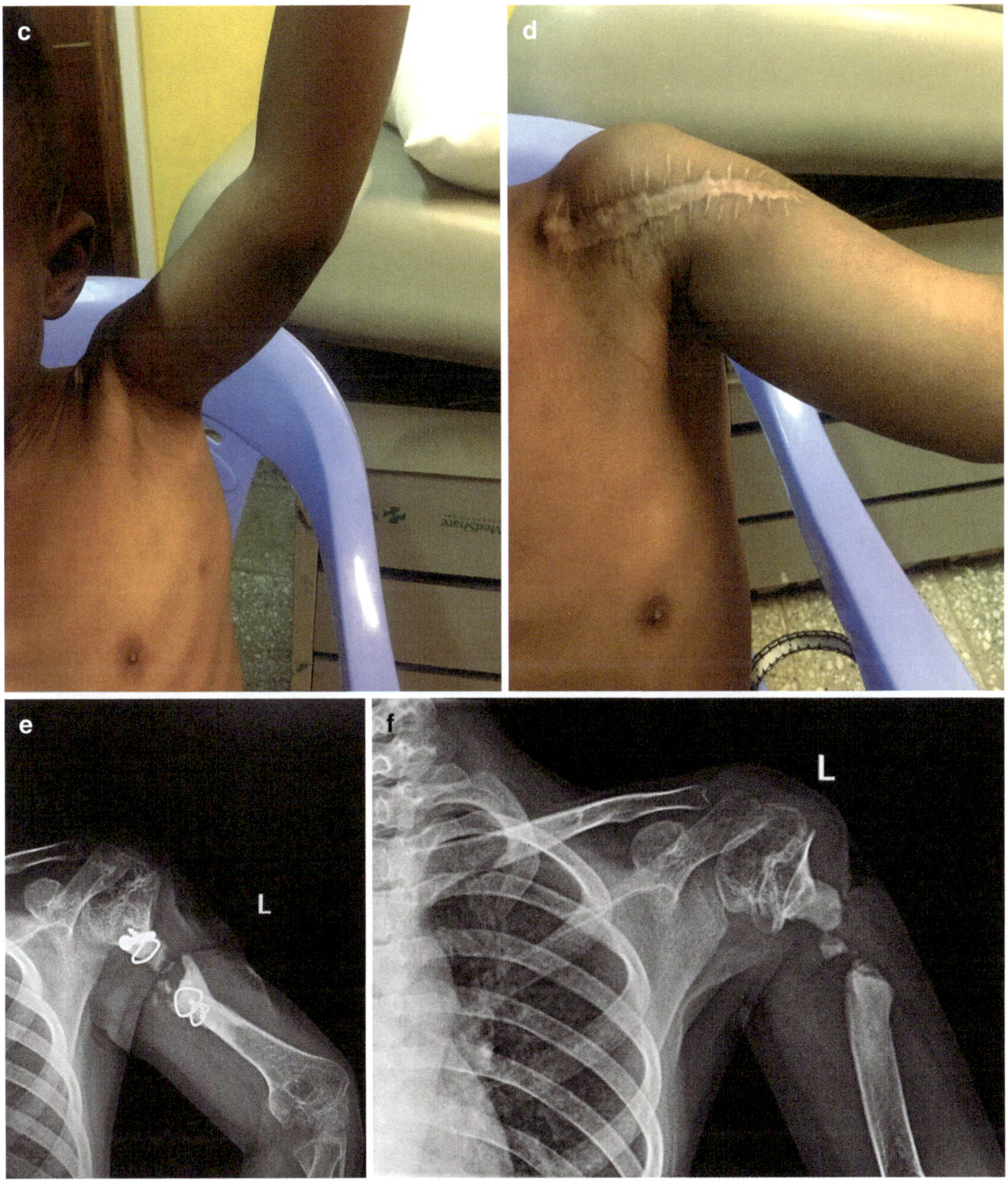

Fig. 25.6 (continued)

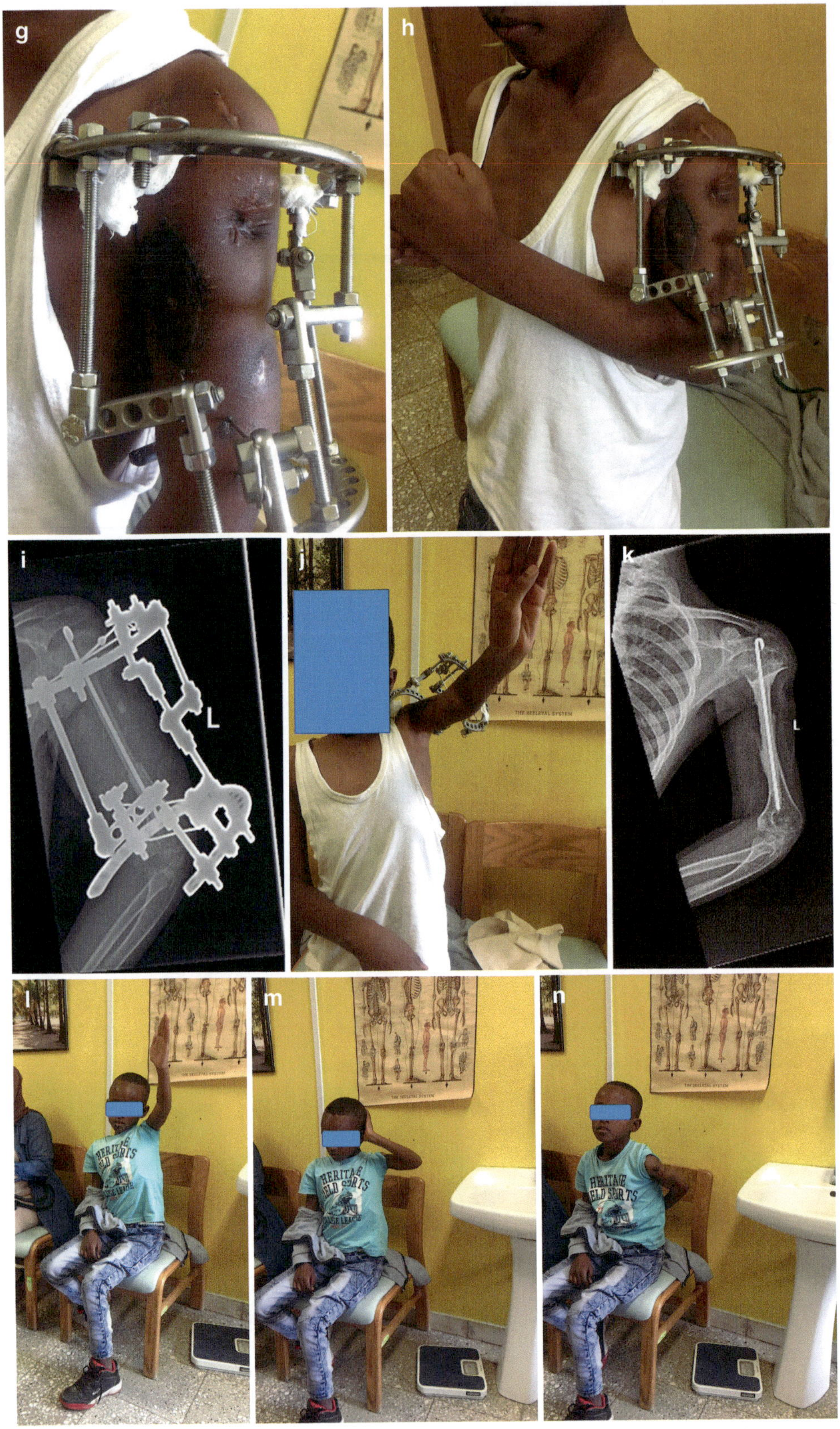

Fig. 25.6 (continued)

good alternative for larger defects. Induced membrane technique involves radical debridement of the infected bone and placement of polymethylmethacrylate (PMMA) cement spacer in the defect. The bone is stabilized with external or internal fixation. After 6–8 weeks, the PMMA spacer is removed with careful preservation of the biologic membrane. The defect is filled with an autologous bone graft, and the bone defect is stabilized. The autologous graft may be combined with graft extenders such as allograft or tricalcium sulfate [37, 38]. In a systematic review of the induced membrane technique in children, the mean rate of the bone union after the two stages of the induced membrane technique was 58%, but this rate increased to 87% after revision surgeries. The complications were non-union in 27%, lysis of the graft in 9%, and fractures of the bone graft in 9% of patients [39]. The Masquelet technique is discussed elaborately in Chap. 27) (Fig. 25.7).

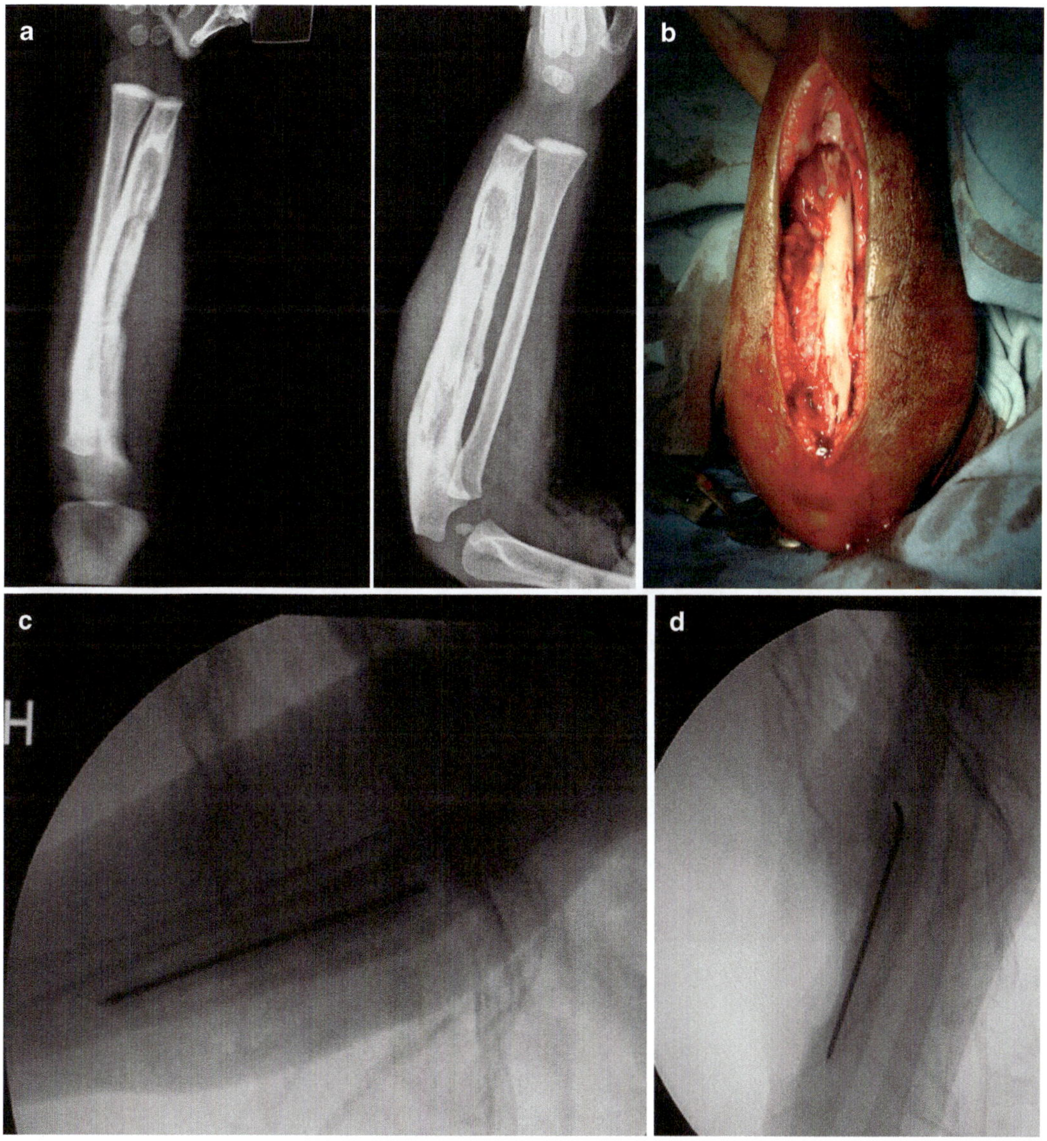

Fig. 25.7 (**a**) A 2-year-6-month old with chronic MRSA osteomyelitis involving the ulna. (**b**) Intraoperative photograph showing sequestrum. (**c, d**) Radiographs showing placement of vancomycin-loaded bone cement K-wire spacer. (**e**) After 6 weeks, the cement spacer was removed. There was no infection and healthy tissue was noted. At this point the incision was closed and the extremity was put in a plaster cast. (**f**) Radiographs at 3-month follow-up. (**g, h**) One-year follow-up showing restoration of the osteomyelitic defect. There was no infection

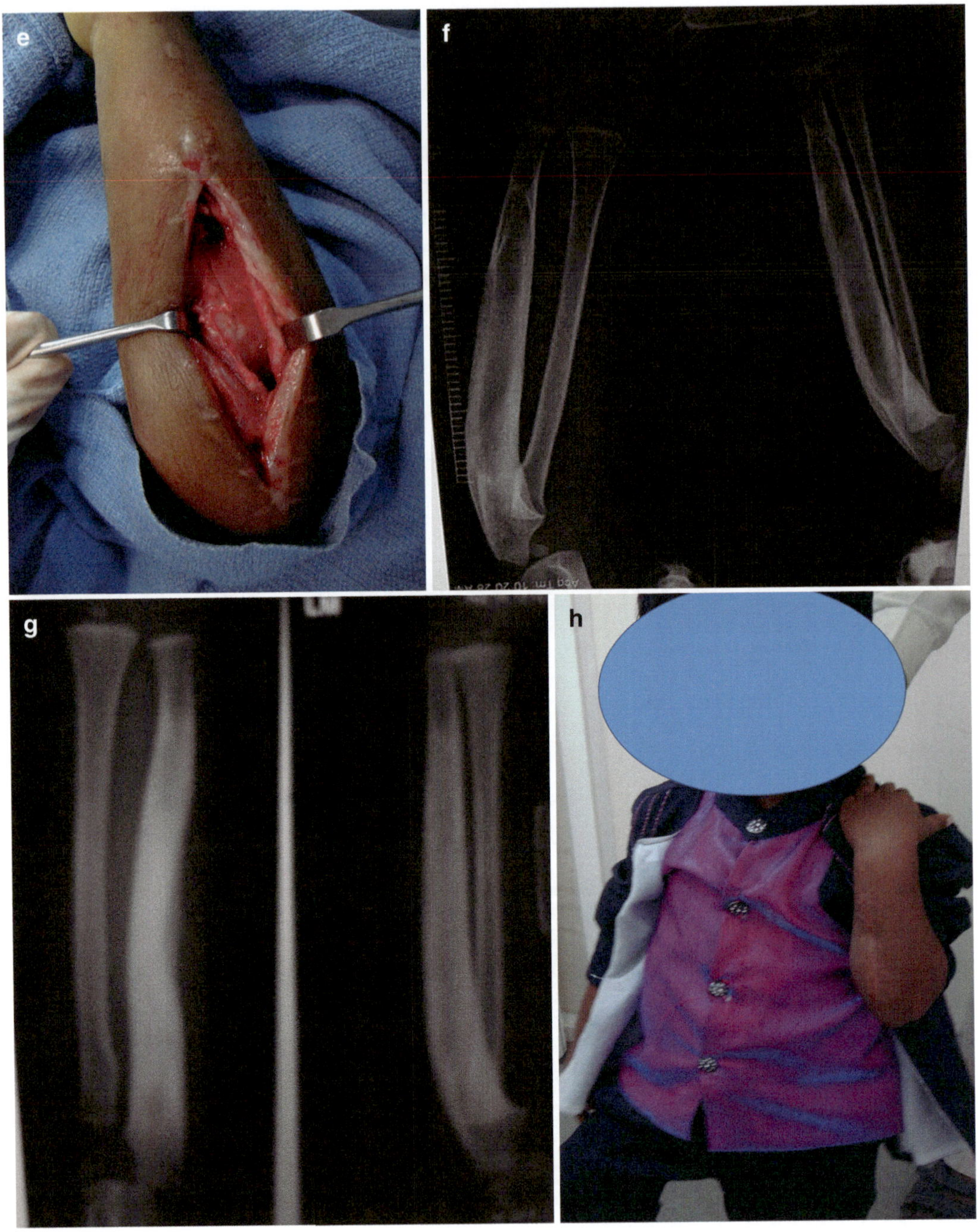

Fig. 25.7 (continued)

Newer technologies such as tissue-engineered bone using various biomaterials are being explored with the hope of providing an alternative to the current treatment options. The ceramic or polymer scaffolds with various osteogenic growth factors are a work in progress and are yet to reach clinical use [7]. Successful use of hydroxyapatite-tricalcium phosphate-tricalcium silicate composite scaffold with autologous bone-marrow-derived mesenchymal stem cells has been described in a case report for treating an 11-year-old with a post-osteomyelitic proximal humeral bone defect [40].

Creation of a Single-Bone Forearm

Large radial or ulnar diaphyseal or articular bone defects can be salvaged by a single-bone forearm procedure. It is most helpful when other reconstructive options may not work. It is based on the principle "ulna makes the elbow and the radius make the wrist." [41] A bony bridge is created between the ulno-humeral joint proximally and the radiocarpal joint distally. This bridge is formed by creating synostosis or creating an "ulnius." [42–44] Creating a single-bone forearm addresses instability and pain from the proximal or distal radioulnar joints. The function of the wrist and elbow are improved, allowing the growth of the forearm to continue. Loss of forearm rotation is compensated through the shoulder. The single-bone forearm procedure results in a cosmetically acceptable forearm and stability at the elbow and the wrist. A vascularized fibular bone graft has been used to bridge the gap between the radius and ulna. A fibular osteocutaneous bone graft also fills the soft tissue defect [45–46]. There is no consensus on the position of the forearm rotation. The forearm position is decided by age, dominance, dexterity, demands, and patient preference. There are no clear guidelines due to the rarity of the treatment. The prognosis depends on the amount of distal radius that was involved by the infective pathology. The duration, the extent of defect, age of the patient, and amount of initial shortening usually dictate the outcome [44]. When the distal radius is destroyed, the carpus is translated and fused to the ulna creating a wrist (ulnocarpal) arthrodesis [44, 47] (Figs. 25.8 and 25.9). Tables 25.2 and 25.3 summarize the various treatment strategies.

Complications and Outcomes

The treatment of a bone gap in the upper extremity can be challenging, is very lengthy, and can take several months. Several surgeries may be required to achieve bony union and restoration of function. Results are successful in salvaging the upper extremity with some loss of function.

In summary, the treatment of post-osteomyelitic upper extremity bone gap is difficult. Modern reconstruction concepts have resulted in the availability of a variety of choices. The therapeutic goals remain the same: repair of the bone defect and re-establishment of joint function. Prospective studies comparing the outcomes and complications of the various methods are still scarce. There is limited data on long-term patient-reported functional outcomes. Pooled data on treatment outcomes will be beneficial from multicenter cooperation (Boxes 25.4 and 25.5).

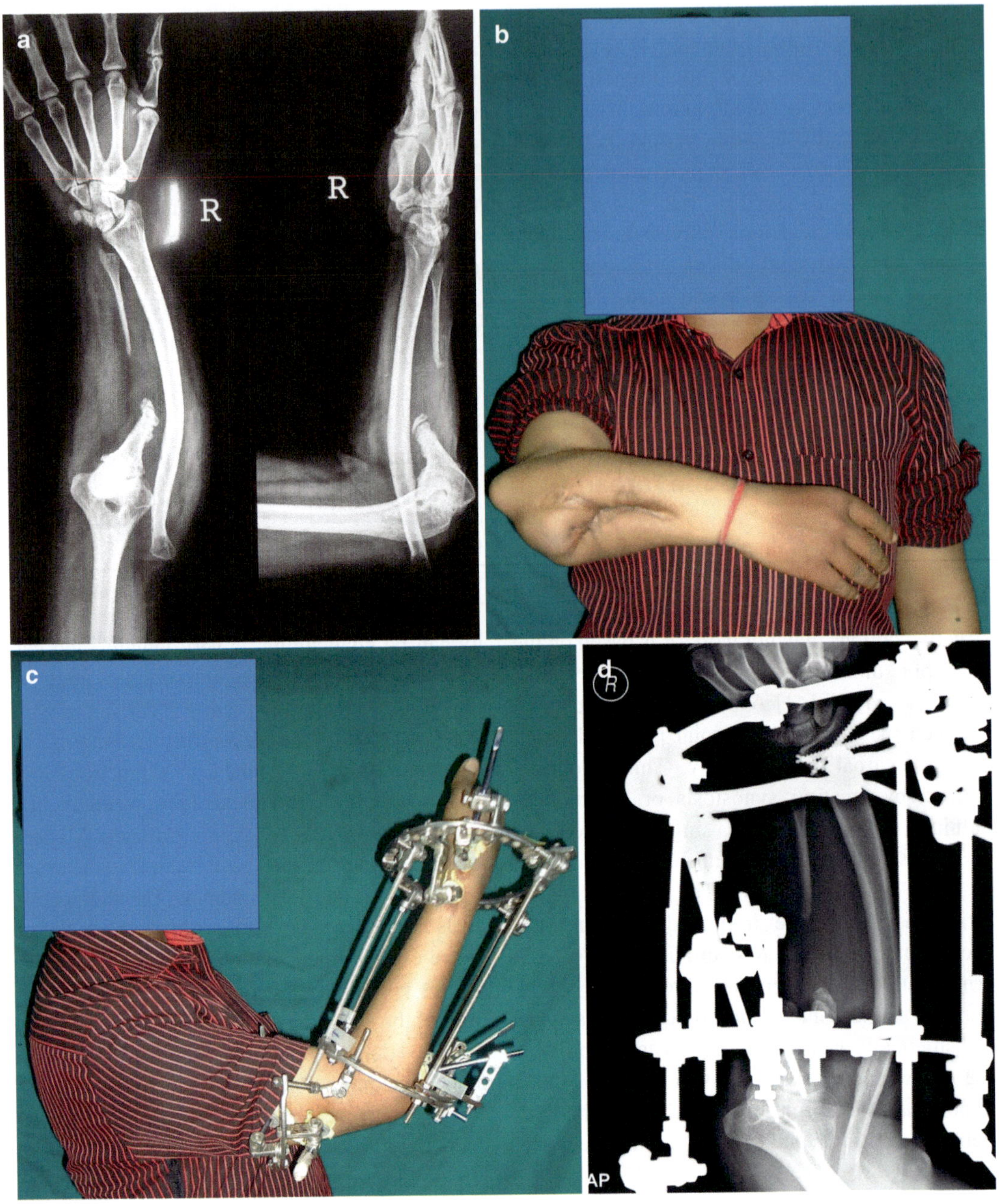

Fig. 25.8 (**a**, **b**) A 28-year-old with residual deformity after hematogenous osteomyelitis of the ulna in childhood and multiple attempts at surgical reconstruction. The proximal ulna is present. The distal ulna is pencil thin. Even if bone transport were attempted or a vascularized fibular graft was done, it would not result in satisfactory function. The proximal radius has migrated 8 cm proximally. (**c**, **d**) The ring fixator was used to fix the distal radius and proximal ulna and the distal humerus with three half-pins each. Hinges at the elbow joint permitted some range of motion during treatment. (**e**, **f**) The radius was pulled down. Once it approached the station, it was fused with the proximal ulna and held in the apparatus till the fusion matured. Elbow ROM continued. (**g**, **h**) Successful completion of single-bone forearm. The forearm length has also increased, and elbow and wrist function are retained. Rotations, as expected, must occur through the shoulder

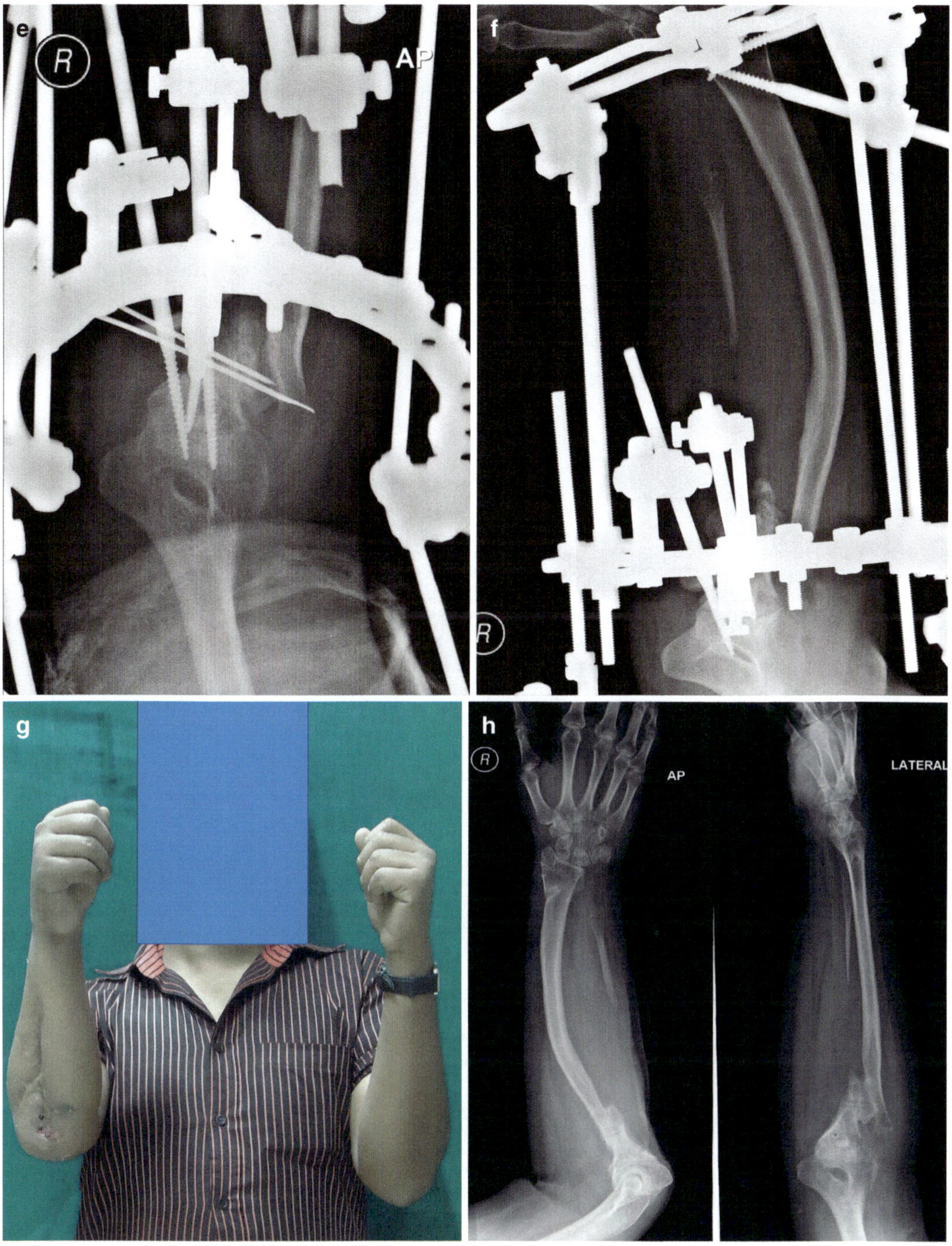

Fig. 25.8 (continued)

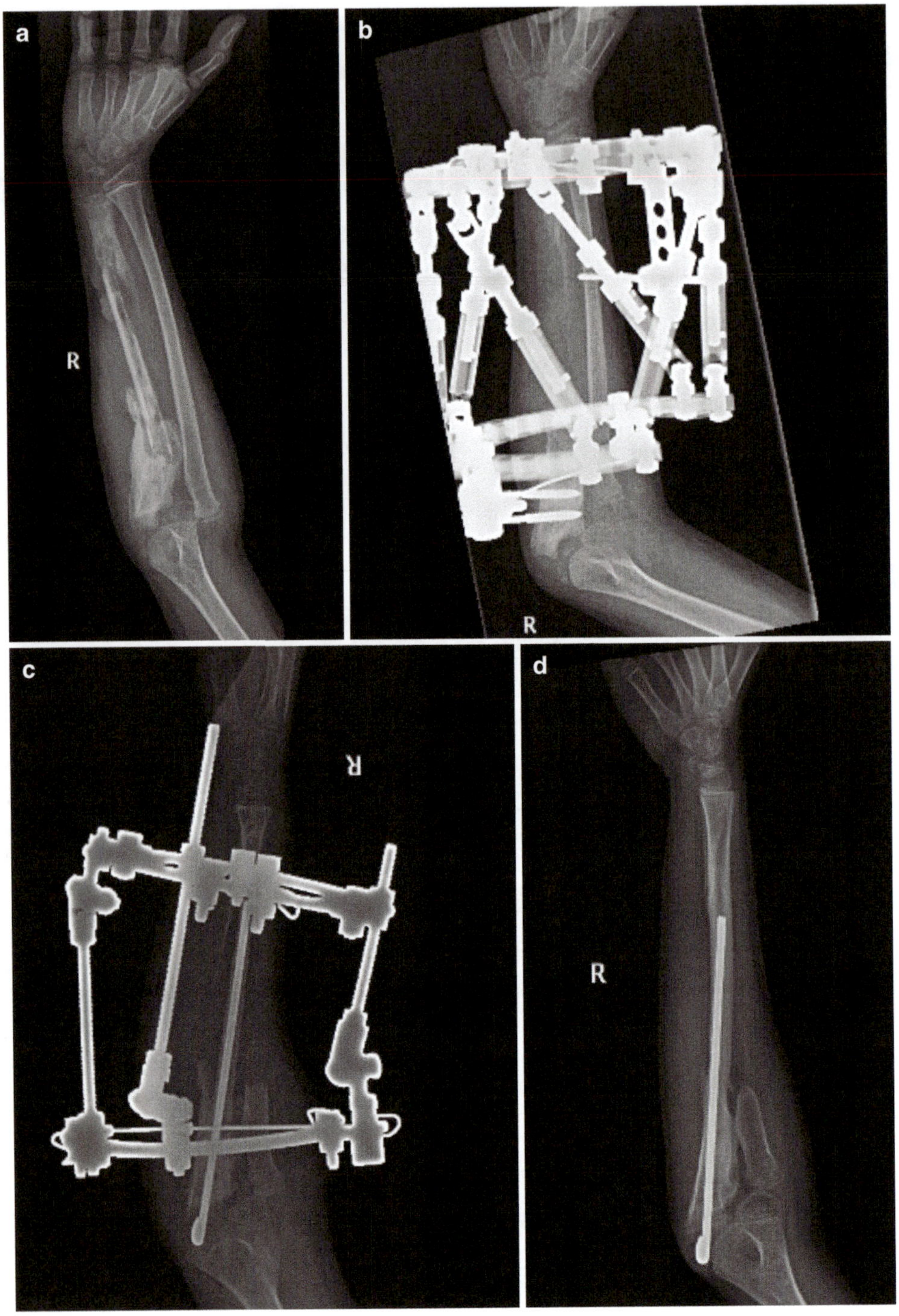

Fig. 25.9 (**a**) Radiograph of a10-year-old male with chronic osteomyelitis of the right ulna (dominant arm) with large sequestrum and radial head dislocation. The elbow range of motion was 20–110 degrees. (**b**) Application of external fixator after sequestrectomy and debridement of the ulna. Distraction was started at a rate of 1 mm/day. (**c**) After second-stage exploration of posterior interosseous nerve, osteotomy with incision of periosteum, and transfer of the osteo-periosteal radius to the ulna, IM rodding and compression frame are shown. The forearm was positioned in semi-pronation. (**d**) Radiograph after 6 weeks of compression by the external fixator. (**e**) Radiograph after the rod removal. The elbow ROM was 10–145 degrees. (**f**) Hypertrophy of the transferred radius and the final position of the forearm. (Images **a**–**f**: Case courtesy: Dr. Tim R. Nunn, FRCS [Tr & Orth], CURE Ethiopia Children's Hospital, Addis Ababa, Ethiopia)

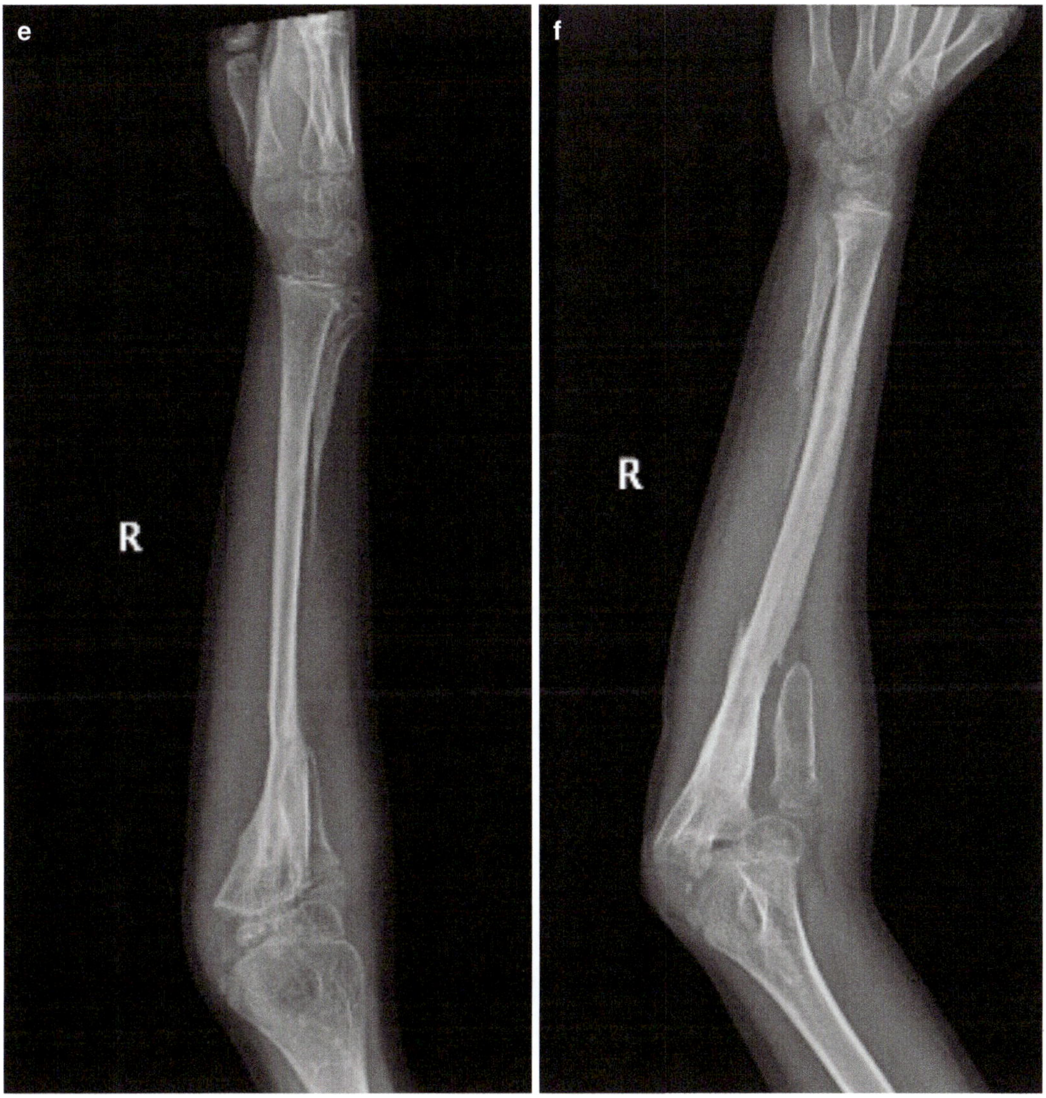

Fig. 25.9 (continued)

Table 25.2 Options for the management of humeral bone defects

Bone defect size	Strategy
<3 cm	Shortening, iliac crest autograft
>3 cm	Non-vascularized fibula, vascularized fibula
Large defects	Bone transport, induced membrane technique

Table 25.3 Options for the management of forearm bone defects

Bone defect size	Strategy
<2 cm	Shortening
2–4 cm	Iliac crest bone graft
2–6 cm	Non-vascularized fibular bone graft
6 cm	Non-vascularized/ vascularized fibular graft
6 cm	Bone transport
Any size	Induced membrane technique
Loss of articular segment of radius or ulna with bone defect	Single-bone forearm

Box 25.4 Tips and Tricks for Successful Outcome

- Start bone defect reconstruction after complete eradication of the infection.
- Non-vascularized fibula forms the mainstay of treatment.
- Use intramedullary K-wire or external fixator to stabilize the NVFG.
- Use additional bone graft at the ends of the non-vascularized fibular graft to avoid non-union.
- In humerus, shortening followed by humeral lengthening can be safely done by device of surgeon's choice.

Box 25.5 Pitfalls to Avoid

- Prolonged protection of the extremity with a splint to avoid fracture of the graft.
- Restore anatomy of the proximal and distal radioulnar joint.
- Leave at least 5–6 cm of fibula distally while obtaining a fibular graft to avoid ankle valgus, and proximal migration of the distal fibula.

References

1. Rasool MN. Pyogenic osteomyelitis of the forearm bones in children. SA Orthopedic J. 2011;10(4):18–24.
2. Stevenson AJ, Jones HW, Chokotho LC, Beckles VL, Harrison WJ. The Beit CURE Classification of Childhood Chronic Haematogenous Osteomyelitis–a guide to treatment. J Orthop Surg Res. 2015; 10:144. https://doi.org/10.1186/s13018-015-0282-9. PMID: 26384208; PMCID: PMC4573297.
3. Meena DK. Post-osteomyelitic-acquired radial club hand deformity in children treated by centralization of Ulna. J Orthop Surg (Hong Kong). 2017 May-Aug;25(2):2309499017718950. doi: 10.1177/2309499017718950. PMID: 28675976.
4. Pawar DP, Ninawe DT, Sheth DBA. A novel technique of ulna strut grafting for post-septic radial clubhand deformity: case series of 4 patients with review of literature. J Clin Orthop Trauma. 2020;11(Suppl 5): S883–8. https://doi.org/10.1016/j.jcot.2020.07.007. Epub 2020 Jul 18. Erratum in: J Clin Orthop Trauma. 2020;11(6):1169–1171. Erratum in: J Clin Orthop Trauma. 2020;11(6):1178. Erratum in: J Clin Orthop Trauma. 2020;11(6):1172–1174. PMID: 32999573; PMCID: PMC7503140.
5. Allsopp BJ, Hunter-Smith DJ, Rozen WM. Vascularized versus nonvascularized bone grafts: what is the evidence? Clin Orthop Relat Res. 2016;474(5):1319–27. https://doi.org/10.1007/s11999-016-4769-4. Epub 2016 Mar 1. PMID: 26932740; PMCID: PMC4814434.
6. Mauffrey C, Barlow BT, Smith W. Management of segmental bone defects. J Am Acad Orthop Surg. 2015;23(3):143–53. https://doi.org/10.5435/JAAOS-D-14-00018. PMID: 25716002.
7. Roddy E, DeBaun MR, Daoud-Gray A, Yang YP, Gardner MJ. Treatment of critical-sized bone defects: clinical and tissue engineering perspectives. Eur J Orthop Surg Traumatol. 2018;28(3):351–62. https://doi.org/10.1007/s00590-017-2063-0. Epub 2017 Oct 28. PMID: 29080923.
8. Netrawichien P. Radial clubhand-like deformity resulting from osteomyelitis of the distal radius. J Pediatr Orthop. 1995;15(2):157–60. PMID: 7745085.
9. Krishna C, Mondal J, Sengupta A. Modified Nicoll's graft for treatment of gap non-union of ulna: a rare case report. J Orthop Case Rep. 2017;7(2):17–20. https://doi.org/10.13107/jocr.2250-0685.730. PMID: 28819594; PMCID: PMC5553827.
10. Gupta DK, Kumar G. Gap non-union of forearm bones treated by modified Nicoll's technique. Indian J Orthop. 2010;44(1):84–8. https://doi.org/10.4103/0019-5413.58611. PMID: 20165682; PMCID: PMC2822425.
11. Dugdale TW 3rd, Pillsbury SL, Cates KL, Ogden JA. Successful autogenous corticocancellous grafting of a radial defect complicating acute hematogenous osteomyelitis in an infant. J Pediatr Orthop. 1985;5(4):479–82. https://doi.org/10.1097/01241398-198507000-00019. PMID: 4019765.
12. Swamy MK, Rathi A, Gupta V. Results of non-vascularised fibular grafting in gap non-union of long bones in paediatric age group. J Clin Orthop Trauma. 2013;4(4):180–4. https://doi.org/10.1016/j.jcot.2013.09.001. Epub 2013 Sep 26. PMID: 26403879; PMCID: PMC3880954.
13. Patwardhan S, Shyam AK, Mody RA, Sancheti PK, Mehta R, Agrawat H. Reconstruction of bone defects after osteomyelitis with nonvascularized fibular graft: a retrospective study in twenty-six children. J Bone Joint Surg Am. 2013;95(9):e56, S1. https://doi.org/10.2106/JBJS.K.01338. PMID: 23636195.
14. Agarwal A, Raj RY, Gupta S, Shanker M. Osteosynthesis of Postosteomyelitic forearm defects in children using a modified bone grafting technique: the fibular intramedullary bridging bone and additional grafting (FIBBAG). J Hand Surg Asian Pac. 2020;25(1):13–9. https://doi.org/10.1142/S2424835520500010. PMID: 32000603.
15. Kaewpornsawan K, Eamsobhana P. Free nonvascularized fibular graft for treatment of large bone defect

around the elbow in pediatric patients. Eur J Orthop Surg Traumatol. 2017;27(7):895–900. https://doi.org/10.1007/s00590-017-1955-3. Epub 2017 Apr 9. PMID: 28393309.
16. Steinlechner CW, Mkandawire NC. Non-vascularised fibular transfer in the management of defects of long bones after sequestrectomy in children. J Bone Joint Surg Br. 2005;87(9):1259–63. https://doi.org/10.1302/0301-620X.87B9.15734. PMID: 16129754.
17. Lucas G, Lopez J, Fraisse B, Marleix S, Violas P. Minimally invasive harvesting of nonvascularized fibular graft in children. Orthop Traumatol Surg Res. 2015;101(4):515–8. https://doi.org/10.1016/j.otsr.2015.02.006. Epub 2015 Apr 15. PMID: 25890811
18. Agarwal A, Kumar D, Agrawal N, Gupta N. Ankle valgus following nonvascularized fibular grafts in children-an outcome evaluation minimum two years after fibular harvest. Int Orthop. 2017;41(5):949–55. https://doi.org/10.1007/s00264-017-3403-8.
19. Al-Zahrani S, Harding MG, Kremli M, Khan FA, Ikram A, Takroni T. Free fibular graft still has a place in the treatment of bone defects. Injury. 1993;24(8):551–4.
20. Soucacos PN, Kokkalis ZT, Piagkou M, Johnson EO. Vascularized bone grafts for the management of skeletal defects in orthopaedic trauma and reconstructive surgery. Injury. 2013;44(Suppl 1):S70–5. https://doi.org/10.1016/S0020-1383(13)70016-0. PMID: 23351876.
21. Bumbasirevic M, Stevanovic M, Bumbasirevic V, Lesic A, Atkinson HD. Free vascularised fibular grafts in orthopaedics. Int Orthop. 2014;38(6):1277–82. https://doi.org/10.1007/s00264-014-2281-6. Epub 2014 Feb 22. PMID: 24562850; PMCID: PMC4037521.
22. del Piñal F, Innocenti M. Evolving concepts in the management of the bone gap in the upper limb. Long and small defects. J Plast Reconstr Aesthet Surg. 2007;60(7):776–92. https://doi.org/10.1016/j.bjps.2007.03.006. Epub 2007 Apr 23. PMID: 17452133.
23. Yajima H, Tamai S, Ono H, et al. Free vascularized fibula grafts in surgery of the upper limb. J Reconstr Microsurg. 1999;15:515e21.
24. Ling XF, Peng X. What is the price to pay for a free fibula flap? A systematic review of donor-site morbidity following free fibula flap surgery. Plast Reconstr Surg. 2012;129:657–74. https://doi.org/10.1097/PRS.0b013e3182402d9a.
25. Pal JN, Banik R. Monoaxial distraction of Ulna to second metacarpal followed by single bone forearm in massive post infective radial bone loss. Indian J Orthop. 2012;46(6):685–9. https://doi.org/10.4103/0019-5413.104214. PMID: 23325973; PMCID: PMC3543888.
26. Villa A, Paley D, Catagni MA, Bell D, Cattaneo R. Lengthening of the forearm by the Ilizarov technique. Clin Orthop Relat Res. 1990;250:125–37. PMID: 2293920.
27. Liu Y, Yushan M, Liu Z, Liu J, Ma C, Yusufu A. Treatment of diaphyseal forearm defects caused by infection using Ilizarov segmental bone transport technique. BMC Musculoskelet Disord. 2021;22(1):36. https://doi.org/10.1186/s12891-020-03896-w. PMID: 33413259; PMCID: PMC7789280.
28. Zhang X, Duan L, Li Z, Chen X. Callus distraction for the treatment of acquired radial club-hand deformity after osteomyelitis. J Bone Joint Surg Br. 2007;89(11):1515–8. https://doi.org/10.1302/0301-620X.89B11.19012. PMID: 17998192.
29. Hosny GA. Humeral lengthening and deformity correction. J Child Orthop. 2016 Dec;10(6):585–92. https://doi.org/10.1007/s11832-016-0789-6. Epub 2016 Nov 8. PMID: 27826910; PMCID: PMC5145839.
30. Liu T, Zhang X, Li Z, Zeng W. Management of chronic radial head dislocation associated with segment bone defect in ulna after osteomyelitis. J Trauma Acute Care Surg. 2012;73(4):1014–7. https://doi.org/10.1097/TA.0b013e318254a933. PMID: 22722824.
31. Smith WR, Elbatrawy YA, Andreassen GS, Philips GC, Guerreschi F, Lovisetti L, Catagni MA. Treatment of traumatic forearm bone loss with Ilizarov ring fixation and bone transport. Int Orthop. 2007;31(2):165–70. https://doi.org/10.1007/s00264-006-0172-1. Epub 2006 Jul 4. PMID: 16821011; PMCID: PMC2267575.
32. Liu T, Zhang X, Li Z, Zeng W, Peng D, Sun C. Callus distraction for humeral non-union with bone loss and limb shortening caused by chronic osteomyelitis. J Bone Joint Surg Br. 2008;90(6):795–800. https://doi.org/10.1302/0301-620X.90B6.20392. PMID: 18539674.
33. Farr S, Mindler G, Ganger R, Girsch W. Bone lengthening in the pediatric upper extremity. J Bone Joint Surg Am. 2016;98(17):1490–503. https://doi.org/10.2106/JBJS.16.00007. PMID: 27605694.
34. Jager T, Popkov D, Lascombes P, Popkov A, Journeau P. Elastic intramedullary nailing as a complement to Ilizarov's method for forearm lengthening: a comparative pediatric prospective study. Orthop Traumatol Surg Res. 2012;98(4):376–82. https://doi.org/10.1016/j.otsr.2012.01.007. Epub 2012 May 2. PMID: 22560591.
35. Kadhim M, Herzenberg JE. Staged humerus lengthening with monolateral fixation followed by a circular frame: Technique of fixator change. J Limb Lengthen Reconstr [serial online] 2018 [cited 2021 Mar 28];4:111–4. Available from: https://www.jlimblengthrecon.org/text.asp?2018/4/2/111/253388
36. Hoel RJ, Novotny SA, Dahl MT. Humeral lengthening using a retrograde motorized intramedullary lengthening nail. J Limb Lengthen Reconstr [serial online] 2018 [cited 2021 Mar 28];4:55–8. Available from: https://www.jlimblengthrecon.org/text.asp?2018/4/1/55/231789

37. Gouron R. Surgical technique and indications of the induced membrane procedure in children. Orthop Traumatol Surg Res. 2016;102(1 Suppl):S133–9. https://doi.org/10.1016/j.otsr.2015.06.027. Epub 2016 Jan 7. PMID: 26774902.
38. Shen J, Sun D, Yu S, Fu J, Wang X, Wang S, Xie Z. Radiological and clinical outcomes using induced membrane technique combined with bone marrow concentrate in the treatment of chronic osteomyelitis of immature patients. Bone Joint Res. 2021;10(1):31–40. https://doi.org/10.1302/2046-3758.101.BJR-2020-0229.R1. PMID: 33380210; PMCID: PMC7845462.
39. Aurégan JC, Bégué T, Rigoulot G, Glorion C, Pannier S. Success rate and risk factors of failure of the induced membrane technique in children: a systematic review. Injury. 2016;47(Suppl 6):S62–7. https://doi.org/10.1016/S0020-1383(16)30841-5. PMID: 28040089.
40. Madhuri V, Ramesh S, Varma H, Sivadasan SB, Sahoo B, John A, Fernandez F, Rajagopal K, Mathews V, Balakumar B, Dinesh VD, Chilbule SK, Gibikote S, Srivastava A; Bone Defect Study Group. First report of a tissue-engineered graft for proximal humerus gap non-union after chronic pyogenic osteomyelitis in a child: a case report. JBJS Case Connect. 2020;10(1):e0031. https://doi.org/10.2106/JBJS.CC.19.00031. PMID: 32224678.
41. Vitale CC. Reconstructive surgery for defects in the shaft of the ulna in children. J Bone Joint Surg Am. 1952;34(4):804–10.
42. Peterson HA. The ulnius: a one-bone forearm in children. J Pediatr Orthop B. 2008;17(2):95–101.
43. Schiffman B, Hanel D. The one bone forearm. Hand Clin. 2020;36(4):531–8. https://doi.org/10.1016/j.hcl.2020.07.007.
44. Rasool MN. Radioulnar fusion for forearm defects in children – a salvage procedure. SA Orthop J. 2008;7(1):60–6.
45. Artiaco S, Ciclamini D, Teodori J, Dutto E, Benigno T, Battiston B. One bone forearm with vascularized fibular graft. Clinical experience and literature review. Injury. 2020;51(12):2962–5. https://doi.org/10.1016/j.injury.2020.06.018. Epub 2020 Jun 15. PMID: 32571550
46. Devendra A, Velmurugesan PS, Dheenadhayalan J, Venkatramani H, Sabapathy SR, Rajasekaran S. One-bone forearm reconstruction: a salvage solution for the forearm with massive bone loss. J Bone Joint Surg Am. 2019;101(15):e74. https://doi.org/10.2106/JBJS.18.01235. PMID: 31393431.
47. Manojlović R, Tulić G, Kadija M, Vucetić C, Tabaković D, Bumbasirević M. Forearm reconstruction after loss of radius: case report. Srp Arh Celok Lek. 2013;141(1–2):100–3. https://doi.org/10.2298/sarh1302100m. PMID: 23539919.

Post Infective Bone Gap Management of the Lower Extremity

26

Timothy Nunn, Sandeep Patwardhan, and Gamal Ahmed Hosny

Introduction

Pathological fractures leading to bone gaps are unusual sequelae of childhood osteomyelitis in healthcare systems that are advanced with good access to care. Data documenting the epidemiology of bone gaps in low- and middle-income countries at the population level are not available. In a large series of children with chronic osteomyelitis (COM) admitted to a tertiary referral hospital in Sub-Saharan Africa, 20% of those admitted were classified as Beit-CURE B4, defined as 'sequestrum present, unstable, inadequate involucrum' or alternatively 'bone gap type' [1]. The tibia was the most commonly involved bone followed by the femur, humerus and forearm bones, respectively. It was noted that the tibia has poor soft tissue cover leaving the periosteum more vulnerable to damage because of sepsis. These data, although relevant for specialist children's orthopaedic hospitals, are not representative of the frequency of bone gaps in cases of chronic osteomyelitis. This chapter will seek to explore the relevant clinical features and the principles of management that are available for the successful treatment of bone gaps following chronic osteomyelitis in childhood. Many reconstruction techniques exist and consensus on the most successful methods is lacking due to a paucity of comparative long-term functional outcome studies. The information below is drawn largely from the authors' combined experience.

T. Nunn (✉)
CURE Children's Hospital, Ethiopia, Addis Ababa, Ethiopia
e-mail: tim.nunn@cureinternational.org

S. Patwardhan
Sancheti Institute for Orthopaedics and Rehabilitation, Pune, India

G. A. Hosny
Benha University, Kalyubia, Egypt

Microbiology and Pathology of Bone Gap Formation

The microbiology of osteomyelitis has yielded *Staphylococcus aureus* (60–90%) as the most common pathogen, especially in haematogenous osteomyelitis. Polymicrobial infections are commonly seen with secondary or exogenous osteomyelitis with compound fractures and/or surgical implants. *Pseudomonas*, *Staphylococcus epidermidis*, methicillin-resistant *Staphylococcus aureus*, *Escherichia coli* and *Haemophilus influenzae* are other common organisms in decreasing order of frequency. *Mycobacterium tuberculosis* is more frequently seen in low- and middle-income settings and successful drug treatment of skeletal tuberculosis can lead to bone gaps with no attendant sinuses. *Salmonella* is often isolated in children with Sickle cell disease; however, *Staphylococcus aureus* is still the commonest

© Springer Nature Switzerland AG 2022
M. V. Belthur et al. (eds.), *Pediatric Musculoskeletal Infections*,
https://doi.org/10.1007/978-3-030-95794-0_26

pathogen. Primary epiphyseal or apophyseal subacute osteomyelitis in children has yielded *Kingella kingae* as the common pathogen in children less than 4 years old [2].

Two characteristics of *Staphylococci* species that increase its toxicity to bone, cartilage and periosteum include:

1. Ability to produce and reside in a biofilm
2. Intracellular infection of bone components

Staphylococcus aureus is an important human pathogen that causes a variety of infections, including serious conditions such as osteomyelitis, pneumonia and necrotising fasciitis. Biofilm-associated infections such as chronic osteomyelitis are difficult to treat because the biofilm itself confers intrinsic resistance to antibiotics. Biofilm-associated infections cannot be treated by oral or intravenous antibiotic administration [3]. This is important as surgery in the form of radical debridement of the infected bone is often required to eliminate infection and this leads to bone loss or gaps requiring reconstruction.

In childhood it is the periosteum that is the key regenerative structure of bone, and children have excellent remodelling potential compared to adults [4, 5]. Inhibition or destruction of the periosteum accompanying a pathological fracture with instability of a segment causes involucrum failure [4]. The periosteum, just like in fracture healing, requires stability, healthy cells, adequate blood supply, nutrition and the absence of toxic substances such as inflammatory mediators to generate extracellular bone matrix.

Clinical Presentation and Examination

The relevant assessment of the history, examination and investigations help to establish answers to the following points:

1. Presence or absence of continued infection: This is most obviously detected by the presence of a persistent draining sinus tract.
2. Biology of the periosteum and the bone above and below the bone gap: Failure of periosteum that leads to a bone gap and laying down of poor involucrum is often seen where stability is inadequate and sepsis overwhelming.
3. The state and involvement of the physes: Physeal involvement often leads to growth disturbance manifesting as angular or length discrepancy of the bone segment. The effects of bone loss along with physeal growth potential can pose significant challenges for reconstruction.
4. Size of the bone defect following debridement: Whilst it is wise to drain focal pus collections, widely laying-open infected diaphysis leads to periosteal desiccation and poor involucrum formation. Such treatments are often evidenced by long surgical scars, particularly along the subcutaneous tibia.
5. Adequacy of the soft tissue envelope: Soft tissue abscess can necrose large amounts of skin and fat tissue leading to exposed dead bone. In addition, where a bone defect has been present for a long time, a cord of thick fibrous tissue may form in the gap.
6. Extent of deformity present: Malunited fractures, partial growth disturbances, weight bearing exclusively through the fibula all lead to complex deformities that should be characterised in detail prior to reconstruction.
7. Presence of feeding vascular supply: Vessels in a post-septic limb may become shrouded with significant soft tissue scarring, making the vessels difficult to identify and vulnerable to injury.
8. Joint stiffness and position: Accompanying joint sepsis may make the joint stiff and in mycobacterial infection may lead to joint ankylosis.
9. Nutritional status: Height and weight and the mid-upper arm circumference are helpful to review. The effect of the septic focus added to the background of pre-existing malnutrition can be a challenge for the surgeon. The periosteum will not respond well in such circumstances; nutritional support is a key pillar of successful treatment.

10. Social setup and remoteness: Reconstruction of a bone defect will often require extensive periods of in-patient stay and multiple procedures, a significant social and economic burden for working parents.
11. Views of amputation as a fall-back option: In many cultures the taboo of amputation and the availability of quality prostheses are factors that can heavily influence decision-making in reconstruction attempts.

Box 26.1 Examination of a Child with a Bone Gap

Look:

- General condition of the child
- Gait
- Signs of active infection – swelling, heat and sinuses
- Deformity in the bone segments
- Signs for previous surgical treatments
- Limb length discrepancy

Feel:

- Soft tissue adequacy
- Pulses and neurological function
- The contralateral leg

Move:

- Mobility at the non-union site
- Joints above and below the defect
- Motor units
- Rotational profile

Investigations and Work-Up

In the presence of active infection, a debridement can be combined with sampling deep tissue samples for microbiological analysis, culture and sensitivities. This is superior to swabbing sinuses for microbiology, which often yields mixed growth as contaminants from the sinus tract are often detected. The diagnosis of tuberculous osteomyelitis should also be considered. A deep tissue sample for additional histology and a Mantoux test may be needed.

Sequestra may be identified on plain radiographs, and over-penetrated radiographs may help better identify sclerotic avascular fragments, which are more densely seen as compared to vascularised cortex [6]. In planning for sequestrectomy, particularly in the femur, it is helpful to have axial imaging to define the surgical approach and fragments that are not well seen on plain radiographs.

Bone gaps often signify severe infection since the infection has overwhelmed the periosteal sleeve. The frequency of physeal damage is high in these cases. Imaging of the physes if suspicious of a bony bar and growth disturbance is important to determine and may alter the surgical strategy. Although magnetic resonance imaging (MRI) is the best and most sensitive and specific for diagnosing a physeal arrest, fine cut computed tomography (CT) is reasonable if MRI is not available or not practical and can quantify the site and extent of a bony bar.

Inflammatory serum markers can be helpful in determining if there is any residual infection, and trends do help in evaluating responses to treatment. However, clinical appearance and sinus closure are also good measures of whether the surgical debridement was sufficient.

Finally, vascular assessments with a handheld Doppler ultrasound are useful where a free vascularised fibular graft is to be inserted. Recipient vessels may be poor and surrounded in scar tissue on the affected leg. The peroneal artery must be present in the donor leg and at least one other good vessel to the foot.

Bone Defect Treatment Options in the Presence of Ongoing Sepsis

The principles of bone gap management are to improve the mechanical environment and the biology of the bone. This can be conveniently remembered as the four S's: 'sterilising' and 'stimulating' the bone to heal (biological) and 'straightening' and 'stabilising' the bone segments (mechanical).

Mechanical environment	Biological environment
Stabilising Adequate fixation with sufficient bone fragment control	**'Sterilising'** Pus drainage Adequate debridement of dead bone and biofilm to remove infective load Local antibiotic therapies
Straightening Reducing bone ends Deformity correction (angular and translational correction)	**'Stimulating'** Weight bearing Nutrition Distraction histogenesis Biologics (autologous or synthetic, once infection is under control)

The treatment options should address the following issues as indicated:

Preventing a Bone Gap

A bone gap may be impending if an unstable or non-structural involucrum is found. This occurs often with a fracture between the pathological bone and the vascularised bone. In these impending cases, the periosteum should be given a chance to declare itself as insufficient. Debridement of dead bone along with the biofilm, providing stability with cast, external fixation or traction (as appropriate), nutritional support and monitoring with serial radiographs over a 6–12-week period are helpful in identifying periosteal failure. In most cases of chronic osteomyelitis (COM), even with a pathological fracture, an involucrum forms, and waiting for this to become structurally sound is important. In the author's experience, the femur, the radius and the fibula are bones that have excellent biological activity. Up to the age of 5 years, rapid involucrum will reliably form in these sites given the correct mechanical and biological environment. This is exemplified in the case below (Fig. 26.1).

If after 3 months of systemic treatment with high protein and energy rehabilitation, no substantial involucrum is seen, proceeding to a debridement with stabilisation is indicated.

Surgical Debridement of an Established Septic Gap

Surgical debridement is a key step in the management of established septic bone gaps. Systemic antibiotics are not effective and will serve to select out resistant strains. Surgical debridement is considered important to address both the offending biofilm and the dead bone tissue. Radical resection of the infected bone in adults

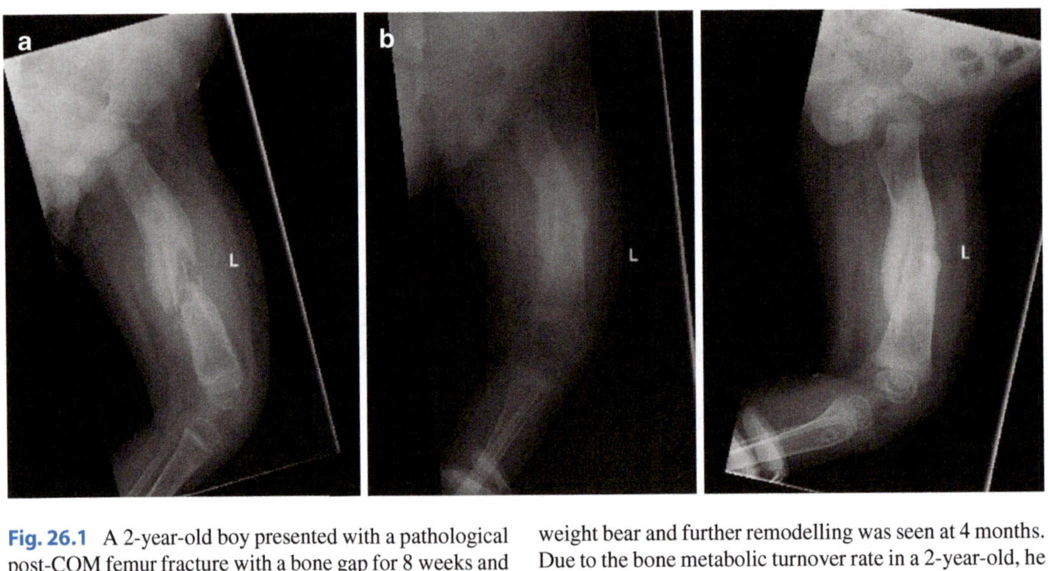

Fig. 26.1 A 2-year-old boy presented with a pathological post-COM femur fracture with a bone gap for 8 weeks and a dry sinus (**a**). He was immobilised in a Spica cast for 6 weeks following which union occurred (**b**). He started to weight bear and further remodelling was seen at 4 months. Due to the bone metabolic turnover rate in a 2-year-old, he is expected to resorb the sequestra without surgical intervention

was considered as key to obtain infection control. However, it may be considered as a double-edged sword, with the possibility of eradication of the infection and at the same time sacrificing segments of living bone. In this sense, aggressive debridement eradicates infection more effectively at the expense of creating a larger bone defect.

Younger children's bones have a remarkable osteogenic biological power. The addition of corticotomy followed by distraction improves the blood supply significantly, which increases the potential of controlling infection. Minimal debridement with excision of dead bone and necrotic tissues would be enough to achieve good results without unnecessary excision of healthy bone. Hosny and Ahmed (2019) reported 36 cases with paediatric infected tibial non-union, treated without radical or aggressive debridement [7]. The limited debridement was done by removal of the clinically evident necrotic bone and soft tissues without excision of any healthy part. At the last follow-up, there was only one case of infection recurrence despite limited debridement. No corticotomy site became infected. This technique was thus named the 'corticotomy first technique' (Fig. 26.2).

Appropriate Dead Space Management

The combined use of locally delivered antibiotics in carriers such as bone cement and calcium sulphate materials is an established and effective part of treatment of bone gaps in adults. Stability and local antibiotic delivery by incorporating heat-stable antibiotics may improve outcomes following surgical debridement in childhood too [8, 9]. Routine availability of such carrier material is limiting for many healthcare providers.

Gap Management Strategies Once Septic Foci Have Been Removed

Gap Shortening and Compression

Acute shortening of bone gaps can pose challenges due to non-compliance of soft tissues. Bunching of skin leading to difficulty in closure and the potential of kinking of neurovascular structures is challenging. As a proportion of limb length, children tend to tolerate acute shortening better than adults but care must be taken whenever greater than 4 cm is acutely shortened [10, 11].

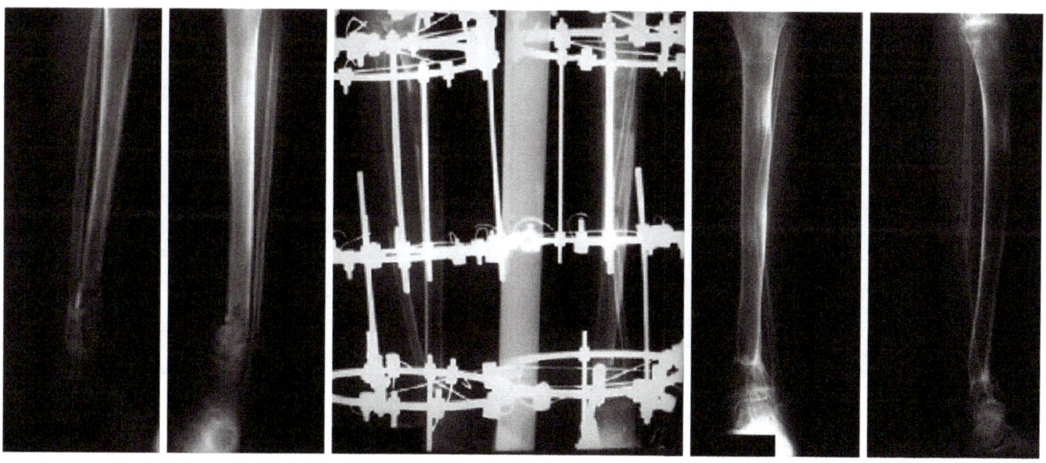

Fig. 26.2 Distal tibial post-traumatic infected non-union. Minimal debridement, application of an Ilizarov fixator with a careful proximal corticotomy and transport into the gap resulted in sound union

Gap Grafting

Simple Bone Grafting

Many gaps following osteomyelitis are relatively small but the quality of the bone on each side of the gap is often poor, sclerotic and thin (Fig. 26.3). Grafting of these defects can be done creating a synostosis with the fibula [12]. This confers strength by increasing the cross-sectional area of bone, which resists re-fracture. Such grafting is often not easy to do as large volumes are required; in addition, stable fixation of the fibula to the tibia is required to allow incorporation of such a graft (Fig. 26.3). Careful preparation of the adjacent cortices is also required to allow optimal incorporation.

> Gap grafting principle: Grafting along the interosseous membrane can create a fusion mass that is strong. Further surgical interventions are needed to correct deformities.

Staged Grafting

The Masquelet induced membrane technique is a tried and trusted technique for gap management [9, 13–16, 31]. An induced membrane is formed by the foreign body response to polymethylmethacrylate. Cannulation of the medullary canal with a rod and bone grafting into the defect once the vascularised membrane has formed will in time yield bony integrity (Fig. 26.4). The Masquelet technique requires an

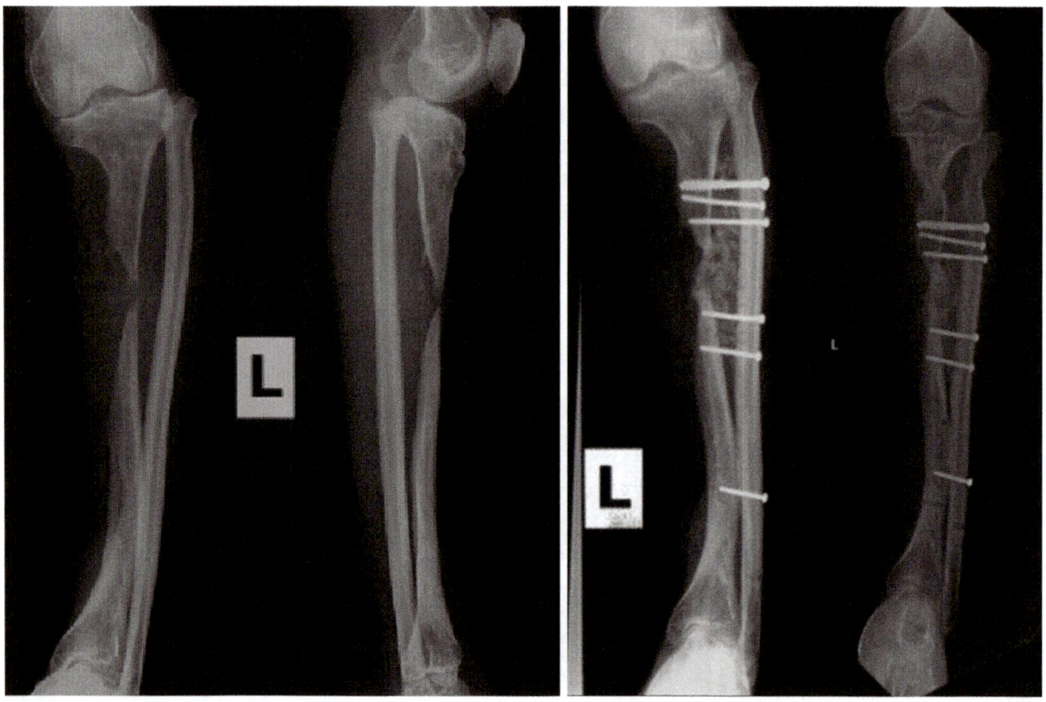

Fig. 26.3 This case illustration is in an adolescent boy who, although had a small gap, received decortication, iliac crest bone grafting and screw stabilisation across the interosseous membrane. Soft tissue precluded an antero-lateral approach, so postero-lateral grafting was performed. Scar tissue around the tibia was dense and this required an extensive dissection. Bone graft incorporation took approximately 3 months. The residual deformities of length, proximal tibial recurvatum and varus were dealt with following union. The distal deformity is being addressed. Further lengthening is not being considered as distraction osteogenesis would be in sclerotic bone that has previously been affected by chronic osteomyelitis and would not be optimal biologically for lengthening

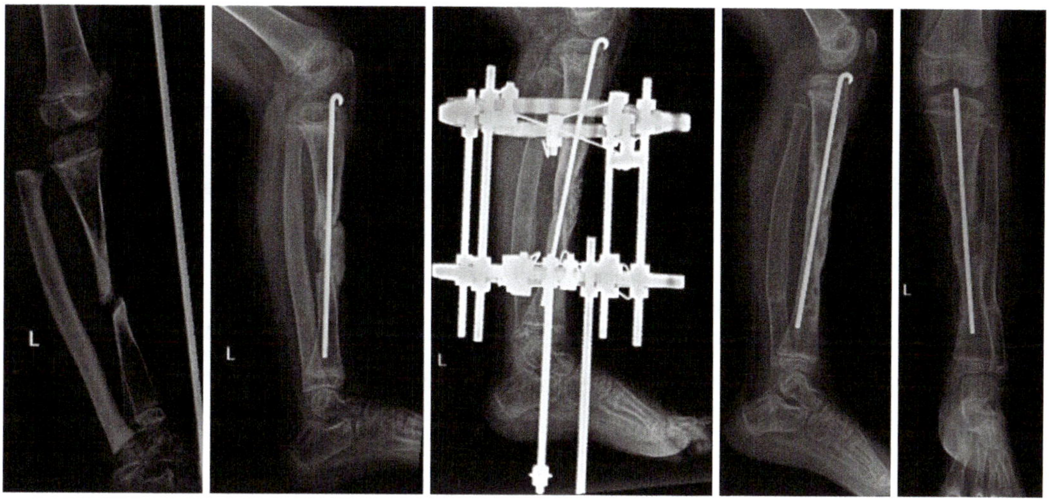

Fig. 26.4 Bone gap is temporarily bridged by an antibiotic impregnated cement spacer. The cement is removed preserving its surrounding membrane. The void is grafted. Additional stability against shearing forces is provided here by the two-ring fine wire circular fixator to allow rapid incorporation and weight bearing through an attached foot plate

excellent soft tissue envelope. An infective biofilm growing on the cement will likely cause graft loss. A full selection of heat-stable and systemic antibiotics along with good microbiological culture services is required. In childhood, obtaining adequate volume of graft can be problematic. In addition, graft extenders such as calcium sulphate and tri-calcium phosphate may not be available, making harvest of sufficient autograft difficult. Biologics such as Bone Morphogenic Proteins (BMPs) are unlicensed for such methods and are very expensive.

> Masquelet technique principle: An induced membrane can act as a pseudo-periosteum. The technique works well where there is excellent soft tissue envelope, access to bone cement, sufficient graft, and ideally access to heat-stable antibiotics and good microbiological facilities.

Immediate Bone Transport (Grafting Ipsilateral Tibia)

In 2018, a case report of an ‘immediate bone transport’ was published in a young patient who had focal bone defect with good periosteal sleeve in most of the diaphysis [17]. The principle is that in the young child, bone regeneration through rapid periosteal recovery can take place. A cylinder of bone can thus be stripped of its periosteum, moved into the gap and fixed leaving a defect from where it came, which will rapidly fill in. The concept demonstrates the activity of periosteum in a young child. The preferred age of the child is less than 5 years. For this to succeed, compression between the cylinder of graft and the metaphyseal segment should be present with good bone apposition to incorporate the cylinder. The length of a good periosteal sleeve must exceed the gap to be immediately transported into or shortening of the bone is required (Figs. 26.5 and 26.6).

> Immediate transport principle: The technique relies on a healthy periosteum from the donor area. It suits younger children with an active bone metabolic turnover.

Non-vascularised Fibula Graft Transfer

Gap non-unions in diaphyseal region of long bones are commonly seen as a complication after radical debridement in chronic osteomyeli-

Fig. 26.5 Schematic diagram of the concept of immediate transport

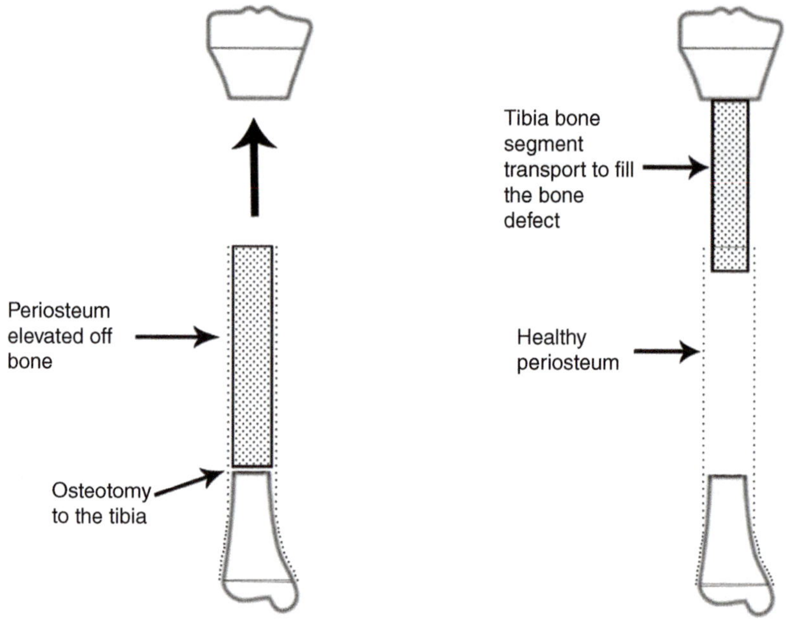

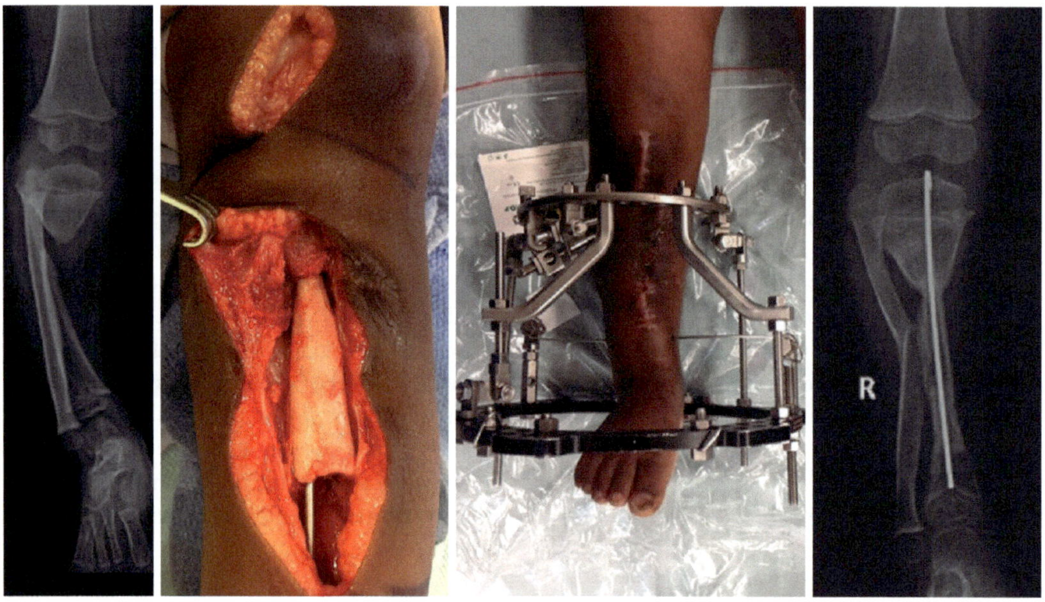

Fig. 26.6 Immediate transport case illustration. The fixator was removed at 6 weeks, there being an excellent solid bony gap regeneration. The indications for this technique is that it is best performed in very young one with high regenerative potential and a good periosteal sleeve. Physeal growth inhibition is noted at the ankle prior to this reconstruction, which will require a future attempt at physiolysis

tis or because of sequestration of large dead bone segments in the course of the disease process and pose a significant challenge to the orthopaedic surgeon, with respect to reconstructive options. The commonest bones involved are the tibia, femur, radius, ulna and rarely the clavicle. Amongst various methods described, reconstruction with non-vascularised fibular grafts (ipsilateral or contralateral) is a reliable option [18–20].

The first stage of the process involves thorough debridement of all dead bone granulation tissue and excision of sinuses through a direct extensile approach over the bone. After a thorough lavage with betadine, hydrogen peroxide or saline, negative suction drains are kept for 48–72 hours and appropriate immobilisation of limb with plaster slab is required. Sutures are removed after 3 weeks, and all patients are given functional cast braces to encourage use of the limb. A knee ankle foot orthosis is used in lower limbs with an ischial weight bearing socket to encourage walking for a period of 3 months. This allows us to observe for recurrence of infection and gives proprioceptive feedback that helps rehabilitation of a longstanding unused limb. We also believe it helps improve muscle blood flow and enhances integration of the graft used for reconstruction.

We repeat radiographs and C Reactive Protein (CRP) after 3 months to ensure absence of active infection, and plan reconstruction after radiological and haematological parameters are normalised.

Under general anaesthesia and tourniquet control, after exposing the gap through a direct approach, all interposed fibrous tissue is excised, and the proximal and distal bone stumps are trimmed transversely allowing the graft to contact and seat well. We routinely use a mini distractor to stretch out soft tissue contractures and restore appropriate length to the gap such that the graft can be inserted snugly. After measuring the defect, through a lateral incision, the contralateral fibula of the required length is harvested sub-periosteally protecting the branches of the peroneal nerve. The graft is then inserted over a 2 mm 'K' wire passing through the medulla of the fibular graft and fixing across the distal and proximal bone stumps. The mini distractor may be used for additional stability depending on the bone segment being treated. Closure is done after tourniquet is released and haemostasis achieved in layers over a drain with absorbable sub-cuticular sutures. Additional immobilisation is given with a plaster slab for 3 weeks till suture removal, followed by appropriate cast for 3 months.

The 'K' wire is removed at 3 months and functional bracing is used until graft consolidation is seen. We have observed hypertrophic delayed union at one end of the host-bone graft interface, especially where there was mechanical instability (lower femur, upper tibia). Addition of compression plating has resulted in complete healing of delayed unions.

In children aged 3–12 years with post-osteomyelitic gap non-unions, we found 100% healing of all gaps within 5 months. Slower healing was found in the longer gaps. Excellent alignment of the mechanical axis was found. However, some additional procedures for limb length discrepancies were required.

We believe this is a good low-cost option in low- and middle-income countries where childhood bone gaps are prevalent. This technique does not need any microsurgical expertise needed for vascularised fibular grafts; it does not need expensive instrumentation or implants, and does not need specialised training in Ilizarov techniques to reconstruct even large defects.

The technique provides a simple solution for achieving union but some residual problems such as shortening of affected limb, appearance of coronal plane deformities on long follow-up (due to infection across physis) [21] and donor site morbidity in the form of ankle valgus [22] need to be addressed in time.

It is important to follow the prerequisites for a successful outcome, which we believe are:

1. Radical debridement of septic foci
2. Functional rehabilitation to enhance muscle blood flow
3. Ensuring no residual infection at the time of reconstruction
4. Proper bed preparation and perfect graft fit
5. Adding stability with plates as needed
6. Prolonged immobilisation/protection till graft consolidation

We present a representative case (Fig. 26.7).

Free non-vascularised fibular transfer graft takes longer for the bone graft to incorporate and hypertrophy, as compared to a vascularised free flap. Failure to incorporate the segment leads to

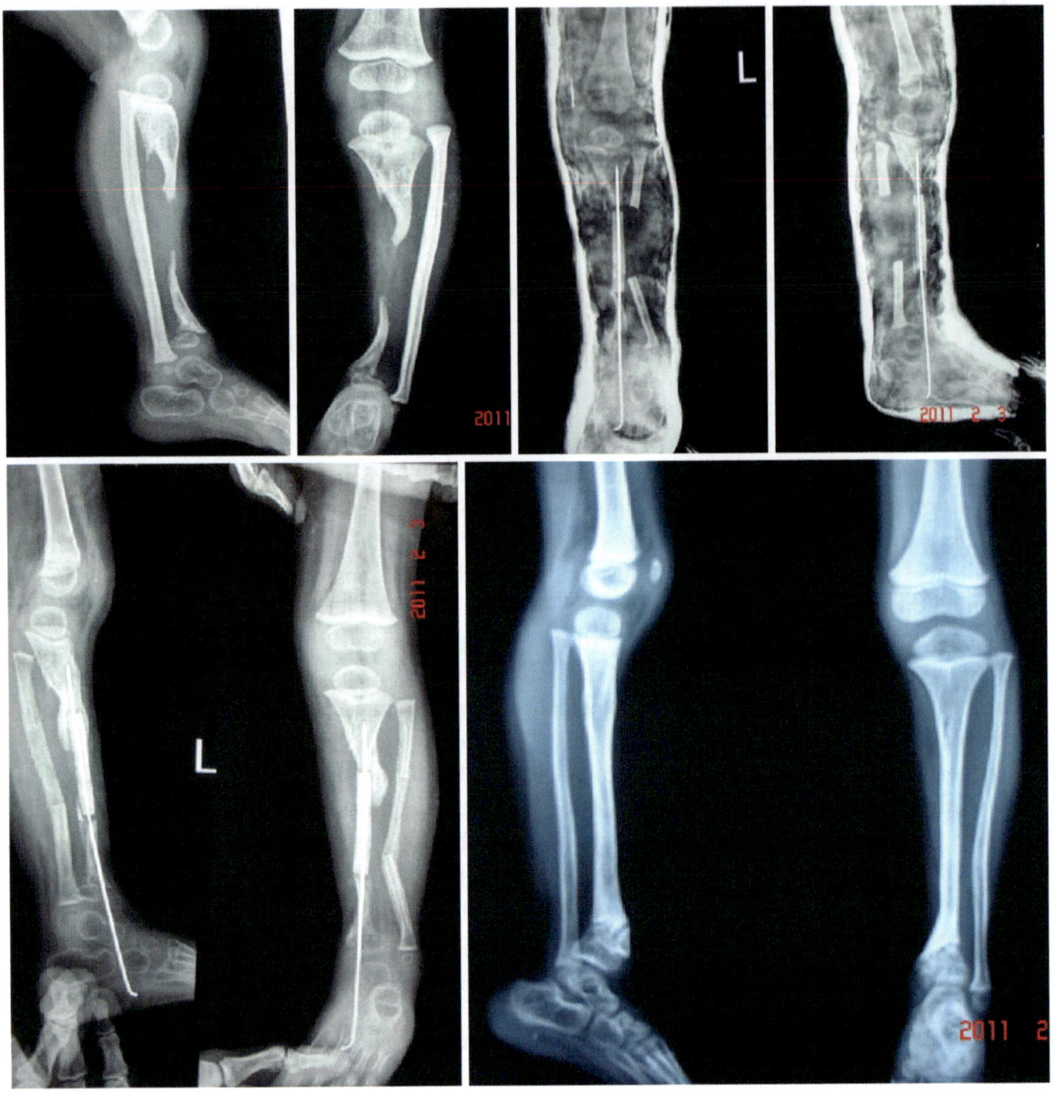

Fig. 26.7 Case illustration managed with an ipsilateral non-vascularised fibular graft showing healing in 3 months and remodelling over 6 months

non-union. Fracture of a slender piece of fibula is also seen where hypertrophy is slow. The use of orthotics until significant hypertrophy has occurred is helpful as well as internal splinting with an intramedullary device.

> Contralateral fibula transfer principle: Requires healthy bone ends to incorporate a long avascular graft. Meticulous technique is necessary, with better results expected in younger children.

Good results have also been reported using the ipsilateral fibular non-vascularised grafts to bridge bone defects of the tibia [19, 20].

Ilizarov Transport

Tibial corticotomy and transport has the benefit of greatly increasing the vascular environment of the limb. This aids resolution of any infective process as well as helping to preserve length [23–27]. A circular fixator has many mechanical advantages as compared to a monolateral, and

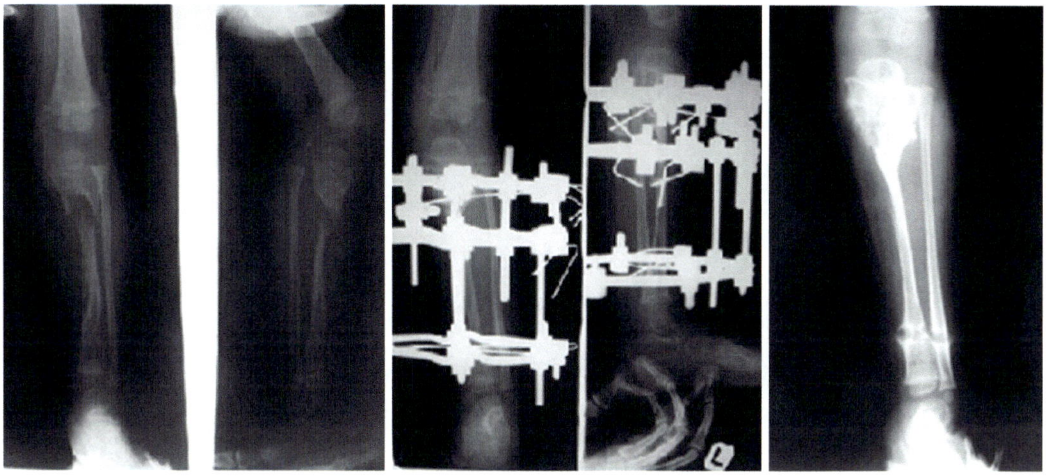

Fig. 26.8 High tibial osteotomy with transport of a segment of bone across a bone gap

care must be taken to adequately control all segments, and prevent entrapment of skin and other tissue into the docking site. Scar releases and other soft tissue procedures are sometimes required to create a 'channel' for the segment to transport through. Figure 26.8 demonstrates the use of Ilizarov tibial transport to treat a post-septic bone gap.

In the childhood femur, transport of a segment is possible, but the length discrepancy can be easier addressed on the long side with a timed physiodesis. Close to or following skeletal maturity, transport can be used to make up a gap and improve blood supply to optimise the biological situation. This can be seen in Fig. 26.9.

> Bone transport principle: Distraction histiogenesis is helpful in prior sepsis cases through stimulation of vascularity and length preservation. The technique is best tolerated in the tibia and prolonged fixator times are expected.

Vascularised Ipsilateral Fibula Transfer

This technique was described as a two-stage technique by Huntington and re-evaluated by Gupta et al. [28–30]. The segment of fibula is sequentially transferred preserving vascular supply. Proximally, a twin incision allows protection of the common peroneal nerve and branches whilst the fibular shaft is medialised and brought anterior. This is fixed whilst union occurs. A second-stage distal transfer is then performed and stabilised until distal union has occurred. Where the ipsilateral fibula is taken, it will usually unite back with its native fibula creating a double synostosis in the lower limb segment. This seems a particularly good option if the ipsilateral fibula is hypertrophied already (Fig. 26.10). Where significant deformity exists in the fibula, such as in chronic cases where unprotected weight bearing through the laterally placed fibula produces recurvatum and varus deformity, these deformities can make reconstruction more challenging.

Ipsilateral fibular transfer is best staged to allow union and vascularisation prior to the second site. Done in one sitting, the entire fibula may lose vascular supply, especially if the segment is not long. Particular care is required in mobilising the fibula proximally. Two incisions are preferred by the authors to visualise and protect the common peroneal nerve, and then adequate exposure to visualise and protect the deep peroneal nerve and the anterior tibial vessel as it runs down close to the interosseous membrane. The dissection can be challenging in the presence of significant scar tissue. An amount of necessary tibial shortening is expected so that the fibula can be translated anterior and medially to dock onto the tibial

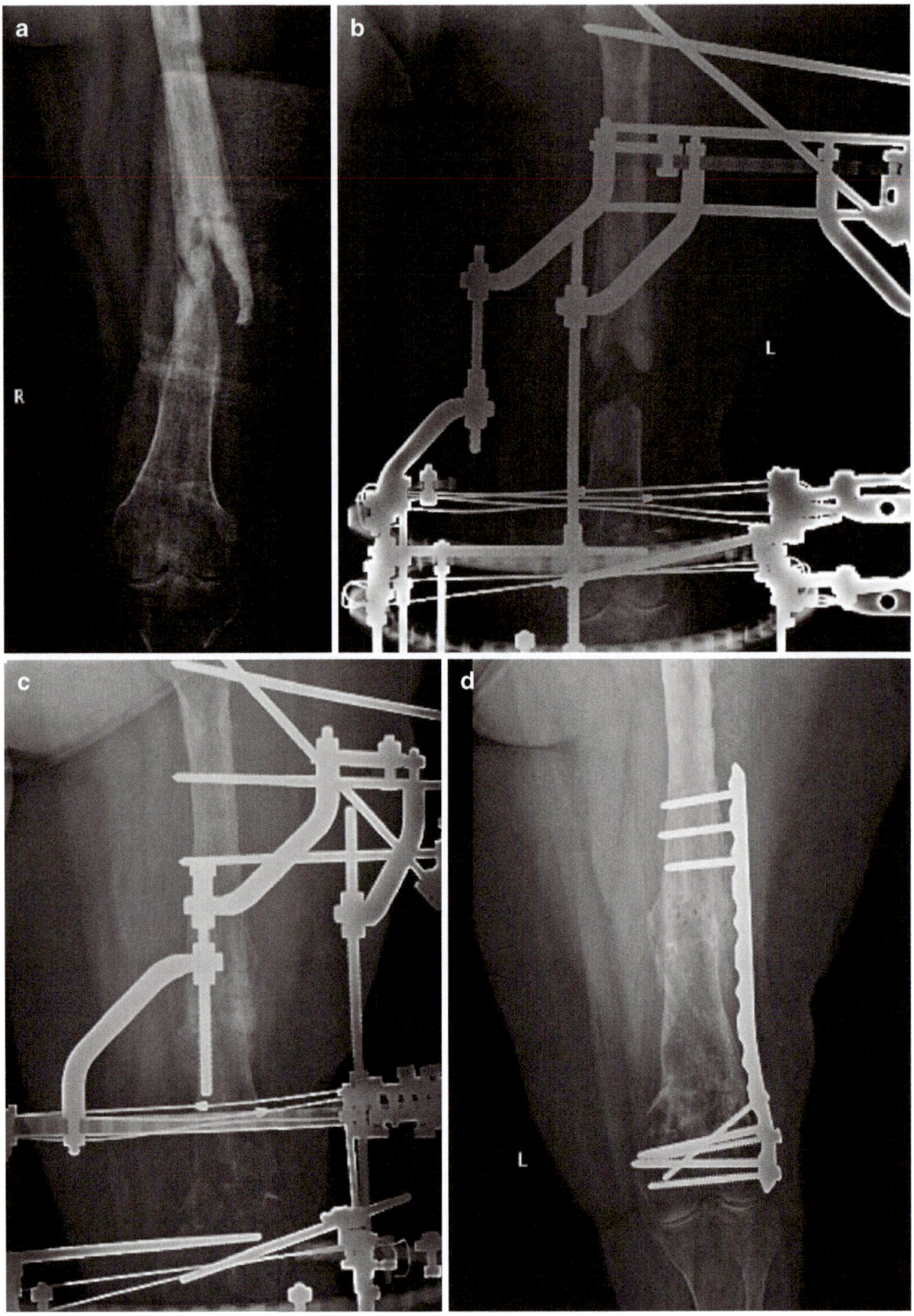

Fig. 26.9 A post-traumatic (open femur fracture) non-union in a 15-year old present for 2 years following medullary sepsis that complicated a retrograde femoral nailing procedure. An external fixator was removed as it became loose. The knee was stiff in extension and there were multiple draining sinuses (**a**). Body mass index was high. Debridement to bleeding bone with a distal corticotomy and retrograde transport (**b**) with a docking grafting procedure (**c**) followed by an interval stabilisation of the segment was performed (**d**). As the knee was stiff in extension (intra-articular and extra-articular causes) and the distal femoral bone stock poor, the fixator for transport was extended across the knee joint to improve the distal fixation

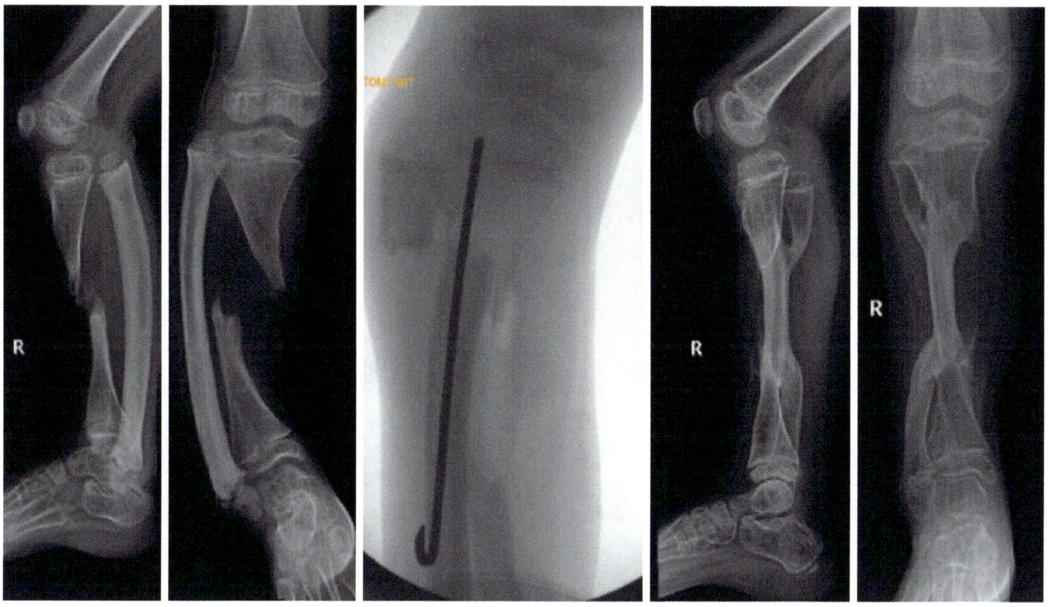

Fig. 26.10 Staged ipsilateral fibula transfer. The fibula was fixed using a Rush pin into the proximal segment. Following incorporation, the distal fragment is transferred across the path of the interosseous membrane and fixed using wires

stumps. If length is critical, then this can be achieved by distraction histogenesis at one or both sites of the fibula osteotomy (Fig. 26.13). The lower site is easier and does not put the common peroneal nerve under undue tension.

> Vascularised ipsilateral fibula transfer principle: An already hypertrophied fibula is a good donor to transfer.

> Tip: Careful soft tissue dissection is necessary with preservation of the fibula middle segment periosteum

Vascularised Contralateral Fibula Transfer as a Composite Free Flap

Where large limb length discrepancies exist and periosteum in the diaphysis has produced wispy poor regenerate, large, long defects can be reconstructed using a free vascularised fibula flap [31–33]. This has several advantages over a non-vascularised graft as firstly the incorporation speed is rapid and secondly it will hypertrophy quickly. It is particularly useful for lengthening and the slender fibula can be telescoped down the tibia and gradually pulled out to length after a latency of some 10 days to allow the vessel anastomoses to have soundly healed (Fig. 26.11). Concerns exist regarding donor site morbidity. Donor site fibular length insufficiency and ankle valgus is often noted on a radiograph. This can be mitigated by placement of screws to augment the interosseous membrane/syndesmosis whilst scar tissue forms. Our observation is that this entity is asymptomatic in childhood. However, this might pose a problem later in life. In low- and middle-income countries, microvascular services are often not available. The usefulness in chronic osteomyelitic bone gaps is limited in many settings as many of the preceding described techniques are successful and simpler to perform.

A free vascularised transfer success rate is typically 85% and will vary according to the unit. It requires microvascular training and equipment, usually with two teams of surgeons. Long surgical times are required with intraoperative maintenance of blood pressure without the use of inotropes/pressor agents. Post-operative high-level care is essential.

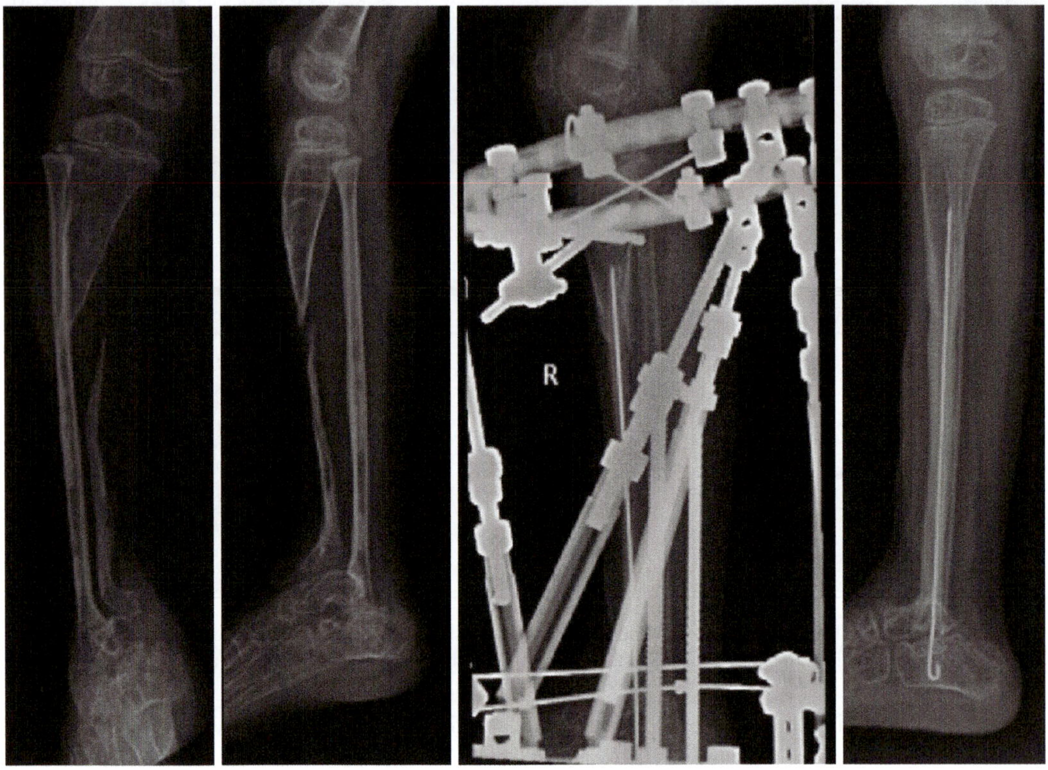

Fig. 26.11 The case illustration is of a large bone defect where distal sequestrum was excised; the disease process included the distal tibial plafond and the destroyed growth plate. The free fibula enabled a tibio-talar fusion with lengthening. The lengthened segment is fed inside the capacious proximal tibia and lengthening was stopped when the desired amount was achieved

Vascularised free fibula transfer principle: A successful vascularised fibula flap incorporates quickly. Best indication is where length and/or soft tissue envelope is problematic in an older child. A technically difficult multidisciplinary reconstruction, with recognized donor site morbidities.

Treatment of Limb Length Discrepancy/Angular Deformity Following Successful Bone Continuity

Physiolysis

Whilst physiolysis is recognised as more challenging in a post-sepsis physeal bar, a small bar in a young child would certainly be worth an attempt of physiolysis once the bone gap has been successfully treated.

Physiodesis of Contralateral Physes

Where a complete growth arrest is produced, all remaining growth from that plate is lost and a predictable amount of shortening at maturity can be calculated by using the multiplier method for 'growth remaining'. If the predicted height minus this amount of anticipated shortening because of the treatment is reasonable, then long-leg epiphysiodesis can be considered. Historically, the threshold for considering this was 5 cm, but sclerotic post-chronic osteomyelitis bone may not be wise to lengthen. This means that larger shortenings can be accepted should the patient be happy with this. Physiodesis can be in the same segment as in the contralateral shorter limb or a combination of segments timed to correct the limb length inequality. Using a combination of segments will produce a discrepancy in knee height but this is probably very acceptable up to 5 cm, making little changes to gait patterns. In the author's practice, the long-leg proximal fibular physis is also fused if the proximal tibia is halted in growth before the age of 11 years.

Complete Physiodesis

Angular deformity is often a sequela of severe chronic osteomyelitis due to focal physeal damage. Premature closure of the anterior proximal tibial physis produces a recurvatum deformity and a clinically apparent knee hyperextension (Fig. 26.12).

Soft Tissue Deficiency

Once all dead tissue has been removed, dressing changes on an old sinus is all that is often required in a child to achieve closure, which occurs by granulation tissue and epithelialisation. This requires good nutrition and regular wound care. Other techniques to achieve closure are shortening and the use of flaps. These should be used on a debrided bed where no dead bone remains.

Combinations of Above Techniques

One of the more difficult challenges is restoration of length in larger defects. Correction of length and angulation with distraction histogenesis and ipsilateral fibular transfer can be performed and are a good choice if the fibula is hypertrophied

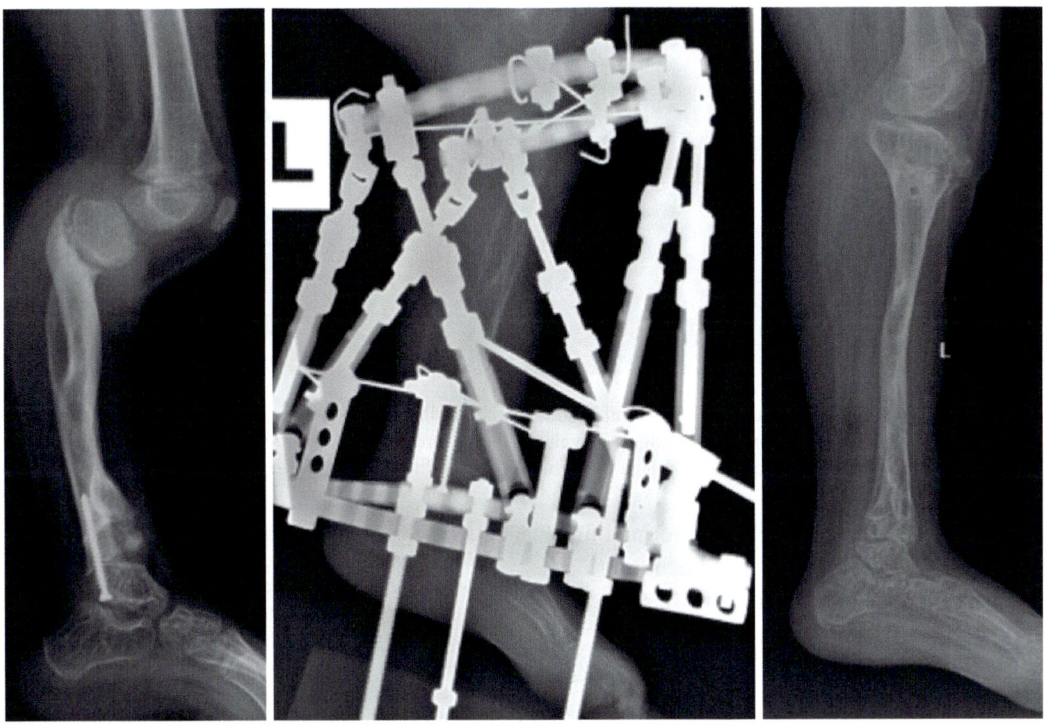

Fig. 26.12 The case illustration below shows combined complete physiodesis with recurvatum deformity correction with a hexapod fixator

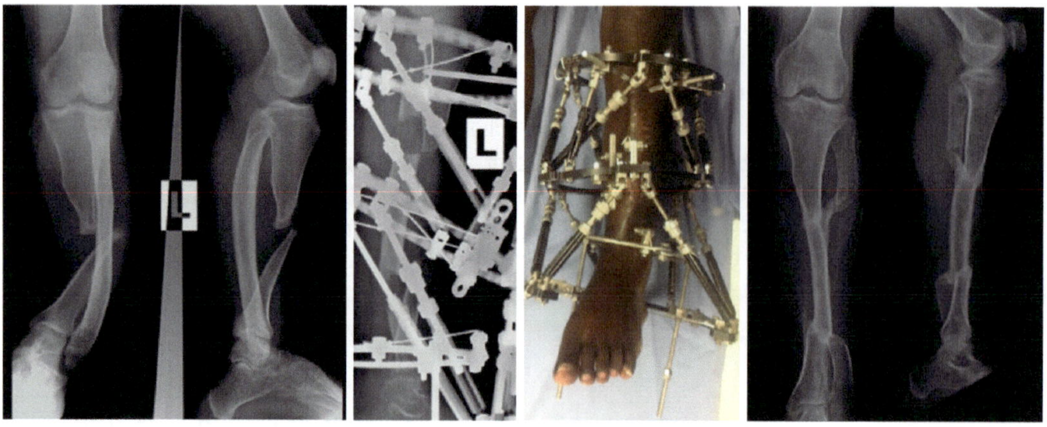

Fig. 26.13 A tibial segment that was 6 cm short with an old chronic osteomyelitis bone gap. The hypertrophied fibula was osteotomised in two places: the leg slightly over-lengthened on both sites and the fibula brought into the gap using a hexapod fixator. Grafting and docking procedures were required at both sites to ensure rapid union

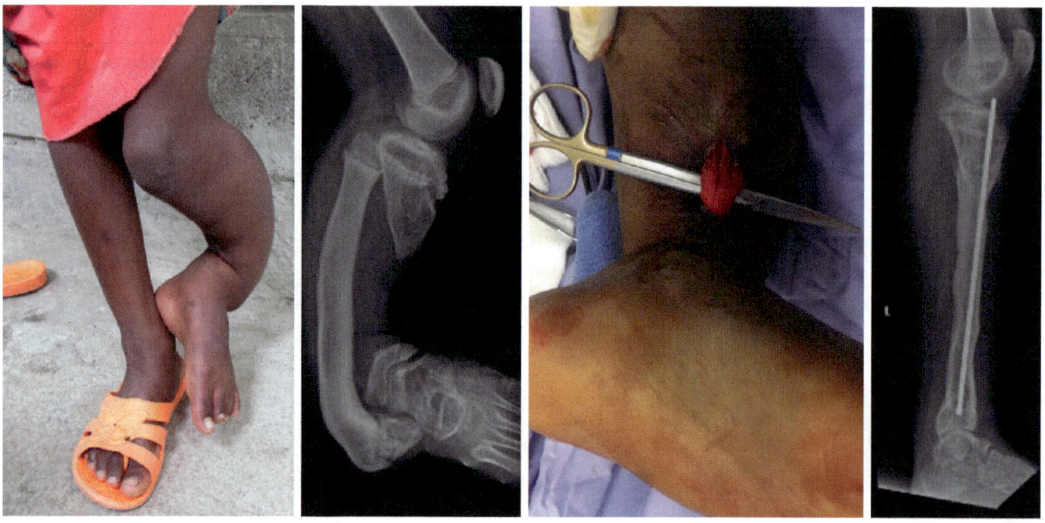

Fig. 26.14 Subtotal tibial defect with ipsilateral graduated fibular deformity correction and transfer. Note the subcutaneous thick soft tissue scar band (image c) in the place of the tibia, which was palpable and likely contributing to produce this severe fibular deformity. This was resected first to allow easier lower-leg distraction

(Fig. 26.13). The hypertrophied deformed fibula may require initial deformity correction prior to transfer and tibialisation (Fig. 26.14).

References

1. Stevenson AJ, Wynn Jones H, Chokotho LC, Beckles VLL, Harrison WJ. The Beit CURE Classification of Childhood Chronic Haematogenous Osteomyelitis—a guide to treatment. J Orthop Surg Res. 2015; 10: 144. Published online 2015 Sep 17. https://doi.org/10.1186/s13018-015-0282-9
2. Dartnell J, Ramachandran M, Katchburian M. Haematogenous acute and subacute paediatric osteomyelitis: a systematic review of the literature. J Bone Joint Surg (Br). 2012;94(5):584–95. https://doi.org/10.1302/0301-620X.94B5.28523.
3. Moormeier DE, Bayles KW. Staphylococcus aureus biofilm: a complex developmental organism. Molecular Microbiology. 2017;104(3):365–376. https://doi.org/10.1111/mmi.13634.
4. Daoud A, Saighi-Bouaouina A. Treatment of sequestra, pseudarthroses, and defects in the long bones of children who have chronic hematogenous osteomyelitis. J Bone Joint Surg Am. 1989;71(10):1448–68.
5. Jain AK, Sharma DK, Kumar S, Sethi A, Arora A, Tuli SM. Incorporation of diaphyseal sequestra in

chronic haematogenous osteomyelitis. Int Orthop. 1995;19(4):238–41.
6. Wynn Jones H, Bates J, Harrison WJ. The use of over-penetrated radiographs for assessment of chronic osteomyelitis in children. Ann R Coll Surg Engl. 2007;89(8):821–2. https://doi.org/10.1308/003588407X232143h.
7. Hosny GA, Ahmed AA. Infected tibial nonunion in children: is radical debridement mandatory? Injury. 2019;50(2):590–7.
8. Ellur V, Kumar G, Sampath JS. Treatment of chronic hematogenous osteomyelitis in children with antibiotic impregnated calcium sulphate. J Pediatr Orthop. 2021;41(2):127–31.
9. Canavese F, Corradin M, Khan A, Mansour M, Rousset M, Samba A. Successful treatment of chronic osteomyelitis in children with debridement, antibiotic-laden cement spacer and bone graft substitute. Eur J Orthop Surg Traumatol. 2017;27:221–8.
10. Wen H, Zhu S, Li C, Xu Y. Bone transport versus acute shortening for the management of infected tibial bone defects: a meta-analysis. BMC Musculoskelet Disord. 2020;21(1):80.
11. Pierrie SN, Hsu JR. Shortening and angulation strategies to address composite bone and soft tissue defects. J Orthop Trauma. 2017;31(Suppl 5):S32–5.
12. Ryzewicz M, Morgan SJ, Linford E, Thwing JI, de Resende GV, Smith WR. Central bone grafting for nonunion of fractures of the tibia: a retrospective series. J Bone Joint Surg Br. 2009;91(4):522–9.
13. Masquelet AC, Begue T. The concept of induced membrane for reconstruction of long bone defects. Orthop Clin North Am. 2010;41(1):27–37.
14. Morelli I, Drago L, George DA, Romanò D, Romanò CL. Managing large bone defects in children: a systematic review of the 'induced membrane technique'. J Pediatr Orthop B. 2018;27(5):443–55.
15. Gouron R, Deroussen F, Plancq M-C, Collet L-M. Bone defect reconstruction in children using the induced membrane technique: a series of 14 cases. Orthop Traumatol Surg Res. 2013;99(7):837–43.
16. Rousset M, Walle M, Cambou L, et al. Chronic infection and infected non-union of the long bones in paediatric patients: preliminary results of bone versus beta-tricalcium phosphate grafting after induced membrane formation. Int Orthop. 2018;42(2):385–93.
17. Cruickshank JA, Graham M, Harrison WJ. Immediate bone transport: a novel technique for the management of bone defects after chronic osteomyelitis in children. Trop Dr. 2018;48(1):64–6. https://doi.org/10.1177/0049475517717361.
18. Patwardhan S, Shyam AK, Mody RA, Sancheti PK, Mehta R, Agrawat H. Reconstruction of bone defects after osteomyelitis with nonvascularized fibular graft: a retrospective study in twenty-six children. J Bone Joint Surg Am. 2013;95:e56(1–6).
19. Tuli SM. Tibialization of the fibula. Clin Orthop Relat Res. 2005;431:80–4.
20. Steinlechner CWB, Mkandawire NC. Non-vascularised fibular transfer in the management of defects of long bones after sequestrectomy in children. JBJS-Br. 2005; 87-B(9). https://doi.org/10.1302/0301-620X.87B9.15734
21. Agarwal A, Kumar D, Agrawal N, Gupta N. Ankle valgus following non-vascularized fibular grafts in children-an outcome evaluation minimum two years after fibular harvest. Int Orthop. 2017;41(5):949–55. https://doi.org/10.1007/s00264-017-3403-8. Epub 2017 Feb 16. PMID: 28210804.
22. Agarwal A. Fibular donor site following non vascularized harvest: clinico-radiological outcome at minimal five-year follow-up. Int Orthop. 2019;43(8):1927–31. https://doi.org/10.1007/s00264-018-4086-5. Epub 2018 Aug 7. PMID: 30088054.
23. Ilizarov GA, Ledyaev VI. The replacement of long tubular bone defects by lengthening distraction osteotomy of one of the fragments. 1969. Clin Orthop Relat Res. 1992;(280):7–10.
24. Kucukkaya M, Kabukcuoglu Y, Tezer M, Kuzgun U. Management of childhood chronic tibial osteomyelitis with the Ilizarov method. J Pediatr Orthop. 2002;22(5):632–7.
25. Yeargan SA 3rd, Nakasone CK, Shaieb MD, Montgomery WP, Reinker KA. Treatment of chronic osteomyelitis in children resistant to previous therapy. J Pediatr Orthop. 2004;24(1):109–22.
26. El-Rosasy MA. Ilizarov treatment for pseudarthrosis of the tibia due to haematogenous osteomyelitis. J Pediatr Orthop B. 2013;22(3):200–6.
27. Abdelkhalek M, El-Alfy B, Ali AM. Ilizarov bone transport versus fibular graft for reconstruction of tibial bone defects in children. J PediatrOrthop B. 2016;25(6):556–60. https://doi.org/10.1097/BPB.0000000000000334.
28. Huntington TW. Case of bone transference: use of a segment of fibula to supply a defect in the tibia. Ann Surg. 1905;41:249e251.
29. Gupta SP, Garg G. The Huntington procedure: still a reasonable option for large tibial defects in paediatric patients. J Child Orthop. 2014;8(5):413–21. https://doi.org/10.1007/s11832-014-0618-8.
30. Khan AQ, Siddiqui YS. Julfiqar, Abbas M, Sabir AB. Role of Huntington procedure as a limb salvage surgery for complex gap nonunion of tibia in children. J Clin Orthop Trauma. 2021;18:20–4.
31. Zalavras CG, Femino D, Triche R, Zionts L, Stevanovic M. Reconstruction of large skeletal defects due to osteomyelitis with the vascularized fibular graft in children. J Bone Joint Surg Am. 2007;89:2233–40.
32. Sun Y, Zhang C, Jin D, Sheng J, Cheng X, Liu X, Chen S, Zeng B. Free vascularised fibular grafting in the treatment of large skeletal defects due to osteomyelitis. Int Orthop. 2010;34:425–30.
33. Loro A, Hodges A, Galiwango GW, Loro F. Vascularized fibula flap in the management of segmental bone loss following osteomyelitis in children at a Ugandan hospital. J Bone Jt Infect. 2021;6(6):179–87. https://doi.org/10.5194/jbji-6-179-2021.

Post Infective Bone Gap Management: Induced Membrane Technique

27

Richard Gouron

Introduction

The induced membrane technique for bone reconstruction was first described by Masquelet [1] in the context of multitissue repair of the tibia after chronic bone infection in adults. The technique involves two distinct surgical sessions. After infected tissue and necrotic bone have been removed, the bone defect is filled with polymethylmethacrylate (PMMA) cement. The segment is stabilization with a screwed plate, a nail, or an external fixator, depending on the overlying tissue coverage (fascia, muscle and/or skin). Once the infection has been cleared and local wounds have healed (typically by 6 weeks after the first operation), the second operation can be undertaken. An incision is carefully created in the membrane that has formed around the surgical cement. The cement is then carefully broken up and removed, that is, without damaging the membrane. Fragmented, corticocancellous bone is then grafted into the membrane, which serves as a mold for reconstruction. Graft expansion (using an allograft or a bone substitute) is possible but should not exceed 30% of the total graft volume. Once the bone has stabilized, the membrane is sutured tightly, and the surgical site is closed. Provided that the infection does not recur, the bone will consolidate over the following weeks or months.

In children, the Masquelet technique was first used to treat long bone loss following the surgical resection of bone sarcomas [2]. The indication was then extended to reconstructions necessitated by congenital abnormalities, such as congenital pseudarthrosis and the treatment of bone infections [3]. Use of this technique in young children and in the context of residual bone growth involves a few technical challenges [4], which will be described in more detail below.

Most acute bone infections in children are hematogenous and are usually cured with antibiotic therapy. However, some infections can become chronic; this may result in bone sequestration or necrosis that requires reconstruction in the long term. In other cases, posttraumatic or postoperative bone infections (Fig. 27.1) may lead to bone loss. However, the implementation of the Masquelet technique does not depend on the source or cause of the infection.

The Physiology of the Masquelet Technique

The Masquelet technique is increasingly used for reconstruction because it is easy to perform and has a high success rate. This biological method

R. Gouron (✉)
Department of Pediatric Orthopedic Surgery, Amiens University Medical Center and Jules Verne University of Picardie, Amiens, France

Service d'Orthopédie Pédiatrique, CHU Amiens, Groupe Hospitalier Sud, Amiens, France
e-mail: gouron.richard@chu-amiens.fr

© Springer Nature Switzerland AG 2022
M. V. Belthur et al. (eds.), *Pediatric Musculoskeletal Infections*,
https://doi.org/10.1007/978-3-030-95794-0_27

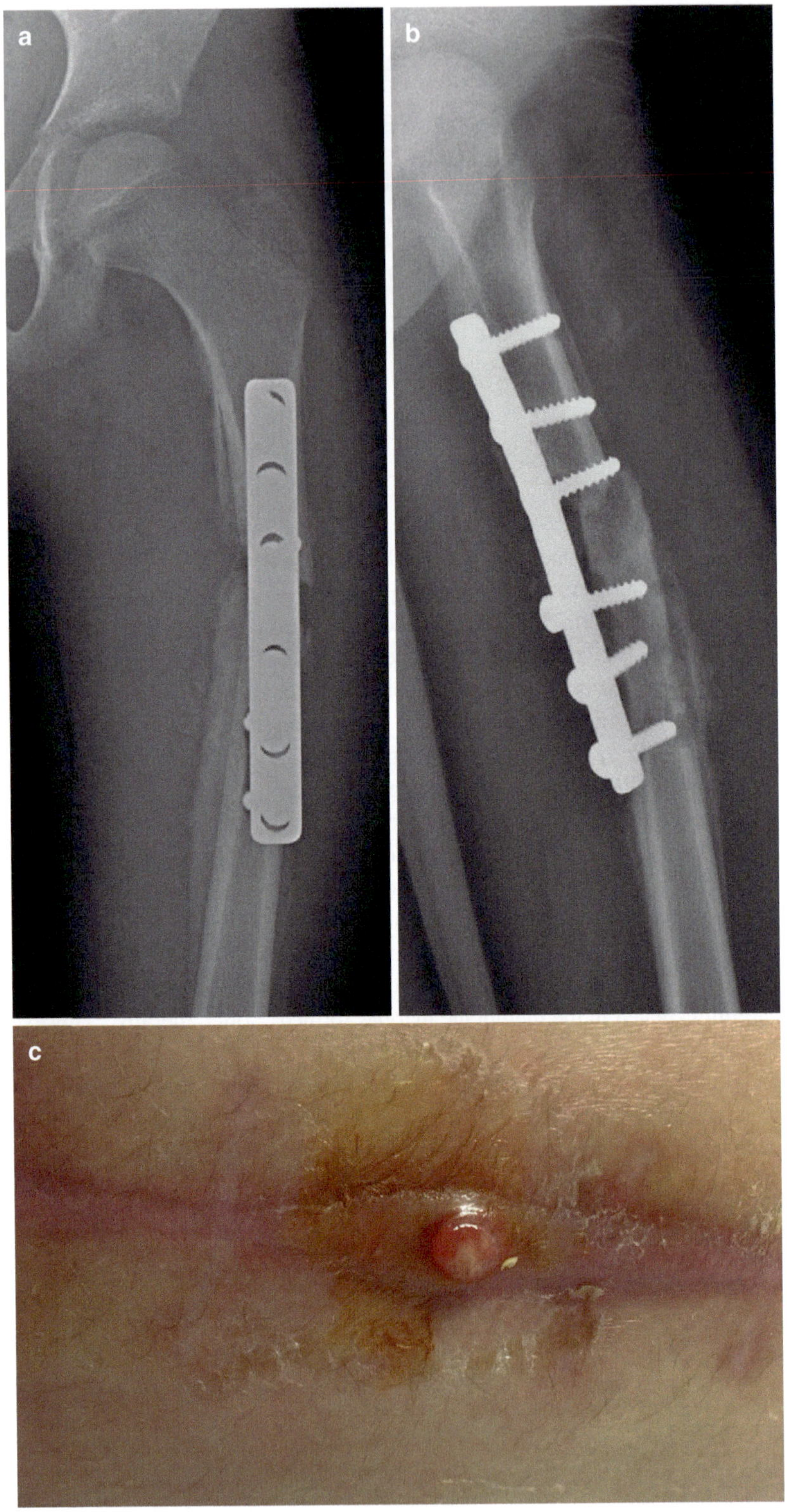

Fig. 27.1 Femoral osteomyelitis after fracture treatment in an eight-year-old girl. Antero-posterior X-ray view (**a**) and lateral X-ray view (**b**). Septic fistula on the scar (**c**)

meets all the present criteria for bone reconstruction. Corticocancellous bone is grafted into a mechanically stable, growth-factor-rich, well-vascularized environment [5]. Indeed, it has been shown that the membrane that forms in response to the presence of a foreign body (the PMMA cement) contains many different growth factors [6]. The membrane is well vascularized and can protect the morcelized corticocancellous graft from resorption. Osteoclasts accumulate at the interface with the cement [7], which enables rapid remodeling of the graft via creeping substitution. The membrane is also rich in mesenchymal stem cells, which can differentiate into osteoblasts. Thus, the graft remodels and consolidates very quickly. The membrane itself may calcify.

Description of the Technique [4]

The induced membrane technique enables the reconstruction of diaphyseal or metaphyseal defects in long bones. It also helps to control bone infections through the broad excision of infected tissues.

The First Surgical Session

Surgical Site Preparation

For obvious reasons, implementation of this procedure can only be considered after optimal infection control and the full excision of contaminated or necrotic tissue. Biopsies must be cultured to identify the bacterium or fungus (mucormycosis) responsible for osteomyelitis. Necrotic or pseudarthrotic bone must be pared back to healthy areas (Fig. 27.2). To avoid leaving devascularized bone in place, it is better to remove too much bone than too little [8].

It is essential to plan skin/muscle coverage at this stage because the cement spacer cannot be left uncovered. This may involve the creation of local or regional muscle flaps or free muscle flaps and can be combined with negative pressure therapy.

Bone Stabilization

The bone must be stabilized prior to insertion of the cement spacer. The gap between the bone fragments must be maintained. This step is particularly delicate in children because of the presence of the growth plate at each end of the long bone. In cases of severe sepsis, it is not always appropriate to stabilize the bone with in situ material; this might perpetuate the infection and thus compromise reconstruction. If the osteomyelitis is severe, it is preferable to stabilize the operating area via external fixation. An external ring fixation is usually preferred (especially for the tibia) because it avoids the shear stresses associated with single-plane fixation and favors the compressive stresses that facilitate consolidation (Fig. 27.3). External fixation is also easy to use in children because it can be positioned outside the growth zones. Single-plane fixation is more feasible for the femur and the humerus.

If the infection is not severe, the bone can be stabilized directly. In very young children, elastic, stable, intramedullary nails can be used, although additional cast immobilization is required for sufficient stabilization. Plate stabilization is more rigid but is cumbersome for children, and it is often not possible to insert the plate near to growth areas. However, plate stabilization is perfectly applicable for older children and adolescents. Nail fixation can be applied in older children once the bones have stopped growing. It enables the resumption of weight-bearing activity even when the bone has not fully consolidated. Nail fixation also has the advantage of taking up a lot of space, and so filling the bone defect requires a much smaller graft volume.

Installation of the Spacer

The spacer can now be installed in the bone defect. The PMMA cement contains antibiotics, which will spread locally in the 6 weeks prior to the graft. Installation of the spacer requires some preparation; the surgical site must be prepared by the installation of a mold that will shape the spacer. Syringes cut in half can be placed on each end of the bone end and are then sutured together to mold the entire length of the bone defect. To

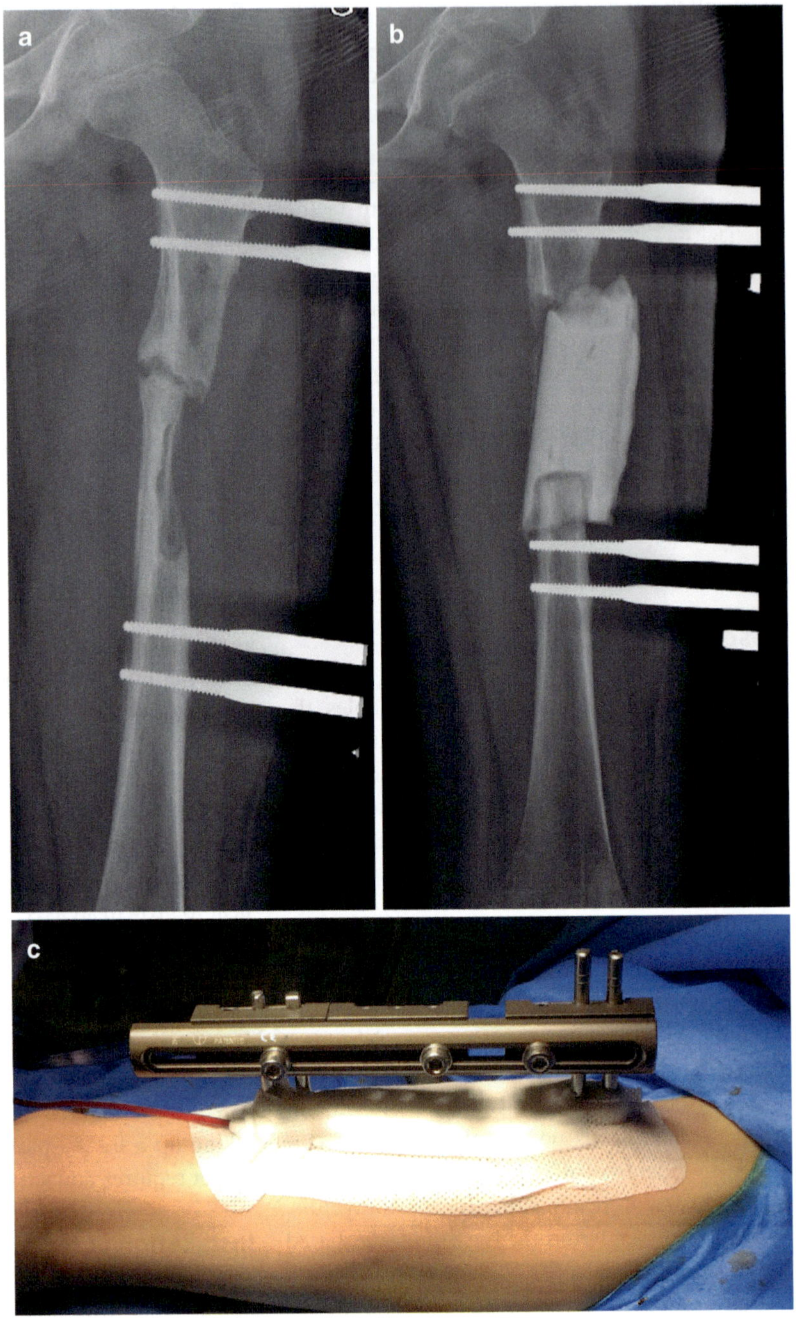

Fig. 27.2 Necrotic bone after plate removal (same patient as in Fig. 27.1) and stabilization using external fixation (**a**). Necrotic bone pared back to healthy areas and cement interposition (**b**) after biological control of the infection using appropriate antibiotics. Stabilization using single-plane fixation (**c**)

facilitate introduction of the cement installation and to maintain spacing, tractor wires can be installed in the syringes (Fig. 27.4). If the bone can be stabilized with a locked screw plate, locked screws can be installed in the defect; they will maintain the space between the syringes and help to give the right shape to the reconstructed bone (Fig. 27.5). Furthermore, the syringes usefully protect the surrounding tissue from the heat released by formation of the PMMA.

The cement is still malleable at this stage and is applied so that it covers each end of the bone inside the syringes. Enough cement is used to recreate the shape of the bone to be reconstructed.

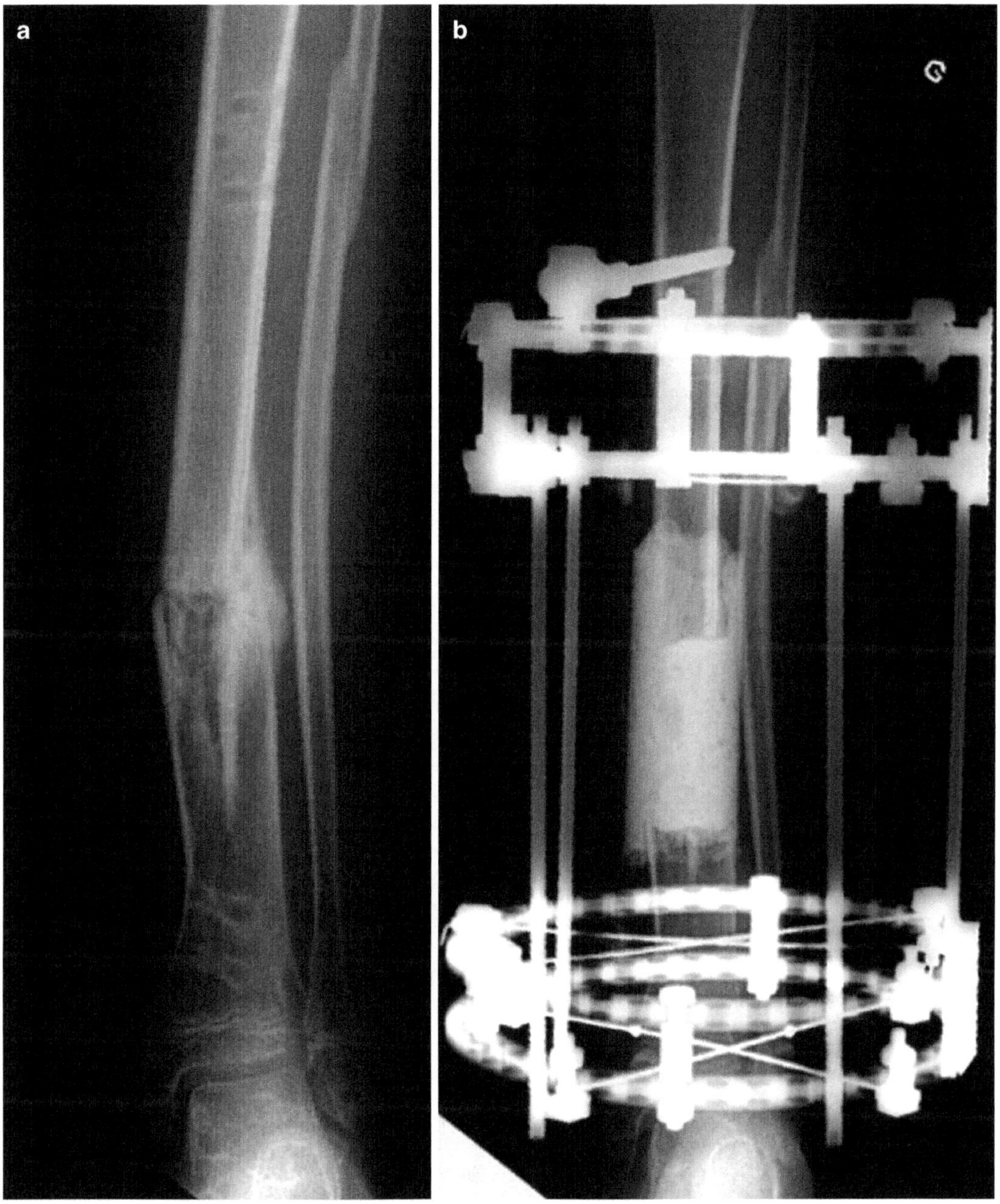

Fig. 27.3 Septic pseudarthrosis after open tibial fracture (**a**). Cement interposition after septic bone removal and stabilization using an external ring fixation (**b**)

The surgical site is washed with saline regularly in order to dissipate the heat released during polymerization. Once the cement has set, the syringes can be easily removed by pulling on the previously installed tractor wires.

Wound Closure

The muscle layer is sutured over the cement spacer. If necessary, a muscle flap is formed so that the cement is completely covered. The skin is closed with a tight suture.

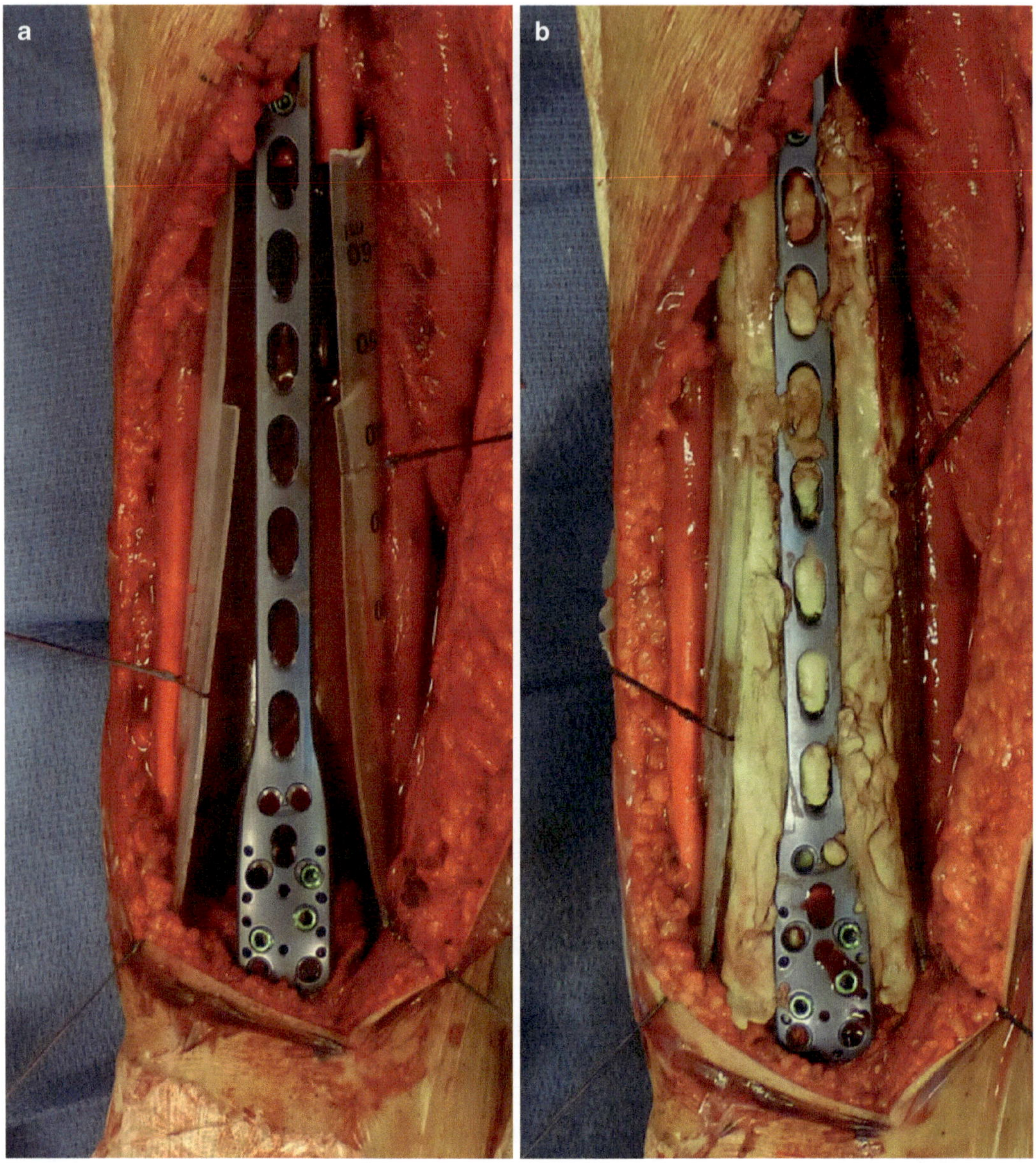

Fig. 27.4 Example of a tibial reconstruction. Syringes cut in half placed on each end of the bone end and sutured together to mold the entire length of the bone defect. To facilitate introduction of the cement installation and to maintain spacing, tractor wires are installed in the syringes (**a**). The cement spacer installed in the bone defect (**b**)

Postoperative Care

Empiric intravenous antibiotic therapy is initiated and can then be adjusted according to the results of the bacterial cultures of intraoperative samples. The antibiotic therapy can often be continued per os once levels of inflammation markers have normalized for at least 3 months.

Weight must not be placed on the limb with the bone defect.

The Second Surgical Session

The second surgical step can be performed about 45 days after the first. Levels of C-reactive protein must have normalized, and local (surgical site) wounds must have healed.

If local discharge or inflammation is present, reoperation, debridement, tissue sampling, removal of the cement, washing of the surgical

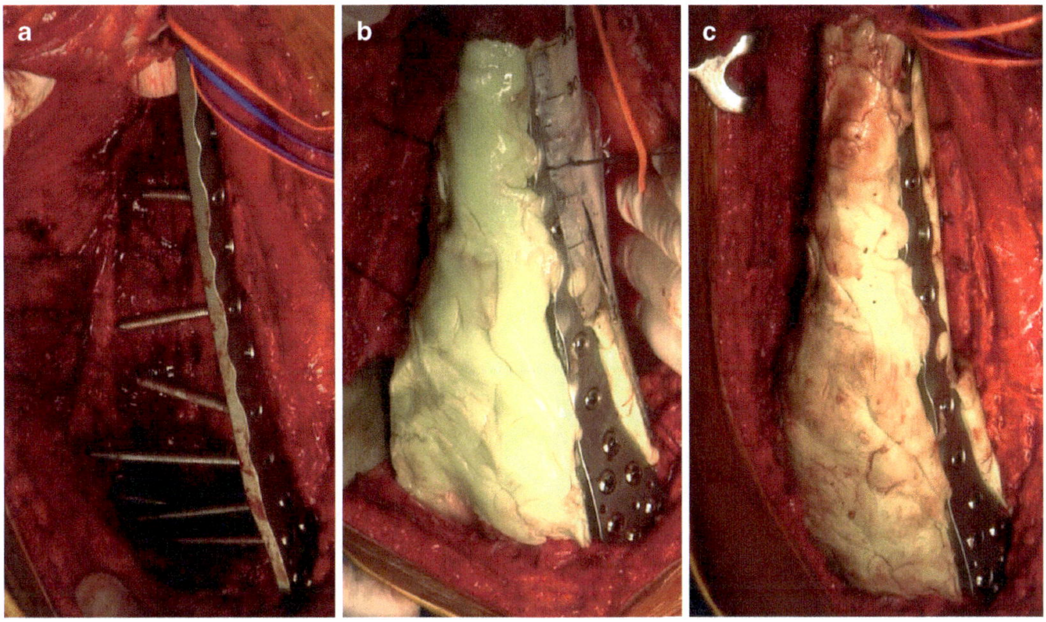

Fig. 27.5 Example of a distal femoral reconstruction. Stabilization with a locked screw plate. Locked screws installed in the defect (**a**) to maintain the space between the syringes and help to give the right shape to the reconstructed bone. Cement installation in the syringes (**b**). Once the cement has set, the syringes are easily removed by pulling on the previously installed tractor wires (**c**)

site, and re-application of cement (as described above) are required. A further course of antibiotic therapy is then initiated and should be adjusted according to the results of the bacterial cultures. The site is then left to heal for a further 6 weeks. The cement serves as a sentinel for resolution of the infection.

If the surgical site is clean 45 days later, the second stage can be initiated.

Preparation of the Graft

The graft must be planned and prepared before further intervention at the defect site. It will mainly be composed of morselized corticocancellous bone; this is why the posterior iliac crests are typically used. Each posterior crest enables the reconstruction of about 5 cm of diaphyseal bone.

The bone is harvested with the patient in the prone position. An oblique incision is made on the posterior iliac crest. The periosteum on the lateral surface of the crest is lifted. Flaps of cortical bone are harvested with a gouge chisel. Flaps of cancellous bone are then harvested until the inner cortical surface can be seen. Bone marrow from this site is removed with a syringe and mixed with the waiting graft. Bone wax is applied lightly to the harvesting site before closure. The periosteum is repositioned and sutured over the crest. Wound closure does not require drainage.

The second crest is harvested in the same manner, if necessary.

The graft is then divided up evenly with an electric grinder. Graft expansion may be necessary if the volume to be filled is large; if so, a fragmented allograft is mixed with the harvested graft and bone marrow. The allograft volume should not exceed one-third of the total graft volume.

This graft volume is often sufficient (Fig. 27.6). In femoral and metaphyseal locations, it is prudent to add a bone strut (taken from the contralateral tibia) for mechanical reinforcement and expansion of the graft volume. The strut is usually harvested later in the surgical session (see the description below), once the exact dimensions have been established.

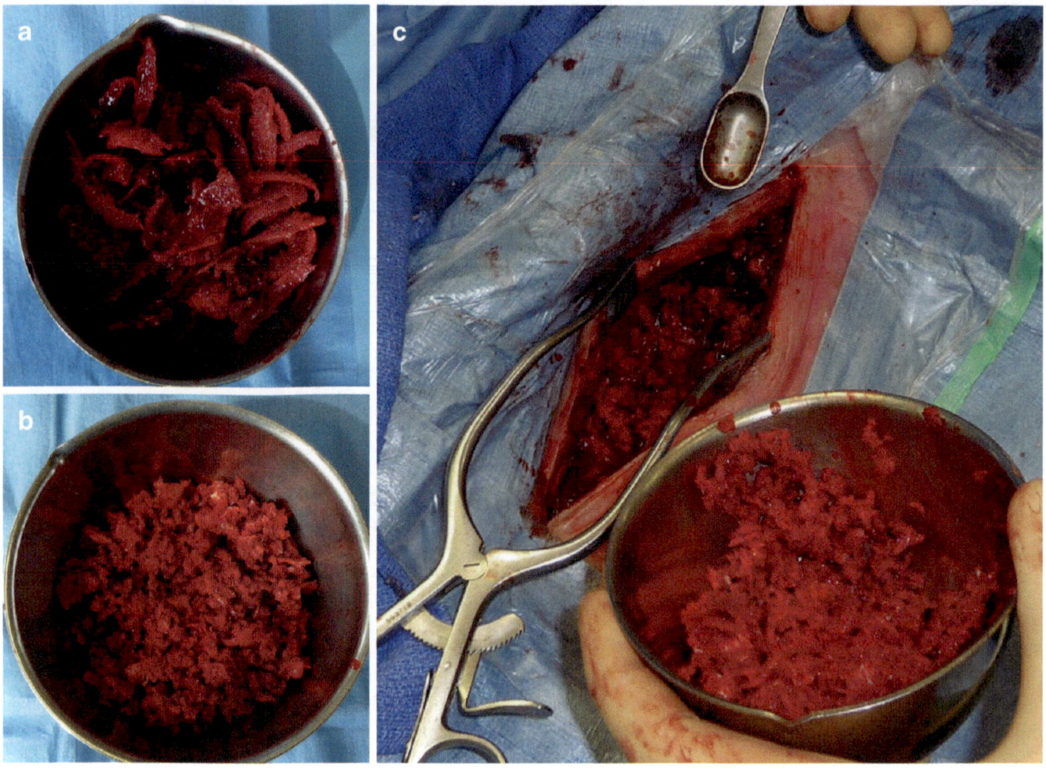

Fig. 27.6 Flaps of cancellous bone harvested from posterior iliac crests (**a**). The graft after been divided up evenly with an electric grinder (**b**) inserted in the defect into the induced membrane (**c**)

The whole graft is kept on a sterile table as the patient changes position for the second surgical step.

The Surgical Approach

The skin is incised over the old scar, and the cement spacer is approached longitudinally and directly. If a muscle flap had been created, it can be lifted at this point. Tissue samples are again collected for bacteriological analysis and confirmation of the absence of infection.

Clear discharge is always observed in contact with the cement; a very thick, non-adherent membrane will have formed at the interface with the cement. The membrane is carefully lifted up and moved away, which thus fully exposes the cement spacer.

The cement is then removed. It is first weakened with a motorized drill and then fragmented with a chisel. It is essential not to damage the membrane at this stage. Any residual cement debris is then washed out of the operating site. If any screws had been placed in the defect void, they are removed and kept to hand for later use.

Bone Repermeabilization

At this stage, it is important to repermeabilize the upstream and downstream diaphyseal bone using a square awl or a drill bit. It is also important to sharpen and shear the upstream and downstream bone, to facilitate its consolidation.

Checking Bone Stabilization

At this point, the surgeon must check that the bone has been fully stabilized. The external fixator must be stable but can be supplemented with pins if required. If a plate is present, the screws must still be tight.

The Graft

A tibial strut can be installed in the diaphyseal and metaphyseal areas, opposite a plate or external fixator. The strut is harvested from the concomitantly prepared contralateral tibia. The strut should be 2 cm longer than the void to be filled. It is embedded in the metaphysis, placed along a diaphysis, fixed firmly, and (if possible) screwed back onto the plate using the screws that were initially placed in the void (Fig. 27.7). The strut maintains the width of the reconstructed bone. The whole graft and its expansion are then placed into the membrane (Fig. 27.8), with special attention paid to the bone ends.

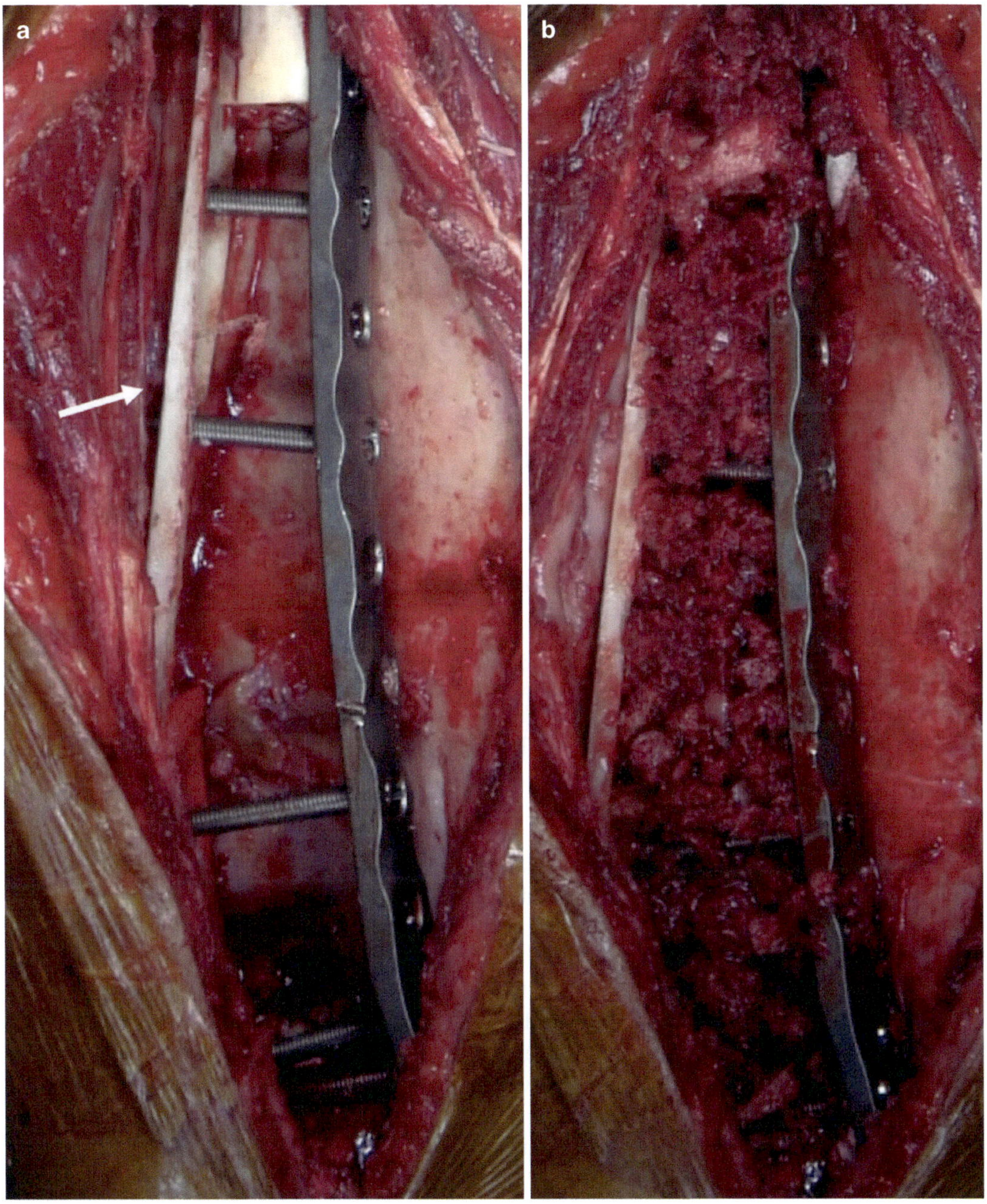

Fig. 27.7 Tibial strut (white arrow) fixed firmly and screwed back onto the plate using the screws that were initially placed in the void (**a**). The whole graft and its expansion are then placed into the membrane (**b**)

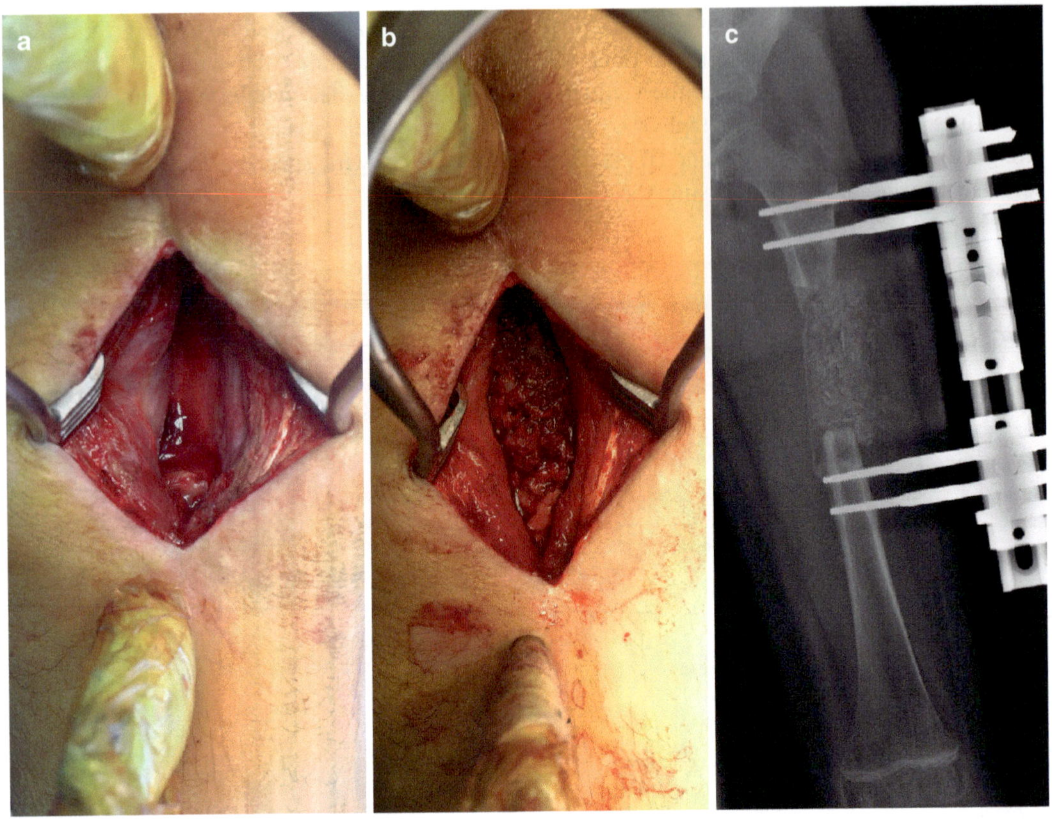

Fig. 27.8 Bone defect (same patient as in Fig. 27.1) after cement removal (**a**). The whole graft placed into the membrane (**b**). Antero-posterior X-ray view with graft in place (**c**) after the second surgical session

Closure

The membrane is then closed using a tight overlocking suture. The muscle is also sutured, and the skin is closed. No drainage is required.

Postoperative Care

Any ongoing antibiotic therapy is continued. Weight must not be placed on the operated limb. It is usual to see discharge, but this will stop spontaneously after a few days.

The graft is checked on an X-ray every month. The healing at the ends of the graft (the most delicate) must be monitored carefully. Weight-bearing is not allowed until the extremities have consolidated fully; this usually takes between 2 and 6 months, depending on the bone's length and site (Fig. 27.9).

Complications

The main complication of this reconstruction technique is pseudarthrosis at each end of the reconstructed area [3, 9]. If the surgical technique has been implemented rigorously (i.e., with sharpening of the edges and repermeabilization of the medullary canal), pseudarthrosis should not occur. If the extremities have not consolidated 6 months after the graft placement, iterative grafting and decortication surgery must be performed. In some cases, a different bone stabilization technique must be used to stiffen the assembly. For example, a screwed plate can be installed 3–4 weeks after the removal of an external fixator when all the skin orifices have healed. This procedure can only be performed during

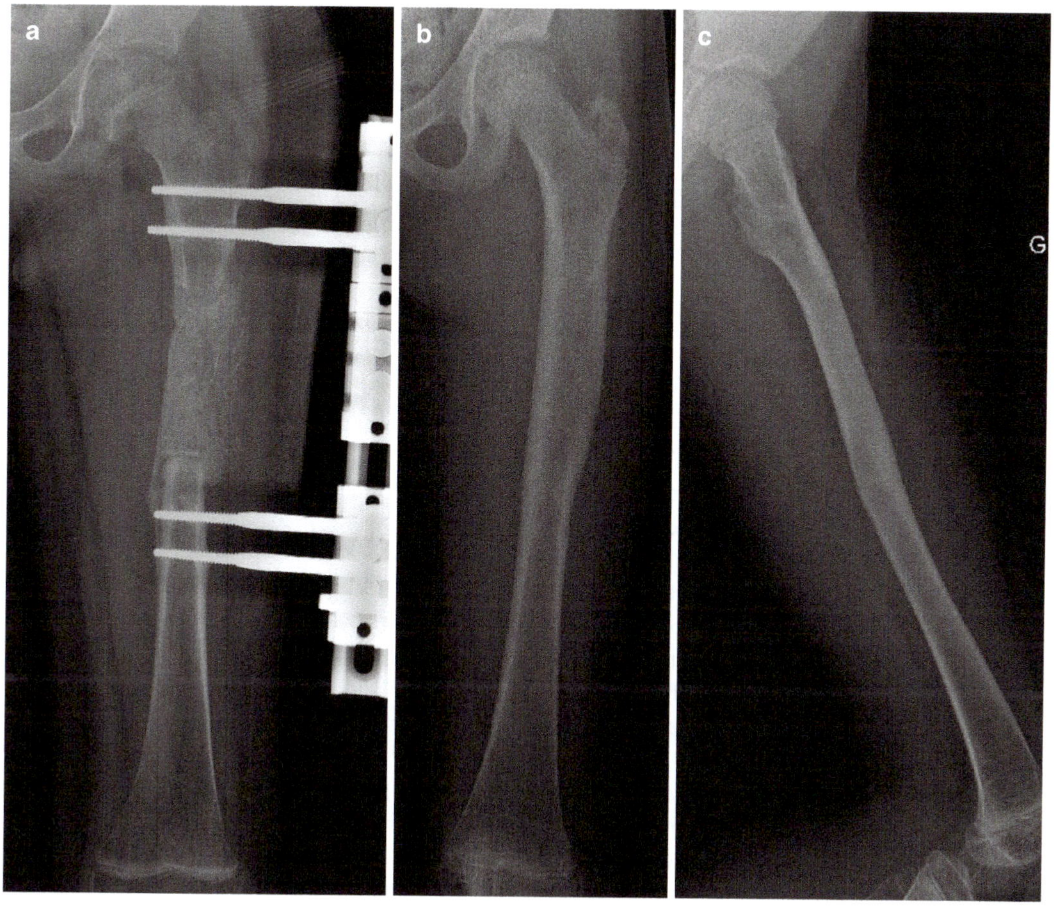

Fig. 27.9 Antero-posterior X-ray view (same patient as in Fig. 27.1) 45 days after the second surgical session (**a**) showing bone healing. Antero-posterior X-ray view (**b**) and lateral X-ray view (**c**) 6 months after the second surgical session showing total bone remodeling

prophylactic antibiotic treatment and once the initial infection has healed.

Slow bone healing is common and should not be classified as a complication per se. Patients must be aware that they will not be able to place weight on the limb for a long time—up to 12 months, in some cases. This is not always easily achievable in pediatric patients but must be explained clearly. The patient must receive appropriate supportive care.

Failure of the stabilization equipment is a typical complication; bone healing is always long, and the equipment is subject to high levels of stress. Osteolysis may occur around an external fixator's pins and will require the latter's revision. Screws in a plate may break and will have to be replaced. The type of stabilization can be changed, if necessary. In very young children, stabilization via elastic stable intramedullary nailing should always be accompanied by plaster cast immobilization for as long as required.

Graft resorptions (i.e., complete disappearance of the graft) have been described in cases of tumor reconstruction but not during the treatment of an infection [10]. Nevertheless, the physician should screen for this complication because it may mean that an infection has recurred. Deep tissue samples should be collected. Use of a different reconstruction technique (such as bone transport or vascularized bone grafting) should then be considered.

Lastly, failure might result from the induced membrane's inherent composition and the patient's genetic predispositions (e.g., the metalloproteinase-9/tissue inhibitor of metalloproteinases-1 gene expression ratio) [11].

Discussion of the Technique in the Literature

The induced membrane (Masquelet) reconstruction technique gives good results and failures are rare [12]. It generally gives a better functional result than the other techniques with a return to normal function in most cases [6, 13, 14]. This technique is also a good choice for the reconstruction of periarticular bone defects [13].

However, the quantity of the graft obtained in children is subject to debate. In adults, use of a reamer/irrigator/aspirator makes it possible to obtain a large amount of graft material without removing the posterior iliac crests. This procedure goes through the growth cartilage and is therefore prohibited in a pediatric setting. However, the amount of graft material is usually the limiting factor in pediatric cases [4], especially in very young children. This is why graft expansion may be required. The fragmented allograft described above is one possible option. Rousset et al. [15] reported that beta-tricalcium-phosphate graft expansion was associated with high-quality reconstructed bone and, above all, a shorter consolidation time. Larger-scale studies of these aspects are now warranted (Boxes 27.1–27.3).

Outcomes

The induced membrane technique has been utilized more frequently over the last decade to treat pediatric post-infective bone defects. This technique offers promising early/midterm functional outcomes. However, the graft volume in children remains a challenge. Induced membrane technique with the addition of bone graft expanders and biological enhancement may provide a promising solution while treating post-infective bone defects in children.

Box 27.1 Key Learning Points

- All infected tissue (including bone) must be excised.
- The cement spacer must cover each end of the bone completely and must be larger than the bone defect.
- The bone must be stabilized as firmly as possible.
- The infection must be controlled, using appropriate antibiotics.

Box 27.2 Tips and Tricks

- Syringes cut in half can be used as molds to facilitate installation of the spacer.
- Screws can be placed in the bone defect to help maintain the bone width for plate osteosynthesis.
- Each posterior iliac crest will provide 5 cm of diaphyseal bone for reconstruction.

Box 27.3 Pitfalls to Avoid

- Filling the defect when the infection is not under control.
- Not covering the cement sufficiently with tissue or muscle (i.e., an increased risk of exposure).
- Forgetting to decorticate the bone ends and repermeabilize the medullary canal in areas at risk of pseudarthrosis.

References

1. Masquelet AC, Fitoussi F, Begue T, Muller GP. Reconstruction des os longs par membrane induite et autogreffe spongieuse. Ann Chir Plast Esthét. 2000;45:346–53.

2. Villemagne T, Bonnard C, Accadbled F, L'kaissi M, de Billy B, Sales de Gauzy J. Intercalary segmental reconstruction of long bones after malignant bone tumor resection using primary methyl methacrylate cement spacer interposition and secondary bone grafting: the induced membrane technique. J Pediatr Orthop. 2011;31:570–6.
3. Gouron R, Deroussen F, Plancq M-C, Collet L-M. Bone defect reconstruction in children using the induced membrane technique: a series of 14 cases. Orthop Traumatol Surg Res. 2013;99:837–43.
4. Gouron R. Surgical technique and indications of the induced membrane procedure in children. Orthop Traumatol Surg Res. 2016;102:S133–9.
5. Masquelet AC, Begue T. The concept of induced membrane for reconstruction of long bone defects. Orthop Clin North Am. 2010;41:27–37.
6. Careri S, Vitiello R, Oliva MS, Ziranu A, Maccauro G, Perisano C. Masquelet technique and osteomyelitis: innovations and literature review. Eur Rev Med Pharmacol Sci. 2019;23:210–6.
7. Gouron R, Petit L, Boudot C, Six I, Brazier M, Kamel S, Mentaverri R. Osteoclasts and their precursors are present in the induced-membrane during bone reconstruction using the Masquelet technique. J Tissue Eng Regen Med. 2017;11:382–9.
8. Chadayammuri V, Hake M, Mauffrey C. Innovative strategies for the management of long bone infection: a review of the Masquelet technique. Patient Saf Surg. 2015;9:32.
9. Mathieu L, Durand M, Collombet J-M, de Rousiers A, de l'Escalopier N, Masquelet A-C. Induced membrane technique: a critical literature analysis and proposal for a failure classification scheme. Eur J Trauma Emerg Surg. 2020. https://doi.org/10.1007/s00068-020-01540-9.
10. Accadbled F, Mazeau P, Chotel F, Cottalorda J, Sales de Gauzy J, Kohler R. Induced-membrane femur reconstruction after resection of bone malignancies: three cases of massive graft resorption in children. Orthop Traumatol Surg Res. 2013;99:479–83.
11. Durand M, Barbier L, Mathieu L, Poyot T, Demoures T, Souraud J-B, Masquelet A-C, Collombet J-M. Towards understanding therapeutic failures in Masquelet surgery: first evidence that defective induced membrane properties are associated with clinical failures. J Clin Med. 2020;9:450.
12. Canavese F, Corradin M, Khan A, Mansour M, Rousset M, Samba A. Successful treatment of chronic osteomyelitis in children with debridement, antibiotic-laden cement spacer and bone graft substitute. Eur J Orthop Surg Traumatol. 2017;27:221–8.
13. Tong K, Zhong Z, Peng Y, Lin C, Cao S, Yang Y, Wang G. Masquelet technique versus Ilizarov bone transport for reconstruction of lower extremity bone defects following posttraumatic osteomyelitis. Injury. 2017;48:1616–22.
14. Sales de Gauzy J, Fitoussi F, Jouve J-L, Karger C, Badina A, Masquelet A-C. Traumatic diaphyseal bone defects in children. Orthop Traumatol Surg Res. 2012;98:220–6.
15. Rousset M, Walle M, Cambou L, Mansour M, Samba A, Pereira B, Ghanem I, Canavese F. Chronic infection and infected non-union of the long bones in paediatric patients: preliminary results of bone versus beta-tricalcium phosphate grafting after induced membrane formation. Int Orthop. 2018;42:385–93.

Part IV

Region Specific Musculoskeletal Infections

Epiphyseal Osteomyelitis

28

Maulin M. Shah, Anil Agarwal,
and Prateek Rastogi

Introduction

The metaphyseal region due to peculiar blood vessel arrangement is a common site for osteomyelitis and in children, epiphyseal involvement through tranphyseal vessels is known. Primary epiphyseal osteomyelitis (PEO) and primary epiphyseal sub-acute osteomyelitis (PESAO) are comparatively rarer conditions whereby the primary focus of infection is in the epiphysis. They are more common in epiphyses around the knee joint due to larger epiphyseal vessels. Virulent organisms like Staphylococcus cause acute disease with severe pain, local tenderness, swelling, and fever but the more common sub-acute form caused by Mycobacterium species or Kingella kingae may present with painless limp, some swelling, and little functional impairment. X-ray changes may appear late and MRI (preferably contrast-enhanced) helps in localization and delineation of the lesion, differentiation from tumors or other similar-looking lesions as well as planning of the surgical exploration. Surgical management is recommended for decompression of the abscess and for obtaining tissue samples for cultures, histopathology, and molecular assays. Long-term observation is required because late sequelae due to physeal or articular involvement are common.

Definitions

Various terminologies and phrases have been used in the literature to describe epiphyseal osteomyelitis. Primary epiphyseal osteomyelitis (PEO) is defined as isolated infection of epiphysis without metaphyseal involvement. The term primary epiphyseal osteomyelitis is used to cover all the epiphyseal infection varieties, whether acute or subacute, irrespective of the causative organism.

The terms primary epiphyseal sub-acute osteomyelitis (PESAO) and primary epiphyseal or apophyseal sub-acute osteomyelitis (PEASAO) have been used for the insidious variety with minimal inflammatory signs. They are more commonly caused by *Mycobacterium* species but other bacteria have also been implicated [1–3].

Pathogenesis

Trueta and Morgan in the late 1950s, in their studies by injecting various dyes, described in detail the vascular anatomy of the growing ends of bones [4]. Apart from the last ramifications of the nutrient artery (4/5th epiphysis), the metaphysis and the metaphyseal side of growth plate (up to hyper-

M. M. Shah (✉)
Orthokids Clinic, Ahmedabad, Gujarat, India

A. Agarwal · P. Rastogi
Department of Paediatric Orthopaedics, Chacha Nehru Bal Chikitsalaya, Delhi, India

© Springer Nature Switzerland AG 2022
M. V. Belthur et al. (eds.), *Pediatric Musculoskeletal Infections*,
https://doi.org/10.1007/978-3-030-95794-0_28

trophic zone) are also supplied by direct perforating metaphyseal arteries (1/5th). On the other side, a separate system of epiphyseal arteries penetrates the epiphysis close to the capsular insertion near the growth plate. These vessels form an anastomosis just above the physeal line and may enter the growth plate sometimes reaching up to the proliferation zone. The sluggish blood flow in these epiphyseal anastomoses above the growth plate provides an opportunity to the bacteria to colonise and therefore makes epiphysis prone to infection. This arrangement of vessels is present independent of the transphyseal vessels of infancy and thus primary epiphyseal osteomyelitis (PEO) can occur irrespective of the age of the child [1, 4, 5].

Microbiology

Commonly described pathogenic organisms are *Staphylococcus* species mainly *Staphylococcus aureus*. *Mycobacterium* is another important pathogen in developing countries as well as in countries where tuberculosis is endemic. *Streptococcus pneumonia, Pseudomonas aeruginosa* and *Brucella* sp. are other organisms reported but in many cases no organism may be isolated. With the advent of more specific molecular assays, *Kingella kingae* is being identified as a causative organism of many orthopaedic infections in general and epiphyseal osteomyelitis in particular [1–3, 6–8]. Fungal osteomyelitis of the distal femoral epiphysis has also been reported [11].

Epidemiology

Males are more commonly affected than females, with reported male to female ratio ranging between 1.5 and 2 [1, 2, 6, 8].

As stated earlier, PEO can occur in children of all age groups but it is more commonly reported in children less than 4 years of age, with incidence peaking between 1 and 2 years [1, 2, 6]. Epiphyseal osteomyelitis caused by *Mycobacterium* species has a comparatively older age of presentation, averaging around 8 years [6, 8]. *Kingella kingae* is more common in children aged less than 4 years as compared to older children [3].

The commonest involvement is around the knee joint. Distal femoral epiphysis is the most common epiphysis involved followed by upper tibial epiphysis. Large size of these epiphyses with increased blood supply may be the reason for this pattern of distribution. Other less commonly reported areas of involvement include greater trochanter, proximal humerus, proximal femur, distal fibula and distal radius [1, 3, 8] (Fig. 28.1).

Clinical Manifestations

Epiphyseal osteomyelitis can have an *acute* presentation with rapid disease onset and progression. Local pain and tenderness are severe. Swelling is usually present. There might be a limp or gross inability to bear weight on the affected extremity. Systemic signs like fever may

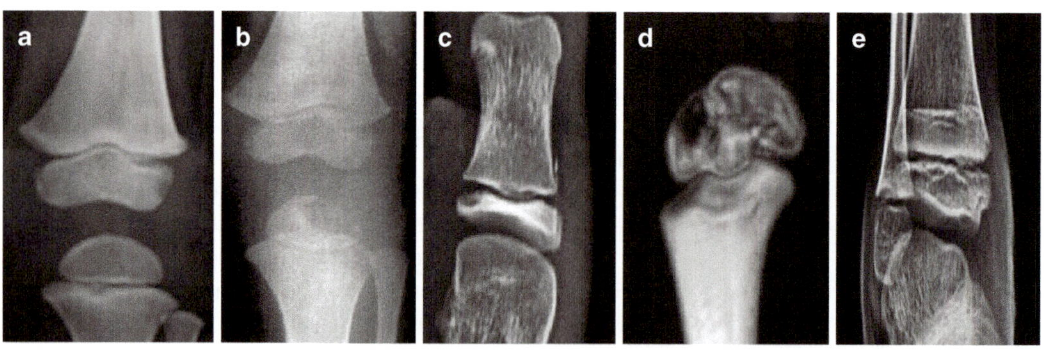

Fig. 28.1 Different sites of affection: (**a**) distal femoral condyle; (**b**) proximal tibia; (**c**) proximal phalanx; (**d**) proximal humerus; and (**e**) distal tibia

be present. The children usually present between 5 and 14 days post onset of disease [9].

More common variety (80%) is *subacute* presentation. They typically present approximately 2 weeks after disease onset. Symptoms appear more insidiously and progression of disease is slow and gradual. Mild local pain with tenderness is present. Symptoms are exaggerated by activities. Systemic features like fever are usually absent (80%) or minimal [1, 2].

Painless limp with swelling and little functional impairment is the usual presentation for subacute epiphyseal osteomyelitis caused by *Mycobacterium* species or *Kingella kingae*. Other features that may be present are discharging sinuses, muscle atrophy in the affected region and enlarged regional lymph nodes. A subacute disease is thought to be a result of an atypical host–pathogen relationship that may comprise any combination of increased host resistance, decreased virulence of the causative organism and/or prior antibiotic exposure. The children with tubercular osteomyelitis should also be evaluated for pulmonary involvement, which is commonly associated [8]. A recent study observed that patients with tubercular epiphyseal osteomyelitis presented later with predominant symptoms of limp and swelling and mild or no pain, whereas the patients with *Staphylococcus* epiphyseal osteomyelitis presented comparatively earlier (within 3 weeks) with predominant complaint of severe pain and inability to bear weight over the affected limb [1] (Box 28.1 Key Learning Points).

Box 28.1 Key Learning Points

1. Primary epiphyseal osteomyelitis (PEO) is defined as isolated infection of epiphysis without metaphyseal involvement. Epiphyseal blood supply is independent of the transphyseal vessels of infancy and thus PEO can occur irrespective of the age of the child. About 80% cases of PEO are seen around knee joint.
2. Primary bacterial osteomyelitis is usually diagnosed early, with pain and inability to bear weight as the main presenting symptoms. Primary tuberculous osteomyelitis is usually diagnosed late and they have swelling and limp as the main complaints.
3. Early diagnosis of PEO is crucial, as diagnostic delay may lead to articular cartilage penetration, joint and adjacent bone involvement and permanent articular cartilage thinning.

Laboratory Findings

Total leucocyte count (TLC), erythrocyte sedimentation rates (ESR: 30–40 mm/h) and C-reactive protein (CRP: <10 mg/L) may be elevated (20–30% cases) in acute setting but are usually non-contributory in most of the cases.

In *Kingella kingae* infections, TLC and CRP are abnormal only in 20% cases. Elevated ESR and platelet count are more sensitive indicators for *Kingella* [3].

Blood cultures are usually negative or may sometimes show growth, most commonly of *Staphylococcus aureus*. Polymerase chain reaction (PCR) test has become an important tool in the diagnosis of *Mycobacterium* species. *Kingella kingae* may require high index of suspicion, fastidious culture methods and *Kingella*-specific molecular assays/PCR [1–3].

Histopathology of biopsy material reveals non-specific features of inflammation in case of bacterial infections. In tubercular infections, granulomatous inflammation, Langhans giant cells, lymphocytes, epithelioid cells and necrotic caseous formation are the findings that might be expected. But these features may be absent in cartilage-rich lesions [1, 2].

Radiological Findings

Plain Radiographs

Initial X-rays especially in acute and subacute presentation are usually benign with minimal or no abnormality. Earliest change to appear may be of regional osteopenia. Joint space is usually preserved unless there is joint penetration of the abscess. Lesion may be missed in first X-rays in as much as 50% patients [1, 2]. X-rays usually reveal rarefaction of the periphery of the ossified part of epiphysis with irregularities. Comparison with opposite epiphysis can help in differentiating it from a normal variety of epiphyseal anatomy.

Two distinct radiological patterns in epiphyseal osteomyelitis have been described. The 'localised' variety can be [1] purely epiphyseal or [2] transphyseal and shaped like 'hourglass'. The 'diffuse' transphyseal variety had more extensive growth plate involvement and bony destruction [8].

In the transphyseal varieties, there is always a possibility that the lesion was an primarily metaphyseal with a secondary spread to epiphysis. During the healing phase, osteopenia is the first to recover as it is slowly replaced by sclerosis. Areas of lucency may persist for years, even after active infection has been successfully treated.

Ultrasonography

Ultrasound may be helpful to identify and localise concomitant soft tissue abscesses. It may also be helpful to diagnose and quantify collection in the adjoining joint, if present.

Computed Tomography (CT)

Computed tomography (CT) scan in epiphyseal osteomyelitis has very few indications. It is helpful in localising and defining the lesions in three dimensions. During follow-up, CT scans may be used to confirm presence and location of any osseous physeal bar.

Magnetic Resonance Imaging (MRI)

Magnetic resonance imaging (MRI) has become the gold standard imaging technique in the diagnosis of epiphyseal osteomyelitis. It is the modality of choice when plain radiographs are apparently normal [6]. It helps in localising the lesion and delineating the extent of the lesion. It is also important for pre-operative planning and helps to differentiate it from various other conditions like tumours. Many a times, joint penetration can be visualised on MRI and thus decisions regarding surgical approach and arthrotomy can be taken [1]. Gadolinium-enhanced MRI is more sensitive than non-contrast MRI [6].

Radioisotope Scans

Bone scan may confirm the diagnosis as early as 12–24 hours. The bone scan reflects increased bone mineral turnover in general, and not specifically infection. The incongruence of the spatial distribution of gallium and bone uptake is considered reliable indicator of osteomyelitis [9].

Differential Diagnosis

Various other lesions that may mimic epiphyseal osteomyelitis and should be considered as differential diagnosis are chondroblastoma, chondromyxoid fibroma, eosinophilic granuloma and malignant tumours like Ewing's sarcoma and leukaemia; some rare fungal infections may also be present as epiphyseal infection [8, 10] (Box 28.2 DD of PEO).

Box 28.2 Differential Diagnosis of PEO

1. Chondroblastoma.
2. Chondromyxoid fibroma.
3. Eosinophilic granuloma.
4. Ewing's sarcoma.
5. Leukaemia.

Treatment

Treatment should be started as early as possible. A delay in treatment can lead to joint destruction and is associated with poorer prognosis (Box 28.3 Tips and Tricks).

Box 28.3 Tips and Tricks

1. PEO is one of the important differential diagnoses of swelling around the knee joint in children.
2. MRI of the affected part will help in locating the lesion, defining its extent and studying its morphology.
3. Joint communication of the lesion should be checked with a blunt probe. Most of the tuberculous PEO have the articular cartilage penetration, while bacterial PEO are confined to the epiphysis.

Medical Treatment

Medical treatment alone is not recommended for PEO except for the acute cases with minimal swelling, where relief is expected with antibiotic therapy and surgical exploration can be delayed. In all cases, it is preferable to start antibiotic therapy only after obtaining tissue samples.

For acute PEO, antibiotics are recommended for 4–6 weeks. Intravenous cloxacillin for 5 days followed by oral for 6 weeks is recommended for methicillin-sensitive *Staphylococcus aureus*. *Kingella kingae* is sensitive to wide range of antibiotics. Oral ampicillin or cefuroxime for 4 weeks is usually sufficient to treat these infections. [1, 2]

For *Mycobacterium tuberculosis*, anti-tubercular therapy is recommended for 16–18 months, or at least for a minimum of 12 months. All patients must receive an intensive phase multidrug anti-tubercular treatment (isoniazid: 10 mg/kg/day; rifampicin: 10 mg/kg/day; pyrazinamide: 25 mg/kg/day; and ethambutol: 20 mg/kg/day) for 2 months and continuation phase (isoniazid: 10 mg/kg/day; rifampicin: 10 mg/kg/day; and ethambutol: 20 mg/kg/day) for 10–16 months as per the institutional protocol [8].

Surgical Interventions

Surgical drainage is recommended for all patients of PEO except for select acute presentation as described above.

For subacute cases, surgery is recommended for decompression of the abscess and for obtaining tissue samples. MRI is helpful in preoperative planning of incision and approach. Under C-arm guidance, incision is given just above the lesion in the bone. Window is made by multiple drill holes. Thorough curettage is done and samples are obtained for histopathological examinations, cultures and molecular assays. Inadequate curettage may lead to unfavourable results [6]. A probe may be used to identify joint penetration and if present arthrotomy and joint lavage should be performed. In a series of 11 patients with primary tubercular epiphyseal osteomyelitis, 1 study found 9 patients had articular cartilage penetration [1]. Depending upon the size of lesion, a negative suction drain may be left inside before closure is done (Figs. 28.2 and 28.3).

For transphyseal hourglass lesions, recent advances have recommended a minimally invasive endoscopic technique to minimise physeal damage. To prevent future bar formation in the physis, a pad of fat may be placed in the physeal defect. Other indications of surgical exploration are poor clinical response to antibiotics, concomitant septic arthritis or progression on serial X-rays.

Supportive Treatment

Post-operative immobilisation and a splint support are recommended for 4–6 weeks depending

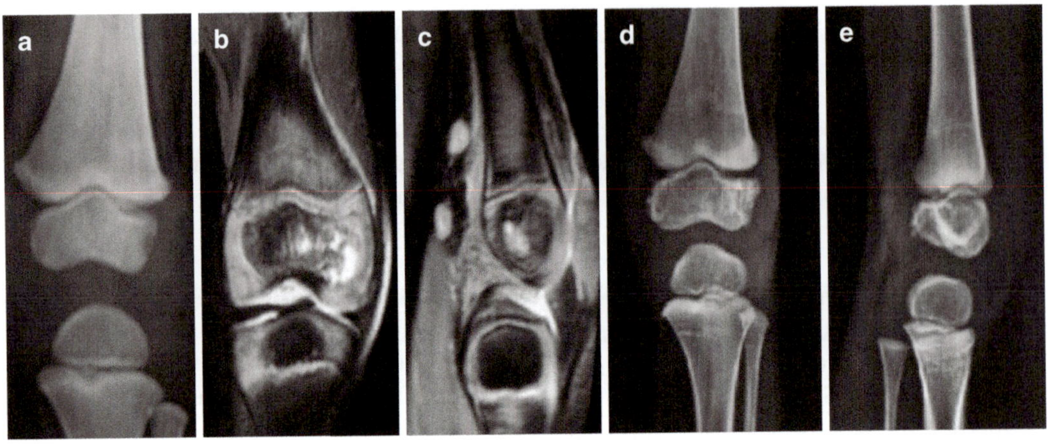

Fig. 28.2 Primary epiphyseal osteomyelitis of distal femur. (**a**) X-ray knee: antero-posterior (AP) view at the time of presentation. (**b**, **c**) MRI knee: coronal and sagittal sections. (**d**, **e**) Two-year follow-up X-ray knee: antero-posterior and lateral views

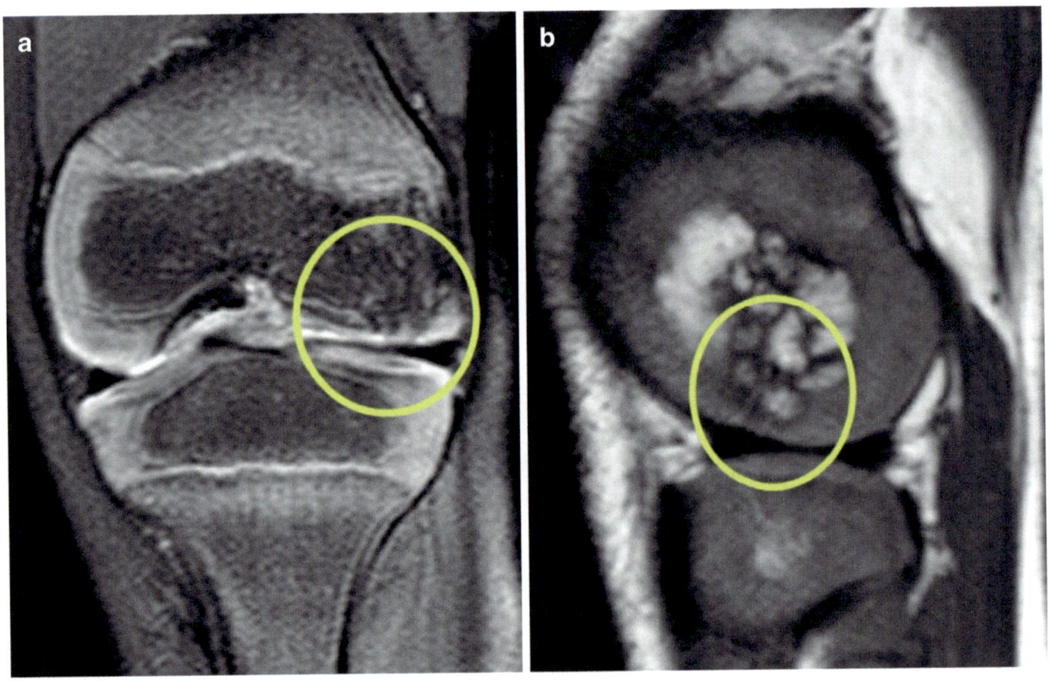

Fig. 28.3 Two-year follow-up of case shown in Fig. 28.2. (**a**, **b**) MRI coronal and sagittal sections at two-year follow-up showing thinning of articular cartilage

on the site and extent of the lesion. Range of motion exercises are then commenced gradually. Weight-bearing should be delayed for 2–3 months, especially in patients in whom articular cartilage penetration has been observed. Analgesics may be used appropriately.

Follow-Up

Regular follow-up is recommended in initial 6 months to evaluate pain, range of motion, healing response in X-rays and any recurrence of lesion and infection. Long-term follow-up is also desirable for possible angular or limb length discrepancy. Status of physis must be seen for remodelling of growth plate and development of any physeal bar [8].

MRI is an important modality in follow-up to visualise physeal damage and bar formation.

Complications

Orthopaedic complications are seen in approximately 30–40% patients with PEO [1, 2]. An abscess localised to epiphyses may spread to metaphysis through a transphyseal spread. Early weight bearing can lead to collapse and deformity. Both physeal stimulation and premature physeal arrest have been reported leading to limb length/alignment discrepancies. Loss of range of movement can occur as a complication of concomitant septic arthritis [6] (Figs. 28.4 and 28.5).

Children under 2 years of age are at a much higher risk for developing disseminated disease and severe complications [9].

Summary

Primary epiphyseal osteomyelitis is a rare entity and thus a high index of suspicion should be kept in mind to diagnose it. *Staphylococcus aureus* is the most common infective organism. Uncommon causative organisms like *Kingella kingae* and *Mycobacterium tuberculosis* should be kept in causative aetiology. Specific molecular assays are available, when these are suspected. Clinical manifestations can be varied and presentation and diagnosis are usually delayed. Epiphyses around knee are most commonly affected. MRI is the imaging modality of choice. Surgical decompression, curettage and tissue sampling for cultures and histopathological examination are

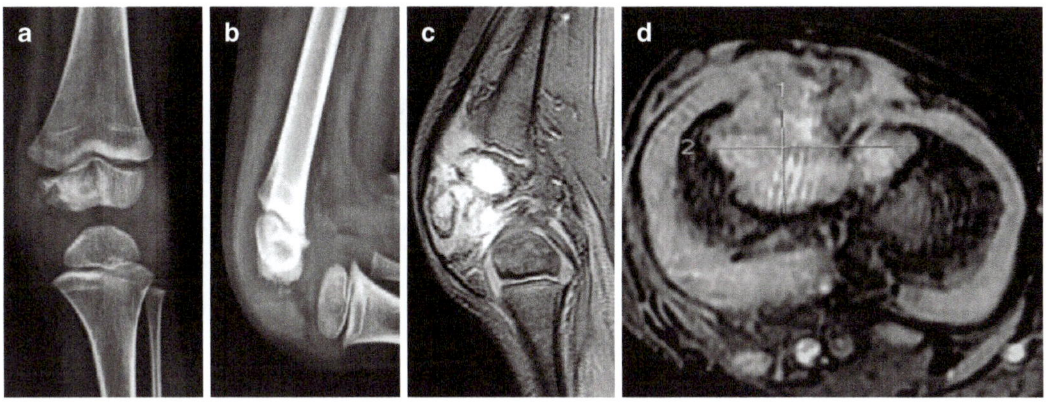

Fig. 28.4 This 5-year-old girl initially presented to us with complaint of limp and swelling over right knee since 3 months. X-ray of the right knee showed lytic lesion in the distal femoral epiphysis (**a**, **b**). Patient was advised MRI of the involved joint followed by biopsy and debridement, but patient denied surgery and was lost to follow-up. After 3 years, patient again presented to us with complaint of right knee fixed flexion deformity of 40 degrees. MRI revealed lytic lesion of right distal femoral epiphysis penetrating the right knee joint along with complete erosion of articular cartilage of femoral trochlea and corresponding surface of the patella (**c**, **d**). On exploring the joint, we found purulent collection and breech in the femoral articular surface communicating with epiphysis. There was severe erosion of femoral trochlea and patellar medial facet. The joint was thoroughly lavaged and debrided. A blunt probe was passed from the articular surface of femur into the femoral epiphysis and surrounding area was curetted out. Pus culture was positive for *Mycobacterium tuberculosis*. The child was given four-drug anti-tubercular treatment for 3 months followed by three drugs for further 9 months. Splint was removed after 2 weeks at the time of suture removal and gentle exercises were started. Gradual weight bearing was started after 1 month. After 8 years of follow-up, the child has full range of motion and function with no limb length discrepancy. This case suggests that untreated PEO of tubercular aetiology can lead to severe destruction of the joint

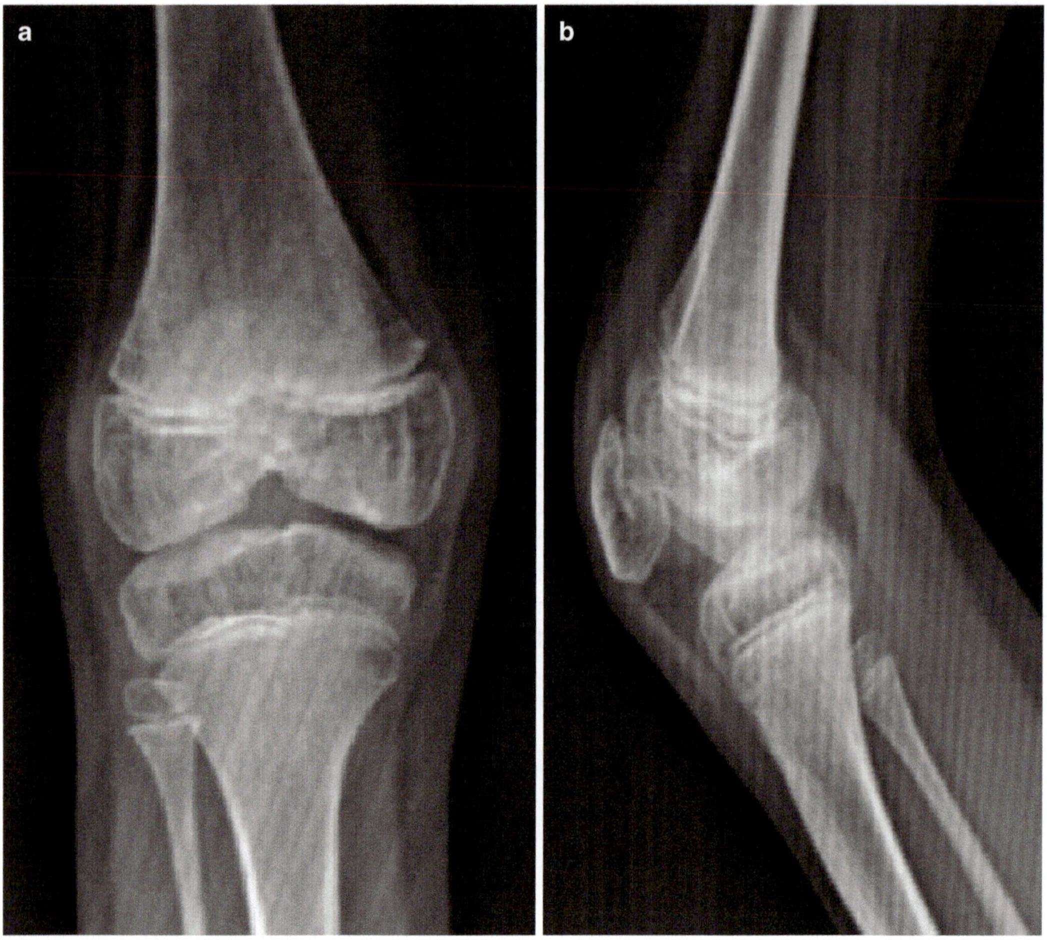

Fig. 28.5 Seven-year follow-up of case shown in Fig. 28.4. (**a**, **b**) Antero-posterior and lateral X-rays of affected knee at 7-year follow-up

recommended. Limb length/alignment discrepancies are common complications due to physeal arrest or stimulation. Failure to diagnose the PEO in time may lead to joint penetration and articular cartilage thinning (Box 28.4 Pitfalls to Avoid).

Box 28.4 Pitfalls to Avoid

1. Acquire adequate imaging to make an early diagnosis.
2. Aim for adequate bacteriological and histopathological diagnoses.
3. Regular follow-up of PEO is required to identify any angular deformity or articular cartilage thinning early in its course.

References

1. Shah MM, Gupta G, Makadia AK, Rabbi Q. Primary epiphyseal osteomyelitis (PEO) in 18 children: a rare entity with atypical features. J Pediatr Orthop. 2020;40:361–6.
2. El Houmami N, Minodier P, Bouvier C, Seligmann H, Jouve L, Raoult D, Fournier E. Primary subacute epiphyseal osteomyelitis caused by mycobacterium species in young children: a modern diagnostic approach. Eur J Clin Microbiol Infect Dis. 2017;36:771–7.
3. Ceroni D, Belaieff W, Cherkaoui A, Lascombes P, Schrenzel J, Coulon G, Dubois-Ferrière V, Dayer R. Primary epiphyseal or apophyseal subacute osteomyelitis in the pediatric population: a report of fourteen cases and a systematic review of the literature. J Bone Joint Surg Am. 2014;96:1570–5.

4. Trueta J, Morgan JD. The vascular contribution to osteogenesis. I. Studies by the injection method. J Bone Joint Surg Br. 1960;42:97–109.
5. Trueta J. The three types of acute haematogenous osteomyelitis: a clinical and vascular study. J Bone Joint Surg Br. 1959;41:671–80.
6. Yoo WJ, Choi IH, Yun YH, Cho TJ, Cheon JE, Song MH, Chung CY, Park MS, Choi E, Lee HJ, Park KU. Primary epiphyseal osteomyelitis caused by mycobacterium species in otherwise healthy toddlers. J Bone Joint Surg Am. 2014;96:e145.1–9.
7. Hempfing A, Placzek R, Göttsche T, Meiss AL. Primary subacute epiphyseal and metaepiphyseal osteomyelitis in children diagnosis and treatment guided by MRI. J Bone Joint Surg Br. 2003;85:559–64.
8. Agarwal A, Gupta N, Mishra M, Agrawal N, Kumar D. Primary epiphyseal and metaepiphyseal tubercular osteomyelitis in children – a series of 8 cases. Acta Orthop Belg. 2016;82:797–805.
9. Kao FC, Lee ZL, Kao HC, Hung SS, Huang YC. Acute primary hematogenous osteomyelitis of the epiphysis: report of two cases. Chang Gung Med J. 2003;26:851–6.
10. Gardner DJ, Azouz EM. Solitary lucent epiphyseal lesions inchildren. Skelet Radiol. 1988;17:497–504.
11. Nissen TP, Lehman CR, Otsuka NY, Cerruti DM. Fungal osteomyelitis of the distal femoral epiphysis. Orthopedics. 2001;24(11):1083–4.

29 Pediatric Hand Infections

Casey M. Codd, Scott H. Kozin, and Joshua M. Abzug

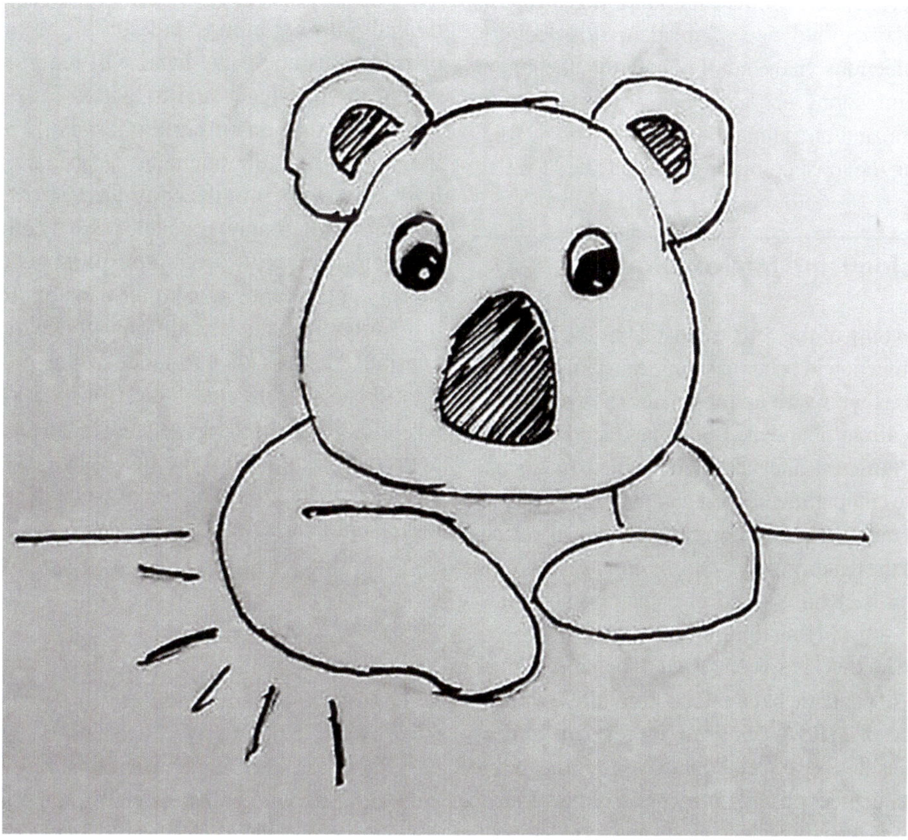

C. M. Codd · J. M. Abzug (✉)
Department of Orthopaedics, University of Maryland School of Medicine, Baltimore, MD, USA
e-mail: ccodd@som.umaryland.edu; jabzug@som.umaryland.edu

S. H. Kozin
Department of Orthopedics, Shriners Hospital, Philadelphia, PA, USA
e-mail: skozin@shrinenet.org

© Springer Nature Switzerland AG 2022
M. V. Belthur et al. (eds.), *Pediatric Musculoskeletal Infections*,
https://doi.org/10.1007/978-3-030-95794-0_29

Introduction and Epidemiology in Brief

Touch is one of the first senses to develop in children and, as a result, the pediatric patient explores their world around them utilizing their hands. This exploration aids in developing tactile perception, fine motor skills, depth perception, and interacting with their surroundings. As a result, hand injuries are common in the pediatric population, some of which lead to subsequent infections. The epidemiology of infections of the hand varies based on the type of infection present and the age of the child. Therefore, there is limited literature regarding the epidemiology and rate of incidence of pediatric hand infections. In the adult population, the majority of infections are secondary to a laceration, puncture, and/or trauma to the hand, with the digits being the most common infection site [1, 2].

Pathology and Microbiology

The anatomy of the pediatric hand has the potential for an infection to occur in a wide range of locations as well as with various presentations of the infection. With an abundance of bones, tendons, ligaments, muscles, and nerves contained in a small area, the compartmentalized nature of the hand provides a unique presentation of infections in various parts of the hand. *Staphylococcus aureus* is the most common bacteria isolated in pediatric hand infections [1–4]. Methicillin-resistant *Staphylococcus aureus* (MRSA) has been found to be present in up to 30% of pediatric hand infection cultures, with the presence of MRSA being more prevalent in deep infections that have formed abscesses compared to superficial infections [5]. *Streptococcus* bacteria are the second most prevalent organisms found in pediatric hand infections [1–4].

Clinical Presentation, Examination, Investigation, and Treatment

When a patient presents with concern for a hand infection (bacterial, viral, or fungal), one of the most crucial steps is to obtain a complete and robust patient history. This history should include, but not be limited to, patient hobbies, recent activities and/or travel, recent hospitalizations or procedures, vaccination status, patient guardian occupations, exposure to animals, immunocompetency, and any previous infections, regardless of anatomic location. All of these factors can provide clues as to the potential type of infection present as well as the underlying responsible organism. With this information, a correct diagnosis and course of treatment can be determined more swiftly and lead to better patient outcomes. While some infections, particularly those with an early presentation, can be treated with antibiotics and soaks, the majority of infections about the hand will require drainage of the purulence and irrigation followed by the administration of antibiotics. Following an irrigation and debridement procedure, it is imperative to permit the continued egress of any purulence that may redevelop by leaving the incision open, with or without packing, or very loosely approximating a larger incision. Routine utilization of soaks is common practice to permit continued egress of purulence while providing dilution to the affected area. Consultation with an infectious disease colleagues ensures that appropriate antibiotics are prescribed as well as appropriate length of treatment when deep infection, septic arthritis, and/or osteomyelitis are present (Box 29.1).

Box 29.1 Key Learning Points

- An in-depth patient history in the early diagnosis and treatment of hand infections is vital to the ultimate diagnosis.
- An infectious origin to a hand abnormality should be on almost every differential diagnosis list.
- Prompt recognition and treatment of hand infections is crucial to avoiding complications.
- Complications of hand infections often result due to a delayed diagnosis and treatment.

Paronychia

A paronychia is an infection that occurs about the nail complex at the lateral nail fold and adjacent tissue. These infections can present as either acute (i.e., present for less than 6 weeks), or chronic (present for more than 6 weeks) [6]. Presentation of a paronychia is characterized by eponychial or paronychial swelling, tenderness at the infection site, and erythema. Spontaneous drainage of purulent material may occur [6, 7].

In pediatric patients, this infection, particularly the acute presentation, may be the result of nail biting and sucking on their fingers [6, 7]. Chronic presentation of a paronychia is more commonly attributed to excessive and prolonged exposure to moisture [7]. Paronychia infections can be caused by a mixture of anaerobic and aerobic organisms [2, 3, 6, 7]. The most common organism isolated from paronychia infections is *Staphylococcus aureus*, followed by *Streptococcus pyogenes* [1, 3, 6, 7]. Additional organisms that are less commonly identified in paronychia infections include *Pseudomonas pyocyanea*, *Proteus vulgaris*, and *Candida albicans* (more common in chronic presentations) [1, 3, 6, 7]. Methicillin-resistant *Staphylococcus aureus* can be present in, under, and around pediatric patients' fingernails and should be tested for when a culture swab is obtained [5, 9]. Fungal paronychia has been noted to occur most commonly in chronic cases of paronychia, and therefore fungal cultures should be included in the analysis of any purulence [7]. Culture swabs should be routinely obtained to identify the organism(s) present if purulence is able to be drained from the infection site.

The initial treatment of a paronychia infection should include broad-spectrum antibiotics, such as dicloxacillin, amoxicillin clavulanate, or clindamycin [6, 7]. In the acute stage and without the presence of an abscess/purulence, warm soaks should accompany the oral antibiotics [6, 7]. The soaks can consist of equal parts of hydrogen peroxide and sterile saline and should occur multiple times (three to four) throughout the day. If the infection is a result of MRSA, antibiotic treatment should include vancomycin, linezolid, or clindamycin coupled with trimethoprim/sulfamethoxazole [6, 7]. If there is fluctuance or frank purulence present, the area should be drained. The surgical approach to draining the purulence is dependent on the location and spread of the infection in the affected tissues. Incisions for acute paronychia can include resection/removal of the nail plate adjacent to the infection, a single incision at the infection site to allow for drainage of the purulence, or a double incision on either side of the infection if the infection has spread to warrant two incisions [10]. Depending on the patient's age and compliance, the drainage of a paronychia can be done utilizing a proximal digital block with or without sedation or general anesthesia in the young child [11]. It may be required to remove a portion of the nail plate via eponychial marsupialization to decompress the site of infection adequately [9, 12].

During an acute presentation, draining the infection coupled with oral antibiotic treatment is typically curative [6, 7]. The addition of soaks to the regimen permits continued egress of the purulence until the antibiotics can overcome the causative organisms. In the case of fungal paronychia, an antifungal topical ointment with steroids can aid in the treatment of the infection [8, 9] (Box 29.2).

Box 29.2 Paronychia

- Clinical signs include erythema, swelling, and/or tenderness of the eponychia or paronychia and possibly spontaneous drainage of purulent material.
- Warm soaks may aid in decreasing swelling, bringing the infection to a head, and/or continued egress of purulence if it is already draining.
- Broad-spectrum antibiotics should be initiated until culture swab specificities are returned.
- Surgical approach for drainage of purulence varies based on infection location but typically involves elevation of the paronychia/eponychia from the nail plate at the infection location.
- If infection is fungal, a topical antifungal ointment with steroids can aid in treatment.

Felon

A felon is an infection of the digital pad, or pulp, of the distal fingertip. If the felon presents prior to the development of an abscess, the infection may be adequately treated with antibiotics alone, though it is uncommon for the infection to present at this stage [11]. Soaking the digit may cause the infection to come to a head and spontaneously drain or permit a smaller incision if drainage is necessary. Most commonly, a felon will present at the abscess stage, which will require surgical intervention to facilitate drainage. Presentation will often involve considerable pain, rapid swelling, and erythema due to the pressure the abscess creates in a relatively small and constrained area [8, 12, 13].

Felons are most commonly the result of a *Staphylococcus aureus* infection. The infection should be initially treated with broad-spectrum antibiotics and, depending on the results of the culture swab during drainage, the antibiotic course can be adjusted accordingly [14].

The surgical approach for draining a felon can vary depending on the primary location of tenderness and the severity of the abscess. A longitudinal and lateral incision on the less-utilized side of the digit is the typically recommended method of drainage [10, 14]. Other approaches include a volar transverse, a volar longitudinal, and the fish-mouth and hockey-stick incisions [10, 14]. The fish-mouth incision is associated with high rates of complications and the hockey-stick incision is only indicated in cases of severe and extensive abscesses [10, 15]. The volar transverse incision poses a higher risk of damaging the neurovascular structures compared to the lateral longitudinal and volar longitudinal incisions [10, 14, 15]. Once the incision is made, a thorough debridement is necessary to ensure an adequate drainage has occurred. This includes breaking through the numerous septa that are present that attach the finger pulp to the distal phalanx. Failure to break through the septa will result in persistence of the infection in isolated compartments within the finger pulp. Following the debridement and drainage, the area should be irrigated thoroughly and soaked in equal parts of sterile saline and hydrogen peroxide. Packing can be utilized to aid in egress of the purulent material. It is imperative to leave the incision open to permit drainage and continued irrigation of the area.

Surgical drainage of a felon infection in a timely manner is crucial to avoid complications such as osteomyelitis, septic arthritis, and/or flexor tenosynovitis. When an adequate drainage is performed and appropriate antibiotics are utilized, the typical result is complete resolution of the infection without any long-term complications.

Herpetic Whitlow

Herpetic whitlow is a viral infection caused by the herpes simplex virus. Typically the virus type-1 strain is the causative organism in pediatric patients due to them putting their fingers/hands in their mouths [16]. The clinical presentation of herpetic whitlow is either a single vesicle or cluster of vesicles on the distal aspect of the finger [8, 12, 16]. The vesicles typically present as clear vesicles that progress to yellow and purulent [8]. Associated symptoms can include erythema, swelling, pain, tingling, and numbness [16]. Pain typically precedes the presentation of vesicles and the pain may seem disproportionate to the appearance [17].

Testing for herpetic whitlow involves obtaining skin scrapings and viral swabbing of the vesicles [8, 12, 16]. Testing may also include a Tzanck smear and serum antibody cultures [12, 17]. The vesicles are typically de-roofed and then samples are collected. A felon and/or a paronychia can present similarly to herpetic whitlow and therefore it is necessary to obtain both bacterial and viral cultures to determine the diagnosis. Herpetic whitlow typically appears on only one digit and if multiple digits are affected with vesicles, coxsackievirus or human enterovirus, also known as hand, foot, and mouth disease, should be considered and tested for in the viral culture [8, 18].

Treatment for herpetic whitlow is typically conservative in nature. Rest, elevation, and anti-inflammatory agents prescribed to treat any associated pain are the common measures utilized [8]. De-roofing the vesicles may provide some relief of symptoms; however, surgical intervention and drainage of these lesions is contraindicated as this approach may introduce a secondary bacterial infection and does not improve patient outcomes [12, 16]. Herpetic whitlow can reoccur, with approximately 20% of patients experiencing recurrence. If recurrence is persistent or if the patient is immunocompromised, acyclovir or valacyclovir may be prescribed to aid in achieving remission [19]. The viral lesions can also present with a secondary bacterial infection and, in these cases, antibiotics should be prescribed to eradicate the bacterial infection. However, the bacterial nature of the secondary infection should be confirmed prior to prescribing antibiotics [16].

Flexor Tenosynovitis

Flexor tenosynovitis most commonly presents with tenderness over the flexor tendon sheath, substantial swelling of the affected digit, the finger being held in a partially flexed position, and pain with passive extension of the digit (Kanavel's signs) (Fig. 29.1). The infection is often secondary to a puncture wound involving the tendon sheath. Due to the closed system nature of the tendon sheath and the presence of synovial fluid, the infection and any purulence that develops will travel the length of the tendon sheath very quickly [9, 12, 13]. Ultrasound can be utilized to compare the affected digit to the contralateral side to determine if there is any noted thickening of the affected flexor tendon or fluid present in the tendon sheath [20]. Flexor tenosynovitis is an emergent condition and therefore the diagnosis should be swift so that treatment can be administered. Failure to quickly obtain the accurate diagnose can result in flexor tendon rupture and/or scarring of the flexor tendon sheath.

The most common organisms involved in flexor tenosynovitis are *Streptococcus* and *Staphylococcus* strains of bacteria [12, 21]. Fungi, mycobacterium, and gonococcus strains can also lead to flexor tenosynovitis [12, 21]. During the surgical treatment of the infection, culture swabs should be procured to

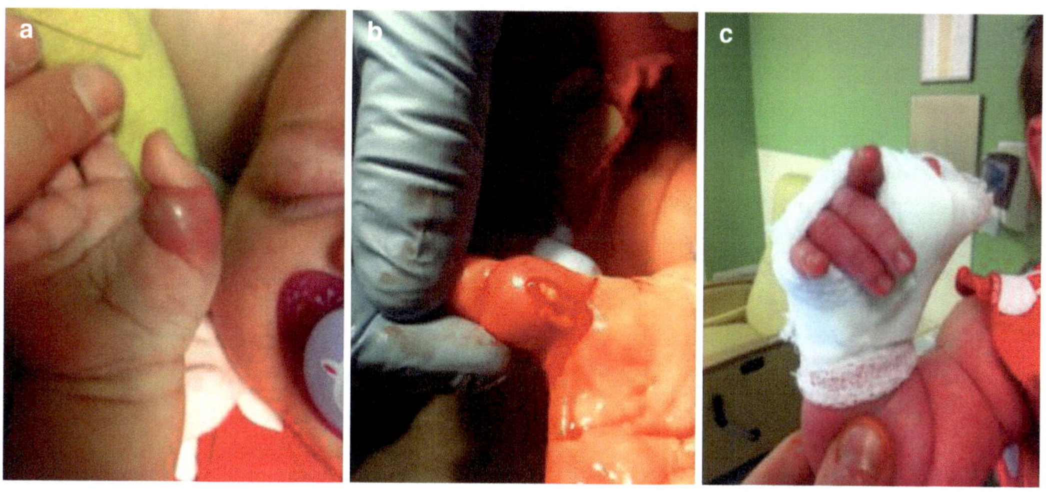

Fig. 29.1 (**a**) A 10-week-old presenting with an abscess on the volar aspect of the proximal phalanx of the thumb, who underwent emergent operative intervention. (**b**) Intraoperative findings of purulent drainage from the abscess and extension into the flexor tendon sheath. (**c**) Postoperative dressing placing the thumb into maximal extension to try to prevent a flexion contracture from occurring. (Courtesy of Joshua M. Abzug, MD)

determine the organism(s) responsible for the infection.

An emergent irrigation and debridement procedure is necessary to treat these infections except for the rare case of an extremely early presentation that can be treated with antibiotics and close observation. Repeated washouts are commonly necessary [22]. Typically, a Bruner zig-zag incision is utilized to open the tendon sheath and drain the infection, followed by a thorough irrigation. Alternatively, a closed tendon sheath irrigation approach may be utilized with the insertion of a catheter into the proximal tendon sheath for irrigation and utilization of a distal incision to permit egress of the purulence and fluid [22, 23]. Close observation is required following intervention and the patient should be splinted with the digit in full extension to prevent a contracture. Early active range of motion will aid in restoring full motion and function as scarring and stiffness are common complications associated with this infection (Box 29.3).

Box 29.3 Flexor Tenosynovitis

- Emergent diagnosis is key to preventing complications.
- Clinical signs include tenderness over the flexor tendon sheath, substantial swelling of the affected digit, the finger being held in a partially flexed position, and pain with passive extension of the digit (Kanavel's signs).
- Emergent irrigation and debridement are often necessary for successful outcomes.
- Multiple repeat procedures may be necessary.
- Splinting in full extension and early active range of motion will aid in restoration of motion and function.
- Delays in diagnosis or treatment can lead to tendon rupture, scarring, and contractures.

Deep Space Infection

Deep space infections of the hand most commonly occur secondary to a puncture introducing the infection or a contiguous spread of infection. The most common organisms involved with deep space infections are *Staphylococcus aureus*, *Streptococci*, and coliform [12]. A deep space infection of the hand can occur at the thenar, midpalmar, hypothenar, or interdigit web spaces. Following the initial drainage, debridement, and irrigation, the patient should be admitted for close observation, administration of antibiotics, and isolation of the causative organism(s). Repeat drainage and irrigation procedures may be necessary until the antibiotics are able to adequately defeat the causative organism(s).

The thenar space is superficial to the adductor pollicis muscle and connects the radial and ulnar bursae. An infection in the thenar space may present with swelling as well as the thumb in abduction to accommodate the presence of fluid and minimize the pain of the abscess forming in this space [9, 12]. Drainage of an abscess in the thenar space can occur via a variety of incisions including dorsal, palmar, dorsal/palmar combined, and transcommissural, with the dorsal/palmar combined approach being preferred by most surgeons [8, 12]. Adequate drainage of the infection with subsequent irrigation is necessary.

Mid-palmar space infections will present with tenderness and swelling about the volar aspect of the palm, often to the point of loss of palmar concavity; however, the swelling may be substantial enough that there is abundant swelling present on the dorsal aspect of the hand as well (Fig. 29.2). Patients with mid-palmar space infections will present, in addition to tenderness and swelling, with pain at passive movement of the long and ring fingers [8, 9, 12]. In mid-palmar space infections, drainage of the abscess is typically performed via a transverse or oblique incision to enter the volar aspect of the space [8, 12].

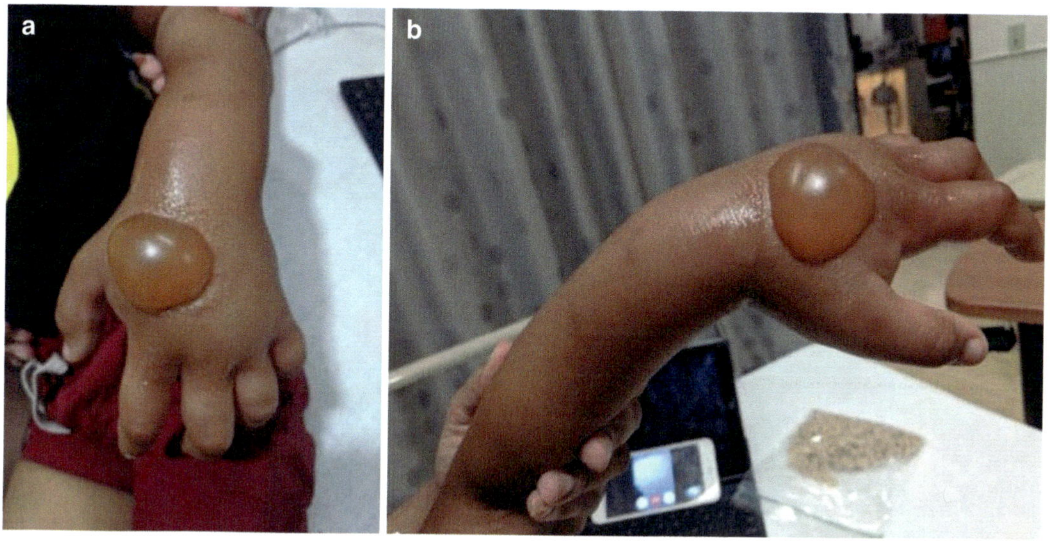

Fig. 29.2 A 3-year-old presenting with a mid-palmar infection that had substantial swelling on the dorsal aspect of the hand. A large blister developed due to the rapid, extensive swelling. (**a**) Dorsal view. (**b**) Radial view. (Courtesy of Joshua M. Abzug, MD)

Hypothenar infections may present with swelling and tenderness about the hypothenar space and may cause pain with movement of the small finger [8, 9]. Drainage of infections to the hypothenar space can occur utilizing a volar longitudinal incision [8].

Parona space infections are typically infections that have spread from elsewhere in the hand through the radial or ulnar bursae. The space lies between the fascia of the pronator quadratus muscle and the flexor digitorum profundus tendon sheath. Patients who present with parona space infections may have symptoms consistent with acute carpal tunnel syndrome and may have pain with any flexor movement of the digits [12]. Incisions for drainage of a parona space infection must be mindful of the surrounding anatomy and avoid injury to the structures in the area, particularly the flexor tendons, the median nerve, and the palmar cutaneous branch of the median nerve.

Interdigit web space infections will present with swelling in the web space. These infections are also commonly referred to as a collar-button abscess. This abscess presents with both volar and dorsal components of the swelling at the affected web space [8]. The adjacent digits will likely be in an abducted position relative to the affected web space (Fig. 29.3). Drainage of these infections should be carried out utilizing both a volar and dorsal incision to drain both sides of the abscess [8]. Transverse incisions are contraindicated due to their propensity of forming web space contractures [12].

Following drainage of all deep space infections, the incision should be left open or if reapproximated it should be done loosely. Utilization of packing or a drain is warranted when substantial purulence is present [12]. Repeat procedures are common and a more formal closure of the incision can be performed once the infection is adequately controlled. A scar revision can always be performed in the future if needed. Postoperatively, the hand and wrist should be splinted in a functional posi-

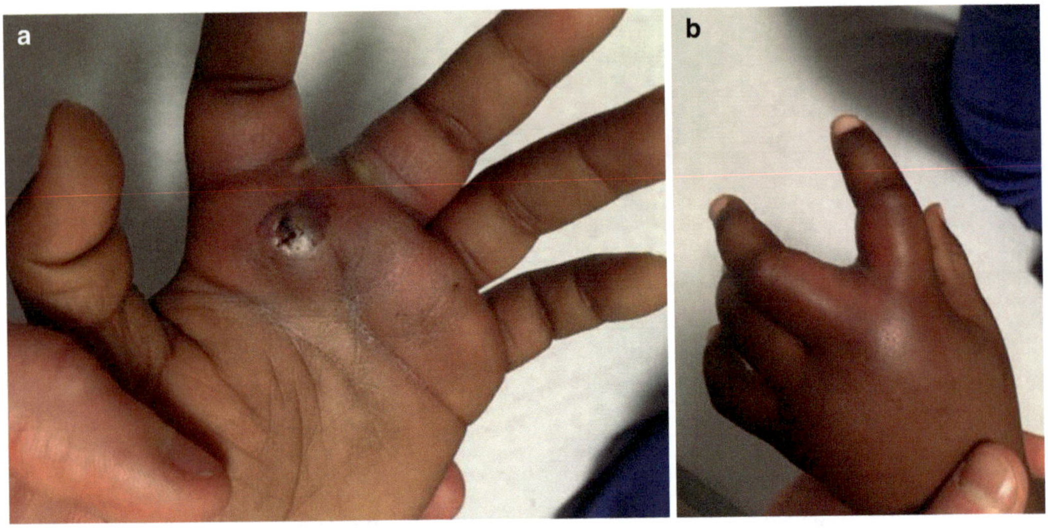

Fig. 29.3 An 8-year-old presenting with a collar-button abscess infection of the interdigit web space. Note the presence of the swelling both volarly and dorsally as well as the abducted positioning of the digits. (**a**) Volar view. (**b**) Dorsal view. (Courtesy of Joshua M. Abzug, MD) bird bite

tion to minimize the risk of contracture formation [10] (Box 29.4).

Box 29.4 Deep Space Infections

- Patients can present with hand swelling that is volar, dorsal, or both.
- Volar swelling may be recognized by loss of the hand concavity.
- Operative intervention is warranted to drain the purulence.
- Thorough irrigation and debridement is necessary.
- The incision should be left open/loosely approximated and packed or a drain placed to promote egress of the purulence.
- Multiple repeat procedures are often necessary.
- Soaks throughout the day may aid in continued egress of the purulence.
- Between procedures and soaks, the hand should splinted in the position of function to minimize stiffness and contracture formation.

Septic Arthritis

Septic arthritis, though rare in the hand and digits, typically occurs through a direct puncture of the joint leading to an infection. This can result from bite wounds, particularly if the bite wounds occur on the digit, but the infections can occasionally be atraumatic in nature [24, 25]. The clinical presentation is in line with most infections, presenting with swelling, erythema, and pain about the affected joint that is increased with passive movement. If septic arthritis is suspected, the joint needs to be aspirated and the aspirated fluid sent for a cell count and cultures.

The most common organisms identified in septic arthritis are *Staphylococcus aureus* and *Beta-hemolytic Streptococcus*. [24, 25] *Kingella kingae* has been reported to be responsible for septic arthritis in pediatric patients, particularly younger pediatric patients [25]. In pediatric patients that have not been vaccinated, *Hemophilus influenza* has also been isolated as the culprit in some septic arthritis cases [12, 25]. In rare instances, *Neisseria gonorrhoeae* has been noted to cause septic arthritis and, if suspected, should be tested for by growing a culture sample on chocolate agar [11].

Pediatric patients are unlikely to present with crystalline arthropathies in the hand, such as gout and pseudogout, Lyme disease, and rheumatologic arthritis, all of which are common differential diagnoses in the adult population. While uncommon, if the patient has any known history of rheumatoid diseases, exposure to Lyme, or crystalline arthropathies, these diagnoses can be ruled out by analysis of the aspirated fluid from the affected joint [9].

The majority of septic arthritis cases will require surgical intervention in the form of irrigation and debridement. The incision location will vary based on the joint affected by the infection. After the affected joint has been irrigated, a catheter or drain may be left in place if there is the need for continued drainage of purulence.

Animal Bites

Animal bites are common in the pediatric population with the hand being a frequent location of these bites. Dog bites occur far more frequently than cat bites; however, approximately 50% of all cat bites become infected whereas only around 4–20% of dog bites become infected [27, 28]. This is likely due to the mechanical differences in the animal teeth and the wounds they leave behind. Dog teeth and bites tend to leave more open puncture wounds that allow for any bacteria and/or organisms from the bite to drain, which results in fewer infections. In contrast, cat teeth and bites are smaller and do not leave as large of puncture wounds thus allowing the bacteria and organisms to remain in the wound site and develop into infections.

Infections from animal bites can be caused by a range of bacterial organisms. These include *Pasteurella multocida*, *Staphylococcus aureus*, *Streptococcus* species, and anaerobes [8, 12, 15, 27]. Antibiotic treatment should be broad-spectrum if administered prior to obtaining culture results and cover *Pasteurella multocida*, such as penicillin, amoxicillin clavulanate, or doxycycline [8, 12, 15, 27].

Domestic animal bites are not limited to cat and dog bites. Birds that are kept as pets can deliver bite wounds that present with a range of organisms depending on the species of bird. (Fig. 29.4) Akin to other animal bites, bird bites can present with *Pasteurella multocida*, *Staphylococcus* species, and *Streptococcus* species [29]. In addition to these more common

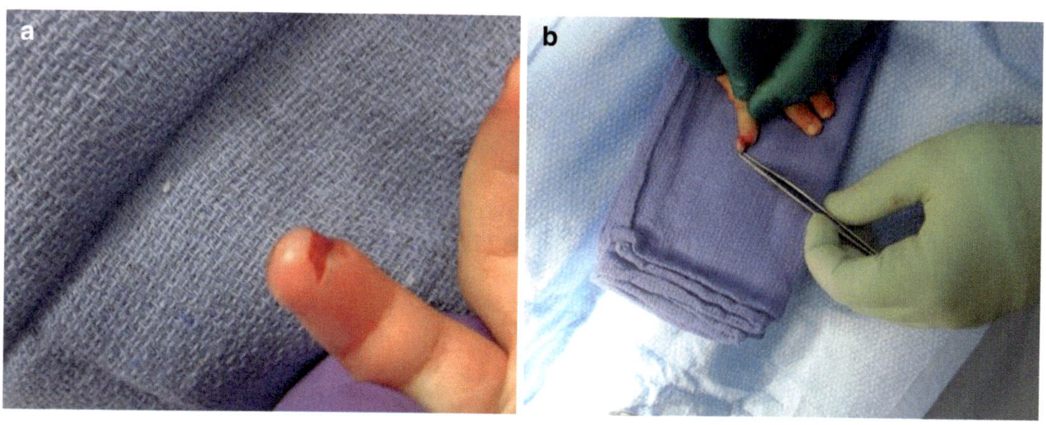

Fig. 29.4 (**a**) Volar view. Note the angular shape of the laceration caused by the bird's beak. (**b**) Dorsal view. Note the near amputation of the digit caused by the amount of force present in the bird's beak. (Courtesy of Joshua M. Abzug, MD)

organisms, bird bites can present with *Escherichia coli*, *Salmonella*, *Proteus*, *Lactobacillus*, *Corynebacterium*, *Pseudomonas*, *Klebsiella*, and *Acinetobacter* organisms [29]. Cultures of the bite site should be obtained to determine which organism(s) are present. Bird bites should be treated in a similar fashion to cat bites with debridement of the wound and utilization of the appropriate antibiotic treatment. Ciprofloxacin is commonly prescribed to cover for *Salmonella*, *Pseudomonas*, and *Klebsiella* species [29]. Bird bites can be delivered with an immense amount of force, up to 200 psi, and the bite site should be evaluated for possible fractures, nail bed injuries, and distal digit amputation [29] (Fig. 29.4).

If a patient presents to the emergency department or physician's office with an animal bite, every effort should be made to open and irrigate the wound, either under local or general anesthesia. If the wound has not reached the point of forming an abscess and there is no concern of tendon or joint space involvement when it is opened and irrigated, wounds that are treated with both irrigation and antibiotics have better outcomes than wounds treated with irrigation/debridement alone [27] (Box 29.5).

Box 29.5 Animal Bites

- The hands are common locations for domestic animal bites due to children's curiosity or the hand being used as a defense mechanism.
- Dog bites create larger breaks in the skin due to the tooth structure of the dog.
- Cat bites are typically puncture wounds that lead to deeper infections due to the shape of their teeth.
- Bird bites are crushing injuries due to their powerful beaks.
- All bites should be treated with prompt irrigation and debridement as well as antibiotics to improve outcomes.

Human Bites

Bite wounds from humans fall into two categories including a closed fist/fight bite and an occlusive bite injury. Closed fist/fight bite injuries occur when the hand, while in a fist shape, comes into contact with another human's teeth/mouth. This infection will typically present as a wound over the metacarpal head. There may be an associated injury to the extensor mechanism and violation of the joint capsule. Therefore, a formal and thorough assessment is mandatory.

If a patient presents with a bite wound, radiographs should be obtained to assess for any retained foreign bodies (i.e., tooth fragments) and for any underlying damage to the bone and cartilage at the site of impact. Culture swabs should be collected from the bite site and sent for analysis with testing for both anaerobic and aerobic bacteria. At presentation, a broad-spectrum antibiotic should be administered until the wound cultures are finalized and specific organisms have been identified. Additionally, the patient's tetanus vaccination status should be assessed and updated if necessary. If the bite wound has formed an abscess, surgical intervention including an irrigation and debridement procedure is necessary coupled with antibiotic treatment. Exploration of the joint capsule and extensor mechanism is mandatory during this procedure.

Due to the plethora of organisms that live in the human mouth, the bacteria most commonly responsible for infection following a human bite are both anaerobic and aerobic in nature. Common anaerobic organisms are *Bacteroides*, *Prevotella*, *Propionibacterium*, *Fusobacterium*, *Veillonella*, *Enterobacteriaceae*, and *Clostridum* [27]. Aerobic bacteria are both alpha- and beta-hemolytic *Streptococci*, *Staphylococcus aureus*, *Staphylococcus epidermis*, *Corynebacterium*, and *Eikenella corrodens* [26, 27]

Osteomyelitis

Osteomyelitis is uncommon in the hand but may present as a secondary complication following a hand infection, particularly if the initial infection had a delay in diagnosis, went undiagnosed, or was misdiagnosed. Osteomyelitis has been reported following Seymour fractures, particularly when there is involvement of the nail plate [31]. The clinical manifestation of osteomyelitis typically includes pain, erythema, and warmth at the affected site [25, 30]. Radiographs may aid in determining the presence of osteomyelitis (Fig. 29.5); however, if the infection is in the early stages, radiographs may not show any appreciable changes in the affected bone [25]. Magnetic resonance imaging (MRI) can aid in diagnosing osteomyelitis and an MRI study should be ordered if there is a high index of suspicion for osteomyelitis that is not apparent on X-ray [25].

Some cases of osteomyelitis may be treated with antibiotics alone while others will necessitate surgical intervention with irrigation and debridement. Discussion of the treatment options with an infectious disease colleague as well as the presence or absence of any bony abscesses will aid in the decision-making process. If surgical intervention is warranted, samples of the affected bone should be obtained and sent for culture and pathological assessment to confirm the diagnosis and attempt to isolate the infecting organism. An extended course of antibiotic treatment, ranging from 4 to 8 weeks, should be prescribed until all symptoms and signs of the osteomyelitis have resolved [25]. In some cases where the osteomyelitis infection has progressed substantially, amputation may be necessitated if the bone is beyond salvage [25, 30].

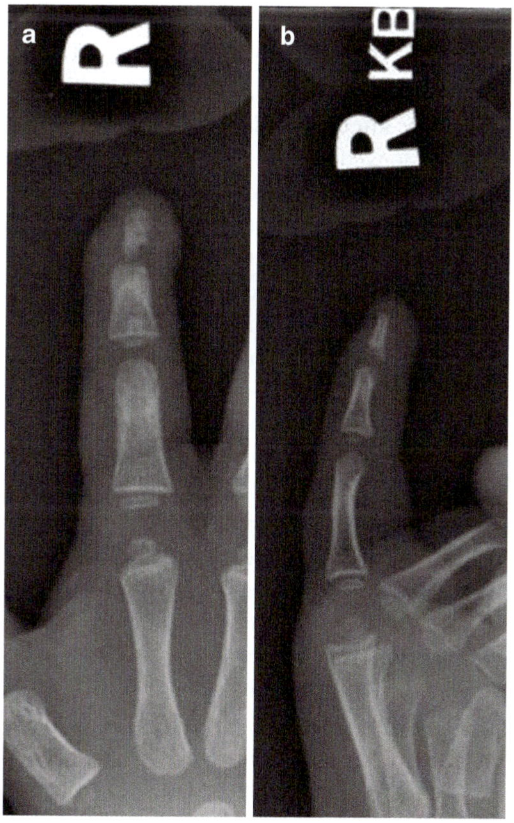

Fig. 29.5 Radiographs showing osteomyelitis of the distal phalanx in a 2-year-old patient. (**a**) Posterioranterior (PA) view. (**b**) Lateral view. (Courtesy of Joshua M. Abzug, MD)

Cellulitis

Cellulitis is a superficial infection of the soft tissues, typically due to *Staphylococcus aureus* or beta-hemolytic *Streptococcus*. Clinically, cellulitis will present with erythema, pain, and swelling. Upon presentation, the erythema should be marked and monitored for progression of the infection. Radiographs of the affected area can be obtained to rule out or identify any foreign bodies, osteomyelitis, gas in the soft tissues, and/or associated fractures.

The early presentation of cellulitis can be managed with a course of empiric antibiotics, elevation, and close observation. If the infection worsens, then an investigation into the progression of the infection to deeper structures is warranted. In addition, a change in the antibiotic regimen may be warranted. If the cellulitis is left untreated, it can progress into the deeper structures and/or cause skin necrosis necessitating operative intervention. If an abscess has formed, surgical intervention with irrigation and debridement is necessary to drain the infection. If skin necrosis occurs, a skin graft may be needed to cover the affected area [10]. The typical outcome of cellulitis with appropriate treatment is complete resolution of the infection without any long-term complications.

Necrotizing Fasciitis

Necrotizing fasciitis is a rare but aggressive and life-threatening bacterial infection of the skin and soft tissues. Patients with necrotizing fasciitis typically present with erythema, edema, purulence, necrosis, and/or substantial and disproportionate pain. Patients may present with systemic symptoms of fever, signs of shock, and/or toxicity [32]. Imaging studies may show gas in the soft tissues that has been produced by the bacteria. Laboratory values consistent with necrotizing fasciitis include a C-reactive protein ≥150 mg/L, a white blood cell count of >15,000/μL, hemoglobin <13.5 g/dL, sodium <135 mmol/L, creatinine >1.6 mg/dL, and/or glucose >180 mg/dL, which may aid in diagnosing necrotizing fasciitis [33].

Group A beta-hemolytic *Streptococcus* bacteria is the most common cause of necrotizing fasciitis in the upper extremity including young and non-immunocompromised patients. Other microbial culprits of necrotizing fasciitis include *Staphylococcus aureus* and a polymicrobial mixture of aerobic and anaerobic bacteria.

Treatment for necrotizing fasciitis is aggressive surgical irrigation and debridement. Intraoperative findings include the presence of purulence, often described as looking like dishwater fluid, and necrosis of the fascia [32]. Necrotizing fasciitis patients are likely to require multiple surgeries to determine if the debridement has been sufficient in removing the affected tissue and halt the spread of the infection. In addition to operative intervention, patients should be treated with intravenous antibiotics beginning with broad-spectrum and empiric and, as culture results are available, tailored to the identified bacterial organism(s).

Rare Infections

Mycobacterial infections are relatively rare but occur most commonly in the hand. Mycobacterial infections can present in numerous ways including as a skin infection, tenosynovitis, septic arthritis, and osteomyelitis. One common, though not universal, aspect of mycobacterial infections is the presence of granulomas. Patient history can help to identify possible mycobacterial infection strains. *Mycobacterium marinum*, the most common mycobacterial infection, is found in patients who have had recent contact with aquatic life. Many mycobacteria are endemic in nature, so it is important to assess the patient's recent travel history. Testing for mycobacterial infections can be accomplished by acid-fast stains of the affected tissue and cultures for mycobacterial infections can be grown on Lowenstein-Jensen media between 30° and 42° Celsius [34, 35]. Most courses of treatment involve lengthy antibiotic courses, typically of 2–6 months with some treatment lasting for up to 18 months [35]. If the infection is deep, surgical intervention is warranted with an irrigation and debridement of the affected area.

Papillomavirus causes warts to form on the skin. These are primarily a cosmetic concern and can be treated by dermatologists as well as hand surgeons. In most pediatric patients, these warts are self-limiting [35]. Common treatments include topically removing the wart via acid application, freezing the wart with liquid nitrogen, or the application of electric currents to destroy the affected cells. Placement of duct tape for a prolonged period over the wart has also been shown to be effective [36]. Surgical removal can be considered if these topical approaches fail or if there is a frequent recurrence of the warts; however, caution must be taken as surgical intervention may cause a greater spread of the infection and lead to recurrent and, at times, satellite lesions [35].

Orf is a purulent papule caused by parapoxvirus. The infection is typically associated with exposure to an animal that is infected with parapoxvirus, particularly sheep. The infection is self-limiting in most patients but patients who are immunocompromised may need a topical antiviral treatment, such as topical imiquimod [37, 38].

Sporotrichosis infections result from *Sporothrix schenckii*, a type of fungus typically found in plant and soil material [39, 40]. The infection typically manifests after a puncture wound is inoculated with the fungus, most commonly from sources such as thorns that provide both the puncture mechanism and inoculation source [39–41]. The mechanism of inoculation results in a subcutaneous infection that presents as a purulent, ulcerative lesion at the site of injury

[39, 41]. Cultures for *Sporothrix schenckii* can be grown on modified Sabouraud agar at 30° Celsius and the infection can be treated with itraconazole for a duration of 3–6 months at a dosage of 200 mg per day [41].

Molluscum contagiosum is a viral infection that results in small, dome-shaped, shiny lesions [42, 43]. The lesions are typically pink to skin-toned in color and can range in size from 3 to 5 mm [42, 43]. The virus is usually transmitted through skin-to-skin contact with the infection lesions [42, 43]. The infection is self-limiting in the majority of patients and the lesions do not require treatment unless they are irritating [42, 43]. If there is persistent itchiness at the site of the active infection, a topical steroid cream can be applied to mitigate the itchiness [43]. Topical treatments of the infection include topical application of cantharidin, imiquimod, potassium hydroxide solution, or salicylic and lactic acid solution [42–44]. Physical methods of treatment include cryotherapy and curettage [42, 43]. Immunocompromised patients who present with *Molluscum contagiosum* can be treated with either topical or intravenous cidofovir, which aids in treating the infection; however, there is a risk of renal toxicity with the intravenous delivery of cidofovir and, due to the immunocompromised status of the patient, the viral lesions may persist [42].

Overall Complications

Complications of infections of the hand are typically due to delayed or missed diagnoses of the infections. These complications depend on the location, type, and severity of the initial infection as well as the treatment that was provided. Scarring and stiffness are the most common complications associated with the treatment of pediatric hand infections. The most common complications from delayed or missed diagnoses include tenosynovitis, osteomyelitis, cellulitis, septic arthritis, and compartment syndrome. Prompt diagnosis and treatment of the vast majority of pediatric hand infections results in optimal outcomes without long-term complications or functional limitations (Box 29.6).

Box 29.6 Pitfalls to Avoid

- It is imperative not to obtain a cursory history as an in-depth history is crucial to narrowing down the possible type of infection and subsequent course of treatment.
- Do not delay; if there is suspicion of a hand infection, act and do not wait.
- Prompt diagnosis and treatment provides the best outcomes in all cases of infection; therefore do not be a passive observer.
- Culture swabs of any purulence can aid in identifying the pathogenic culprit of the infection and can guide treatment for that infection, so make sure to follow-up on any cultures obtained.

Bibliography

1. Fowler JR, Ilyas AM. Epidemiology of adult acute hand infections at an urban medical center. J Hand Surg Am. 2013;38(6):1189–93.
2. Houshian S, Seyedipour S, Wedderkopp N. Epidemiology of bacterial hand infections. Int J Infect Dis. 2006;10(4):315–9.
3. Fuchsjäger N, Winterleitner H, Krause R, Feierl G, Koch H. Susceptibility of microorganisms causing acute hand infections. PLoS One. 2019;14(8):e0220555.
4. Harness N, Blazar PE. Causative microorganisms in surgically treated pediatric hand infections. J Hand Surg Am. 2005;30(6):1294–7.
5. Chung MT, Wilson P, Rinker B. Community-acquired methicillin-resistant Staphylococcus aureus hand infections in the pediatric population. J Hand Surg Am. 2012;37(2):326–31.
6. Leggit JC. Acute and chronic paronychia. Am Fam Physician. 2017;96(1):44–51.
7. Shafritz AB, Coppage JM. Acute and chronic paronychia of the hand. J Am Acad Orthop Surg. 2014;22(3):165–74.
8. Teo WZW, Chung KC. Hand infections. Clin Plast Surg. 2019;46(3):371–81.
9. Koshy JC, Bell B. Hand infections. J Hand Surg Am. 2019;44(1):46–54.
10. Belcher HJCR, Clare TD. Hand infections. Curr Orthop. 2003;17:28–43.
11. Styron JF. Pediatric hand infections. Hand Clin. 2020;36(3):381–6.
12. Franko OI, Abrams RA. Hand infections. Orthop Clin North Am. 2013;44(4):625–34.

13. Kieffer WK, Gallagher K, Rogers BA, Leonard L. Hand infections. Br J Hosp Med (Lond). 2013;74(8):C124–7.
14. McCarthy JJ, Dormans JP, Kozin SH, Pizzutillo PD. Musculoskeletal infections in children: basic treatment principles and recent advancements. Instr Course Lect. 2005;54:515–28.
15. Arango CA. How best to approach these acute hand infections. J Fam Pract. 2020;69(1):E1–8.
16. Wu IB, Schwartz RA. Herpetic whitlow. Cutis. 2007;79(3):193–6.
17. Rubright JH, Shafritz AB. The herpetic whitlow. J Hand Surg Am. 2011;36(2):340–2.
18. Smith C, Scott J. Necrotising fasciitis complicating hand, foot and mouth disease. BMJ Case Rep. 2019;12(8):e228581.
19. Patel R, Kumar H, More B, Patricolo M. Paediatric recurrent herpetic whitlow. BMJ Case Rep. 2013;2013:bcr2013010207.
20. Cohen SG, Beck SC. Point-of-care ultrasound in the evaluation of pyogenic flexor tenosynovitis. Pediatr Emerg Care. 2015;31(11):805–7.
21. Brusalis CM, Thibaudeau S, Carrigan RB, Lin IC, Chang B, Shah AS. Clinical characteristics of pyogenic flexor tenosynovitis in pediatric patients. J Hand Surg Am. 2017;42(5):388.e1–5.
22. Giladi AM, Malay S, Chung KC. A systematic review of the management of acute pyogenic flexor tenosynovitis. J Hand Surg Eur. 2015;40(7):720–8.
23. Draeger RW, Bynum DK Jr. Flexor tendon sheath infections of the hand. J Am Acad Orthop Surg. 2012;20(6):373–82.
24. Okubo Y, Nochioka K, Marcia T. Nationwide survey of pediatric septic arthritis in the United States. J Orthop. 2017;14(3):342–6.
25. Dodwell ER. Osteomyelitis and septic arthritis in children: current concepts. Curr Opin Pediatr. 2013;25(1):58–63.
26. Griego RD, Rosen T, Orengo IF, Wolf JE. Dog, cat, and human bites: a review. J Am Acad Dermatol. 1995;33(6):1019–29.
27. Bula-Rudas FJ, Olcott JL. Human and animal bites. Pediatr Rev. 2018;39(10):490–500.
28. Flevas DA, Syngouna S, Fandridis E, Tsiodras S, Mavrogenis AF. Infections of the hand: an overview. EFORT Open Rev. 2019;4(5):183–93.
29. Meyer CL, Abzug JM. Domestic bird bites. J Hand Surg Am. 2012;37(9):1925–7.
30. Okubo Y, Nochioka K, Testa M. Nationwide survey of pediatric acute osteomyelitis in the USA. J Pediatr Orthop B. 2017;26(6):501–6.
31. Lankachandra M, Wells CR, Cheng CJ, Hutchison RL. Complications of distal phalanx fractures in children. J Hand Surg Am. 2017;42(7):574.e1–6.
32. Leiblein M, Marzi I, Sander AL, Barker JH, Ebert F, Frank J. Necrotizing fasciitis: treatment concepts and clinical results. Eur J Trauma Emerg Surg. 2018;44(2):279–90.
33. Wong CH, Khin LW, Heng KS, Tan KC, Low CO. The LRINEC (Laboratory Risk Indicator for Necrotizing Fasciitis) score: a tool for distinguishing necrotizing fasciitis from other soft tissue infections. Crit Care Med. 2004;32(7):1535–41.
34. Tuan J, Spichler-Moffarah A, Ogbuagu O. *Mycobacterium marinum*: nodular hand lesions after a fishing expedition. BMJ Case Rep. 2020;13(12):e238835.
35. Chan E, Bagg M. Atypical hand infections. Orthop Clin North Am. 2017;48(2):229–40.
36. Abzug JM, Cappel MA. Benign acquired superficial skin lesions of the hand. J Hand Surg Am. 2012;37(2):378–93.
37. Al-Qattan MM. Orf infection of the hand. J Hand Surg Am. 2011;36(11):1855–8.
38. Erbağci Z, Erbağci I, Almila TA. Rapid improvement of human orf (ecthyma contagiosum) with topical imiquimod cream: report of four complicated cases. J Dermatolog Treat. 2005;16(5–6):353–6.
39. Carr MM, Fielding JC, Sibbald G, Freiberg A. Sporotrichosis of the hand: an urban experience. J Hand Surg Am. 1995;20(1):66–70.
40. Kieselova K, Santiago F, Henrique M. Rose thorn injury. BMJ Case Rep. 2017;2017:bcr2017221757.
41. Fox MP, Jacoby SM. Fungal infections of the hand. Hand Clin. 2020;36(3):355–60.
42. Chen X, Anstey AV, Bugert JJ. Molluscum contagiosum virus infection. Lancet Infect Dis. 2013;13(10):877–88.
43. Schaffer JV, Berger EM. Molluscum contagiosum. JAMA Dermatol. 2016;152(9):1072.
44. van der Wouden JC, Koning S, Katz KA. Interventions for nongenital molluscum contagiosum in persons without immune deficiency. JAMA Dermatol. 2018;154(2):203–4.

Pediatric Foot Infections

30

Laurence Wicks, Vrisha Madhuri,
and Richard Gardner

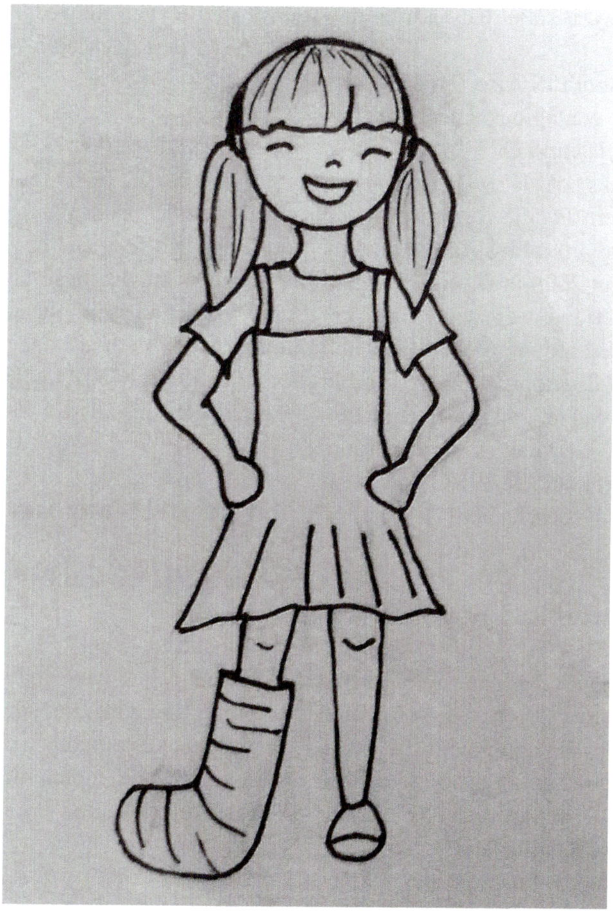

L. Wicks (✉) · R. Gardner
CURE International, Grand Rapids, MI, USA
e-mail: laurence.wicks@cureinternational.org;
richard.gardner@cureinternational.org

V. Madhuri
Paediatric Orthopaedic Department, Ida Scudder Chair for Clinical Research, Adjunct Scientist, Centre for Stem Cell Research, Christian Medical College and Hospital, Vellore, Tamil Nadu, India
e-mail: madhuriwalter@cmcvellore.ac.in

© Springer Nature Switzerland AG 2022
M. V. Belthur et al. (eds.), *Pediatric Musculoskeletal Infections*,
https://doi.org/10.1007/978-3-030-95794-0_30

This chapter begins with a brief discussion of infectious diseases of the foot that do not require surgical management, but are globally common and therefore justify their inclusion. Following this, infections of varying severity are included along with clinical cases.

Hand, Foot and Mouth Disease

Introduction and Epidemiology

There is extensive literature on this condition. Although it is not strictly a foot infection, because of its potential severity, it should at least be discussed in brief.

Hand, foot and mouth disease (HFMD) is a common and highly contagious infectious disease that mainly affects children.

Repeated outbreaks of HFMD have been reported in the Western Pacific Region in many countries. For example, an outbreak of Enterovirus 71 (EV71) in China in 2009 involved 1,155,525 cases, including 13,810 that were severe and 353 deaths. This had led to the World Health Organisation (WHO) developing guidance in an attempt to control spread and optimise treatment. For a comprehensive overview of the condition, please read the freely available WHO document referenced at the end of this chapter [1].

Pathology and Microbiology

HFMD is caused by a group of enteroviruses that include Coxsackievirus A16 (CA16) and Enterovirus 71 (EV71). Infection with EV71 can cause severe disease in children, with central nervous system (CNS) involvement (including aseptic meningitis, encephalitis and acute flaccid paralysis), myocardial dysfunction and pulmonary oedema; it is sometimes fatal.

Clinical Presentation and Examination

HFMD can present with a range of signs and symptoms that include:

- Fever
- Sore throat
- General malaise, or irritability in younger children
- Painful, red, blister-like lesions on the tongue, gums and inside of the cheeks
- A red rash, without itching, but sometimes with blistering, on the palms of hands, soles of feet and the buttocks
- Loss of appetite

The usual incubation period is 3–6 days, often with non-specific fever being the first sign. Lesions in the mouth and throat develop 1 or 2 days after fever, followed by lesions on the hands and feet 1 or 2 days later.

Investigations/Work-Up

Swab samples from the throat, or from vesicles on hands and feet, can be processed in a laboratory to confirm diagnosis and then isolate the specific virus that is implicated in an outbreak. A number of methods for testing samples are described in the WHO guidance and are beyond the scope of this chapter.

Differential Diagnoses

- Chickenpox (varicella)
- Measles
- Rubella
- Herpetic gingivostomatitis (if predominantly presenting with a mouth infection)
- Aphthous stomatitis (if predominantly presenting with a mouth infection)
- Scabies infestation

Treatment Options

The majority of cases of HFMD are self-limiting and will be managed at home. Cases that will go on to develop severe complications and require hospitalisation, including those with CNS involvement, are hard to initially identify. Therefore careful clinical evaluation is required, with regular monitoring in the early stages. If CNS involvement is suspected, a cerebrospinal fluid sample is required. In severe cases that require hospitalisation, management will largely be supportive, but there is some evidence to support use of intravenous (IV) immunoglobulin in severe cases during an epidemic.

When an outbreak occurs, a wide range of measures will need to be employed to limit spread of the disease. Again, this is beyond the scope of this chapter and the reader should refer to WHO guidance if further information is required.

Viral Warts

Introduction and Epidemiology

Also termed verrucas, or verruca vulgaris, these foot lesions are incredibly common the world over [2, 3]. Reported prevalence rates vary, with up to 22% of school age children affected in one study from Australia [4]. They are commonest around the age of 12 years [5].

Pathology and Microbiology

Human papillomavirus causes these warty lesions, of which there are more than 80 serotypes. Direct contact leads to infection, and therefore they are associated with regularly walking barefoot, often in swimming pools, and if another family member at home also has viral warts [2].

Clinical Presentation and Examination

Viral warts on the hands are almost equally as common as those on the feet [2]. The warty lesion has a fairly typical appearance with a skin callosity and underlying central black area. The majority of children with viral warts will be relatively unbothered by the lesions, but location on a weight-bearing area may cause pain, and their appearance may be unacceptable to some.

Differential Diagnoses

- Foreign body
- Insect/spider bites
- Tick bite

Treatment Options

The majority will have resolved within 5 years of presentation [4] and are very unusual beyond the age of 16. For those with persistent and symptomatic warts, various treatment options have been described to try and ablate the symptomatic wart. Options described include cryotherapy (liquid nitrogen), topical salicylic acid and electrocautery. No treatment has been shown to be significantly superior to another and none guarantee complete resolution in all patients [2, 5].

Athlete's Foot

Introduction and Epidemiology

Also termed tinea pedis, athlete's foot is the commonest fungal infection of skin. It can occur concurrently with fungal infections of toenails, which is also known as onychomycosis.

Pathology and Microbiology

Both athlete's foot and fungal toenail infections are caused by a group of fungi termed dermatophytes. There are three main types: Microsporum, Epidermophyton and Trichophyton [6].

Tinea pedis is more common in those who have regular contact with the spores in humid environments, where fungal spores are able to survive for long periods. Therefore, regular use of swimming pools, communal showers, athletic shoes and locker rooms will put an individual at risk. Other skin conditions, such as psoriasis or atopic dermatitis, can increase the risk of also developing this fungal infection.

Clinical Presentation and Examination

Interdigital tinea pedis is what is conventionally referred to as athlete's foot, but there are three other recognised variations of tinea pedis with different clinical presentations: moccasin (chronic hyperkeratotic) tinea pedis; inflammatory or vesicular tinea pedis; and ulcerative tinea pedis [6].

Patients usually present with symptoms of itching, small blisters, burning and malodour. Appearance is typically of white, macerated skin with painful fissuring in the interdigital spaces, usually of the third, fourth and the fifth toes. The condition may also present with scaling plaques and slight erythema on the soles, heels and lateral aspect of the feet. The dorsal surface of the foot is usually unaffected.

Chronic fungal infection of nails causes thickened brittle nails with a yellow discolouration.

Investigations/Work-Up

Diagnosis is usually made based on typical clinical appearance, as described above. However, laboratory testing can confirm diagnosis, which may be necessary before commencing therapies in persistent severe cases.

Laboratory diagnosis requires a scraped-off sample from an active area, ideally from the peripheral, raised border; direct microscopic examination can then be performed. The test is easy and quick, and is highly specific and sensitive for dermatophyte identification. Alternative methods of identification include the use of dermatophyte test strips and performing a fungal culture [6].

Differential Diagnoses

- Alternative infections, such as with *Candida* species or bacterial cellulitis
- Contact or atopic dermatitis
- Psoriasis

Treatment Options

Simple measures are probably most important:

- Keep feet dry, using a separate towel for the feet after washing.
- Take off socks and shoes when at home.
- Wear clean socks each day.
- Do not walk barefoot in communal areas.
- Try to rotate shoe wear, especially sports shoes, to allow them to dry out.

Antifungal therapies can also help, but a high recurrence rate is likely unless the preventive measures outlined above are observed. Topical antifungal agents (examples include terbinafine or butenafine 1%) applied directly to the affected areas for 2 weeks are usually effective. In severe cases, or those unresponsive to topical treatment, systemic treatment may be needed. Examples include terbinafine 250 mg once daily for 2 weeks, or fluconazole 150 mg once weekly for 3 weeks [7].

Summary Points: Most foot infections are superficial, easily diagnosed and do not require complex management.

Non-surgical infectious diseases are common, often caused by viruses and fungi.

Ingrown Toenails

Introduction and Epidemiology

Ingrown toenail, also referred to as onychocryptosis or unguis incarnates, is not an infective condition in itself, but is mentioned here as it is associated with repeated infections of the surrounding soft tissue (paronychia) until definitive treatment is provided.

In a large observational study of paediatric ingrown toenails, 23% were considered infected at the time of presentation, and 34% were being given antibiotics in the week prior to their surgical treatment [8].

Pathology and Microbiology

Traditionally this is thought to be a problem with the toenail, growing into the adjacent soft tissue. However, there is increasing recognition that it is in fact overgrowth of the nail fold through repeated microtrauma, leading to localised inflammation and excessive granulation tissue formation. Superinfection is typically a result, caused by common *Staphylococcus* species found on the skin.

Clinical Presentation and Examination

An infected ingrown toenail can be exquisitely painful with localised swelling and erythema, normally on the lateral border of the great toenail, although both sides of the nail may be affected. There may also be purulent discharge from under the nail fold. It is typically seen in teenagers and is twice as common in males.

Investigations/Work-Up

Consider the possibility of undiagnosed diabetes mellitus in patients with recurrent foot infections, as paronychia associated with ingrown toenails is more common in diabetics [9].

X-rays may show evidence of a periosteal reaction. However, often this is not representative of a true osteomyelitis, but rather periosteal inflammation adjacent to the nail fold. True osteomyelitis of the underlying distal phalanx is possible but rare [10].

Differential Diagnoses

- Other nail conditions, such as fungal nail infections (although typically the nail will appear abnormal but the adjacent soft tissue relatively unaffected).

Treatment Options

Active acute infection of the skinfold is treated with antibiotics targeting staphylococcal species and encouraging the patient to clean the foot regularly in a foot bath. If recurrent episodes of infection occur, then surgical intervention is recommended. Performing definitive surgery at a time when there is an acute exacerbation of the infection may lead to excessive debridement. Theoretically, it also risks the introduction of microorganisms into previously uninvolved underlying bone. This may lead to a more protracted recovery with infection that is more difficult to eradicate. Give antibiotics, therefore, to treat acute infective exacerbations and perform surgery once the situation is more settled.

Traditionally, a surgical strategy involved partial nail excision, with or without partial germinal matrix ablation. The germinal matrix ablation may be performed by surgical excision or chemical ablation using phenol. Recurrence is a well-recognised problem, though, occurring in around 20% of patients. Patients may eventually require total nail excision with complete ablation of the germinal matrix. Furthermore, traditional surgery is associated with a 6% post-operative infection rate [8].

More recently, a move away from nail excision has become popular, with a focus rather on excision of the overgrown and inflamed fold of soft tissue. The Vandenbos procedure for ingrown toenails consists of extensive excision of the surrounding skinfold, to expose the whole of the side of the nail, and then allowing the wound to heal by secondary intention [11]. The wide margin of soft tissue excision may initially seem dramatic but reports suggest this is a more satisfactory method of definitive treatment. In a study of 39 children (59 ingrown toenails) treated in this way, there were no recurrences recorded, with median time of 7 days to return to school and 23 days to wear enclosed shoes again [12].

Penetrating Injuries and Subsequent Infections

Introduction and Epidemiology

Whilst penetrating injuries to the foot are a common occurrence in children, caused by, among other mechanisms, stepping onto an object whilst running and playing outside barefoot, the majority will not become infected if appropriate early prophylactic treatment is given. In a study of children presenting to an emergency department following penetrating foot injuries, just 6% required hospitalisation for either parental antibiotics alone, or in combination with formal surgical debridement [13]. In another observational study, no patients developed infection when oral antibiotics were given within 24 hours of sustaining the injury [14].

Pathology and Microbiology

Penetrating injuries can result in contamination through all muscle layers of the sole of the foot, bones and joints, leading to subsequent infection. *Pseudomonas aeruginosa* is a typical infecting organism associated with contaminated foot wounds [14], although multiple microorganisms may be cultured in established infections [15].

Clinical Presentation and Examination

Assess the plantar for signs of puncture wounds or visible foreign bodies and focal swelling. Like the hand, the dorsal skin of the foot is loosely connected to underlying structures and so dorsal swelling from oedema may be even more evident than plantar swelling, despite an infection that is focused in the more tightly packed plantar structures.

As with all infections, assess the patient for systemic signs of sepsis. Also, look for evidence of ascending lymphangitis, or lymphadenopathy in the popliteal fossa and groin.

Investigations/Work-Up

If a retained foreign body is suspected, it is useful to obtain imaging to look for foreign material – typically three x-ray views of the foot and ultrasound of the plantar foot. If a foreign body is causative, it typically is found within a cavity of pus. Also, the presence of bony changes from osteomyelitis or gas in the soft tissues on plain radiographs may give an indication of the severity and extent of the infection. If there is doubt about the presence of a collection with or without a foreign body, ultrasound or magnetic resonance imaging (MRI) will further aid diagnosis.

Differential Diagnoses

- Foreign body reaction without associated infection
- Necrosis from cytotoxic venomous bites

Treatment Options

Appropriate prophylaxis should be given for all patients who present with a penetrating foot injury, regardless of whether there is evidence of infection [13]. If the wound looks relatively clean and there is no significant soft tissue injury, broad-spectrum antibiotics can be given along with a tetanus booster; the patient may be discharged and instructed to follow-up in the outpatient office within several days. For a clear and detailed guide on the management of wounds, please see the freely available and excellent WHO guidance on general principles for the 'Prevention and Management of Wound Infection', which is referenced at the end of this chapter [16].

If there is any concern of infection at the time of presentation, we would suggest at least a period of observation with the limb elevated and parental antibiotics initiated. Where to observe the patient (i.e. the emergency department versus a main hospital ward) will depend on the healthcare setting you are in, but the child should not be sent home unless the treating team is happy that the treatment is systemically well and that the infection is not spreading. If this is the beginning of gas gangrene or necrotising fasciitis, the patient may quickly deteriorate. In the absence of an obvious collection, surgery might be avoided. Broad-spectrum antibiotics should be administered, with continued limb elevation and close monitoring for either improvement of worsening infection. Any areas of erythema should be mapped out with a permanent marker along with date and time. Also, consider oxygen and intravenous fluids if signs of sepsis are present. If available, arrange imaging as described above.

The aims of any surgical intervention should be to adequately drain pus and debride necrotic tissue, whilst protecting important structures and limiting scarring. When washing and debriding infected wounds, do not use high-pressure lavage, as this may force microorganisms and contamination into other tissue planes that have not previously been violated. Use extensile longitudinal incisions that will permit adequate exposure to the cavity of infection and do not close wounds primarily; it is also preferable to avoid plantar incisions over weight-bearing areas when possible.

Complications

Persistent or recurrent infection is a concern, especially if there is unrecognised bone or joint contamination.

Gas gangrene, or gas forming myonecrosis (often caused by *Clostridium perfringens*), and necrotising fasciitis, can both develop as a result of deep contamination in untreated foot wounds. The onset of these life-threatening conditions may initially be subtle. A systematic review of available literature on necrotising fasciitis in children found that Group-A streptococci accounted for 44.8% of cases, Gram-negative rods in 29.8% and polymicrobial infections occurred in 17.3%. Extremities were affected in 45.6%, of which 73.5% occurred in the lower extremities [17].

> Summary Points: Penetrating injuries are easily managed if they present early, but in established infection thorough debridement may be needed to eradicate *Pseudomonas*.

> Following minor trauma, be diligent to avoid missing early presentation of rare but devastating infections, such as gas gangrene or necrotising fasciitis.

Osteomyelitis of the Hindfoot

Introduction and Epidemiology

The calcaneus is a common site of infection in the hindfoot, accounting for nearly one-third of such infections in one series [18]. Osteomyelitis of the calcaneus accounts for 3–10% of all paediatric bone infections [19]. It is an uncommon but important emergent condition in a limping child [20]. This infection's importance lies in the fact that its clinical and laboratory presentation is sometimes slow-developing or misleading, causing a delay in the diagnosis, which seriously impacts the outcome, resulting in chronicity and sequelae [21].

Age related incidence varies in different series, with the age of peak incidence ranging from neonates (from heel pricks) to 2- and 9-year olds. Males are predominant, and most patients acquire their infections by haematogenous spread.

Pathology and Microbiology

Repetitive trauma to the heel during ambulation possibly makes this region more susceptible to osteomyelitis through haematogenous spread. Penetrating injuries (thorns, foreign bodies) is an additional risk factor for direct contamination of the calcaneus. Another well-established predisposing cause is taking blood samples in neonates by heel prick (Guthrie test) technique. The penetrating injuries commonly result in pseudomonas osteomyelitis.

Success in isolating organisms from blood or local aspirate varies and is usually less than 60% [21, 22]. The microbiological isolates reveal infection most commonly with *Staphylococcus aureus* (usually methicillin-sensitive. although there are recent reports of methicillin-resistant organisms). Other reported organisms include *Streptococcus pyogenes* and Group D streptococci [22]. Rare infections from the osteomyelitis site have been reported in the literature. They include *Salmonella* Livingstone, *Pasteurella pneumotropica* and *Kingella kingae* from puncture wounds, and delayed presentations from penetrating injuries, including *Serratia marcescens* (chicken bone penetration) and *Mycobacterium fortuitum* (rake puncture).

The calcaneus infection can breach the cortex and growth plate in the early stages, causing soft tissue oedema and abscess around the joints adjacent to calcaneus, and leads to arthritis of the subtalar joint and other foot bones in late cases.

Clinical Presentation and Examination

Calcaneal infections are rare, and, in the early stage, present with a limping child holding the foot in the equinus and avoiding weight-bearing on the heel. There may be a delay of nearly 1 week before presentation, with only 40% giving a history of trauma [22]. The pain may not be localised to the calcaneus in the early stages, causing misdiagnosis of nearby joint infection, such as the subtalar or ankle joints. Fever, a cardinal symptom of acute osteomyelitis, may be absent, with only 22% presenting a temperature above 38 °C in a large series [22].

Findings of infection in the foot, such as swelling, erythema and warmth, lack in more than half of the cases, making localisation to the calcaneus difficult. However, in late presenting cases, the local findings are more visible with swelling, marked equinus posture of the foot, and painful, restricted ankle and subtalar joints movements.

Investigations/Work-Up

Diagnosis is delayed, with a correct diagnosis initially in only 63% of the Crawford case series [22].

Blood Work

White blood cell (WBC) counts are often not useful, as mean WBC counts are not elevated in many cases. In suspect paediatric bone infections, elevations of erythrocyte sedimentation rate (ESR) and C-reactive protein (CRP) typically have a sensitivity of 94 and 95%. However, in calcaneal cases, this is decreased to 81–95% and 47–71%, respectively [20]. Between the two, ESR elevation above 20 mm/hour is more reliable, especially for late cases. Prior antibiotic use and the small size of the calcaneus are probably the cause for a less vigorous inflammatory response compared to osteomyelitis in other sites such as long bones or the pelvis.

Imaging

Ultrasound examination is helpful when the lesion extends beyond the cortex. Subperiosteal elevation, fluid collections and soft tissue oedema have been noted [21]. Radiographic changes are present, but typically only after 7 days; hence this investigation is not diagnostic of osteomyelitis in early cases but is useful to rule out other diagnoses such as fractures. When the changes are present, osteolysis, cavitation and sequestration within the calcaneus may be noted. In late cases, breach of the physis and physeal damage may be noted, in addition to sclerosis, growth arrest and widening of the bone. Radiographic changes are present in 14–71% of the patients. Magnetic resonance imaging, however, is the most sensitive modality for diagnosing calcaneal osteomyelitis.Changes are seen in nearly 100% of cases, with lesions showing a high signal on T2 short tau inversion recovery (STIR) images and low signal in T1. Computed tomography (CT) scan is useful for delineating cortical breach and sequestrum formation, assisting in preoperative planning, in particular if surgical debridement is indicated [20].

Differential Diagnoses

The differential diagnosis of calcaneal osteomyelitis in a child includes causes of limp attributable to hindfoot conditions, such as traumatic injuries and overuse conditions. When the symptoms are mild to moderate, Sever's disease has frequently been misdiagnosed in children with calcaneal osteomyelitis, and several such cases have been reported [23, 24].

Common differential diagnoses to consider, aside from Sever's disease and osteomyelitis, include calcaneal stress fracture, retrocalcaneal bursitis and Achilles tendinopathy. Ankle and subtalar joint synovitis/septic arthritis, either concomitant with calcaneal osteomyelitis or as other important differential diagnoses, must also be considered in a child with systemic and laboratory features of infections; arthrotomy may be necessary in some cases (Fig. 30.1). Osteomyelitis of adjacent bones can be confirmed or ruled out by a bone scan or MRI in the early stages. Reactive arthritis or Reiter's syndrome requires appropriate rheumatologic work-up. An osteoid osteoma or other bone tumours (osteoblastoma, osteosarcoma, haematological malignancy or Ewing's) are other possible diagnoses that need to be considered and ruled out appropriately by imaging and biopsy.

Treatment Options

Treatment follows the principles of osteomyelitis management in children with osteomyelitis elsewhere in the skeleton. When diagnosed early based on blood and fluid culture, IV antibiotics for 72 hours, followed by an oral antibiotic course using a broad-spectrum cephalosporin or clindamycin, is recommended by Pääkkönen et al. [25]. Antibiotics are combined with trepanation (decompress by drilling a hole) in cases where intraosseous abscess has occurred. Other alternatives include chloramphenicol- and penicillin-based antibiotics [26]. About one-third of the cases required a change to specific antibiotics after culture report in Mooney's series [26].

In the early stage of intraosseous disease, an open trepanation with drainage of the abscess is sufficient. However, neglected and chronic cases with subperiosteal and soft tissue abscess require formal irrigation and debridement. The approach depends on the location of the soft tissue collection and the extent of breach in the osseous structure.

In predominantly plantar, chronic calcaneal osteomyelitis, a modified Gaenslen's approach is preferred for debridement. In this procedure, the heel is split in the middle. However, in children, unlike the traditional Ganselen's approach, the incision is restricted to the sole and not extended proximally to the back of the heel. This modification avoids any physeal damage [27]. The approach has the disadvantage of broadening the heel profile but provides excellent access; the incision heals well and does not affect walking.

Eradicating the infection in chronic and recurrent osteomyelitis is sometimes a challenge. Vancomycin- and gentamicin-loaded beads of calcium sulphate have been used to fill

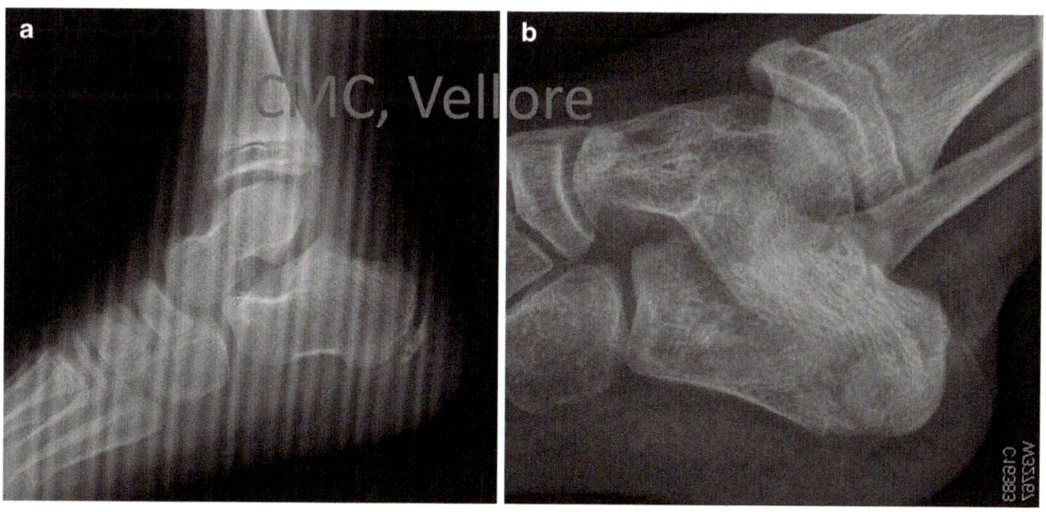

Fig. 30.1 (**a**, **b**) Case example: Hindfoot osteomyelitis. (Source: CMC Vellore)

the cavity and left in place after performing an eggshell debridement through acortical window. This technique has the advantage that the beads need not be removed. This technique was performed in a series of 34 patients, with eradication of infection in 29 cases, when combined with systemic antibiotics of appropriate sensitivity [28]. A significant complication of this procedure in this superficial location is aseptic leakage, seen in 11 patients, which required removal of the beads.

For neglected cases with multiple recurrences, deformity and pain, total calcanectomy has been carried out [29]. The same series also reported talectomy, which could address pain, mobility and deformity in an avascular talus.

Complications

Early diagnosis and treatment is the key to successful management in calcaneal osteomyelitis [25]. Good outcomes are reported, with no complications, when an early diagnosis was made, and a short course of IV antibiotics for 3 days, followed by a month of oral antibiotics, was given. However, recurrence rates of 17% have been reported by Crawford [22]. The older series of Jenzri et al. reports 27% sequelae with significant joint motion restriction, fistulae and painful arthritis [21]. Complication rates are even higher in published literature series, especially when there are significant delays to commencing treatment [19, 29]. The most common sequela is recurrent osteomyelitis [9]. Other problems include calcaneal apophyseal premature closure and surgical scar sensitivity. Spontaneous fusion of the adjacent subtalar and other joints and hindfoot varus deformity have also been reported [18].

Severe neglected infections have also been reported, resulting in equinus and calcaneal deformities, subtalar septic arthritis, Brodie's abscess formation, and avascular necrosis of the talus.

In conclusion, awareness of this rare infection as a cause of limp is essential. However, whilst the good outcome is the rule in early cases, the condition is often misdiagnosed; delays in diagnosis could seriously damage walking ability and lead to chronic infections and permanent disability.

High clinical suspicion of calcaneal osteomyelitis is warranted in a limping child.

When atraumatic hindfoot symptoms are present, suspect osteomyelitis is present, even if systemic features are minimal, and laboratory tests and radiographs are normal.

Advanced imaging, such as MRI, may be required to aid diagnosis and localise infection in early presentations.

Case Example: Hindfoot Osteomyelitis (Fig. 30.1)

With a limp of 10 days and an inability to bear on the right heel, an 8-year-old child presented with intense pain and fever and swelling around the hindfoot.

The total WBC count was 16,900/mm^3. The initial CRP was 4.63 mg/L (normal for the lab).

The initial radiographs were normal. However, serosanguinous fluid was obtained from the ankle and subtalar joint on emergency arthrotomy. An abscess overlying the lateral calcaneus drained 15 mL of pus. Pus culture from the abscess revealed oxacillin-sensitive *Staphylococcus aureus*. A CRP at 6 weeks had increased to 7.9 mg/L, and the wound continued to discharge pus. The radiographs show lytic and sclerotic areas in the calcaneus and the talus at 6 months, suggesting established chronic osteomyelitis.

Case Example: Limping Child with Delayed Diagnosis of Osteomyelitis of the Talus (Figs. 30.2, 30.3, 30.4, 30.5, and 30.6)

This 2-year-old child presented to the clinic with a limp and reluctance to weight-bear. There was no definite history of trauma, and he was systemically well. An X-ray of his lower leg showed no obvious abnormality, and a working diagnosis of presumed toddlers fracture was made.

At his follow-up visit, he remained symptomatic, refusing to bear weight. Repeat X-ray was performed a month later. By this time, a lesion had become visible in the talar dome. Erythrocyte sedimentation rate was 35 mm/hour, but he remained systemically well. There was no swelling of note.

An MRI was performed, which showed a distinct subchondral lesion within the talar dome. Also noted was an associated high signal suggestive of synovitis around the cuboid. The findings were considered consistent with a diagnosis of subacute osteomyelitis of the talus.

Following discussion with the infectious diseases team, a decision was made to treat him empirically with oral co-amoxiclav, which was continued for 6 weeks. His symptoms recovered relatively quickly, and serial X-rays demonstrated gradual resolution of the lesion in the talus over the following 12 months.

Take Home Point: In a small case series of 11 patients with primary subacute haematogenous osteomyelitis (PSHO) of the foot, all presented with a limp. Nine were under three years of age. The talus was involved in 36%. All patients except one were cured with antibiotics [30].

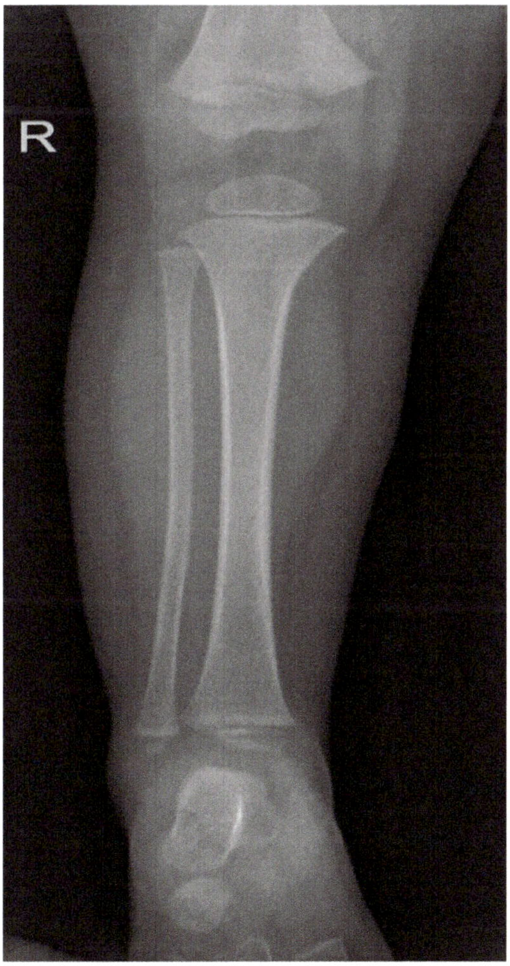

Fig. 30.2 X-ray at initial presentation of limping child. (Source: Sheffield Children's Hospital)

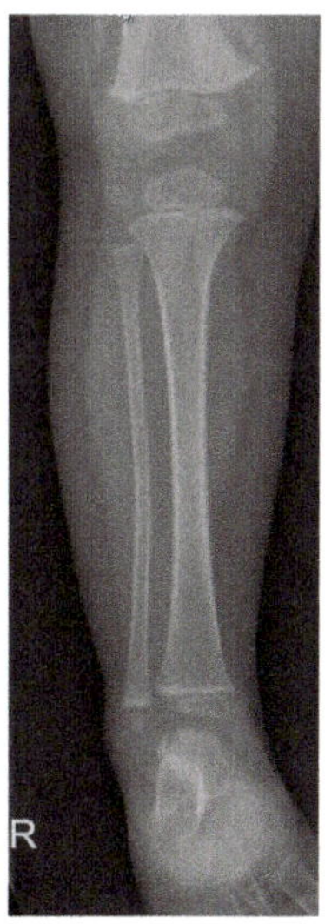

Fig. 30.3 X-ray at 1-month follow-up, with persistent limp, and lesion in talus now visible. (Source: Sheffield Children's Hospital)

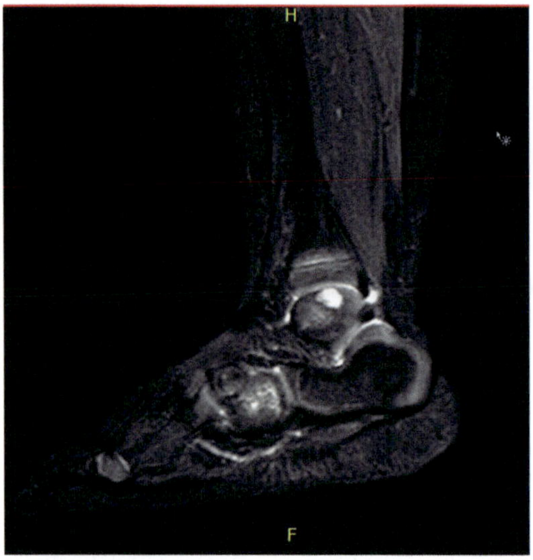

Fig. 30.4 Lateral MRI of foot ankle, defining lesion in talus. (Source: Sheffield Children's Hospital)

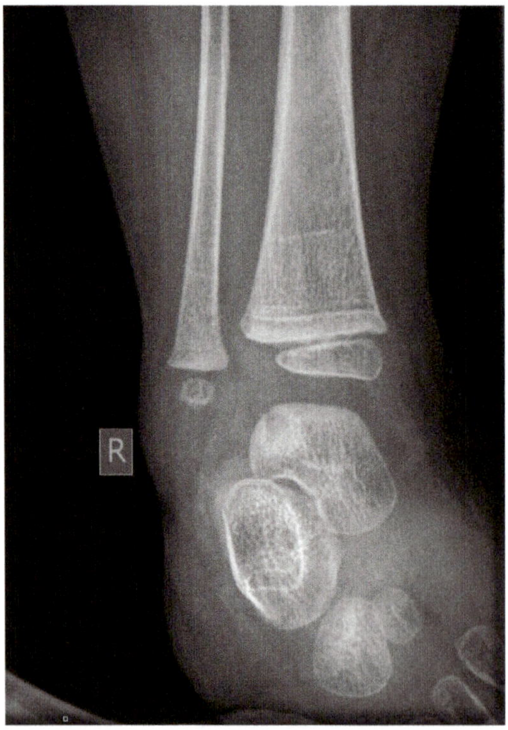

Fig. 30.5 X-ray at follow-up, with resolving lesion, following antibiotic treatment. (Source: Sheffield Children's Hospital)

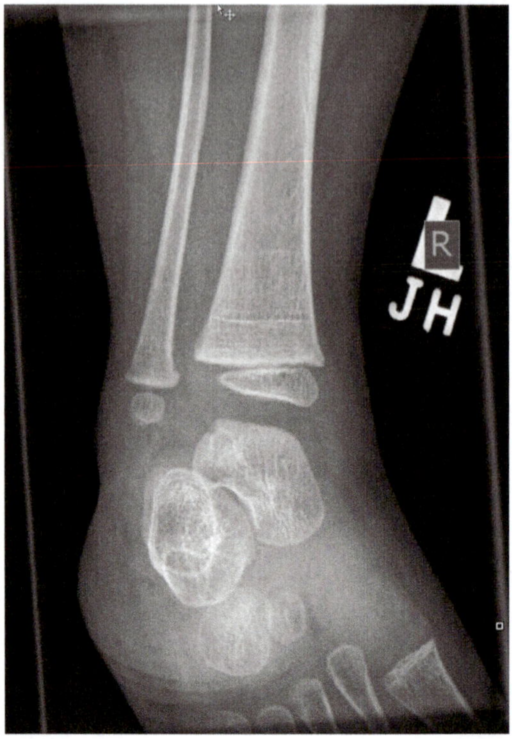

Fig. 30.6 X-ray showing continued resolution of talar lesion. (Source: Sheffield Children's Hospital)

Case Example: Osteomyelitis Leading to Growth Arrest (Figs. 30.7, 30.8, 30.9, 30.10, 30.11, 30.12, and 30.13)

This boy presented to the hospital at the age of ten. He had been treated 6 months earlier by incision and drainage of infection around his left ankle. Both medial and lateral incisions had been performed at the referring treatment centre.

At follow-up, he was having discharge from a medial sinus. X-rays confirmed the presence of a distal tibial metaphyseal sequestrum with medial physeal arrest. The lateral physis and distal fibula seemed unaffected, with fibula overgrowth and a varus deformity.

Initially, a sequestrectomy was performed. Once active infection had resolved, and there was sufficient consolidation of the distal tibia, drill epiphysiodesis of the distal fibula and lateral distal tibia was performed.

Nearly 2 years after he first presented, the residual distal tibia varus deformity was not causing any symptoms, but it was decided to treat the resultant leg length discrepancy through drill epiphysiodesis of the contralateral proximal tibia.

At the most recent follow-up, he reports no pain. He will continue to be monitored until skeletal maturity.

Pyogenic osteomyelitis may cross the physis more often than has been thought historically (possibly in up to 81% of cases). Both valgus and varus ankle alignments may occur, depending on what area of involvement of the physis has occurred [31].

Take Home Point: Treat any active ongoing infection. After treating an infection around the ankle, continue to follow-up the patient annually until skeletal maturity, looking for physeal integrity and any evidence of progressive deformity in the radiographs, as fibrous physeal bars caused by infection may present clinically several years later. Consider completing the epiphysiodesis of the damaged growth plate rather than bar excision in older children as the growth rate is slow at the distal tibial physis. Contralateral epiphysiodesis to avoid or manage a limb length discrepancy should also be considered. This is easier to perform in the proximal tibia. If a persistent deformity of the ankle is significant or symptomatic, a supra-malleolar osteotomy may be required to correct angular malalignment.

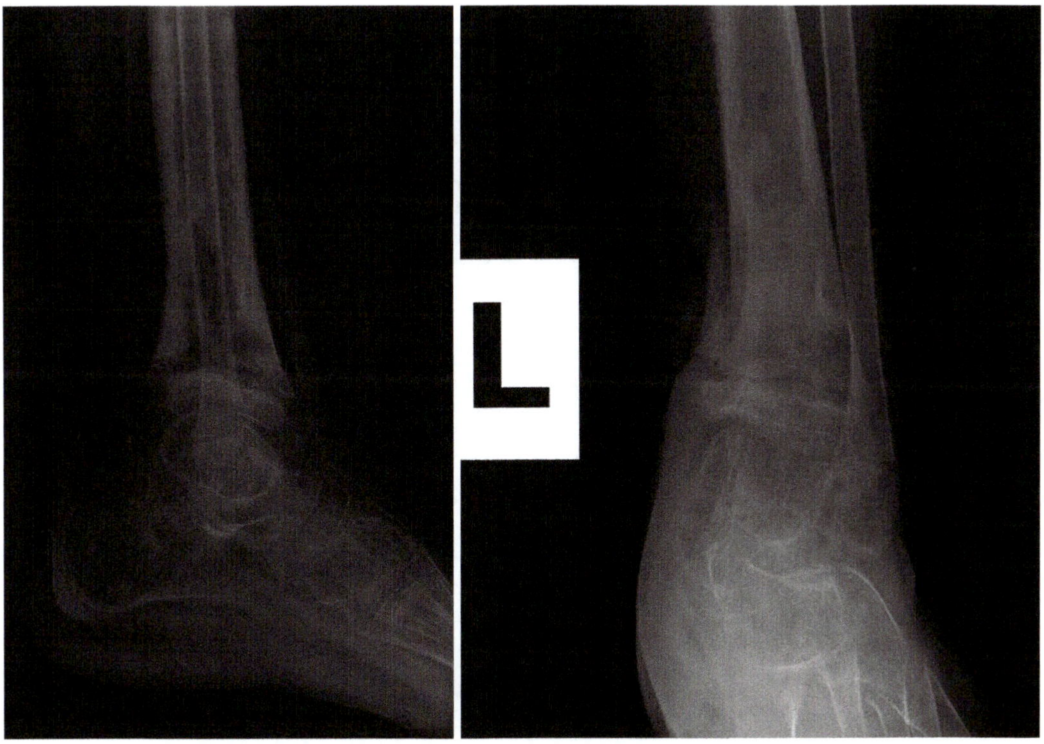

Fig. 30.7 X-ray of ankle of a 10-year-old, 6 months after incision and debridement of acute osteomyelitis. (Source: CURE Ethiopia)

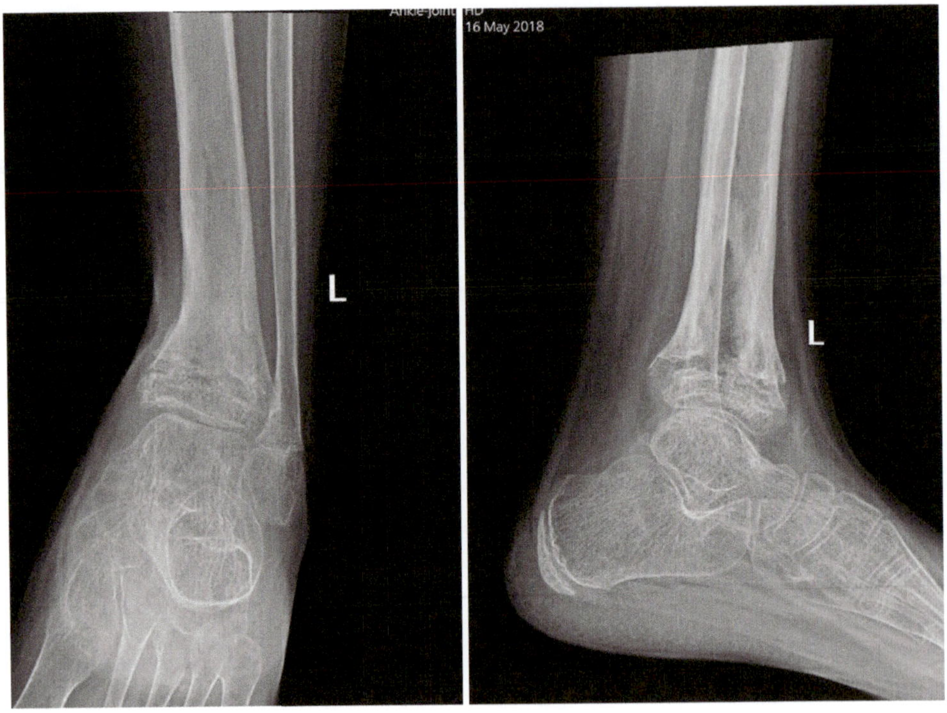

Fig. 30.8 X-ray of ankle after further debridement and sequestrectomy. (Source: CURE Ethiopia)

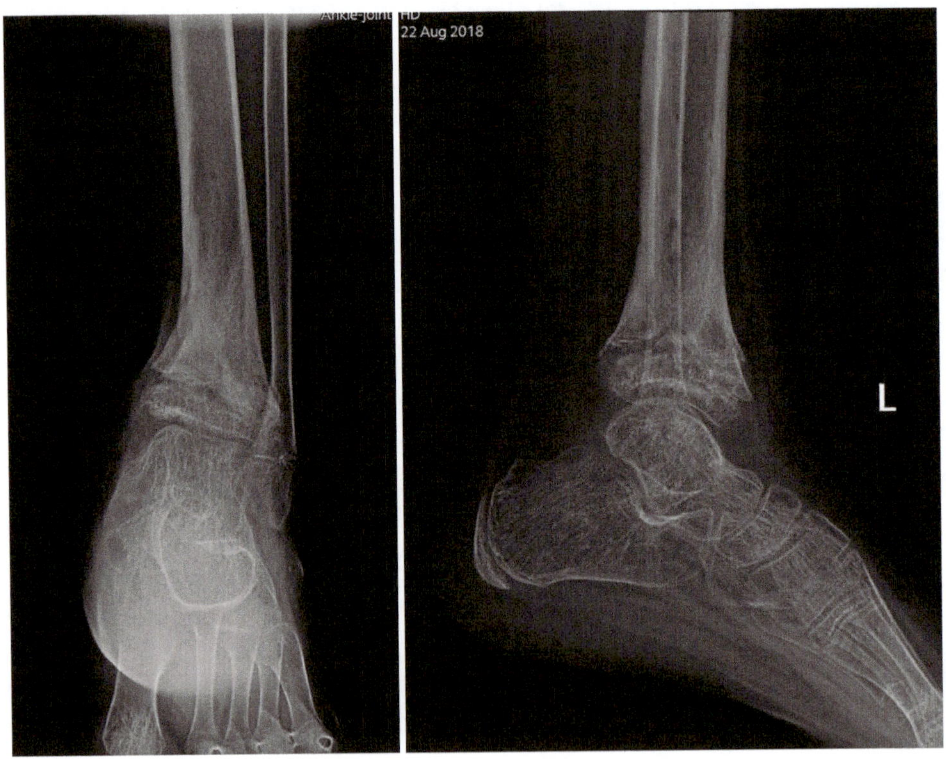

Fig. 30.9 X-ray of ankle showing consolidation but persistent ankle varus. (Source: CURE Ethiopia)

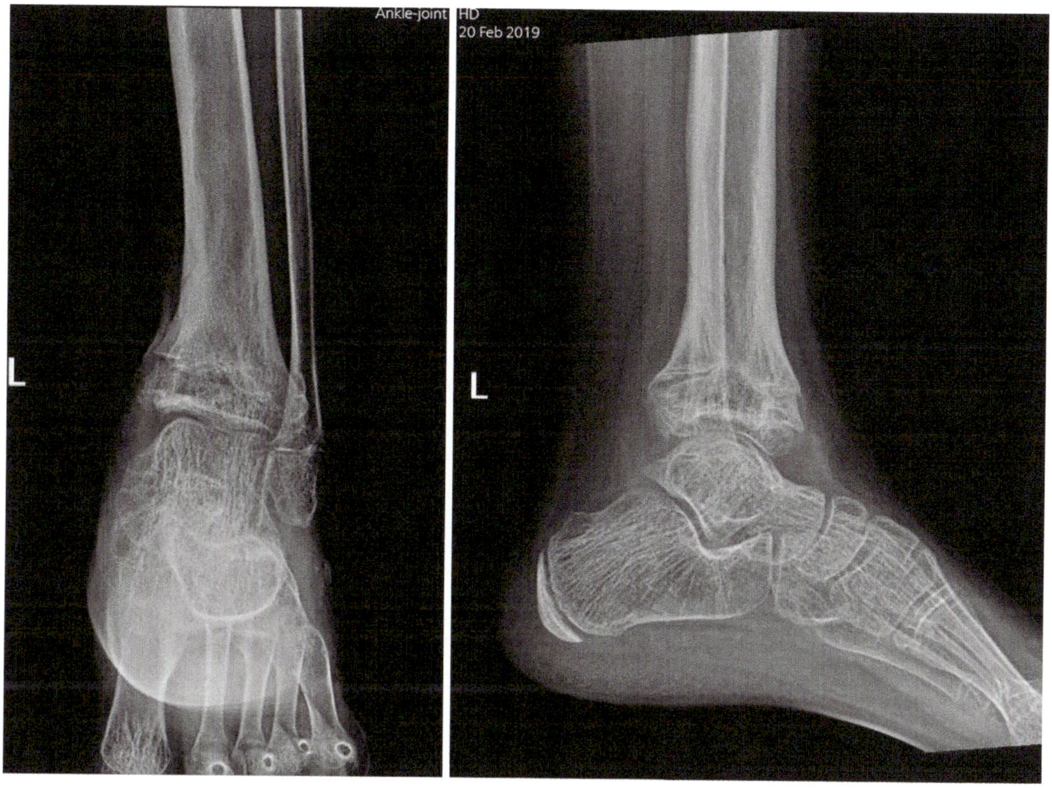

Fig. 30.10 X-ray of ankle showing consolidation but persistent ankle varus. (Source: CURE Ethiopia)

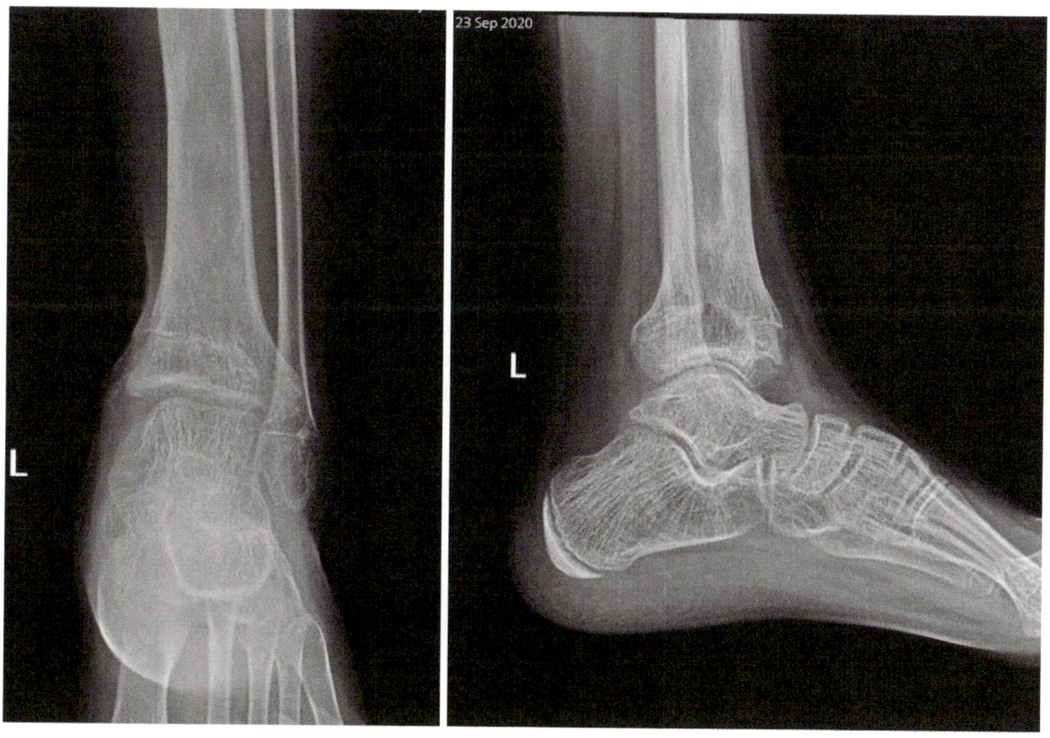

Fig. 30.11 X-ray of ankle after epiphysiodesis of distal tibia. (Source: CURE Ethiopia)

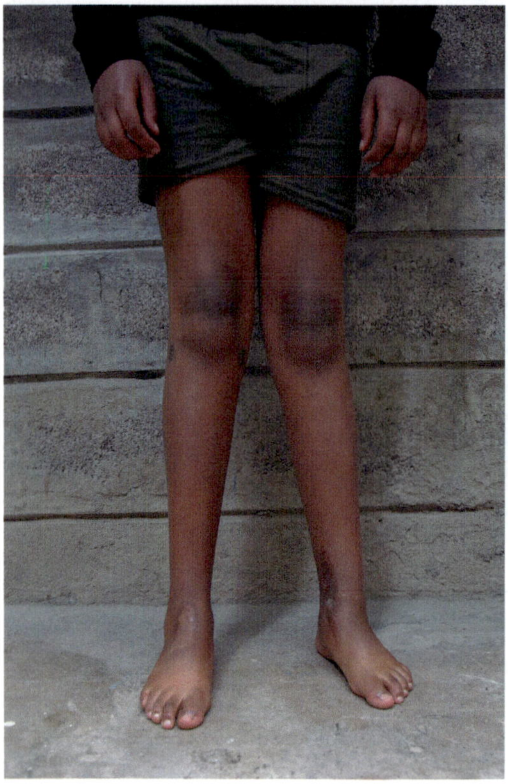

Fig. 30.12 Clinical photos of lower limbs, after infection control, distal tibia epiphysiodesis and contralateral epiphysiodesis to control limb length discrepancy. (Source: CURE Ethiopia)

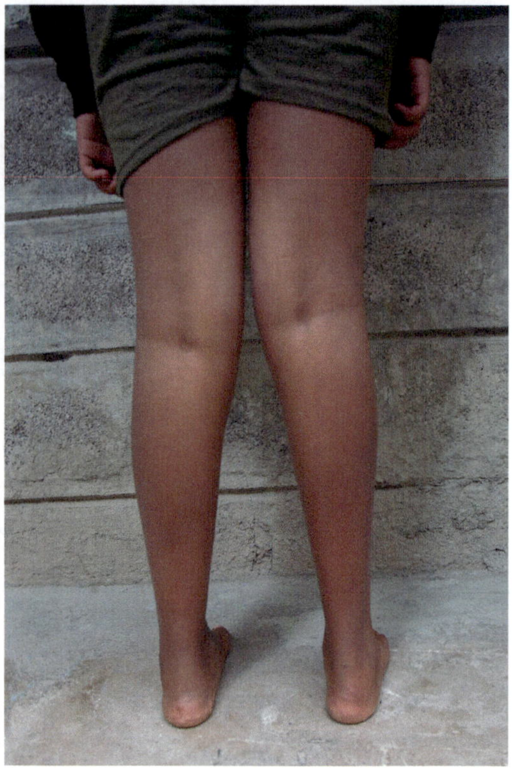

Fig. 30.13 Clinical photos of lower limbs, after infection control, distal tibia epiphysiodesis and contralateral epiphysiodesis to control limb length discrepancy. (Source: CURE Ethiopia)

Tuberculosis of the Foot and Ankle

Introduction and Epidemiology

Tuberculosis (TB) of the foot and ankle is uncommon. It constitutes less than 10% of the osteoarticular and 0.1–0.3% of all extrapulmonary tuberculosis [32]. It tends to occur in young children. These infections occur even in the very young [33, 34] and can present on the first visit as a limp. When the lesion is primarily osseous, the initial presentation is a swelling, and the presentation is delayed for several months [33]. Osseous lesions that have penetrated the cortex and present as abscesses and articular lesions cause pain, soft tissue swelling and a limp.

Pathology and Microbiology

In the foot, tuberculosis can present in many different ways [32].

1. *Granulomatous juxta-articular infection*: These may spread to adjacent joints in the midfoot and Lisfranc joints, with the potential for adjacent joint infections throughout the foot.
2. *An intraosseous central granuloma involving the metatarsals or phalanges causing surrounding expansion of the cortex (Spina ventosa)*: These lesions may also occur in tarsal bones and the distal tibia, and often are multicentric. Isolated bony involvement is frequent in the calcaneus but is also reported in other

tarsal bones such as talus, cuboid, navicular and cuneiform.

3. *Primary synovial infection*: These are typically seen in the ankle joint; an example is seen in Fig. 30.17.
4. *Tenosynovitic or bursal tuberculosis*: More common in adults, these conditions in children are rare.

Clinical Presentation and Examination

The duration before presentation varies with the lesion site and can be from weeks to several years [2–4]. Subperiosteal lesions and infections of weight-bearing joints tend to present early because of the development of superficial abscesses or pain on loading the joint. Insidious onset and course are typical, with a slight rise in temperature and malaise. There may be a misleading history of trauma that draws attention to the bony lesions at the affected site. Significant family history is elicited, especially in the younger children, who often have tuberculous contact from a primary caregiver.

Clinical examination reveals an ankle joint in a position of plantarflexion when the primary site is the ankle joint itself. The skin overlying the affected area may be mildly warm to touch but not erythematous like in acute infections. The effusion is seen as an anterior bulge, initially below the extensor retinaculum, followed by swelling on either side of the Achilles tendon posteriorly, with a fluid wave or fluctuance palpable. The synovial thickening, when present, has a doughy consistency to touch.

The mild pain experienced in the early effusion and synovitic stages is followed by progressive limb wasting and impaired movement. In those with tuberculous arthritis, restriction of movement in all directions is seen, resulting from associated protective muscle spasm. In the foot, involvement of multiple joints, such as the subtalar, midtarsal or Lisfranc joints, is suggestive of the diagnosis. In late stage disease, fractures through large juxta-articular cavities cause collapse of the longitudinal arch resulting in a rocker bottom foot. The muscle spasm in the foot can give the appearance of a peroneal spastic foot, with the heel locked in eversion.

Bony swelling is typically metadiaphyseal in position, diffuse and ill-defined; radiographically these lesions can be seen breaching the physis. In the os calcis, the bone's thickening is appreciated by pressing the calcaneal tuberosity mediolaterally between the thumb and forefingers; when affected, the calcaneus is tender and feels broader or thicker than the unaffected side. The presence of cold abscesses (collection of pus without sign of inflammation) or sinus tracts is pathognomonic of tuberculosis. Unlike in septic lesions, sinuses of tuberculosis are classically undermined at the edges with a pale ulcer and a lack of granulation tissue.

> Diffuse foot osteoporosis is the hallmark of midfoot tuberculous disease.

> A tuberculous osteomyelitis lesion may breach the cortex and physis, damaging the physis or even eroding into the joint.

> Metadiaphyseal lytic bone lesions with expansion of the cortex (spina ventosa) in short bones are classic radiographic findings of tuberculous osteomyelitis.

Investigations/Work-Up

Diagnosis can be difficult [35] but the work-up for a suspected tuberculous-related lesion is similar to that for other sites of potential osteoarticular tuberculosis and includes a Mantoux test and chest radiograph. Findings supportive of the diagnosis seen on chest radiographs are hilar lymphadenopathy, cavities (especially in the apical lobes), nodular infiltration of the lung paren-

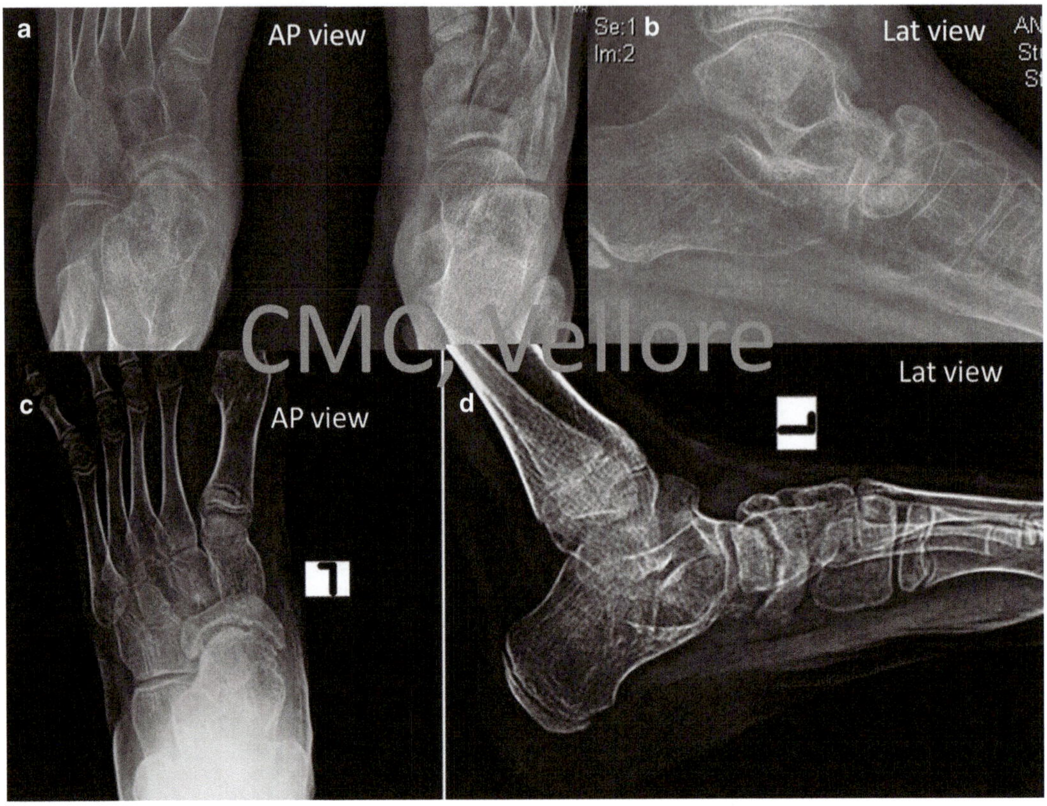

Fig. 30.14 TB of talonavicular joint-different views of the foot demonstrating peri-articular erosion and subsequent arthritis. (Source: CMC Vellore)

chyma and consolidation. Aspirate of the synovial fluid or abscess, or a small tissue biopsy, sent for microbiological and histopathological examination often confirms the diagnosis. White blood cell counts are not useful; an erythrocyte sedimentation rate (ESR) > 20 mm/hour and CRP > 6 mg/mL suggest an infection.

Radiographs often show diffuse and periarticular osteoporosis, a hallmark of tuberculosis in the synovial disease; decreased or obliterated joint spaces, with periarticular erosions, indicate arthritis (Fig. 30.14). Abscess formation in juxta-periosteal or late cases is seen as a soft tissue shadow on radiographs; ultrasound examination is often used to define the abscess's extent better. Some bony lesions are present as osteolytic metadiaphyseal lesions, with an expansion of the medullary canal but minimal periosteal reaction on radiographs. The changes are often most pronounced in the metatarsals and phalanges, giving a ballooned appearance known as *spina ventosa*. Large juxta-articular destructive lesions and periosteal breaks may also be seen (Fig. 30.16). Sequestrum formation (necrotic bone), though rare, is seen in tuberculosis. It appears as bone flakes also described as feathery in appearance. These do not require removal and get absorbed spontaneously on antituberculous treatment. Magnetic resonance imaging [36] shows intense marrow oedema, seen as a high signal on T2-weighted images. MRI is also useful for demonstrating cortical breaks, early cavitations and soft tissue abscesses [32].

Microbiological Techniques

The molecular diagnosis of tuberculosis can be established by a tissue or pus polymerase chain reaction (PCR) test, such as Xpert MTB/RIF [37], which also determines rifampicin resistance. Serological tests such as QuantiFERON-TB Gold for tuberculosis have a high false-positive rate and are not recommended.

Acid-fast bacillus or AFB (Ziehl-Neelsen) stain is a special bacteriological stain used to identify acid-fast organisms, such as *Mycobacterium tuberculosis*. It can be used on the pus or histological slides of the specimen to demonstrate the acid-fast bacillus causing tuberculosis.

A standard culture using Löwenstein-Jensen medium, which took 3–4 weeks to detect *Mycobacterium tuberculosis* and 6–8 weeks for its sensitivity patterns to antituberculous agents to be determined, was commonly used before. It is now replaced by rapid methods of detecting *Mycobacterium tuberculosis* in the extracted samples, such as BACTEC assay, which takes 5–10 days, and MGIT (Mycobacteria growth indicator tube) growth, which yields results in 7–12 days.

> Tuberculous osteomyelitis is a great mimic of other disease processes; lesions may be missed for years and are often diagnosed as osteochondrosis, avascular necrosis and cysts, especially when minimally symptomatic.

> The supporting evidence for tuberculosis such as ESR, Mantoux test and chest X-ray (CXR) may be normal.

Differential Diagnoses

Very often in children, the diagnosis is made by the presence of a raised ESR, a positive Mantoux test, a chest radiograph showing sentinel tuberculous lesions in the presence of clinical signs of localised painful swelling in the bones around the ankle and foot or evidence of synovitis or arthritis with osteoporosis. In non-endemic areas, or when the diagnosis is equivocal, a histological or bacteriological proof is mandatory [38].

The bone lesions of acute osteomyelitis, Brodie's abscess and enchondroma form the differential diagnosis. Tuberculous lesions have also masqueraded as avascular necrosis of the talus and navicular, as well as other osteochondroses [39, 40]. It is noteworthy that the supporting parameters, such as ESR, have been normal in many instances. Histopathologically, granulomatous inflammation with or without caseation or the presence of acid-fast bacilli in the isolates from the lesions is confirmatory. A PCR test positive from tissue isolates is also critical in establishing the diagnosis.

Pyogenic arthritis forms a vital differential diagnosis. Mixed infections are not uncommon, so a tuberculous confirmation should still be looked for even if a pyogenic organism is isolated. Pigmented villonodular synovitis affecting joints and the tendon sheath shows haemosiderin deposition in the joint and synovium, a distinct histological finding. Neoplastic lesions of the bones and synovium also need to be differentiated histologically. Warm foot of tuberculosis has been mistaken for Kaposi sarcoma. Amyloidosis deposition in the foot is associated with swelling and can be mistaken for tuberculosis; neurological and skin changes can help to differentiate this condition from tuberculosis, in addition to histological findings.

Treatment Options

Treatment of foot and ankle tuberculous infection aims to provide biological control of the disease and maintain painless stable weight-bearing lower extremity, preserving mobility whenever possible.

Medical treatment is started once a culture or histological diagnosis is made. Most published series have used antituberculous regimens ranging from 12 to 18 months with no existing evidence for shorter drug regimens in these lesions. The suggested regimen [41] is 2 months of 4 drugs (rifampicin, isoniazid with pyridoxine, ethambutol, and pyrazinamide) followed by 10–16 months of 3 drugs (rifampicin, isoniazid, and ethambutol). The paediatric dosages for these are isoniazid 10–20 (300) mg/kg/day, rifampicin 10–20 (600) mg/kg/day, pyrazinamide 15–30 (2000) mg/kg/day and ethambutol 15–25 mg/kg/day (Table 30.1). Treatment is monitored by improving the local symptoms and systemic features, weight gain and lowering of ESR, or returning to normal ESR. Improvement in osteoporosis of the foot and ankle region takes longer than 3 months. However, increased bone density should be seen by 6 months in patients with good response to treatment [32]. When a clinical and laboratory response is not present, a resistant tuberculosis, or other alternative diagnoses, should be considered and investigated.

Surgery is not the rule for foot and ankle lesions, though a diagnostic aspiration or biopsy may be required in most cases. Surgery is indicated for open biopsy to obtain a tissue diagnosis or for surgical debridement in a clinically non-responsive case. Intervention is also required for deformity of the feet in neglected cases, juxta-articular lesions, which are likely to invade the joint, and for large cavities and abscesses to improve drug access (Fig. 30.15). Synovial resection, excision of the lesion or arthrodesis to avoid painful sequelae in articular lesions, and pre-emptive surgery involving temporary external fix-

Table 30.1 Standard antituberculous therapy for foot and ankle tuberculosis in children

Drug	Daily dose	Maximum dose	Duration in months
Rifampicin	10–20 mg/kg	600 mg	12–18
Isoniazid (isonicotinic acid hydrazide: INH)	10–20 mg/kg	300 mg	12–18
Pyridoxine (vitamin B6) to avoid peripheral neuropathy of INH therapy in susceptible individuals	25–100 mg	100 mg	12–18
Ethambutol	25 mg/kg 15 mg/kg		2 (initial) 10–16 (maintenance)
Pyrazinamide	15–30 mg/kg	2000 mg	2

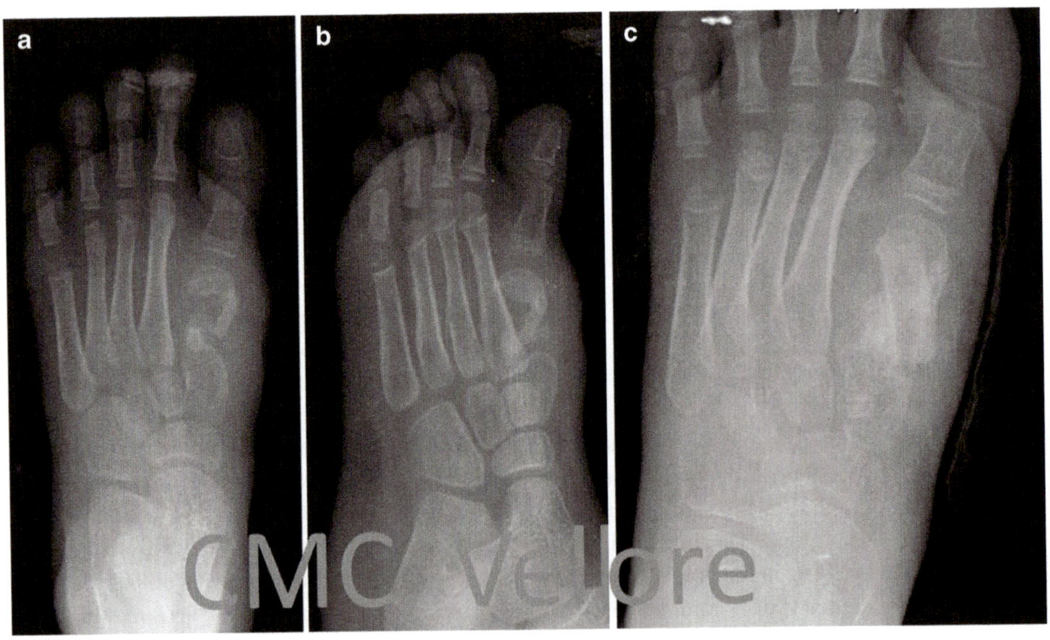

Fig. 30.15 (**a–c**) Case example: TB of first metatarsal. (Source: CMC Vellore)

ation in an impending collapse in midfoot lesions have been described [32]. In addition, arthrodesis such as triple arthrodesis, Lisfranc joint arthrodesis and limited talonavicular arthrodesis have been described to stabilise damaged joints.

Three to four weeks are sufficient for postoperative cast immobilisation after synovectomy, joint debridement and curettage of bony lesions. Triple arthrodesis and limited arthrodesis require 10 weeks of a below-knee plaster cast followed by protection with an ankle–foot orthosis, based on radiological fusion progress and to assist with progressive weight-bearing.

Summary Points: Antituberculous therapy is the mainstay of treatment of ankle and foot tuberculosis.

Protected weight-bearing in a cast is required to avoid subchondral collapse in cases of hind- or mid-foot osteomyelitis or tuberculosis.

Indications for surgery are obtaining tissue and pus samples for diagnosis, draining abscesses, achieving painless stable joints without deformity and preventing a collapse of juxta-articular lesions.

Reconstructive surgery may be required to stabilise joints with arthritis, aiming for fusion to achieve stable, plantigrade feet.

Complications

Adverse outcomes include painful deformities and ankyloses. In the midfoot, large juxta-articular lesions may result in a collapse of the longitudinal arch, resulting in a rocker bottom foot. Painful, healed arthritic lesions of the foot may cause peroneal spastic feet. All painful lesions require solid fusion with correction of deformities to achieve a plantigrade foot. Secondary infections with pyogenic organisms are known to occur in chronic, neglected lesions and can worsen articular damage.

In conclusion, ankle and foot tuberculosis requires care in the diagnosis, especially for bony lesions, lesions with mixed infections, and bacteriological and histological confirmation. Medical treatment with antituberculous therapy is the mainstay, with surgical intervention used primarily to manage the severe disease and maintain the foot's biomechanical integrity.

Box 30.1 Case Example: Tuberculous Arthritis of the Talonavicular Joint (Fig. 30.14)

An 11-year-old had a history of insidious foot pain for 2.5 years. His walking and playing were restricted. He had a normal CRP and an ESR of 31 mm/hour. The foot antero-posterior (AP) and lateral (A & B) radiographs showed diffuse foot osteoporosis, irregular joint space, and juxta-articular destruction of talus and navicular. Biopsy from the talonavicular joint revealed necrotising granulomas. An Xpert MTB/RIF PCR on the tissue sample showed *Mycobacterium tuberculosis* with intermediate rifampicin resistance. There was no growth in the rapid MGIT culture medium.

He was treated with pyrazinamide for 2 months and with rifampicin INH and ethambutol for 1 year. At 6 months he could walk pain-free, had gained 3 kg weight and had normal ESR. The foot AP and lateral (C & D) radiographs showed increased sclerosis with well-defined bone outlines and irregular talonavicular joint space.

Box 30.2 Case Example: TB of First Metatarsal (Fig. 30.15)

An 8-year-old with a 6-month history of discharging sinus, no warmth, but enlargement and thickening in the first metatarsal area was confirmed to have caseous granulomatous inflammation on histology. ESR, CRP and culture for mycobacteria were negative; QuantiFERON-TB Gold was positive at 6.8. Radiographs show bone loss in the first metatarsal diaphysis and generalised osteoporosis with no new bone formation (A & B). After 6 weeks of antituberculous therapy, a cancellous bone grafting was carried out to restore bony continuity. At 1 year (C), the AP radiograph shows bony continuity and sclerosis and restoration of the weight-bearing column on the medial side.

Box 30.3 Case Example: TB of Subarticular Second Metatarsal (Fig. 30.16)

A 14-year-old girl with a limp has a histologically confirmed lesion of the second metatarsal head. Note the cavity formation with an articular breach and no reaction of the surrounding bone in the AP view (A). The lesion has wholly healed without surgery after antituberculous treatment as evident in the radiographs 18 months later (B).

Box 30.4 Case Example: TB of Ankle (Fig. 30.17)

Magnetic resonance imaging (MRI) of a 15-year-old girl shows features of tuberculosis of the ankle joint. This child's diagnosis was confirmed on histology and microbial culture.

The T2-STIR sagittal MRI shows that the talus and distal tibial epiphysis have hyper-intense areas with the talus showing irregular geographic areas of signal change. Multiple areas of cortical break and small well-defined hyper-intense outpouchings are seen along the margins of the talar dome and tibial articular surfaces. Adjacent tissues are oedematous.

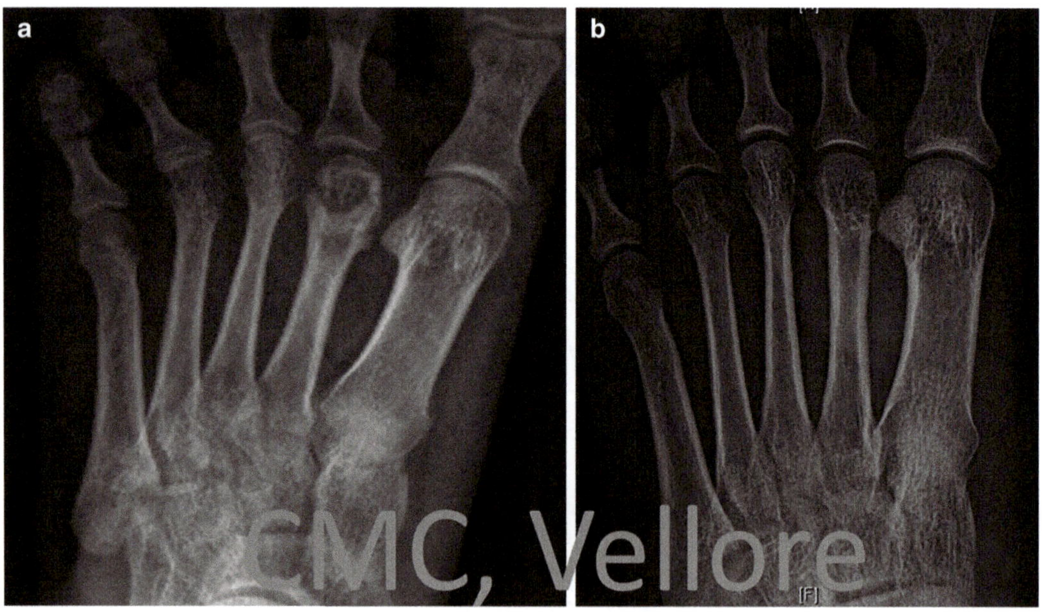

Fig. 30.16 (**a**, **b**) Case example: TB of second metatarsal (subarticular). (Source: CMC Vellore)

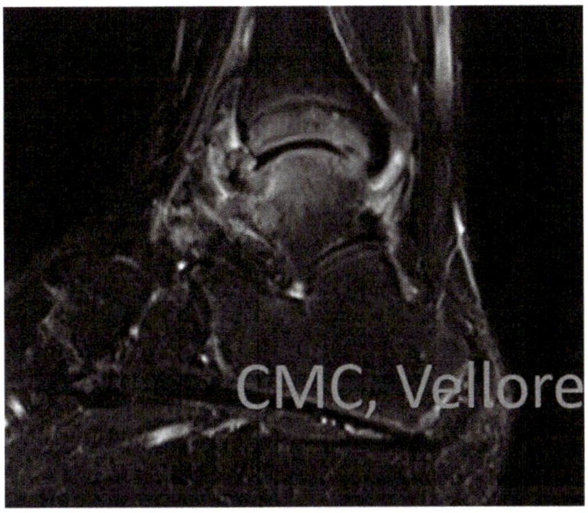

Fig. 30.17 TB of ankle. (Source: CMC Vellore)

Madura Foot

Introduction and Epidemiology

Madura foot, or mycetoma, is an uncommon chronic infection of the skin and subcutaneous tissues that, if untreated, can cause substantial bone erosion and disability. The condition typically affects the foot and is characterised by a triad of chronic induration, draining sinuses and with small black granules found in the exudate. A detailed description from Madurai district in Tamil Nadu, India, led to the name, Madura foot. It is also termed mycetoma due to its aetiology.

The condition is found in tropical, subtropical and equatorial regions. It most commonly affects the foot in male agricultural workers who walk barefoot [42].

Pathology and Microbiology

The granules are composed of colonies of either Gram-positive actinomycotic bacteria (60% of cases), e.g. *Nippostrongylus brasiliensis* and *Streptomyces madurae*, or eucomycotic fungi, e.g. *Madurella mycetomatis* and *Madurella griesia*. The differentiation between the aetiologies of the causative organism is needed as the management differs.

Infection is typically associated with repeated minor trauma, typically abrasions or thorn pricks that cause direct inoculation of the infecting organisms. Abscesses containing the black granular material develop with localised fibrosis and granulation tissue.

Clinical Presentation and Examination

Mycetoma is a chronic infection that presents with multiple nodules that discharge pus that contain granules. After the initial inoculation, the incubation period can last up to several months. A small, painless subcutaneous nodule develops that slowly enlarges. Subcutaneous abscesses develop and over the following months sinuses develop that drain a purulent, granular exudate. Deeper extension can develop that, over time, can result in extensive bone erosion. Actinomycetoma typically has a more rapid and destructive course than eumycetoma [43].

Investigations/Work-Up

The history of a chronic infectious condition affecting the foot in equatorial regions is suggestive. Multiple sinuses discharging granular material that may be black, white or red can occur. Obtaining microbiological culture is a key part of the diagnosis. Dark grains are found in the eumycotic mycetoma (typically *M. mycetomatis*), whilst red and yellow grains suggest actinomycetoma (e.g. *Actinomadura pelletieri*, *Streptomyces* and *Nocardia species*). Gram-stain of the exudate containing granules differentiates between actinomycetoma (granules of the bacteria consist of fine filaments, approximately 1 micron thick and are Gram-positive) and eumycetoma (fungal hyphae filaments that are around 5 microns thick and are Gram-negative) [44].

Culture can be performed of the granules, obtained ideally by a clean surgical biopsy. The granules should be put into normal saline before being inoculated onto a culture media. A number of different culture media can be used. Antibiotic-free culture media is required for the isolation of actinomycetes, whereas a culture media with antibiotics is required to identify eumycetes. Antibiotics used include penicillin G, gentamicin sulphate, streptomycin and chloramphenicol [45].

Radiographs in the early stages reveal soft tissue swelling. Over time, periosteal reaction and later cortical erosion may be seen. In an advanced case, there is substantial erosion of several rays of the foot and midfoot [46].

Differential Diagnoses

- Chronic bacterial osteomyelitis
- Tuberculosis
- Buruli ulcer
- Syphilis
- Yaws (chronic skin infection)

Treatment Options

Differentiation between eumycetoma and actinomycetoma is needed to effect proper treatment, based on laboratory findings including Gram-stain and culture:

Eumycetoma: A combination of medical therapy and surgical excision is often needed. Surgical debridement of the grossly infected tissues, combined with a prolonged antifungal medication regimen (e.g. ketoconazole and itraconazole), is required. The recommended course is 9–12 months in a tapered dose. Because antifungal therapy can cause hepatotoxicity, liver function tests should be performed every 8 weeks [47].

Actinomycetoma: This condition typically responds well to pharmaceutical therapy alone but surgical debridement is often necessary. Combination therapy with trimethoprim-sulfamethoxazole, dapsone and streptomycin has been used effectively.

Surgical management involves removal of the infected, unhealthy tissue, debriding back to a small cuff of normal tissue. Where the bone is involved, curettage is performed. Iodine lavage may help destroy missed granules. Repeated returns to the operating theatre are often necessary to remove any diseased tissue and granules until the wound is clean. Wound closure may be a problem, requiring serial dressings and skin grafting. A vacuum dressing, changed every 2–3 days, can help shrink the dead space and allow for effective secondary closure.

Complications

In some advanced cases, secondary bacterial infection can supervene and the foot may not be salvageable. Amputation is necessary for such cases to prevent overwhelming sepsis [48].

Box 30.5 Case Example: Madura Foot (Figs. 30.18 and 30.19)

A 12-year-old child referred with Madura foot. Surgical drainage had been attempted but had failed to control the infection.

Radiographs demonstrate progressive, severe erosion of the central rays and midfoot.

Repeated surgical debridement and curettage was performed with vacuum dressings to close the dead space. Black granules were initially found, suggestive of eumycetoma. The infection resolved with a combination of repeated surgical debridement, vacuum therapy and a prolonged course of antifungal medication. The child mobilised well with the use of an ankle–foot orthosis to support the foot.

Summary

The commonest infections of the foot are superficial and many do not require surgical intervention, although they can be highly contagious. Deep infections, that require surgical exploration and drainage, may be hard to localise without the use of MRI or ultrasound. Foot infections should

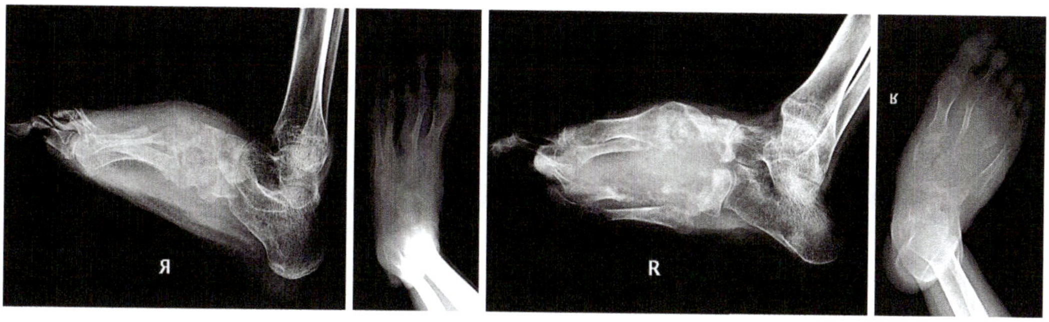

Fig. 30.18 X-ray of Madura foot, with extensive bony destruction. (Source: CURE Ethiopia)

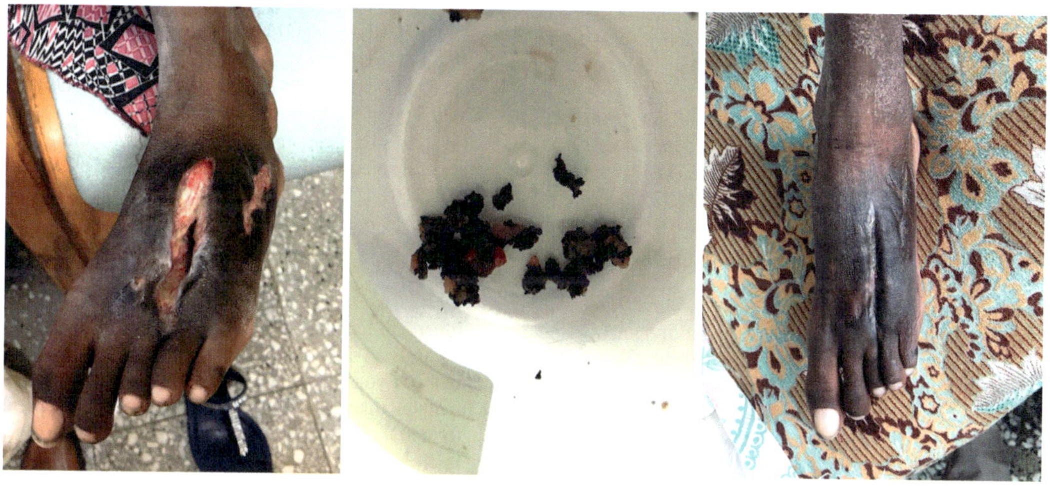

Fig. 30.19 Clinical photos of Madura foot; extensive debridement required; classic appearance of black granules shown. (Source: CURE Ethiopia)

always be considered as a differential diagnosis in the limping child. Destructive infections of the foot will be rarely seen in the developed world but advanced osteomyelitis, tuberculosis and, occasionally, Madura foot will be encountered in low- and middle-income countries.

References

1. World Health Organization. A guide to clinical management and public health response for hand, foot and mouth disease (HFMD). 2011. https://apps.who.int/iris/bitstream/handle/10665/207490/9789290615255_eng.pdf.
2. Al-Mutairi N, AlKhalaf M. Mucocutaneous warts in children: clinical presentations, risk factors, and response to treatment. Acta Dermatovenerologica. 2012;21:69–72.
3. Williams HC, Pottier A, Strachan D. The descriptive epidemiology of warts in British schoolchildren. Br J Dermatol. 1993;128(5):504–11.
4. Kilkenny M, Merlin K, Young R, Marks R. The prevalence of common skin conditions in Australian school students: 1. Common, plane and plantar viral warts. Br J Dermatol. 1998;138(5):840–5.
5. Theng TS, Goh BK, Chong WS, Chan YC, Giam YC. Viral warts in children seen at a tertiary referral centre. Annals-Acad Med Singapore. 2004;33(1):53–6.
6. Makola NF, Magongwa NM, Matsaung B, Schellack G, Schellack N. Managing athlete's foot. S Afr Fam Pract. 2018;60(5):37–41.
7. Andrews MD, Burns M. Common tinea infections in children. Am Fam Physician. 2008;77(10):1415.
8. Yang G, Yanchar NL, Lo AY, Jones SA. Treatment of ingrown toenails in the pediatric population. J Pediatr Surg. 2008;43(5):931–5.
9. Kapellen TM, Galler A, Kiess W. Higher frequency of paronychia (nail bed infections) in pediatric and adolescent patients with type 1 diabetes mellitus than

in non-diabetic peers. J Pediatr Endocrinol Metab. 2003;16(5):751–8.
10. Majcen ME, Wilfinger CC, Pilhatsch A. Interpretation of radiologic abnormalities in patients with chronically infected ingrown toenails with regard to a possible exogenic osteomyelitis. J Pediatr Surg. 2009;44(11):2179–83.
11. Chapeskie H, Kovac JR. Soft-tissue nail-fold excision: a definitive treatment for ingrown toenails. Can J Surg. 2010;53(4):282.
12. Livingston MH, Coriolano K, Jones SA. Nonrandomized assessment of ingrown toenails treated with excision of skinfold rather than toenail (NAILTEST): an observational study of the Vandenbos procedure. J Pediatr Surg. 2017;52(5):832–6.
13. Volk A, Zebda M, Abdelgawad AA. Plantar and pedal puncture wounds in children: a case series study from a single level I trauma center. Pediatr Emerg Care. 2017;33(11):724–9.
14. Pennycook A, Makower R, O'Donnell AM. Puncture wounds of the foot: can infective complications be avoided? J R Soc Med. 1994;87(10):581.
15. Jacobs RF, McCarthy RE, Elser JM. Pseudomonas osteochondritis complicating puncture wounds of the foot in children: a 10-year evaluation. J Infect Dis. 1989;160(4):657–61.
16. Prevention and management of wound infection. Guidance from 'WHO's Department of Violence and Injury Prevention and Disability and the Department of Essential Health Technologies. https://www.who.int/hac/techguidance/tools/guidelines_prevention_and_management_wound_infection.pdf, published 2nd March 2013.
17. Schroder A, Gerin A, Firth GB, Hoffmann KS, Grieve A, von Sochaczewski CO. A systematic review of necrotising fasciitis in children from its first description in 1930 to 2018. BMC Infect Dis. 2019;19(1):317.
18. Nadau E, Joseph C, Haraux E, Deroussen F, Gouron R, Klein C. Clinical features and outcomes in children with bone and joint infections of the ankle or foot. Arch Pediatr. 2020;27(8):464–8.
19. Puffinbarger WR, Gruel CR, Herndon WA, Sullivan JA. Osteomyelitis of the calcaneus in children. J Pediatr Orthop. 1996;16(2):224–30.
20. Ingersoll J, Halliday M, Adams DJ, Auten JD, Morrison PD. Inflammatory markers limitations in the diagnosis of pediatric calcaneal osteomyelitis. Am J Emerg Med. 2019;37(11):2119 e3–5.
21. Jenzri M, Safi H, Nessib MN, Smida M, Jalel C, Ammar C, et al. Hematogenous osteomyelitis of the calcaneus in children: 26 cases. Rev Chir Orthop Reparatrice Appar Mot. 2008;94(5):434–42.
22. Leigh W, Crawford H, Street M, Huang M, Manners S, Puna R. Pediatric calcaneal osteomyelitis. J Pediatr Orthop. 2010;30(8):888–92.
23. Pepper M, Willick S, Beals T, Randall RL. An unusual cause of heel pain in a young athlete: a case report. PM R. 2010;2(12):1145–8.
24. Kumar S, Jain N, Karpe P, Limaye R. Osteomyelitis complicating Sever's disease: a report of two cases. J Clin Orthop Trauma. 2020;11(2):310–3.
25. Paakkonen M, Kallio MJ, Peltola H, Kallio PE. Antibiotic treatment and surgery for acute Hematogenous calcaneal osteomyelitis of childhood. J Foot Ankle Surg. 2015;54(5):840–3.
26. Mooney ML, Haidet K, Liu J, Ebraheim NA. Hematogenous calcaneal osteomyelitis in children: a systematic review of the literature. Foot Ankle Spec. 2017;10(1):63–8.
27. Wang E, Zhao Q, Zhang L, Ji S, Li J. The split-heel technique in the management of chronic calcaneal osteomyelitis in children. J Pediatr Orthop B. 2009;18(1):23–7.
28. Jiang N, Zhao XQ, Wang L, Lin QR, Hu YJ, Yu B. Single-stage debridement with implantation of antibiotic-loaded calcium sulphate in 34 cases of localized calcaneal osteomyelitis. Acta Orthop. 2020;91(3):353–9.
29. Rasool MN. Hematogenous osteomyelitis of the calcaneus in children. J Pediatr Orthop. 2001;21(6):738–43.
30. Ezra E, Wientroub S. Primary subacute haematogenous osteomyelitis of the tarsal bones in children. J Bone Joint Surg. British volume. 1997;79(6):983–6.
31. Gilbertson-Dahdal D, Wright JE, Krupinski E, McCurdy WE, Taljanovic MS. Transphyseal involvement of pyogenic osteomyelitis is considerably more common than classically taught. Am J Roentgenol. 2014;203(1):190–5.
32. Dhillon MS, Nagi ON. Tuberculosis of the foot and ankle. Clin Orthop Relat Res. 2002;398:107–13.
33. Agarwal A, Qureshi NA, Khan SA, Kumar P, Samaiya S. Tuberculosis of the foot and ankle in children. J Orthop Surg (Hong Kong). 2011;19(2):213–7.
34. Maqungo M, Kaur M, Kwofie SK, Radovanovic A, Schaefer U, Schmeier S, et al. DDPC: dragon database of genes associated with prostate cancer. Nucleic Acids Res. 2011;39(Database issue):D980–5.
35. Choi WJ, Han SH, Joo JH, Kim BS, Lee JW. Diagnostic dilemma of tuberculosis in the foot and ankle. Foot Ankle Int. 2008;29(7):711–5.
36. Kaushik SK, Khan A, Mathur M, Jaiswal M, Jadon D. Role of PRP injection in delayed union and non union of long bone fractures. Indian J Orthop. 2020;6(1):35–40.
37. Dheda K. Tuberculosis and Poncet's disease: the many faces of an old enemy. Lancet. 2016;387(10018):618.
38. Vohra R, Kang HS, Dogra S, Saggar RR, Sharma R. Tuberculous osteomyelitis. J Bone Joint Surg. 1997;79(4):562–6.
39. Anand A, Sood LK. Isolated tuberculosis of talus without ankle and subtalar joint involvement. Med J Malaysia. 2002;57(3):371–3.

40. Bozkurt M, Dogan M, Sesen H, Turanli S, Basbozkurt M. Isolated medial cuneiform tuberculosis: a case report. J Foot Ankle Surg. 2005;44(1):60–3.
41. Sharma SK, Ryan H, Khaparde S, Sachdeva KS, Singh AD, Mohan A, et al. Index-TB guidelines: guidelines on extrapulmonary tuberculosis for India. Indian J Med Res. 2017;145(4):448–63.
42. Emery D, Denning DW. The global distribution of actinomycetoma and eumycetoma. PLoSNegl Trop Dis. 2020;14(9):e0008397. https://doi.org/10.1371/journal.pntd.0008397. PMID: 32970667; PMCID: PMC7514014
43. Venkatswami S, Sankarasubramanian A, Subramanyam S. The madura foot: looking deep. Int J Low Extrem Wounds. 2012;11(1):31–42. https://doi.org/10.1177/1534734612438549. Epub 2012 Feb 14. PMID: 22334597
44. Alam K, Maheshwari V, Bhargava S, Jain A, Fatima U, Haq EU. Histological diagnosis of madura foot (mycetoma): a must for definitive treatment. J Glob Infect Dis. 2009;1(1):64–7. https://doi.org/10.4103/0974-777X.52985. PMID: 20300390; PMCID: PMC2840937
45. Ahmed AA, van de Sande W, Fahal AH. Mycetoma laboratory diagnosis. PLoS Negl Trop Dis. 2017;11(8):e0005638.
46. Sharif HS, Clark DC, Aabed MY, Aideyan OA, Mattsson TA, Haddad MC, Ohman SO, Joshi RK, Hasan HA, Haleem A. Mycetoma: comparison of MR imaging with CT. Radiology. 1991;178(3):865–70. https://doi.org/10.1148/radiology.178.3.1994434. PMID: 1994434
47. Fahal AH, Rahman IA, El-Hassan AM, Rahman ME, Zijlstra EE. The safety and efficacy of itraconazole for the treatment of patients with eumycetoma due to Madurellamycetomatis. Trans R Soc Trop Med Hyg. 2011;105(3):127–32. https://doi.org/10.1016/j.trstmh.2010.11.008. Epub 2011 Jan 17. PMID: 21247608
48. Ahmed AO, Abugroun ES. Unexpected high prevalence of secondary bacterial infection in patients with mycetoma. J Clin Microbiol. 1998;36(3):850–1. https://doi.org/10.1128/JCM.36.3.850-851.1998. PMID: 9508332; PMCID: PMC104645

Tuberculosis of the Axial Skeleton

31

Arjun Dhawale, K. Venugopal Menon, and Anil K. Jain

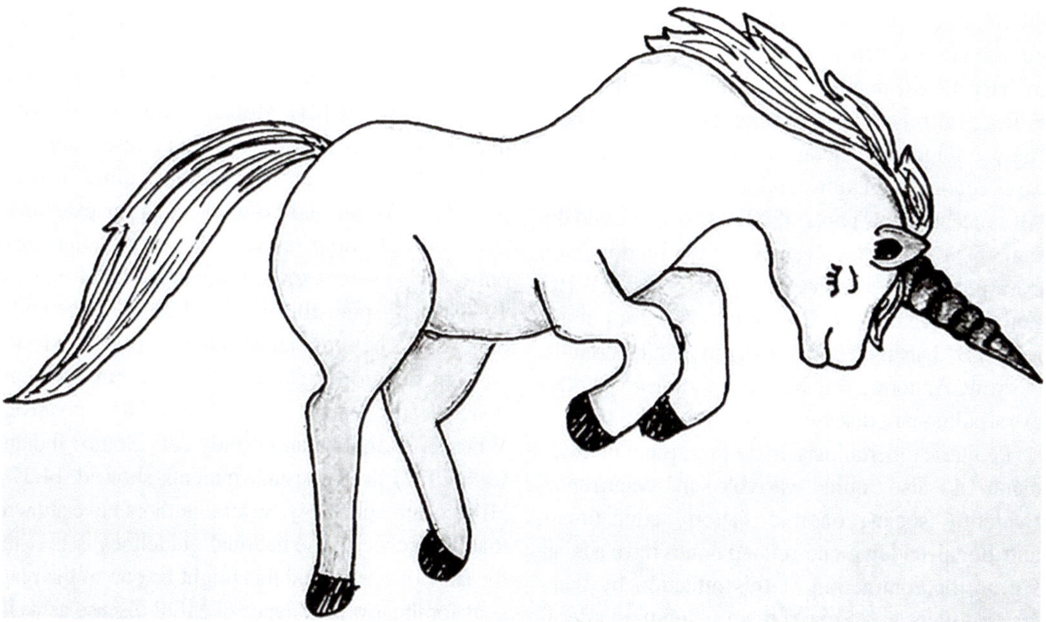

A. Dhawale (✉)
Department of Orthopaedics, Bai Jerbai Wadia Hospital for Children, Mumbai, India

Department of Orthopaedics, Sir H.N. Reliance Foundation Hospital, Mumbai, India

K. Venugopal Menon
Department of Orthopaedics, Bharati Vidyapeeth University, Pune, India

A. K. Jain
Department of Orthopaedics, University College of Medical Sciences, New Delhi, India

© Springer Nature Switzerland AG 2022
M. V. Belthur et al. (eds.), *Pediatric Musculoskeletal Infections*,
https://doi.org/10.1007/978-3-030-95794-0_31

Epidemiology

The WHO estimated annual incidence of tuberculosis is 10.4 million cases worldwide (2016) of which over 4.7 million occur in India, China, and Indonesia alone [1, 2]. The CDC data suggests that 1/3rd of the world population might be afflicted with TB [3]. The proportion of musculoskeletal affections also varies with the population sample. It has been estimated that 5–10% of the pediatric spine infections are primary (occurring within 1 year of infection) while 90–95% become latent infections only to be reactivated during phases of immune compromise (like poor nutrition or intercurrent illness) [5]. The prevalence of Pott's disease is also quite variable in different parts of the world [1–16]. Spinal TB is reported to occur in 10% of the cases of extra-pulmonary disease in Nepal [12] while in South Africa Polley et al. report 15–20% cases [13]. Tuli's classic study on Indian patients reports 50% spinal TB cases among the extra-pulmonary affections [14]. Ali's recent review paper of 2019 also suggested the same 50% spinal involvement as the predominant extra-pulmonary affection [15]. The WHO European region has recorded 17% extra-pulmonary TB, barring United Kingdom, Netherlands, Norway, Andorra, and Malta reporting over 40% extra-pulmonary disease [1].

Pediatric tuberculosis, including spinal involvement, is also quite variable in occurrence. Evidently socio-economic factors, educational, nutritional, and hygiene-related issues have a bearing on the contracting of this infection by these factors often fail to explain some unique patterns of the disease. Elsen reported 21 patients from the United Kingdom in 15 years of which only one was Caucasian [17]. Mann's study of 4 years from South Africa reported 393 cases with 74 children (18%). Other studies report between 5% and 15% children. In the same region du Preez showed that 19% of the children were HIV positive and 34% malnourished [18]. Govender also reports nutritional depletion in 67% of the South African children with spinal TB [19]. Perhaps it is interesting to note that in an endemic country like India the southern state of Kerala alone has virtually no pediatric spinal TB cases over the last several years where lymph node TB seems to be the commoner extra-pulmonary manifestation [4]. While the global prevalence seems to be increasing or at best stable, in Kerala pediatric TB cases are sharply declining at the rate of 7.5% per year [4]. The results of positivity in TB testing in this region by the Cartridge Based Nucleic Acid Amplification Test (CBNAAT) were 1% against the national average of 10% (*The Hindu*, January 13, 2020). It might be interesting to postulate how this has been achieved in an endemic country in the face of steady global rise of the burden of TB.

Another major issue is the prevalence of various strains of drug resistant Tubercular bacteria. The WHO estimates 650,000 cases of MDR-TB globally with 20% children in high burden areas [20, 21]. It is also suggested that 3.5% of all fresh cases are reportedly MDR [20]. Goyal has shown that western India has the highest prevalence and previously treated patients rather than fresh cases had higher prevalence [21]. Mohan's study also showed that in drug resistant spinal TB (111 cases) approx. 40% had previous anti-TB therapy, often incomplete [22]. Desai and co-workers in an extensive study of 1743 drug resistant TB cases found that only 4.4% were extra-pulmonary TB of which 19.7% were spine affections and 30.3% were children [23]. The remarkable feature of this study in western Indian population from Mumbai was that none in the entire cohort were HIV positive. Whereas Rajasekeran's study on South Indian (n = 2927) drug-resistant patients showed 14.2% HIV co-infection [24]. Several authors have shown that adherence to the national guidelines is best in the state of Kerala and this might be one of the reasons for the low prevalence of MDR disease as well as the better cure rates [25]. Yadav et al. have shown that majority of the private doctors do not follow the Revised National Tuberculosis Control Programme (RNTPC) guidelines resulting in MDR-TB in western India [26, 27]. Babu has established that the main cause of MDR-TB in India is inappropriate treatment of the primary infection [28].

The prevalence of HIV has significantly impacted TB in many parts of the world. In 2016 South Africa reported a prevalence of 18% pediatric TB with the highest incidence of 38.5% HIV co-infection [6, 7]. The WHO report of 2014 also suggests that Latin America has a prevalence of 28 TB cases per 100,000 population of which 13% are co-infected with HIV [8]. In contrast, Kumar's population sample consisted of North Indian children with Pott's spine, none with HIV positivity [9]. Garcia reports 1400 cases from Spain of which 25.2% cases were extra-pulmonary and only 14 spinal disease (4% approximately) [10]. They also found that it was rare even in HIV affected population. Thailand reports a rather small 2% cases of pediatric TB as against the global average of 10% [11] but a high rate (27%) of HIV co-infections and rare drug resistance. Kerala in India also reports a unique dual burden of diabetes in TB patients with 44% prevalence [16]. Sayi and colleagues from Tanzania have reported that BCG vaccination does not seem to protect their cases against spinal TB [29]. Similarly, a group of authors from Morocco have suggested that genetically pre-determined immunological dysfunctions might be implicated in the spinal TB cases from their country [30] (Box 31.1).

Box 31.1 Epidemiology

- The prevalence of spinal TB is very much region dependent; it is rare in the South Indian state of Kerala.
- Co-infection with HIV is high in South Africa, Latin America, Thailand, and Western India.
- Drug resistance is also frequent in western India and appears to be related to inadequacy of previous therapy.

Pathology

The organism causing TB has often been described as *Mycobacterium tuberculosis* complex due to the various strains that might cause disease in humans directly or via domestic animals. *M. tuberculosis* is the most frequent pathogen while a small number of cases are caused by atypical Mycobacteria such as *M. bovis*, *M. intercellulaire*, *M. kansasi*, *M. avium*, *M. marinum*, *M. abscessus*, *M. africanum*, *M. microti*, *M. caneti*, etc. Such atypical organisms are relatively rare and difficult to isolate in culture and do often present diagnostic and therapeutic dilemmas [31, 32]. It is a slow growing strictly aerobic organism showing as gram stain neutral, acid fast bacilli of non-sporing non-motile variety. It has a high content of Mycolic acid and the cell wall is lipid and proteoglycan rich making it difficult to digest. It is resistant to most surface disinfectants [2].

Primary infection typically occurs in the lung but also the gut, genitourinary system, rarely the skin/eye, tonsils, etc., may be affected. Spread to the spine has been suggested to be predominantly hematogenous, though lymphatic spread and direct spread by contiguity is also possible [33]. The valveless venous system in the spine—the Batson's plexus—is particularly conducive to the wide spread of the bacterium from its site of origin into the entire vertebral column. Tuli has also proposed a possible arterial spread [14]. Previous studies had suggested that up to 60% of the cases would reveal positive lung lesions [14, 34, 35] whereas current studies fail to reveal such an association or rather the numbers are much smaller. The primary site is more often concealed than not, reinforcing the hypothesis that musculoskeletal TB is possibly reactivation of a latent infection.

The pathognomonic lesion of TB is called a tubercle. The typical histological features are an area of central necrosis and caseation surrounded by chronic inflammatory cells consisting of lymphocytes, epithelioid cells which are morphosed macrophages which coalesce to form Langerhans giant cells. Figure 31.1 shows the histopathological features and Fig. 31.2 shows the central type of TB with vertebral collapse. Unlike pyogenic infections where the bacteria generate proteolytic enzymes causing destruction of the surrounding tissues, *M. tuberculosis* causes tissue damage by a delayed hypersensitivity reaction where the host immune response is the source of tissue destruction. Figure 31.3 is an example of features of pyogenic versus tuberculous infection.

Most publications describe the commonest site of affection as the thoracolumbar spine followed by the thoracic spine [36]. The authors' experience is that this is true in endemic regions, whereas in non-endemic areas the lesions are often equally distributed along the spine. Classically five patterns of vertebral affection have been described. The commonest is the paradiscal type of lesion where the disease starts under the end plates of both sides of discs, progresses along the cancellous vertebral bone and eventually destroys the entire vertebra, often multiple

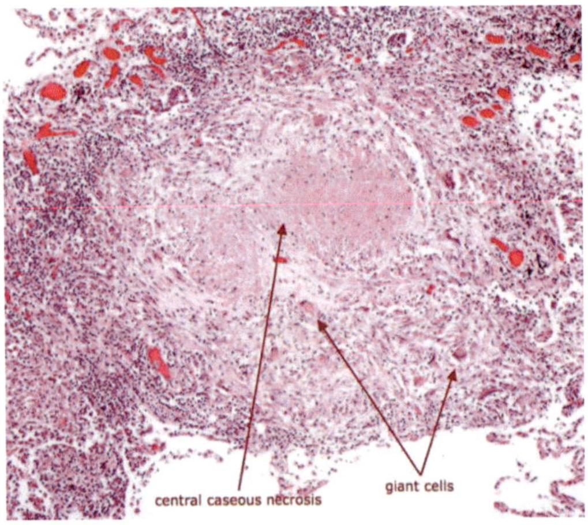

Fig. 31.1 The essential lesion of tuberculosis is a tubercle—an area of central caseation necrosis surrounded by lymphocytes, epithelioid cells, and Langerhans giant cells

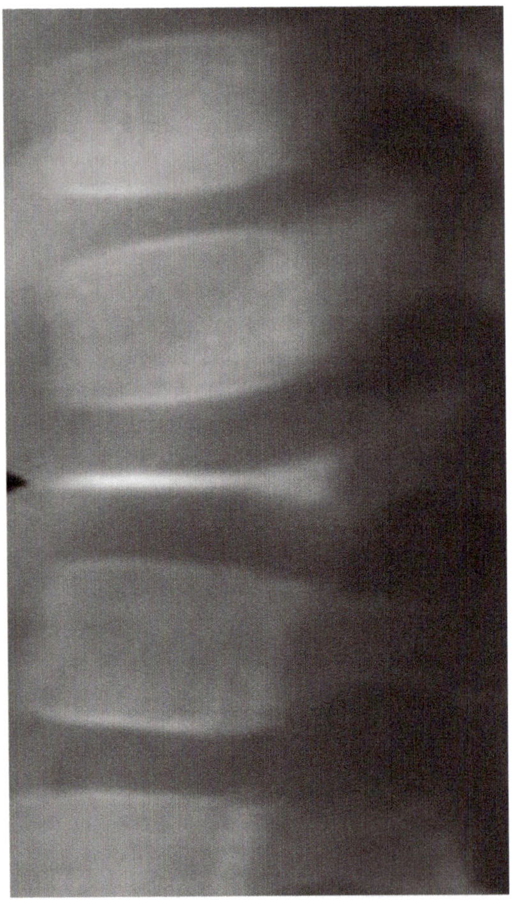

Fig. 31.2 Vertebra plana in a child due to Tubercular spondylitis

contiguous vertebrae, resulting in collapse and kyphosis. Typically, the discs are spared till late in the evolution of the disease. Anterior disease is the next common pattern where segments of the vertebra, classically anterior, are affected; this is best appreciated on MRI scans [37]. In advanced disease the distinction disappears and most forms appear with kyphosis and collapse. Posterior element disease is quite a rare form of vertebral affection and occurs in approximately 1–2% of cases [38]. Tuli's study reported 7% multicentric (skip lesions) disease but it must be emphasized that this was during the period where X-rays were the main diagnostic imaging tool; Isotope scans have revealed 25% skip lesions and MRI scans have picked up over 40% lesions as multicentric [39]. Figure 31.4 is an example of multicentric involvement. This suggests that spinal TB is a localized manifestation of systemic disease. Bone scintigraphy is currently not recommended for the diagnosis of TB spine though it is eminently suitable in pyogenic spinal infections. Children may present with central disease. Here, the vertebra is destroyed, often with complete collapse and little or no pus formation and a "vertebra plana" type of radiological lesion ensues. The adjoining discs usually remain intact. A non-osseous form has also been described where a cold psoas abscess or epidural abscess is detected on imaging with little signal change in the vertebrae. Often these latter lesions are associated with sacroiliac joint affection or retropharyngeal affection (Box 31.2).

Box 31.2 Pathology

- Extra-pulmonary TB is typically paucibacillary; ZN stains and cultures may often be negative.
- The typical lesion is a Tubercle that is the histological hallmark.
- Spread occurs by hematological and lymphatic routes, and direct contiguity.
- Central lesions occur in children though they may be paradiscal, anterior, posterior, or non-osseous.
- MRI whole spine is mandatory since multicentric lesions occur more frequently than previously thought.

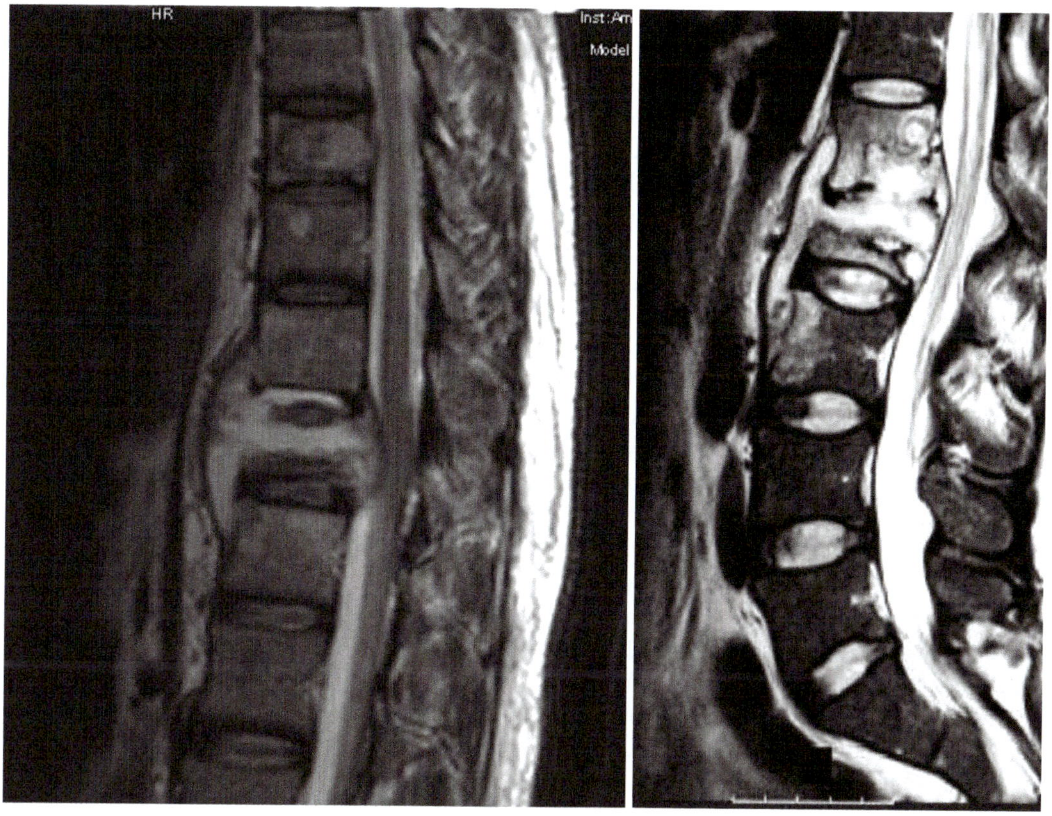

Fig. 31.3 The left side image shows a tubercular infection where the disc is intact despite advanced vertebral disease. The right side shows a pyogenic infection for comparison—note that the disc is destroyed early in the disease

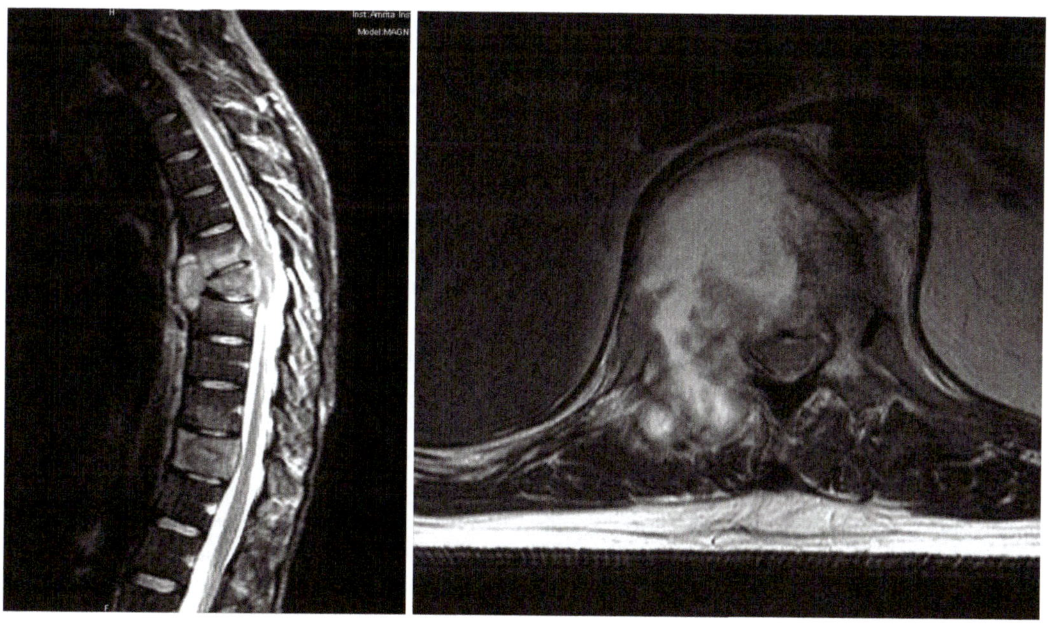

Fig. 31.4 Multicentric TB and posterior element disease are not infrequent

Clinical Features

There are substantial differences between pulmonary and skeletal TB affections as well as persons from endemic and non-endemic areas. The patient is typically a malnourished child living in an overcrowded urban area of poorly educated family, and less hygienic environment. Classic systemic features of intermittent fever, weight loss, malaise, anorexia evening rise of temperature, night sweats have been described for pulmonary TB in endemic areas. Spinal TB in non-endemic regions may not demonstrate the above signs and present with local symptoms alone. The disease evolves slowly and pain is often the main feature. Deformity, typically kyphosis, slowly progressive neurological symptoms and abscess formation are described as the classic tetrad (along with pain) [38].

The pain of Pott's spine is characteristically axial pain, aggravated by rest and diminished by activity and associated with muscle spasm. Night cries are described as typical and is due to the relaxation of the spastic muscles leading to segmental mobility and pain. Instability pattern of pain is typically seen when destruction of bony elements leads to abnormal mobility of adjacent segments. Three signs have been described in relation to spinal instability—Gower's sign—wherein forward flexion of the spine is often painless but extension from flexion is painful and needs support by placing the hands on the knee, often "climbing up" the legs. The Tripod sign is demonstrated as the child sits but needs to support the trunk by placing the hands on either side of the seat. The third sign is supporting the head in the hands is seen in cervical spine affection or occipito-cervical affection.

Deformity is often the presenting feature usually accompanied by axial spine pain. Torticollis if the disease is cervical, particularly C1–C2 rotary subluxation produces the characteristic Cock Robbin sign [37]. Cervical or cervico-thoracic kyphosis needing hand support for the head is also common. Cervico-thoracic, thoracic, and thoraco lumbar lesions present as angular kyphosis. Single vertebral destruction usually produces a "knuckle deformity" whereas multiple vertebral collapse causes a "gibbus." Spinal deformity in children is viewed with concern compared to corresponding lesions in adults for many reasons. The bone being softer and cartilaginous tends to cause greater collapse and structural changes than in adults during the active phase of the infection [39]. Additionally, even after the infective process heals the deformity can progress due to biological or mechanical reasons, often with disastrous consequences like neurological dysfunction [40, 41]. The late biological sequel is growth arrest occurring of the cartilaginous apophysis of the vertebra resulting in asymmetric growth and progressive kyphosis. The mechanical effect is inefficiency of the anterior column support resulting in "buckling collapse" of the spine. Rajasekaran et al. have reported the natural history of tubercular kyphosis in children and observed that 44% of spinal deformity in the acute phase will resolve with healing and subsequent growth, whereas 39% will worsen and 17% will remain static with no change in the sagittal plane measurements [39]. Age less than 10 years, kyphosis more than 30°, loss of more than 1–1.5 vertebral heights, lesion at junctions (cervico-thoracic and thoraco-lumbar) predicted significant progression in later life. These authors also described 4 radiological signs called spine at risk signs (Fig. 31.5) that predicts progression of kyphosis in children with Pott's disease [39]. They are facet widening, retropulsion of the diseased body, coronal plane lateral translation of the affected segments, and toppling of the spine at the involved segment. Most authors would recommend that children who are at risk be followed till skeletal maturity with regular radiological and clinical examination [39, 40].

Neurological dysfunction is obviously one of the most dreaded complications of Pott's disease. Jain has reported that neurological deficits occur in 32–76% Pott's spine cases [41]. Neurological dysfunction can occur during the acute phase of the disease or during the healed phase of spinal tuberculosis [41–43]. Acute phase paralysis is mostly due to infected bone detritus or pus compressing the neural tissues. Vaishnav et al. have recently described a series of 100 cases with acute phase neurological compromise (91 paraplegias and 9 quadriplegias) [42]. They suggest that vertebral body destruction and retropulsion seemed to be the commonest cause (69%). MRI findings in the others were

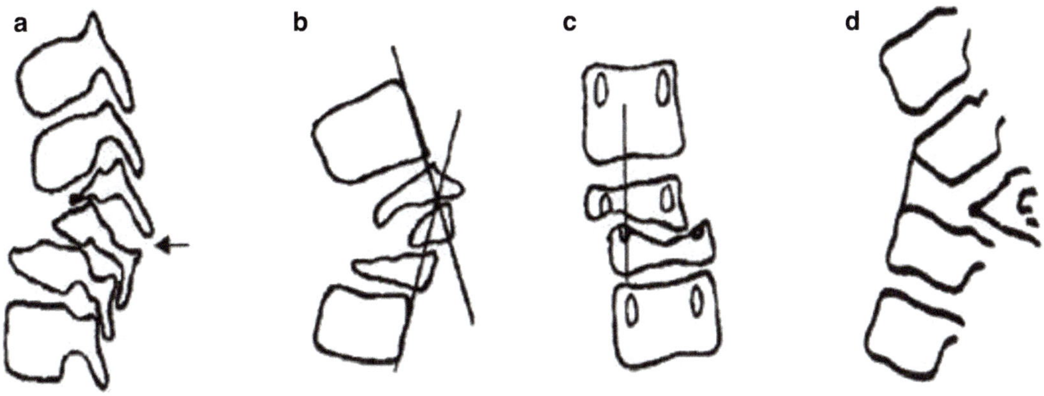

Fig. 31.5 (**a**) facet widening, (**b**) retropulsion of the diseased body, (**c**) coronal plane lateral translation of the affected segments, and (**d**) toppling of the spine at the involved segment

of epidural abscess, myelitis, meningitis, arachnoiditis, intramedullary tuberculoma. Late onset neurological deficit is almost always due to progressive severe deformity causing an internal gibbus and draping the spinal cord around the knuckle. The latter occurs in late childhood and adolescence and is typically insidious in onset and gradually progressive resulting in spastic paraplegia [41–43].

While the results of surgical decompression in acute phase neurological dysfunction in active disease are often encouraging, the outcomes in surgery for neurological deficit for late onset is less rewarding. In acute disease 88% of grade A&B and 92.8% of grade C neurological deficits will improve by two grades [43]. Whereas in late deformity patients with grades A–C paralysis Ha's study has demonstrated 44.4% recovery by two grades [44]. Jain has suggested that MRI findings of wet lesions with cord edema and myelitis is a good prognostic indicator while dry lesions with myelomalacia and reduced cord volume reflect poor prognosis for neural recovery [41].

Another typical feature of spinal TB is the presence of cold abscess. The frequency of identifying such collections is variable—Kanna [38] records 50% while Kotil's study records 100% abscess formation [45]. Absence of the characteristic warmth of pyogenic abscess has led to the name of cold abscess. Pathologically the lesion consists of inflammatory exudate and necrotic caseous material [46]. These collections progressively grow and track along fascial planes and extend into far regions of the body. Anterior cervical paravertebral, retropharyngeal, sub occipital, posterior paravertebral, pleural, peritoneal, perinephric, inguinal, obturator, gluteal, and the most frequent psoas abscess are the frequently described locations besides the catastrophic epidural abscess with its neurological consequences. Traditionally, it was believed that pus collection is an indication for surgical drainage, yet in tubercular abscess formation it has been established that most of them can be treated non-operatively (unless there are other indications for the surgery). Even epidural abscess formation can be conservatively managed in adults with Pott's spine [47–49] (Box 31.3).

Box 31.3 Clinical Features

- Systemic features of classic pulmonary TB may not be present in spinal TB in children in non-endemic areas.
- Local pain, deformity, neurological dysfunction, and abscess formation form the classic tetrad of the disease.
- Approx. 39% of deformities progress with growth even after attaining healed status and they are best predicted by the "spine at risk signs."
- Acute phase neurological dysfunction has better surgical prognosis than that due to delayed kyphosis.
- Cold abscess need not necessarily be surgically drained; it can be treated medically.

Investigations/Workup

Radiographs

Anteroposterior and lateral spine radiographs are the initial investigation. Disc space narrowing and end plate irregular margins are early changes. Progressive changes include vertebral collapse and kyphosis [50]. A soft tissue abscess will be detected by an increase in the retropharyngeal space in the cervical spine, a paraspinal fusiform abscess in the thoracic spine or a fullness of the psoas in the lumbar spine. However, the diagnosis may be missed if the lesion is in the cervicodorsal or junctional region or in case of posterior element involvement [51]. Calcification may be seen in older lesions.

Evidence of healing on follow-up radiographs is reduction in osteopenia (remineralization) and paravertebral shadows, sharpening of disc margins, and appearance of sclerosis [2, 35, 46].

MRI

MRI is the investigation of choice for diagnosing spinal TB and can pick up early changes.

Spinal involvement may be paradiscal, central, posterior element, or subligamentous. Typical findings are contiguous vertebral body involvement, disc space preservation, marrow edema, pre- and para-vertebral collections, end-plate erosions, with intra-osseous abscesses extending into epidural space [2, 46, 50]. It is also useful to differentiate soft epidural compression like abscess which is and granulation tissue hyperintense on T2 and hypointense on T1 from hard compression like disc and bone which will be hypointense on T1 and T2 [35, 51, 52]. It is important to evaluate the entire spine for skipped lesions. MRI is very useful for assessing cord changes of myelopathy, myelomalacia, and cord edema which are predictors of neurological recovery in patients with deficit [52]. MRI signs of healing are partial or complete resolution of abscesses with replacement of bone marrow edema by normal fatty marrow [50, 52].

Figures 31.5, 31.6, 31.7, 31.8, 31.9, 31.10, 31.11, 31.12, and 31.13 are case examples with different case scenarios and MRI changes.

CT

CT is necessary to accurately assess bony destruction and differentiate bony and soft tissue compression as the causes of canal encroachment. It is helpful for pre-surgical planning [51] (Box 31.4).

Box 31.4 Investigations for a Child Suspected to Have Spinal Tuberculosis

- Radiographs—Spine and chest
- MRI spine
- CT spine
- Ultrasound abdomen—psoas abscess
- Labs—Complete Blood Count (CBC), Erytrocyte Sedimentation Rate (ESR), CRP
- HIV
- Liver and renal function tests—baseline before initiation of treatment

Differential diagnoses are listed in Box 31.5.

Box 31.5 Differential Diagnoses

- Pyogenic discitis
- Brucellosis
- Fungal osteomyelitis
- Lymphoma
- Spinal tumors
- Eosinophilic granuloma

Fig. 31.6 An 11-year-old female came with neck pain in neck for the last 3 months and weakness in both upper and lower limb for the last 15 days. Patient had a previous consultation at another facility, MRI was done, and ATT was started on empirical basis but pain didn't subside. (**a**) X-ray shows subluxation of C2 over C3 with loss of cervical lordosis. Also, a large retropharyngeal shadow on the lateral view. (**b**) MRI retropharyngeal abscess extending into epidural space with cord compression. Patient was managed conservatively with anterior drainage of abscess. Sample was sent for Gen Xpert, TB-MGIT, Histopathology, Culture sensitivity. Gen Xpert was S/O rifampicin resistant MTB. Patient was started on the second-line ATT and was put on cervical traction for 1 month. Subsequently the patient was given a Total Contact CTLSO brace. Patient responded to treatment and recovered neurologically completely. (**c**) Follow-up radiograph shows reduction in subluxation and reduction in retropharyngeal space. (**d**) Follow-up MRI also shows complete reduction in size of abscess in retropharyngeal and epidural abscess

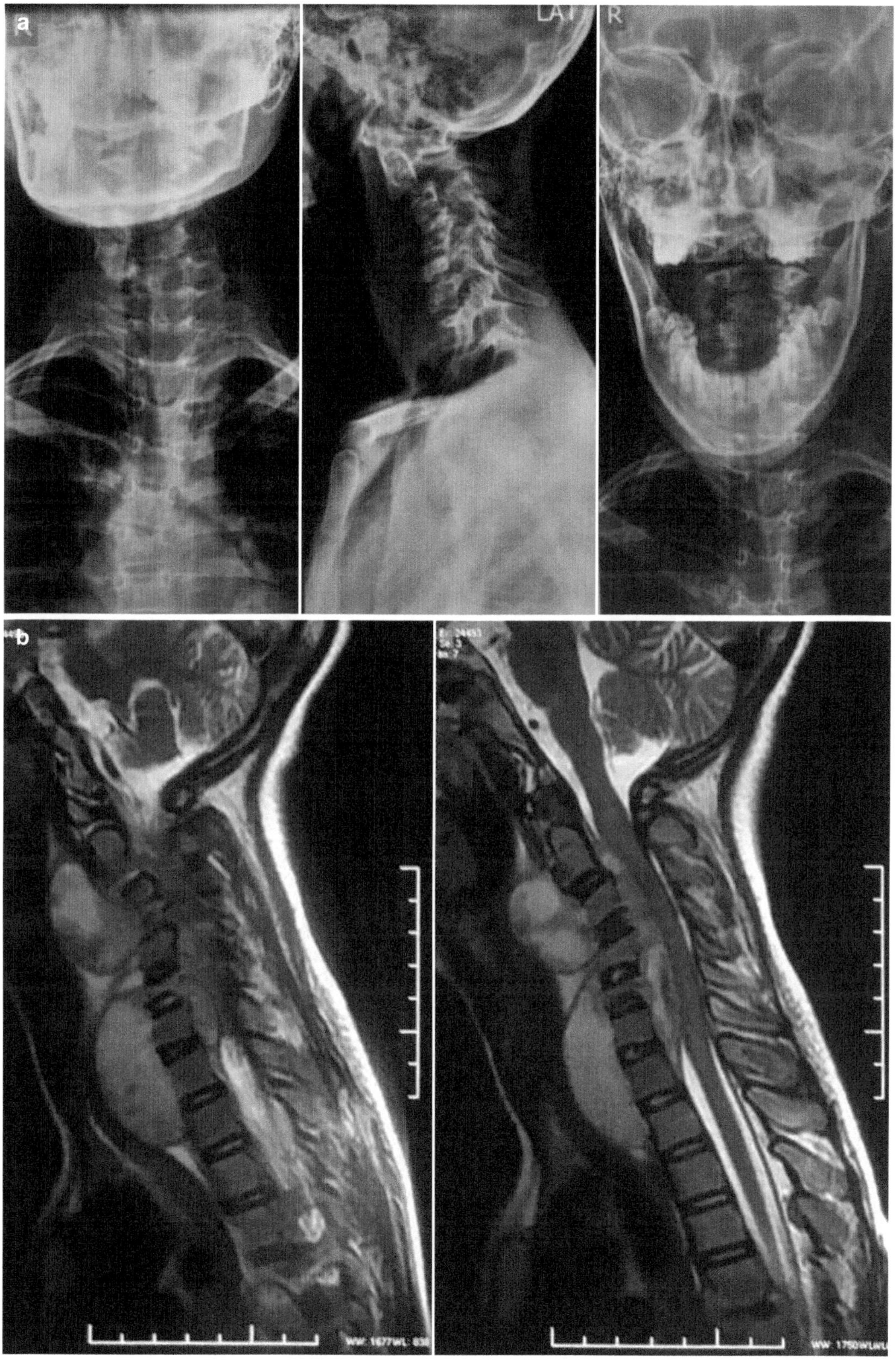
a
LAT
R
b

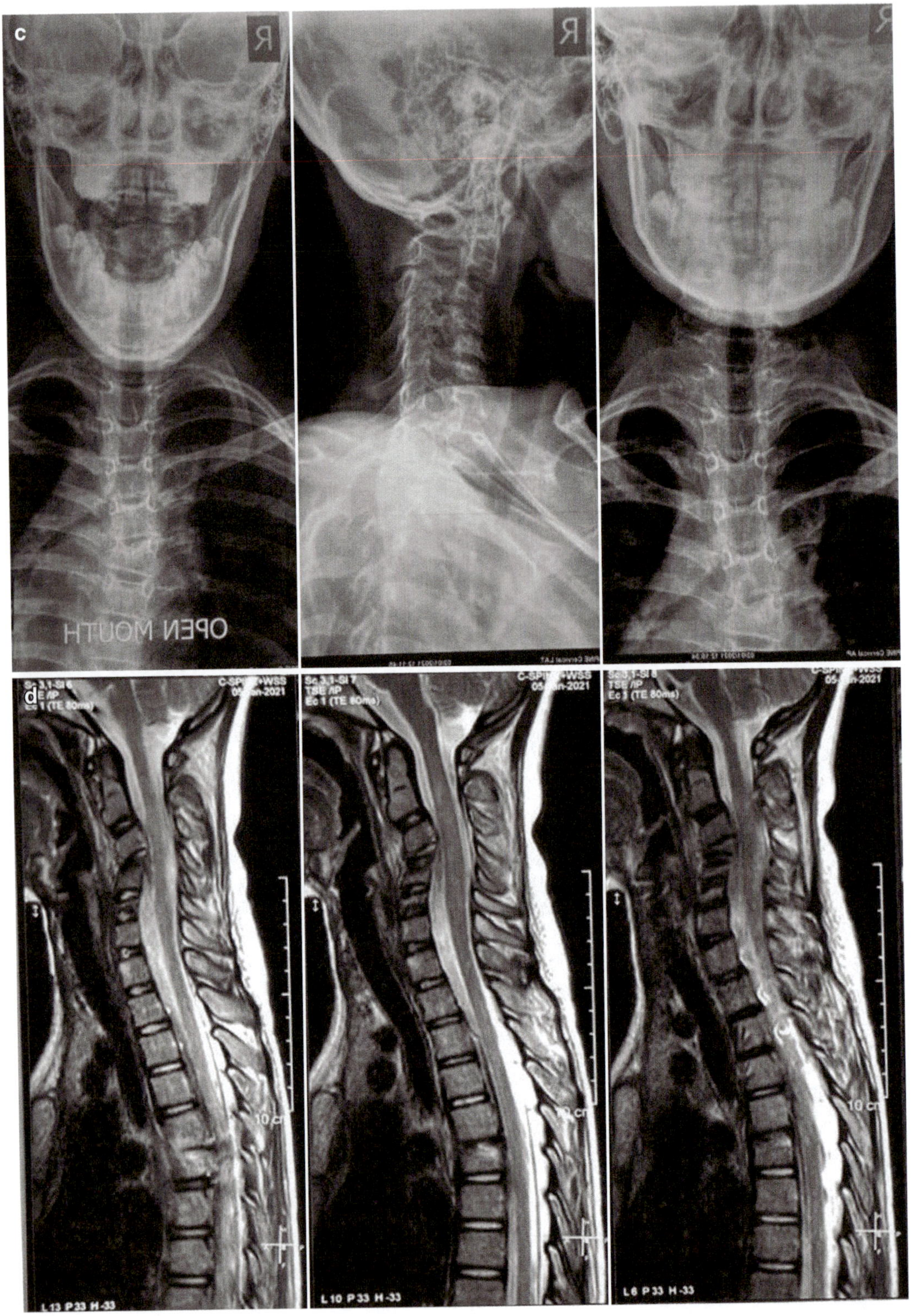

Fig. 31.6 (continued)

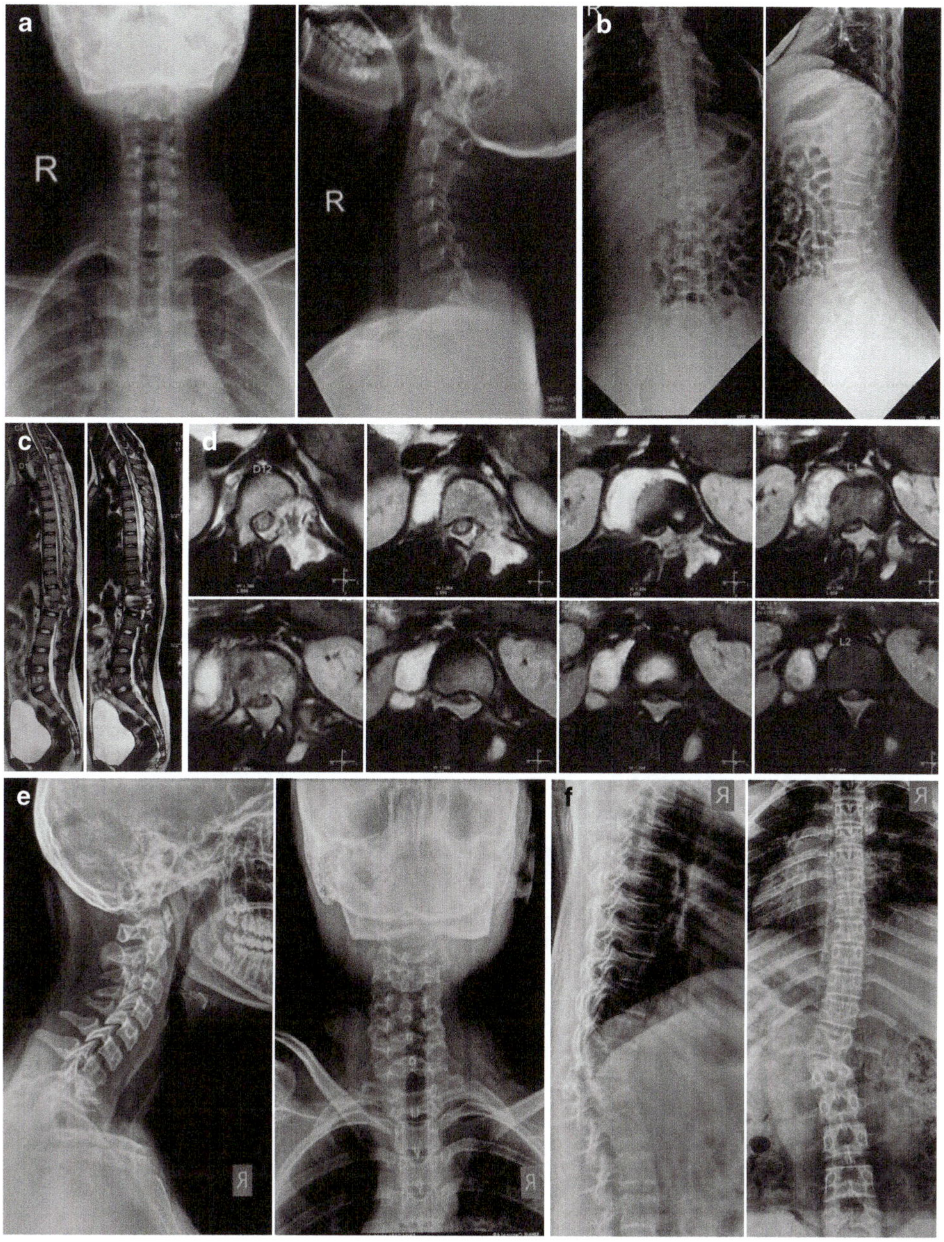

Fig. 31.7 A 12-year-old female came with C/o pain in mid back for the last 5 months and weakness in right lower limb for the last 7 days. The patient was initially treated elsewhere, MRI was done, and ATT was started on empirical basis. But pain didn't subside, and the patient developed weakness in the right lower limb, so she was referred for further management. (**a**, **b**) Radiograph shows loss of cervical lordosis with increased retropharyngeal space in front of C7 vertebra and decreased disc space between D12-L1 vertebrae with toppling of D12 vertebra over L1. Cervicodorsal TB can be missed as it is difficult to discern on plain radiographs. (**c**, **d**) MRI shows C7-D1 decreased disc space with anterior abscess and decreased disc space between D12-L1 with abscess extending anteriorly and with some posterior extension. Patient underwent a USG guided biopsy. Sample was sent for Gen Xpert, TB-MGIT, Culture sensitivity, Histopathology. Gen Xpert came negative. TB-MGIT showed no growth. Histopathology s/o Chronic granulomatous inflammation s/o TB. Patient was started on first-line ATT with dose readjustment by the ID team. The patient was given a CTLSO brace. Patient improved clinically. Power improved in the right lower limb to 5/5. Pain gradually subsided. (**e**, **f**) X-ray shows radiological healing in the form of sclerosis at the D12-L1 level. (**g**, **h**) MRI also shows resolution of collection at C7-D1 level and D12- L1 level

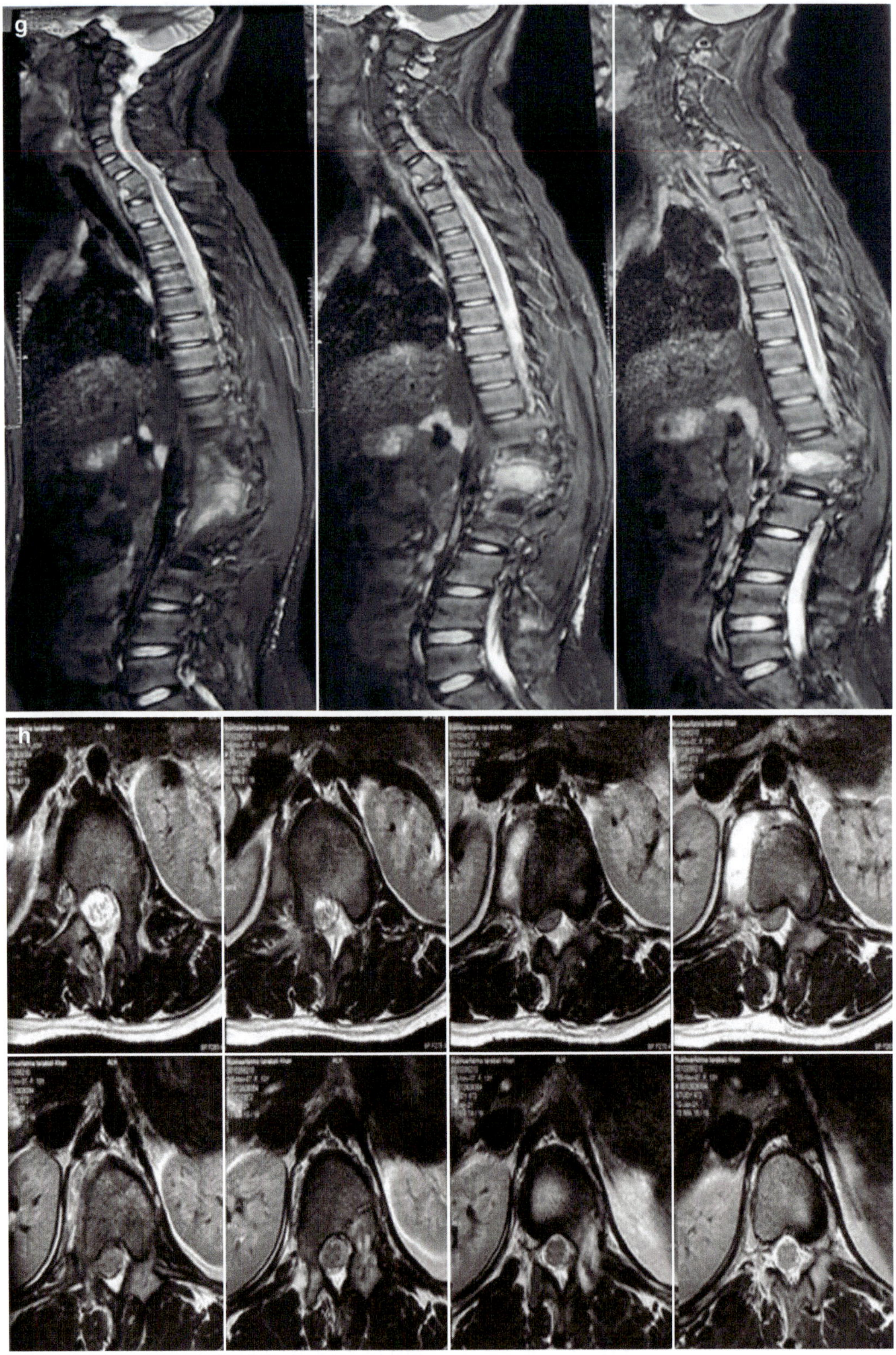

Fig. 31.7 (continued)

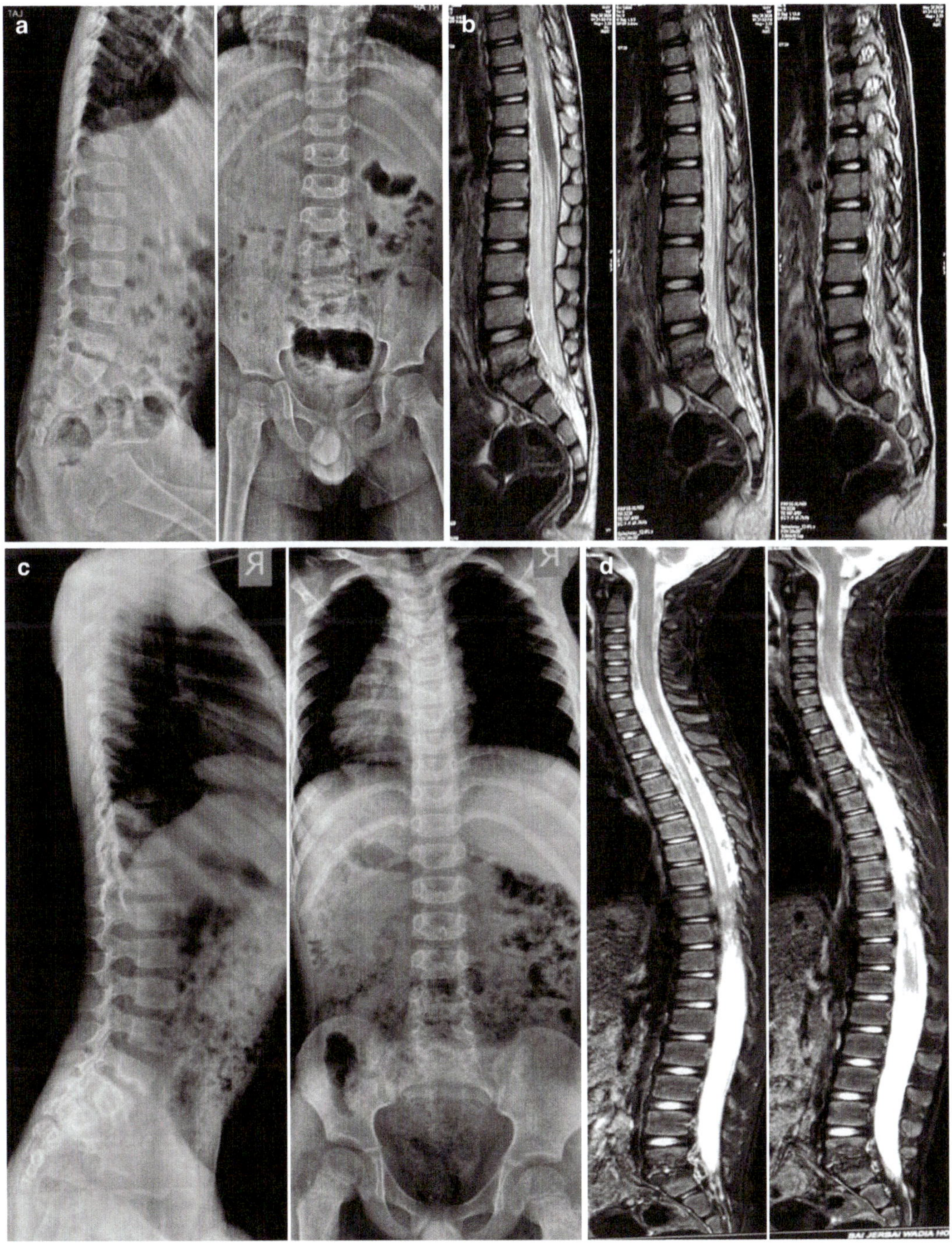

Fig. 31.8 A 5-year boy, C/o pain in lower back for the last 4 months. Pain was insidious in onset, gradually progressing over a period of 4 months. Not associated with any weakness but associated with constitutional features of weight loss, evening rise of fever. History of contact with TB present. (**a**) X-ray was done, S/o end plate erosion of L5-S1 with decreased disc space between L5-S1. (**b**) MRI end-plate erosion of L5-S1 with decreased disc space with peri-discal edema present. Patient was started on first-line ATT on empirical basis as facilities for biopsy were not available and responded to the treatment. Pain gradually subsided. Constitutional symptoms improved. (**c, d**) X-ray and MRI pictures showed improvement on subsequent follow up. Peri-discal edema completely resolved with X-ray showing sclerosis of end plates of L5-S1

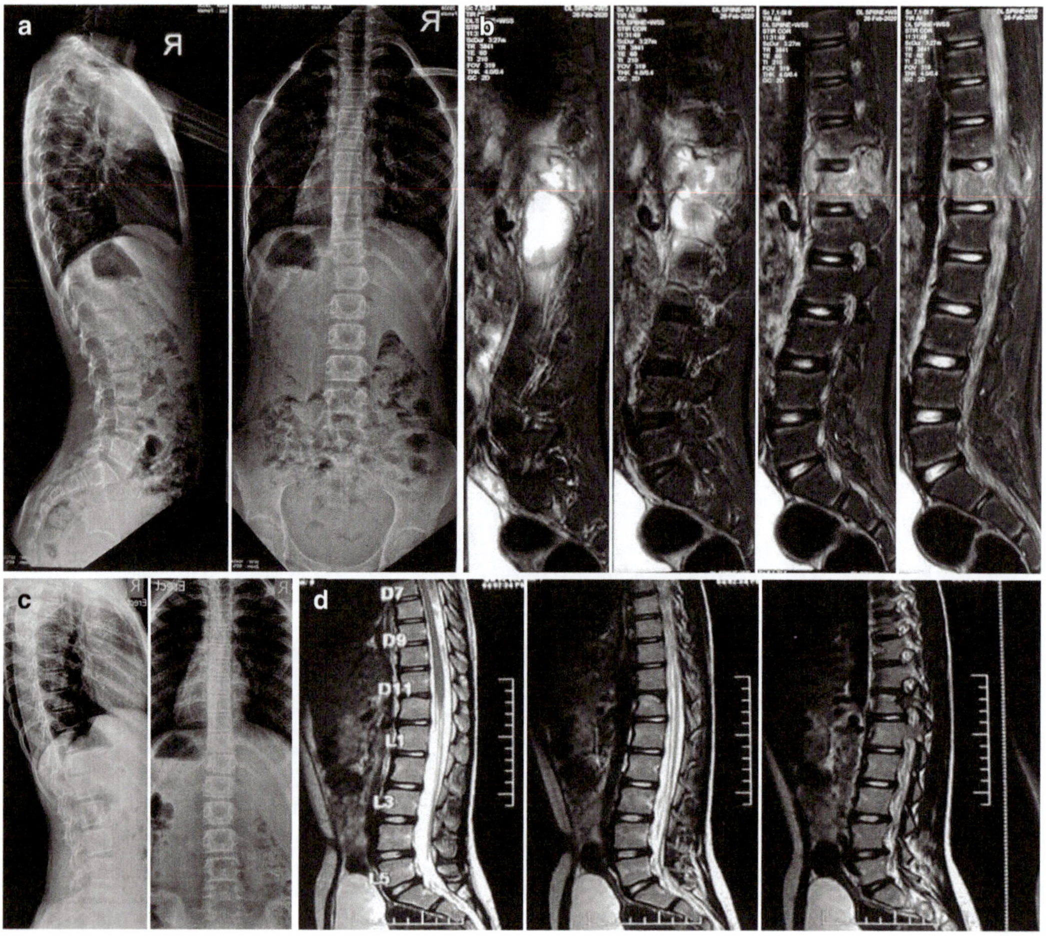

Fig. 31.9 An 11-year-old female with pain in mid-back for the last 6 months. Pain was insidious in onset which gradually progressed over a period of 6 months. Not associated with any constitutional symptoms. No H/o contact. (**a**) X-ray was done which was S/o erosion of pedicle of D12 vertebra with decreased disc space between D11 and D12. (**b**) MRI-decreased disc space between D11 and D12 with D12 body involvement and collection around D11–D12. Patient underwent a CT guided biopsy. Sample was sent for Gen Xpert, TB-MGIT, culture sensitivity, histopathology. Gen Xpert rifampicin sensitive MTB. Histopathology chronic granulomatous inflammation. Patient was started on first-line ATT and was given a TLSO brace. (**c**, **d**) Follow up X-ray showing sclerosis of D12 pedicle and MRI showing complete resolution of peri-vertebral collection

Biopsy

Diagnosis of spinal TB should be ascertained on histopathological, AFB smear, molecular methods (CBNAAT and LPA) Line Probe Assay and microbiological culture examination [2, 4, 17]. The two important reasons are that the imaging findings are not specific and there is increasing incidence of MDR-TB so the culture and drug sensitivity is important for treatment planning with appropriate chemotherapy [20, 22, 28, 48, 50]. Biopsy yield depends on the technical skill of the radiologist/surgeon, accurate and adequate sample obtained from pathological foci, microbiology laboratory facilities, and previous ATT treatment [50, 51].

Biopsy can be obtained with image guided modalities—CT, C-arm, or sometimes ultrasound guided and in patients undergoing surgery, tissue and pus samples can be obtained at the time of surgical debridement of the lesion. In the thora-

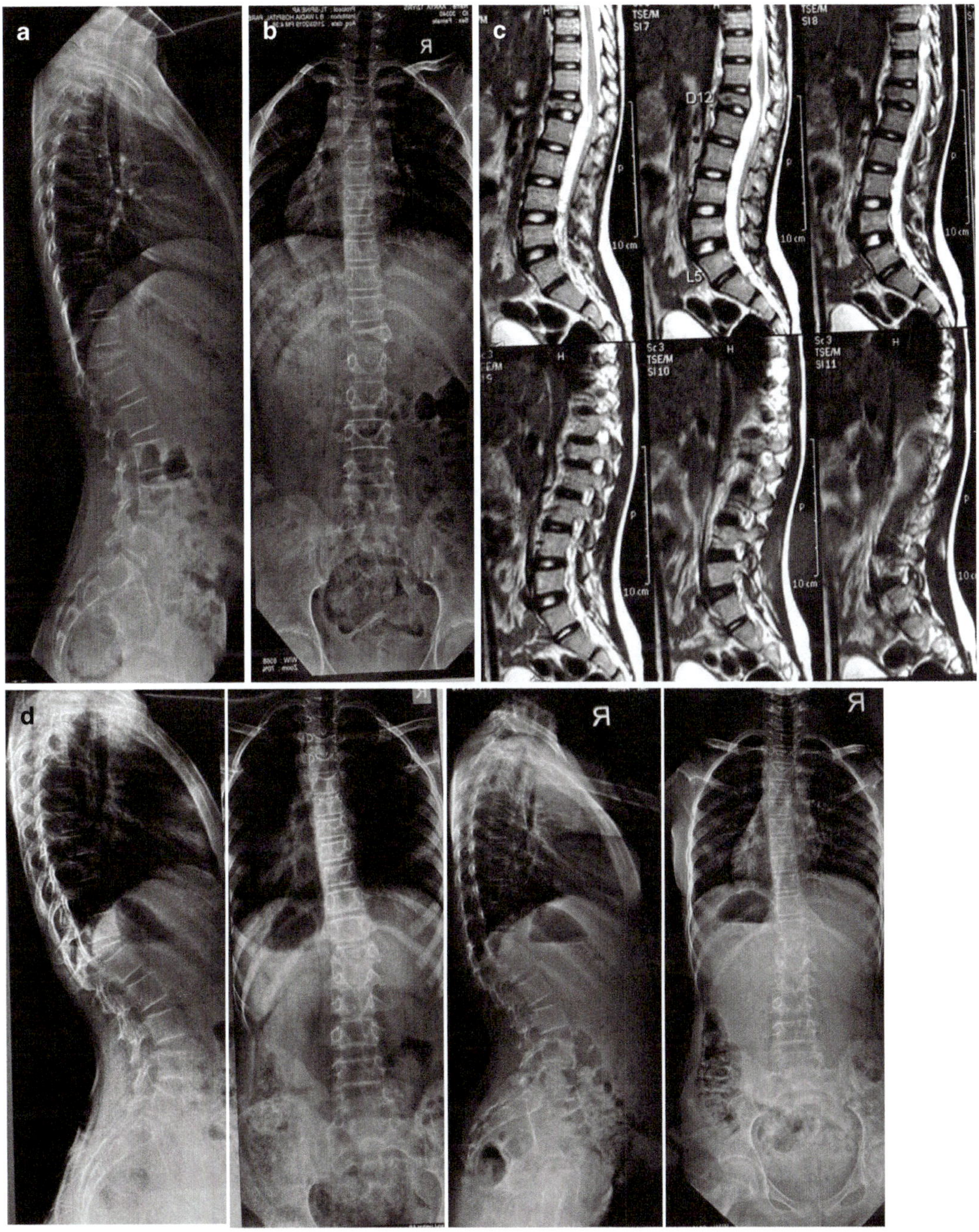

Fig. 31.10 A 12-year-old female came with pain in mid-back and deformity in mid-back noticed for the last 4–5 months. H/o of constitutional symptoms present. No H/o contact. (**a**) X-ray shows central collapse of D12 vertebra with decreased disc space between D12-L1 vertebra. (**b**) MRI shows central collapse of D12 vertebra with minimal collection. Patient underwent open biopsy and a sample was sent for Gen Xpert, TB-MGIT, Histopathology and culture sensitivity. Investigations are S/o rifampicin sensitive MTB. Patient was started on the first-line ATT. (**c–e**) Gradual progression of deformity and K angle. (**f**) X-ray at completion of treatment which shows further progress of deformity with progression of K angle with sclerosis of end plates. (**g**) MRI at completion of treatment showing healed lesion with internal gibbus

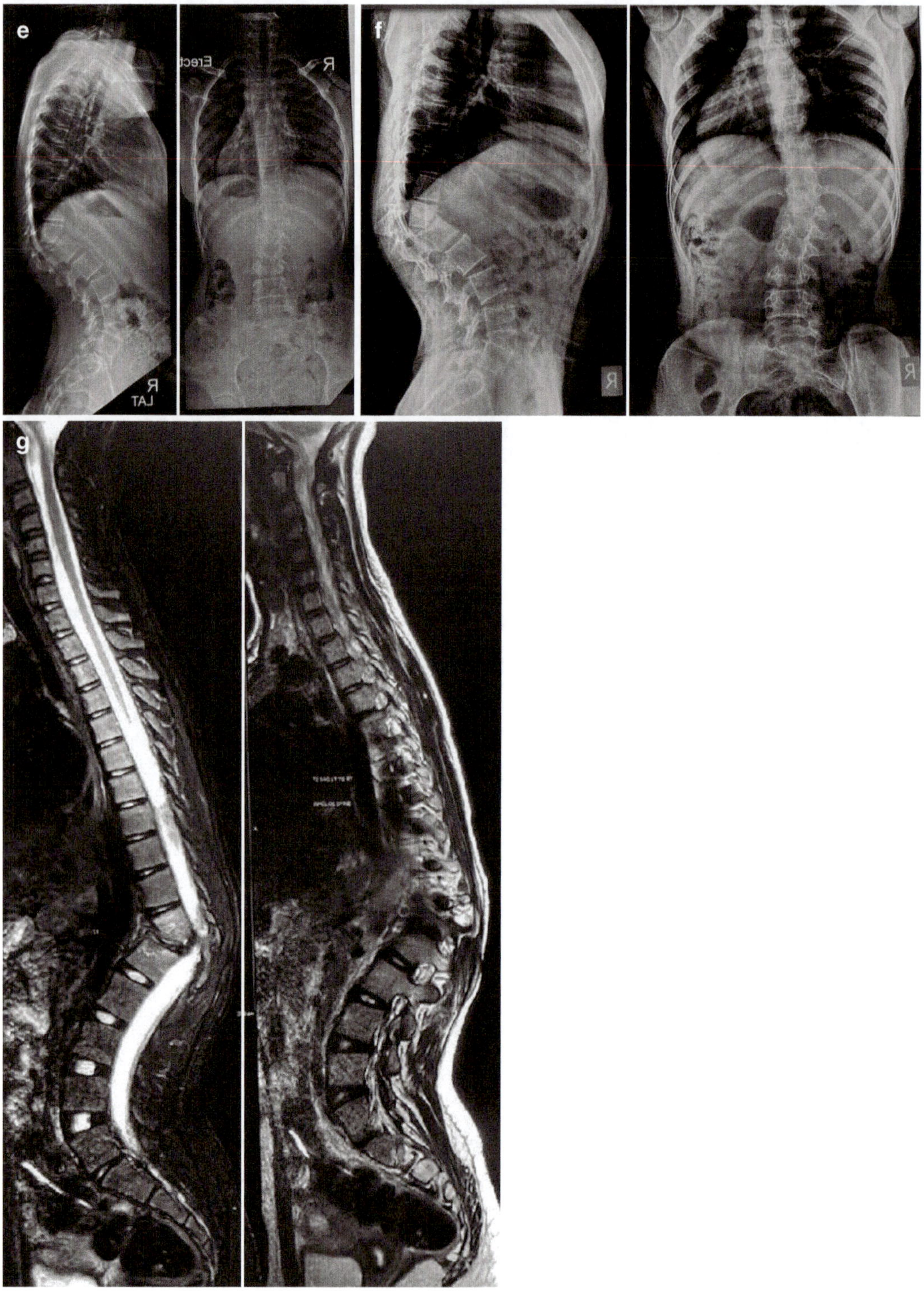

Fig. 31.10 (continued)

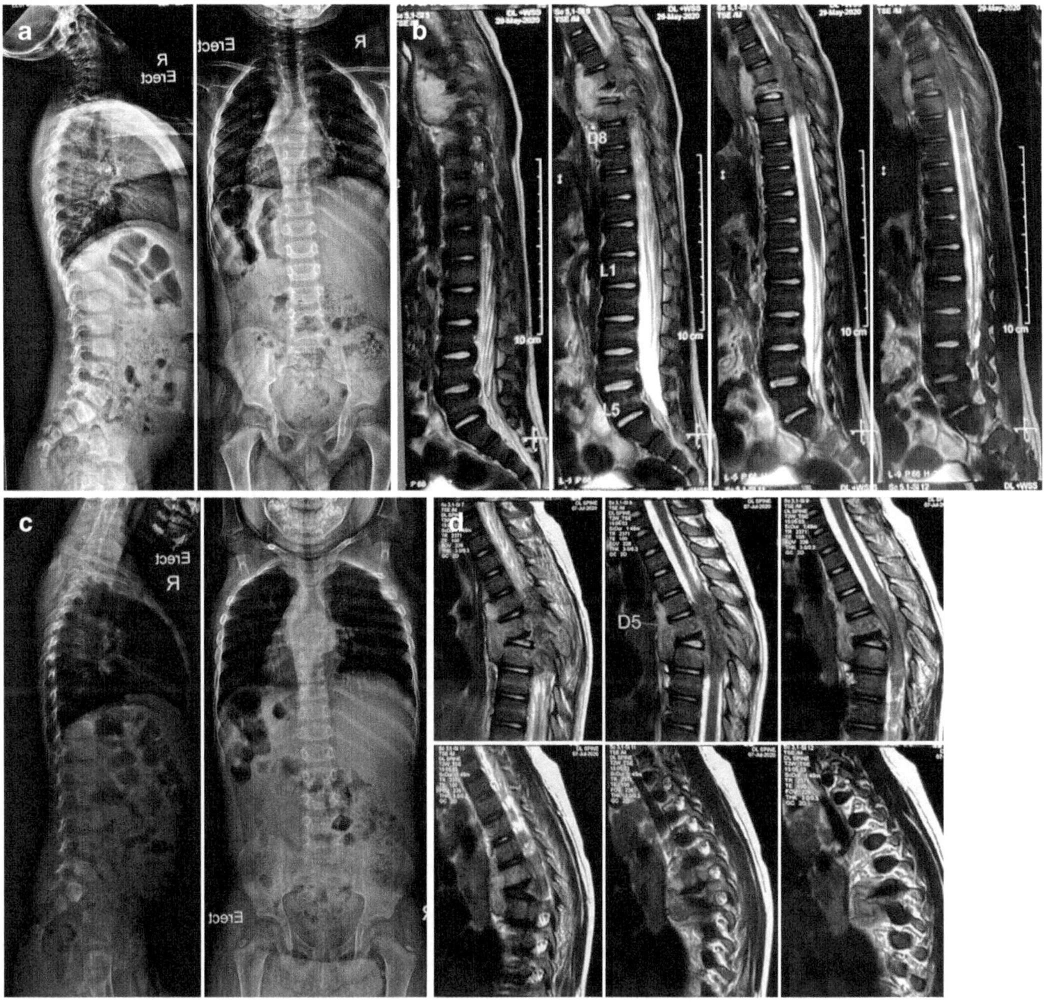

Fig. 31.11 A 4-year-old boy came with pain in upper back for 3–4 months. H/o Contact present. H/o constitutional symptoms present. (**a**) X-ray shows partial collapse of D6 vertebra with decreased disc space of D6-D7 vertebrae. AP view shows bird nest appearance. (**b**) MRI showing partial collapse of D6 vertebra with abscess extending from D5 to D7 vertebrae anteriorly. Patient was started on empirical ATT as the facility for biopsy was not available. One month down the line patient presented with paraplegia in extension without bowel bladder involvement. (**c**) X-ray shows further collapse of D6 vertebra with increased K angle. AP view shows increase in size of bird nest appearance. (**d**) MRI shows complete collapse of D6 vertebra with abscess anteriorly extending into epidural space with cord compression at the level of D5–D6 vertebrae. Patient underwent posterior decompression and instrumentation. Sample obtained was sent for Gen Xpert, TB-MGIT, Histopathology, Culture and sensitivity. Investigations S/o rifampicin sensitive MTB. Patient was started on the first-line ATT. Postoperatively patient recovered neurologically with power 3/5 at the end of 1 week and 5/5 at the end of 1 month. (**e**) Post-op X-ray of the patient. (**f**) Subsequent follow-up X-ray at 1 year. (**g**) Follow-up MRI shows complete resolution of abscess anteriorly and in epidural space

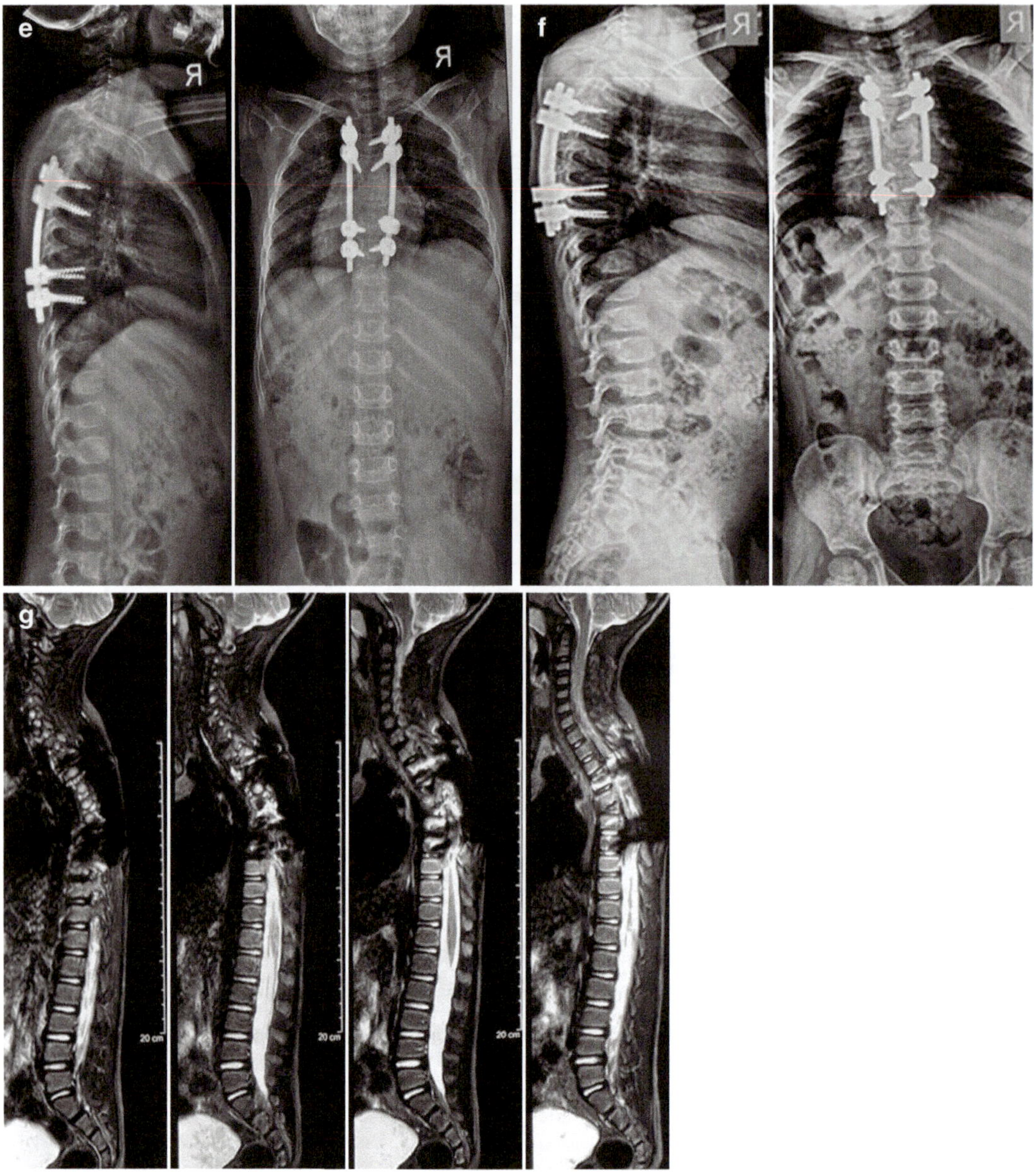

Fig. 31.11 (continued)

columbar spine, transpedicular biopsy or paravertebral tissue is usually obtained, while in the subaxial cervical spine an anterolateral approach is used [2, 46, 50, 51].

A core needle biopsy is used to obtain bony tissue and pus, usually the abscess pus has higher microbiological yield than the bone sample [2, 28, 46, 50, 51]. Culture samples should be collected in normal saline and histopathology samples in formalin 10%.

Microbiological samples are processed with BACTEC Mycobacteria Growth Indicator Tube (MGIT) cultures as TB is paucibacillary and will mostly not be seen on initial Ziehl–Neelsen stain smear [38, 46]. PCR is a molecular diagnostic test that amplifies the DNA of *M. tuberculosis* and provides results within hours [38, 37]. MTB GenXpert rifampin sensitivity is useful to diagnose rifampin drug resistance early without waiting for the culture and sensitivity results which

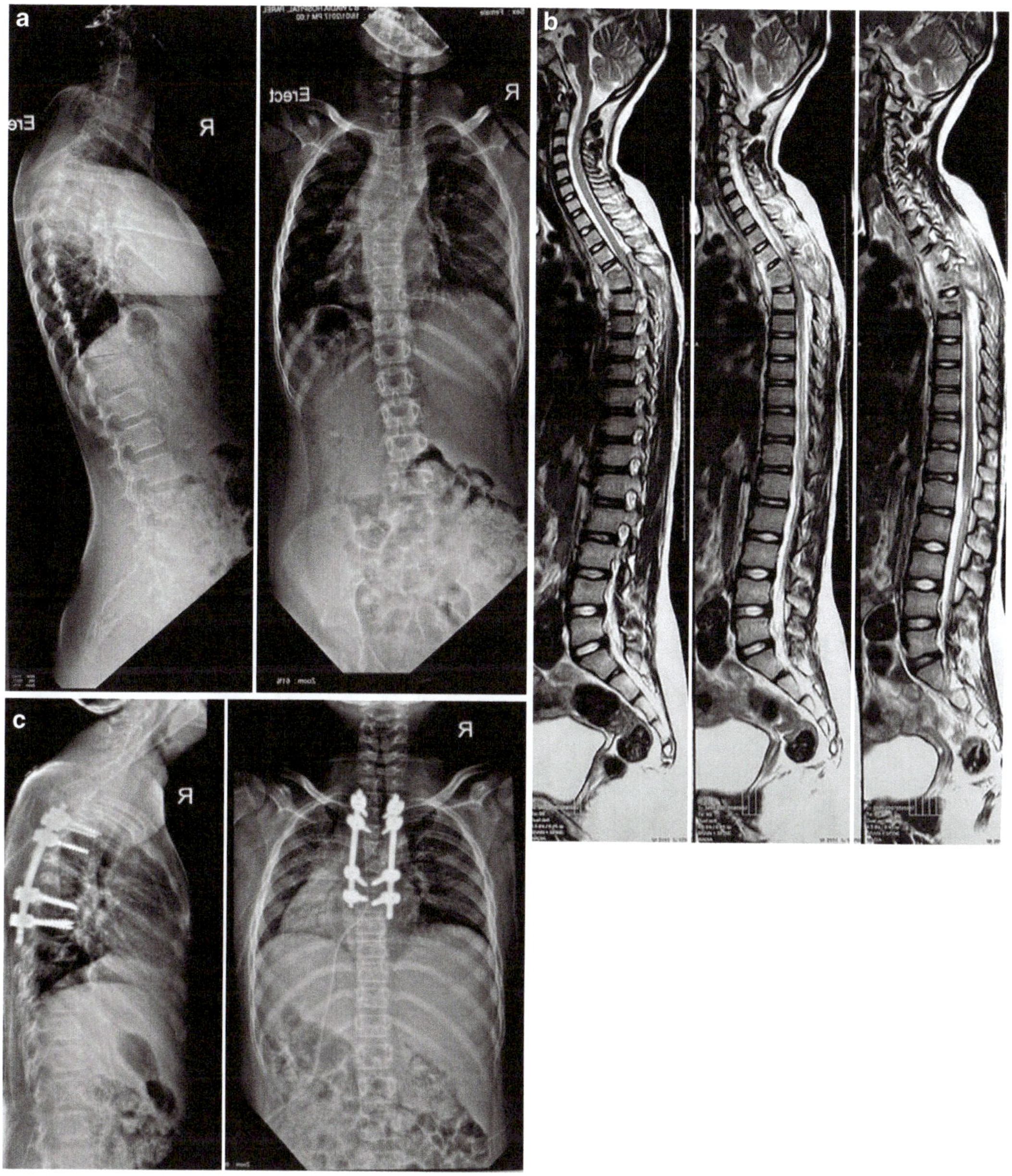

Fig. 31.12 An 11-year-old girl came with pain in upper back for the last 4 months and weakness in both lower limbs for the last 5 days. No H/O constitutional symptoms. No H/o contact. O/e kyphotic deformity present over the upper dorsal region with tenderness. The patient presented with paraplegia in extension with bowel and bladder involvement. (**a**) X-ray shows collapse of D4-D5 with reduction in disc space. AP view shows lateral translation at D4–D5 level. (**b**) MRI shows collapse of D4–D5 vertebra with collection anteriorly with extension into epidural space with cord compression. Patient underwent transpedicular decompression and posterior instrumentation. Sample obtained was sent for Gen Xpert, TB-MGIT, Histopathology, Culture, and sensitivity. Investigations S/o rifampicin sensitive MTB. Patient was started on the first-line ATT. Postoperatively patient recovered neurologically. (**c**) Post-op X-ray of patient. (**d**) Follow-up X-ray of the patient showing healing. (**e**) MRI showing post-op status with complete resolution of abscess

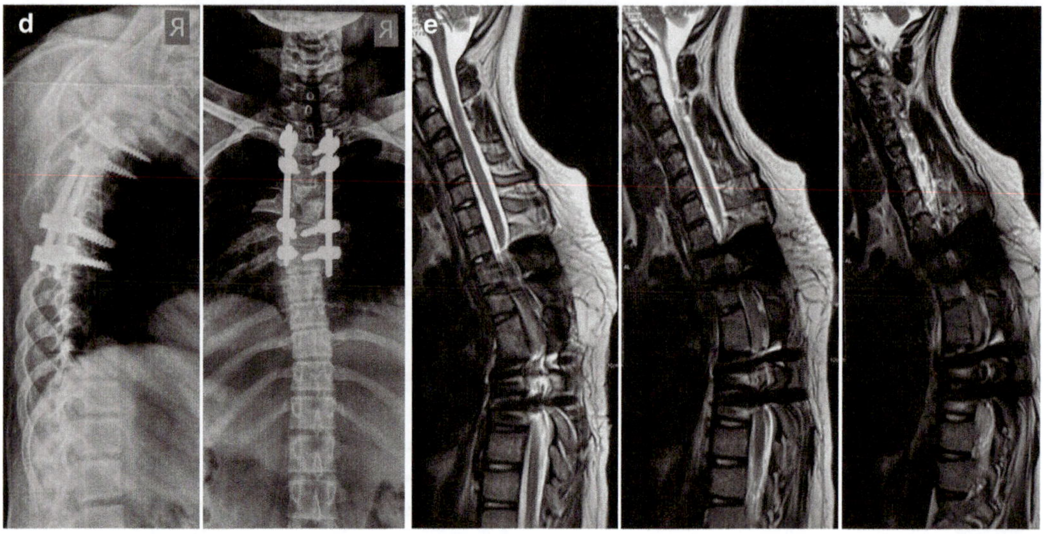

Fig. 31.12 (continued)

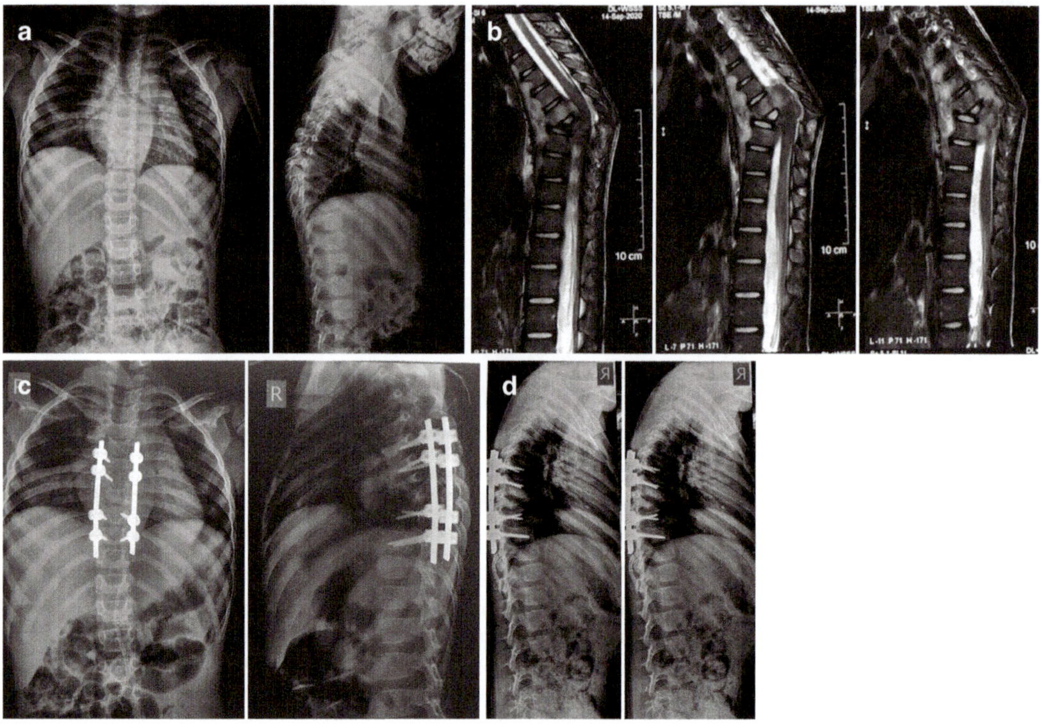

Fig. 31.13 A 7-year-old boy with D6–D8 Pott's spine started on first-line ATT on empirical basis. Patient took drugs for 3 months and stopped (defaulter). Came to emergency with paraplegia in extension. (**a**) X-ray showing collapse of D7–D8 vertebra with kyphotic deformity. (**b**) MRI showing complete collapse of D7 vertebra with abscess extending anteriorly and in epidural space with cord compression. (**c**) Post-op X-ray of the patient underwent transpedicular decompression and posterior instrumentation with anterior bone grafting. Sample obtained was sent for Gen Xpert, TB-MGIT, Histopathology, Culture and sensitivity. Rifampicin resistant MTB. Patient was started on second line ATT. Post-operatively patient recovered neurologically. (**d**) X-ray at subsequent follow-up at 2 years

takes a few weeks [2, 38, 46, 50, 51]. Positive results obtained on MGIT should be processed for phenotypic drug sensitivity testing or line probe assay testing for first-line drugs and for second-line drugs if GenXpert is positive for rifampicin resistance or there is suspicion of drug resistance based on previous history, close contact history with a proven drug resistant case, and therapeutically refractory disease with clinical and radiological deterioration on first-line ATT drugs [50]. Clearly population samples from different parts of India show different trends depending on the local culture, and practice settings [50] (Box 31.6).

Box 31.6 Investigations to be Done on Biopsy Specimen

- Histopathology—granulomatous inflammation, epitheloid giant cells, caseous necrosis, AFB smear, PCR
- GenXpert (2 hours) for Rifampin sensitivity: reported in 24–48 hours
- MGIT TB cultures: reported at 48 hours, 3 weeks and 6 weeks.
- Aerobic bacterial cultures
- Drug sensitivity testing for first line and second line ATT drugs

Treatment Options

Medical Management

Medical management with appropriate chemotherapy is the cornerstone for successful treatment of spinal TB. Initial MRC trials were performed with 18 months of combined chemotherapy and then over time reduced to 6–12 months with the first-line drug regimens and results of shorter regimens are comparable [53]. Second-line drug regimens need to be administered for 18 months to 2 years [22–24, 54–56]. With the advent of multidrug resistance, medical management has become more challenging and chemotherapy regimen prescriptions should preferably involve a pediatrician or chest/infectious disease specialist [50, 51].

The first-line drugs include isoniazid, rifampicin, ethambutol, pyrazinamide, and streptomycin [2, 3, 50, 54]. Baseline liver function and renal function tests should be checked prior to initiation of ATT. Usually first-line ATT is initiated immediately after clinicoimaging diagnosis of TB and biopsy is obtained, culture, and ATT sensitivity reports are followed to confirm the efficacy of the drugs administered. In case of neurological deficit, first-line ATT may be initiated even before biopsy is obtained and steroids may be administered short term although this is controversial as there is some evidence [14, 41, 50]. Four drugs (isoniazid, rifampicin, ethambutol, and pyrazinamide) are used in the initial intensive phase and subsequently 3 drugs (isoniazid, rifampicin, and ethambutol) in the continuation phase [2, 3, 50]. There are national health programs like the RNTCP in India through which these drugs are administered free of cost and in a supervised fashion to ensure patient compliance [1, 24, 51, 54] (Box 31.7).

Box 31.7 First-Line Drugs of the Anti-Tuberculous Treatment (ATT)

- Isoniazid dosage 5 mg/kg PO
- Rifampicin dosage 10 mg/kg PO
- Ethambutol dosage 15 mg/kg PO
- Pyrazinamide 25 mg/kg PO
- Streptomycin 15 mg/kg IM

Second-line ATT should be initiated in cases of GenXpert-/culture-proven MDR-TB or in case of therapeutically refractory disease which has been described as poor clinical and radiological response, appearance of fresh lesion, deterioration of spinal deformity, new discharging sinus, and wound dehiscence after first-line ATT >5 months [49–51]. The incidence of secondary drug resistance is increasing in endemic regions as a result of patient non-compliance with a correctly prescribed first-line regimen, or due to an incorrectly prescribed regimen by the physician [20–24, 50, 54–56]. Infection with a primary drug resistant strain may occur in children due to contact history with other family members who were infected with MDR-TB previously and should be obtained during the initial consultation [25–28] (Box 31.8).

Box 31.8 Second-Line Drugs of the Anti-tuberculous Treatment (ATT)

- *MDR-TB*: Resistance to both Isoniazid and Rifampicin
- *Extensively Drug Resistant TB (XDR-TB)*: Resistance to any fluoroquinolone and one injectable second line antibiotic along with Isoniazid and Rifampicin
- *Total Drug Resistant TB (TDR)*
- *Second line Drugs*
  - *Group A:* Flouroquinolones (Levofloxacin, Moxifloxacin, Gatifloxacin)
  - *Group B:* Injectables (Kanamycin, Amikacin, Careomycin)
  - *Group C:* Other second-line drugs (Ethionomide, Prothonamide, Cycloserine, Terizidone, Linezolid, Clofazimine)
  - *Group D* (Add-on agents): Pyrazinamide, Ethambutol, INH high dose, Betaquiline, Delamanid, PAS, Imipenem-Cilastatin, Meropenem, Amoxicillin-Clavulanate, Thioacetazone

A commonly used ATT second-line regimen should consist of 5–6 drugs and includes 4 second-line drugs with one drug from group A and B each and two from group C with add on agents from group D. It is important to combine bactericidal or bacteriostatic drugs [50, 51, 56]. An example of a second-line regimen is injection amikacin for 6 months and moxifloxacin, cycloserine, clofazimine, and para-aminosalicylic acid (PAS) for 18 months [50]. Second-line regimens are expensive, need to be closely monitored for adverse effects and compliance. Clinical improvement and follow-up radiographs and MRI are used for assessing healing.

Bed Rest, Traction and Bracing—Some of the initial MRC trials involved prolonged bed rest. Presently the role of bed rest is limited to patients presenting with neurology and craniovertebral and cervical tuberculosis where Sayer's cervical traction may be used for a few weeks followed by a well-fitting Miami J collar or CTO. For thoracic or thoracolumbar TB, a TLSO is used in the initial months.

Figure 31.7 is a case example of a child with multifocal TB with monoparesis treated conservatively.

Figures 31.8, 31.9, and 31.10 are examples of conservatively treated patients.

Surgical Management

Broadly indications for surgical treatment in pediatric spinal tuberculosis are gross or worsening neurological deficit, deficit not improving with ATT, significant early or late kyphosis, spinal instability, open biopsy when image guided biopsy has been inconclusive, and rarely large abscesses with lack of response to chemotherapy [2, 46, 50]. The medical treatment remains the mainstay for successful outcomes while surgical treatment is for complications. The additional factor of spinal growth in a child is an important consideration and prevention of kyphosis due to asymmetric growth of the anterior and posterior columns if there is multilevel vertebral body destruction should be taken into account [39, 40, 50] (Box 31.9).

Box 31.9 Indications for Surgery

- Active TB with neurological deficit
- Active TB with kyphosis
- Active TB with instability
- Active TB with inadequate response to AKT
- Old TB with kyphosis
- Healed TB with kyphosis

The decision making for the surgical approach depends on the region of pathology, location of epidural compression (anterior or posterior), presence of kyphosis, number of vertebral levels involved, instability and technical comfort level and training [51].

The goals of surgical treatment are debridement of the abscess, involved vertebra and disc, adequate cord decompression, reconstruction if the anterior column is damaged with more than one vertebral body destroyed and posterior instrumentation and stabilization when there is spinal instability and kyphosis [2, 14, 46, 50, 51]. The flowchart below can be a guide for thoracic and thoracolumbar disease with associated myelopathy.

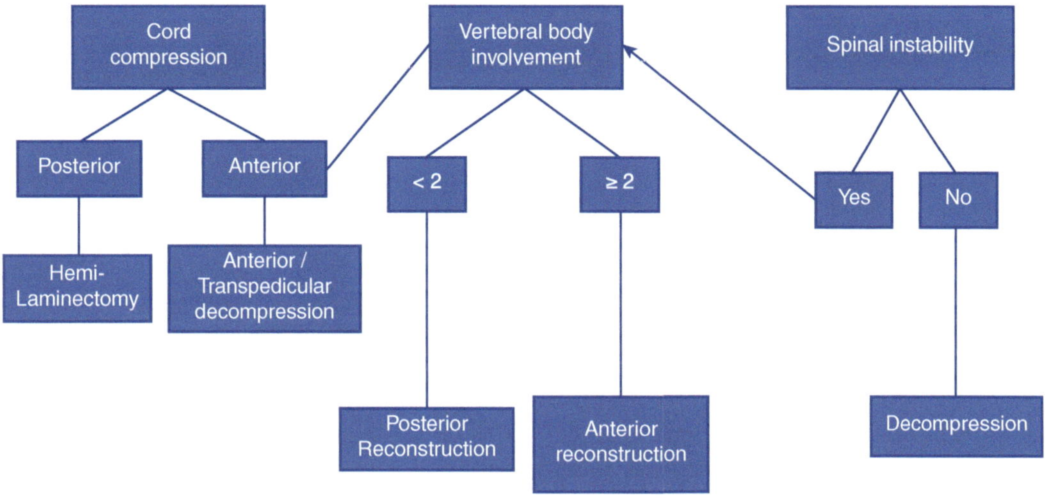

Cervical Spinal Tuberculosis

Surgery is recommended surgery for dysphagia for solids due to a retropharyngeal abscess, neurological deficit, instability of the atlanto-axial joint on flexion/extension views, and progressive kyphosis (>30°) while on orthotic treatment [19]. Occipitocervical or C1-2 fusion is indicated if there is C1-2 instability, destruction of one or both C1 lateral masses, basilar invagination, rotatory subluxation, and myelopathy [57]. An anterior approach is preferred when there is a large retropharyngeal abscess and anterior epidural abscess, reconstruction with strut graft and plating can be used in the subaxial cervical region [19]. Multilevel corpectomy often needs to be supplemented with a posterior instrumented fusion. Post-operative cervical brace is recommended.

Figure 31.6 is a case example of cervical TB treated with ATT, anterior abscess decompression and traction.

Cervicodorsal Tuberculosis

Cervicodorsal junction is a challenging region to approach anteriorly due to the anatomical structures, vessels, and the manubrium which makes the inferior vertebral body exposure difficult. A low anterior cervical approach can be used in a patient with a long neck after checking the vertebral level corresponding with the manubrium or a manubrium splitting approach can be used when the lesion is below the level of the manubrium [58]. An all posterior approach is suitable for a circumferential decompression and anterior reconstruction with posterior instrumentation [59]. The cervical anchor points can be subaxial lateral mass screws, sublaminar wires with C7 pedicle screws.

Figure 31.14 is an example of upper dorsal kyphosis with neurological deficit treated with all posterior transpedicular approach.

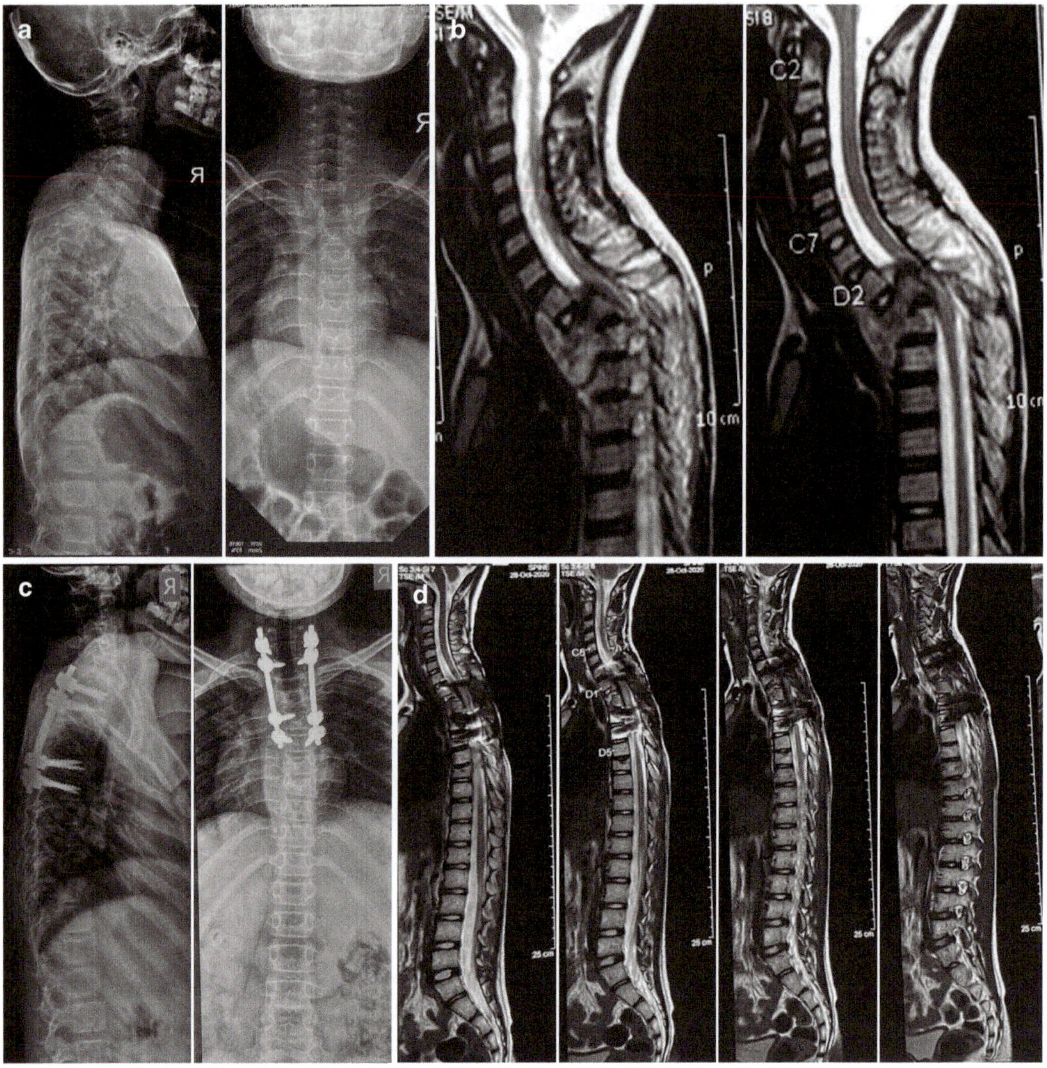

Fig. 31.14 An 11-year-old boy came with pain in the upper back for 4 months and weakness in both lower limbs for the last 15 days. Bowel and bladder were also involved. (**a**) X-ray shows complete destruction of D3 vertebra with crowding of ribs in AP view and subluxation in lateral view. And reduction of disc space between D2–D4 vertebrae. (**b**) MRI shows complete destruction of D3 vertebra with patient underwent surgery. Posterior decompression and fixation with reduction of subluxation was done. Patient improved clinically post operatively and attended complete bowel and bladder control and complete recovery in power by the end of 6 weeks. Paravertebral and epidural abscess with cord compression. (**c**) Patient underwent surgery. Posterior transpedicular decompression and fixation with reduction of subluxation. Patient improved clinically post operatively and attended complete bowel and bladder control and complete recovery in power by the end of 6 weeks. (**d**) Follow-up MRI of patient showing complete resolution of abscess and post-op status

Thoracic and Thoracolumbar Tuberculosis

Hodgson advocated anterior transthoracic surgery for spinal tuberculosis with debridement and fibular grafting as posterior decompression resulted in inadequate decompression and anterior debridement without graft placement resulted in kyphosis [60].

A combined approach with transthoracic/retroperitoneal decompression and reconstruction and posterior instrumented fusion can be used when there are more than two vertebral bodies involved [50, 61].

The all-posterior approach can be used to address the anterior pathology with a transpedicular/costotransversectomy with decompression of the abscess and removal of the involved disc and retropulsed fragments and diseased bone with anterior reconstruction with a strut graft or titanium mesh cage filled with autograft [2, 14, 46, 50, 51, 62]. Kyphosis correction should be achieved without having an anterior gap to prevent rigid instrumentation failure. Posterior pedicle screw fixation and fusion two levels above and below the lesion is usually adequate. Sublaminar wires may be used to supplement the fixation or as an alternative to pedicle screws as they allow some collapse. Intra-operative neurological monitoring with SSEP and MEP should be used during the surgery especially in neurologically intact patients and for late deformity corrections.

Figures 31.11, 31.12, and 31.13 are case examples of thoracic TB treated surgically.

Complications

Complications are more likely to occur in MDR-TB [48, 50]. In a cohort of 26 surgically treated children for spinal TB a higher complication rate was observed in MDR-TB patients with increased kyphosis, vertebral collapse, revision surgeries and wound dehiscence [50] (Box 31.10).

Box 31.10 Complications

- Wound complications—more often in MDR-TB
- Implant failure
- Neurological deterioration
- Systemic complications
- Miliary tuberculosis—immunocompromised children
- Late kyphosis
- Late neurological deficit
- Reactivation of disease

Worsening of kyphosis with age and growth and cord compression can result in severe kyphosis and late myelopathy in the cervicodorsal, thoracic, and thoracolumbar regions [39, 40]. It is important to monitor these children during their growth and intervene before the deformity becomes severe [39].

A posterior vertebral column resection osteotomy or pedicle subtraction osteotomy is used [63, 64]. Halo traction may be utilized for very severe kyphosis followed by staged surgery [64]. Rajasekeran et al. have described a classification for management of the spectrum of late presenting kyphotic deformity ranging from posterior fusion, posterior column osteotomies, pedicle subtraction osteotomies, three column osteotomies, and anterior palisade grafting in very severe kyphosis [2, 39, 63, 64]. Figure 31.10 is an example of thoracolumbar kyphosis developing on follow-up.

Figure 31.15 is an example of thoracic TB with kyphosis and myelopathy treated with vertebral column resection.

The aim should be early detection and treatment and avoid grotesque deformities, neurological deterioration, and the superadded risk of surgical complications with close monitoring and appropriately timed intervention (Box 31.11).

Box 31.11 Key Learning Points

- Socioeconomic disease which needs robust public health programs.
- Early diagnosis confirmed radiologically and on biopsy and culture.
- Medical management mainstay with appropriate chemotherapy.
- Rising drug resistance needs attention.
- Deformity progression to be monitored with growth during follow-up.
- Surgical treatment supportive and for limited indications.
- Avoid late kyphosis and neurological deficit.

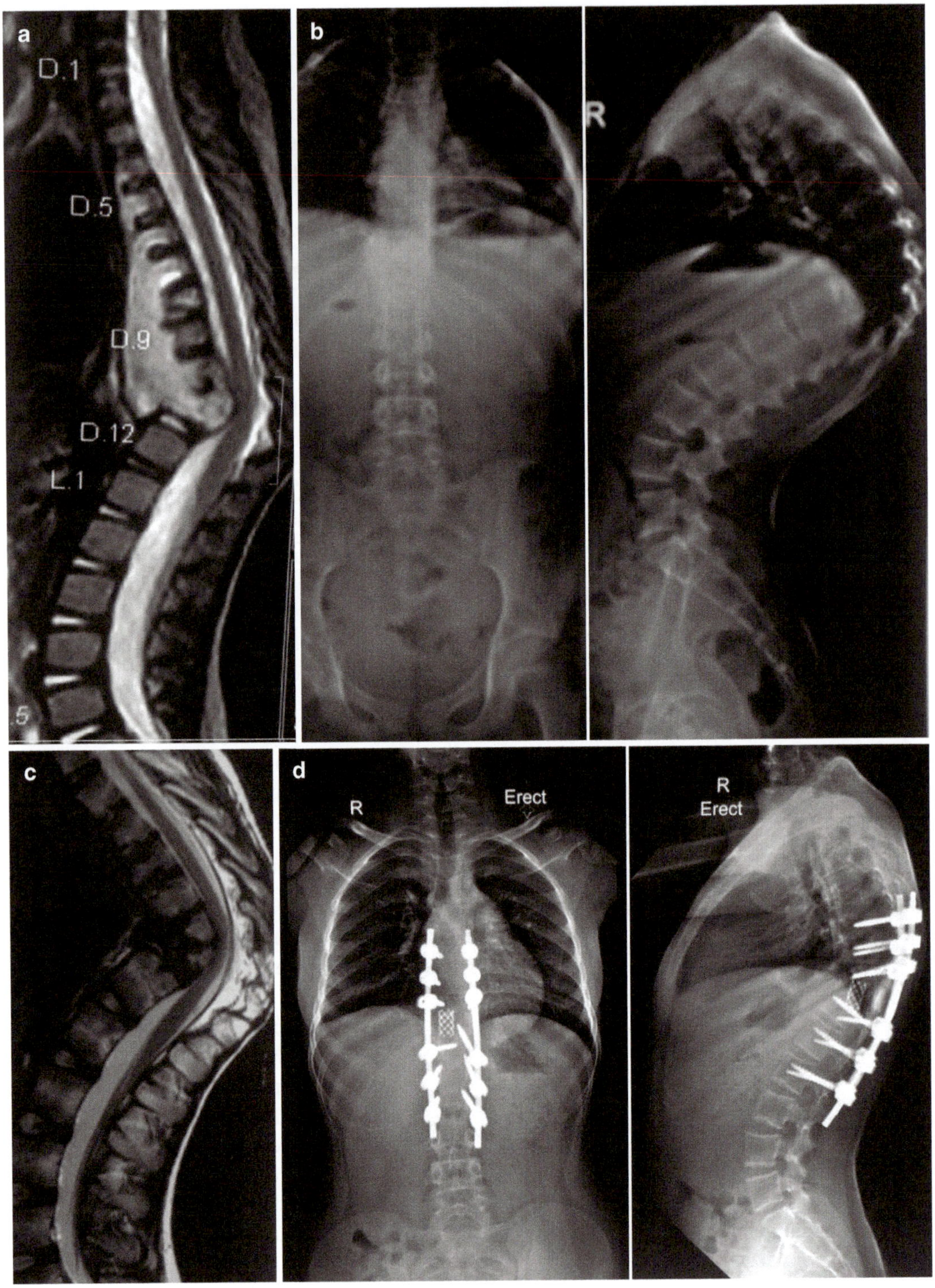

Fig. 31.15 (**a**) MRI at 2 years age showing multiple body involvement treated with first-line ATT. (**b**) Progression of kyphosis at 10 years age. (**c**) MRI at 10 years showing cord tenting with early myelopathy signs. (**d**) Vertebral column resection done and child improved and doing well. (**e**, **f**) Pre-op and post-op clinical picture

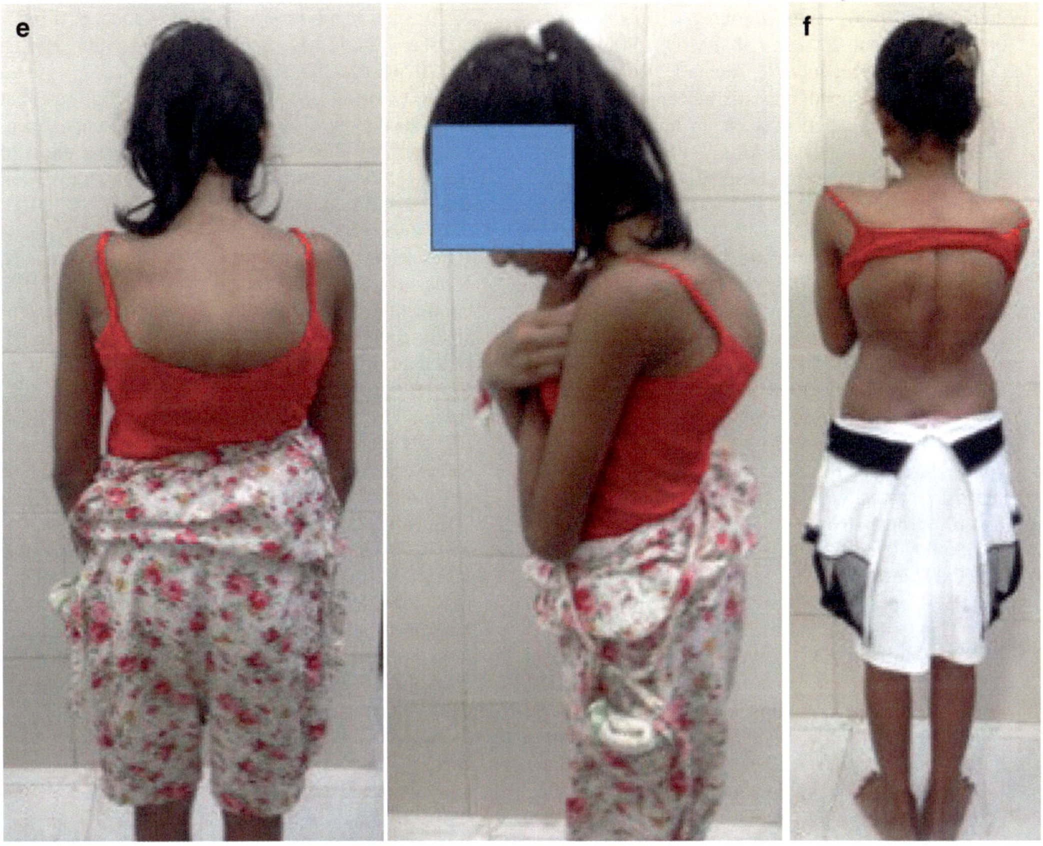

Fig. 31.15 (continued)

References

1. Dara M, Dadu A, Kremer K, Zaleskis R, Kluge HH. Epidemiology of tuberculosis in WHO European Region and public health response. Eur Spine J. 2013;22(Suppl 4):549–55. https://doi.org/10.1007/s00586-012-2339-3.
2. Jain AK, Rajasekaran S, Jaggi KR, Myneedu VP. Tuberculosis of the spine. J Bone Joint Surg. 2020;102(7):617–28. https://doi.org/10.2106/JBJS.19.00001.
3. Nahid P, Dorman SE, Alipanah N, et al. Official American Thoracic Society/Centers for Disease Control and Prevention/Infectious Diseases Society of America Clinical Practice Guidelines: treatment of drug-susceptible tuberculosis. Clin Infect Dis. 2016;63(7):e147–95. https://doi.org/10.1093/cid/ciw37.
4. Sanker P, Satheesan A, Ambika AP, Balakrishnan R, Moosan H, Mrithunjayan SK. Role of line probe assay in detection of extra-pulmonary tuberculosis/multidrug-resistant tuberculosis: the experience from Kerala state, India. J Acad Clin Microbiol. 2017;19:12–8.
5. Getahun H, Matteelli A, Chaisson RE, Raviglione M. Latent mycobacterium tuberculosis infection. N Engl J Med. 2015;372(22):2127–35.
6. Mann TN, Schaaf HS, Dunn RN, Dix-Peek S, du Preez K, Lamberts RP, du Toit J, Davis JH. Child and adult spinal tuberculosis at tertiary hospitals in the Western Cape, South Africa: 4-year burden and trend. Epidemiol Infect. 2018;146(16):2107–15. https://doi.org/10.1017/S0950268818002649. Epub 2018 Sep 28. PMID: 30264687; PMCID: PMC6453008.
7. Massyn N, Day C, Peer N, Padarath N, Barron P, English R. District health barometer 2013/14. Durban: Health Systems Trust; 2014.
8. Rendon A, Fuentes Z, Torres-Duque CA, del Granado M, Victoria J, Duarte R, Migliori GB. Roadmap for tuberculosis elimination in Latin American and Caribbean countries: a strategic alliance. Eur Respir J. 2016;48:1282–7. https://doi.org/10.1183/13993003.01549-2016.
9. Kumar R. Spinal tuberculosis: with reference to the children of northern India. Childs Nerv Syst.

2005;21(1):19–26. https://doi.org/10.1007/s00381-004-1029-9. Epub 2004 Sep 30. PMID: 15459785.
10. García-Lechuz JM, Julve R, Alcalá L, Ruiz-Serrano MJ, Muñoz P. Espondilodiscitis tuberculosa o enfermedad de Pott: experiencia en un hospital general [Tuberculous spondylodiskitis (Pott's disease): Experience in a general hospital]. Enferm Infecc Microbiol Clin. 2002;20(1):5–9. Spanish. PMID: 11820973.
11. Lolekha R, Anuwatnonthakate A, Nateniyom S, et al. Childhood TB epidemiology and treatment outcomes in Thailand: a TB active surveillance network, 2004 to 2006. BMC Infect Dis. 2008;8:94. Published 2008 Jul 18. https://doi.org/10.1186/1471-2334-8-94.
12. Gautam MP, Karki P, Rijal S, Singh R. Pott's spine and paraplegia. JNMA J Nepal Med Assoc. 2005;44(159):106–15. PMID: 16570378.
13. Polley P, Dunn R. Noncontiguous spinal tuberculosis: incidence and management. Eur Spine J. 2009;18(8):1096–101. https://doi.org/10.1007/s00586-009-0966-0. Epub 2009 Apr 9. PMID: 19357878; PMCID: PMC2899513.
14. Tuli SM. General principles of osteoarticular tuberculosis. Clin Orthop Relat Res. 2002;(398):11–9.
15. Ali A, Musbahi O, White VLC, Montgomery AS. Spinal tuberculosis: a literature review. JBJS Rev. 2019;7(1):e9. https://doi.org/10.2106/JBJS.RVW.18.00035. PMID: 30694877.
16. Balakrishnan S, Vijayan S, Nair S, Subramoniapillai J, Mrithyunjayan S. High diabetes prevalence among tuberculosis cases in Kerala, India. PLoS One. 2012;7(10):e46502.
17. Eisen S, Honywood L, Shingadia D, Novelli V. Spinal tuberculosis in children. Arch Dis Child. 2012;97(8):724–9. https://doi.org/10.1136/archdischild-2011-301571. Epub 2012 Jun 25. PMID: 22734017.
18. du Preez K, du Plessis L, O'Connell N, Hesseling AC. Burden, spectrum and outcomes of children with tuberculosis diagnosed at a district-level hospital in South Africa. Int J Tuberc Lung Dis. 2018;22(9):1037–43. https://doi.org/10.5588/ijtld.17.0893. PMID: 30092869.
19. Govender S, Ramnarain A, Danaviah S. Cervical spine tuberculosis in children. Clin Orthop Relat Res. 2007;460:78–85. https://doi.org/10.1097/BLO.0b013e31806a915f.
20. Kendall EA, Fofana MO, Dowdy DW. Burden of transmitted multidrug resistance in epidemics of tuberculosis: a transmission modelling analysis. Lancet Respir Med. 2015;3:963–72.
21. Goyal V, Kadam V, Narang P, Singh V. Prevalence of drug-resistant pulmonary tuberculosis in India: systematic review and meta-analysis. BMC Public Health. 2017;17(1):817. https://doi.org/10.1186/s12889-017-4779-5. PMID: 29041901; PMCID: PMC5645895.
22. Mohan K, Rawall S, Pawar UM, Sadani M, Nagad P, Nene A, Nene A. Drug resistance patterns in 111 cases of drug-resistant tuberculosis spine. Eur Spine J. 2013;22(Suppl 4):647–52. https://doi.org/10.1007/s00586-012-2154-x. Epub 2012 Jan 20. PMID: 22270244; PMCID: PMC3691404.
23. Desai U, Joshi JM. Extrapulmonary drug-resistant tuberculosis at a drug-resistant tuberculosis center, Mumbai: our experience – hope in the midst of despair! Lung India. 2019;36(1):3–7. https://doi.org/10.4103/lungindia.lungindia_192_18. PMID: 30604698; PMCID: PMC6330803.
24. Rajasekaran S, Chandrasekar C, Mahilmaran A, Kanakaraj K, Karthikeyan DS, Suriakumar J. HIV coinfection among multidrug resistant and extensively drug resistant tuberculosis patients--a trend. J Indian Med Assoc. 2009;107(5):281–2, 284–6. PMID: 19886382.
25. Rakesh PS, Balakrishnan S, Jayasankar S, Asokan RV. TB management by private practitioners - is it bad everywhere? Indian J Tuberc. 2016;63(4):251–4. https://doi.org/10.1016/j.ijTB.2016.09.009. Epub 2016 Nov 22. PMID: 27998498.
26. Yadav A, Garg SK, Chopra H, Bajpai SK, Bano T, Jain S, Kumar A. Treatment practices in pulmonary tuberculosis by private sector physicians of Meerut, Uttar Pradesh. Indian J Chest Dis Allied Sci. 2012;54(3):161–3. PMID: 23008922.
27. Udwadia ZF, Pinto LM, Uplekar MW. Tuberculosis management by private practitioners in Mumbai, India: has anything changed in two decades? PLoS One. 2010;5(8):e12023. https://doi.org/10.1371/journal.pone.0012023. PMID: 20711502; PMCID: PMC2918510.
28. Babu GR, Laxminarayan R. The unsurprising story of MDR-TB resistance in India. Tuberculosis (Edinb). 2012;92(4):301–6. https://doi.org/10.1016/j.tube.2012.02.009. Epub 2012 Apr 14. PMID: 22504008.
29. Sayi EN, Mlay SM. Tuberculosis of the spine in children at Muhimbili Medical Centre, Dar es Salaam. East Afr Med J. 1995;72(1):46–8. PMID: 7781556.
30. El Azbaoui S, Alaoui Mrani N, Sabri A, Jouhadi Z, Ailal F, Bousfiha AA, Najib J, El Hafidi N, Deswarte C, Schurr E, Bustamante J, Boisson-Dupuis S, Casanova JL, Abel L, El Baghdadi J. Pott's disease in Moroccan children: clinical features and investigation of the interleukin-12/interferon-γ pathway. Int J Tuberc Lung Dis. 2015;19(12):1455–62. https://doi.org/10.5588/ijtld.15.0290. PMID: 26614186; PMCID: PMC4959462.
31. Park JW, Kim YS, Yoon JO, Kim JS, Chang JS, Kim JM, Chun JM, Jeon IH. Non-tuberculous mycobacterial infection of the musculoskeletal system: pattern of infection and efficacy of combined surgical/antimicrobial treatment. Bone Joint J. 2014;96-B(11):1561–5. https://doi.org/10.1302/0301-620X.96B11.33427. PMID: 25371475.
32. Pande KC, Babhulkar SS. Atypical spinal tuberculosis. Clin Orthop Relat Res. 2002;398:67–74.
33. Almeida A. Tuberculosis of the spine and spinal cord. Eur J Radiol. 2005;55:193–201. https://doi.org/10.1016/j.ejrad.2005.04.018.

34. De Tavera MP, De Leon EP. Tuberculosis of the lymphatics in children; its relation to spinal tuberculosis: a clinico-radiological study. Dis Chest. 1967;52(4):469–77. ISSN 0096-0217. https://doi.org/10.1378/chest.52.4.469.
35. Moorthy S, Prabhu NK. Spectrum of MR imaging findings in spinal tuberculosis. Am J Roentgenol. 2002;179:979–83. https://doi.org/10.2214/ajr.179.4.1790979. https://www.ajronline.org/doi/abs/10.2214/ajr.179.4.1790979.
36. Pandit HG, Sonsale PD, Shikare SS, Bhojraj SY. Bone scintigraphy in tuberculous spondylodiscitis. Eur Spine J. 1999;8:205–9.
37. Rahimizadeh A, Williamson W, Rahimizadeh S, Amirzadeh M. Painful torticollis due to tubercular atlantoaxial rotatory fixation: a case report. Surg Neurol Int. 2020;11:440. https://doi.org/10.25259/SNI_663_2020.
38. Kanna RM, Shetty AP, Rajasekaran S. Spinal tuberculosis: pathogenesis, clinical features and investigations. In: Vialle RL, editor. AOSpine Master series, Spinal infections, vol. 10. New York: Thieme; 2018.
39. Rajasekaran S. Natural history of Pott's kyphosis. Eur Spine J. 2013;22(Suppl 4):634–40. https://doi.org/10.1007/s00586-012-2336-6. Epub 2012 May 15. PMID: 22584918; PMCID: PMC3691402.
40. Moon MS, Kim SJ, Kim MS, Kim DS. Most reliable time in predicting residual kyphosis and stability: pediatric spinal tuberculosis. Asian Spine J. 2018;12(6):1069–77. https://doi.org/10.31616/asj.2018.12.6.1069.
41. Jain AK, Kumar J. Tuberculosis of spine: neurological deficit. Eur Spine J. 2013;22(Suppl 4):624–33. https://doi.org/10.1007/s00586-012-2335-7. Epub 2012 May 8. PMID: 22565802; PMCID: PMC3691413.
42. Vaishnav B, Suthar N, Shaikh S, Tambile R. Clinical study of spinal tuberculosis presenting with neuro-deficits in Western India. Indian J Tuberc. 2019;66(1):81–6. https://doi.org/10.1016/j.ijTB.2018.04.009. Epub 2018 Apr 13. PMID: 30797289.
43. Sai Kiran NA, Vaishya S, Kale SS, Sharma BS, Mahapatra AK. Surgical results in patients with tuberculosis of the spine and severe lower-extremity motor deficits: a retrospective study of 48 patients. J Neurosurg Spine. 2007;6(4):320–6. https://doi.org/10.3171/spi.2007.6.4.6. PMID: 17436920.
44. Ha KY, Kim YH. Late onset of progressive neurological deficits in severe angular kyphosis related to tuberculosis spondylitis. Eur Spine J. 2016;25(4):1039–46. https://doi.org/10.1007/s00586-015-3997-8. Epub 2015 May 19. PMID: 25987452.
45. Kotil K, Alan MS, Bilge T. Medical management of Pott disease in the thoracic and lumbar spine: a prospective clinical study. J Neurosurg Spine. 2007;6(3):222–8. https://doi.org/10.3171/spi.2007.6.3.222. PMID: 17355021.
46. Khanna K, Sabharwal S. Spinal tuberculosis: a comprehensive review for the modern spine surgeon. Spine J. 2019;19(11):1858–70. https://doi.org/10.1016/j.spinee.2019.05.002. Epub 2019 May 15. PMID: 31102727.
47. Nene A, Bhojraj S. Results of nonsurgical treatment of thoracic spinal tuberculosis in adults. Spine J. 2005;5(1):79–84. https://doi.org/10.1016/j.spinee.2004.05.255. PMID: 15653088.
48. Seddon JA, Donald PR, Vlok GJ, Schaaf HS. Multidrug-resistant tuberculosis of the spine in children: characteristics from a high burden setting. J Trop Pediatr. 2012;58:341–7.
49. Jain AK, Dhammi IK, Modi P, Kumar J, Sreenivasan R, Saini NS. Tuberculosis spine: therapeutically refractory disease. Indian J Orthop. 2012;46:171–8.
50. Pinto D, Dhawale A, Shah I, Rokade S, Shah A, Chaudhary K, Aroojis A, Mehta R, Nene A. Tuberculosis of the spine in children - does drug resistance affect surgical outcomes? Spine J. 2021;21(12):1973–84, S1529-9430(21)00722-1. https://doi.org/10.1016/j.spinee.2021.06.001.
51. Chaudhary K, Dhawale A, Chaddha R, Laheri V. Spinal tuberculosis – an update. J Clin Orthopaed. 2017;2(1):31–42.
52. Jain AK, Sreenivasan R, Saini NS, Kumar S, Jain S, Dhammi IK. Magnetic resonance evaluation of tubercular lesion in spine. Int Orthop. 2012;36(2):261–9.
53. Luk KD. Tuberculosis of the spine in the new millennium. Eur Spine J. 1999;8(5):338–45.
54. Lan X, Xu JZ, Liu XM, Ge BF. Drug susceptibility testing guided treatment for drug-resistant spinal tuberculosis: a retrospective analysis of 19 patients. Int Surg. 2013;98:175–80. https://doi.org/10.9738/INTSURG-D-12-00004.1.
55. Arockiaraj J, Robert M, Rose W, Amritanand R, David KS, Krishnan V. Early detection and analysis of children with multidrug-resistant tuberculosis of the spine. Asian Spine J. 2019;13:77–85. https://doi.org/10.31616/ASJ.2017.0217.
56. Ramachandran G, Swaminathan S. Safety and tolerability profile of second-line anti-tuberculosis medications. Drug Saf. 2015;38:253–69. https://doi.org/10.1007/s40264-015-0267-y.
57. Mehrotra A, Das KK, Nair AP, Kumar R, Srivastava AK, Sahu RN, Kumar R. Pediatric cranio-vertebral junction tuberculosis: management and outcome. Childs Nerv Syst. 2013;29(5):809–14.
58. Mihir B, Vinod L, Umesh M, Chaudhary K. Anterior instrumentation of the cervicothoracic vertebrae: approach based on clinical and radiologic criteria. Spine (Phila Pa 1976). 2006;31(9):E244–9. https://doi.org/10.1097/01.brs.0000214883.11874.80.
59. Zhang HQ, Wang YX, Guo CF, Zhao D, Deng A, Wu JH, Liu JY. One-stage posterior focus debridement, fusion, and instrumentation in the surgical treatment of cervicothoracic spinal tuberculosis with kyphosis in children: a preliminary report. Childs Nerv Syst. 2011;27(5):735–42. https://doi.org/10.1007/s00381-010-1319-3.

60. Bailey HL, Gabriel SMG, Hodgson AR, Shin JS. Tuberculosis of the spine in children. J Bone Joint Surg Am. 1972;54:1633–57.
61. Sundararaj GD, Behera S, Ravi V, Venkatesh K, Cherian VM, Lee V. Role of posterior stabilisation in the management of tuberculosis of the dorsal and lumbar spine. J Bone Joint Surg Br. 2003;85(1):100–6. https://doi.org/10.1302/0301-620x.85b1.13300.
62. Dalal S, Modi J, Soman S, Patel H, Dhanani S. Results of single-staged posterior decompression and circumferential fusion using a Transpedicular approach to correct a kyphotic deformity due to thoracolumbar spinal tuberculosis. Asian Spine J. 2016;10(6):1106–14. https://doi.org/10.4184/asj.2016.10.6.1106.
63. Bakaloudis G, Lolli F, Di Silvestre M, Greggi T, Astolfi S, Martikos K, Vommaro F, Barbanti-Brodano G, Cioni A, Giacomini S. Thoracic pedicle subtraction osteotomy in the treatment of severe pediatric deformities. Eur Spine J. 2011;20(Suppl 1):S95–104. https://doi.org/10.1007/s00586-011-1749-y. Epub 2011 Apr 6.
64. Rajasekaran S, Rajoli SR, Aiyer SN, Kanna R, Shetty AP. A classification for kyphosis based on column deficiency, curve magnitude, and osteotomy requirement. J Bone Joint Surg Am. 2018;100(13):1147–56. https://doi.org/10.2106/JBJS.17.01127.

Tuberculosis of the Appendicular Skeleton

32

Chang Ho Shin and Won Joon Yoo

Introduction and Epidemiology

Tuberculosis (TB) is a chronic granulomatous infection caused by *Mycobacterium tuberculosis*. Evidence of TB in humans' dates back to 3400 BC, as Egyptian mummies have been shown to have signs of the disease in their spines. In 1882, Robert Koch first demonstrated the causal agent of TB by applying a new staining method to a sputum sample obtained from a patient with TB.

TB remains a major cause of skeletal infections in many developing countries. According to a global TB report, an estimated 10.0 million (range, 8.9–11.0 million) people contracted TB worldwide in 2019 and 10% of them were children [1]. There has been a resurgence in the incidence of TB in developed countries, with increasing numbers of patients with acquired immunodeficiency syndrome and multidrug-resistant TB, intravenous drug abusers, immigrant populations, and other socioeconomic factors (e.g., changing elderly population demographics) [2]. Young children, particularly those younger than 3 years, have a high incidence of progression from latent TB infection to TB disease (up to 40%) [3].

TB can involve almost any organ. Extrapulmonary TB is estimated to account for 8–24% of all TB infections, occurring more commonly in children than in adults [1, 4]. The most common extrapulmonary TB is TB lymphadenitis (35%) [5, 6]. Approximately 1–3% of TB cases may have an osteoarticular involvement, which represents approximately 10–20% of extrapulmonary TB forms [7, 8]. The most common skeletal manifestation is spondylodiscitis (50%). The other 50% of cases are extraspinal manifestations, of which peripheral arthritis accounts for 60%; osteomyelitis, for 38%; and tenosynovitis and bursitis, for 2% (Table 32.1) [7–9]. Osteoarticular TB is usually a monoarticular or monostotic disease, with frequent involvement of the hips and knees [4]. The bones of the hands are involved approximately eight times more frequently than bones of the feet. The proximal phalanges of the index and middle fingers are the most often affected bones in the TB of the hand in children [10]. The calcaneus is the most common bone involved in the TB of the foot [11]. A multifocal disease occurs in only approximately 5–10% of patients with TB [4, 7, 12].

C. H. Shin · W. J. Yoo (✉)
Division of Pediatric Orthopaedics, Seoul National University Children's Hospital, Seoul, Republic of Korea

Department of Orthopaedic Surgery, Seoul National University College of Medicine, Seoul, Republic of Korea
e-mail: yoowj@snu.ac.kr

© Springer Nature Switzerland AG 2022
M. V. Belthur et al. (eds.), *Pediatric Musculoskeletal Infections*,
https://doi.org/10.1007/978-3-030-95794-0_32

Table 32.1 Different types of TB of the appendicular skeleton

Type of TB of the appendicular skeleton	Frequency	Treatment[a]	Outcome
TB arthritis	60%	Open biopsy	Early stage: good or excellent Advanced stage: fair or poor
TB osteomyelitis (cystic, infiltrative, erosive, spina ventosa forms)	38%	Curettage without bone grafting	Generally good or excellent
TB tenosynovitis and bursitis	2%	Tenosynovectomy, bursectomy	Unknown in pediatric patients

[a]Multiple antitubercular chemotherapy should be combined.

Pathology and Microbiology

Mycobacterium is an aerobic, nonmotile, facultative, slender, curved intracellular rod (bacillus), measuring 0.2–0.5 μm by 2–4 μm in size (Fig. 32.1). The mycobacterial cell wall consists of mycolic acids, complex waxes, and specific glycolipids. The cell wall structure enables mycobacteria to resist to dehydration, acids, and alkalis, enabling differential staining methods (e.g., Ziehl–Neelsen staining) in contaminated clinical specimens [13]. In Ziehl–Neelsen staining, carbol fuchsin initially stains every cell. Following de-staining with acid-alcohol, only non-acid-fast bacteria are decolorized, and *Mycobacterium* resists decolorization owing to its cell wall structure. When a counter stain is applied, non-acid-fast bacteria are stained with methylene blue or malachite green. Eventually, *Mycobacterium*, which is an acid-fast bacterium retaining carbol fuchsin, appears in deep pink-red when viewed under a microscope (Fig. 32.2).

Nowadays, most TB infections are initiated by the respiratory route of exposure. Several factors determine the probability of TB transmission, including infectiousness of the source patient, host susceptibility of the contact, infectiousness of the TB strain, environment in which the exposure occurs, and duration of the exposure of the contact to the source patient [14]. First, after inhalation, *M. tuberculosis* contained in inhaled aerosols is carried down the bronchial tree and implants in a respiratory bronchiole or alveolus. Whether inhaled *M. tuberculosis* can establish an infection or not depends on both host-related and microbial factors. Implanted tubercle bacteria are

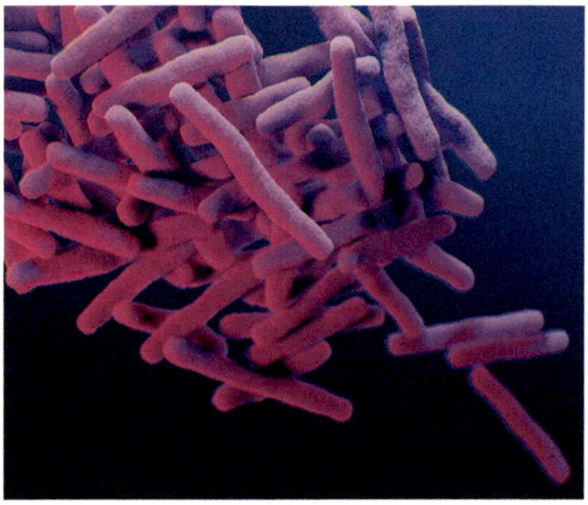

Fig. 32.1 An illustration of drug-resistant *Mycobacterium tuberculosis* bacteria presented in the Centers for Disease Control and Prevention publication entitled *Antibiotic Resistance Threats in the United States, 2019*. (Figure from Public Health Image Library, Centers for Disease Control and Prevention. https://phil.cdc.gov/Details.aspx?pid=23254)

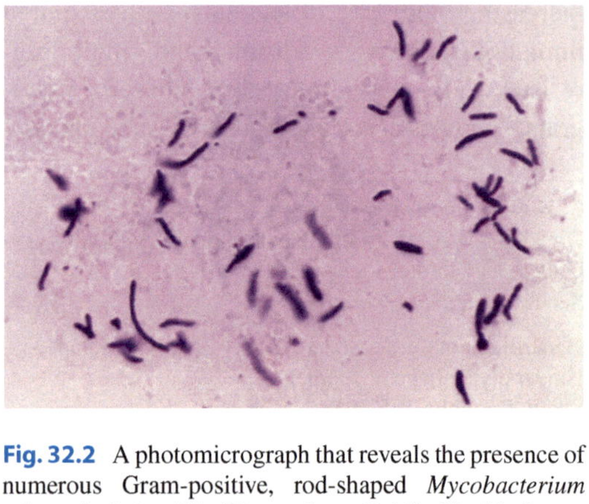

Fig. 32.2 A photomicrograph that reveals the presence of numerous Gram-positive, rod-shaped *Mycobacterium tuberculosis* bacilli. (Figure from Public Health Image Library, Centers for Disease Control and Prevention. https://phil.cdc.gov/Details.aspx?pid=21462)

disseminated by the lymphatic circulation to the regional lymph nodes of the lung. Subsequently, tubercle bacteria are distributed via a hematogenous route to many organs, including other parts of the lung [15].

In the early events of the infectious process, when *M. tuberculosis* enters the alveolus, it first contacts resident macrophages and alveolar epithelial type II pneumocytes. The bacteria are phagocytosed in a process initiated by the bacterial contact with macrophage mannose and/or complement receptors. In later events of the infectious process, infected macrophages recruit inactivated monocytes, neutrophils, and lymphocytes, none of which efficiently kills *M. tuberculosis*. Then, granulomatous lesions consisting of macrophage-derived giant cells (Langhans giant cells) and lymphocytes begin to form. This process effectively hinders the spread of *M. tuberculosis* in general. As cellular immunity develops, macrophages loaded with *M. tuberculosis* are killed, resulting in the formation of the caseous center of the granuloma, surrounded by a cellular zone of lymphocytes, blood-derived monocytes, and fibroblasts. In individuals with competent cell-mediated immunity, the granulomas subsequently heal, leaving small fibrous and calcified lesions. However, in case of compromised immune systems, the granuloma center can become liquefied and serves as a medium in which the revived *M. tuberculosis* cells can replicate. At this time, viable *M. tuberculosis* can escape from the granuloma and spread within the lung (active pulmonary TB) and to other organs via the blood and lymphatic route (extrapulmonary or miliary TB) [15].

TB osteomyelitis usually starts in the metaphysis but can also begin in the epiphysis [16]. Growth plates and joints have little resistance to the spread of *M. tuberculosis*. TB arthritis can result from transphyseal spread from the adjacent metaphyseal TB into the joint or from hematogenous dissemination. Synovial hypertrophy causes peripheral and central erosions by pressure necrosis [17]. Subsequently, subchondral bone and articular cartilage destruction and joint space narrowing occur as relatively late complications. Reactive hyperemia leads to demineralization and local bone destruction.

Some studies have suggested the important role of vitamin D during the immune system regulation in TB [18–20]. In a prospective Indian study, patients with osteoarticular TB had significantly lower vitamin D levels than healthy individuals, irrespective of sex or age differences [19]. Vitamin D promotes intracellular killing of *M. tuberculosis* by enhancing the fusion of phagosomes and lysosomes in infected macrophages. It leads to the expression of cathelicidin, an enzyme involved in the first line of macrophage-initiated defense in the prevention of infections, including TB. Vitamin D also increases the activity of natural killer cells and regulatory T cells and suppresses the effector T-cell activation.

Moreover, studies have demonstrated an association between genetic polymorphisms and susceptibility to pediatric TB [21–23]. Malik et al. reported that allelic variants of the natural resistance-associated macrophage protein gene 1 (NRAMP1) are significantly associated with pediatric TB [22]. A Chinese study revealed that a functional promoter polymorphism of IFITM3 influences the risk of pediatric TB in the Han Chinese population [23].

Clinical Presentation and Examination

Although most TB infections are initiated through the respiratory exposure, Hosalkar et al. reported that only 22% of patients had a possible history of contact with a likely case of chronic cough/possible lung infection during the onset-preceding months [24]. According to a systematic review of tuberculous dactylitis in children and adolescents, concurrent pulmonary TB is present in approximately 20% of patients [25].

Usually, children with osteoarticular TB show insidious onset and vague symptoms [26–28]. An abscess developed by TB is referred to as “cold abscess,” as it involves relatively low inflammation and develops slowly and becomes painful only when there is pressure on the surrounding area. The most common symptoms of osteoarticular TB are pain and swelling [24, 28].

However, there may be no complaints of pain in some children. Local warmth and redness are usually absent. Fever is also not definite, although some children have low-grade fever, mainly in late afternoons or evenings. Some children show night sweating and "night cries." The latter is thought to be due to the decrease in voluntary muscle tone when the child goes to sleep, permitting the painful joint to be moved more than when the child is awake with joint stiffness caused by muscle spasms [29]. TB of the lower limbs can cause antalgic gait [30]. Some patients can experience the enlargement of draining lymph nodes and matted lymph nodes may be noted on examination [26]. As the disease develops, swelling and limitation of motion may be observed. Muscle atrophy, draining sinus, and systemic symptoms such as loss of appetite, fatigue, anemia, and weight loss are symptoms of advanced disease. The draining sinus may heal with a puckered scar [31].

Patients with TB arthritis may have swelling, redness, pain, and tenderness of the involved joints, which are caused by synovitis. In patients with infection of the superficial joint such as the knee or elbow, joint swelling caused by synovial hypertrophy and effusion is easily recognized. TB of the shoulder can be of two forms, a dry form (caries sicca) and an abscess form (caries exudata). The dry form manifests as marked wasting and painful movement limitation, whereas the abscess form manifests as cold abscesses and swelling and is more common in children [27].

Multifocal osteoarticular TB is observed mostly in immunocompromised patients, but it may occur in immunocompetent patients with normal pulmonary findings as well [12, 31]. Pain and swelling around the lesions are the main symptoms, and fever, weight loss, or night sweats are not common, even in these patients.

TB tenosynovitis and bursitis are extremely rare in children. TB tenosynovitis is more common in hand and wrist than foot and ankle and in flexor apparatus than extensor apparatus [32]. Its clinical presentation is painful swelling, slow-growing mass, and limitation-of-motion [33, 34]. Tendon rupture and carpal tunnel syndrome can occur as complications [32, 34]. During operation, rice bodies are sometimes found although they are not pathognomonic sign of TB [32]. TB of trochanteric bursa is the most common form of TB bursitis [35–38]. It can cause swelling with or without pain. There would be no heat or redness. As the disease progresses, destruction of greater trochanter may advance from the outermost part to the central region [37].

Box 32.1 Diagnosis of Osteoarticular TB

- The key to the diagnosis is a high index of suspicion.
- The most common symptoms are pain and swelling.
- Systemic symptoms can be absent even in multifocal osteoarticular TB.
- Interferon-gamma release assays and nucleic acid amplification test have become more widely adopted in recent years.

Investigations/Workup

The diagnosis of TB in children is a challenge because early manifestations are subtle, and advanced disease can be confused with other pathologies such as tumors and trauma. The key to the diagnosis of osteoarticular TB is a high index of suspicion, even in children without associated medical conditions that cause immunosuppression. Also, a detailed family history to identify adult contacts with active TB is helpful.

General tests for inflammation markers are neither specific nor reliable. Leukocyte count, erythrocyte sedimentation rate (ESR), and C-reactive protein (CRP) levels in the peripheral blood can be normal in some patients [16, 28] but can be elevated in others [7, 16, 24, 27, 39]. According to previous studies, in those with elevated ESR, the ESR was 27–74 mm/h [7, 24, 27, 39]. Leukocyte and polymorphonuclear cell counts from the joint fluid in patients with TB arthritis range from 40 to 136,000/mm^3 and from 10% to 99%, respectively [40, 41]. Predominance of lymphocytes in the joint fluid is found in some patients [40], but not in others [41].

The tuberculin skin test (TST) has been used to detect latent TB infections [14]. TST detects cell-mediated immunity to *M. tuberculosis* through a delayed-type hypersensitivity reaction using a protein precipitate of the heat-inactivated tubercle bacilli. TST is inexpensive, simple to perform, and does not require special laboratory equipment. However, it is prone to show false-positive results due to the cross-reactivity of the antigens within the purified protein derivative tuberculin to both Bacillus Calmette-Guérin (BCG) vaccine and nontuberculous mycobacteria. It also shows false-negative results in patients with malnutrition and congenital or acquired immunodeficiency.

Interferon-gamma release assays (IGRA) are T cell-based assays that measure interferon gamma release by sensitized T cells in response to highly specific *M. tuberculosis* antigens. IGRA is more specific for *M. tuberculosis* detection than TST, particularly in the setting of BCG immunization.

Nowadays, nucleic acid amplification tests such as the Xpert MTB/RIF assay are used for rapid diagnosis of TB and detection of rifampicin resistance [8, 42, 43]. The Xpert MTB/RIF assay detects not only the TB bacillus DNA but also the presence of mutations responsible for resistance to rifampicin. In the meta-analyses on the efficiency of the Xpert MTB/RIF assay, the sensitivity ranged from 60% to 97% and the specificity ranged from 82% to 100% in the bone or joint tissue [42, 44–46].

Biopsy can be used for TB diagnosis. If a biopsy specimen is taken from a joint, tissues from adjacent cystic lesions and synovial tissue should also be collected [4]. Epithelioid cell granulomas accompanied by Langhans multinucleated giant cells and enclosing caseating necrosis are a typical pathological feature of TB (Fig. 32.3). In a previous study using bone tissue, eight of nine *M. tuberculosis* culture-positive patients showed one or both chronic granulomatous inflammation or caseating necrosis [47]. However, the specificity of mycobacterial microscopy tends to be low because necrotizing and non-necrotizing granulomas are found in other infectious and noninfectious diseases [14].

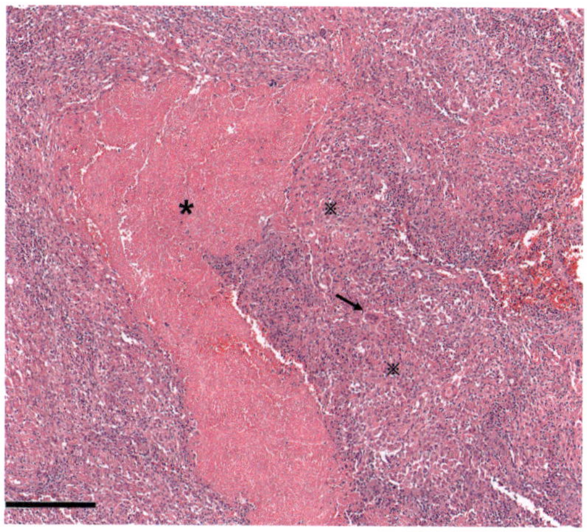

Fig. 32.3 Histopathology of tuberculosis. Epithelioid cell granulomas (reference mark) accompanied by Langhans multinucleated giant cells (arrow) and enclosing caseating necrosis (asterisk) are a typical pathological feature of tuberculosis. Bar = 300 μm

Traditional Ziehl–Neelsen staining for acid-fast bacteria is a rapid and inexpensive method. However, because of the paucibacillary nature of osteoarticular TB, it may produce false-negative results, especially in children [48, 49]. Multiple sample aspirations and the use of fluorescence microscopy techniques with fluorochrome dyes such as auramine-O staining may possess higher sensitivity and specificity [49].

Culture examination is the gold standard of mycobacteriological diagnosis. Mycobacteria isolation is important not only for definitive diagnosis but also for determining the phenotypic drug susceptibility. However, the method has low sensitivity (64–73%) due to the paucibacillary characteristics of pediatric TB [7, 43, 48], and it requires prolonged incubation at a temperature of 35–37 °C for up to 6–8 weeks before the sample can be considered negative [8]. In patients with positive cultures, it is necessary to identify the species or at least differentiate non-tubercular mycobacteria from those belonging to the *M. tuberculosis* complex because both are able to grow in the most frequently used media.

There are no specific radiographic features that are pathognomonic of TB arthritis or osteomyelitis. In the early stage of TB arthritis, the joint space is preserved due to the lack of proteolytic enzymes in *M. tuberculosis*. With disease progression, a gradual decrease in the joint space is observed. The Phemister's triad of juxta-articular osteoporosis, marginal bony erosions, and gradual narrowing of the joint space suggest TB arthritis (Figs. 32.4 and 32.5). Soft tissue swelling can also be observed. Reactive hyperemia may lead to epiphyseal overgrowth. In the hip joint, subluxation or dislocation of the femoral head may be observed. In TB of the elbow, an "ice cream scoop" appearance of the proximal ulnar metaphysis may be seen on radiographs [28]. MRI can detect synovial thickening, pannus, joint effusion, articular erosions, subchondral bone destruction, and marrow changes [9, 50]. These changes are typically low on T1- and high on T2-weighted images. Gradient-echo sequences are useful for evaluating cartilage destruction. After Gd-DTPA administration, acute synovitis often results in marked enhancement, whereas chronic synovitis may show no enhancement at all [9].

TB osteomyelitis can be situated at the metaphysis or epiphysis or both by abscess spreading through the growth plate from its original location (Fig. 32.6). Four different types of TB osteomyelitis have been described—cystic, infiltrative, local erosive and spina ventosa. The cystic form is the most common on radiographs, visible as round-to-ovoid radiolucent lesions with slight marginal sclerosis in some patients. The cavity of the cyst may contain a sequestrum. Expansion of the bones and honeycombing are sometimes present. In infiltrative forms, diffuse areas of bone destruction with permeation may sometimes be observed [2]. Compared with pyogenic osteomyelitis, TB osteomyelitis has less periosteal reaction and sequestrum [3, 17]. In

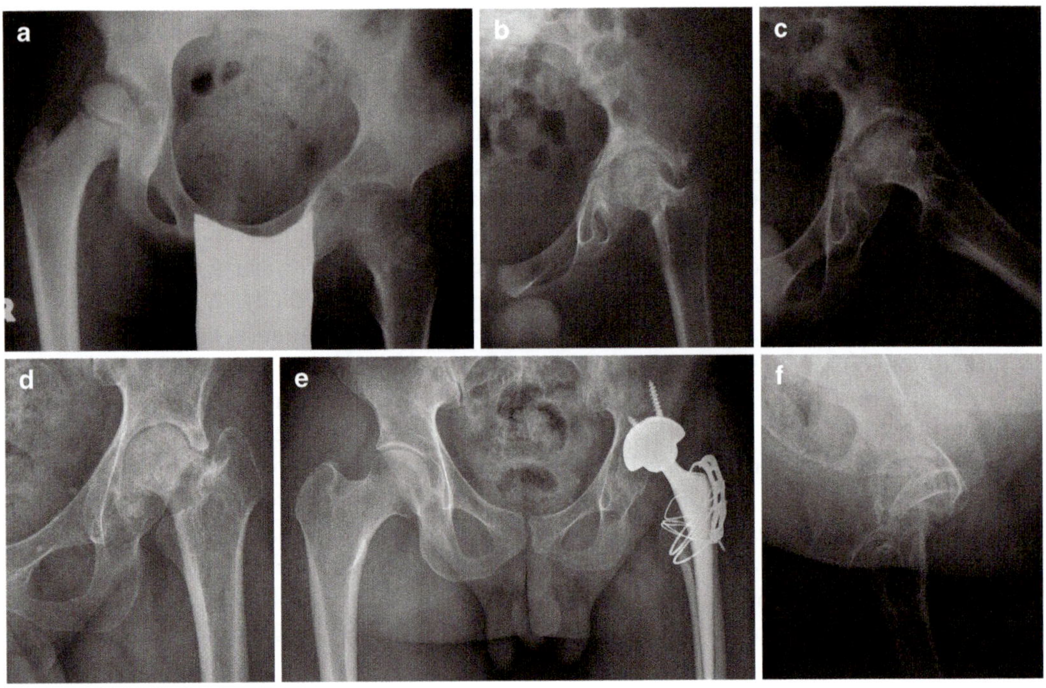

Fig. 32.4 Tuberculosis of the left hip. (**a**) Pelvic radiography showing an example of the relatively advanced stage of tuberculosis of the left hip in an 8-year-old boy. Juxta-articular osteoporosis and marginal bony erosions are seen both in the proximal femur and pelvis. Atrophy of the femoral head, small volume acetabular cavity, and acetabular overcoverage, which results in pincer-type femoroacetabular impingement, are observed in (**b**) the anteroposterior and (**c**) frog-leg lateral hip radiographs recorded at 14 years. Shanmugasundaram named this type of deformity as "mortar and pestle" (Shanmugasundaram [70]). (**d**, **e**) Owing to pain and limited motion of the left hip, (**f**) total hip replacement arthroplasty was performed at the age of 28 years

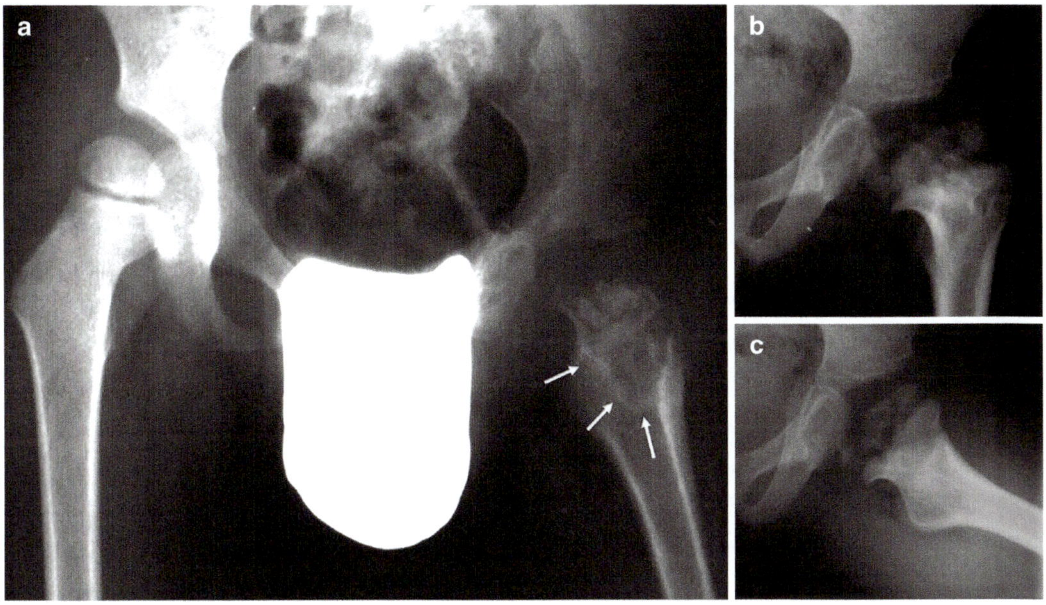

Fig. 32.5 Tuberculosis of the left hip. (**a**) Hip radiography of a 3.5-year-old boy showing destructed femoral neck, juxta-articular osteoporosis, and marginal sclerosis at the proximal femoral metaphysis (arrows) on the left side. Left proximal femoral epiphysis is not visible. Legg–Calvé–Perthes disease-like changes such as fragmented capital femoral epiphysis, coxa magna, and coxa breva are seen on (**b**) the anteroposterior and (**c**) frog-leg lateral hip radiographs at the age of 5.2 years

local erosive form, a small, localized area of osteolysis, usually positioned eccentrically, may be observed with or without destruction of cortex [2]. Spina ventosa (a spine-like projection puffed with air) is a term used to describe the ballooned-out appearance of the bone with an internal cyst-like cavity in TB dactylitis.

Primary diaphyseal TB of the long bone is very rare. It probably results from a tuberculous embolus that remains lodged in the nutrient vessel and thus fails to spread to the metaphysis [51]. Radiographs may mimic Brodie's abscess, pyogenic or fungal osteomyelitis, tumors, or granulomatous lesions [52, 53].

MRI is the imaging modality of choice for early TB detection. In general, infected areas can be seen as low signals on T1- and high signals on T2-weighted images. Some patients show heterogeneous signal intensity on T2 images. The degree of hyperintensity on T2-weighted images may provide hints concerning caseating necrosis. After Gd-DTPA administration, marked peripheral rim-like enhancement is then observed. In young children with largely unossified epiphyses and suspected of having epiphyseal osteomyelitis, MRI should be performed because cartilage destruction may not be evident on plain radiographs (Fig. 32.7) [16, 54].

Technetium bone scans can be obtained to exclude multifocal osseous lesions.

Box 32.2 Radiographic Findings of Osteoarticular TB

- Radiographic findings become evident as the disease progresses.
- Phemister's triad of juxta-articular osteoporosis, marginal bony erosions, and gradual narrowing of joint space suggest TB arthritis.
- The cystic form, seen as round-to-ovoid radiolucent lesion, is the most common form in TB osteomyelitis.
- TB osteomyelitis has less periosteal reaction and sequestrum, compared to pyogenic osteomyelitis.

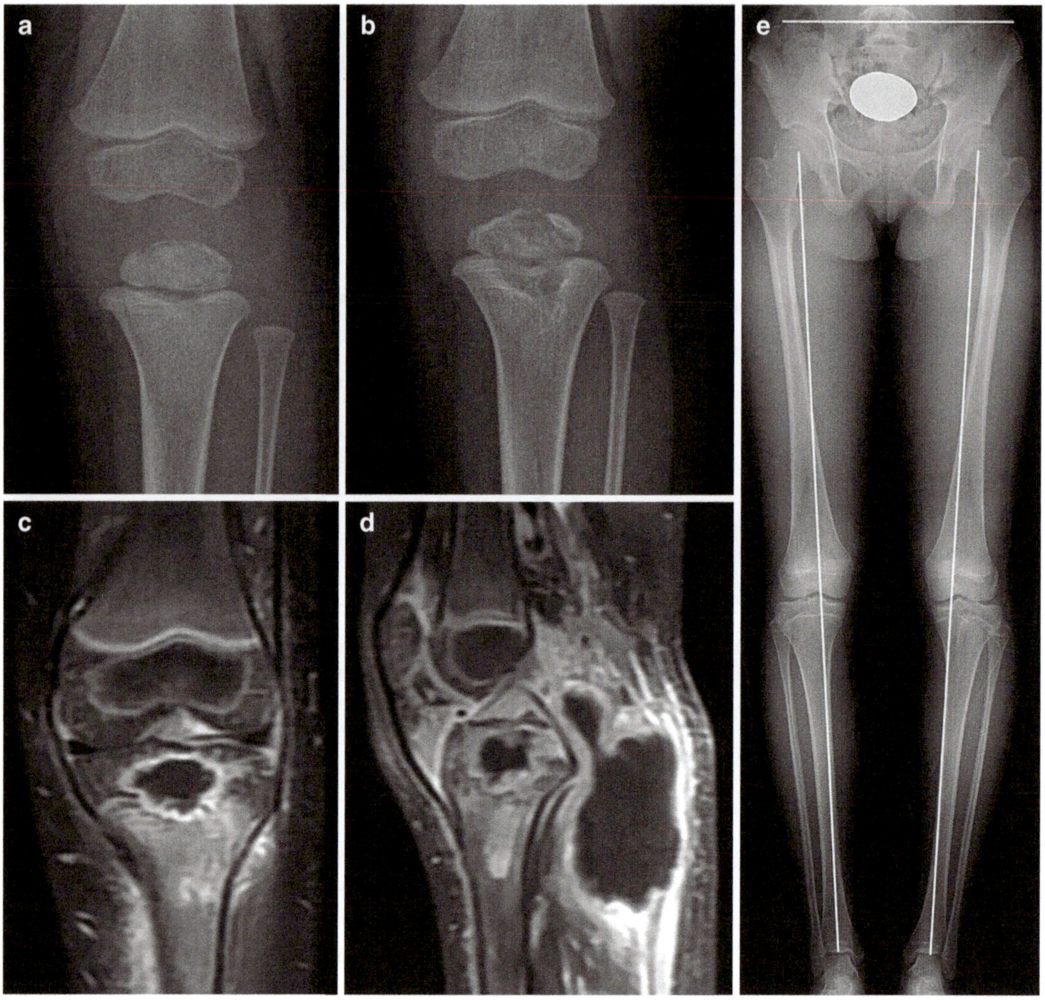

Fig. 32.6 Tuberculosis osteomyelitis of the left proximal femur tibia. (**a**) The radiolucent lesion is confined to the left proximal tibial epiphysis on a knee anteroposterior radiograph of a 2-year-old girl. (**b**) This lesion extends to the proximal metaphysis through the growth plate at the age of 2.2 years. (**c**) Coronal and (**d**) sagittal contrast-enhanced T1-weighted magnetic resonance imaging showing cold abscess formation in the left posterior calf associated with tuberculosis osteomyelitis. (**e**) Deformities other than mild genu varum of the left lower limb are not observed on a standing anteroposterior hip-to-ankle radiograph at the age of 12 years

Differential Diagnoses

The radiological appearance of osteoarticular TB arthritis and osteomyelitis can mimic various conditions in children. TB osteomyelitis must be differentiated from fungal and subacute pyogenic osteomyelitis; benign bone tumors, including Langerhans' cell histiocytosis, non-ossifying fibroma, osteoblastoma, unicameral or aneurysmal bone cyst, and chondroblastoma; and malignant conditions, including osteosarcoma, Ewing's sarcoma, lymphoma, and metastatic lesions from undiagnosed solid tumors originating elsewhere in the body. TB arthritis must be differentiated from pyogenic, hemophilic, and juvenile idiopathic arthritis.

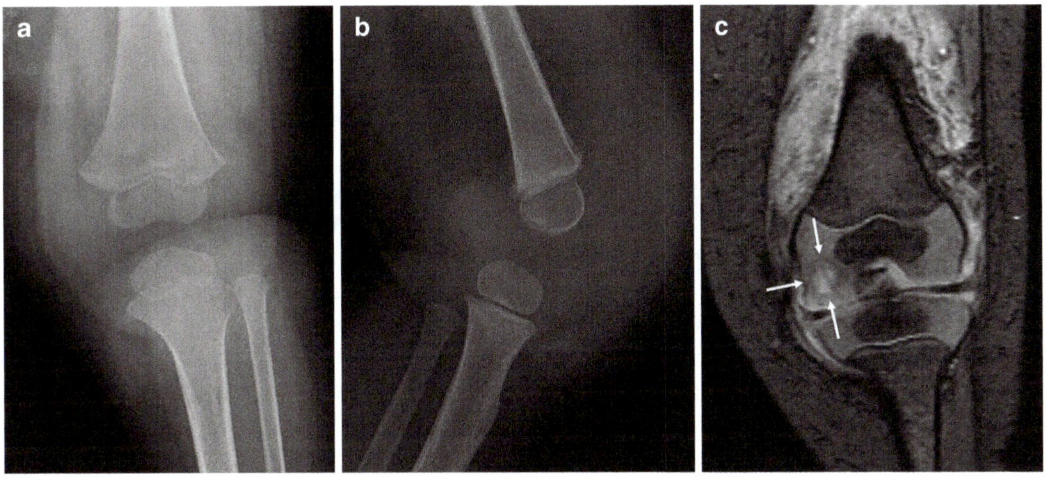

Fig. 32.7 Tuberculosis of the cartilaginous epiphysis of the left distal femur. (**a**, **b**) A 13-month-old boy has a painful swelling of the left knee with limited range of motion. Radiography showing no osseous lesion. (**c**) Gradient-echo sequence of magnetic resonance imaging showing the lesion (arrows), which involves only the epiphyseal cartilage near the secondary ossification center of the distal femur

Treatment Options

The basic treatment for osteoarticular TB involves adequate and prolonged chemotherapy with multiple antitubercular agents. The treatment regimen often includes isoniazid, rifampicin, ethambutol, and pyrazinamide. Streptomycin and quinolones are sometimes used. Streptomycin and ethambutol concentrations in the cold abscess are much higher than the minimum inhibitory concentration required for *M. tuberculosis* [55]. The medications need to be continued for 12–15 months based on clinical and hematological responses (Table 32.2).

Surgical intervention plays a limited role in the treatment of TB of the appendicular skeleton. The role of surgery could be in the form of biopsy when the diagnosis is uncertain, or debridement and drainage in patients who do not respond to antitubercular medications. Indications for surgery in a previous study included (1) lack of early response to medications (i.e., no evidence of early healing in 6–8 weeks) and (2) severity of skeletal involvement that leads its mechanical weakening [24]. In the past, bone grafting after

Table 32.2 Mechanism of action and adverse effects of antituberculosis drugs

Drug	Mechanism of action	Adverse effects
Isoniazid	Inhibit the cell wall synthesis	Peripheral neuritis, muscle twitching, insomnia, skin rash, hepatitis (rare in children)
Rifampicin	Inhibit the nucleic acid synthesis	Abdominal pain, nausea, vomiting, hepatitis, thrombocytopenic purpura, skin rash
Ethambutol	Inhibit the cell wall synthesis	Visual disturbances including optic neuritis and retinal damage, headache, confusion, hyperuricemia
Pyrazinamide	Inhibit and deplete the membrane energy	Arthralgia, hyperuricemia, myalgia, abdominal pain, nausea, hepatitis, photosensitivity reactions
Streptomycin	Inhibit protein synthesis	Vestibular and auditory nerve damage, renal damage, allergic reactions

curettage of the lesion was advocated for patients with TB osteomyelitis [56]. Currently, curettage alone has been reported to produce favorable results in most children [2, 57, 58]. In another study, surgical intervention was needed in 11 (28.2%) patients of which 5 (45.5%) underwent curettage, drainage was done in 1 (9.1%), arthrotomy in 4 (36.4%), and spinal surgery in 1 (9.1%) patient [7].

Although synovectomy and curettage of periarticular erosions were advocated as the treatment of TB arthritis in the past [59, 60], multidrug antitubercular medications following open biopsy have been the mainstay of treatment for TB arthritis in hip, knee, shoulder, and elbow joints nowadays [27, 28, 61–63]. Some authors prefer synovectomy and debridement for advanced-stage TB arthritis [64]. Long-term immobilization is not indicated in early-stage TB arthritis [61].

Tenosynovectomy and bursectomy combined with antitubercular medications have often been used for TB tenosynovitis and bursitis, respectively, in adult patients [32–37]. Nonetheless, there is little evidence to support it in pediatric patients because of their rarity.

Outcomes

Treatment outcome of TB osteomyelitis is generally good [2, 24, 57, 58, 65]. Antitubercular chemotherapy has a high success rate provided compliance with treatment regimen is maintained. Clinical and radiographic improvement is usually noted within 4–8 weeks [2, 58, 65], and complete radiographic resolution takes up to 1–2 years [24, 57, 58, 65]. Recurrence of TB osteomyelitis is rare [2, 24, 57, 58, 65]. Treatment outcome of TB arthritis depends on the radiographic disease stage [66]. Joints with just osteopenia, soft-tissue swelling, and epiphyseal or metaphyseal erosions have a generally good or excellent outcome [61–64]. However, joints with narrow joint space or gross anatomical destruction show a fair or poor outcome. A previous study reported that, depending on the extent of joint destruction, some degree of motion restriction always persisted in TB elbow after the treatment, despite the improvement in the range of motion [28].

Complications

In the TB of the appendicular skeleton, deformity and joint stiffness may occur in patients with an advanced disease stage. Limb length discrepancy can also develop in the patients who have large area of physeal damage. Although abscess easily spreads from metaphysis to epiphysis across the growth plate in the metaphyseal TB osteomyelitis, physeal growth disturbances are reportedly not as frequent as in pyogenic osteomyelitis [57, 67] (Figs. 32.6 and 32.8).

BCG Osteomyelitis

BCG vaccine contains live bacteria that have been attenuated and is developed from the serial passage of *Mycobacterium bovis*. BCG vaccination is recommended to prevent extrapulmonary TB and disseminated TB in young children. The incidence of dissemination of BCG is estimated to be 0.19–1.56 per million vaccinations [68]. Acute pyogenic osteomyelitis can develop at any age in children, while BCG osteomyelitis usually develops from 6 months to 5 years of age, with 14 months of median symptom onset from BCG immunization (Fig. 32.9) [69]. Clinical symptoms and laboratory findings of BCG osteomyelitis are also usually vague and not severe. In a previous study, fever was only observed in 19% of the affected patients. The femur was the most commonly affected site (33%), and the epiphysis was affected in 50% of patients (Fig. 32.10) [69]. The most common radiographic findings included demarcated osteolytic lesions and cortical breakage. BCG-specific PCR is required for correct diagnosis. Although surgery is frequently performed, BCG osteomyelitis patients usually have a good prognosis, and the disease is well con-

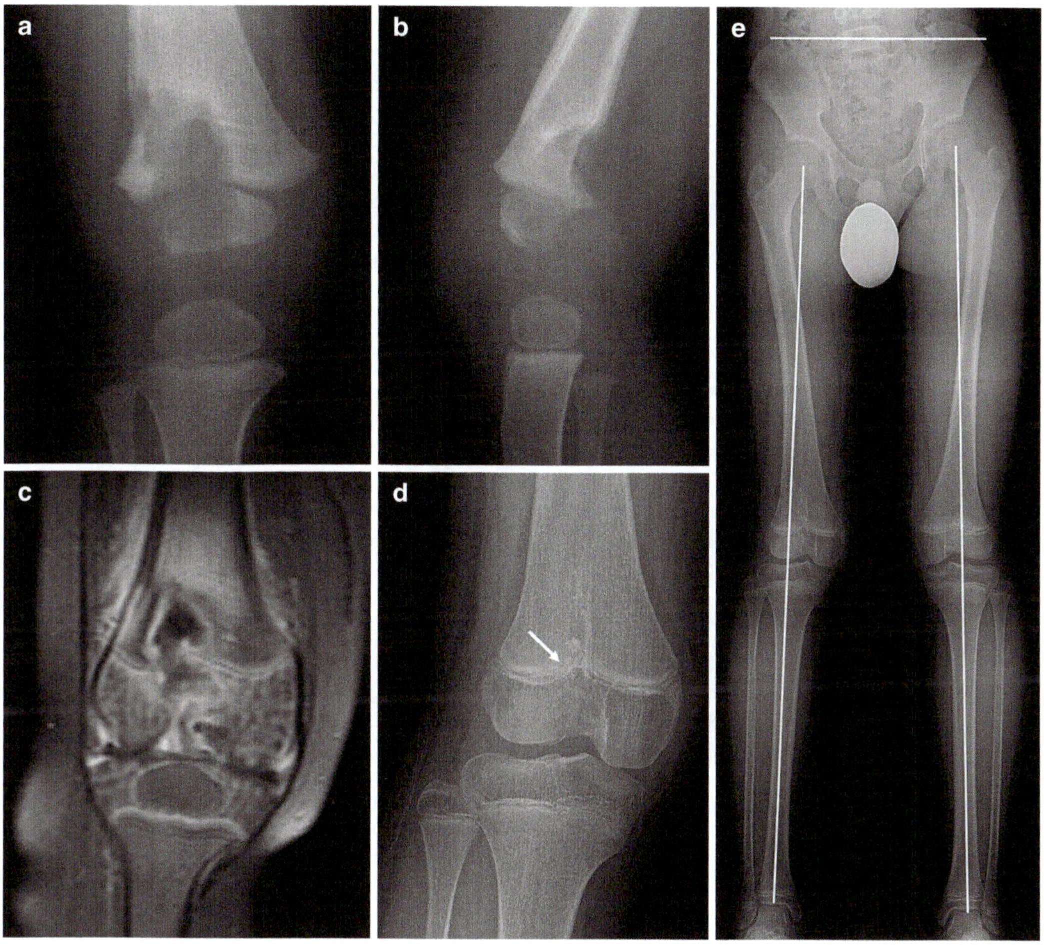

Fig. 32.8 Tuberculosis osteomyelitis of the right distal femur. A large radiolucent lesion extending from the right distal femoral metaphysis to the epiphysis is observed on the knee (**a**) anteroposterior and (**b**) lateral radiographs of a 1.3-year-old boy. (**c**) Physeal damage is evident on a contrast-enhanced T1-weighted magnetic resonance image recorded at 1.3 years. (**d**) Although evidence of physeal damage (arrow) is noticeable on a knee anteroposterior radiograph, (**e**) a valgus deformity of the right knee and leg length discrepancy are not severe on a standing anteroposterior hip-to-ankle radiograph at 12 years, considering the age when tuberculosis impaired the growth plate

trolled with medications of isoniazid and rifampicin for a median duration of 12 months, which is different from TB osteomyelitis, which requires 4 antitubercular medications. Recurrence is rare after the completion of antimycobacterial medications. In a recent study, however, an unfavorable clinical course was reported in young children who had mycobacterial infection primarily in the epiphysis [16].

Box 32.3 BCG Osteomyelitis

- BCG osteomyelitis usually develops from 6 months to 5 years of age.
- Epiphysis is more commonly affected, compared to pyogenic osteomyelitis.
- For diagnosis, BCG-specific PCR is required.

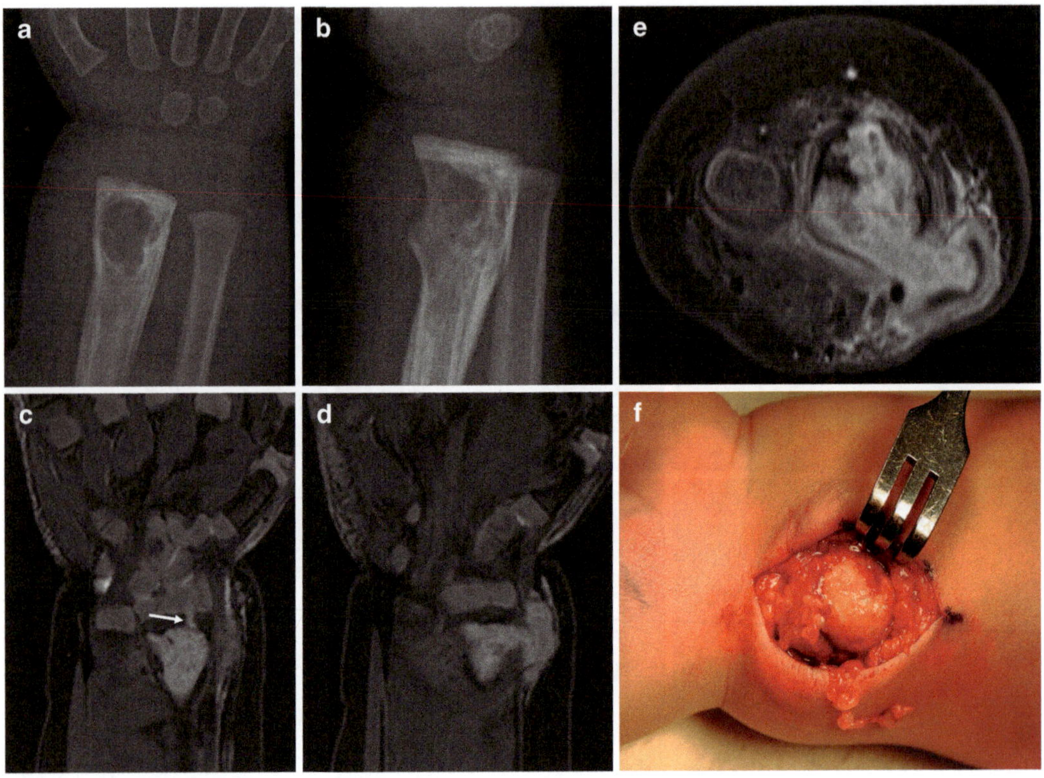

Fig. 32.9 Bacille Calmette–Guérin vaccine-associated osteomyelitis of the left distal radius. An ill-defined radiolucent lesion with a ventral cortical defect in the left distal radius and soft tissue bugling shadow at the volar aspect of the left wrist is observed on (**a**) the anteroposterior and (**b**) lateral wrist radiographs of a 1-year-old boy. There is a diffuse periosteal reaction in the left distal radius. Magnetic resonance imaging showing (**c**) epiphyseal extension of this lesion through the growth plate (arrow) and (**d**, **e**) cortical destruction with subcutaneous abscess formation. (**f**) The subcutaneous abscess is easily detected intraoperatively

Conclusion

Early diagnosis and treatment of TB of the appendicular skeleton can lead to favorable outcome. However, early diagnosis of osteoarticular TB is often difficult because of its insidious onset, vague symptom, and no specific radiographic features. Therefore, the key to correct diagnosis is a high index of suspicion. Although biopsy and mycobacterial cultures are acceptable diagnostic tools, nucleic acid amplification tests are commonly used nowadays for rapid diagnosis. Adequate and prolonged multiple antitubercular chemotherapy combined with appropriate surgical intervention are necessary for the effective treatment of osteoarticular TB.

Box 32.4 Key Learning Points

- Early diagnosis and treatment of osteoarticular TB by having a high index of suspicion can lead to favorable outcome.
- Osteoarticular TB must be ruled out in patients with symptoms that appear less severe, compared to the size of pus and the degree of radiographic abnormalities.
- Surgical intervention is not necessary in many patients.

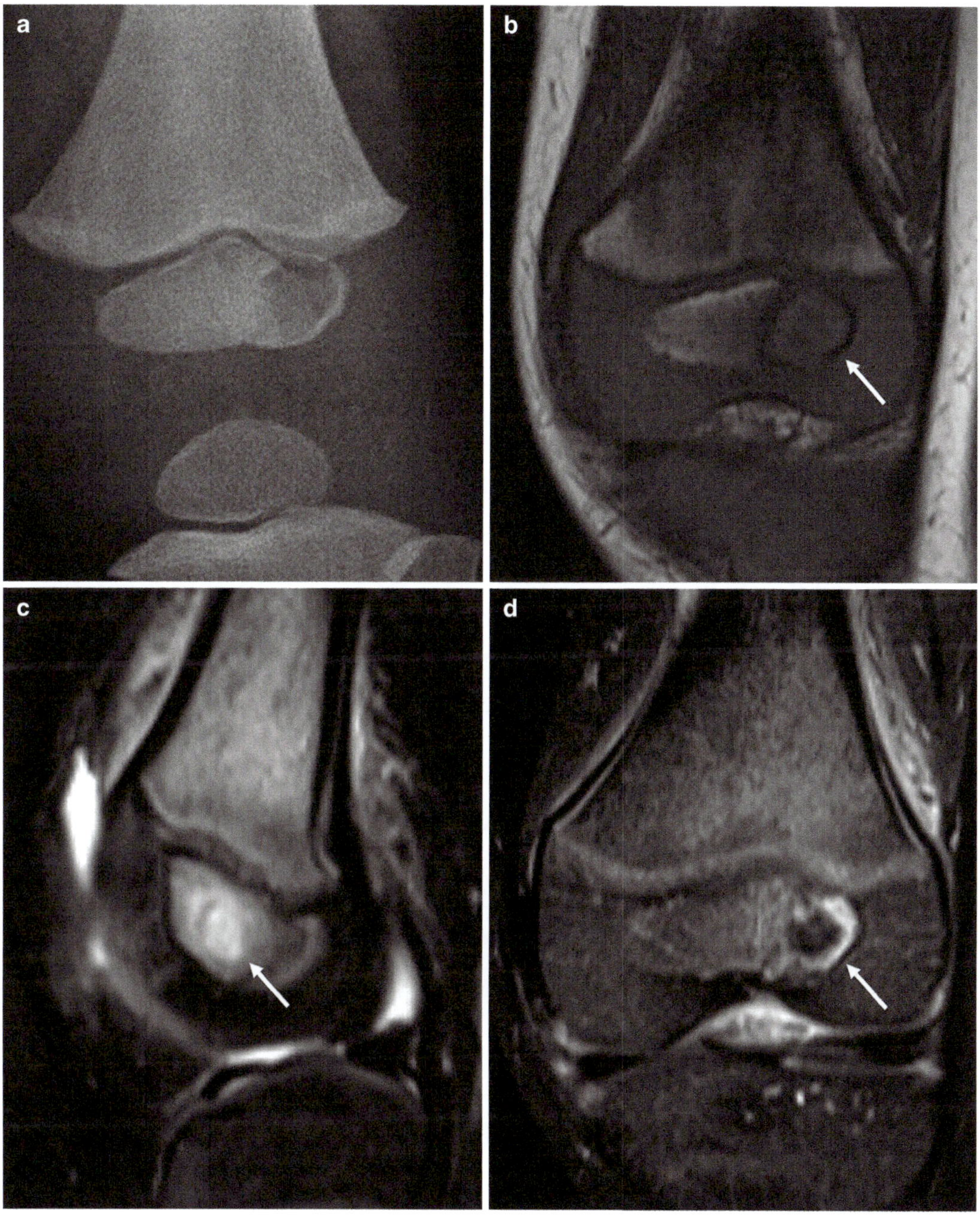

Fig. 32.10 Bacille Calmette–Guérin vaccine-associated osteomyelitis of the left distal femur. (**a**) A radiolucent lesion confined to the left distal femoral epiphysis is observed on a radiograph of a 2.2-year-old boy. This lesion (arrows) has low and high signal intensity on (**b**) T1-weighted and (**c**) T2-weighted magnetic resonance imaging, respectively. (**d**) Marked peripheral rim-like enhancement is evident on contrast-enhanced T1-weighted images

Box 32.5 Pitfalls to Avoid

- In immunocompromised patients, the possibility of multifocal osteoarticular TB has to be ruled out.
- The tuberculin skin test is prone to show false-positive results due to the cross-reactivity of the antigens within the purified protein derivative tuberculin to both BCG vaccine and nontuberculous mycobacteria.
- Compliance with antitubercular medications needs to be monitored.

References

1. World Health Organization. Global Tuberculosis Report 2017. Geneva: World Health Organization; 2020. https://www.who.int/publications/i/item/9789240013131. Accessed 15 Dec 2020.
2. Rasool MN. Osseous manifestations of tuberculosis in children. J Pediatr Orthop. 2001;21(6):749–55.
3. Kritsaneepaiboon S, Andres MM, Tatco VR, Lim CCQ, Concepcion NDP. Extrapulmonary involvement in pediatric tuberculosis. Pediatr Radiol. 2017;47(10):1249–59.
4. Watts HG, Lifeso RM. Tuberculosis of bones and joints. J Bone Joint Surg Am. 1996;78(2):288–98.
5. Santiago-Garcia B, Blazquez-Gamero D, Baquero-Artigao F, Ruiz-Contreras J, Bellon JM, Munoz-Fernandez MA, et al. Pediatric extrapulmonary tuberculosis: clinical spectrum, risk factors and diagnostic challenges in a low prevalence region. Pediatr Infect Dis J. 2016;35(11):1175–81.
6. Mete Yesil A, Yalcin E, Ademhan Turhal D, Emiralioglu N, Dogru D, Ozcelik U, et al. From diagnosis to treatment of pediatric tuberculosis: ten years experience in a single institution. Clin Pediatr (Phila). 2020;59(4–5):476–82.
7. Shah I, Dani S, Shetty NS, Mehta R, Nene A. Profile of osteoarticular tuberculosis in children. Indian J Tuberc. 2020;67(1):43–5.
8. Chiappini E, Lo Vecchio A, Garazzino S, Marseglia GL, Bernardi F, Castagnola E, et al. Recommendations for the diagnosis of pediatric tuberculosis. Eur J Clin Microbiol Infect Dis. 2016;35(1):1–18.
9. Teo HE, Peh WC. Skeletal tuberculosis in children. Pediatr Radiol. 2004;34(11):853–60.
10. Hardy JB, Hartmann JR. Tuberculous dactylitis in childhood; a prognosis. J Pediatr. 1947;30(2):146–56.
11. Mittal R, Gupta V, Rastogi S. Tuberculosis of the foot. J Bone Joint Surg Br. 1999;81(6):997–1000.
12. Agarwal A, Khan SA, Qureshi NA. Multifocal osteoarticular tuberculosis in children. J Orthop Surg (Hong Kong). 2011;19(3):336–40.
13. McMurray DN. Mycobacteria and nocardia. In: Baron S, editor. Medical microbiology. 4th ed. Galveston: University of Texas Medical Branch at Galveston; 1996.
14. Lewinsohn DM, Leonard MK, LoBue PA, Cohn DL, Daley CL, Desmond E, et al. Official American Thoracic Society/Infectious Diseases Society of America/Centers for Disease Control and Prevention clinical practice guidelines: diagnosis of tuberculosis in adults and children. Clin Infect Dis. 2017;64(2):e1–e33.
15. Smith I. Mycobacterium tuberculosis pathogenesis and molecular determinants of virulence. Clin Microbiol Rev. 2003;16(3):463–96.
16. Yoo WJ, Choi IH, Yun YH, Cho TJ, Cheon JE, Song MH, et al. Primary epiphyseal osteomyelitis caused by mycobacterium species in otherwise healthy toddlers. J Bone Joint Surg Am. 2014;96(17):e145.
17. Morris BS, Varma R, Garg A, Awasthi M, Maheshwari M. Multifocal musculoskeletal tuberculosis in children: appearances on computed tomography. Skeletal Radiol. 2002;31(1):1–8.
18. Chocano-Bedoya P, Ronnenberg AG. Vitamin D and tuberculosis. Nutr Rev. 2009;67(5):289–93.
19. Dabla PK, Agarwal A, Mishra M, Sharma S. Vitamin D deficiency among pediatric osteoarticular tuberculosis patients. J Clin Orthop Trauma. 2016;7(Suppl 2):147–9.
20. Maruthai K, Sankar S, Subramanian M. Methylation status of VDR gene and its association with vitamin D status and VDR gene expression in pediatric tuberculosis disease. Immunol Invest. 2020:1–16.
21. Shen C, Wu XR, Wang BB, Sun L, Jiao WW, Wang J, et al. ALOX5 is associated with tuberculosis in a subset of the pediatric population of North China. Genet Test Mol Biomarkers. 2013;17(4):284–8.
22. Malik S, Abel L, Tooker H, Poon A, Simkin L, Girard M, et al. Alleles of the NRAMP1 gene are risk factors for pediatric tuberculosis disease. Proc Natl Acad Sci U S A. 2005;102(34):12183–8.
23. Shen C, Wu XR, Jiao WW, Sun L, Feng WX, Xiao J, et al. A functional promoter polymorphism of IFITM3 is associated with susceptibility to pediatric tuberculosis in Han Chinese population. PLoS One. 2013;8(7):e67816.
24. Hosalkar HS, Agrawal N, Reddy S, Sehgal K, Fox EJ, Hill RA. Skeletal tuberculosis in children in the Western world: 18 new cases with a review of the literature. J Child Orthop. 2009;3(4):319–24.
25. Ritz N, Connell TG, Tebruegge M, Johnstone BR, Curtis N. Tuberculous dactylitis--an easily missed diagnosis. Eur J Clin Microbiol Infect Dis. 2011;30(11):1303–10.
26. Agarwal A, Rastogi A. Tuberculosis of the elbow region in pediatric age group - experiences from a single centre. J Hand Surg Asian Pac. 2017;22(4):457–63.

27. Agarwal A, Kumar A, Shaharyar A, Bhat MS. Shoulder tuberculosis in children: a report of two cases. J Orthop Surg (Hong Kong). 2015;23(3):398–401.
28. Agarwal A, Mumtaz I, Kumar P, Khan S, Qureshi NA. Tuberculosis of the elbow joint in children: a review of ten patients who were managed nonoperatively. J Bone Joint Surg Am. 2010;92(2):436–41.
29. Leavitt HL. Bone and joint tuberculosis; a serious complication of a systemic infection. Am J Nurs. 1948;48(3):213–5.
30. Agarwal A, Qureshi NA, Khan SA, Kumar P, Samaiya S. Tuberculosis of the foot and ankle in children. J Orthop Surg (Hong Kong). 2011;19(2):213–7.
31. Dhammi IK, Jain AK, Singh S, Aggarwal A, Kumar S. Multifocal skeletal tuberculosis in children: a retrospective study of 18 cases. Scand J Infect Dis. 2003;35(11–12):797–9.
32. Matta Ramos RF, Cancian L, Calcagnotto F, Zeni R, Varela G, Burgues T, et al. Synovial tuberculosis of the hand: an ancient disease in an unusual localisation. Indian J Plast Surg. 2017;50(2):130–7.
33. Mansour O, Moussa MK, Khalaf Z, Zreik H, Bou RR. Tuberculous extensor tenosynovitis presenting as huge mass on the dorsum of the hand. Cureus. 2020;12(9):e10236.
34. Kriegs-Au G, Ganger R, Petje G. The sequelae of late diagnosis in tuberculous flexor tenosynovitis of the hand--a report of 2 cases. Acta Orthop Scand. 2003;74(2):221–4.
35. Kim ST, Moon MS, Yoon MG, Park WS, Heo JH. Tuberculosis of the trochanteric bursa: a case report. J Orthop Surg (Hong Kong). 2014;22(1):126–9.
36. Crespo M, Pigrau C, Flores X, Almirante B, Falco V, Vidal R, et al. Tuberculous trochanteric bursitis: report of 5 cases and literature review. Scand J Infect Dis. 2004;36(8):552–8.
37. Briede PC. Tuberculosis of the greater trochanter and its bursa. Radiology. 1945;44(1):32–6.
38. Abdelwahab IF, Bianchi S, Martinoli C, Klein M, Hermann G. Atypical extraspinal musculoskeletal tuberculosis in immunocompetent patients: part II, tuberculous myositis, tuberculous bursitis, and tuberculous tenosynovites. Can Assoc Radiol J. 2006;57(5):278–86.
39. Carender CN, Akoh CC, Kowalski HR. Mycobacterium tuberculosis monoarthritis of the knee in children: a case report. Iowa Orthop J. 2018;38:17–23.
40. Wallace R, Cohen AS. Tuberculous arthritis: a report of two cases with review of biopsy and synovial fluid findings. Am J Med. 1976;61(2):277–82.
41. Allali F, Mahfoud-Filali S, Hajjaj-Hassouni N. Lymphocytic joint fluid in tuberculous arthritis. A review of 30 cases. Joint Bone Spine. 2005;72(4):319–21.
42. Seo YS, Kang JM, Kim DS, Ahn JG. Xpert MTB/RIF assay for diagnosis of extrapulmonary tuberculosis in children: a systematic review and meta-analysis. BMC Infect Dis. 2020;20(1):14.
43. Held M, Laubscher M, Mears S, Dix-Peek S, Workman L, Zar H, et al. Diagnostic accuracy of the Xpert MTB/RIF assay for extrapulmonary tuberculosis in children with musculoskeletal infections. Pediatr Infect Dis J. 2016;35(11):1165–8.
44. Kohli M, Schiller I, Dendukuri N, Dheda K, Denkinger CM, Schumacher SG, et al. Xpert(®) MTB/RIF assay for extrapulmonary tuberculosis and rifampicin resistance. Cochrane Database Syst Rev. 2018;8(8):Cd012768.
45. Shen Y, Yu G, Zhong F, Kong X. Diagnostic accuracy of the Xpert MTB/RIF assay for bone and joint tuberculosis: a meta-analysis. PLoS One. 2019;14(8):e0221427.
46. Allahyartorkaman M, Mirsaeidi M, Hamzehloo G, Amini S, Zakiloo M, Nasiri MJ. Low diagnostic accuracy of Xpert MTB/RIF assay for extrapulmonary tuberculosis: a multicenter surveillance. Sci Rep. 2019;9(1):18515.
47. Bae KM, Lim S-C, Kim HH, Lee WJ, Yun NR, Kim C-M, et al. The relevance of biopsy in tuberculosis patients without human immunodeficiency virus infection. Am J Trop Med Hyg. 2015;92(3):636–40.
48. Mousa HA. Tuberculosis of bones and joints: diagnostic approaches. Int Orthop. 1998;22(4):245–6.
49. Agarwal A, Singh S, Agarwal S, Gupta S. Needle aspiration and cytology for suspected osteoarticular tuberculosis in children. Malays Orthop J. 2018;12(3):31–7.
50. Dawani A, Gupta AK, Jana M. Imaging in pediatric extra-pulmonary tuberculosis. Indian J Pediatr. 2019;86(5):459–67.
51. Abdelwahab IF, Bianchi S, Martinoli C, Klein M, Hermann G. Atypical extraspinal musculoskeletal tuberculosis in immunocompetent patients, a review. Part I: atypical osteoarticular tuberculosis and tuberculous osteomyelitis. Can Assoc Radiol J. 2006;57(2):86–94.
52. Chattopadhyay P, Bandyopadhyay A, Ghosh S, Kundu AJ. Primary diaphyseal tuberculosis of the tibia. Singapore Med J. 2009;50(6):e226–8.
53. Gahlot N, Saini UC, Chouhan DK. Diaphyseal tuberculosis - a rare manifestation. BMJ Case Rep. 2017;2017:bcr2017221617.
54. Prasad A, Manchanda S, Sachdev N, Baruah BP, Manchanda V. Imaging features of pediatric musculoskeletal tuberculosis. Pediatr Radiol. 2012;42(10):1235–49.
55. Tuli SM, Kumar K, Sen PC. Penetration of antitubercular drugs in clinical osteoarticular tubercular lesions. Acta Orthop Scand. 1977;48(4):362–8.
56. Kumar K, Saxena MBL. Multifocal osteoarticular tuberculosis. Int Orthop. 1988;12(2):135–8.
57. Erol B, Topkar MO, Basar H, Caliskan E, Okay E. Solitary cystic tuberculosis of the distal femur and proximal tibia in children. J Pediatr Orthop B. 2015;24(4):315–20.

58. Eren A, Atay EF, Omeroğlu H, Altintaş F. Solitary cystic tuberculosis of long tubular bones in children. J Pediatr Orthop B. 2003;12(1):72–5.
59. Katayama R, Itami Y, Marumo E. Treatment of hip and knee-joint tuberculosis: an attempt to retain motion. JBJS. 1962;44(5):897–917.
60. Wilkinson MC. Tuberculosis of the hip and knee treated by chemotherapy, synovectomy, and débridement. A follow-up study. J Bone Joint Surg Am. 1969;51(7):1343–59.
61. Dix-Peek SI, Vrettos BC, Hoffman EB. Tuberculosis of the elbow in children. J Shoulder Elbow Surg. 2003;12(3):282–6.
62. Campbell JA, Hoffman EB. Tuberculosis of the hip in children. J Bone Joint Surg Br. 1995;77(2):319–26.
63. Lee AS, Campbell JA, Hoffman EB. Tuberculosis of the knee in children. J Bone Joint Surg Br. 1995;77(2):313–8.
64. Chen WS, Wang CJ, Eng HL. Tuberculous arthritis of the elbow. Int Orthop. 1998;21(6):367–70.
65. Wang MN, Chen WM, Lee KS, Chin LS, Lo WH. Tuberculous osteomyelitis in young children. J Pediatr Orthop. 1999;19(2):151–5.
66. Kerri O, Martini M. Tuberculosis of the knee. Int Orthop. 1985;9(3):153–7.
67. Kao HK, Yang WE, Shih HN, Chang CH. Physeal change after tuberculous osteomyelitis of the long bone in children. Chang Gung Med J. 2010;33(4):453–60.
68. World Health Organization. BCG vaccine. WHO position paper. Wkly Epidemiol Rec. 2004;79(4):27–38.
69. Choi YY, Han MS, Lee HJ, Yun KW, Shin CH, Yoo WJ, et al. Mycobacterium bovis osteitis following immunization with Bacille Calmette-Guerin (BCG) in Korea. J Korean Med Sci. 2019;34(1):e3.
70. Shanmugasundaram TK. Current concepts in bone and joint tuberculosis. Madras, India: Proceedings of Combined Congress of International Bone and Joint Tuberculosis Club and the Indian Orthop Assoc; 1983. p. 60.

Non-tuberculous Infections of the Spine

33

Kelly Gillock, Archana Malik, and Martin J. Herman

Non-tuberculous Infections of the Pediatric Spine

Spinal infections are estimated to occur in 0.3 cases per 100,000 each year in children younger than 20 years old, with an average age of occurrence between 2 and 7 years of age [1]. These infections occur in many locations of the spinal tract including the spinal cord, meninges, nerve roots, intervertebral discs, vertebra, and epidural space (Table 33.1) [1]. Spinal infections can be categorized as pyogenic or non-pyogenic, with pathogens ranging from bacterial, fungal, viral, and parasitic origins. Although spinal infections rarely occur, they remain a significant cause of morbidity due to their non-specific symptoms resulting in treatment delays and further progression of infection. This chapter will provide you with the necessary tools to recognize and treat pediatric spinal infections of various etiologies, focusing on the most common infections: the spectrum of spondylodiscitis and spinal abscesses.

Table 33.1 Risk factors associated with spinal infections in children [1]

Type of infection	*Risk factor*
All infections	Hematologic seeding from infectious focus in skin, genitourinary tract, gastrointestinal tract, oral cavity, respiratory tract
Spinal epidural abscesses	Underlying disease (in one-third of children)
	Immunocompromised states (sickle cell anemia, polymyositis, leukemia)
	Tuberculosis
	Vertebral osteomyelitis
	Trauma and hematoma (in 17–24% of cases)
Spinal subdural abscesses	Midline congenital dermal sinuses and hematogenous spread of infection
Intramedullary spinal cord abscesses	Dermal sinus tracts (53% of cases)
	Hematogenous spread of infection from foci in vulva, urinary tract, lungs, middle ear, endocardium, kidney, and sagittal sinus
	Intramedullary spinal cord tumors, trauma, bacterial meningitis

Spondylodiscitis

Spondylodiscitis (SD) is a broad term encompassing many variations of the same pathological process including discitis, vertebral osteomyeli-

K. Gillock (✉)
Drexel University College of Medicine in Philadelphia, Philadelphia, PA, USA
e-mail: Kjg93@drexel.edu

A. Malik
St. Christopher's Hospital for Children, Department of Radiology, Philadelphia, PA, USA

M. J. Herman
Drexel University College of Medicine, Philadelphia, PA, USA

Orthopedic Surgery, St. Christopher's Hospital for Children, Philadelphia, PA, USA

© Springer Nature Switzerland AG 2022
M. V. Belthur et al. (eds.), *Pediatric Musculoskeletal Infections*,
https://doi.org/10.1007/978-3-030-95794-0_33

tis, spondylitis, and pyogenic spondylitis. It is commonly divided into the following groups based upon causative pathogens: pyogenic, tuberculous, fungal, and parasitic [1]. Viral, fungal, and parasitic organisms can cause SD, but bacterial organisms are a common cause of pyogenic SD. Fortunately, most patients fully recover, although many do experience benign long-term outcomes. Below, pyogenic SD will be discussed, covering etiology, radiographic imaging, and treatment.

Pathogenesis

SD is rare, occurring in 1–2 cases in 30,000 at one New Mexico hospital [2]. On average, it affects children between 2 and 8 years of age, with three peaks emerging upon the age distribution in infants a few weeks to few months old, children aged 6 months to 4 years, and school aged children [3]. The most severe cases have been shown to occur in children less than 6 months old, associated with multiple foci of infection and septicemia. *Staphylococcus aureus*, the most common causative agent, is most prevalent among infants and older children; however, *Kingella kingae*, an opportunistic organism part of the normal oropharyngeal flora [4], has been shown to be the most common pathogen occurring in children between 6 months and 4 years [5]. Other pathogens (Table 33.2) [1] identified less frequently include: *Staphylococcus*, alpha-hemolytic *Streptococcus*, *Streptococcus pneumoniae*, *Escherichia coli*, and *Salmonella* spp.

Table 33.2 Common pathogens associated with spinal infections in children [1]

Category	*Name of pathogen*
Bacteria	*Staphylococcus aureus* (including Methicillin Resistant *Staphylococcus aureus*, MRSA)
	Group B streptococci
	Escherichia coli
	Listeria spp.
	Haemophilus influenzae
	Neisseria meningitides
	Pneumococcus
	Neisseria meningitides
	Brucella spp.
	Kingella kingae
Viral	*Herpes viruses*
	Polio viruses
	Cytomegalovirus
Fungal	*Aspergillus* spp.
	Candida spp.
Parasitic	*Taenia solium*
	Schistosoma

SD commonly occurs most commonly in the lumbar spine, specifically at L3–4 and L4–5 levels, followed by thoracic and cervical spine locations [1, 3, 6–10]. Transmission can occur via three mechanisms including hematogenous spread, direct contiguous spread from adjacent tissue and iatrogenic spread through various procedures and surgery. Hematological transmission occurs most frequently, and although not completely understood, it is thought to occur due the presence of a septic emboli traveling from a focus of infection and reaching the intervertebral (IV) disc through the blood vessels still present in the cartilaginous end plates surrounding the IV disc. Until the age of 7–8 years, children possess increased vascularity in the end plates until their disappearance with only the peripheral vasculature remaining [3, 5–8, 10, 11]. While this increases ease of access for infectious pathogens, it also leads to good outcomes of antibiotic treatment.

In addition to traditional hematogenous transmission, SD has been identified as a rare complication of button battery ingestion, a peculiar form of transmission. Ingestion of foreign bodies in children often occurs among ages less than 6 years. Due to increased utilization of electronics and their shiny, metallic appearance, battery ingestion among children has increased recently. Event after as little as a few hours, esophageal burns can occur from cathode to anode current discharge and alkali leakage leading to subsequent micro-perforations and upper gastrointestinal bacteria access to the spinal tract [11].

Clinical Evaluation

History

Symptoms of SD are often variable and nonspecific including fever, back pain, abdominal pain, difficulty in walking, new-onset spinal deformity such as scoliosis or torticollis, neck pain, dysphagia, discomfort in all positions except when lying supine and avoiding activity [1–3, 7–9, 12]. Neurological symptoms such as radiating buttock or leg pain, weakness, and bowel or bladder dysfunction may also occur but are generally not common [1, 5, 10]. Delays in diagnosis, some recorded as long as 4–6 months, commonly occur due to the non-specific nature of symptoms and inability to verbalize symptoms among younger patients unless a high index of suspicion is present [1, 3, 5–7, 9, 10].

Physical Exam

Local tenderness, paraspinal spasm and decreased spinal range of motion, and scoliosis may be present upon exam. In children able to walk, movement may be less fluid with the spine held rigid and a gait that is asymmetric or antalgic-appearing (Table 33.3). Though neurological examination findings may not be present, a positive straight leg test and some non-specific clinical signs have been noted such as the "quarter sign" (pain while bending forward and picking up a coin, such as a quarter) and "log-roll sign" (stretching of the psoas muscle during leg extension causes pain in the hip and groin) [1, 5, 9] (Box 33.1).

Table 33.3 Clinical signs and symptoms of patients with discitis seen at Santa Casa de Misericórdia de São Paulo [9]

Clinical signs and symptoms	*No. of complaints*	*Percentage (%)*
Difficulty walking	4	15
Lumbago	4	15
Claudication	1	4
Abdominal pain	1	4
Radiation to lower limbs	1	4
Back pain	1	4
Correction of lumbar lordosis	3	12
Decompensation of the trunk of the belly	1	4
Pain on palpation of the spine	8	31
Fever	2	7
Neurological dysfunction	0	0
Total	26	100

Box 33.1 Spondylodiscitis differential diagnoses

Differential diagnoses

- Spinal tumor
- Vertebral osteomyelitis
- Spinal tuberculosis
- Scheuermann disease
- Progressive ventral fusion of vertebral endplates
- Langerhans cell granulomatosis of the spine (LCGS)

Diagnostic Tests

In pediatric patients with suspected SD, a complete blood count (CBC), blood and urine cultures, and the inflammatory markers C-reactive protein (CRP) erythrocyte sedimentation rate (ESR) are recommended [3–8]. In a majority of cases, a normal white blood cell (WBC) was found with elevated inflammatory markers. Commonly, ESR is markedly elevated and CRP is normally or only slightly elevated; however, in severe cases of SD, much higher values can occur. Although most frequently within the normal range, WBC can also be elevated with instances of left shift or mild leukocytosis. In adult populations, procalcitonin has been shown to be a better marker than WBC, CRP, and ESR, but no data is present in pediatric SD patients [3, 5].

Anaerobic blood cultures may be helpful in identification of the disease-causing pathogen; however, on average, organisms are identified only 50% of the time [9]. It is also important to recognize that *K. kingae* can be difficult to isolate through solid cultures of blood or synovial fluid and is more readily identified through polymerase chain reaction from pharyngeal swabs [4].

Imaging

Magnetic Resonance Imaging

The modality of choice (Fig. 33.1), magnetic resonance imaging (MRI), with and without gadolinium, has a sensitivity and specificity for SD greater than 90% and the ability to visualize the

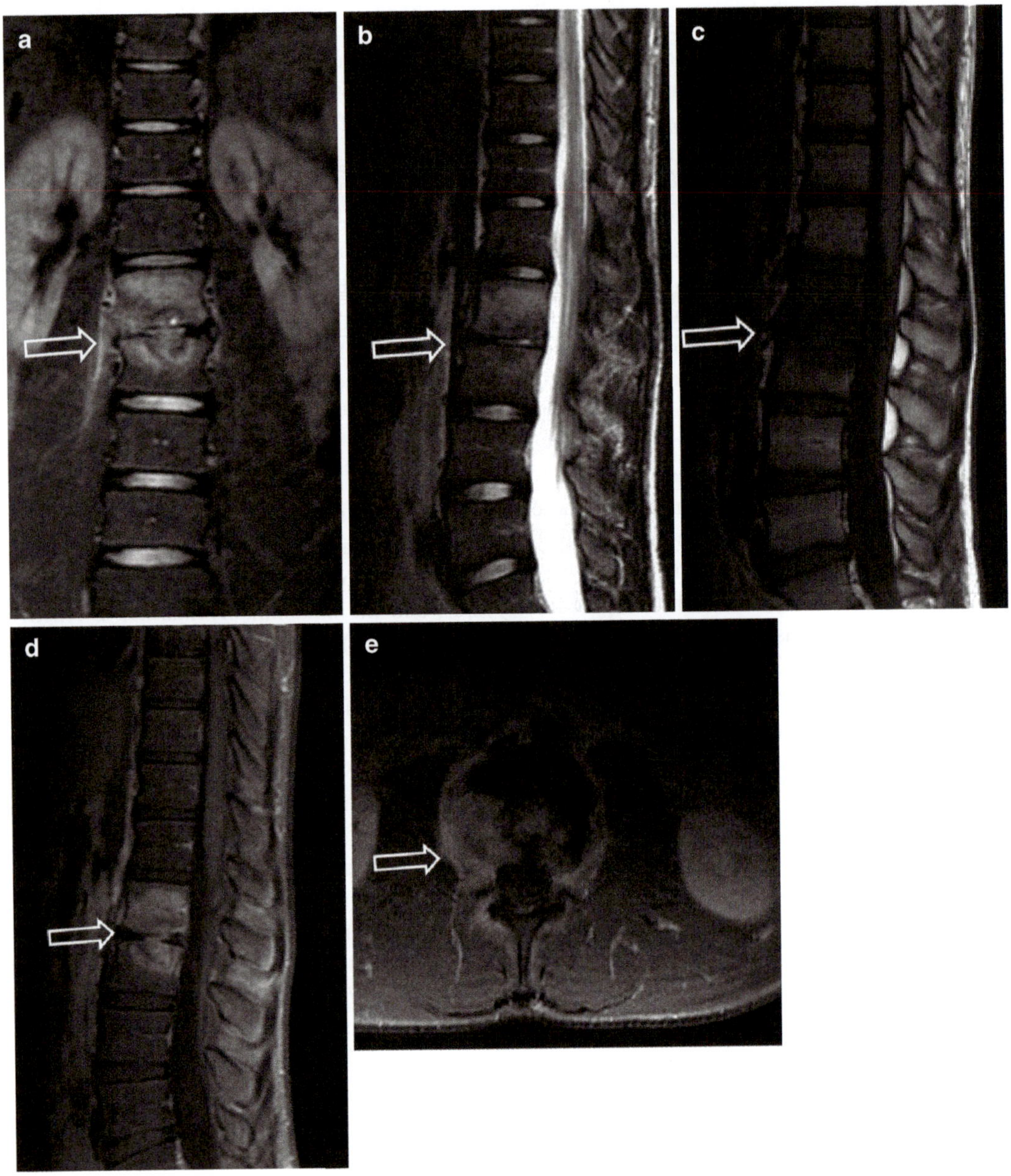

Fig. 33.1 Discitis-osteomyelitis. A 17-year-old boy presented with back pain and high inflammatory markers. (**a**) Coronal short-T1 inversion recovery (STIR) and (**b**) sagittal T2 fat saturated sequences demonstrate T2 hyperintense signal abnormality centered at the L2–3 disc with associated narrowing, destruction and irregularity of the end plates (arrows). (**c**) There is corresponding hypointense T1 signal abnormality as seen on sagittal T1-weighted sequence. (**d**, **e**) Sagittal and axial post-contrast T1-fat saturated sequences show marrow and soft tissue enhancement in the prevertebral region (arrow). There is no evidence of intraspinal extension or drainable collection

disc and associated disc space reduction or end plate erosion, vertebra, nervous tissues, and surrounding soft tissues [3, 6, 8–10]. Magnetic resonance imaging (MRI) is capable of distinguishing discitis from vertebral osteomyelitis, the former includes an infection of the IV disc and latter is an infection of the IV disc and associated vertebra. MRI is also useful for identifying paraspinal and epidural abscesses.

X-Ray

Initial imaging typically consists of standing posteroanterior (PA)/lateral radiographs of the entire spine (Figs. 33.2 and 33.3). Disc space narrowing, scoliosis, and other spinal deformities such as saw-tooth endplates, scalloping or block vertebra may appear early in the disease process [2, 9]. Endplate erosion, disc space collapse, and cortical disruption can be seen 10 days to 3 weeks after onset of infection [5, 6]. In patients with a suspected battery ingestion, it is especially important to evaluate both and anteroposterior (AP) and lateral views to also allow for location of the foreign object [11].

Nuclear Bone Scan

Gallium and technetium nuclear bone scans (Fig. 33.3) are sometimes recommended in young children with a non-specific physical exam when attempting to localize inflammation [1, 8]. However, nuclear scans typically provide non-specific findings and do not reliably differentiate between discitis and vertebral osteomyelitis. Its use is also associated with radiation exposure, leading many surgeons to abandon this modality for MRI.

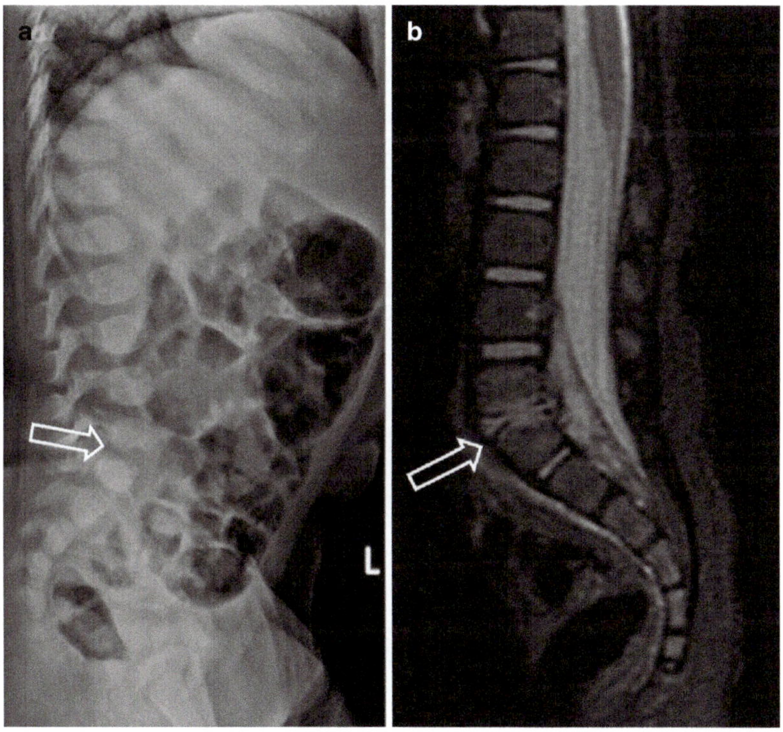

Fig. 33.2 Discitis-osteomyelitis with spinal canal extension. A 14-month-old female presented to the emergency department with back pain, non-weight bearing, fever, and high inflammatory markers. (**a**) Plain radiograph of the lumbar spine shows subtle end plate irregularity at L5-S1 with disc space narrowing (arrow). (**b, c**) Subsequent MRI of the lumbar spine shows disc destruction and T2 hyperintense (arrow) and T1 hypointense signal abnormality at L5-S1 with subjacent marrow signal abnormality of the vertebral bodies on sagittal STIR and T1 fluid-attenuated inversion recovery (FLAIR) sequences respectively. (**d, e**) There is associated abnormal enhancement with extension of phlegmonous changes to the epidural space in the spinal canal (arrow), as seen on sagittal and axial T1 fat saturated sequences. These findings are consistent with discitis-osteomyelitis and extension into the spinal canal

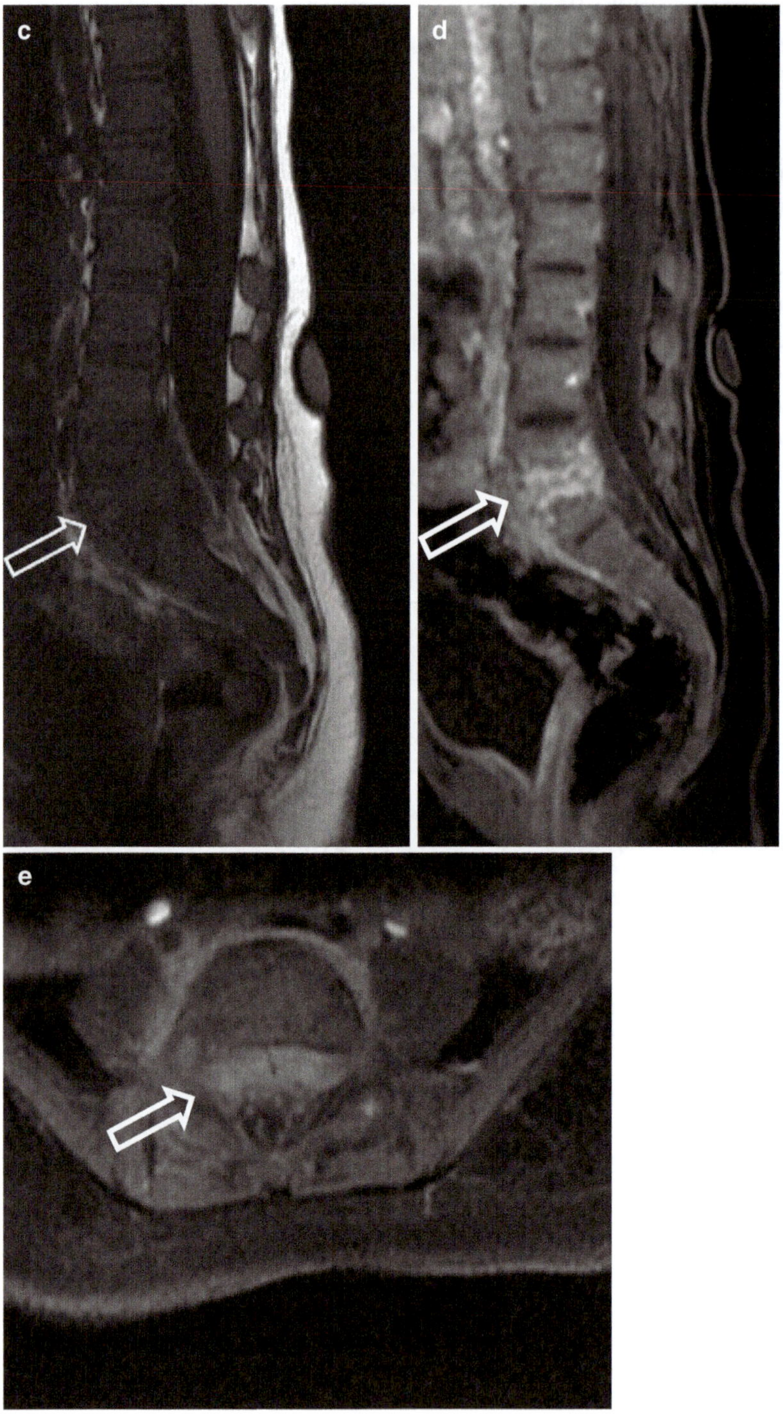

Fig. 33.2 (continued)

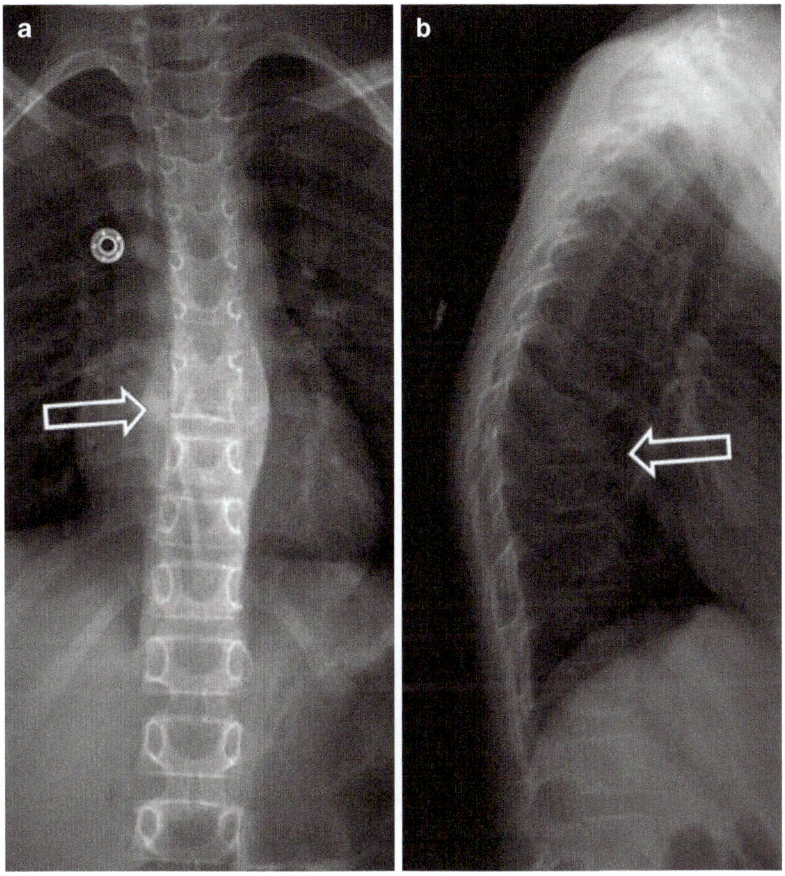

Fig. 33.3 Chronic recurrent multifocal osteomyelitis (CRMO). An 8-year-old female presented with back pain for approximately 2-month duration. Initial work up included plain radiographs of the thoracic spine (**a**, **b**) which demonstrate marked flattening of T9 vertebral body (arrow), consistent with vertebra plana. Better seen on the (**c**) magnified lateral radiograph of the thoracic spine. There is associated focal kyphotic deformity of the thoracic spine. Subsequent MRI of the thoracic spine. (**d**, **e**) Sagittal T1 FLAIR and STIR sequences of the thoracic spine. There is abnormal marrow signal abnormality with T2 hyperintense and T1 hypointense signal involving contiguous distal thoracic vertebrae extending from T7-T10 (arrows), with anterior wedging of T8, vertebra plana at T9, and involvement of disc space at T8–9. (**f**, **g**) Axial T2 fast recovery fast spin echo (FRFSE) and T1 fat saturated post-contrast sequences demonstrate mild effacement and compression of the thoracic spinal cord with epidural enhancement at T8/9 due to retropulsion of the compressed disc and vertebral body (arrow). No cord signal abnormality. Differentials included non-pyogenic discitis-osteomyelitis, and Langerhans cell histiocytosis. (**h**) A follow-up bone scan shows increased activity in the known thoracic spine, with additional areas of increased activity in right anterior sixth rib, left anterior third and seventh ribs. Rib biopsy was in concordance with chronic recurrent multifocal osteomyelitis (CRMO), also known as chronic non-bacterial osteomyelitis (CNO)

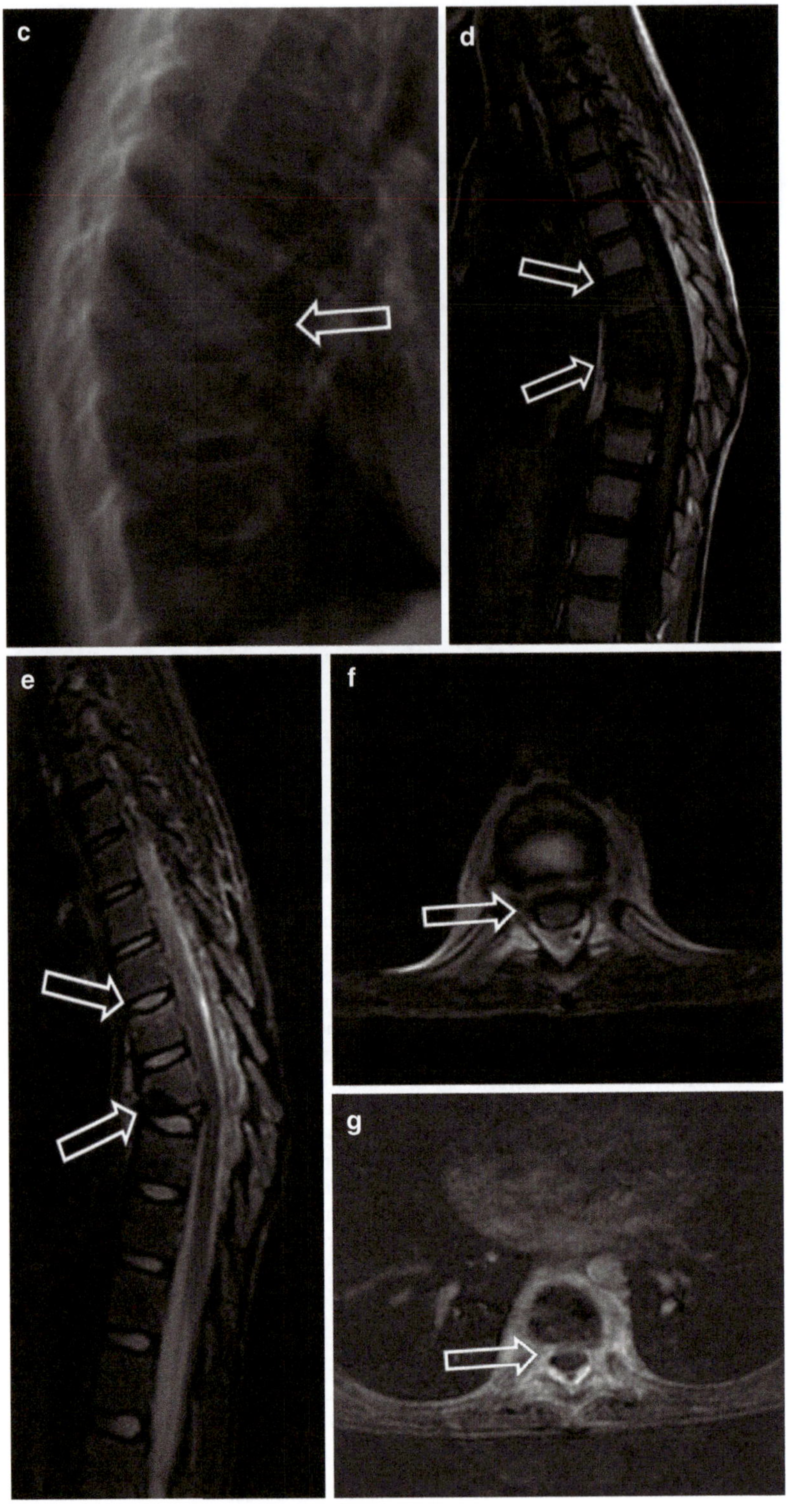

Fig. 33.3 (continued)

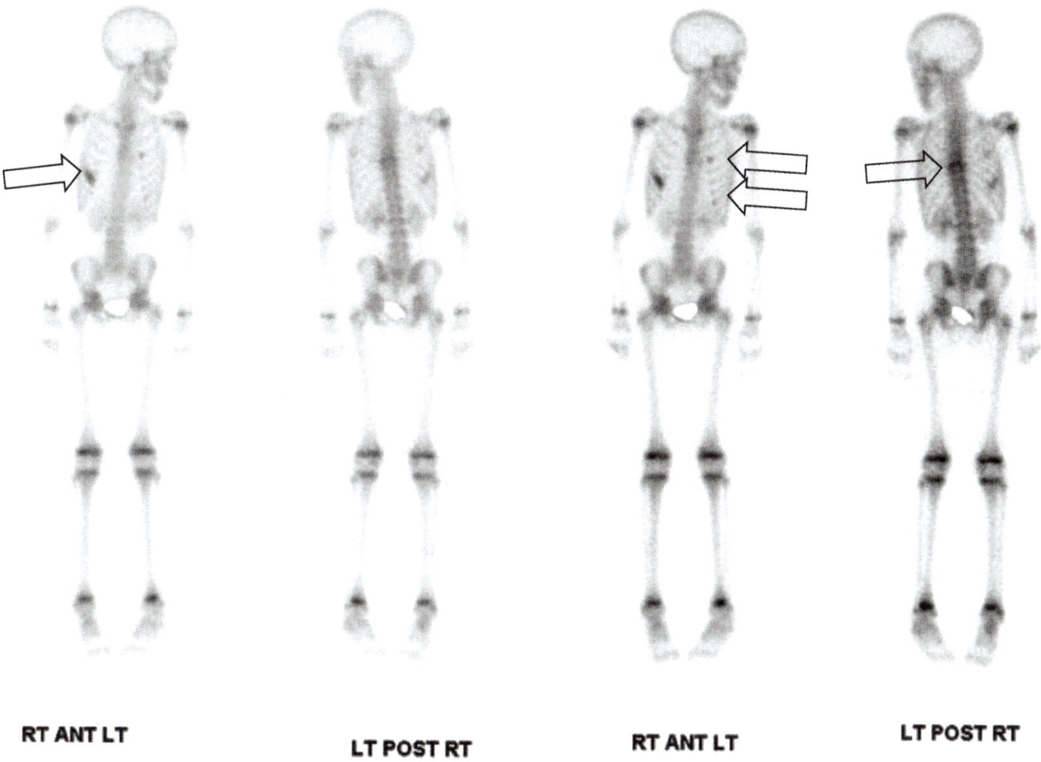

Fig. 33.3 (continued)

Computed Tomography

Computed tomography (CT) also does not provide reliable diagnosis in SD, but bone erosion, subluxation, and the presence of pathological fractures can be shown. Additionally, CT-guided aspiration has been utilized to help identify the causative pathogen in SD although most cultures unfortunately fail [9].

Treatment

Antibiotic therapy is the treatment of choice for SD; however, treatment guidelines have not been established for pediatric patients as they have been for adults. In years past, SD treatment was considered controversial as some cases (studies with fewer patients) have shown the infection to be self-limiting with bed rest and various modes of immobilization including braces to decrease pain and minimize deformity [1–3, 6, 7, 10]. Nonetheless, most patients who did not recover after self-limiting therapy were administered anti-staphylococcal therapy and showed marked improvement. With a goal of eliminating infection while also preserving function, Chandrasenan et al. [6] and Fucs et al. [9] both identify the importance of conservative treatment involving pathogen sensitive antibiotics as the appropriate course of action in modern era treatment. Duration of antibiotic therapy is also unclear, although most recommend intervertebral antibiotic therapy for 2 weeks with subsequent oral antibiotics ranging from 2 weeks to 6 months (Box 33.2) [5, 10]. Discontinuation of medications typically occurs once the inflammatory markers (CRP and ESR) are within normal ranges and symptoms have been resolved.

Box 33.2 Spondylodiscitis antibiotic treatment

Typical antibiotic management

1. Empiric antibiotic treatment
2. Identify the pathogen and perform sensitivity testing
3. Treat with appropriate antibiotics
4. Immobilize the spine for comfort
5. Trent WBC, CRP, and ESR

Surgical treatment for pyogenic SD is uncommon. If interventional radiologic services are available, CT-guided needle aspiration for biopsy/culture is indicated for those patients in whom the diagnosis is in question or for those who have failed a trial of empiric antibiotic therapy; open bone biopsy/culture may be performed posteriorly via a transpedicular approach or anteriorly via limited open or thoracoscopic techniques, but ideally is done as minimally invasively as possible [2, 3, 5, 8, 12]. Incision and drainage procedures are indicated for SD associated with an epidural abscess or other collections not amenable to interventional radiologic drainage or minimally invasive techniques because of extent of the abscess, presence of necrotic tissue or location [1, 5, 10]. It is also important to consider atypical etiologies of SD when the response to standard empiric antibiotic regimens is poor, including multiple organisms, fungi, and mycobacteria.

Outcomes and Complications

Among patients diagnosed with SD, Mohanty et al. [5] found that most completely recover with a mortality less than 5%. Additionally, Chandrasenan et al. [6] noted evidence of early degenerative changes that can be identified at a mean follow-up of 24 months. In another retrospective study spanning 23 years, Kayser et al. [10] found residual radiological abnormalities (e.g., narrowed disc space or block vertebra) after many years post-diagnosis. Other rarer complications may arise including secondary spinal deformities, recurrent vertebral osteomyelitis, or abscesses and neurological deficits; the majority of these complications are associated with neglected cases or those with a significant delay in diagnosis [3, 5, 10].

Spinal Abscesses

Spinal abscesses (SA) are categorized upon location in relation to the dura: epidural and intradural. The intradural abscesses are then sub-categorized into intramedullary and subdural extramedullary spinal abscesses [5]. In children, epidural abscesses are the most common type. SA formation is rare in children and adolescents with no antecedent medical risk factors or behaviors (such as intervertebral (IV) drug use) [1, 5, 13–16].

Pathogenesis

SA are suppurative lesions of inflammatory tissue present within various locations of the vertebral canal. Compared to adults, children are more frequently diagnosed with a specific subtype, spinal epidural abscesses, which are commonly associated with SD [1, 5, 15, 17]. Infection leading to abscess formation is commonly caused by *Staphylococcus* and *Streptococcus* spp. through hematogenous and lymphatic spread. SA occurs most often in the thoracic spine. Other pathogens that may cause SA include *E. coli*, *Salmonella enteritis*, *Bartonella henselae*, *Aspergillus*, and *Candida*; however, in some instances, no source of infection can be identified [5, 16]. Risk factors for SA formation can include immunocompromised hosts such as those with sickle cell anemia and leukemia, previous trauma, long-term steroid use, bacterial meningitis, spinal dysraphisms, and the presence of spinal implants such as for scoliosis [1, 5, 13].

Clinical Evaluation

History

Many symptoms can occur in SA, including fever, back and neck pain, and neurological deficits including limb weakness, paraplegia, paraparesis, or bowel and bladder incontinence [1, 5,

13–19]. In addition to an antecedent history of infection elsewhere, other non-specific symptoms have been reported, such as radicular hip pain instead of back pain typical for adults, headache, neck stiffness, and gastrointestinal symptoms [15, 19]. Spennato et al. [14] described a staging system for clinical diagnosis to aid in determining prognosis for the disease; the clinical stages are (1) fever, back pain, and spinal tenderness; (2) beginning signs of neurological changes such as decreased reflexes and neck stiffness; (3) neurological symptoms including bowel and bladder incontinence; and (4) indications of total spinal cord injury [14].

Physical Exam

Unfortunately, diagnosis is frequently delayed due to the non-specificity of symptoms and physical exam findings [1, 5, 13–16, 18, 19]. Findings are similar to those for SD and include the presence of fever, a palpable paraspinal mass or spasm, spinal tenderness, limited spinal ROM and occasionally spine deformity [5, 14, 15, 17, 18]. Neurological deficits, such as extremity weakness or abnormal reflexes, are uncommon and are typically identified later in the disease course. The differential diagnosis is limited and includes other serious conditions (Box 33.3) [13–15, 17–19].

Box 33.3 Spinal abscess differential diagnoses

Differential diagnoses

- SD with abscess formation
- Neoplasm
- Meningitis

Diagnostic Tests

Although non-specific, an elevated ESR, CRP, WBC will be often be present. Additionally, blood, urine, and spinal abscess cultures should be obtained in order to identify the pathogen. Lumbar puncture is not generally performed for several reasons including possible damage to a low-lying cord, potential to seed new bacteria and inability to differentiate from meningitis. This procedure is indicated only after MRI has ruled out abscess formation at the site selected for the puncture and when meningitis is the leading diagnosis; cerebral spinal fluid (CSF) has also been shown, however, to be sterile in most instances of SA [5, 15, 17]. While blood cultures may not be helpful due to avascularity, specifically within the subdural space, it is worthwhile to obtain these with the goal of identifying the causative organism [5, 17].

Imaging

Ultrasonography

Ultrasonography (US) can be used quickly at bedside for infants <9 or so months of age to aid in diagnosis but its specificity is limited [5]. US may be able to identify paraspinal abscesses in the soft tissue but cannot reliably identify SA.

X-Ray and Computed Tomography

Plain radiographs and CT scan are indicated to assess for concomitant changes in the disc spaces or vertebral bodies but cannot fully define the extent of SA involvement [5, 16, 19].

Magnetic Resonance Imaging

Diagnostically, MRI with and without contrast is the gold standard. Findings include T2 hyperintense and T1 hypointense changes with peripheral rim enhancement (Fig. 33.4) and possible associated signs of spinal cord edema and expansion, fat suppression, dura thickening, narrowing of subarachnoid space [5, 14, 18, 19]. Additionally, MRI allows for exclusion of other differential diagnoses such as an astrocytoma or demyelinating diseases.

Treatment

A combination of surgical evacuation and appropriate antibiotic therapy is regarded as the treatment of choice. Laminectomy or laminoplasty is performed and a catheter is used to obtain specimens for culture, drain the abscess and irrigate the epidural space with saline and/or an antibiotic solution, taking care to avoid dural or nerve root

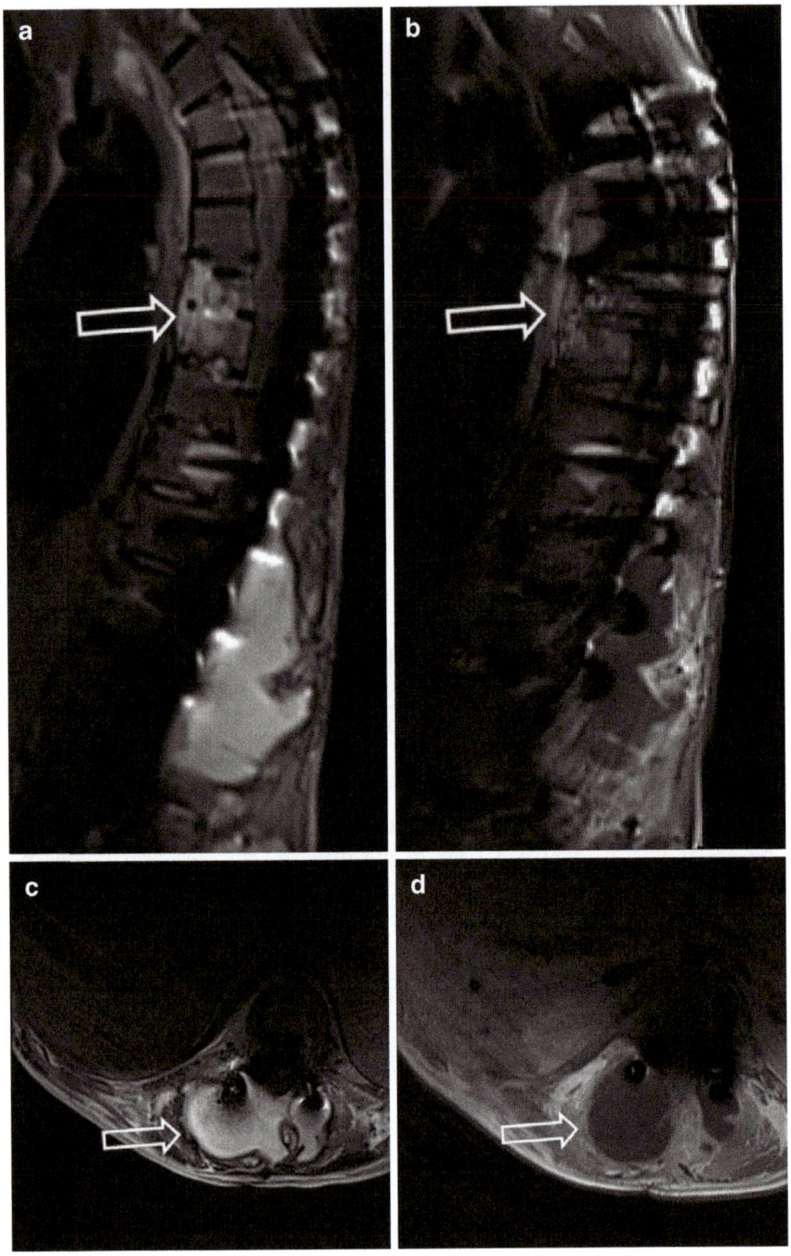

Fig. 33.4 Discitis-osteomyelitis with secondary large paraspinal abscess. A 18-year-old female with remote history of posterior spinal fixation for thoracolumbar scoliosis presented with back pain, fever, and increased inflammatory markers. MRI of the thoracolumbar spine was performed. (**a**) Sagittal STIR sequence shows abnormal hyperintense bone marrow signal abnormality involving T6 and T7 vertebral bodies, with destruction of the intervening disc space. There is associated heterogeneous marrow enhancement on the (**b**) post-contrast sagittal T1 fat saturated sequence (arrows). Phlegmonous changes are noted along the prevertebral soft tissues. A large T2 hyperintense rim enhancing complex fluid collection is noted in the dorsal paraspinal musculature on (**c**) axial T2 fat saturated and (**d**) post-contrast axial T1 fat saturated sequence, consistent with paraspinal abscess. These findings are consistent with discitis-osteomyelitis and complication of paraspinal abscess

injury [5, 14–17, 19]. Intraoperatively, multimodal electrophysiology monitoring for evoked motor and somatosensory potentials are recommended for those patients with neurological deficits. Intraoperative US can be used to assess possible dural infiltration, in which case an US-guided durotomy may be indicated [5]. Appropriate IV and oral antibiotics are continued after surgery until normalization of CBC and inflammatory markers are witnessed; the choice of antibiotic is based on the organism and its sensitivities identified from cultures.

In some rare instances, non-surgical measures such as CT-guided drainage combined with appropriate antibiotic therapy may be indicated in patients with risk factors for anesthesia, no neurological deficits or signs of sepsis; however, surgical drainage is recommended for most cases

[5, 16]. If a non-surgical approach is taken, it is critical that progression is documented with frequent repeat neurological examinations, serial checking of inflammatory markers and repeats MRI until full resolution of the abscess is documented [15].

Outcomes and Complications

With timely diagnosis and effective treatment, patients with spinal epidural abscesses generally have good outcomes [5, 13–15]. Significant morbidity and mortality, however, may occur in patients with intradural abscesses, mostly related to incomplete recovery of neurological function [5, 17, 19]. Neurological deficits present preoperatively and delay in treatment time lengths are strong outcome prognosticators [15].

Other Uncommon Spinal Infections

Blastomycosis

Granulomatous infections are caused by many pathogens including fungi, bacteria, and spirochetes [20]. Caused by *Blastomyces dermatitidis* (Fig. 33.5) [21, 22], blastomycosis is a fungal infection common in Mississippi and the Ohio River Valley but uncommon in children. Because Blastomycosis normally presents as a pulmonary infection, the diagnosis of central nervous system (CNS) blastomycosis is often delayed and associated with increased mortality. Symptoms can include headache, seizures, and neurological sequelae. Additionally, in diagnosing Blastomycosis, cerebral spinal fluid identifies the organism in the less than half of patients reported, necessitating tissue samples in obtaining diagnosis. Unfortunately, limited data exists in regard to treatment guidelines for children, but liposomal amphotericin is the recommended treatment in adults. In evaluating treatment, serial urine antigen levels have been used in pediatric populations, but further study is needed [23] (see Chap. 27 for further details).

Acute Flaccid Myelitis

Many viruses can cause infection within the spine leading to myelitis such as poliovirus, herpes virus, enteroviruses, and cytomegalovirus [20]. Enteroviruses and Japanese encephalitis virus (JEV) have both be implicated in acute flaccid myelitis in children. Transmitted by mosquitos, JEV most commonly occurs in children of Vietnam but is also endemic to Asia and the

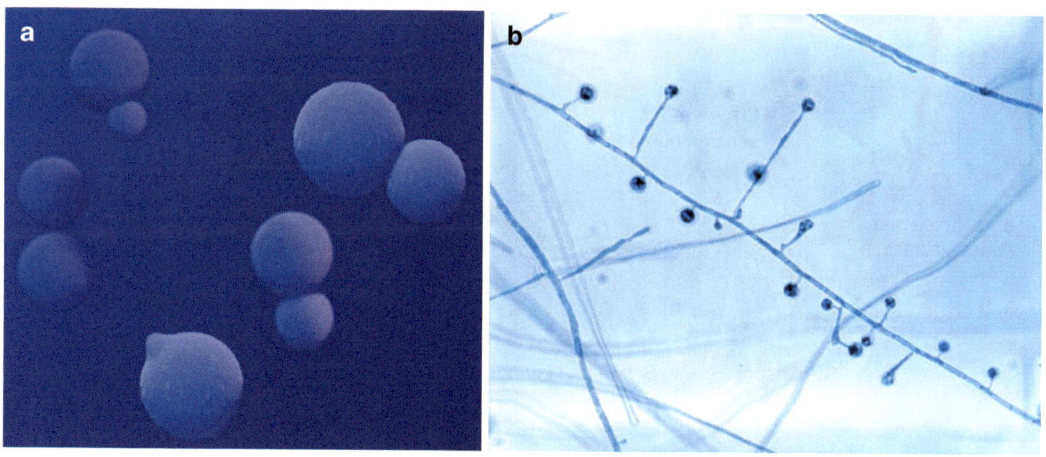

Fig. 33.5 An illustration of blastomycosis fungus (**a**) exhibiting broad based budding of yeast cells. ID # 24210, Centers for Disease Control and Prevention (2020) Public Health Image Library. (Courtesy CDC/Pooja Gandhi/ Stephanie Rossow, MSMI). (**b**) An 800× magnification of the ultrastructure displaying septate hyphae with perpendicular sprouting conidiophore. ID# 20210, Centers for Disease Control and Prevention (1967) Public Health Image Library. (Courtesy CDC/Dr. Libero Ajello)

Western Pacific. Although frequently asymptomatic, invasion of the CNS can affect the anterior horns of the spinal cord, leading to acute flaccid paralysis acutely [24].

Additionally, initial symptoms of enterovirus infection present with respiratory symptoms, but on average, acute onset of flaccid paralysis occurs days later. Children of all ages can be affected from infancy or older, but children ranging from 5 to 9 years are more commonly seen [25]. T2 hyperintensity of longitudinal central gray matter on MRI imaging is apparent [20]. CSF commonly displays elevated WBC with increased lymphocytes and cannot confirm identification of the virus. Respiratory swabs have an increased chance of identifying the offending pathogen, but this may not be likely 1-week post-symptom onset. Treatment can involve antiviral and immunomodulatory treatment; however, most patients continue to display weakness after treatment [25].

Schistosomiasis

Common in tropical and subtropical areas of developing countries, Schistosomiasis occurs as a result of the *Schistosoma* spp.: *Schistosoma japonicum*, *S. haematobium*, and *S. mansoni* (Fig. 33.6) [26–28]. Manifestation of physical

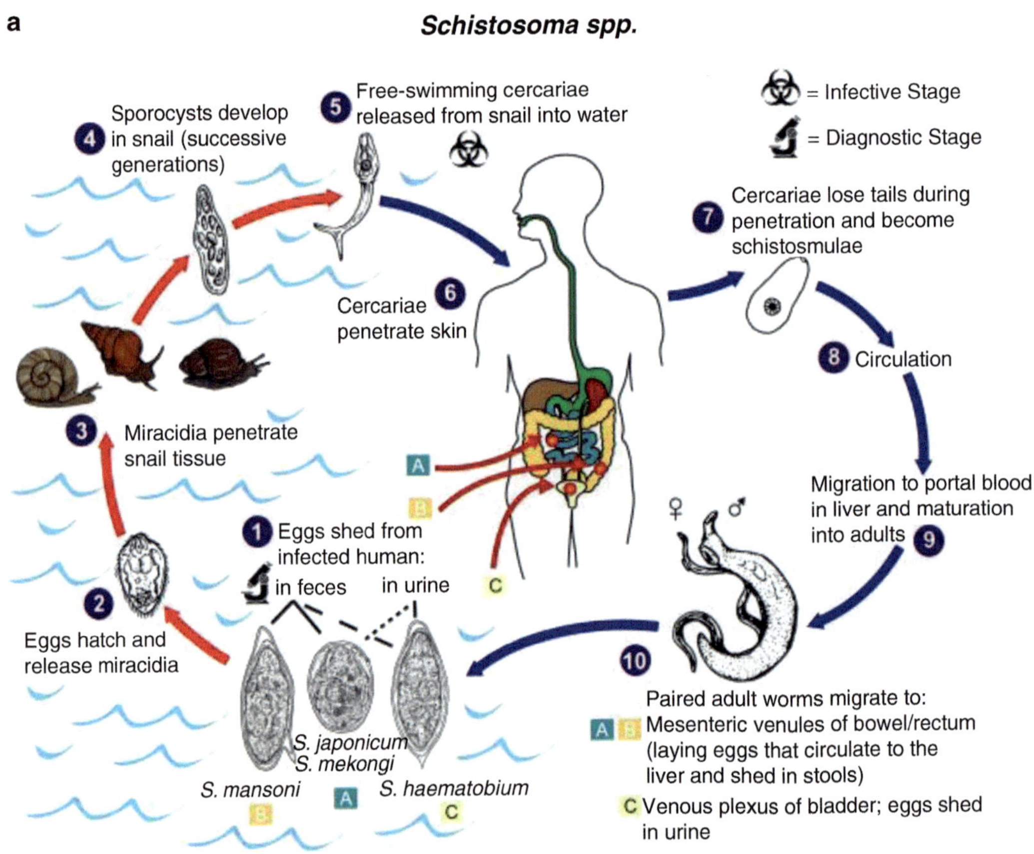

Fig. 33.6 An illustration of the Schistosoma species life cycle (**a**) exhibiting demonstrates the infective and diagnostic stages and differences between species ova. ID # 3417, Centers for Disease Control and Prevention (2002) Public Health Image Library. (Courtesy CDC/Alexander J. da Silva, PhD; Melanie Moser). (**b**) A photomicrograph of each species ova. *S. mansoni* exhibits a lateral spine, *S. japonicum* an absent or rudimentary spine, and *S. haematobium* a terminal spine. ID # 21017, Centers for Disease Control and Prevention (1965) Public Health Image Library. (Courtesy CDC/Dr. Brodsky). (**c**) A 200× micrograph displays the larval stage of *S. mansoni* species. ID # 21586, Centers for Disease Control and Prevention (1966) Public Health Image Library. (Courtesy CDC/Dr. D.S. Martin)

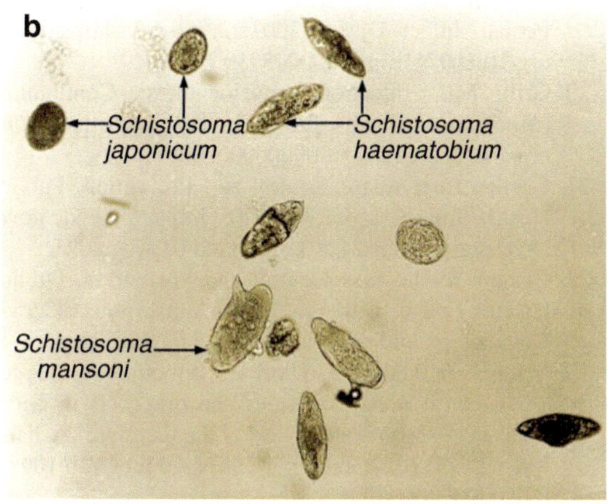

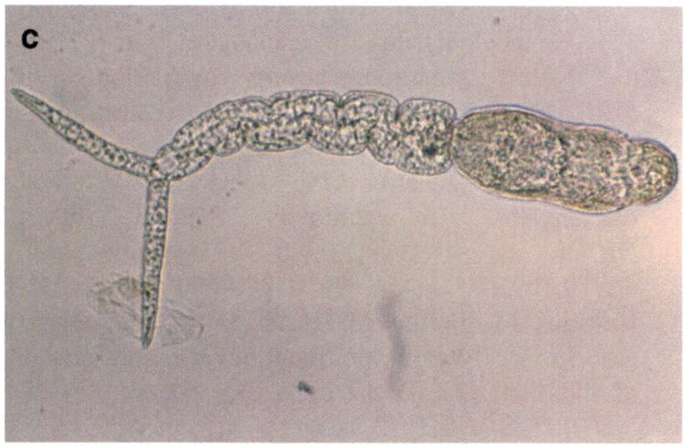

Fig. 33.6 (continued)

pathology is the result of mated adults' egg deposition following venous blood flow to the CNS instead of exiting through the gastrointestinal or urinary tracts [29]. Although all species interact with the CNS, *S. haematobium* and *S. mansoni* act more specifically on the spinal cord and *S. japonicum* on the brain and spinal cord. Described as occurring in both acute and chronic forms, Schistosomiasis is more frequently identified in adults, however, older children and infant cases have been reported [1]. In acute cases, symptoms may manifest as fever, arthralgias, urticaria, abdominal pain, vomiting, and diarrhea. Additionally, within the second phase of acute cases or patients chronically infected, neurological symptoms become apparent as a result of granuloma or nodule formation on the spinal cord, such as seizures, ataxia, muscle weakness, hemiparesis, spastic or flaccid paraplegia, and sphincter dysfunction among others [29, 30]. Although spinal lesions and intracerebral eggs can be visualized by CT and MRI, respectively, clinical history is important in diagnosing patients with Schistosomiasis. Typically, praziquantel is the drug of choice with extended use with CNS involvement in addition to corticosteroids [30]. Surgical removal or laminectomy may be indicated for spinal cord lesions; however, standardization of such practices has not been achieved [29].

Bibliography

1. Tyagi R. Spinal infections in children: a review. J Orthop. 2016;13:254–8. https://doi.org/10.1016/j.jor.2016.06.005.
2. Cushing AH. Diskitis in children. Clin Infect Dis. 1993;17(1):1–6. https://doi.org/10.1093/clinids/17.1.1.
3. Principi N, Esposito S. Infectious discitis and spondylodiscitis in children. Int J Mol Sci. 2016;17. https://doi.org/10.3390/ijms17040539.
4. Principi N, Esposito S. Kingella kingae infections in children. BMC Infect Dis. 2015;15:260. https://doi.org/10.1186/s12879-015-0986-9.
5. Mohanty CB, Fieggen G, Deopujari CE. Pediatric spinal infections—a review of non-tuberculous infections. Childs Nerv Syst. 2018;34:1947–56. https://doi.org/10.1007/s00381-018-3885-8.
6. Chandrasenan J, Klezl Z, Bommireddy R, Calthorpe D. Spondylodiscitis in children. J Bone Joint Surg Br. 2011;93:1122–5. https://doi.org/10.1302/0301-620X.93B8.25588.
7. Kang HM, Choi EH, Lee HJ, et al. The etiology, clinical presentation and long-term outcome of spondylodiscitis in children. Pediatr Infect Dis J. 2016;35:e102–6. https://doi.org/10.1097/INF.0000000000001043.
8. Fernandez M, Carrol CL, Baker CJ. Discitis and vertebral osteomyelitis in children: an 18-year review. Pediatrics. 2000;105:1299–304. https://doi.org/10.1542/peds.105.6.1299.
9. Fucs PM, Meves R, Yamada HH. Spinal infections in children: a review. Int Orthop. 2012;36:387–95. https://doi.org/10.1007/s00264-011-1388-2.
10. Kayser R, Mahlfeld K, Greulich M, Grasshoff H. Spondylodiscitis in childhood: results of a long-term study. Spine. 2005;30:318–23. https://doi.org/10.1097/01.brs.0000152097.57891.98.

11. Young A, Tekes A, Huisman TAGM, Bosemani T. Spondylodiscitis associated with button battery ingestion: prompt evaluation with MRI. Neuroradiol J. 2015;28:504–7. https://doi.org/10.1177/1971400915611142.
12. Correa AG, Edwards MS, Baker CJ. Vertebral osteomyelitis in children. Pediatr Infect Dis J. 1993;12:228–33. https://doi.org/10.1097/00006454-199303000-00011.
13. Hawkins M, Bolton M. Pediatric spinal epidural abscess: a 9-year institutional review and review of the literature. Pediatrics. 2013;132. https://doi.org/10.1542/peds.2012-3805.
14. Spennato P, Renedo D, Cascone D, et al. Spinal epidural abscess in children: a case-based review. Childs Nerv Syst. 2020;36:1385–92. https://doi.org/10.1007/s00381-020-04609-3.
15. Fotaki A, Anatoliotaki M, Tritou I, Tzagaraki A, Kampitaki M, Vlachaki G. Review and case report demonstrate that spontaneous spinal epidural abscesses are rare but dangerous in childhood. Acta Paediatr. 2019;108:28–36. https://doi.org/10.1111/apa.14579.
16. Auletta JJ, John CC. Spinal epidural abscesses in children: a 15-year experience and review of the literature. Clin Infect Dis. 2001;32:9–16. https://doi.org/10.1086/317527.
17. Sandler AL, Thompson D, Goodrich JT, et al. Infections of the spinal subdural space in children: a series of 11 contemporary cases and review of all published reports. A multinational collaborative effort. Childs Nerv Syst. 2013;29:105–17. https://doi.org/10.1007/s00381-012-1916-4.
18. Kim M, Simon J, Mirza K, et al. Spinal Intradural Escherichia coli abscess masquerading as a neoplasm in a pediatric patient with history of neonatal E. coli meningitis: a case report and literature review. World Neurosurg. 2019;126:619–23. https://doi.org/10.1016/j.wneu.2019.02.243.
19. Simon JK, Lazareff JA, Diament MJ, Kennedy WA. Intramedullary abscess of the spinal cord in children: a case report and review of the literature. Pediatr Infect Dis J. 2003;22:186–92. https://doi.org/10.1097/01.inf.0000048910.19136.49.
20. Grill MF. Infectious myelopathies. Continuum (Minneap Minn). 2018;24:441–73. https://doi.org/10.1212/CON.0000000000000597.
21. Centers for Disease Control and Prevention. Public Health Image Library. 2020. https://phil.cdc.gov/Details.aspx?pid=24210. Accessed 01 Aug 2021.
22. Centers for Disease Control and Prevention. Public Health Image Library. 1967. https://phil.cdc.gov/Details.aspx?pid=20210. Accessed 01 Aug 2021.
23. Madigan T, Fatemi Y, Theel ES, Moodley A, Boyce TG. Central nervous system blastomycosis in children: a case report and review of the literature. Pediatr Infect Dis J. 2017;36:679–84. https://doi.org/10.1097/INF.0000000000001523.
24. Tiroumourougane SV, Raghava P, Srinivasan S. Japanese viral encephalitis. Postgrad Med J. 2002;78:205–15. https://doi.org/10.1136/pmj.78.918.205.
25. Theroux LM, Brenton JN. Acute transverse and flaccid myelitis in children. Curr Treat Options Neurol. 2019;21(12):64. https://doi.org/10.1007/s11940-019-0603-0.
26. Centers for Disease Control and Prevention. Public Health Image Library. 2002. https://phil.cdc.gov/Details.aspx?pid=3417. Accessed 01 Aug 2021.
27. Centers for Disease Control and Prevention. Public Health Image Library. 1965. https://phil.cdc.gov/Details.aspx?pid=21017. Accessed 01 Aug 2021.
28. Centers for Disease Control and Prevention. Public Health Image Library. 1966. https://phil.cdc.gov/Details.aspx?pid=21586. Accessed 01 Aug 2021.
29. Lowichik A, Ruff AJ. Topical Review Parasitic Infections of the Central Nervous System in Children. Part III: Space-Occupying Lesions. 1995;10.
30. Newton CR, Preux PM, Singhi P. Parasitic disorders. In: Handbook of clinical neurology, vol. 112. Elsevier B.V.; 2013. p. 1139–52. https://doi.org/10.1016/B978-0-444-52910-7.00034-9.

Part V

Uncommon Musculoskeletal Infections

Musculoskeletal Infections in Immunocompromised Children

34

Sara Louise Dorman, John P. Cashman, and William James Harrison

Introduction

Musculoskeletal (MSK) infections in the immunocompromised child can provide significant diagnostic and treatment challenges. Presentation is frequently atypical or delayed and may involve unusual pathogens. Furthermore, the presence of complex pre-existing or undiagnosed medical conditions often complicates the treatment of acute and established infections.

The majority of infections within the musculoskeletal system can be broadly divided into those affecting joints (septic arthritis), bones (osteomyelitis) and muscles (pyomyositis). The cardinal features of musculoskeletal infections include pain, swelling, restricted movement and inability to weight bear, combined with features of infection such as malaise, pyrexia, tachycardia, hypotension and raised inflammatory markers.

In immunocompromised patients, the clinical presentation may be atypical. Without a competent immune system, there may not be release of inflammatory cytokines and subsequent pyrexia, and, with absent or deficient white cell lines, there may not be a perceivable rise in white cell count (WCC). As such, a high index of suspicion must be used in order to achieve early diagnosis and prompt management [1].

Immunodeficiency in children can be broadly considered as primary or acquired. Primary immunodeficiency typically results from a genetic mutation in the immunological system creating defective, absent cell lines or ineffective complement production. Acquired or secondary immunodeficiencies are a distinct group that may result from many causes, such as coexisting viral or bacterial infections, malnutrition, autoimmune disease, chronic illness including malignancy or drug-induced immunosuppression.

The immunocompromised child is not only more prone to infection but, even with appropriate treatment, will have more difficulty in eradicating infection and is at increased risk of developing chronic or recurrent infection with significant morbidity. Long-term sequelae are more common as well, including physical disability due to chronic pain, deformity, and residual infection, as well as the psychological and socio-economic impact to the whole family due to repeated hospital admissions, loss of earnings and the educational impact for the child.

S. L. Dorman (✉) · J. P. Cashman
Sheffield Childrens Hospital, Sheffield, UK
e-mail: sara.dorman@nhs.net; john.cashman@sch.nhs.uk

W. J. Harrison
Countess of Chester Hospital NHS Foundation Trust, Chester, UK

AO Alliance, Musculoskeletal Biology, University of Liverpool, Liverpool, UK
e-mail: jharrison@ao-alliance.org

© Springer Nature Switzerland AG 2022
M. V. Belthur et al. (eds.), *Pediatric Musculoskeletal Infections*,
https://doi.org/10.1007/978-3-030-95794-0_34

Recognizing an Immunocompromised Child

The clinical presentation of an immunocompromised child is highly variable. As with treatment of any infection, having a high index of suspicion combined with a thorough history and clinical examination of the child is crucial.

The majority of children, even if currently undiagnosed, will have systemic features in the clinical history or abnormal signs on clinical examination. These symptoms or signs may be subtle and may not necessarily be musculoskeletal in nature.

A hallmark presentation is faltering growth with early onset of recurrent infections, which may be bacterial, viral or fungal in nature [2]. Common infective organisms include encapsulated bacteria and opportunistic pathogens such as *Pneumocystis jirovecii* or persistent candida. There may be a history of severe 'reaction', increased symptoms or failure to clear live vaccines due to uncontrolled replication that caused vaccine-induced disease in childhood.

There is often a delay in diagnosis, and in hindsight, systemic features are often identified. Clinicians should take care to perform a holistic assessment and ensure that potentially relevant features in the personal or family history are not dismissed. A high index of suspicion should be aroused, particularly in unusual or atypical presentations.

In fact, many primary or secondary immunodeficiencies initially present as 'routine' infections (typically otitis media, sinusitis or pneumonia) and, therefore, may go undetected in the primary-care setting for some time.

The Jeffrey Modell Foundation [3, 4] (Fig. 34.1) has reported 10 warning signs that raise suspicion of an underlying Primary Immune Deficiency (PID). For patients with PID, the first presentation is usually with non-musculoskeletal infections. However, bone and joint infections are seen more commonly in patients with some immune deficiencies, including common variable immunodeficiency (CVID) and X-linked agammaglobulinemia (XLA) [5].

Severe genetic causes of PID tend to present within the first year of life, although milder forms may present in late childhood or adolescence. The most common presenting complaint is recurrent infection; however, parents will often give a history of co-existing systemic features depending on the underlying cause (see Table 34.1 for symptoms associated with PID) which may include chronic diarrhoea, thrush, skin rashes, stomatitis and mouth ulcers. PID is often X-linked and so there may be a family history of PID or a history of male relatives with a propensity for recurrent infections [4].

Secondary causes of immunodeficiency may present at any age and symptoms may vary depending on the underlying pathology.

A full assessment should be undertaken to identify any other potential sources of infection. Whilst musculoskeletal infection may be the primary presenting complaint, it may also present as a secondary infection following haematogenous spread or as part of a multifocal infection.

Examination should involve a head-to-toe examination for clinical signs of immunosuppression. Musculoskeletal features may include short stature, failure to thrive, evidence of chronic infections including discharging sinuses, scar-

Fig. 34.1 Key clinical warning signs of potential underlying Primary Immune Deficiency

1. ≥ 8 new ear infections within1 year.
2. ≥ 2 serious sinus infections within 1 year.
3. ≥ 2 months on antibiotics for infection of any cause with poor response
4. ≥ 2 pneumonias within 1 year.
5. Failure of an infant to gain weight or grow normally.
6. Recurrent, deep skin or organ abscesses.
7. Persistent thrush in mouth or elsewhere on skin, after age 1.
8. Need for intravenous antibiotics to clear infections.
9. ≥ 2 deep-seated infections.
10. A family history of PID.

Table 34.1 Immune system defects, subtypes of PID and common features of clinical presentation

Immune system	Subtype	Example	Common features
Adaptive	T cell	Interferon-gamma (IFN-g)/IL-12 Autoimmune regulator (AIRE) mutations	Atypical mycobacterium or salmonella infections *Mucocutaneous candidiasis*, autoimmune-mediated endocrinopathy
	B cell	X-linked Agammaglobinaemia (XLA)	X-linked recessive. Recurrent sinopulmonary infections with encapsulated bacteria
		Common Variable Immune Deficiency (CVID)	Autoimmune disease and increased risk of malignancy
		IgA	Most common (1 in 500) and often asymptomatic. History of recurrent minor respiratory and GI infections. Associated with autoimmune conditions and coeliac disease
	Combined	Wiskott–Aldrich syndrome	X-linked recessive. Associated with thrombocytopenia and clotting disorders, eczema, autoimmune disease and immune-mediated organ dysfunction
		Ataxia telangiectasia	Autosomal recessive neurodegenerative disorder characterized by chronic sinopulmonary disease; cerebellar ataxia, endocrine disorders, lymphoma and leukaemia increased
		Di George syndrome	Di George also known as 22q11.2 deletion syndrome. Associated with significant comorbidities including cardiac abnormalities, dysmorphic facial features and endocrine disorders (hypoparathyroid, hypocalcaemia)
		Severe CID	Usually autosomal recessive. Severe, recurrent opportunistic infections; failure to thrive; chronic diarrhoea; rash
Innate	Phagocyte	Chronic granulomatous	Majority X-linked recessive. Secondary to defect in NAPH enzyme produces hydrogen peroxide required for intracellular bacterial death. Characterized by recurrent deep-seated pyogenic soft tissue abscesses, osteomyelitis and pneumonia. Other systemic features include chronic granulomas, chronic diarrhoea, hepatosplenomegaly, failure to thrive, short stature, defective osteoclast function and bone remodelling. The most commonly implicated organisms include *Staphylococcus aureus*, *Aspergillus*, *Nocardia* and *Serratia*
		Hyper IgE	Chronic pustular dermatitis, osteomyelitis, soft tissue abscess and recurrent pyogenic pneumonia. Usually *Staphylococcus aureus*. Associated with STAT3 mutation, a defect which affects phagocytic cell recognition of *Staphylococcus* as well as osteoclast function involved in bone remodelling, with associated complications of osteopenia, low energy fracture and scoliosis.
	Complement	Early, late or regulatory pathways	Usually autosomal recessive. Associated with SLE–like syndrome, rheumatoid disease, multiple autoimmune diseases. Prone to infections caused by encapsulated bacteria and in particular *Neisseria* species and severe meningococcal infection

Adapted from McCusker [4]

ring, loss of joint motion, muscle atrophy, limb length discrepancy or deformity. Local growth disturbance may include limb shortening, secondary to physis damage, or more commonly overgrowth of the infected limb secondary to prolonged chronic inflammation and hyperaemia causing stimulation of the immature physis [6] (Fig. 34.2).

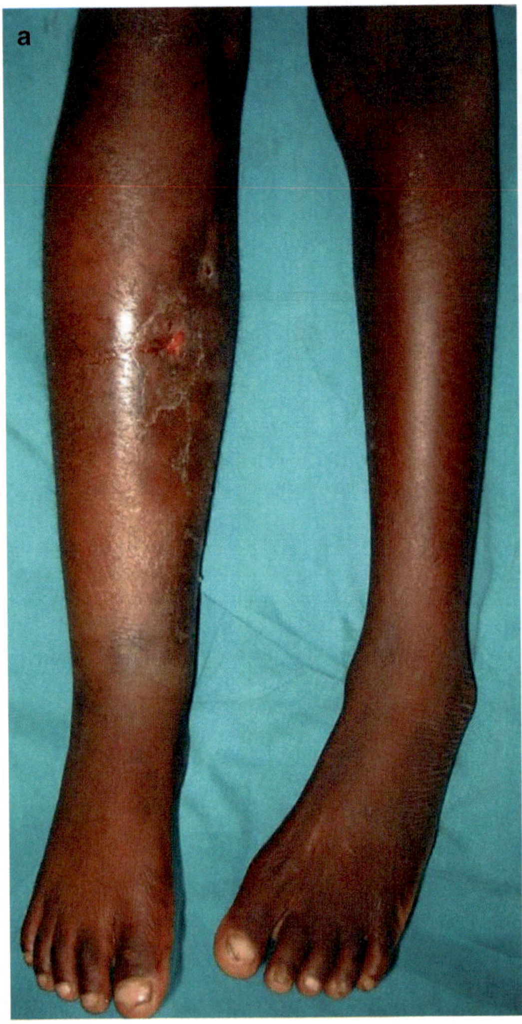

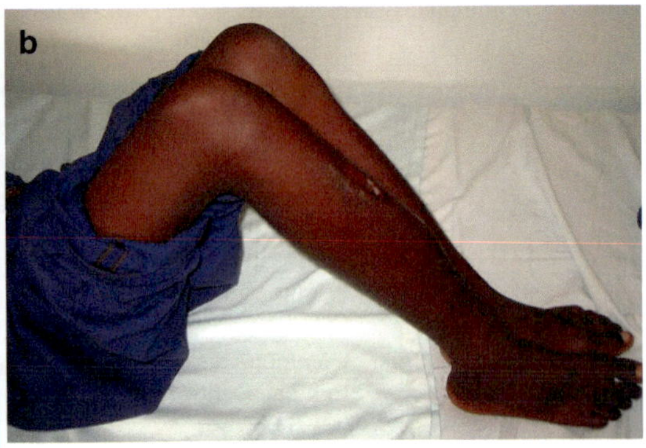

Fig. 34.2 (**a**) Clinical images of a child with tuberculosis. Note that general malnutrition has led to atrophy and a thin 'normal' left leg. The right leg, chronic TB osteomyelitis, shows skin changes, scarring and multiple chronic sinus tracts on the medial tibia. (**b**) Galeazzi test demonstrating subsequent leg length discrepancy and an apex anterior tibial deformity

Caregivers should be asked specifically about child development, including learning and motor milestones, with particular attention paid to growth in young children. If concerns are raised, then formal assessment of height and weight should be undertaken to assess the growth centile matched to age and gender. If available, routine childhood health records should be cross-referenced to ascertain whether the child has been growing steadily along a centile range or, more concerning, whether they have been crossing into lower centiles due to poor growth, or a one-off reading shows that they are below the second centile.

If immunodeficiency is suspected, consultation with a paediatrician or, if available, a clinical immunologist who is experienced in the evaluation and management of immunodeficiencies is essential. Early diagnosis and treatment are critical for preventing significant disease-associated morbidity and improving patient outcomes.

Differential Diagnosis

Primary Immunodeficiency Disease

Primary Immunodeficiency Disease (PID) is an umbrella term used to describe a heterogeneous group of immunodeficiency disorders of genetic cause with over 406 distinct disorders with 430 different gene defects listed in the 2019 International Union of Immunological Societies (IUIS) classical classification [7]. PID can be due to a defect in the adaptive or innate immune system and has five main subtypes (Table 34.1) [4, 8, 9].

The estimated prevalence of these disorders is poorly understood and typically under-reported. As such, rates are highly variable with a minimum reported prevalence of 6 per 100,000 in UK registries [10], 2–6 per 100,000 in mainland Europe [11] and 1 in 1200 in the United States (with IGA deficiencies reported to be as high as 1 in 300–600) [12, 13]. Little or no data exists in low-income countries. There are no known differences in racial distribution; however, PIDs are more common in areas with high rates of consanguineous marriage since most of these conditions display an autosomal recessive mode of inheritance [14].

T cells and B cells are the primary cells of the adaptive immune system. B cells mediate antibody production and, therefore, defects in these cell lines cause an antibody deficiency disorder. T cells govern cell-mediated immune responses so that defects occurring at any stage of T-cell development, differentiation or maturation lead to a cellular immunodeficiency. Due to the complex nature of the immune system, B-cell-mediated antibody production also requires intact T-cell function. Therefore, many T-cell defects are referred to as combined (B- and T-cell) immunodeficiency disorders (CID) [4].

In addition to the adaptive system, the innate immune responses provide the first line of defence against invading organisms. Appropriate recognition of threats and induction of the inflammatory cascade are essential steps for removal of potentially harmful organisms. Failure of the innate system to identify pathogens delays the induction of the immune response and may worsen outcomes of infection.Numerous cells and proteins are involved in the innate immune response including phagocytes, dendritic cells and complement proteins. Phagocytes are primarily responsible for phagocytosis, the process by which cells engulf and eliminate invading pathogens. Complement proteins function to identify and opsonize foreign antigens, rendering them susceptible to phagocytosis. Defects in the development and function of any of these elements of innate immunity may lead to PIDs [4].

Mendelian susceptibility to mycobacterial disease (MSMD) is another rare genetic immunodeficiency in an otherwise healthy child. It is characterized by a selective vulnerability to low virulence mycobacteria including Bacillus Calmette Guerin (BCG) vaccine, non-tuberculous environmental mycobacterium, TB and non-typhoidal salmonella.

The clinical phenotype extends beyond mycobacterial diseases, and children with MSMD are also more prone to infection with unusual organisms such as typhoidal salmonella, intramacrophagic bacteria (listeriosis, nocardia, klebsiella), as well as fungal (candidiasis, histoplasma), parasitic (leishmaniasis, toxoplasma) and viral infections (CMV, Varicella zoster, human herpes virus and parainfluenza).

MSMD arises due to a defect in interferon gamma receptor 1 and 2. Nine MSMD genes have been identified with variable penetrance; 7 autosomal recessive and 2 milder X-linked forms. These conditions can cause serious and disseminated infections of soft tissue, bone, skin and respiratory tracts. Interestingly, these disease entities may have no overt abnormalities on haematological or immunological blood tests [15].

Secondary or Acquired Immunodeficiency

Secondary or acquired immunodeficiency is much more common than PID. Common causes include malnutrition, chronic health conditions such as diabetes, malignancy and autoimmune disorders as well as end organ failure such as renal failure, liver failure or asplenia. A summary of common secondary causes and the underlying mechanisms of action can be seen in Table 34.2.

Malnutrition

Malnutrition can be considered in three broad categories: (1) undernutrition, leading to acute or chronic weight loss, wasting and failure to thrive, (2) micronutrient deficiency of essential vitamins and minerals and (3) poor diet leading to obesity [20].

Chronic malnutrition and poverty are closely linked to infection and high levels of musculoskeletal sepsis. There is a bi-directional relationship between malnutrition and infection; malnourished children are at increased risk of infection, and chronic, repeat or recurrent infections contribute to reduced appetite, increased catabolism and increased nutrient demand [16, 21] (Fig. 34.3).

Globally the most common cause of childhood immunodeficiency is malnutrition. The WHO estimates that worldwide 52 million children under 5 years of age suffer from wasting malnutrition, 14.3 million are severely wasted, 144 million are stunted and 38.3 million are overweight or obese.

Malnutrition also exists as a major cause of immunosuppression in developed countries. In the first half of 2020, 2500 children were admitted to hospitals in England with malnutrition, double that of the same time period in the previous year [22].

Ideally nutritional status should be measured and assessed over a period of time. However, in an emergency situation, a crude one-time assessment of nutrition can be assessed using height, weight, age and presence of edema. This can be correlated against WHO standard growth charts to calculate the age and sex-matched Z score. A Z score of −3 indicates severe undernutrition, −2 indicates under nutrition, −1 to 1 is within normal range, +2 indicates the child is overweight and +3 indicates obesity. In situations with limited resources, the mid-upper arm circumference can also be used [23].

Common micronutrient deficiencies such as vitamins A, C, B, as well as iron and zinc, often co-exist and should be investigated appropriately. In the absence of available laboratory testing, useful clinical signs of specific deficiencies may include night blindness (vitamin A), tiredness or pallor (iron), goitre or cretinism (iodine), easy bruising, bleeding or swollen gums (vitamin C) and pellagra (vitamin B3) [23].

Vitamin D deficiency in particular is well known to have negative effects on skeletal health, including bone fragility, increased susceptibility to fractures, rickets and growth disturbance. It also plays a role in the maturation of macrophages, production of macrophage-specific surface antigens, and the secretion of the lysosomal enzymes. These important features of antimicrobial function are impaired in the setting of vitamin D deficiency and increase susceptibility to infection, particularly those of bacterial origin [24].

Co-existing Infection

The global burden of human immunodeficiency virus (HIV) in children (aged 0–19 years) has been declining due to education and interventions, with a 70% decline reported in total paediatric cases between 2010 and 2015. Despite this, however, the global numbers still currently exceed 2.8 million and, in particular, the diagnosis and treatment of children with HIV is less well established than the adult global AIDS response. It is estimated that 47% (850,000) children currently are living with undiagnosed HIV, and are without access to treatment. In 2019 alone, over 110,000 children died of AIDS-related causes, and a 50% mortality is expected by age 2 in those infected around the time of birth. In addition, the wider social and psychological impact may be profound, with 13.8 million children having lost one or both parents to AIDS-related causes [25]. Early recognition, diagnosis and initiation of antiretroviral treatment are essential in suppression of the viral load and improving long-term morbidity and mortality. It is recommended that counselling and an HIV test should be offered for children with atypical MSK infection, failure to thrive or who present with recurrent or multifocal infections.

Table 34.2 Acquired causes of immunosuppression, examples and underlying impact on immune system function

Acquired immunodeficiencies	Examples	Impact on immune system
Malnutrition	Undernutrition	Skin atrophy, hyperpigmentation, dermatitis and skin breakdown can provide an entry portal for infection. Gastrointestinal findings include reduced gastric acid secretion, thinning of the intestinal mucosa, reduced villous height and morphology and increased permeability leading to increasing risk of bacterial translocation. Abnormal mucosal secretions: Secretory IgA and lysozymes are reduced in tears, urine and saliva in malnourished children. Reduced complement levels often associated with low albumin levels. Serum CD4 counts and B-lymphocyte malfunction leading to reduction in ability to produce immunoglobulins. Reduction in seroconversion rate for vaccinations [16].
Co-existing infection	HIV	Reduced CD4 count and adaptive immune response
	Malaria	Acute lymphopenia, decreased levels of CD4+ T cells and a functional immunosuppression greater than the quantitative fall in CD4+ cells
	Hydatid	Parasitic infection, space occupying cystic lesions with end organ dysfunction (respiratory and hepatic) and secondary malnutrition.
	Bilharzia	Parasitic infection with egg deposits causing granulomatous reactions in soft tissues and end organ dysfunction (liver, brain, intestinal tract, spleen) leading to secondary anaemia and malnutrition.
Chronic health diseases	Renal failure	Renal disease results in a reduction of B-lymphocytes via increased apoptosis, combined with protein energy wasting, thereby reducing the production of complements and immunoglobulin complexes [17].
	Hepatic failure	Reduced capacity of the liver for production of protein complexes such as complements
	Asplenia	Reduced capacity to identify and phagocytose encapsulated organisms [18]
	Diabetes	Creates a resource rich environment for bacteria (hyperglycaemia) reduced blood flow (atherosclerosis) and neuropathic injury to soft tissues. Associated insult of end organ renal and liver impairment [19].
Drug induced	Steroids	Sequestration of CD4+ T-lymphocytes in the reticuloendothelial system and by inhibiting the transcription of cytokines
	Rheumatological DMARDS & biologics	DMARDS: Interfere with critical pathways in inflammatory cascadeBiologics: Interfere with cytokine function or production, inhibition of T-cell activation or depletion of B-cells or inhibiting factors that activate B-cells.
	Chemotherapy	Variable mechanism of action but cause profound temporary immunosuppression secondary to inhibition of mitosis or induction of DNA damage and apoptosis.

In the context of HIV and a painful joint, it is important to consider juvenile arthritis as a differential diagnosis, particularly if repeated tissue samples have failed to demonstrate infection. Arthritis is a common presenting feature of HIV in the child or young person, although the exact role of viral replication and immune dysregulation in pathogenesis remains unclear.

Although less commonly encountered in the Western setting, the presence of other co-existing infections such as tuberculosis, malaria, hydatids, worms and many others can have profound

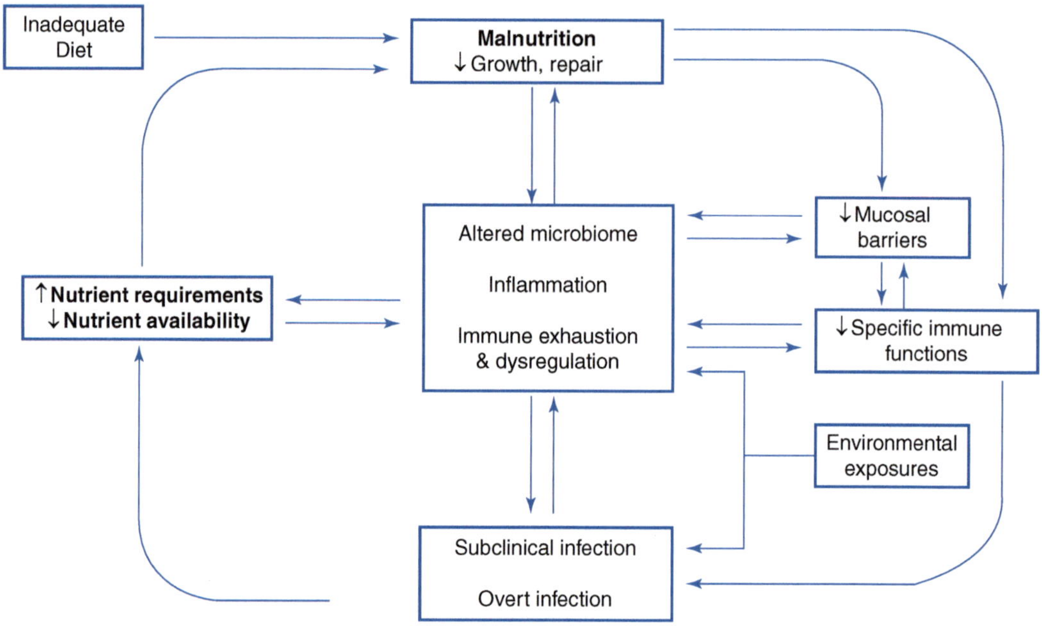

Fig. 34.3 The 'vicious cycle': interactions between malnutrition, infection and intestinal dysfunction. From: The impact of malnutrition on childhood infections. Walson & Berkley [21]

effects on children originating from Sub-Saharan Africa and Asia. TB, whilst not necessarily indicative of an immune deficiency merits an HIV test to rule out co-existing infection. Chronic infections have negative effects on the immune system function at a cellular level and cause reduced physiological reserves due to secondary wasting and malnutrition.

Chemotherapy and Cancer

Every year 400,000 children worldwide are diagnosed with cancer, and it is estimated that approximately 1 in 6700 children will develop cancer in childhood. The most common childhood cancers include leukaemia, lymphoma, brain tumours and solid tumours, such as neuroblastoma and Wilms tumour. The majority of these involve treatment with chemotherapy, which causes a temporary, profound immunocompromised state [26].

In high-income countries, more than 80% of children with cancer are cured, but in many low- and middle-income countries (LMICs) only about 20% are cured, leading to a prolonged, chronic disease state and increased susceptibility to infection [27].

Diagnosis of infection in these children has added complexity due to potential differential diagnoses including musculoskeletal metastasis or avascular necrosis, which may present with musculoskeletal pain, and atypical or non-specific MSK features.

Drug-Induced Immune Incompetence

In addition to chronic disease itself, many children may have iatrogenic secondary immunocompetence due to a drug-induced state. Common pharmaceutical causes include chemotherapy for malignancy, long-term steroid use, disease-modifying therapy or biological agents for rheumatological disease and some anticonvulsant agents.

Sclerosing Bone Dysplasia

Sclerosing bone dysplasias (SBD) such as osteopetrosis and pycnodysostosis are associated with increased risk of infection such as osteomyelitis. Osteopetrosis is an inherited metabolic bone disease that results from defective osteoclastic resorption of immature bone due to defects in carbonic anhydrase or chloride channels.

Pycnodysostosis is a rare inherited genetic disorder resulting from a mutation in the cathepsin K (*CTSK*) gene that causes abnormal storage of toxic material within lysosomes [30, 31].

In both cases the resultant bone is abnormally dense with obliteration of the medullary canal leading to lack of bone marrow. This causes locally impaired bone vascularity and systemic dysfunction due to pancytopenia, which in severe cases may cause bone marrow failure in early childhood. Pancytopenia and reduced bone vascularity are associated with increased risk of osteomyelitis of long bones in children. Infections may be difficult to treat and surgical debridement is often required. Other general features of SBD may include short stature, dental problems including dental abscesses and mandibular osteomyelitis, recurrent or low energy fractures [32].

The material properties of the skeleton in SBD make orthopaedic surgery particularly challenging; the combined hardness and brittleness is resistant to drilling, generates heat and bone necrosis, reduces the bone's ability to hold screws and may reduce the overall stability of any fixation. These factors combined with reduced vascularity and systematic immunocompromise may increase the risk of postoperative delayed union, non-union, and surgical site infection. Awareness of surgical strategies including meticulous technique including bone cooling with saline, intermittent drilling, sharpened instruments, achieving stable fixation and careful soft tissue handing may help preserve local biology as much as possible and reduce the risk of iatrogenic surgical infection [33].

Sickle Cell Disease

Sickle cell disease (SCD) is an inherited autosomal recessive disorder due to a mutation in the *HBB* gene resulting in an abnormal haemoglobin, characterized by chronic haemolytic anaemia and recurrent infections. Erythrocytes are abnormal, stiff and 'sickle-shaped' which become lodged typically within small, low flow blood vessels causing microvascular vaso-occlusion and activation of acute inflammatory cascades. Due to the presence of low flow vasculature, bone and joints are susceptible to infection in sickle cell anaemia. In addition, in young children autoinfarction of the spleen may lead to resultant hyposplenia and increased susceptibility to encapsulated bacteria [34].

This often presents a diagnostic dilemma, as acute vaso-occlusive episodes can often be difficult to distinguish from an acute infection. In the general population, *Staphylococcus aureus* is the most common organism associated with osteomyelitis. However other atypical bacteria such as Gram-negative enteric bacilli including *Salmonella* are well documented. It has been hypothesized that enteric bacterial infections may result from micro-occlusive episode and ischemic bowel infarction during vaso-occlusive episode that leads to hematogenous bacterial spread to distant sites [34].

Management of suspected osteomyelitis in SCD includes maintenance of good intravenous (IV) hydration, oxygenation and adequate pain control to prevent further complication or bone infarcts. Empirical antibiotic therapy followed by targeted antibiotic treatment after blood cultures or biopsies are the mainstay of treatment. In cases that do not respond to medical management and antibiotics therapy alone surgical treatment may be required. This may include surgical debridement, combined local and systemic antibiotics delivery and in cases of large bone defects after debridement a two-stage induced membrane technique (Masquelet) using an antibiotic cement loaded spacer such as Masquelet may be employed [35] (Fig. 34.4a–m).

Investigations

Routine investigations for musculoskeletal infection typically involve a combination of baseline blood tests (full blood count, CRP or ESR, blood cultures), plain film radiographs, ultrasound or advanced imaging (Fig. 34.5) as per standard treatment outlined in the previous chapters.

Typical laboratory investigations suggestive of MSK infection may include elevated CRP, ESR or a positive joint aspirate (>50,000 WBC/ml and >90% polymorphs). The severity of the immunocompromised state may impair the ability of the child to mount a normal immune response to infection, and blood responses may be atypical [1].

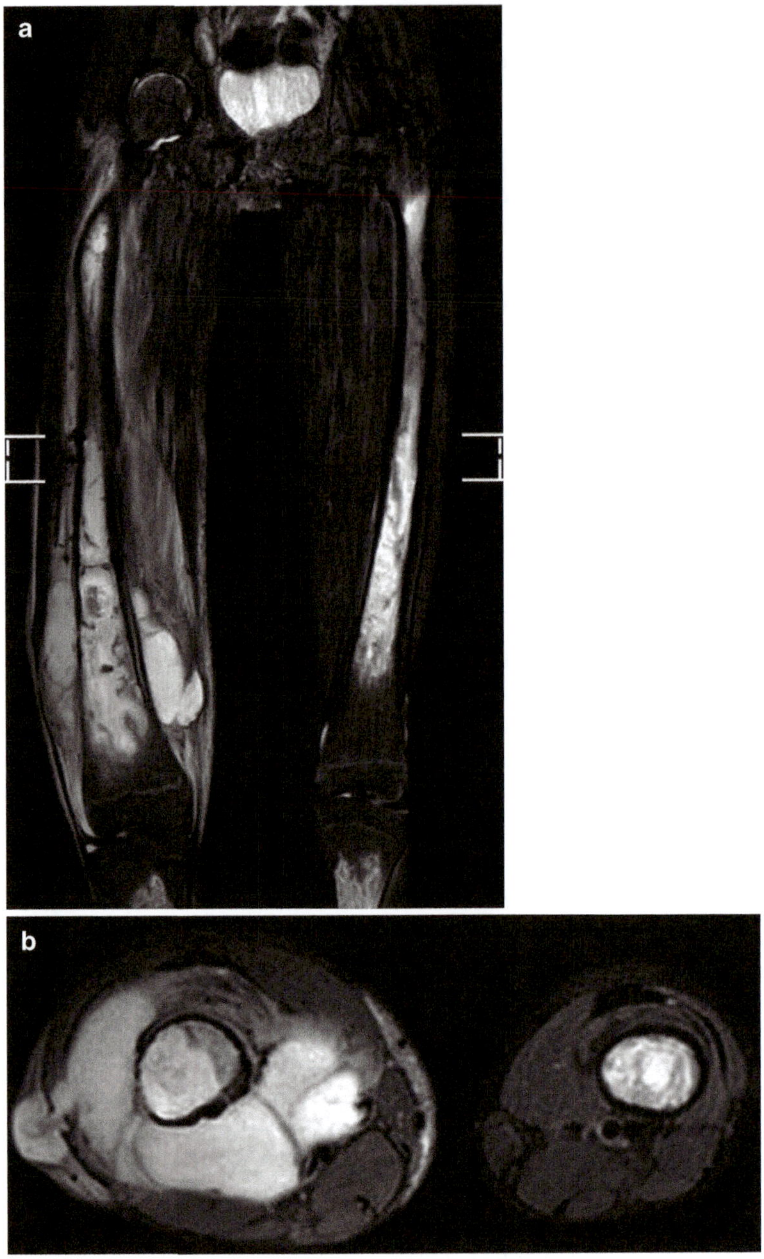

Fig. 34.4 (**a**, **b**) Cor and axial T2 mDIX MR images in a 15 yo male showing a large right femoral intraosseous abscess and osteomyelitis change in background of marrow infarction. Bony breach seen laterally with associated large partially surrounding soft tissue abscess. Inflammation of the vastus musculature with a soft tissue abscess extending to the subcutaneous tissue. Red marrow hyperplasia noted, findings consistent with patient's history of sickle cell disease. Extensive marrow infarction left femoral shaft and areas of marrow infarction proximal tibial metadiaphyses. (**c**, **d**) Radiographs of Rt femur AP, Lateral done 3 months later showing resolved osteomyelitis following incision and drainage, with residual multiapical deformity of femur in 2 planes with areas of infarction in distal femur consistent with sickle cell disease. (**e–g**) AP, lat radiographs of Right femur showing a pathologic fracture with a sequestrum, angulation and healing periosteal reaction in the same patient 3 years later. (h, i) Radiographs of the Rt distal femur AP, lat showing a pseudoarthrosis of the distal right femur secondary to osteomyelitis. (**j**, **k**) CT scan with 3D reconstruction showing progression of right distal femoral diaphysis pseudoarthrosis formation. Expansion of the previously reported sequestrum, now containing bony fragments consistent with involucrum with multi-apical biplanar deformity. (**l**, **m**) AP, Lateral radiographs of the Right femur showing well aligned Rt femur following wound debridement + 2 stage Induced membrane technique with RIA femur autograft, bifocal osteotomy, IM nail + Plating

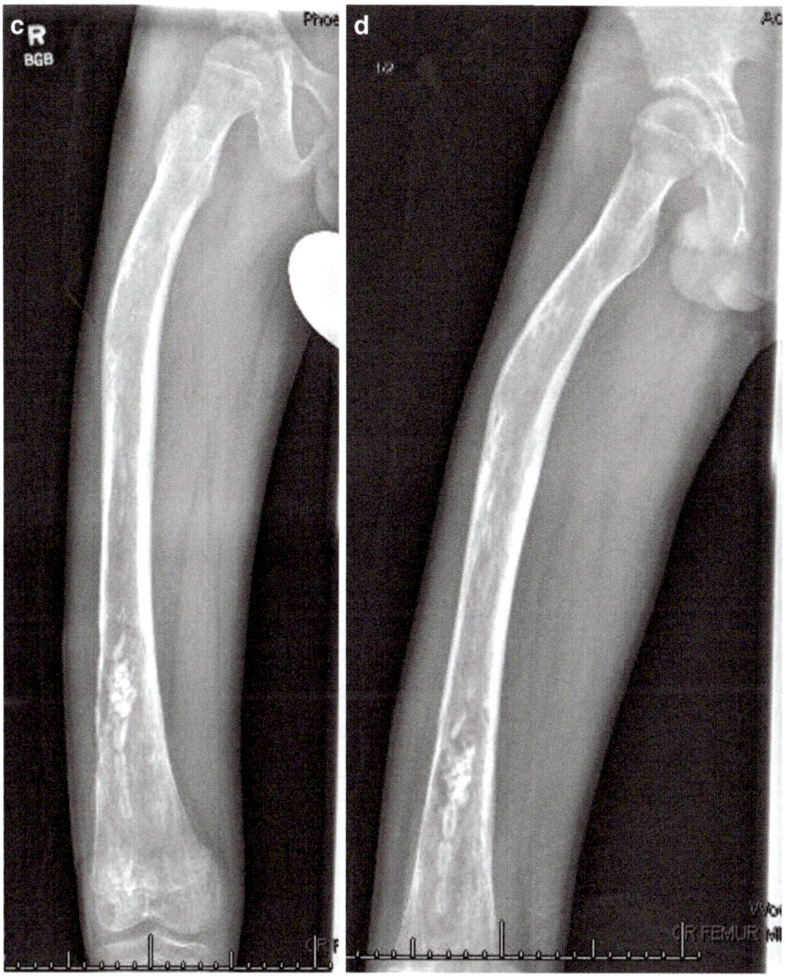

Fig. 34.4 (continued)

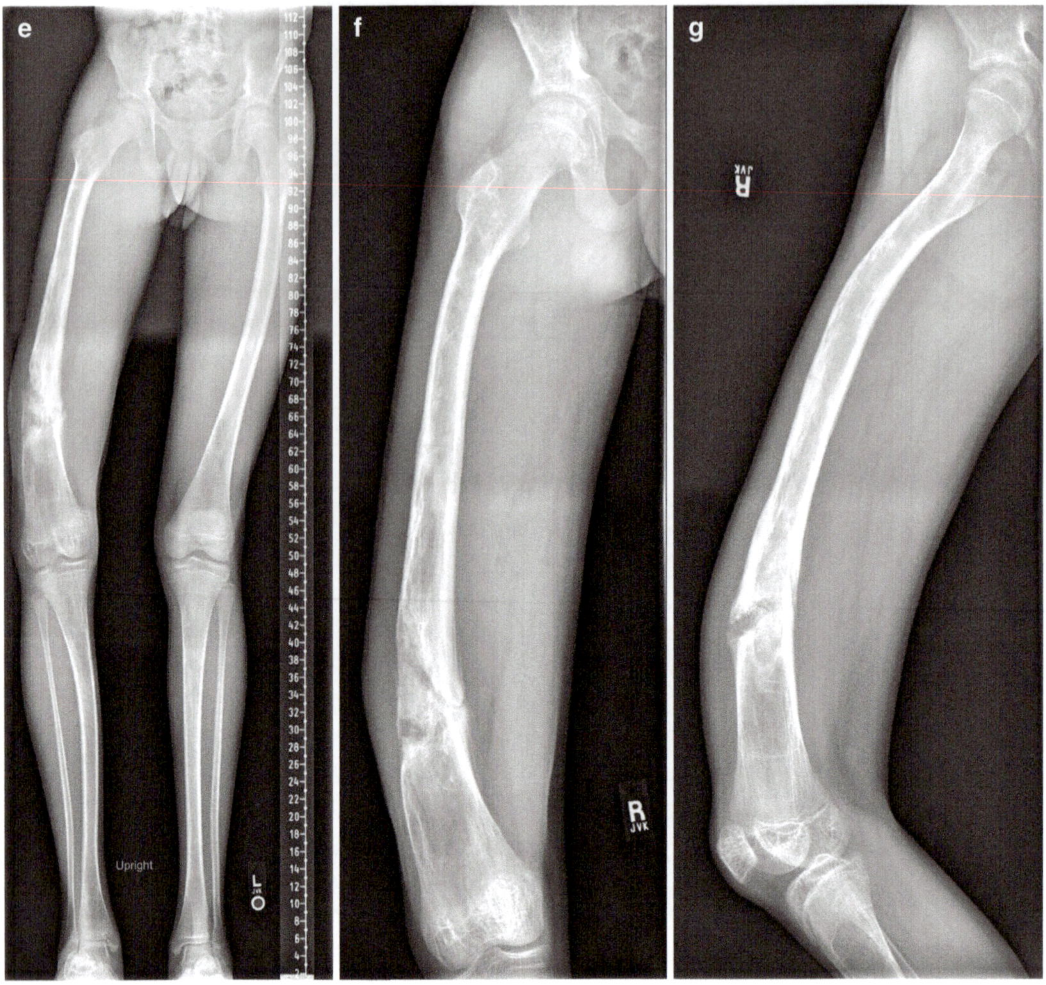

Fig. 34.4 (continued)

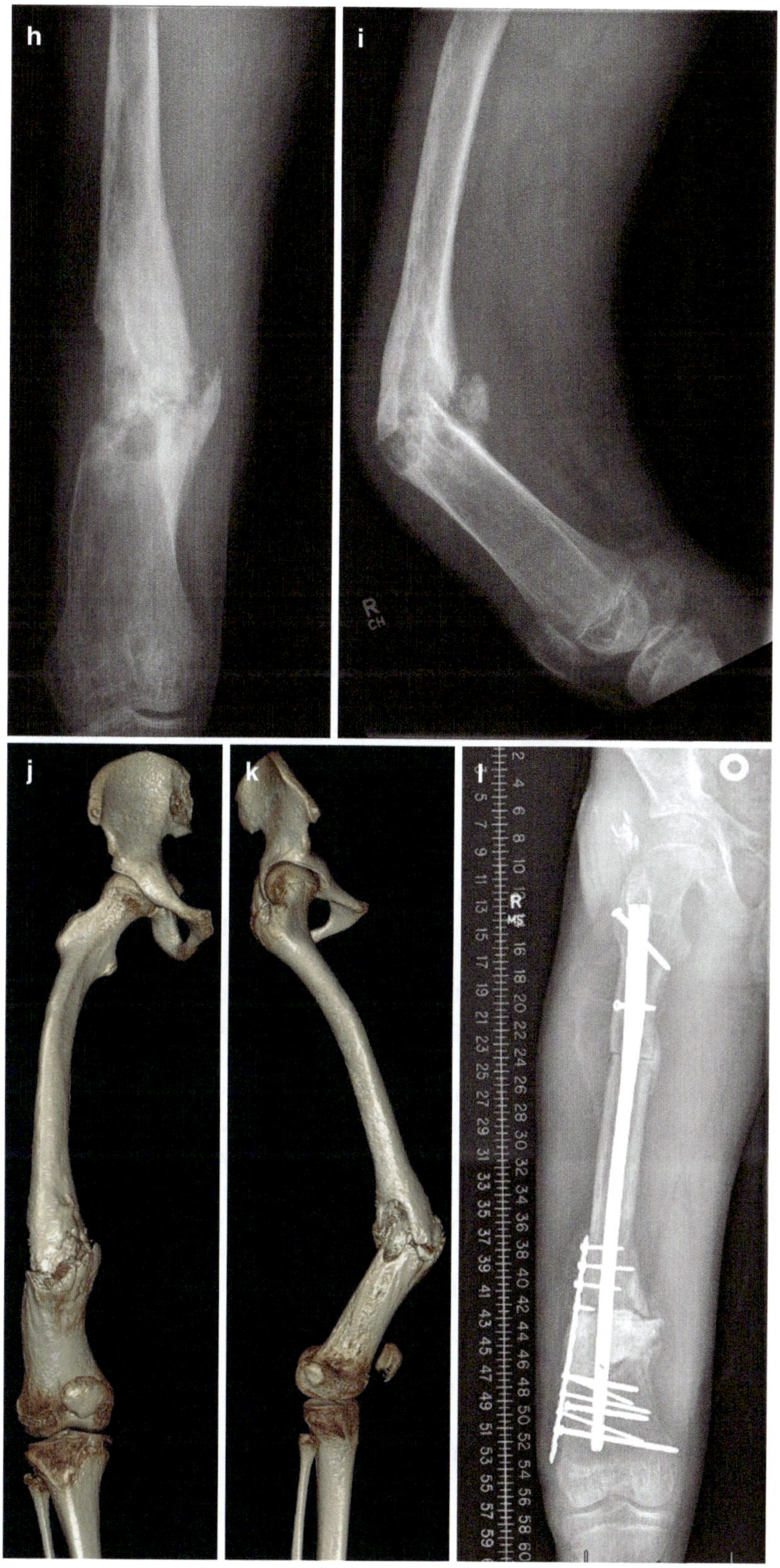

Fig. 34.4 (continued)

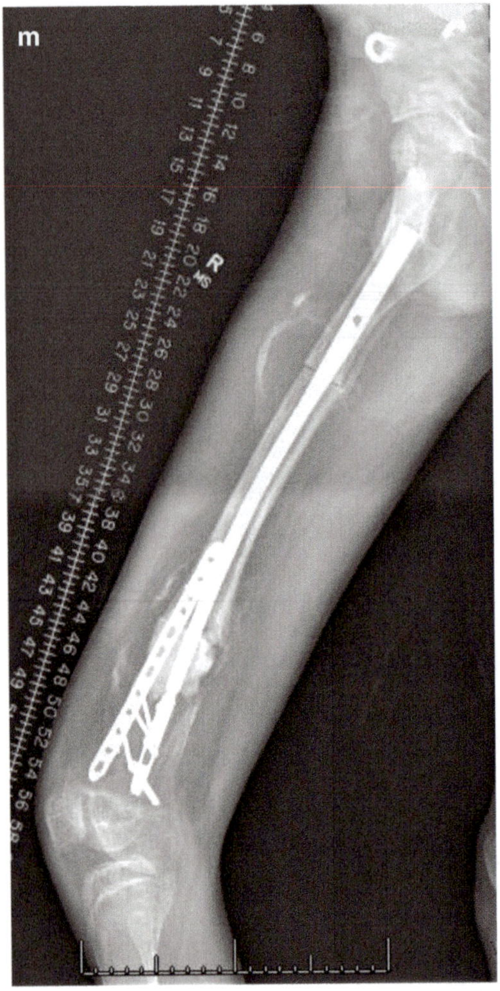

Fig. 34.4 (continued)

In addition, if immunosuppression is known or suspected, baseline investigations should include a peripheral blood smear. These tests will assess for the presence of lymphopenia, abnormal or unusual lymphocytes or phagocytic cells, and any associated gross hematologic abnormalities that may be indicative of a primary immune deficiency or underlying haematological malignancy. Full blood count and clotting studies are essential in identifying any pre-existing anaemia, thrombocytopenia or clotting disorder which may have an impact on surgical decision-making, timing of intervention and precautions that may need to be taken in the treatment of emergent infection. Baseline electrolytes and liver function including albumin should be performed to assess end organ function and as a surrogate marker for nutritional status.

Other diagnostic tools that may be considered for assessment of PID, after discussion with an immunologist, may include complement studies (C3, C4, CH50, APCH50), lymphocyte proliferation assays and flow cytometry, which allow for the enumeration of B-cells, T-cells and Natural Killer (NK) cells, and the evaluation of lymphocyte markers, T-cell variability and adhesion receptors that may be associated with specific immune defects [2].

Multiple peripheral blood cultures and tissue samples should be sent as soon as possible to allow identification of a pathogen. Atypical organisms are difficult to grow, often need extended culture and repeat sampling. Early discussion with a microbiologist is recommended, and utilization of polymerase chain reaction testing, if available, should be considered.

Mycobacterium tuberculosis infection should be actively considered and tested for separately, as it is not expected to grow on the standard culture medium. It is important to note that in the context of an immune deficiency, typical TB granuloma formation may be absent and may lead to histological ambiguity. It is recommended that the presence of mycobacterium infection should prompt investigation for co-existing HIV infection.

In patients with PID, early suspicion of atypical infection is crucial to ensure that appropriate culture media for organisms such as mycoplasmas and ureaplasmas are considered. Certain organisms may need special culture conditions or additional non-culture methods, such as polymerase chain reaction (PCR), 16S rRNA sequence analysis or DNA hybridization to identify the specific organism. Cultures may need to be incubated for a minimum of 6 weeks [5].

Treatment

Acute Infection

Infection in the immunocompromised child is associated with significant morbidity and mortality if not diagnosed and treated early. Due

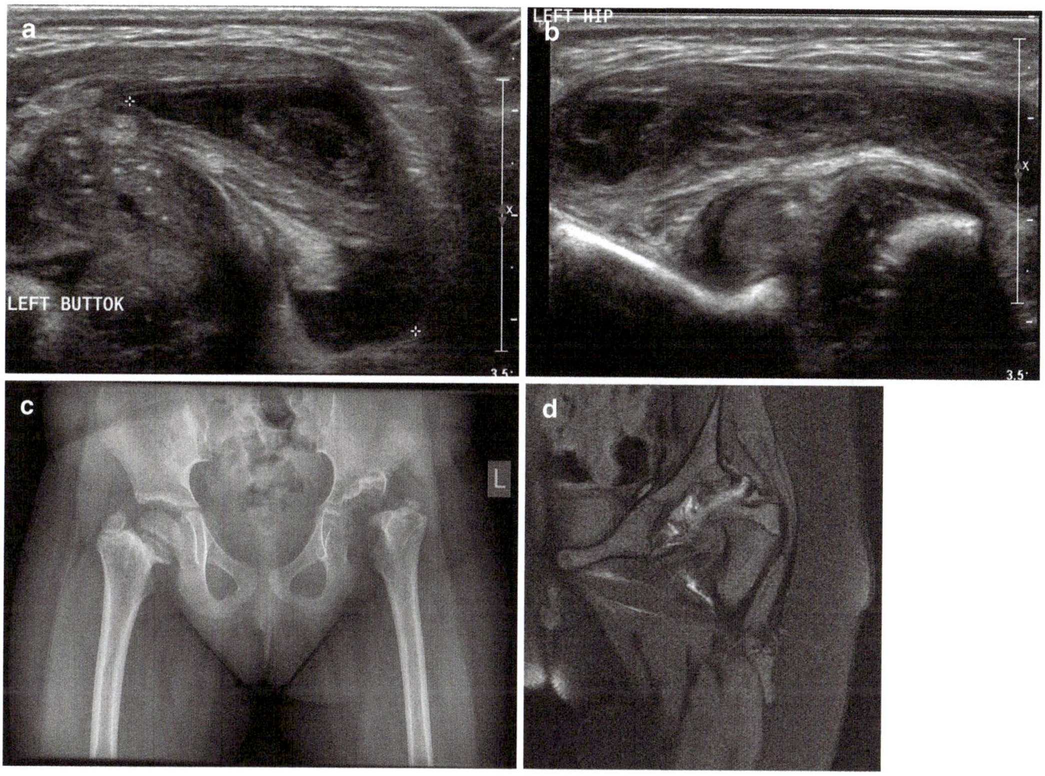

Fig. 34.5 Secondary haemophagocytic lymphohistiocytosis (HLH) in early infancy with undetectable IgA and group A Streptococcus multifocal infection, associated left buttock abscess, septic arthritis and late sequela affecting left hip. (**a**) Ultrasound of left buttock and (**b**) left hip demonstrating collections requiring surgical intervention. Late sequela can be seen on (**c**) plain radiograph and (**d**) coronal MRI scan demonstrating superior subluxation of femoral head, articulation with lateral acetabulum, relative overgrowth of greater trochanter and lack of femoral head ossification

to diminished immune response, systemic features of infection may be more subtle at presentation, infection may present at a much more established phase, and children may decompensate quickly.

Treatment is highly variable, and dependent on the type of MSK infection as well as the underlying cause of immunosuppression. The treatment principles and surgical intervention for acute MSK infection, such as septic arthritis and osteomyelitis, follow the same pathways as for an immune-competent child.

The treatment of the immunocompromised child, however, differs from that for the immunocompetent child in that the threshold for early and more aggressive intervention should be lower. Such children require emergent treatment, prompt assessment, resuscitation with adequate venous access, culturing and early broad-spectrum antimicrobial therapy, ideally given in consultation with a microbiologist's advice to ensure appropriate cover. Surgical intervention, if indicated, should not be delayed.

In severe cases, the child may need specialized critical care with prolonged treatment. Early involvement of a multidisciplinary team, including critical care, immunology, microbiology and paediatrics, is helpful to ensure a rapid diagnosis and to establish an appropriate individualized treatment plan for both the acute infective period and in long-term prevention of recurrence.

A broader range of organisms, including fungal infections, may be involved and, as such, the need for samples for culture is even greater. Initially, a broad spectrum of initial antibiotic therapy will be required until the exact organism is identified, and consideration should be given to the addition of antifungal cover. Typically, a longer duration of treatment is also required.

Specific Considerations for Surgery

Additional measures may need to be taken in the short term to medically optimize the child and, should they require surgical intervention, a number of specialist considerations must be taken into account.

Perioperative Care

Children with immune deficiencies may have pre-existing anaemia that, in some cases, may require pre- or post-operative blood transfusion. In some cases, irradiated, CMV-negative or leuco-depleted components may be required to prevent these patients from developing transfusion-associated graft versus host disease (TA-GVHD), which is a rare but often fatal complication. This condition may occur following therapy with whole blood, red cells, platelets and granulocytes, and is characterized by fever, maculopapular rash, diarrhoea, hepatitis and occasionally delayed jaundice. Significant tissue damage results, mainly due to the action of viable donor T-lymphocytes that can proliferate in a host with an impaired immune defence. Other haematological disorders, including clotting disorders and platelet dysfunction, may also be present, putting the child at risk of increased intraoperative bleeding unless identified and treated prior to surgical intervention [28].

Early emphasis should be given to establishing reliable venous access. Small children frequently require sedation or general anaesthesia early in treatment for either MRI or for surgery. In such instances it is recommended that early consideration is given to securing central venous access under the same general anaesthetic, as children typically require prolonged courses of intravenous antibiotics. In such children, recurrent peripheral cannulation can be distressing and difficult for both child and physician, leading to missed therapeutic intravenous doses and compromised treatment.

Nutritional Support

Severe infections in any child, regardless of their immune status, will cause a catabolic state and increased nutritional demand. As such, all children should be given adequate nutrition that surpasses their normal daily intake.

In cases of severe malnutrition, poor wound healing, increased surgical site infections, poor response to treatment and wound dehiscence may be exhibited. Early input from a paediatric dietician and nutritional support should be given; albumin may be monitored as a surrogate marker for overall nutrition. In resource-limited environments, pragmatic measures to enhance nutrition include diet supplementation with easily available food such as eggs, whole milk and peanut butter spread.

Micronutrient deficiencies commonly co-exist as part of the picture of global malnutrition. Vitamin and mineral supplementation is useful for those with diets deficient in vitamin C, vitamin D, zinc and other important nutritional elements.

Infection Control

Special consideration should be given to the immediate surroundings. The use of barrier nursing or protective isolation in a side room is essential to prevent risk of secondary infection, cross-infection or hospital-acquired infection. Where possible, a side room with HEPA filtration, lamina flow or positive room air pressure may be considered. Visitors should be limited to essential people only, should use barrier clothing, and should not be unwell [2].

Modification of Correctable Underlying Factors

Underlying risk factors for immunosuppression should be identified and modified where possible. It is recommended that individuals at risk of blood borne viruses undergo appropriate opportunistic screening to permit early diagnosis and treatment. In those with confirmed HIV, urgent review by a doctor with experience in infectious diseases is recommended. Antiretroviral medication should be prescribed to reduce and maintain a low viral load and healthy CD4 count, which is essential in treating established infection, and in reducing the risk of future infections. WHO recommends first-line treatment with dolutegravir-based antiretroviral treatment, which is now available in pediatric friendly dispersible tablets and can be used in children as young as 4 weeks old and who weigh >3 kg [29].

In low-income countries, chronic infections such as malaria and TB, or gastrointestinal infections such as threadworms or Schistosomiasis, are also common and easily treatable. Active infection, dysbiosis and pathogen colonization can cause mucosal dysfunction and inflammatory activation, negatively impacting nutritional status and increasing risk of life-threatening infection [21]. Recognition and eradication of treatable co-existing infection has the potential to improve the child's physiological reserves, and nutritional status, as well as improving overall immunological function.

In cases of iatrogenic drug-induced immunosuppression, it is recommended that a prompt discussion with the primary paediatrician or the MDT regarding whether these drugs should be stopped temporarily, may be stopped permanently, adjusted or replaced with an alternative during the period of acute infection and surgery.

Education of Child and Family

Long-term educational advice should be given to children and families to help promote a positive lifestyle and reduce the risk of recurrent infections. This includes advice on recognition of early signs of infection, when to seek help, modification of hygiene practices including regular washing, prevention of broken skin and an appropriate home environment. Advice on optimizing modifiable conditions, including maintaining a healthy balanced diet, general fitness, treatment compliance and attention to managing chronic disease are also ideally included in patient education discussions.

Family, Social, Educational and Spiritual Support

Immunocompromised children typically have co-existing long-term health conditions that necessitate regular, prolonged treatment and multiple hospital admissions. A holistic approach to both children and families is essential to ensure that they have any additional needs met, which may include educational or cognitive support, as well as physical, emotional or spiritual well-being.

Antibiotics

Antibiotic choice in immunocompromised children with infection is often complex due to a history of recurrent infections, often multiple concurrent sites of infection, and a reduced immune response. It is recommended that these children be discussed with a microbiologist. Often children have had frequent hospital exposures and consideration should be given to initial treatment with empirical antibiotics that include cover for MRSA and anti-fungal cover. Common pathogens include encapsulated bacteria and opportunistic organisms. Less usual organisms include pneumococcus, meningococcus and haemophilus, and warrant further investigations. It is important to note that most invasive haemophilus infections in the United Kingdom are non-type B and are not covered by the HiB vaccine given as part of many childhood immunization programmes.

Multiple peripheral blood cultures and tissue samples should be sent as soon as possible to allow identification of a pathogen, which may be opportunistic or atypical, allow for microbial sensitivity testing and the creation of a targeted treatment plan. Unusual organisms include salmonella, serratus, aspergillus, multifocal staphylococcus infection and atypical mycobacteria (Table 34.3).

Specific Considerations for PID

Severe disorders such as Severe Combined Immunodeficiencies (SCID) require definitive therapy for immune reconstitution with bone marrow transplant (BMT) or haematopoietic stem cell therapy (HSCT) as soon as possible. SCID is fatal unless the underlying defect is corrected and, therefore, definitive therapy with BMT or HSCT should be initiated as quickly as possible [4].

Antibiotic and antifungal prophylaxis is also recommended for many PIDs to prevent the frequency and severity of infections. Other PID treatments vary depending on the type of defect, but may involve antifungal and antibiotic prophylaxis, cytokine replacement, vaccinations and bone marrow transplant. Specific considerations or potential treatments are listed in Table 34.4 [4].

Table 34.4 Specific considerations for long-term treatment of children with PID

Supportive	Immunoglobulin replacement Antibiotics prophylaxis Antifungal prophylaxis Increased infection control measures during hospital admissions Optimization of co-morbidities Vaccinations (live vaccines may be contradicted) Cytokine replacement such as interferon (innate)
Definitive	Bone marrow transplant Haematopoietic stem cell transplant Gene therapies

Table 34.3 Examples of common typical and opportunistic infections to consider in MSK infection in children

MSK infection	Typical organisms	Opportunistic/atypical
Septic arthritis	*Staphylococcus aureus* *Kingella kingae* *Streptococcus pneumoniae* *Streptococcus pyogenes* *Haemophilus influenzae* *Neisseria gonorrhoea* (adolescent)	Pseudomonas, Bacteroides, Fusobacterium Propionibacterium, Salmonella
Osteomyelitis	*S. aureus* *K. kingae* *S. pneumoniae* *S. pyogenes* *H. influenzae*	*Mycobacterium tuberculosis* Bartonella Histoplasma Cryptococcus Salmonella Candida (spondylodiscitis)
Pyomyositis	*S. aureus* Strep including Group A *Escherichia coli* Pseudomonas *M. tuberculosis*	Actinomyces Bacillus Fungal Viral

Conclusion

Treatment of MSK infection in the context of an immune-compromised child presents both diagnostic and management challenges. The mainstay of assessment and surgical treatment is the same as for an immune-competent child. However, treatment of acute infection should be prompt and aggressive to prevent deterioration to severe sepsis or chronic infection, which may be more difficult to treat. A high index of suspicion should be raised by children with atypical presentations, unusual infective organisms, co-existing diseases, or a family history of immune-compromised conditions. Early involvement of the MDT is imperative to allow prompt, accurate diagnosis and reduction in overall morbidity and mortality. In patients with irreversible immune-compromised conditions, long-term measures should be explored to reduce risk of recurrence. Treatment of underlying secondary causes and patient education should be employed to reverse immunocompromised states if possible.

Box 34.1 Key Take Home Points

- Clinical presentation is variable. Atypical clinical presentations, recurrent infections or difficult to eradicate infection should raise suspicion of an underlying immune problem.
- Immune system compromise in children is more common than previously thought.
- Most underlying causes are acquired and modifiable.
- Where possible, early involvement of a multidisciplinary team including a microbiologist and paediatrician is recommended.
- Acute infection can be severe and life-threatening. Rapid assessment and treatment without delay is essential.
- If surgery is required, then specific adjustments to pre-, peri- and post-operative care are likely to be needed.
- Treatment should include education and primary prevention strategies to reduce the risk of future infection.

References

1. Butler BA, Fitz DW, Lawton CD, Li DD, Balderama ES, Stover MD. Early diagnosis of septic arthritis in immunocompromised patients. J Orthop Sci. 2018;23(3):542–5.
2. O'Brien R. Assessment of suspected immunodeficiency in childhood. Paediatr Child Health. 2016; https://doi.org/10.1016/j.paed.2016.10.005. Accessed 21 Nov 2020.
3. Jeffrey Modell Foundation. Primary Immunodeficiency Resource Centre. 2020. http://www.info4pi.org/aboutPI/index.cfm?section=aboutPI&content=warningsigns&TrkId=24&CFID=40303331&CFTOKEN=79353748. Accessed Nov 11 2020.
4. McCusker C, Warrington R. Primary immunodeficiency. Allergy asthma. Clin Immunol. 2011;7(1):S11.
5. Bloom KA, Chung D, Cunningham-Rundles C. Osteoarticular infectious complications in patients with primary immunodeficiencies. Curr Opin Rheumatol. 2008;20(4):480–5.
6. Norrish AR, Bates JHJ, Harrison WJ. Overgrowth causing limb length discrepancy in chronic long bone osteomyelitis: a consecutive series of 42 patients. Orthopaed Proc. 2008;90-B:521–52.
7. Bousfiha A, Jeddane L, Picard C, Al-Herz W, Ailal F, Chatila T, et al. Human inborn errors of immunity: 2019 update of the IUIS phenotypical classification. J Clin Immunol. 2020;40(1):66–81.
8. Bonilla FA, Bernstein IL, Khan DA, Ballas ZK, Chinen J, Frank MM, et al. Practice parameter for the diagnosis and management of primary immunodeficiency. Ann Allergy Asthma Immunol. 2005;94(5,1):S1–63.
9. International Union of Immunological Societies Expert Committee on Primary Immunodeficiencies, Notarangelo LD, Fischer A, Geha RS, Casanova JL, Chapel H, et al. Primary immunodeficiencies: 2009 update. J Allergy Clin Immunol. 2009;124(6):1161–78.
10. Shillitoe B, Bangs C, Guzman D, Gennery AR, Longhurst HJ, Slatter M, et al. The United Kingdom primary immune deficiency (UKPID) registry 2012 to 2017. Clin Exp Immunol. 2018;192(3):284–91.
11. Grimbacher B, ESID Registry Working Party. The European Society for Immunodeficiencies (ESID) registry 2014. Clin Exp Immunol. 2014;178(1):18–20.
12. Boyle JM, Buckley RH. Population prevalence of diagnosed primary immunodeficiency diseases in the United States. J Clin Immunol. 2007;27(5):497–502.
13. Hammarström L, Vorechovsky I, Webster D. Selective IgA deficiency (SIgAD) and common variable immunodeficiency (CVID). Clin Exp Immunol. 2000;120(2):225–31.
14. Al-Mousa H, Al-Saud B. Primary immunodeficiency diseases in highly consanguineous populations from Middle East and North Africa: epidemiology, diagnosis, and care. Front Immunol. 2017;8:678.
15. Bustamante J, Boisson-Dupuis S, Abel L, Casanova JL. Mendelian susceptibility to mycobacterial disease: genetic, immunological, and clinical features of inborn errors of IFN-γ immunity. Semin Immunol. 2014;26(6):454–70.

16. Rytter MJ, Kolte L, Briend A, Friis H, Christensen VB. The immune system in children with malnutrition--a systematic review. PLoS One. 2014;9(8):e105017.
17. Kato S, Chmielewski M, Honda H, Pecoits-Filho R, Matsuo S, Yuzawa Y, Tranaeus A, Stenvinkel P, Lindholm B. Aspects of immune dysfunction in end-stage renal disease. Clin J Am Soc Nephrol. 2008;3(5):1526–33.
18. Ashorobi D, Fernandez R. Asplenia. In: StatPearls [Internet]. Treasure Island: StatPearls Publishing; 2020. https://www.ncbi.nlm.nih.gov/books/NBK538171/. Accessed 29 Dec 2020.
19. Van Crevel R, Van de Vijver S, Moore DAJ. The global diabetes epidemic: what does it mean for infectious diseases in tropical countries? Lancet Diabetes Endocrinol. 2017;5(6):457–68.
20. WHO. Malnutrition is a world health crisis. 2019. https://www.who.int/news/item/26-09-2019-malnutrition-is-a-world-health-crisis. Accessed Nov 08 2020.
21. Walson JL, Berkley JA. The impact of malnutrition on childhood infections. Curr Opin Infect Dis. 2018;31(3):231–6.
22. BAPEN. BAPEN statement: cases of child malnutrition in England double in the last six months. bapen.org.uk. 2020. https://www.bapen.org.uk/bapen-statements/child-malnutrition-in-england-doubles. Accessed 29 Dec 2020.
23. World Health Organisation. Child growth standards. https://www.who.int/tools/child-growth-standards/standards. Accessed 12 Dec 2020.
24. Pludowski P, Holick MF, Pilz S, Wagner CL, Hollis BW, Grant WB, et al. Vitamin D effects on musculoskeletal health, immunity, autoimmunity, cardiovascular disease, cancer, fertility, pregnancy, dementia and mortality-a review of recent evidence. Autoimmun Rev. 2013;12(10):976–89.
25. UNICEF. Global and regional trends. July 2020. https://data.unicef.org/topic/hivaids/global-regional-trends/. Accessed 20 Jan 2021.
26. World Health Organisation. Children and cancer. WHO Training Package for the Health Sector. www.who.int/ceh/capacity/cancer.pdf Accessed 12 Dec 2020.
27. World Health Organisation. Cancer in children. https://www.who.int/news-room/fact-sheets/detail/cancer-in-children. Accessed 12 Dec 2020.
28. Badami KG. The immunocompromised patient and transfusion. Postgrad Med J. 2001;77(906):230–4.
29. UNAIDS. Joint statement calling for urgent country scale-up of access to optimal HIV treatment for infants and children living with HIV. https://www.unaids.org/en/keywords/children. Accessed 20 Jan 2021.
30. National Organisation for Rare Disease. Pyknodysostosis. https://rarediseases.org/rare-diseases/pyknodysostosis/. Accessed 12 July 2020.
31. National Organisation for Rare Disease. https://rarediseases.org/rare-diseases/osteopetrosis/. Accessed 12 July 2020.
32. Ihde L, et al. Sclerosing bone dysplasias: review and differentiation from other causes of osteosclerosis. RadioGraphics. 2011;31(7):1865–82.
33. Bhargava A, Vagela M, Lennox CME. Injury. Int J Care Injured. 2009;40:1167–71.
34. AlDallal SM. Osteomyelitis: a manifestation of sickle cell anemia. Clin Med Invest 2. 2017; https://doi.org/10.15761/CMI.1000132.
35. Farii HA, Zhou S, Albers A. J Am Acad Orthop Surg Glob Res Rev. 2020;4(9):e20.00002.

Fungal Infections

35

Mandar Agashe, Binoti Sheth,
and Mohan V. Belthur

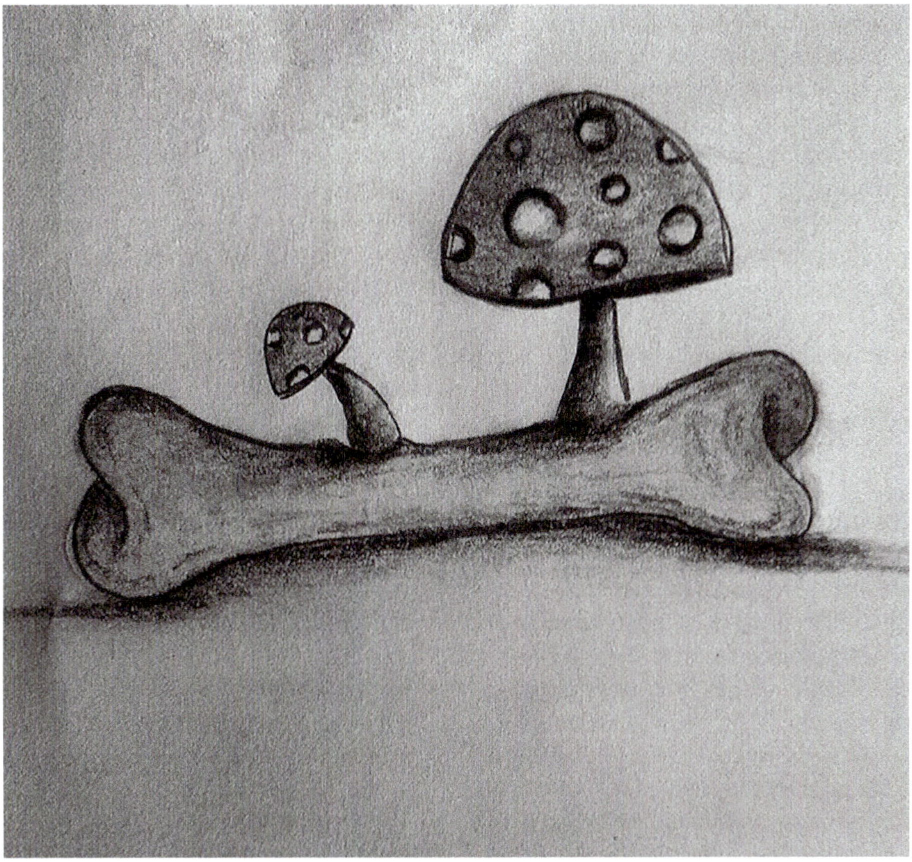

M. Agashe (✉)
Agashe's Paediatric SuperSpeciality Clinic,
Mumbai, India

Childrens' Hip Preservation Services, (CHiPS),
SRCC Childrens' Hospital, Mumbai, India

BJ Wadia Hospital for Children, Mumbai, India

B. Sheth
Department of Orthopaedics, LTMGH and LTM
Medical College, Mumbai, India

M. V. Belthur
Department of Child Health & Orthopedics,
University of Arizona College of Medicine,
Phoenix, AZ, USA

Department of Orthopedics, Phoenix Children's
Hospital, Phoenix, AZ, USA
e-mail: mbelthur@phoenixchildrens.com

© Springer Nature Switzerland AG 2022
M. V. Belthur et al. (eds.), *Pediatric Musculoskeletal Infections*,
https://doi.org/10.1007/978-3-030-95794-0_35

Introduction

A fungus is a member of the group of eukaryotic organisms that includes microorganisms such as yeasts and molds, as well as the more familiar mushrooms [1]. They have a worldwide distribution and about 120,000 species have been described, with over 300 that can be pathogenic to humans [2]. Fungi are an uncommon but important cause of musculoskeletal (MSK) infections in children. The presentation varies widely, ranging from indolent to rapidly destructive, and diagnosis requires a high index of suspicion. Symptoms are often subacute and may masquerade as other disorders, which can lead to substantial delays in treatment. Diagnosis of an indolent infection can be difficult secondary to lack of a significant host response. The severity of the infection depends on the host immune status, pathogenicity of the specific fungus, anatomic site of infection, and presence of foreign bodies [3]. Sometimes, the infection can be potentially life threatening. There is paucity of literature on fungal musculoskeletal infection in children. Hence, diagnosis and management can be challenging at times.

Epidemiology

Although invasive fungal infections contribute substantially to human morbidity and mortality, and their impact on human health is steadily growing, fungal MSK infections are still considered as an uncommon disease [4, 5]. There has been a worldwide increase in the burden of invasive fungal musculoskeletal infections in children in recent times, due to the growing number of patients at risk. Travel and immigration have affected the geographic localization of several important fungal infections, which may be seen in nonendemic areas. The most common fungi causing musculoskeletal infections in children are *Candida* [6, 7], *Aspergillus* [7, 8], dimorphic fungi like *Blastomyces* [8], *Coccidioides* [8], *Histoplasma* [9], and *Cryptococcus* [2, 7]. Less common pathogens include Sporothrix, non-aspergillus filamentous fungi [10] (Hyaline Hyphomycetes, Mucormycetes, Dematiaceous fungi), and eumycetes [11]. There is a wide variation in the geographic distribution of musculoskeletal infection due to various types of fungal species. Table 35.1 provides details of the geographic distribution, environmental microbiology, host characteristics, and annual prevalence of the common fungi causing musculoskeletal infections.

Classification of Fungi

Fungi causing MSK infections can be classified morphologically as belonging to the following groups: (Table 35.1 and Fig. 35.1).

1. *Yeasts:* Fungi that grow as single cells, producing daughter cells either by budding or by binary fission. Sometimes, the bud remains attached to the mother cell, elongates and undergoes repeated budding to form chains of elongated cells known as pseudohyphae.
   (a) Without pseudohyphae: *Cryptococcus* [27]
   (b) With pseudohyphae: *Candida* [3]
2. *Filamentous fungi (Molds):* This subtype is characterized by multinucleated, filamentous fungi composed of *hyphae.* A hypha is an elongated cell producing a tubular thread-like structure. A hypha may be septate or aseptate. A septate hypha is a branching, tubular structure from 2 to 10 μm in diameter and is usually divided into cell-like units divided by cross-walls called *septae*. The total mass of hyphae is termed a *mycelium*. Molds reproduce primarily by means of *asexual reproductive spores.* These spores are disseminated by air, water, animals or objects and, upon landing in a suitable environment, germinate and produce new hyphae.
   (a) *Aseptate hyphae: Rhizopus* spp., *Mucor* spp. [12]
   (b) *Septate hyphae: Aspergillus* spp., *Scedosporium* spp., *Fusarium* spp. [13]
3. *Dimorphic fungi:* Fungi that can exist in the form of both mold and yeast. This is usually brought about by a change in temperature. They exhibit a yeast form in host tissue and enriched media at 37 °C and a mycelial form at 25 °C in vitro. Examples include *Coccidioides* spp. [14], *Blastomyces dermatidis* [15], *Histoplasma capsulatum* [16], *Sporothrix schenkii* [17], and *Paracoccidioides braziliensis.* These fungi show thermal dimorphism. In the soil (22–25 °C), they grow as mold, producing spores that are the infecting particles. Following soil disruption, aerosolized mycelial fragments and

Table 35.1 Epidemiology of common fungal pathogens causing MSK infections

Organism/fungus type	Environmental microbiology	Geographic location	Host characteristics	Frequency of invasive fungal infection
Aspergillus spp (mold) opportunistic	Soil, decaying vegetation	Worldwide	Neutropenia, steroids, transplantations, trauma, primary immune deficiencies	>300,000 cases/year
Blastomyces (dimorphic) Systemic	Soil, Pine forests, beaver dams	Southeast, South Central USA/ Canada, North Central, Mid-Atlantic USA	Usually immunocompetent	1–2/100,000 population in endemic areas
Candida spp (yeast) opportunistic	Normal human Flora	Worldwide	Non-neutropenic, surgical procedures, trauma	>750,000 cases/year
Coccidioides (dimorphic) systemic	Soil, dust,	Southwest USA, Central & South America	Usually immunocompetent	>25–100,000 symptomatic cases/ year
Cryptococcus (yeast) opportunistic	Pigeon droppings, soil	Worldwide, NW USA, Western Canada	Impaired cell-mediated immunity like AIDS, steroids	>200,000 cases/year
Histoplasma (dimorphic) systemic	Soil, bat guano, starling droppings	Mid-western USA, Central & South America	Often immune compromised with impaired cell- mediated immunity	>25–100,000 symptomatic cases/ year
Sporothrix (dimorphic) Subcutaneous	Soil, woody plants,	Worldwide, Mexico, Peru are endemic areas	Impaired cell mediated immunity	1–2 per million population 25/1000 population in endemic areas
Non-aspergillus (dimorphic), opportunistic Hyaline hyphomycetes Mucormycetes Dematiaceous fungi	Soil, decaying vegetation,	Worldwide	Hematologic malignancies, steroids, transplantations	Uncommon with relative frequency of 75, 15 and 10% respectively
Mycetoma Actinomycetes (bacteria) Eumycetes (fungi), Subcutaneous	Soil, decaying vegetation	Tropical & Subtropical Belt, 15° S & 30° N	Agricultural workers, barefoot walkers, trauma	>18,000 cases reported 3–4/100,000 population in endemic areas

spores inhaled into the lungs (37 °C) convert into pathogenic yeast and cause infection.

Classification of Fungal Diseases

Fungal MSK diseases can be categorized into the following clinical types (Table 35.1) [3, 27]:

(a) *Subcutaneous mycoses:* These are the mycotic infections of the skin, subcutaneous tissue and sometimes bone, resulting from inoculation of saprophytic fungi of soil or decaying matter. They are mainly confined to the tropics and subtropics.

(b) *Systemic mycoses:* They involve multiple organs. Most are caused by the saprophytic fungi, which spread by inhalation of spores leading to pulmonary infection. From lungs, they disseminate to cause various systemic manifestations.

(c) *Opportunistic mycoses:* They are caused by fungi that are normally found as human commensals or in the environment but can act as human pathogens in the presence of opportunities, such as an immunocompromised patient.

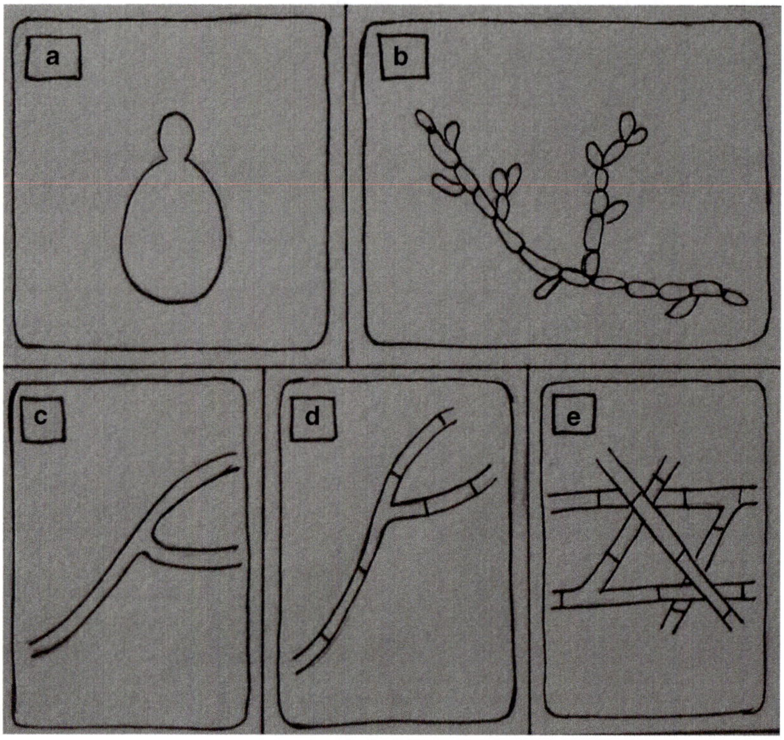

Fig. 35.1 (**a**–**e**) Morphological classification of various fungi causing human infection. (**a**) Budding yeast cell, (**b**) budding yeast with pseudohyphae, (**c**) aseptate hyphae, (**d**) septate hyphae, (**e**) mycelium. (Illustrated by Ms. Rashmi Oka)

Etiopathogenesis

Fungal musculoskeletal infections are caused by a wide variety of commensal, zoonotic and environmental yeasts and molds. Most of these infections occur in immunocompromised hosts, but healthy immunocompetent hosts can also develop these infections at times [1]. Alterations of human flora, disruption of mucocutaneous membranes, and impaired immune function predispose to fungal infections. The outcome of exposure to the pathogen is influenced by the inoculum size, functional integrity of the host cellular immune function, strain-specific virulence factors, and pre-existing immunity. Fungal osteoarticular infection may occur as part of a multisystem process or in isolation [8].

Risk Factors

The risk factors for fungal musculoskeletal infection are as follows: inherited or acquired defects of cell-mediated immunity, immunosuppression secondary to an underlying disease or related to medication, parenteral nutrition, aggressive cancer chemotherapy, presence of an indwelling central venous catheter, use of broad-spectrum antibiotics, HIV infection, substance abuse, alcoholism, presence of foreign bodies or implants, post-organ transplantation, diabetes mellitus, cirrhosis, renal failure, and malignancy [18, 27].

Modes of Spread

There are three possible modes of spread of fungal musculoskeletal infections.

1. Direct inoculation after traumatic injuries that are contaminated with soil via an open wound or post-surgery
2. Contiguous spread from an adjacent focus of infection
3. Hematogenous dissemination, especially in immunocompromised children with fungemia

Bones Involved

Fungal musculoskeletal infection can involve any bone or joint, but the large weight-bearing joints are more commonly involved. The bones commonly involved in children are the femur and humerus, unlike in adults where the vertebrae and ribs are more involved. The femur and humerus are, respectively, 14 and 46 times more likely to be infected in children compared to adults while vertebrae are >7 times less likely to be infected in children compared to adults. Multiple bones are involved in 1% cases [1, 18].

Specific Populations

Certain populations are at increased risk for developing fungal MSK infections. These include:

(a) Neonates: Neonates constitute a vulnerable population for fungal musculoskeletal infection due to additional risk factors like low birth weight, prematurity, NICU stay, umbilical vein catheterization, necrotizing enterocolitis, GI surgery, immunodeficiency, and malignancy. The most common causative organism is *Candida*, mostly *C. albicans* [7, 19].
(b) Patients with Chronic Granulomatous Disease (CGD): CGD is a rare primary immunodeficiency genetic condition in which NADPH (nicotinamide adenine dinucleotide phosphate) oxidase complex fails to generate reactive oxygen species (ROS) in the activated neutrophils, monocytes, and macrophages. Hence, there is an inability to destroy microorganisms. It occurs due to a single gene defect, either X-linked recessive (60%) or autosomal recessive (40%). Two-thirds of the patients <5 years of age present with recurrent bacterial or fungal infections. The overall incidence of fungal infections in CGD patients is 20%. *Aspergillus fumigatus* is responsible for 80–90% of invasive aspergillosis in CGD patients [6, 20].

Diagnosis

The time to diagnosis is typically improved when the clinician considers this entity, and supports the suspicion with a combination of microbiologic, histopathologic, immunologic, or radiographic evidence [6]. Labs are characterized by elevated inflammatory markers [1, 21]. Radiographs are positive 60–70% of the time, are non-specific, showing cortical destruction, periosteal reaction with new bone formation or sclerosis. Magnetic resonance imaging (MRI) is the most accurate diagnostic modality [4, 22]. MRI findings, though non-specific, typically shows an extensive bony involvement with wide zone of transition and subtle burrowing into the medullary cavity. It may also show patchy peripheral hypointensity along with central hypointensity representing an abscess formation. Tissue biopsy is essential for diagnosis and all samples should be sent for culture, smear, and histologic examinations [23].

Differential Diagnosis

Chronic bacterial infections, typical and atypical mycobacterial infections, actinomycetes, Ewing's and osteosarcoma.

Management

The goals of management are eradication of the infection and prevention of future recurrences [7]. Collaboration with an infectious disease specialist is recommended to provide an appropriate antifungal treatment plan and to monitor the patients. Medical management alone may be successful for mild and early disease. A combination of medical and surgical treatment is recommended for advanced disease [24]. Medical management usually involves using antifungal medications (Tables 35.2 and 35.3). Typically, combination therapy is recommended to prevent development of resistance and reduce toxicity [25].

Surgical Management

The surgical recommendations for musculoskeletal fungal infections are relatively nonspecific, but generally follow the principles of surgical treatment of tuberculosis osteomyelitis. Surgery can be a critical component in management of

Table 35.2 Diagnosis and management of common fungal pathogens involved in MSK infections

Fungus type (organism)	Special tests	First-line treatment (Dosage)	Alternative treatment (Dosage)
Aspergillus spp (Mold)	GMS stain may show fungal hyphae. Fungal media required for tissue and synovial fluid culture	Voriconazole IV (6 mg/kg q 12 h for 1 d then 4 mg/kg q 12 h). Voriconazole oral (200 mg q 12 h)	Liposomal AMB (3–5 mg/kg/d); AMB lipid complex (5 mg/kg/d IV)
Blastomyces (dimorphic)	Wet mount microscopy of synovial fluid will be positive for broad-based budding yeast. GMS stain of tissue. Fungal media required for tissue culture	AMB (0.7–1 mg/kg/d for 1–2 week or until improvement) then itraconazole (200 mg tid for 3 d then 200 mg bid for 12 mo)	
Candida spp (yeast)	Grows in routine media used for bacterial cultures. Susceptibility testing may be required if the pathogen is resistant to common antifungals	Fluconazole (400 mg 1 q d) for 6–12 months for osteomyelitis or at least 6 weeks for septic arthritis	AMB (3–5 mg/kg for at least 2 weeks) then fluconazole to make for a full 6–12 months for osteomyelitis or at least 6 weeks for septic arthritis
Coccidioides (dimorphic)	Serum antibody (complement fixation titers 0.1:32)	Fluconazole (400 mg/d); itraconazole (200 mg bid or tid); ketoconazole 400 mg/d	AMB (0.5–1.5 mg/kg/d); liposomal formulation AMB (2–5 mg/kg/d)
Cryptococcus (yeast)	Serum cryptococcal antigen and GMS and periodic acid–Schiff stains of tissue, lumbar puncture to detect occult CNS infection	No meningoencephalitis: Fluconazole (400 mg/d) for 6–12 mo. Meningoencephalitis present: AMB (0.7–1.0 mg/kg/d) 5- flucytosine (100 mg/kg/d) or liposomal AMB (3–4 mg/k/d)	Itraconazole (200 mg PO bid); voriconazole (200 mg PO bid);
Histoplasma (dimorphic)	ELISA, PCR, GMS stain	Liposomal formulation AMB (3–5 mg/kg/d IV) for 1–2 weeks then itraconazole (200 mg tid) for 3 d then 1 q d or bid for 6–12 weeks.	AMB (0.7–1.0 mg/kg/d IV)
Sporothrix (dimorphic)	Mycologic culture is typically required for definitive diagnosis. ELISA, PCR, Sporotrichin skin test	Itraconazole (200 mg PO bid) for at least 12 months	AMB (0.7–1.0 mg/kg/d) then itraconazole (200 mg bid) for 12 months
Non-aspergillus (dimorphic) Hyaline hyphomycetes Mucormycetes Dematiaceous fungi	GMS stain may show fungal hyphae. Fungal media required for tissue and synovial fluid culture	Voriconazole IV (6 mg/kg q 12 h for 1 d then 4 mg/kg q 12 h). Voriconazole oral (200 mg q 12 h) for 6 months	Liposomal AMB (3–5 mg/kg/d); AMB lipid complex (5 mg/kg/d IV)
Mycetoma Actinomycetes (bacteria) Eumycetes (fungi)	Deep tissue biopsy with H& E stain, Immuno-fluorescent antibody and immuno-histochemical techniques are also helpful	Actinomycetes - Amikacin sulfate 15 mg/kg twice daily for 3 weeks and co-trimoxazole 1.5 mg/kg twice daily for 5 weeks. The cycle is repeated until cure is achieved	Eumycetes- itraconazole 200–400 mg per day or voriconazole 300–400 mg per day for a mean of 9–12 months

cases with extensive destructive lesions, large abscesses, progressive tissue destruction, bony sequestrations, vertebral instability, or impingement on critical organs. Surgical debridement should include thorough curettage of all grossly involved bone, and, in cases of spinal disease, radical debridement with drainage of paravertebral/epidural fluid collections and fusion with or without instrumentation [18, 27]. Amphotericin B impregnated cement spacers or beads may be used for dead space management in bone cavities [10]. Synovectomy is beneficial in patients with

Table 35.3 Antifungal medications with common side effects

Class	Drug	Mechanism	Use	Side effects
Antifungal antibiotics				
Polyenes	Amphotericin B	Bind to ergosterol and disrupts fungal cell membranes	Systemic, opportunistic, subcutaneous mycoses	Renal toxicity, febrile reactions
Echinocandins	Capsofungin, micafungin	Inhibits glucan synthesis in fungal cell wall	Aspergillus, candidiasis	Uncommon, nausea, vomiting
Synthetic antifungals				
Azoles – imidazoles	Ketoconazole	Inhibits ergosterol synthesis of fungi	Blastomycosis, candidiasis, Coccidioides, Cryptococcus, histoplasmosis	Hepatotoxicity, nausea, vomiting, adrenal hormone suppression
Azoles – triazoles	Fluconazole, itraconazole, voriconazole Posaconazole	Inhibits ergosterol synthesis of fungi	Aspergillus, blastomycosis, candidiasis, Coccidioides, Cryptococcus, histoplasmosis, Sporothrix	GI toxicity, nausea, vomiting
Antimetabolite	Flucytosine (5 FC)	Inhibits DNA synthesis in fungi; is converted to fluorouracil which inhibits thymidylate synthetase	Candida, Cryptococcus	GI toxicity, hepatotoxicity

septic arthritis. When adjacent bone disease is present, debridement should be performed.

Alternative Antifungal Delivery Methods

Antifungal-impregnated polymethyl methacrylate (PMMA) bone cement has been used clinically for fungal bone and joint infections [10, 27]. The elution of most antifungal agents from PMMA is worse than that of antibacterial agents. Non-bioactive polymers, such as PMMA, typically require surgical removal, whereas bioactive osteoconductive materials do not. Amphotericin B elution levels from all bioactive and non-bioactive cements were found to be consistent for 110 days [27]. Use of other antifungal medications is still being studied.

Common Fungal MSK Infections in Children (Table 35.2)

Candidiasis

This is an opportunistic mycosis and the most common fungal disease in children, caused by *Candida*, a yeast-like fungus that produces pseudohyphae (Fig. 35.2a, b). Over the last few years, with the advent of highly potent anti-bacterial agents being used in bacterial sepsis, candida septic arthritis, and osteomyelitis are recently emerging as relatively common secondary infections [1, 7, 19]. Candida bone and joint infections occur more commonly following disseminated candidemia and may cause significant morbidity if not treated early and effectively [26].

Epidemiology

Candidiasis has a worldwide distribution. Most of the cases of candida MSK infections in children are septic arthritis (SA), and more than 70% occur in the neonatal period [18]. Most of the patients with candida SA occur following hematogenous transmission secondary to underlying immunocompromising conditions like neonatal sepsis, hematological malignancies, and stem cell transplantation [7, 27]. Candida osteomyelitis (OM) is much less common and contiguous spread is more likely [19, 21].

Pathogenesis

Most (almost 60–70%) candidal infections occur due to Candida albicans (*C. albicans*). Other common species are *C. tropicalis (14%),*

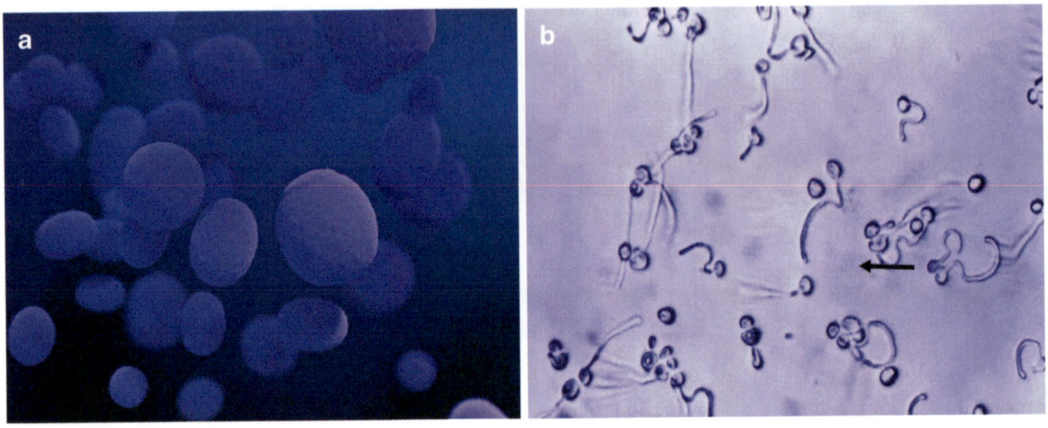

Fig. 35.2 (**a**) Medical illustration of *Candida* sp. organisms. (Source: Public Health Image ID#23240/Stephanie Rossow 2019/Centre for Disease Control and Prevention (Atlanta)/With Permission. (**b**) Photomicrograph of *Candida albicans* spores suspended and allowed to grow in animal serum, giving rise to filamentous spores (Black arrow). (Source: Public Health Image ID#21794/Dr. Lucille K. Georg/Centre for Disease Control and Prevention (Atlanta)/With permission)

C. parapsilosis (11%), C. krusei (4%), C. gibralta (2%), and *C. lusitaniae (2%)*. As previously explained, the commonest population in children with candidal osteoarticular infections are neonates, infants and toddlers. Virulence factors such as adhesins and enzymes (aspartyl and serine proteases) enhance tissue adhesion and invasion. Phenotypic dimorphism enables adaptation to changing conditions in the host and thereby assists the fungus in evading the host defense system [19].

Clinical Features

The common clinical manifestations of candida SA-OM are pain, tenderness and swelling of the affected part/joint, with an onset which is usually sub-acute. The host is usually susceptible secondary to an immunocompromised condition. The typical host is a neonate or an infant who is in the NICU for a long period of time or an NICU graduate with a past history of neonatal bacterial sepsis. The child is currently or in the past has been on multiple antibiotics. The typical features of acute septic arthritis of severe pain and swelling along with fever may not be present due to the sub-acute nature of the illness (Fig. 35.3a, d). In case of OM, there may be some surrounding erythema along with the presence of sinus tracts in a minority of cases.

The most common joints involved for candida SA are knee, hip, shoulder and elbow in that sequence while the femur, tibia, vertebrae, and humerus are the commonest bones involved for candidal OM [7, 19]. Recurrence is common in candidal SA-OM as long as 18 months after successful treatment and, hence, care should be taken to not miss a diagnosis of recurrence.

Imaging Studies

Plain radiographs are usually not sensitive enough to identify changes of candidal infections, especially early in the disease. Late cases of OM may show bony destruction as well as rarefaction, along with joint space widening and dislocations.

Magnetic resonance imaging (MRI) is most sensitive in identifying early disease, though the changes are not specific to candidal SA-OM [23]. Decreased signal intensity on T1-weighted images and increased signal intensity on T2-weighted images is typical of infective processes. In addition, bony destruction, loss of articular cartilage, joint effusion, and cystic changes are seen very commonly.

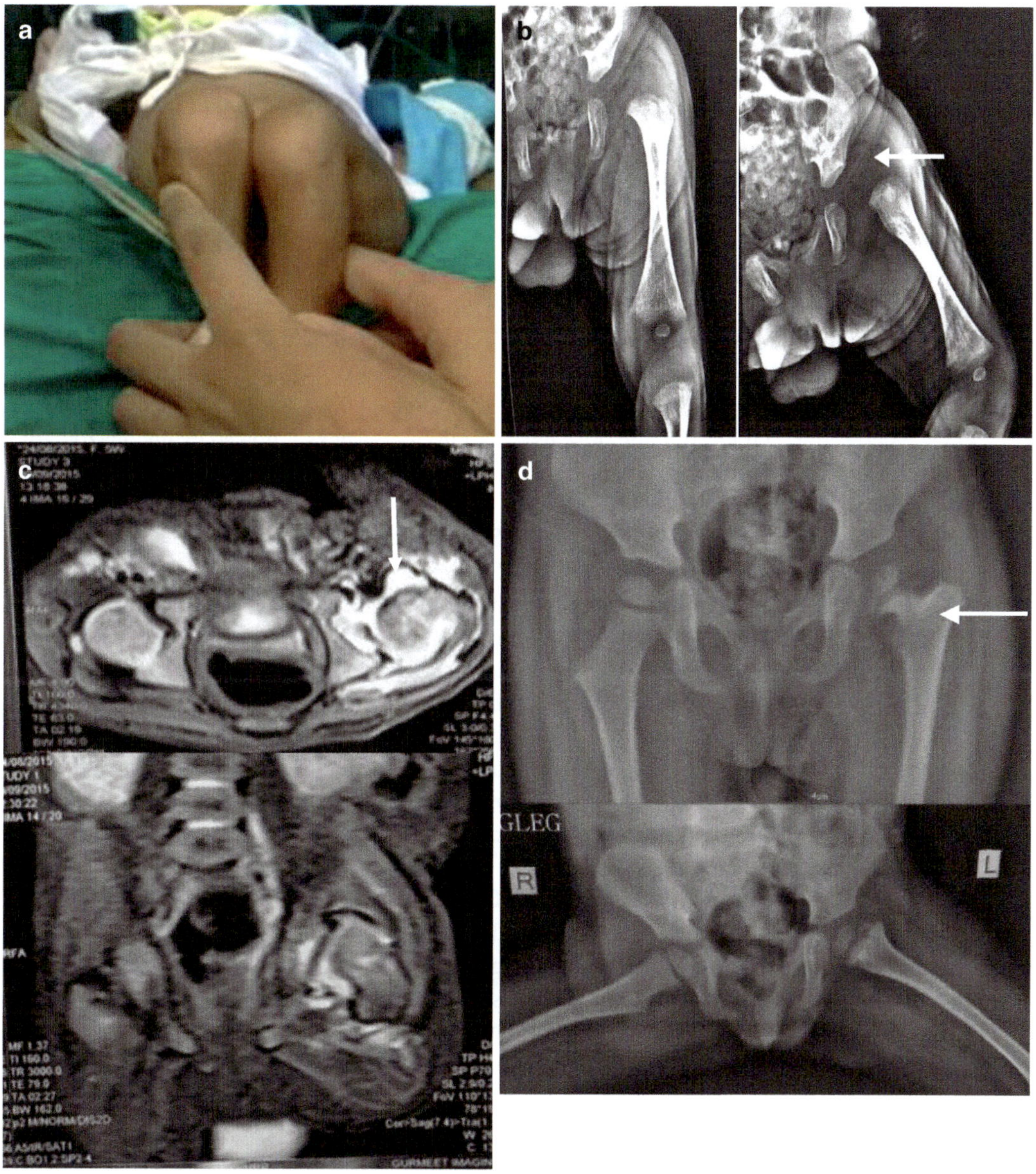

Fig. 35.3 (**a**) Clinical picture of a 5-week-old child (with a known past history of neonatal Bacterial sepsis) with painful left hip movements, showing a positive Galeazzi sign suggestive of dislocated left hip with shortening. (**b**) Anteroposterior and lateral views of the left hip showing an increased medial joint space with soft tissue swelling (white arrow) and a dislocated femoral head. (**c**) Axial and sagittal MRI images of the same child showing left hip effusion (White arrow) with posterior dislocation of femoral head. The child was treated with open reduction, arthrotomy and debridement followed by Pavlik harness application. Fungal culture revealed Candida Albicans for which the child was put on amphotericin B and voriconazole. (**d**) Plain radiograph of the pelvis – Anteroposterior and lateral view of the same child 3 years post-operative showing well-located femoral heads but with changes of old osteomyelitis of proximal femur including coxa vara and coxa breva

Biochemical Investigations

Markers of systemic inflammatory response are minimally, or not elevated, in candidal infections.

Histopathology and Microbiological Diagnosis

Because the clinical and laboratory parameters are extremely non-specific and non-diagnostic, arthrocentesis and diagnostic histopathology and microbiological studies are of paramount importance [7, 19].

(a) Direct Microscopy: Gram staining reveals gram-positive oval budding yeast cells (4–6 μm size) with pseudohyphae.
(b) Culture on SDA (Sabouraud Dextrose Agar): Produces creamy white and pasty colonies at 37 °C. Susceptibility testing helps choose the appropriate antifungal medication.
(c) Immunodiagnosis: Antibody and antigen detection using ELISA test is available.

Treatment

The objective of treatment of candidal SA-OM (as with any other osteoarticular infection) is to obtain source control, eradicate the hematogenous infection, prevent complications, and restore function. These infections, which are often chronic, indolent infections, are usually difficult to control and may have long-term effects on function.

Medical Treatment

Current treatment guidelines recommend a combination of medical and surgical management. The recommended anti-fungal agent is primarily amphotericin B; however, the addition of newer anti-fungals like fluconazole and echinocandins has added a new dimension to the anti-fungal therapy for *Candida* species [1, 25, 28]. The duration of therapy is a matter of debate and ranges from 6 weeks for candida septic arthritis to 6–12 months for candidal osteomyelitis. The typical regimens for candida species are:

1. For neonates: Liposomal amphotericin B 1 mg/kg/day for 2 weeks followed by fluconazole or itraconazole 10 mg/kg/day for 4–6 additional weeks.
2. For older children: Fluconazole 10 mg/kg/day for 6 weeks or a combination of echinocandins (caspofungin, micafungin, or anidulafungin) for 2 weeks followed by fluconazole for 4 more weeks [7].

Surgical Treatment

Surgical treatment is definitely a part of the management of candida septic arthritis as well as osteomyelitis. This helps in decreasing the bacterial load and in achieving good source control, which is difficult with anti-fungal therapy alone. In a few recent studies, it has been shown that good open or arthroscopic joint lavage and debridement helps in reducing complications and decreasing the duration of therapy [1, 18, 23, 25, 28].

Outcome and Complications

The outcome of candidal SA/OM is typically good when the diagnosis is made in the early stages of the disease and appropriate management is instituted. In late presenting cases, there is a chance of recurrence of 10–30%, which can lead to chronic issues like discharging sinuses, deformities, and stiffness. Concomitant bacterial infection can occur in up to 12% of cases, underscoring the need for biopsy and culture. Complete response was obtained in only 30% of OM cases, highlighting the difficulty in treating these infections [1, 18, 23, 25, 28].

Box 35.1 Invasive Candidiasis

- Commonest fungal disease in children
- 70% in neonatal period
- *C. Albicans* > *C. Tropicalis*> *C. parapsilosis*
- Commonest presentation – pseudoparalysis, with localized swelling
- Treatment: Drainage with anti-fungals – Amphotericin B, Itraconazole x 6 weeks
- Outcome: Good. Complete cure possible in most if diagnosed and treated early.

Cryptococcosis

Predominantly an opportunistic infection caused by *Cryptococcus*, a spherical-to-oval, encapsulated, yeast-like fungus that is widespread in spoiled milk, soil, and bird droppings, especially pigeon excreta [29]. It can cause disease in both immune competent as well as immunocompromised individuals [18, 27].

Epidemiology

It has a worldwide distribution. *C. neoformans* var. *grubii* (serotype A) strains are found worldwide; however, *C. neoformans* var. *neoformans* (serotype D) strains are restricted to Europe; *C. gattii* is confined to the tropics and is an emerging pathogen in the NW USA and Western Canada.

Pathogenesis

Infection is acquired by inhalation of aerosolized forms of *Cryptococcus*, but it can also be the result of direct inoculation secondary to trauma, or through the gastrointestinal tract. It is associated with pigeon droppings and can cause meningitis, encephalitis, and pneumonia. Osteomyelitis can occur in 5–10% of patients, and involvement of the spine and hand has been reported. Septic arthritis is a rare manifestation and usually results from contiguous spread of adjacent osteomyelitis. *Cryptococcus* has a polysaccharide capsule, which is the principal virulence factor of the fungus. This capsule is antiphagocytic and also inhibits the host's complement and antibody opsonization mechanisms.

Clinical Features

Patients can develop systemic symptoms, including malaise, weight loss, and fever. MSK symptoms include pain, soft tissue swelling, and joint effusion.

Imaging Studies

Studies are not specific enough to confirm the diagnosis, though MRI may be the best modality for diagnosis. Early on, soft tissue swelling and later bone destruction may be seen on MRI [1].

Biochemical Investigations

Systemic inflammatory markers including ESR and CRP are only mildly elevated.

Histopathologic and Microbiologic Diagnosis

The presence of chronic granulomatous inflammation in tissue should prompt the physician to perform a direct smear and culture to test for fungi or Acid fast bacilli (AFB).

(d) Direct Microscopy: Gram staining reveals gram-positive round budding yeast cells without pseudohyphae. Periodic Acid Schiff (PAS) and Gomori's Methenamine silver (GMS) stain are used to demonstrate the capsule, which appears as refractile delineated clear space surrounding the round, budding yeast cells.

(e) Culture on SDA (Sabouraud Dextrose Agar): *Crypotococcus* produces mucoid, creamy white and yeast-like colonies at 37 °C when cultured on SDA. Susceptibility testing helps choose the appropriate antifungal medication.

(f) Immunodiagnosis: Capsular antigens can be detected from serum or tissue by latex agglutination test. It is a rapid and sensitive (95% sensitivity) and specific method.

Treatment

In the presence of meningoencephalitis infection, amphotericin B is the drug of choice for 2 weeks followed by fluconazole; in the absence of meningoencephalitis, fluconazole alone can be used for 6–12 months [1, 18]. A combined therapy is recommended to be given for shorter duration of therapy, smaller total dosage, reduced likelihood of side effects as well as to prevent secondary drug resistance. According to the Infectious Disease Society of America (IDSA), surgery, which effectively and rapidly eliminates the fungal burden and prevents the contiguous spread of infection, should be performed for patients with persistent or refractory bone disease.

Outcomes

Outcome is good for single site infection in immunocompetent patients. Risk factors for poor prognosis and mortality are immunocompromised status, multiple sites of infection, extraskeletal manifestations and delay in diagnosis.

Box 35.2 Cryptococcosis

- Inhalation of aerosolized form of cryptococcosis
- Sites and presentation – long bone OM, spine, hand
- *Cryptococcus neoformans* > *Cryptococcus gattii* (newer organism)
- *Treatment: Surgery (drainage and debridement) with anti-fungals (Amphotericin B)*

Aspergillosis

Invasive aspergillus osteoarticular infections are some of the most aggressive osteoarticular infections occurring in immunocompromised hosts [6, 20]. There are nearly 35 pathogenic species of *Aspergillus*, with the clinically important ones being *A. fumigatus, A. flavus and A. niger* (Fig. 35.4a, b).

Epidemiology

Most of the cases of osteoarticular aspergillus infections occur in adults and only a small proportion (15–20%) occur in children [6, 21]. It has a worldwide distribution and is frequently associated traditionally with immunocompromised hosts in conditions like prolonged corticosteroid use, chronic granulomatous disease (CGD), neutropenia, primary immunodeficiency, or Acquired Immune Deficiency syndrome (AIDS). However, over the last few years, an increasing number of cases have been described in immunocompetent hosts. Overall aspergillus osteomyelitis is much more common than arthritis, with a ratio of 5:1 [1, 30].

Pathogenesis

The primary associated factor in pediatric aspergillus SA-OM is chronic granulomatous disease (CGD), with CGD diagnosed in almost 3/4th of all pediatric cases [6, 23]. These infections commonly occur due to hematogenous dissemination from a pulmonary focus. The usual pathogen is *Aspergillus fumigatus* which causes around 80% of these infections and has a mortality rate of around 40%. The median age for pediatric Aspergillus infections is 8 years and the most frequently involved bones are the ribs, femur, tibia, and skull [30]. The most commonly involved joints in Aspergillus arthritis are the knee, wrist, intervertebral discs, and hips [6]. Polyarticular involvement occurs in almost 45% of cases.

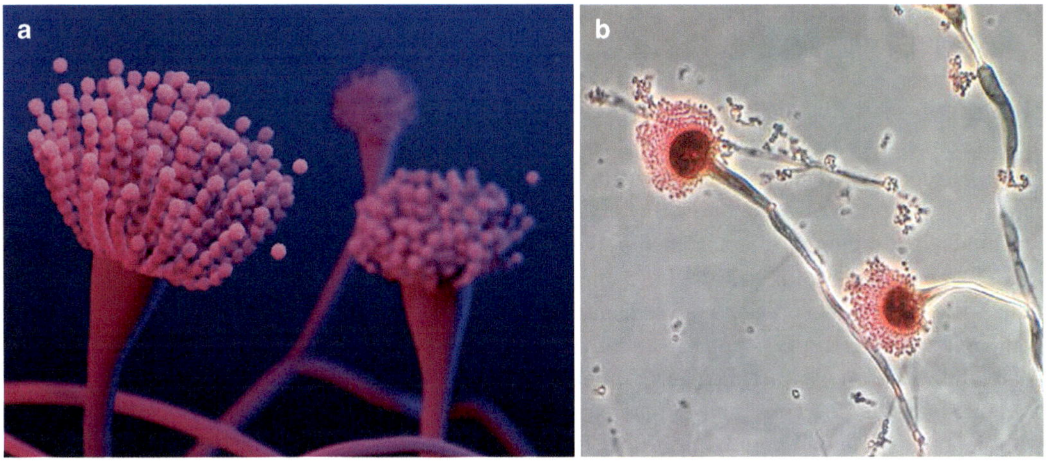

Fig. 35.4 (**a**) Medical illustration of azole-resistant fungus *Aspergillus fumigatus*. (Source: Public Health Image ID#23236/2019/Centre for Disease Control and Prevention (Atlanta)/With Permission). (**b**) Photomicrograph of *Aspergillus fumigatus* showing bulbous filamentous spore. (Source: Public Health Image ID#15145/2012/Centre for Disease Control and Prevention (Atlanta)/With Permission)

Clinical Features

Pain and severe localized tenderness of the affected part are the common clinical features of Aspergillus osteoarticular infection. Fever, local redness, and edema are less common findings. Sinus tract formation occurs in about one-fourth of all cases and is sometimes the presenting symptom. Very rarely in cases of spinal or cranial Aspergillosis, the patients present with neurological manifestations.

Radiological Diagnosis

The X-ray and MRI findings of aspergillus osteomyelitis and septic arthritis are relatively nonspecific [6]. X-ray findings include osteolysis, bony destruction, and enhanced T2- weighted signals, which are similar to other osteoarticular destructive pathologies and not specific to Aspergillosis [30]. Less common manifestations are periosteal reaction, abscess formation and sequestration. Vertebral osteomyelitis is identified by decreased intervertebral space, paraspinal abscesses, and epidural abscesses on MRI.

Biochemical Investigations

The biochemical parameters are typical for any chronic infection, with the mean WBC count found to be mildly elevated. The erythrocyte sedimentation rate (ESR) is characteristically elevated significantly, in the range of 90–100 mm/h, while the CRP is moderately elevated. Synovial fluid usually shows significant leukocytosis, with a high percentage of polymorphonuclear leucocytes (PMN) [23].

Microbiological and Histological Diagnoses

Arthrocentesis and biopsy are the diagnostic modalities of choice for Aspergillus OM-SA. Synovial fluid culture has a very high sensitivity and specificity, ranging between 95% and 100%. In contrast, the histological diagnosis of Aspergillosis is slightly less, with only about 50 and 60% of cases being positive. Gram stain positivity is even less, at approximately 20%. The commonest species of *Aspergillus* is *Aspergillus fumigatus*, followed by *Aspergillus flavus*. KOH mount and H & E staining of specimens reveals characteristic narrow septate hyaline hyphae with acute angle branching [6].

Serological Diagnosis

ELISA detecting *Aspergillus*-specific galactomannan antigen in patient's sera or urine is useful for establishing an early diagnosis. Detection of serum antibodies is very useful for chronic, invasive aspergillosis and to monitor response to treatment [21].

Treatment

The treatment of Aspergillus OM-SA is a combination of surgical and medical management. The Infectious Diseases Society of North America recommends a minimum therapy of 6–8 weeks [1]. The common anti-fungals used are amphotericin-B, itraconazole, and voriconazole. Although amphotericin B is equally effective as compared to the Azoles, its median duration of therapy is almost 12 weeks, and it is associated with nephrotoxicity and vein damage that leads to difficulty in maintaining intravenous access. Because of these factors, amphotericin B is uncommonly used as a single-therapeutic agent. Itraconazole and voriconazole are particularly good alternatives, though voriconazole is more widely used due to its flexibility in having oral as well as intravenous formulations and its good bioavailability. A recently introduced drug, Posaconazole, is increasingly being used, especially as a salvage therapy in intractable invasive Aspergillosis [6, 30].

Surgical management includes debridement, arthrotomy, sequestrectomy and, in some rare cases, life-saving amputations for severe infections. Surgical management is extremely important, as it has been seen that there is almost a 70% recurrence rate in patients managed with medical therapy alone [5, 7]. Surgery decreases the fungal load in infected bone and soft tissues, thus reducing the possibility of recurrence of infection after antifungal therapy is stopped.

Outcome

Bone and joint Aspergillosis is a debilitating infection, with an uncertain course, especially in the presence of immunodeficiency syndromes like CGD. There is a recurrence rate of almost 30% and long-lasting sequelae are common [5, 7].

Box 35.3 Aspergillosis

- Most aggressive osteoarticular fungal infection
- Primarily affects immunocompromised hosts – prolonged corticosteroid use, chronic granulomatous disease, AIDS
- Presentation – pain, swelling, discharging sinuses
- *A. fumigatus* – commonest
- Treatment: Debridement and long-term medical therapy
- Outcome: Poor in disseminated disease (almost 40% mortality)

Coccidiodomycosis

Coccidioidomycosis (valley fever) is an invasive fungal infection caused by the inhalation of aerosolized spores of *Coccidioides* spp., which reside in the arid soil of southwestern United States, northern Mexico and parts of Latin America. This genus comprises two nearly identical species: *Coccidioides immitis* and *Coccidioides posadasii* [9, 14, 31].

Epidemiology

Coccidioidomycosis is a reportable disease in the United States. Of an estimated 150,000 new cases of coccidioidomycosis each year in the United States, most cases (>97%) occur in Arizona and California, where the incidence has increased steadily over the past 20 years. Multiple factors likely explain this rising incidence, including a growing population in the endemic areas, increased physician and laboratory reporting, advances in medical treatment that result in impaired cell-mediated immunity. Risk factors for disseminated disease include race (African or Filipino ancestry), gender (male > female), and suppression of cell-mediated immunity. It can occur at all ages, but incidence in patients younger than 20 years has increased significantly over the last two decades. Travel and tourism to endemic regions have contributed to the increasing presentation of coccidioidomycosis in nonendemic areas such as New York and across the world, making this a disease of national and worldwide importance [32].

Pathogenesis

Coccidioides spp. are dimorphic fungi, existing in a saprophytic mycelial phase in the soil, and the parasitic phase in the infected host [9]. In the soil, extruded endospores develop into the tubular mycelial form. Arthroconidia develop along branching septate hyphae (mycelia) and readily disarticulate as the organism matures. The arthroconidia are barrel-shaped and easily become aerosolized, measuring less than 4 μm in width and 6 μm in width. Once inhaled, the arthroconidia are ingested by pulmonary macrophages and then transform to a round cell that eventually becomes a spherule. The spherule is a thick-walled structure ranging from 8 to 30 μm in diameter that contains hundreds of asexual endospores, each typically measuring 2–4 μm in diameter. Rupture of the spherule leads to dispersion of the contained endospores, inducing an inflammatory response that produces the systemic manifestations of the disease. Endospores may form new spherules and propagate in the lung or spread hematogenously, resulting in disseminated coccidioidomycosis.

The primary infection occurs in the lungs; however, less than 40% of patients are symptomatic. In 1–5% of those infected, primary respiratory infection may progress to disseminated disease and involve any organ system, a serious complication with considerable morbidity. Skeletal coccidioidomycosis occurs in 10–50% of disseminated infections. Skeletal coccidioidomycosis is a chronic and progressive infection that eventually results in bone destruction and loss of function, and often involves adjacent structures such as joints, muscles, tendons and other soft tissues. This infection is frequently multifocal with axial skeletal involvement [24, 32].

In the axial skeleton, the most commonly involved sites are the spine, ribs, pelvis, and skull. In the spine, a single vertebra, multiple contiguous (more common) or noncontiguous vertebrae (less common) may be involved. The lumbar spine is more commonly involved than the thoracic and cervical spine [14]. The intervertebral disc spaces are usually spared and the posterior elements may be involved. Vertebral body collapse, disc space narrowing and gibbus deformity are late manifestations and are not as frequently seen as in tuberculosis [14].

In the appendicular skeleton, the infection has a predilection for the diaphysis of short tubular bones, metaphyses of long bones and for bony protuberances. Joint involvement usually results from direct extension of an adjacent focus of bone infection and less commonly from hematogenous spread. Soft tissue involvement may result in lymphadenitis, abscesses, tenosynovitis, septic bursitis, and pyomyositis [27, 31, 32].

Clinical Features

The clinical presentation can be diverse and nonspecific with bone pain being the most common presenting symptom, and some patients having accompanying pulmonary symptoms. Most patients have normal body temperature; fever is present only in a minority of cases. Disseminated coccidioidomycosis is frequently preceded by an episode consistent with primary pulmonary coccidioidomycosis within the preceding several months (Fig. 35.5a–f). Patients of all ages and both sexes may be involved [32].

Diagnosis

Histologic and Microbiologic Diagnosis

A diagnosis of coccidioidomycosis is confirmed when the organism is either grown in culture or is identified by histopathology [32]. *Coccidioides species* are easily isolated from cultures of infected tissue; this organism grows readily on standard bacterial or fungal medium in about 3–7 days, but fungal media is recommended. Visualization of spherules on histopathologic samples is diagnostic. The spherule is a thick-

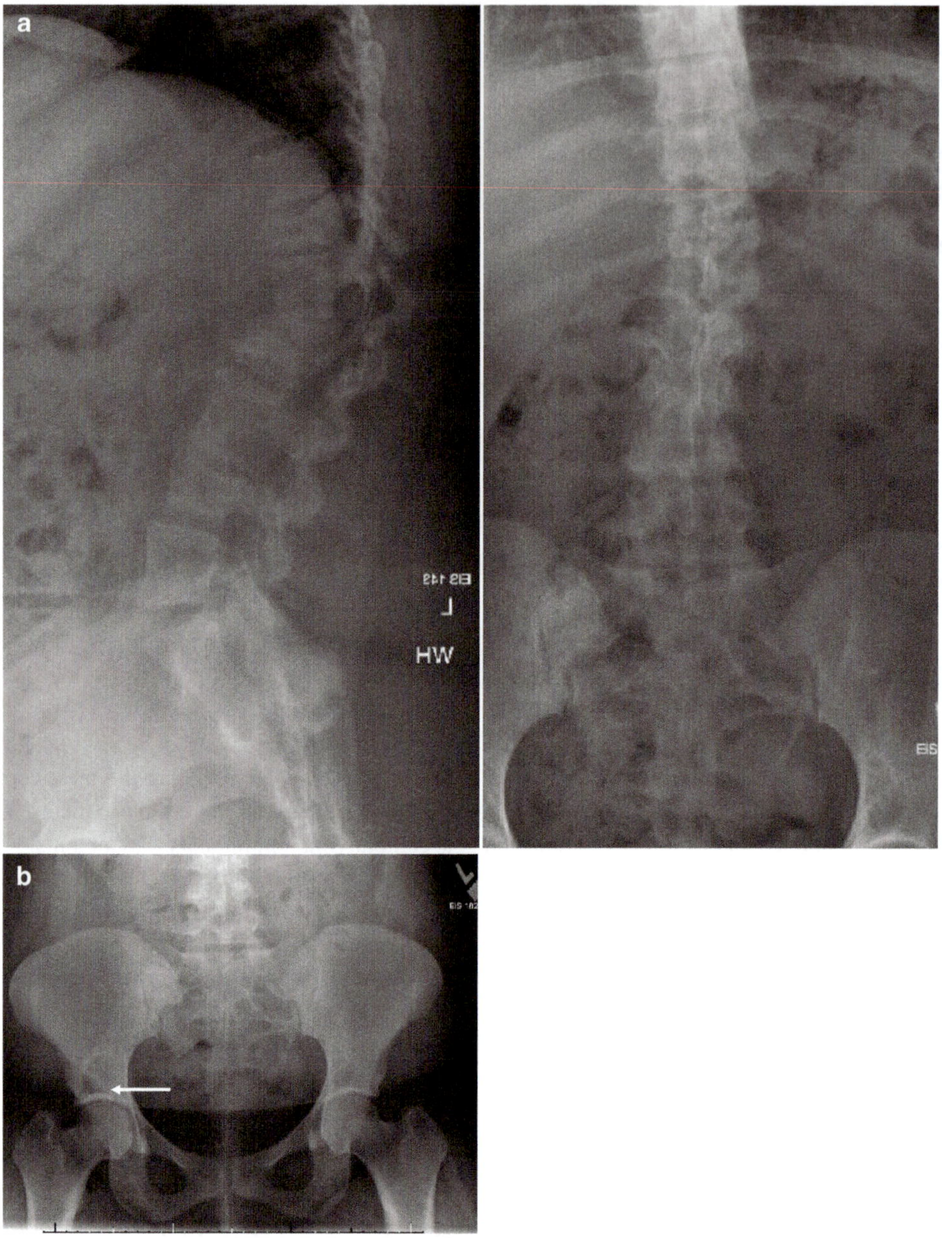

Fig. 35.5 (**a**) Plain radiographs of the lumbosacral spine showing thoracolumbar kyphosis with destruction of multiple vertebral bodies at T12, L1, L2, and L4 with loss of disc space at L1/2, L3/4. (**b**) Anteroposterior radiograph of the Pelvis with both hips showing bilateral supra-acetabular lytic areas Right > left. (**c**) Sagittal and axial T2 W MR images showing severe, destructive changes of the lower thoracic and lumbar spines by disseminated coccidiomycosis infection with multilevel vertebral body destruction, and extension into the spinal canal and narrowing of the thecal sac; the most severe destruction is seen at the L1 and L2 vertebral levels, with extension into bilateral psoas and paravertebral regions. (**d**) CT scan of TL spine with 3D reconstruction showing multilevel, lytic lesions in the lower thoracic and lumbar vertebrae, with a TL kyphotic deformity and partial collapse and fusion of the L1 and L2 vertebral bodies; note retropulsion of the posterior aspect of the body into the central canal with subsequent central canal stenosis. (**e**) MRI (Coronal mDIX TSE T1 and T2 and T1 axial views) showing areas of destruction of the right ilium and supra-acetabular area. (**f**) Spherules of *Coccidioides* (black arrows) demonstrating endospore formation; note the thick wall of the spherules. Infection is often accompanied by inflammatory cell infiltrate that contains multinucleated giant cells (stars) (Hematoxylin and eosin ×400). (Courtesy David Carpenteiri, MD, Phoenix Children's Hospital)

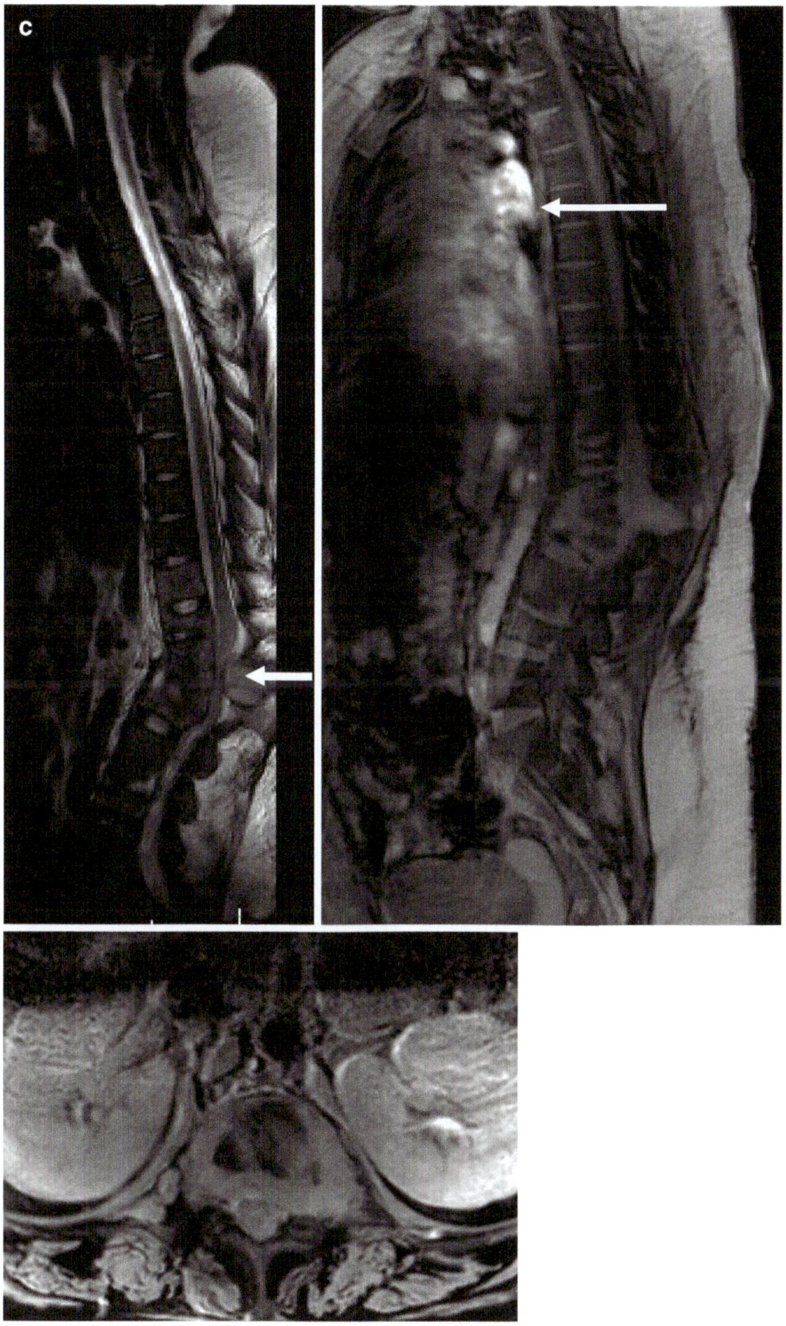

Fig. 35.5 (continued)

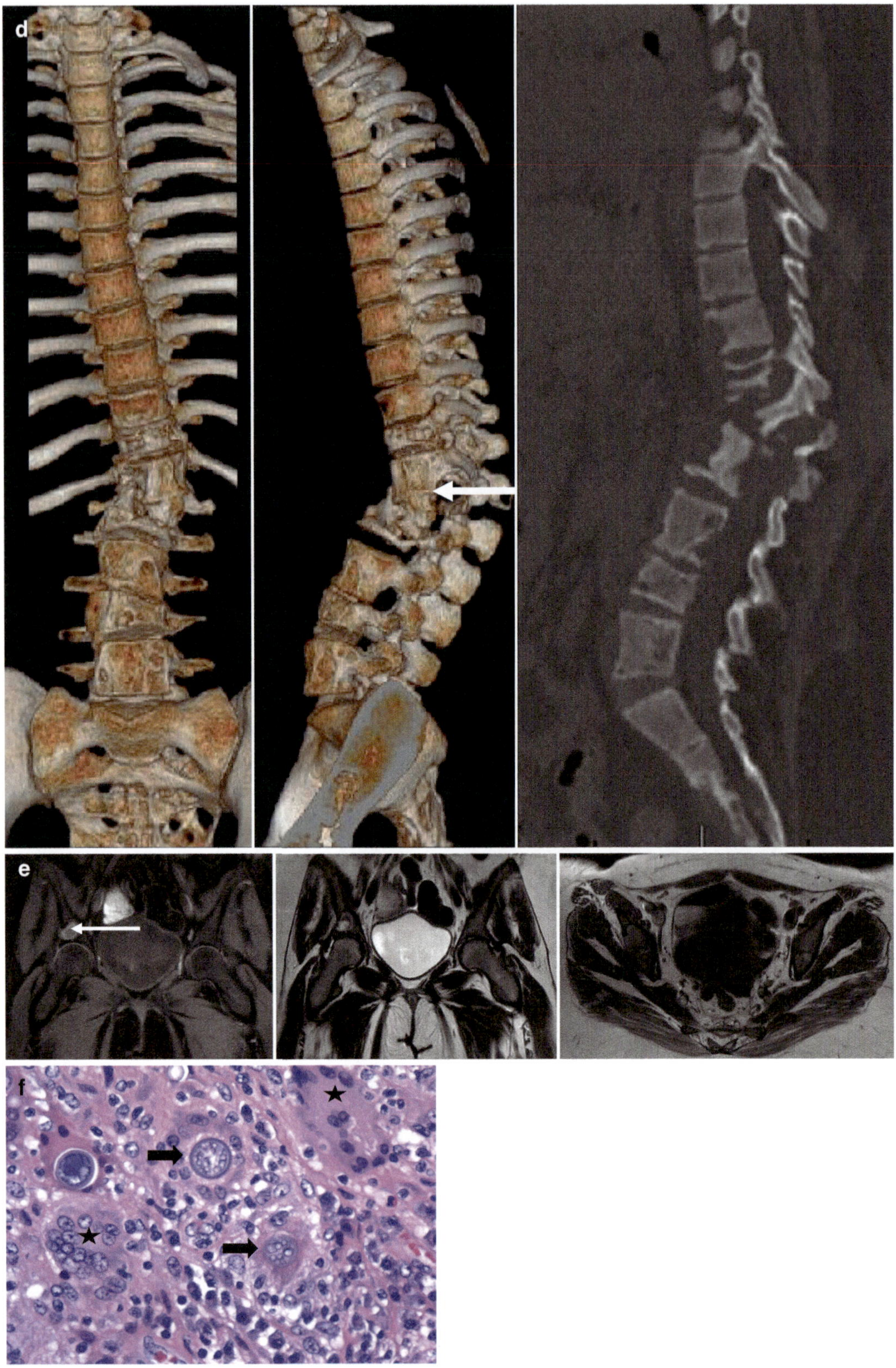

Fig. 35.5 (continued)

walled structure ranging from 8 to 30 μm in diameter that has a doubly refractile capsule containing hundreds of endospores, each typically measuring 2–4 μm in diameter. The endospores produce an acute neutrophilic inflammatory response followed by a chronic granulomatous inflammation characterized by multinucleated giant cells and caseation. The organism is easily identified on standard hematoxylin and eosin stains, although fungal stains may increase the diagnostic yield.

Serologic Diagnosis

Serologic testing for antibodies to *Coccidioides* species can be important in the diagnosis and management of coccidioidomycosis. Antibodies to *Coccidioides* are present only during active infection, and the presence of any antibody by any methodology suggests active infection. The enzyme-linked immunosorbent assay (EIA) for coccidioidal IgG and IgM antibodies is very useful for early diagnosis of primary pulmonary coccidioidomycosis. The complement fixation (CF) antibody test measures IgG antibodies to complement-fixing antigen and usually becomes positive several weeks or months after initial infection [28].

Radiologic Diagnosis

Radiographs can be negative early in the disease course but in some cases may reveal multiple lytic lesions with or without sclerosis, periosteal reaction, and soft tissue swelling. Imaging is effective for evaluation of bone and joint involvement, monitoring of treatment results, and long-term follow-up [33]. Septic arthritis is associated with joint space narrowing, periarticular osteopenia, and destructive bone changes. In the axial skeleton, the intervertebral disc spaces are usually spared, and vertebral collapse is an uncommon and late manifestation. Imaging modalities like radiographs, CT scan, and MRI may identify relevant abnormalities, but they are not pathognomonic.

Treatment

Skeletal coccidioidomycosis is difficult to treat and a combination of medical therapy and surgical debridement is often needed [24, 31]. Early diagnosis and treatment are critical to avoid long-term problems. In patients with skeletal coccidioidomycosis, the triazole antifungals are used as first line therapy while fluconazole is an acceptable alternative. Amphotericin B is used in very severe, life-threatening, or rapidly progressing infections refractory to triazoles and fluconazole [1, 24]. Surgical management should follow principles outlined previously.

Outcomes

Disseminated coccidioidomycosis accounts for most of the mortality compared with <1% mortality in other forms of coccidioidomycosis [24, 31]. A favorable outcome can usually be achieved with combined therapy, but early discontinuation of medical therapy is associated with a high risk of relapse, which can occur years later. Medical treatment must be continued for a prolonged period of time, potentially for a lifetime in some patients.

Box 35.4 Coccidiodomycosis

- Predominantly seen in mid-western USA
- More commonly seen in African-American, Filipino descent, and in immunocompromised
- OA involvement – Chronic progressive destructive disease with involvement of spine, ribs, pelvis, etc.
- Treatment: Debridement + prolonged medical therapy

Blastomycosis

A fungal infection caused by the dimorphic fungus Blastomyces dermatitidis which is ubiquitous in the soil, pine forests, and beaver dams. It is mainly found in the USA, specifically the South East (Alabama, Mississippi), North Central (Illinois, Minnesota, Wisconsin), South Central (Arkansas), and Mid- Atlantic (Maryland, Virginia) regions, as well as South Central Canada [15, 18].

Epidemiology

Only 2–13% of blastomycosis cases occur in children (average 9–11 years), and are seen rarely in newborn and infants. Around 1–2 cases/100,000 population are reported in endemic areas. Most infections are sporadic, but 15 outbreaks have been reported, mostly associated with outdoor activities like camping, hiking, and fishing [27].

Pathogenesis

"Phase transition", that is, the ability of mycelial fragments and spores to convert to yeast in the lung, is a crucial event in the pathogenesis of infection with B. dermatitidis. It enables B. dermatitidis to evade the host immune system and establish the infection. Blastomycosis is usually transmitted via direct inoculation of the soles of the feet, causing subcutaneous soft tissue granulomas and skin sinuses. It can also be transmitted via inhalation, causing an acute respiratory infection. In children with HIV or in those who are transplant recipients, disseminated infection can occur; extra-pulmonary involvement of any organ system can develop in 25–40% patients.

Clinical Features

Clinical disease develops 3 weeks to 3 months following exposure to B. dermatitidis. Asymptomatic or subclinical infection occurs in 50% patients [15, 34]. The most common clinical manifestation of blastomycosis is acute or chronic pneumonia, characterized by pleuritic chest pain, productive cough, and multifocal pulmonary infiltrates. Osteomyelitis commonly presents as pain, soft tissue swelling, sinus tract formation, and ulceration [15]. Commonly involved bones are the ribs, skull, spine, and long bones. Extensive long bone osteomyelitis can result in pathological fracture or septic arthritis. Arthritis due to *Blastomyces* occurs in 30% of cases, mainly involving a single joint either due to hematogenous spread or direct spread from adjacent osteomyelitis. The joint involvement appears as joint space narrowing, joint margin erosions, focal osteopenia, and punched out lesions. In the spine, the infection begins in the vertebral body, mainly in the thoracic and lumbar regions, and eventually spreads to the adjacent discs; further regional spread can lead to paravertebral and psoas abscesses.

Diagnosis

High index of suspicion is required as clinico-radiological features mimic other diseases like tuberculosis, pneumonia, and malignancy. The diagnosis is confirmed by positive wet mount microscopy after histopathological staining of the tissue biopsy specimens, which reveals thick-walled round yeast cells of 8–15 μm size with single round broad-based budding yeasts. Occasionally culture of the synovial fluid or tissue may be positive. Blastomyces antigen test and an antibody test against BAD1 (*B. dermatitidis* adhesin-1) protein have also been developed. A combination of these two tests can increase diagnostic sensitivity to almost 97% [15, 34].

Treatment

For newborns, amphotericin B deoxycholate 1 mg/kg/day is recommended. For children with mild to moderate infection, itraconazole 10 mg/kg/day (maximum 400 mg/day) for 6–12 months is required. For children with severe infection, initial treatment with amphotericin B 0.7–1 mg/kg/day for 7–14 days, followed by itraconazole 10 mg/kg/day for 12 months, is recommended [1, 34].

Box 35.5 Blastomycosis
- Central USA/ Canada – seen in soil, pine forests, and beaver dam areas
- Sub-acute/ chronic course with symptoms 3 weeks–3 months after exposure
- OA involvement – OM of long bones, spine, skull
- Treatment: Primarily medical with prolonged anti-fungal therapy. Surgery for recalcitrant lesions

Histoplasmosis

Histoplasmosis is a systemic granulomatous disease caused by a dimorphic fungus, *Histoplasma capsulatum*, which is prevalent in the regions with soil enriched with bird and bat feces, like the Mississippi and Ohio river basins [9, 16].

Epidemiology

Histoplasma has a worldwide distribution and is one of the commonest endemic mycoses in the United States, commonly seen in the Midwest and Southern US.

Pathogenesis

H. capsulatum is transmitted by inhalation of spores which usually circulate in the air after the contaminated soil is disturbed. Spores are inhaled and attach to the reticuloendothelial system; they subsequently spread to regional lymph nodes, leading to a granulomatous inflammatory reaction, necrosis, and calcification. After the spores enter the lungs, they transform into yeast forms. The intracellular yeasts travel to the lymph nodes and spread to the other parts of the body through the bloodstream. In patients with impaired cell- mediated immunity, disseminated disease develops.

Clinical Features

Primary pulmonary infection presents as a self-limited flu-like illness. Osteomyelitis can present with pain and soft tissue swelling. Septic arthritis is uncommon and usually involves the knee joint.

Diagnosis

Osteomyelitis can present with cortical subperiosteal thickening, a widened medullary canal, osteopenia, and epiphyseal bone destruction on radiographs. Histopathology will demonstrate caseating or non-caseating granulomas and can be used with tissue culture to confirm diagnosis. Histopathological staining (such as PAS or Giemsa) of the specimens reveals tiny oval yeast cells (2–4 μm size), with narrowly based budding within the macrophages, and an underlying granulomatous response. Antibodies in serum can be detected by CFT and immunodiffusion test [16].

Treatment

Amphotericin B is the drug of choice for disseminated histoplasmosis [1, 9].

Box 35.6 Histoplasmosis
- Spore forming organism with worldwide distribution
- Commonest endemic mycosis
- OA infection – extremely rare
- Treatment: Prolonged anti-fungal therapy with Amphotericin B

Sporotrichosis

Sporotrichosis, or Rose gardener's disease, is a rare fungal infection caused by *Sporothrix schenckii* that exhibits temperature dimorphism. It presents as subcutaneous nodulo-ulcerative lesions [17].

Epidemiology

Sporothrix schenckii is found worldwide, but most cases are seen in North and South America, Sub-Himalayan India, and Japan. In the United States, the majority of cases occur in the Midwest, especially along the Mississippi and Missouri rivers. Around 25 cases per 1000 population are reported in endemic areas, where overall prevalence is 1–2 per million population. The fungus is found in decaying vegetation, especially rose bushes, straw, and some types of hay. Transmission in children may be zoonotic, from bites and scratches of animals, mostly by cats and armadillos. In endemic areas of Peru, children are more commonly involved than adults, and the risk factors reported are playing in crop fields, living in houses with dirt floors, and owning a cat [28].

Pathogenesis

Sporothrix schenckii is the cause of the most common deep soft tissue fungal infection of the extremities [17]. Since this fungus contaminates wood, it is inoculated into the hands and feet of agricultural workers, gardeners and children who walk bare feet. Osteoarticular sporotrichosis occurs at single or multiple sites in the setting of local trauma (21%), alcohol abuse (30%), HIV infection, immunosuppression, or diabetes. Sporothrix arthritis mainly involves the knee, hand, wrist, elbow, and ankle and may take up to 17 months from the onset to diagnosis [3].

Clinical Features

Lymphocutaneous sporotrichosis, occurring after traumatic subcutaneous inoculation, is the most common form of disease, accounting for >75% of reported cases in children. After a prolonged incubation period of 1–12 weeks, an isolated painless erythematous papule develops at the inoculation site, most commonly on the face. The original lesion gradually enlarges and ulcerates. Due to lymphatic spread, satellite lesions may occur, appearing as multiple, tender, subcutaneous nodules adherent to the overlying skin with subsequent ulceration, mainly on the hands and feet. Spontaneous healing is rare, and the ulcerated lesions may persist for years. Systemic signs and symptoms are uncommon. Though rare in children, extra-articular sporotrichosis can manifest as osteoarticular infection or chronic pneumonitis. On X-ray, the osteomyelitis appears proliferative or sclerotic in appearance [17].

Diagnosis

Definite diagnosis requires isolation of fungus from the site of infection by culture, but usually the yield is low due to a small number of organisms in the tissues. Special histological staining, such as periodic acid-Schiff and methenamine silver, is required to identify yeast forms in tissues, and reveal cigar-shaped asteroid bodies. An asteroid body consists of a central basophilic yeast cell surrounded by radiating extensions of an eosinophilic mass, which is composed of antigen-antibody complexes. In disseminated cases, identification of serum antibodies against *S. schenckii*-related antigens, identified on a latex agglutination test, can be helpful [17].

Treatment

Treatment with 1 year of oral itraconazole, 200 mg bid, with or without initial amphotericin B, is recommended. The impact of surgery is not well-described, and the relapse rate is high [1, 27].

Box 35.7 Sporotrichosis
- Rare fungal infection – Sporothrix schoneckii
- North/South America, India, Japan
- Presents as subcutaneous nodulo-ulcerative lesions most commonly due to traumatic subcutaneous inoculation
- Treatment: Prolonged medical anti-fungal therapy – 1 year. Surgery – not well described

Mycetoma

Is a chronic slowly progressive granulomatous infection of the skin and subcutaneous tissues. Mycetoma can be caused by actinomycetes (bacteria) or eumycetes (fungi) [2, 20]. Globally, around 42% cases are caused by fungi and 18 different fungal species have been identified as causative agents, but *Madurella mycetomatis* is the most common cause, responsible for around 25% of all cases [11]. *Madura mycetomatis* has recently been included in the WHO's list of neglected diseases.

Epidemiology

More than 18,000 cases of mycetoma have been reported worldwide. The prevalence is 3–4/100,000 population in endemic areas. Though most common in the 20–40 years age group, young children and elderly are also affected, especially in endemic areas. Males are predominantly affected, with a ratio of 3.5:1. It is prevalent in the countries between 30° North and 15° South of the equator, mainly Africa (Sudan), Central & South America (Mexico), and India, with Sudan having the highest prevalence [12, 35].

Pathogenesis

The organism enters the subcutaneous tissue via minor trauma to the foot by thorn, splinter, stone cuts or insect bites. Once within the subcutaneous tissue, the organism organizes itself into small granules called grains. *M. mycetomatis* produces three structural forms of fungal grains: filamentous type, vesicular type (light-colored center with peripheral brown hyphae), and a mix of both. These coalesce into small nodules that gradually grow into a large subcutaneous mass with sinuses that secrete pus and grains. There is gradual invasion of the adjacent bone and joint, with resultant osteomyelitis and arthritis. Finally, a large, mutilating lesion may be formed [10, 12, 35]. Osteoarticular mucormycosis can be highly destructive with poor prognosis if the diagnosis is delayed.

Clinical Features

The commonly involved sites are the lower limb, in 82% of cases, and the hand in 7% of cases, as these sites come into contact with soil during daily activities. In endemic areas, the arm, head and neck, and perineum may also be involved less frequently. Mycetoma presents as enlarging, subcutaneous firm mass (Fig. 35.6a–f) where secondary nodules may develop, suppurate, and drain through interconnecting sinus tracts. The discharge is usually purulent and often contains grains, the color of which depends on the causative organism. As the granuloma enlarges, the overlying skin is tethered and stretched, becoming smooth, pigmented, and shiny, with areas of hyperhidrosis (Fig. 35.7). Eventually the deep structures are invaded, but the tendons and nerves are spared. Mycetoma is usually painless, probably due to a substance produced by the lesion that has an anesthetic effect. Pain and constitutional symptoms may occur if there is secondary bacterial infection. In late cases, cachexia and anemia may develop, due to malnutrition, sepsis, and depression. Mycetoma produces disability and deformity, and can be fatal, especially in cranial cases [12, 20, 35].

Radiographs

An early feature of Madura mycosis is a soft-tissue granuloma, seen as a dense shadow, or several scattered shadows. With progression of the disease, the adjacent cortex may be compressed by the granuloma, leading to scalloping, which is followed by a variable amount of periosteal reaction. Eventually, many punched out cavities are formed, and they are usually filled with solid

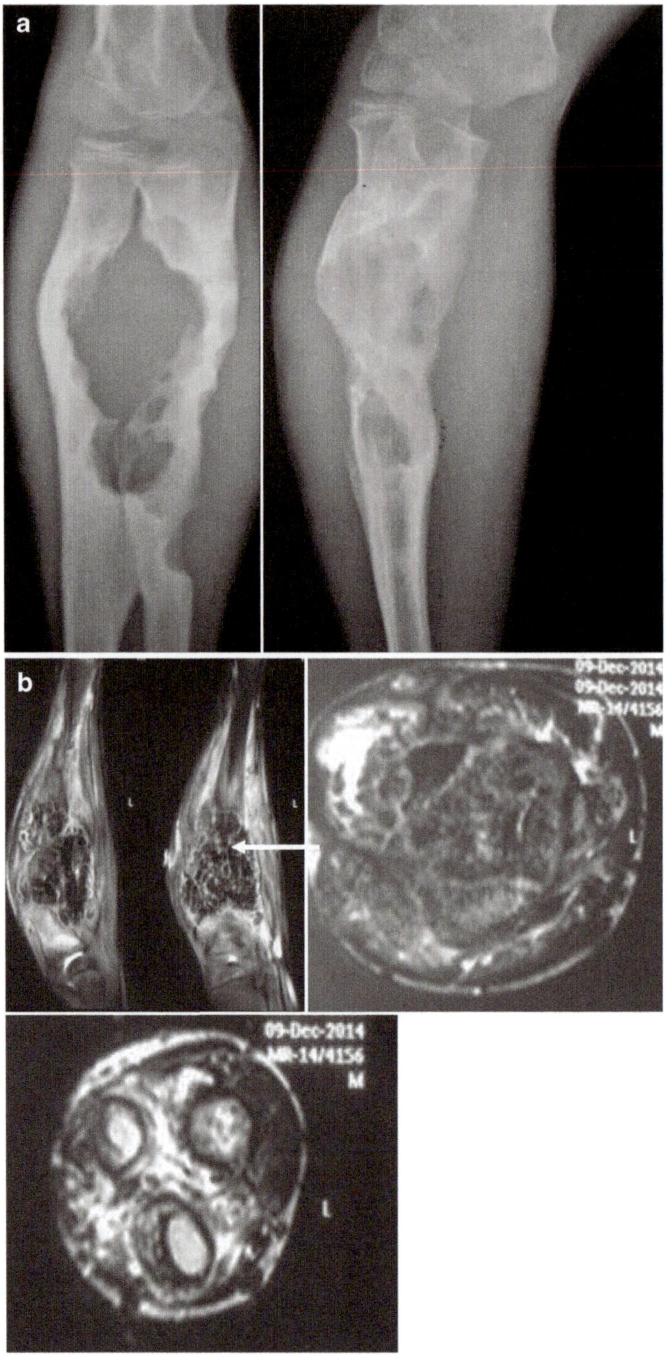

Fig. 35.6 (**a**) Plain radiograph of the forearm of a 10-year-old child with slow growing swelling and pain over the right forearm for 1 year and a discharging sinus for 4 months. The image shows large areas of bony erosions, cortical irregularity, sclerosis, and large soft tissue swelling. (**b**) T2-weighted sagittal and axial MRI images of the right forearm show a large soft tissue collection with a variegated appearance, along with cortical irregularity and surrounding edema. (**c**) Intra-operative clinical images of the right forearm during debridement reveal large brownish-black granules pathognomonic of mycetoma. Post-debridement, a large cavity was seen between the radius and ulna. (**d**) Lactophenol cotton blue mount of M mycetoma showing septate sterile hyphae. (**e**) Clinical photo of the bilateral upper extremities 6 months after surgery showing fair range of motion and completely healed sinus. Radiograph shows synostosis between the radius and ulna

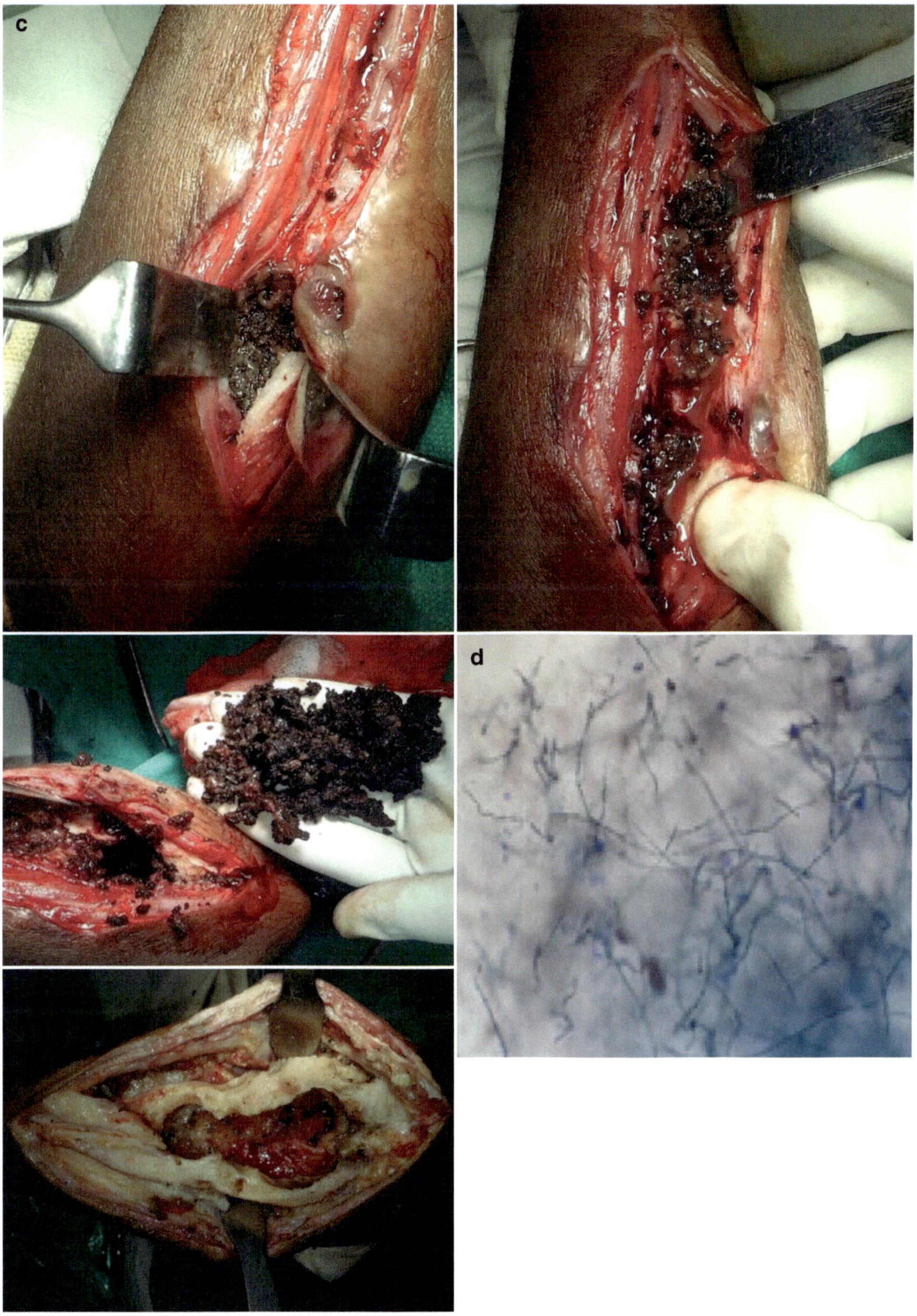

Fig. 35.6 (continued)

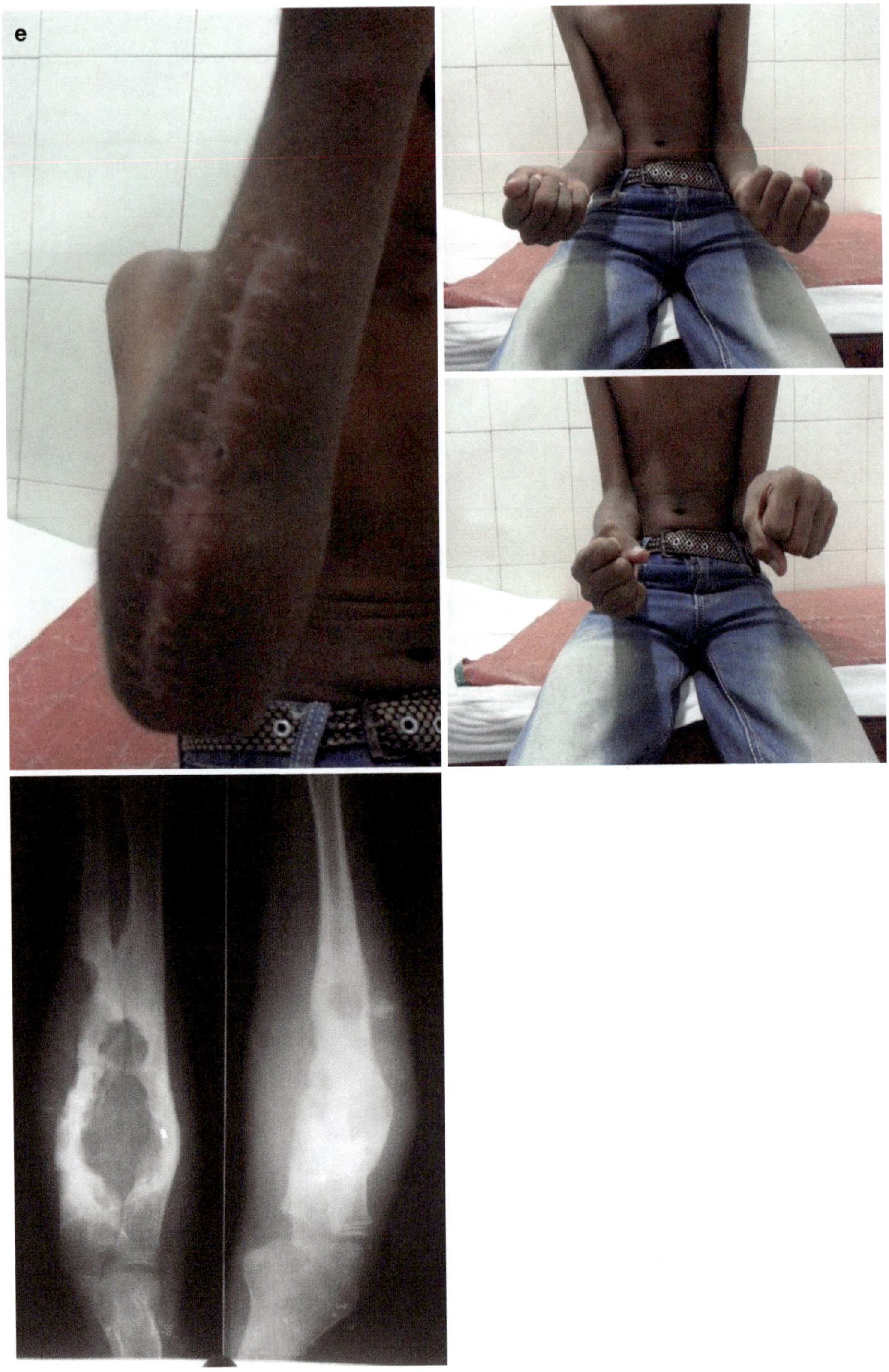

Fig. 35.6 (continued)

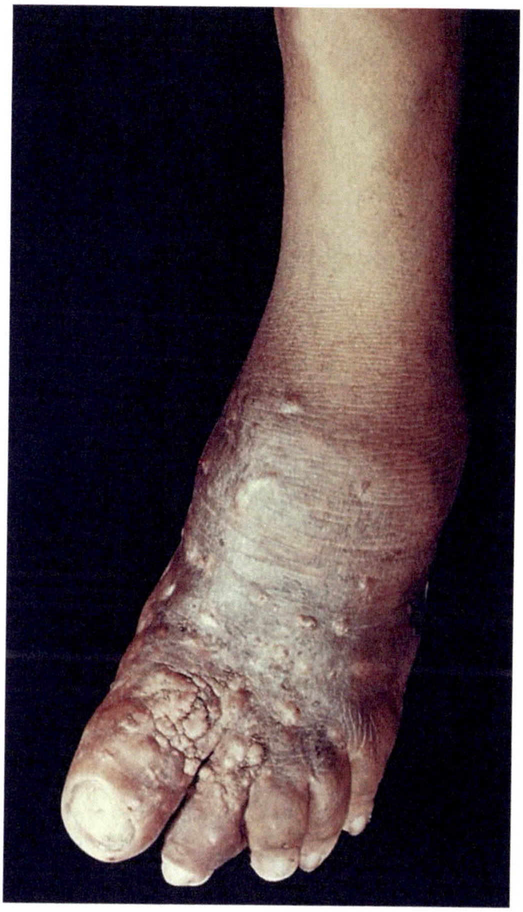

Fig. 35.7 Depicted here, is a dorsal view of a patient's left foot, which exhibited pathologic changes indicative of a mycetoma, due to the cutaneous invasion of the Gram-positive, *Streptomyces somaliensis* bacterial organisms. (Source: Public Health Image # 14816/1971/Dr. Victoria (Mexico); Dr. Lucille K. Georg/Center for Disease Control and Prevention (Atlanta)/with Permission)

masses of grains and fibrous tissue. In some cases, periosteal new bone spicules are laid down at right angles to the cortex to create a sun ray appearance, just like in osteosarcoma [28].

Ultrasonography

This modality may be useful to differentiate eumycetoma from actinomycetoma, based on the specific appearance of the grains and accompanying granuloma. In eumycetoma, the grains produce multiple sharp, bright, hyper-reflective echoes that originate from the cement substance associated with the grains [2].

Magnetic Resonance Imaging

MRI is helpful in assessment of bony and soft-tissue involvement. Within the granuloma, there are many lesions measuring 2–5 mm in diameter of high signal intensity, giving a typical "dot-in-circle" appearance. This represents the grains and is highly specific for mycetoma [2].

Fine Needle Aspiration Cytology

This method is a simple, rapid, and sensitive test for the identification of the organism. Grains are subjected to KOH mount, which reveals hyphae of 2–6 μm width, along with chlamydospores at the margin.

Histopathology

Using a deep surgical biopsy to obtain the grains, identification of the causative organism is done with hematoxylin & eosin stain. Eumycetoma appears as a granulomatous reaction with a palisade arrangement of hyphae in the cement substance.

Microbiology

Deep surgical biopsy is done to obtain the grains, which are then cultured in Sabouraud dextrose agar.

Polymerase Chain Reaction (PCR)

A specific PCR test, amplifying a region of the internal transcribed spacer in the ribosomal gene complex, is available as a diagnostic tool.

Serodiagnosis

The demonstration of significant amounts of antibodies against the causative organism using ELISA is of diagnostic value and important for follow up of patients on medical management.

Treatment

Combined medical and surgical treatment is the gold standard of management. The recommended medical treatment is itraconazole, 200–400 mg per day, or voriconazole, 300–400 mg per day, for 9–12 months. The response to treatment is judged by the disappearance of the mass and healing of sinuses clinically, re-appearance of normal bone pattern radiologically, and absence of grains cytologically. Surgery is needed in all cases, ranging from deep surgical biopsy, wide local excision, or amputation. Amputation is needed in severe disease at a rate of 10 –25% of cases. Wide local excision is recommended for localized early disease. Repeated debridement and debulking may be required for massive infections. In 10–25% cases of advanced mycetoma with extensive bone involvement and severe secondary infection, amputation can be lifesaving [35].

Outcome

Complete cure is difficult to achieve and recurrence rate is 25–50% [12, 35]. Hence long- term follow-up is essential. In general, patients with small lesions are more likely to have a good prognosis and a high rate of cure, whereas patients with massive lesions and long-standing disease are more prone to recurrence. Outcomes can be improved by raising awareness and preventing the disease from causing serious medical, social, and economic impacts.

Box 35.8 Mycetoma

- Chronic slowly progressive granulomatous infection of skin and soft tissues
- *Madurella mycetomasis* – commonest organism
- Predominantly seen in Africa (Sudan), India and Central and south America
- Exposed portions of feet and hands – most common, due to direct thorn pricks – presents as severe, slowly progressive invasive osteomyelitis
- Treatment: Predominantly surgical – with wide local excision, debridement and amputation, with supportive medical management
- Outcome; Complete cure difficult to achieve – with recurrence rate of 25-50 % with long-term morbidity.

Summary

Fungi are an uncommon but important cause of musculoskeletal infections in children. Symptoms are often subacute and may masquerade as other disorders, which can lead to substantial delays in treatment. Diagnosis requires a high index of suspicion. The goals of management are eradication of the infection and prevention of future recurrences. Collaboration with an infectious disease specialist is recommended to provide an appropriate antifungal treatment plan and to monitor the patients.

Acknowledgements Ms. Rashmi Oka for contributing illustrations to the chapter.

References

1. Henry MW, Miller AO, Walsh TJ, Brause BD. Fungal musculoskeletal infections. Infect Dis Clin N Am. 2017;31(2):353–68. https://doi.org/10.1016/j.idc.2017.01.006.
2. Taj-Aldeen SJ, Gamaletsou MN, Rammaert B, et al. Bone and joint infections caused by mucormycetes: a challenging osteoarticular mycosis of the twenty-first century. Med Mycol. 2017;55(7):691–704. https://doi.org/10.1093/mmy/myw136.
3. Arkun R. Parasitic and fungal disease of bones and joints. Semin Musculoskelet Radiol. 2004;8(3):231–42.
4. Monsignore LM, Martinez R, Simão MN, Teixeira SR, Elias J, Nogueira-Barbosa MH. Radiologic findings of osteoarticular infection in paracoccidioidomycosis. Skelet Radiol. 2012;41(2):203–8. https://doi.org/10.1007/s00256-011-1214-3.
5. Gamaletsou MN, Walsh TJSN. Epidemiology of fungal infections. Curr Fungal Infect. 2014;8:262–70.
6. Gamaletsou MN, Rammaert B, Bueno MA, et al. Aspergillus arthritis: analysis of clinical manifestations, diagnosis, and treatment of 31 reported cases. Med Mycol. 2017;55(3):246–54. https://doi.org/10.1093/mmy/myw077.
7. Gamaletsou MN, Rammaert B, Bueno MA, et al. Candida arthritis: analysis of 112 pediatric and adult cases. Open Forum Infect Dis. 2016;3(1):1–10. https://doi.org/10.1093/ofid/ofv207.
8. Rammaert B, Gamaletsou MN, Zeller V, Elie C, Prinapori R, Taj-Aldeen SJ, Roilides E, Kontoyiannis DP, Brause B, Sipsas NV, Walsh TJLO. Dimorphic fungal osteoarticular infections. Eur J Clin Microbiol

Infect Dis. 2014;33(12):2131–40. https://pubmed.ncbi.nlm.nih.gov/24939620/.
9. Rammaert B, Gamaletsou MN, Zeller V, et al. Dimorphic fungal osteoarticular infections. Eur J Clin Microbiol Infect Dis. 2014;33(12):2131–40. https://doi.org/10.1007/s10096-014-2149-0.
10. Arockiaraj J, Balaji G, Ashok A, Kokil G. Amphotericin B cement beads: a good adjunctive treatment for musculoskeletal mucormycosis. Indian J Orthop. 2012;46(3):369–72. https://doi.org/10.4103/0019-5413.96370.
11. Fahal AH, Shaheen SJD. Orthopedic aspects of mycetoma. Bone Joint J. 2014;96-B:420–5.
12. Manesh A, Rupali P, Sullivan MO, Mohanraj P, Rupa V, George BMJ. Mucormycosis-A clinicoepidemiological review of cases over 10 years. Mycoses. 2019;62(4):391–8.
13. Yu OH, Keet AW, Sheppard DC, Brewer T. Articular aspergillosis: case report and review of the literature. Int J Infect Dis. 2010;14(5):e433–5.
14. Ramanathan D, Sahasrabudhe NKE. Disseminated coccidioidomycosis to the spine-case series and review of literature. Brain Sci. 2019;7(9):160.
15. Emamian S, Fox MG, Boatman D, Allard FD, Nacey NC. Spinal blastomycosis: unusual musculoskeletal presentation with literature review. Skelet Radiol. 2019;48(12):2021–7. https://doi.org/10.1007/s00256-019-03234-9.
16. Ravindran S, Sobhanakumari K, Celine M, Palakkal S. African histoplasmosis: the first report of an indigenous case in India. Int J Dermatol. 2015;54(4):451–5.
17. Morris-Jones R. Sporotrichosis. Clin Exp Dermatol. 2002;27(6):427–31. https://pubmed.ncbi.nlm.nih.gov/12372075/.
18. Corr PD. Musculoskeletal fungal infections. Semin Musculoskelet Radiol. 2011;15(5):506–10. https://doi.org/10.1055/s-0031-1293496.
19. Gamaletsou MN, Kontoyiannis DP, Sipsas NV, et al. Candida osteomyelitis: analysis of 207 pediatric and adult cases (1970-2011). Clin Infect Dis. 2012;55(10):1338–51. https://doi.org/10.1093/cid/cis660.
20. Walsh TJ, Gamaletsou MN, McGinnis MR, Hayden RT, Kontoyiannis DP. Early clinical and laboratory diagnosis of invasive pulmonary, extrapulmonary, and disseminated mucormycosis (zygomycosis). Clin Infect Dis. 2012;54(Suppl 1):55–60. https://doi.org/10.1093/cid/cir868.
21. Gamaletsou MN, Walsh TJ, Sipsas NV. Invasive fungal infections in patients with hematological malignancies: emergence of resistant pathogens and new antifungal therapies. Turk J Haematol. 2018;35(1):1–11. https://doi.org/10.4274/tjh.2018.0007.
22. Savarese LG, Monsignore LM, de Andrade Hernandes M, Martinez R, Nogueira-Barbosa MH. Magnetic resonance imaging findings of paracoccidioidomycosis in the musculoskeletal system. Trop Med Int Health. 2015;20(10):1346–54.
23. Yombi JC, Seyler L, Cornu O, et al. Difficult to treat osteoarticulars infections: focus on mycobacterial and fungal infections. Acta Orthop Belg. 2017;83(1):110–23.
24. Blair JE. State-of-the-art treatment of coccidioidomycosis skeletal infections. Ann N Y Acad Sci. 2007;1111:422–33.
25. Pérez-Gómez A, Prieto A, Torresano M, Díez E, Mulero J, Labiano I, Andreu JL. Role of the new azoles in the treatment of fungal osteoarticular infections. Semin Arthritis Rheum. 1998;27(4):226–44.
26. Taneja AK, Torriani M, Simeone FJ. Septic arthritis and osteomyelitis of the hip by Candida albicans. J Rheumatol. 2014;41(11):2270. https://doi.org/10.3899/jrheum.140354.
27. Bariteau JT, Waryasz GR, McDonnell M, Fischer SA, Hayda RA, Born CT. Fungal osteomyelitis and septic arthritis. J Am Acad Orthop Surg. 2014;22(6):390–401. https://doi.org/10.5435/JAAOS-22-06-390.
28. Kohli R, Hadley S. Fungal arthritis and osteomyelitis. Infect Dis Clin N Am. 2005;19(4):831–51. https://doi.org/10.1016/j.idc.2005.08.004.
29. Zhou HX, Lu L, Chu T, et al. Skeletal cryptococcosis from 1977 to 2013. Front Microbiol. 2014;5(Dec):1–18. https://doi.org/10.3389/fmicb.2014.00740.
30. Gamaletsou MN, Rammaert B, Bueno MA, et al. Aspergillus osteomyelitis: epidemiology, clinical manifestations, management, and outcome. J Infect. 2014;68(5):478–93. https://doi.org/10.1016/j.jinf.2013.12.008.
31. Kumar KS, Narasimhan A, Gopalakrishnan R, Geetha N, Thirunarayanan MA, Suryanarayanan P. Coccidioidomycosis in Chennai. J Assoc Physicians India. 2011;59:122–4.
32. Taljanovic MS, Adam RD. Musculoskeletal coccidioidomycosis. Semin Musculoskelet Radiol. 2011;15(5):511–26.
33. Ho AK, Shrader MW, Falk MN, Segal LS. Diagnosis and initial management of musculoskeletal coccidioidomycosis in children. J Pediatr Orthop. 2014;34(5):571–7.
34. Bibbo C, Spellman J. Successful salvage of complicated calcaneal blastomycosis in disseminated disease with staged surgical reconstruction and local-systemic antifungal therapy. J Foot Ankle Surg. 2014;53(4):472–9.
35. Sipsas NV, Gamaletsou MN, Anastasopoulou A, Kontoyiannis DP. Therapy of mucormycosis. J Fungi (Basel). 2018;4(3):1–17. https://doi.org/10.3390/jof4030090.

Necrotising Fasciitis

36

Arne Schröder
and Christina Oetzmann von Sochaczewski

Introduction

Necrotising fasciitis is a chameleon in surgery. It went by a variety of names that changed during history. The term necrotising fasciitis was first coined in 1952 [1] but soon replaced its synonyms. Descriptions of necrotising fasciitis date back to *Hippocrates* in the fifth century before the Common Era [2]. Another name was provided by *Pouteau* in 1783, phagedena, which means "eating-away" [3]. During the American Civil War, necrotising fasciitis was termed hospital gangrene because it affected the wounded and killed them in field hospitals with a higher death toll than the enemy [4]. Another name necrotising fasciitis acquired was *Meleney's* cellulitis as *Meleney* described the first modern cases in both adults [5] and children [6]. To the general public, necrotising fasciitis is equivalent to flesh-eating bacteria, [7] which kind of revives the eighteenth-century term phagadena. Necrotising fasciitis did not appear in paediatric textbooks until 1973 [8]. Although almost 40 years have passed since then, data apart from case reports and case series are scarce. Narrative reviews often derived their recommendations largely from adult data [9–11] because child-centred synthesised evidence is rare [12, 13].

Epidemiology

Incidence rates of necrotising fasciitis are around 2 yearly cases per 100,000 people in Denmark [14] and England [15], whereas 3.26 annual cases per 100,000 persons can be found in Taiwan [16]. Of note, incidence rates of necrotising fasciitis are strongly age dependent and the vast majority of cases occurred in patients above retirement age [14, 16]. Consequently, incidence rates in children are quite small and vary between 0.01 and 0.59 in developed countries (Fig. 36.1) [16–21] (Box 36.1). This focus on developed countries is highly problematic as it is likely to mask the global dimension of the disease: A prospective observational study from only one hospital in Nigeria reported 32 cases of necrotising fasciitis in children within 4 years [22], indicating higher incidence rates in low to middle income countries than in the Western world. This is corroborated by annual incidence rates from Fiji, which were 5.2 per 100,000 children – more than ten times higher than in developed countries [23]. Therefore, necrotising fasciitis – like invasive group-A streptococcal diseases [24] and serious skin infections [25] – is a disease of poverty.

A. Schröder
Klinik für Kinder- und Jugendmedizin, Klinikum Dortmund, Dortmund, Germany

C. Oetzmann von Sochaczewski (✉)
Sektion Kinderchirurgie der Klinik und Poliklinik für Allgemein-, Viszeral-, Thorax- und Gefäßchirurgie, Universitätsklinikum Bonn, Bonn, Germany

© Springer Nature Switzerland AG 2022
M. V. Belthur et al. (eds.), *Pediatric Musculoskeletal Infections*,
https://doi.org/10.1007/978-3-030-95794-0_36

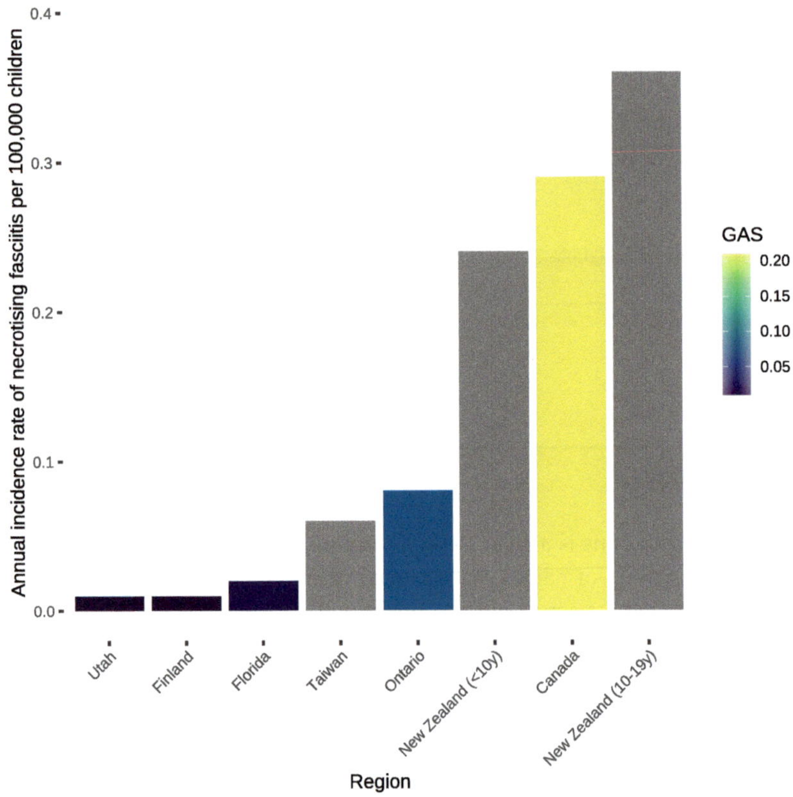

Fig. 36.1 Incidence rates of necrotising fasciitis per 100,000 children per year in developed countries. If incidence rates separate for group-A and non-group-A necrotising fasciitis are provided, the incidence rate of group-A necrotising fasciitis is represented by the colour of the bar graph. Grey bar graphs indicate no information on causative germs

Box 36.1 General Information

- Necrotising fasciitis is a life threatening, rapidly spreading soft tissue infection.
- Annual Incidence rates in developed countries vary between 0.01 and 0.59 cases per 100,000 children, but are much higher in low to middle income countries.
- Cellulitis and abscesses are relevant differential diagnoses and several thousand times more frequent than necrotising fasciitis.
- Group-A streptococci are the most frequent organisms isolated but a shift towards Staphylococcus spp. and Gram-negative bacteria can be expected in countries with a varicella vaccination program and in children with preceding surgery or immunocompromise.

Microbiology

Contrary to many other aspects, the microbiology of necrotising fasciitis in children is well described. A large proportion of cases of necrotising fasciitis were caused by group-A streptococci: 62% in a population-based analysis from Canada [20] and 44.8% in a systematic review of pooled case reports [13]. *Streptococcus* spp. made up only 21.8% of the cases in an analysis of the kid's inpatient database from the United States, in which *Staphylococcus* spp. were top-ranking with 34.5%, attributed to the effects of varicella vaccination [26]. Proportions varied highly between smaller studies, with Streptococcus spp. making up more than three quarters of all cases in some [27, 28], whereas reports with older children and more causative events such as immunosuppression, trauma, and surgery showed a spectrum of causative organisms that was shifted towards *Staphylococcus* spp. and Gram-negative bacteria [29–32]. This was also the case in a prospective evaluation of children treated at paediatric intensive care units in francophone countries [33]. A similar shift of microbiologic isolates towards the Gram-negative spectrum has also been observed in a population-based assessment from England covering all age groups [15]. The analysis of preceding events of necrotising fasciitis and causative organisms revealed a high frequency of group-A streptococci in cases with a varicella infection, but group-A streptococci were also often present in other cases except for immunocompromised children (Fig. 36.2). In contrast, operated cases often had polymicrobial infection and high frequencies of Gram-negative rods, which was also the case in immunocompromised children (Fig. 36.2).

Historically, necrotising fasciitis due to group-A streptococci had been associated with a high mortality rate [4]. In contrast, an analysis of the Paediatric Health Information System database – covering 41 paediatric hospitals in the United States – described a reduced occurrence of mortalities in case of a streptococcal or staphylococcal infection [34]. A result that could be corroborated in adults by a prospective multicentre study from Scandinavia [35]. On the opposite side of the spectrum seems to be necrotising fasciitis caused by fungi: It has been described to increase the chance of death in adults threefold compared to bacteria in the prospectively maintained Acute and Critical Care Surgery database from the United States [36] and also in a smaller retrospective monocentric analysis [37]. A tripled case fatality rate in fungal necrotising fasciitis was present in children too, compared to 10.4% in the overall cohort of 295 cases [13].

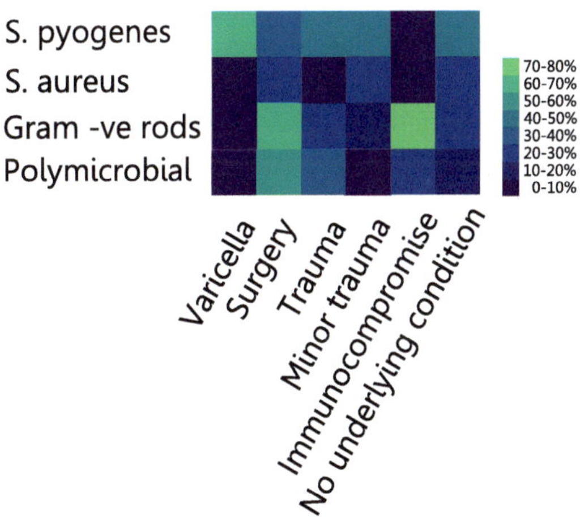

Fig. 36.2 Itemisation of isolated germs for preceding events using the pooled cases from a systematic review [13]

Necrotising fasciitis has been classified in 1977 according to the isolated organisms [38] and extended later on [39] (Table 36.1). Although this classification is widely described in narrative reviews for adults and children [9–11, 40, 41], only two of them [9, 11] point out that the traditional distribution – the vast majority being type I necrotising fasciitis [38, 39] – is not applicable in children. In them polymicrobial infection occurs in less than 20% of cases in systematic reviews [12, 13], whereas Gram-negative germs are more frequent [12, 13]. In addition, the usefulness for differentiating the clinical course or a potential prognostic value of this classification has still to be determined, more than 40 years since its introduction.

Aetiology and Risk Factors

Varicella is the most relevant preceding factor for necrotising fasciitis: Amongst 24 cases of necrotising fasciitis within 7 years in a tertiary hospital in Quebec, 15 were associated with varicella, but none of the cases in the following 7 years after introduction of a varicella vaccine was linked to a varicella infection [42]. A prospective evaluation from Canada [20] and some retrospective studies described similar numbers before the introduc-

Table 36.1 Classification of necrotising fasciitis according to the causative organisms

Type	I	II	III	IV
Mono-/Polymicrobial	Polymicrobial	Poly- or monomicrobial	Monomicrobial	Monomicrobial
Obligate organism	Anaerobes	Throat commensal bacteria	Gram-negative	Fungi

tion of a varicella vaccine [27, 43, 44]. A recent synthesis of 297 cases of necrotising fasciitis from case reports found 26% of them being associated with a varicella infection [13], which is similar to results from small paediatric cohort studies [28–30]. More than 20% of included patients had no associated event [13], followed by minor trauma such as insect bites or bruises in 12.5%, immunocompromised status in 11.8%, preceding surgery in 9.4%, 8.1% experienced significant trauma, and 6.1% of cases had a preexisting skin infection, whereas other causes were rare [13]. Due to the small numbers of included patients, the frequency of the reported contributing factors varied between the case series: In some, preceding surgery was most prominent [31, 33], while in others it was skin infections or trauma [28, 32]. In contrast, necrotising fasciitis in neonates can usually be traced back to omphalitis [27, 29] or mastitis [22], but spontaneous manifestation without any known risk factors may also occur [45]. Although contributing factors for the development of necrotising fasciitis have been described, they are mere associations, but not true risk factors that may guide diagnosis.

Pathophysiology

Necrotising fasciitis is accused of 'pillaging the acute-phase response' [41]. If a preceding event can be found in the patient's history, for example, a traumatic injury, pathogens enter the body. There are two different courses then, either the pathogens get sealed and subsequently eliminated followed by tissue repair or pathogens are able to highjack the acute-phase response and use it in their favour through virulence factors [41, 46, 47]. Sealing of the pathogens is conducted by fibrin and platelet webs due to the activation of the coagulation system, whose signalling colludes with those of the injured tissue alarming the immune system. This process is then aided by neutrophils by their extracellular traps, followed by macrophages killing pathogens and removing cell debris. *Staphylococcus aureus*' strategies for immune evasion are to highjack the coagulation system that effectively allows them to form themselves a shielded compartment within the injured tissues that prevents neutrophils' access [46]. In addition, *Staphylococcus aureus*' enzymes can destroy the neutrophil extracellular traps and produce the extracellular adherence protein, which can at the same time promote the acute-phase response by stimulating immune cells to secrete cytokines and inhibit it by downregulation of the cellular response [46]. These protective effects help *Staphylococcus aureus* to reach quorum in a protected compartment and then destroy it by coordinated release of staphylokinase degrading the protective fibrin capsule, which releases overwhelming amounts of staphylococci into dissemination [46], resulting in necrotising fasciitis.

Streptococcus pyogenes has a different approach: Its streptokinase directly activates plasminogen and some bacterial surface proteins function as plasminogen receptors thereby enhancing streptokinase's activity [46]. This mechanism prevents sequestration of a *Streptococcus pyogenes* inoculation within the body and thereby allows the rapid spread along the fascial planes observed in necrotising fasciitis [46]. However, *Streptococcus pyogenes* also interferes with the coagulation system via streptolysin O, which activates platelets that complex cellular immune effectors and cause microvascular thrombosis [46]. For other germs causing necrotising fasciitis, like *Escherichia coli* and *Pseudomonas aeruginosa*, plasminogen also has a key role for their dissemination, although their mechanisms are different and have a higher degree of similarity to tumour metastasis [46].

Tissue ischaemia, due to micro thrombosis caused by bacterial interference with the coagulation system, does not only hamper the response of the immune system and shield the invading germs [41] but also force the body's metabolism towards anaerobic pathways resulting in accumulation of acidic metabolites and increased osmolality [47]. Acidic pH, elevated temperature, and osmolality have a crucial role in initiation of necrotising fasciitis: They may function as a molecular switch that enables bacteria to transpose themselves from being adapted to the site of injury towards systemic spread [47]. Moreover, ischaemia causes additional tissue damage, thereby optimising the conditions for the invasive bacteria to spread even further and potentiate their destructive potential [47].

Pathology

The combination of macroscopic clinical findings, Gram-staining, and fresh-frozen section has been termed 'triple diagnostics' and is recommended to pathologically establish the diagnosis of necrotising fasciitis based on a retrospective analysis of 21 adult patients [48]. In classical histopathology, the initial phase of necrotising fasciitis may not be differentiated from a much more benign skin infection as epidermal erosions, oedematous thickening of the dermis, and a sparse inflammatory infiltrate represent the only pathologic changes [47]. The inflammation may also include the subcutaneous fat and a superficial hyaline necrosis can develop, which is not discriminatory either [49]. Rapid disease progression of necrotising fasciitis is then characterised by liquefactive necrosis along all tissue layers representing a macroscopic full-thickness necrosis and corresponding to the swollen and dull-greyish discoloured fasciae [49]. Marked inflammatory infiltrates and bacterial colonies accompany necrosis as it spreads along fascial planes [47, 50]. Involvement of underlying muscles via visible myonecrosis correspond to liquefactive necrosis of individual muscle fibres [47]. Obliterative vasculitis causing microangiopathic thrombosis at an earlier stage progresses towards noninflammatory intravascular coagulation with increasing severity of necrotising fasciitis [47, 49]. In contrast to affected tissues, there is minimal bystander inflammation in surrounding tissues [49, 50]. Classifying necrotising fasciitis based on histopathology has only been suggested once [51] without compelling success.

Clinical Presentation

Necrotising fasciitis manifests in around the half of cases in the extremities, with a large preference for the lower extremities [12, 13, 26]. The second most affected region is the trunk followed by the head, and the upper extremity [12, 13]. A recent prospective evaluation from francophone countries however described lower extremities, trunk, and upper extremities to be almost equally affected but included a large proportion of postoperative and trauma patients [33]. Neonates represent a different population in whom the trunk is particularly affected [12], due to the association to omphalitis [22]. As expected, higher frequencies of trunk affections occurred in varicella-related cases, in immunocompromised patients, and in those with preceding surgery (Fig. 36.3). Patients without a preceding event associated with necrotising fasciitis were more frequently affected in the head (Fig. 36.3). However, necrotising fasciitis may occur anywhere in the body.

In Medical School, we were taught that hallmarks of necrotising fasciitis were necrosis, crepitus, and bullae [11]. The first report of paediatric necrotising fasciitis did only mention swelling, bullae, and blisters before the onset of necrosis [6], whereas the first case series describes that 'the affected skin first becomes swollen, erythematous, warm, and painful' [8]. This highlights an important distinction: The signs of early disease are nonspecific, whereas the classic hallmarks of necrotising fasciitis are those of a late-stage infection (Fig. 36.4). Erythema, tenderness, swelling, and pain were common skin signs in a smaller systematic review [12]. In a larger systematic review, the most frequent skin signs were erythema in 58.7%, swelling in 48%, pain in

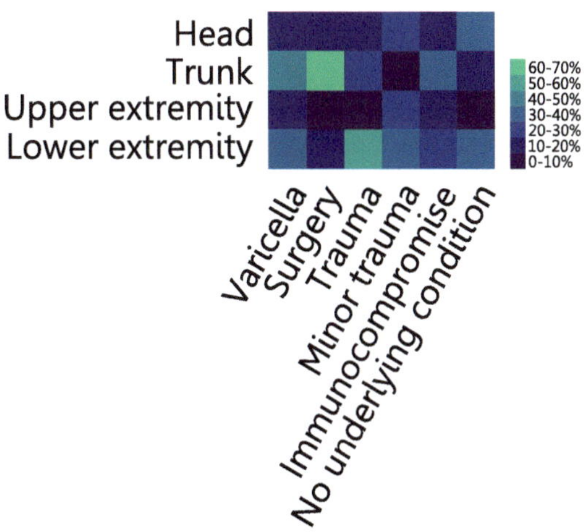

Fig. 36.3 Itemisation of localisations of necrotising fasciitis lesions for preceding events using the pooled cases from a systematic review [13]

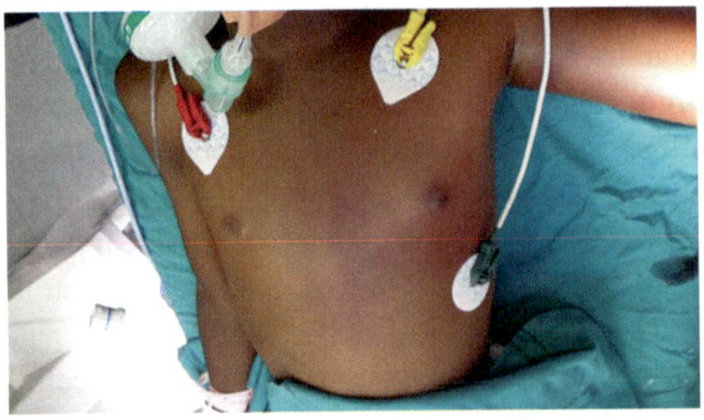

Fig. 36.4 Early stage of skin signs of necrotising fasciitis. Erythema spreading from the arm along the chest extending to the patients right side beyond the sternum, caudally beyond the electrocardiogram-electrode and at the left lateral side towards the back. Also note the beginning discolouration at the left axilla. (The photo has been previously shown in [100] under the licence CC-BY 4.0 with copyright retained by the authors)

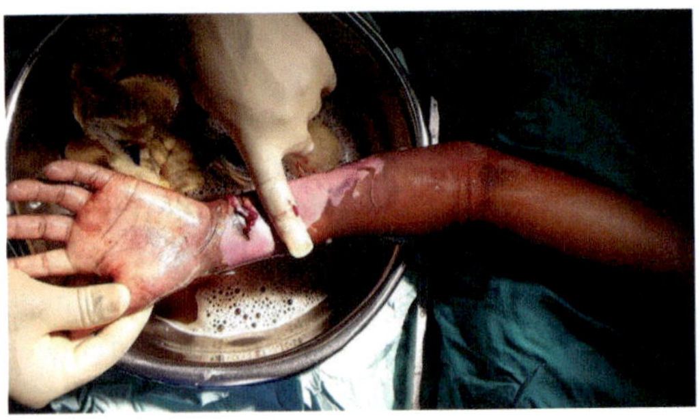

Fig. 36.5 Late stage of skin signs of necrotising fasciitis. Skin necrosis can be observed along the forearm, because it could be easily separated from the underlying subcutis. The forearm and the inside of the elbow also show dark, patchy discolorations that can be observed in the subcutis at the forearm, too

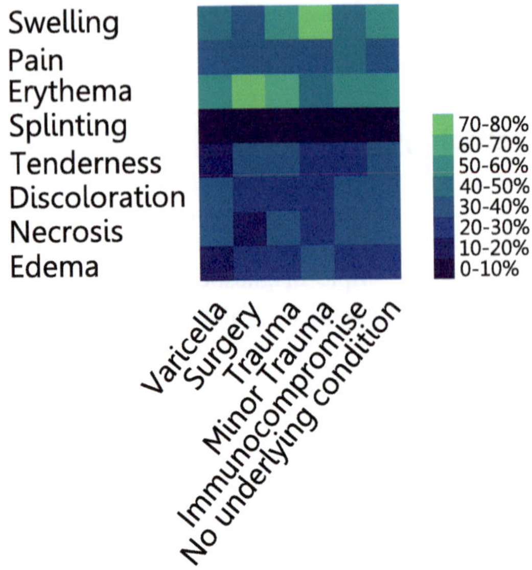

Fig. 36.6 Itemisation of skin signs of necrotising fasciitis for preceding events using the pooled cases from a systematic review [13]

33.6%, oedema in 26.5%, and tenderness in 25.2%, whereas induration in 14.4% and warmth in 10.7% of cases were seldom present [13]. The high frequencies of discoloration in 32.6% and necrosis in 32.2% indicate a relevant proportion of cases with an advanced stage of disease (Fig. 36.5) [13]. Relevant differences in skin signs between the different preceding events seem to be absent (Fig. 36.6). The results of these systematic reviews are likely impaired by recall bias as one retrospective case–control study report a frequency of 87.5% for swelling, pain, and erythema but frequencies of 37.5% for splinting and tenderness [43]. Likewise, another case–control study reported frequencies of 100% for swelling and pain, 95% for erythema, and splinting of an extremity to have been present in 67% of cases [52], whereas signs of advanced disease have not been reported [43, 52].

In adults in whom the diagnosis of necrotising fasciitis had been missed, it has been tried to classify necrotising fasciitis according to skin signs: At day zero, the vast majority of patients had erythema, tenderness, warmth, and swelling, which progressed to blisters or bullae at day two, whereas crepitus, skin anaesthesia, and necrosis did largely appear later at days three and four [53]. However, this classification is far from being perfect and skin signs may not be as selective as they appear: Blisters or bullae were already present in 50% of the included patients at day one as was skin necrosis in 13% of patients [53]. Literature reviews in adults have also shown swelling, erythema, and pain or tenderness to be common symptoms, whereas bullae, crepitus, and necrosis were much less frequent [54–56].

A striking difference between adults and children is fever: While it is not a common symptom in adults [54–57], the vast majority of children have fever, usually around 80% in systematic reviews [12, 13], whereas it was 100% in case–

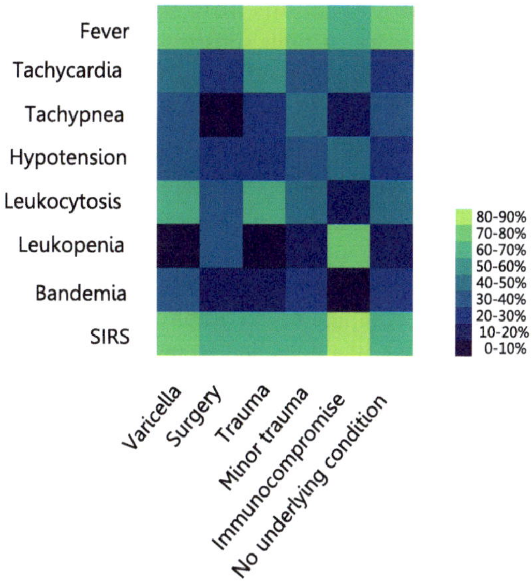

Fig. 36.7 Itemisation of signs of systemic involvement of necrotising fasciitis for preceding events using the pooled cases from a systematic review [13]

control studies [43, 52]. Amongst other signs of systemic illness, tachycardia was much less frequent in a systematic review with 40.7%, but way ahead of tachypnoea with 27.7% [13], whereas both were common in a case–control study [43]. Hypotension can be expected in around 30% of cases [12, 13, 52]. Leucocytosis can be found in half of the cases or in a slight majority [12, 13, 43], but leucopoenia [12, 13, 43, 52] or bandaemia is not unheard of [12, 13, 32, 43], as are toxic shock syndrome [44, 52], acute kidney injury [26, 52], electrolyte disturbances [26, 58], and coagulopathy [30, 52]. A systemic inflammatory response syndrome has seldom been evaluated, but it was present in 65.1% of included cases in a systematic review [13] and in 90% of adult patients [59]. An analysis of systemic illness by preceding events showed that fever was more frequent following trauma, but less frequent in immunocompromised patients, who more frequently had leukopenia, but still were those with the highest number of systemic inflammatory response syndrome (Fig. 36.7). In contrast, leucocytosis did occur more often in patients with a preceding trauma and in those that had varicella, the latter also having bandaemia more frequently (Fig. 36.7).

Taken together, neither skin changes nor laboratory parameters alone are specific for necrotising fasciitis. Consequently, awareness and clinical suspicion is necessary to think of necrotising fasciitis as a differential diagnosis in the early stage of disease (Box 36.2).

Box 36.2 Tips for Establishing Diagnosis

- Think of necrotising fasciitis as a differential diagnosis although it is rare.
- There is neither a key clinical feature nor a specific combination of signs and symptoms that rule in or out the diagnosis.
- Clinical intuition, awareness, and experience of the surgeon guide the diagnosis.
- Imaging should not delay surgical intervention.
- The finger test can be helpful in equivocal cases.
- If in doubt about the possibility of necrotising fasciitis, proceed with surgical exploration – the skin incision of a negative exploration can be sutured, but the damage due to a missed diagnosis will always be much worse.

Investigations/Work-Up

Laboratory Tests There are no standard laboratory parameters that facilitate diagnosis because the suggested instruments may not be reliable. In adults, the laboratory risk indicator for necrotising fasciitis had been proposed [60] but failed to prove its usefulness in further studies [57, 61]. A simplified version, just using low sodium and elevated C-reactive protein, the paediatric laboratory risk indicator for necrotising fasciitis had been proposed [58]. It was based on a case–control study using 20 cases and controls each with predictors identified by stepwise, backward logistic regression and maximisation of the area under the receiver operating characteristic curve. It violated not only sample size criteria but also omitted cross-validation using a validation set. In addition, its results were neither corroborated nor are there any documented cases using this instrument in the literature in the diagnosis of necrotising fasciitis so far; it is only mentioned once in the context of necrotising cellulitis [62]. In order to assess the current status of the patient, a complete blood count, electrolytes, liver and kidney function tests, coagulation parameters – coagulopathy was present in 27.8% in a population-based analysis [20], blood glucose, a blood gas to assess the metabolic status, C-reactive protein, and – if available – procalcitonin should be measured. The latter might be helpful to determine the extent of inflammation [63] and its reduction following surgery [64], based on small studies in adults. Blood cultures need to be drawn before commencement of antimicrobial chemotherapy. Packed red blood cells, fresh frozen or lyophilised plasma, and – in case of a disseminated intravascular coagulation – platelets and coagulation factors need to be available. Transfusions of blood products were reported in 23.1% [34] in one and 15% [26] of cases in another database article, so one needs to be prepared.

Arterial and central venous access should be obtained perioperatively in order to be able to initiate vasopressor therapy in addition to aggressive fluid resuscitation, although this was only reported for 2.2% in a database article, which is conflicting to 22.2% of the patients having had a simultaneous sepsis or septic shock [26]. A Foley catheter is also necessary to monitor the urine output as oliguria and acute kidney injury – 11.1% in a population-based assessment [20] – might be present. An intensive care bed needs to be at hand as 24.6% [34] and 22.1% [26] of patients were ventilated in the database articles, so similar to transfusions, this occurs frequently.

Imaging Studies Studies on imaging for necrotising fasciitis in children have only been case reports with limited value. While plain radiography might be quite specific for necrotising fasciitis [61], this requires the presence of subcutaneous gas, which is seldom the case [65, 66] and thus plain films have no role in diagnosing necrotising fasciitis [61, 67]. Computed tomography has a high sensitivity, specificity, and a positive likelihood ratio of 8.17 for the diagnosis, if fascial gas is present [61], but again, this is not a frequent finding [65, 66]. Consequently, positive likelihood ratio halves if other potential signs of necrotising fasciitis such as fascial oedema or (non)enhancement were included [61]. Additional signs of necrotising fasciitis in computed tomography could be epifascial fluid collections and stranding of subcutaneous fat, all of which represent imaging correlates of necrosis and inflammation [65, 66]. Similar to computed tomography, soft-tissue gas is the hallmark of necrotising fasciitis in magnetic resonance imaging, but seldom present [65, 66]. Typical signs are thickening of deep muscle fasciae, fascial hyperintensity, subfascial fluids, and varying contrast enhancements [65, 66, 68]. While computed tomography requires less time than magnetic resonance imaging, which is also difficult to perform in intensive care patients, both should not be used to verify the clinical diagnosis of necrotising fasciitis: Delays should be avoided to achieve source control if necrotising fasciitis is a possible diagnosis and thus proceed with surgical exploration [61, 65–67].

Special Tests A useful adjunct to diagnosis might be the 'finger test': Diseased skin is incised to the deep fascial plane and blunt dissection along the fascial level is attempted [69]. If the finger meets low resistance, accompanied by minimal bleeding, and dishwater-like fluid at the fascial level, the 'finger test' is considered positive and the diagnosis of necrotising fasciitis is established [69]. A similar explorative method has already been described in children in 1973 by *Wilson & Hatalin*, although with using a probe instead of a finger [8]. The sensitivity of the test was high and the specificity moderate, but it outperformed other tests [69]. As the test may be performed with local anaesthesia or procedural sedation and is less time consuming than imaging studies, it might have some value in supporting the diagnosis without causing a time delay.

Differential Diagnoses

Its differential diagnoses are more common than necrotising fasciitis. The database of a Mormon health insurance has been used to estimate the population-based incidence rate for cellulitis, which was 2460 yearly cases per 100,000 persons [70]. In comparison to necrotising fasciitis, cellulitis is more than 1000 times more frequent in the general population. These numbers are even more striking in children: In a database from commercial insurances [71], the annual incidence rate of cellulitis in childhood per 100,000 persons was 15,100 times higher than that of necrotising fasciitis, if it was assumed to be 0.03 per 100,000 children annually. Consequently, necrotising fasciitis will be exceedingly rare amongst children with skin infections.

Differentiating necrotising fasciitis from cellulitis has been bedevilled by the similarity of the clinical picture in the early phase of necrotising fasciitis. Skin changes are similar and so are fever and white cell counts [43, 44, 52]. In a small retrospective cohort study, it has been suggested that a C-reactive protein elevated above 20 mg/L and a serum sodium below 135 mmol/L were associated with increased likelihood ratios of 3.2 and 5, respectively [58]. This suggestion was based on the laboratory risk indicator for necrotising fasciitis [60], which has not been validated for children and failed to reliably differentiate necrotising fasciitis and cellulitis in a prospective evaluation in adults [57]. In an adult study investigating symptoms and skin changes, pain out of proportion had a positive likelihood ratio of 4.57 for necrotising fasciitis, but of early skin signs, only erythema progressive beyond margins had a relevant positive likelihood ratio of 3.09 [72]. While the other early skin changes were not able to differentiate necrotising fasciitis from cellulitis, only late signs like haemorrhagic bullae had a positive likelihood ratio of 8 and necrosis one of 30 [72], which only confirms textbook knowledge. Pain out of proportion might be helpful in older children and adolescents but not in younger children. Higher C-reactive protein values in necrotising fasciitis compared to cellulitis have not been universally observed in children [44]. This highlights, again, the importance of awareness for subtle signs and clinical intuition to diagnose necrotising fasciitis.

Abscesses are also quite common in the general population with an incidence rate of 450 cases per 100,000 persons per year in England [73], with the only paediatric incidence rate from Fiji with 283.9 annual cases per 100,000 children [23]. However, the abscess is a clinical diagnosis based on a tender and painful induration surrounded by erythematous skin that is often accompanied by a central pustule [74]. Early stages have a characteristically fixed swelling, whereas it becomes fluctuant in later stages with a thinned out skin above the fluctuating area [74]. Contrary to cellulitis and necrotising fasciitis, signs of systemic illness are rare [74] and ultrasound may be helpful to rule in an abscess in those patients with an indistinctive physical examination combined with a medium pre-test probability for an abscess [75]. Hence, differentiating an abscess from necrotising fasciitis is much less of a diagnostic challenge than it is for cellulitis. This is also true for erysipelas that manifest with a rapidly spreading erythema in salmon-red colour and well demarcated margins [74]. Another differential diagnosis is the non-bullous form of impetigo – papules or vesicles with surrounding erythema progressing to pustules and crusts [74].

Treatment Options

Treatment of necrotising fasciitis is surgery (Box 36.3). Conservative treatment of necrotising fasciitis had been described in four small series consisting largely neonates [76–79]. Delays to surgical interventions had a relevant negative effect in adults: Surgery within 6 or 12 hours after first assessment halved the chance of a lethal outcome of necrotising fasciitis [80]. In children, a delay in surgical intervention has also been associated with mortality in necrotising fasciitis [34], whereas surgery was associated with a reduced risk of death [26]. Transfer to a higher-level hospital is associated with mortality [81, 82] and should not be undertaken before debridement due to the time delay [83] and the associated worsened outcome.

Box 36.3 Key Treatment Principles

- Obtain blood cultures before starting intravenous antimicrobial chemotherapy according to local protocols.
- Have an intensive care bed available for the patient and establish invasive blood pressure monitoring and central venous access.
- Excise all necrotic skin and continue skin excision until regular bleeding occurs.
- Achieve wide exposure into clearly healthy tissue and excise all affected fasciae including a margin of healthy fascia.
- Prioritise debridement before referral as surgical source control is the mainstay of therapy.

The classical approach to surgery of necrotising fasciitis in children is fasciotomy and wide debridement [8], which has remained the mainstay of therapy [9, 10, 27, 29, 30, 40, 84]. Recently, a skin-sparing approach has been described in adults that did remove necrotic skin, but instead of removing viable skin above underlying fascial pathology, left the intact skin above the removed fascia to ease reconstruction [85]. A similar approach has also been proposed in children – in a small case series – that conducted small skin excisions of less than 1% total body surface area, which represent around 10% the extent of fascial debridement [86]. Both approaches lift the skin in its full thickness to achieve adequate exposure of the fascial plane [85, 86]. This approach was based on frozen section biopsies of macroscopically intact tissue to determine the correct margin of resection. However, the traditional approach of wide resection of macroscopically affected tissues is advocated by the same group if a pathologist is not available [86]. In both adults [85] and children [86], a skin-sparing approach seems to be associated with a higher number of surgeries than expected from prospective evaluations [14, 34]. In addition, the children treated via this approach [86] presented earlier compared to other cohorts [44, 52] and had their first debridement earlier than reported in other series [34] too.

Technically, the approach to excise all erythematous skin (Fig. 36.8a) irrespective of signs of its disease involvement or viability [87] is too radical because it would sacrifice too much viable tissue. On the contrary, the excision of only the clearly necrotic skin without further explorative skin incision (Fig. 36.8c) has a relevant risk for incomplete source control. Availability of – potentially

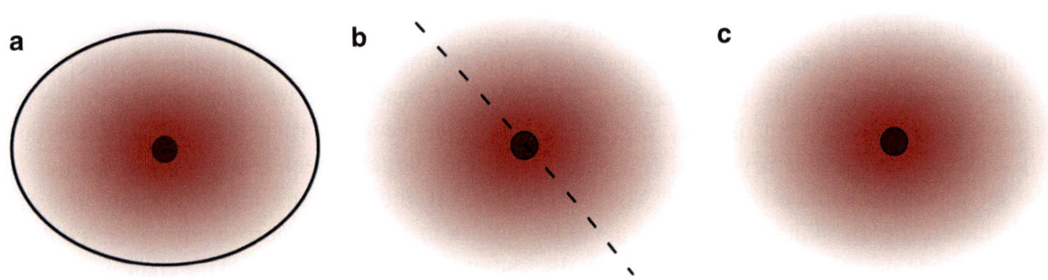

Fig. 36.8 Schematic representation of the different approaches to skin excision during debridement and fasciotomy. Drawings represent a central area of necrosis (brown-grey) with surrounding, radially fading erythema. (**a**) Radical full-thickness excision of all affected skin and underlying fascial planes (solid black circle) as recommended in [87]. (**b**) Full-thickness excision of necrotic skin (solid black circle) and incision into healthy skin (dashed black line) to achieve wide exposure of potentially affected tissues as recommended in [89]. (**c**) Excision of necrotic skin (solid black circle) and full-thickness lift of the non-necrotic skin to inspect and excise the affected fascial planes as described in [86].

unreliable [48, 88] – frozen section biopsies all day and night is rather the exception than reality for the vast majority of hospitals even in the developed world [86]. The preferable approach is wide skin incision into healthy tissue in order to obtain adequate exposure of the potentially diseased area (Fig. 36.8b) [89]. Full thickness specimens are obtained and sent for wound culture and histopathology. Diseased fascia – dull, soft, and friable – is excised exposing underlying muscles and tendons (Fig. 36.9) until only healthy glistening and tough fascia remains below unaffected skin and then a wide margin of a centimetre of healthy fascia is resected, too [89]. The same principle laid out in the finger test is also applicable to exploration along fascial planes: If the overlying subcutaneous tissues can be easily separated from the fascia, it is affected and needs to be excised. Following radical fasciotomy, all necrotic skin and subcutaneous tissues are excised until regular dermal bleeding occurs because poorly bleeding tissues are the correlate of poor microcirculation due to angiitis. In addition, the subcutaneous tissue needs to be examined for signs of necrosis such as liquefaction of fat (Fig. 36.9) and thrombosis of vessels, as they need to be resected too [89]. Radical removal of affected tissues is necessary for two reasons (Fig. 36.10): The liquefactive necrosis and angiitis seen in histopathology are correlates of a poor perfusion that precludes sufficient levels of antimicrobial chemotherapy to reach diseased tissues. In addition, group-A streptococci are able to form a biofilm in necrotising fasciitis in affected tissues, which further promotes bacterial persistence, evasion from antimicrobial chemotherapy, and may increase disease severity [90]. Consequently, be rather too radical in achieving source control to avoid additional debridement than being forced into unplanned redebridement due to disease progression as they will inflict debilitating damage (Fig. 36.11) [89].

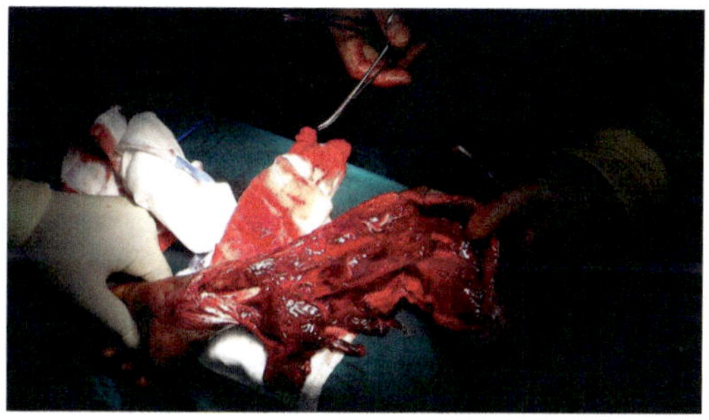

Fig. 36.10 Liquefactive necrosis of the subcutis, fascia, and muscles of the forearm. Maximum exposure of the affected left arm with visible necrosis extending into the muscles for which an amputation was performed to achieve source control

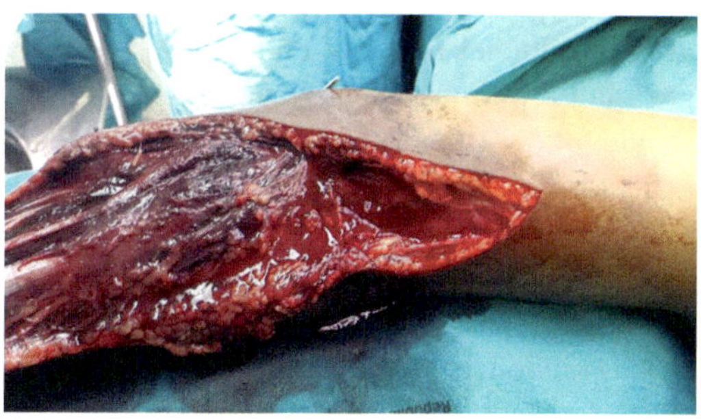

Fig. 36.9 Distinction between affected and healthy tissues. The muscles and the rest of their fascia have a dusky-greyish colour corresponding to fascial and myonecrosis that is also exemplified by liquefaction necrosis of the distal parts of the muscle close to beginning of the tendons. The subcutaneous tissues also show liquefaction necrosis, which is not present above the elbow. There is regular bleeding above the elbow at the cut surface of the skin, but not below the elbow. Note the patchy discoloration proximal to the incision, so it needs to be widened

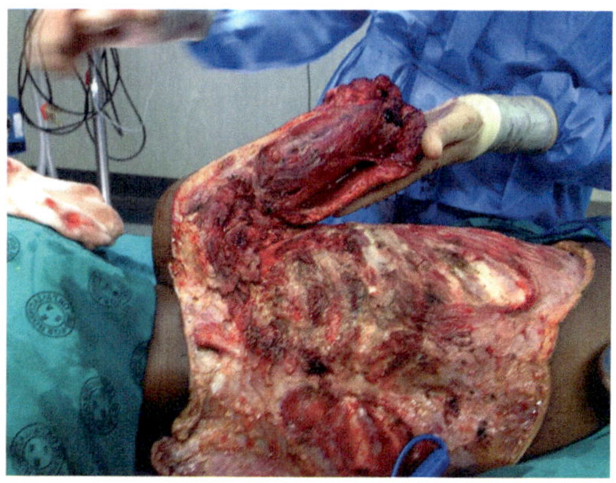

Fig. 36.11 Necessary radical debridement after incomplete source control in first surgery. Debridement extends from the amputation at the left arm towards the beginning of the neck rostrally, to the right clavicle, and caudally towards half the distance to the umbilicus. (The photo has been previously shown in [100] under the licence CC-BY 4.0 with copyright retained by the authors)

Broad-spectrum intravenous antimicrobial chemotherapy is an important adjunct to control the infection and usually continued for weeks, with a median length of 21 days in one study [44]. No data on the duration of antimicrobial chemotherapy either in children or in adults are available, but the World Society of Emergency Surgery recommends to continue antimicrobial agents until surgical interventions are not necessary anymore and fever has resolved for at least 48 hours [67]. In high-resource countries, a procalcitonin-guided approach [64] might provide additional information to support discontinuation of antimicrobial chemotherapy [67]. Usually, combination therapy is used [12, 26, 28, 34, 44], but there is no established gold-standard. Appropriate choice of antimicrobial chemotherapy for necrotising fasciitis depends on the presentation, previous antimicrobial therapy in the last weeks, risk factors for special cases such as health care-associated organisms, and the local resistance profile. Therefore, regional protocols for (necrotising) soft-tissue infections should be followed. This is also true for the use of negative-pressure wound therapy systems, whose use in children is only anecdotally reported [12]. In adults, negative-pressure wound therapy has been evaluated in a clinical trial once but did not show a difference [91]. A retrospective multicentric analysis of negative-pressure wound therapy for Fournier's gangrene in adults showed that only those patients with large skin lesions had higher rates of wound closure after 10 weeks [92]. Thus, evidence for negative-pressure wound therapy in adults is scarce at best, but evidence for its harm or benefit in children is absent.

Intensive care support is another cornerstone of therapy: Many children with necrotising soft tissue infections will need paediatric intensive care; in a recent prospective evaluation from francophone countries, 58% had mechanical ventilation, 54% needed vasopressors, and spend a median of 12.5 days at the paediatric intensive care unit with an overall hospital stay longer than a month [33]. Earlier retrospective studies reported shorter hospital stays for their overall cohorts [20, 26, 34], but noted that those children whose causative germ were non group-A streptococci had a much longer hospital stay [20], being similar to those of the prospective study, in which group-A streptococci were seldom present [33]. Consequently, respiratory support was less frequently used, 17.4% [26] of cases in one and 24.6% [34] in another study, again ventilation was more often necessary in non-group-A streptococci necrotising fasciitis [20]. Likewise, transfusions or albumin replacement are common, too: Half of the cases in the prospective evaluation needed them [33], so did the cases in one retrospective study [20], whereas it was 23% [34] and 15% [26] in others, respectively. While surgery's aim is to stop the infection by achieving source control, supported by antimicrobial chemotherapy, paediatric intensive care and its interventions buy the time to consolidate the trauma due to the infection and its aggressive surgical therapy.

Nutritional support is frequently needed, around 12% of all cases, even more in those of a higher disease severity [34]. In a report on paediatric naso-enteric feeding tubes, there were one patient suffering from necrotising fasciitis and four from severe burns [93], which are much more frequent than necrotising fasciitis. But even without the need for parenteral nutrition, the post-aggression metabolism of the child with necrotising fasciitis is comparable to a child who suffered severe burns: Severe inflammatory response, high levels of oxidative stress, and prolonged hyper catabolism accompanied by the usual nutritional needs of children due to body growth [93]. Consequently, nutritional support should follow established local protocols for burn patients.

Hyperbaric oxygen therapy has been suggested as an adjunct to surgical therapy based on earlier and small case series [94], but a Cochrane Review failed to identify any meaningful evidence for the use of hyperbaric oxygen therapy [95], which did not change if retrospective studies were included, too [96]. In addition, centres offering hyperbaric oxygen therapy are rare and even rarer are those that can treat a child in intensive care environments [97]. Consequently, hyperbaric oxygen therapy was used in 1% in a large paediatric database article [26] and not even mentioned in others [20, 34, 44]. Even in the most recent prospective evaluation of children treated in intensive care units of high-income francophone countries, hyperbaric oxygen therapy was seldom used [33]. This was also true for intravenous immune globulins that were used in 1.9% in the same paediatric database article [26], in 83.2% in a small series [44], and in 36% of the aforementioned prospective study in children [33], but not mentioned elsewhere [12, 20, 34]. Again, a Cochrane Review on data from adults found no relevant effect [98]. Thus, both adjuncts have no compelling role in treatment of necrotising fasciitis at present.

For reconstructive procedures, a transfer towards a higher-level hospital with the availability of a burn centre and a paediatric plastic surgery unit seems useful if extensive reconstructions are necessary, although superior outcomes have not been proven in adults [99]. In one database article, reconstructive procedures were reported for 29.3% of cases [34], 41.7% in a recent series [28], whereas 51.6% of cases had a skin graft in a systematic review and another 10.5% of the included cases had a flap procedure performed [13]. Delayed primary closure was less frequent than healing by secondary intention with 17.3% and 20.4%, respectively [13]. Flap coverage and secondary closure of necrotising fasciitis lesions where more frequent in immunocompromised patients, whereas those that had surgery as an inciting event were more frequently treated via skin graft (Fig. 36.12).

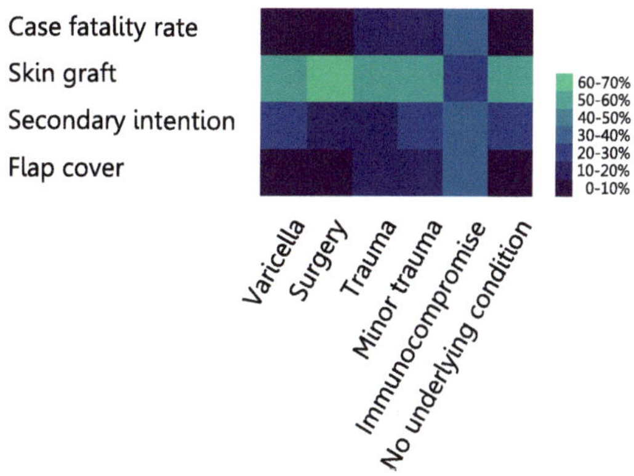

Fig. 36.12 Itemisation of outcomes of necrotising fasciitis for preceding events using the pooled cases from a systematic review [13]

Outcomes and Complications

Necrotising fasciitis has several dreadful complications, the first of which is death, although the chance of death in children is less than one tenth compared to a person at retirement age [15]. In the only prospective multicentric study involving children from francophone countries, the mortality was 6% [33], whereas it was 18% in a prospective multicentric study in adults from Scandinavia [35], indicating a paediatric risk of death around one third of the adult population. In the kid's inpatient database from the United States, the case fatality rate was 6% [26], 6.6% in the Paediatric Health System Information database, also from the United States [34], 5.6% in a monocentric study from Quebec [44], and 10.4% in a systematic review [13]. The latter demonstrated an increased frequency of fatalities in those with severe septicaemic shock and immunocompromised patients (Fig. 36.12) [13, 41]. Missed diagnosis is common [83] and a relevant contributor for fatalities [34, 80] (Box 36.4). Severe septicaemic shock and compartment syndrome were reported in 22.2% and 4.4% of patients [41]. Other complications include amputations, but these were less frequent than death with 3.8% in one series [20], 2.9% [26], and 4.2% [34] in large database articles. An often neglected consequence of necrotising fasciitis seems to be the significant long-term morbidity, indicated by 29.3% of survivors that were discharged to a nursing home or needed home health care (Fig. 36.13) [26].

Box 36.4 Pitfalls to Avoid

- Missed diagnosis occurs often and has devastating effects due to the rapidly progressing infection.
- Insufficient first debridement that does not resect all affected tissues will not stop the rapid spread of necrotising fasciitis.

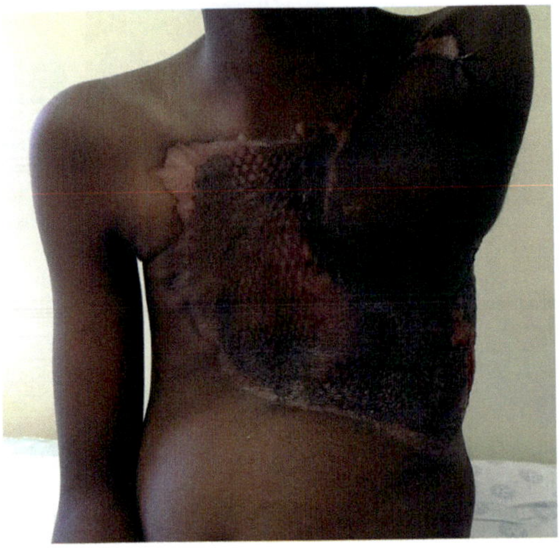

Fig. 36.13 Final situation after necrotising fasciitis with relevant morbidity. The patient had an above elbow amputation and a shoulder dislocation due to extensive myonecrosis and a large skin defect at the trunk that was covered via split-thickness skin grafting. (The photo has been previously shown in [100] under the licence CC-BY 4.0 with copyright retained by the authors)

References

1. Wilson B. Necrotizing fasciitis. Am Surg. 1952;18:416–31.
2. Descamps V, Aitken J, Lee MG. Hippocrates on necrotising fasciitis. Lancet. 1994;344:556.
3. Loudon I. Necrotising fasciitis, hospital gangrene, and phagedena. Lancet. 1994;344:1416–9.
4. Lamb LEM, Sriskandan S, Tan LKK. Bromine, bear-claw scratch fasciotomies, and the Eagle effect: management of group A streptococcal necrotising fasciitis and its association with trauma. Lancet Infect Dis. 2015;15:109–21.
5. Meleney FL. Hemolytic streptococcus gangrene. Arch Surg. 1924;9:317.
6. Meleney FL. Haemolytic streptococcus gangrene following the administration of scarlet fever antitoxin. Ann Surg. 1930;91:287–9.
7. Nowak R. Flesh-eating bacteria: not new, but still worrisome. Science. 1994;264:1665.
8. Wilson HD, Hatalin KC. Acute necrotizing fasciitis in childhood: report of 11 cases. Am J Dis Child. 1973;125:591.
9. Frank G, Mahoney HM, Eppes SC. Musculoskeletal infections in children. Pediatr Clin N Am. 2005;52:1083–106.
10. Jamal N, Teach SJ. Necrotizing fasciitis. Pediatr Emerg Care. 2011;27:1195–9; quiz 1200–1202.
11. Pandey A, Gangopadhyay AN, Upadhyaya VD. Necrotising fasciitis in children and neonates: current concepts. J Wound Care. 2008;17:5–10.
12. Zundel S, Lemaréchal A, Kaiser P, Szavay P. Diagnosis and treatment of pediatric necrotizing fasciitis: a systematic review of the literature. Eur J Pediatr Surg. 2017;27:127–37.
13. Schröder A, Gerin A, Firth GB, Hoffmann KS, Grieve A, Oetzmann von Sochaczewski C. A systematic review of necrotising fasciitis in children from its first description in 1930 to 2018. BMC Infect Dis. 2019;19:317.
14. Hedetoft M, Madsen MB, Madsen LB, Hyldegaard O. Incidence, comorbidity and mortality in patients with necrotising soft-tissue infections, 2005–2018: a Danish nationwide register-based cohort study. BMJ Open. 2020;10:e041302.
15. Bodansky DMS, Begaj I, Evison F, Webber M, Woodman CB, Tucker ON. A 16-year longitudinal cohort study of incidence and bacteriology of necrotising fasciitis in England. World J Surg. 2020;44:2580–91.
16. Liu TJ, Tai H-C, Chien K-L, Cheng N-C. Predisposing factors of necrotizing fasciitis with comparison to cellulitis in Taiwan: a nationwide population-based case–control study. J Formos Med Assoc. 2020;119:18–25.
17. Stockmann C, Ampofo K, Hersh AL, Blaschke AJ, Kendall BA, Korgenski K, Daly J, Hill HR, Byington CL, Pavia AT. Evolving epidemiologic characteristics of invasive group a streptococcal disease in Utah, 2002–2010. Clin Infect Dis. 2012;55:479–87.
18. Mulla ZD. Clinical and epidemiologic features of invasive group A streptococcal infections in children. Pediatr Int. 2007;49:355–8.
19. Laupland KB, Davies HD, Low DE, Schwartz B, Green K, the Ontario Group A Streptococcal Study Group, McGeer A. Invasive group A streptococcal disease in children and association with varicella-zoster virus infection. Pediatrics. 2000;105:e60.
20. Eneli I, Davies HD. Epidemiology and outcome of necrotizing fasciitis in children: An active surveillance study of the Canadian Paediatric surveillance program. J Pediatr. 2007;151:79–84.e1.
21. Das DK, Baker MG, Venugopal K. Increasing incidence of necrotizing fasciitis in New Zealand: a nationwide study over the period 1990 to 2006. J Infect. 2011;63:429–33.
22. Legbo JN, Shehu BB. Necrotising fasciitis: experience with 32 children. Ann Trop Paediatr. 2005;25:183–9.
23. Thean LJ, Jenney A, Engelman D, et al. Hospital admissions for skin and soft tissue infections in a population with endemic scabies: a prospective study in Fiji, 2018–2019. PLoS Negl Trop Dis. 2020;14:e0008887.
24. Ralph AP, Carapetis JR. Group A streptococcal diseases and their global burden. In: Chhatwal GS, editor. Host-pathogen interactions in streptococcal diseases. Berlin, Heidelberg: Springer Berlin Heidelberg; 2012. p. 1–27.
25. O'Sullivan CE, Baker MG, Zhang J. Increasing hospitalizations for serious skin infections in New

Zealand children, 1990–2007. Epidemiol Infect. 2011;139:1794–804.
26. Totapally BR. Epidemiology and outcomes of hospitalized children with necrotizing soft-tissue infections. Pediatr Infect Dis J. 2017;36:641–4.
27. Bingöl-Koloğlu M, Yıldız RV, Alper B, Yağmurlu A, Çiftçi E, Gökçora İH, İnce E, Emiroğlu M, Dindar H. Necrotizing fasciitis in children: diagnostic and therapeutic aspects. J Pediatr Surg. 2007;42:1892–7.
28. VanderMeulen H, Pernica JM, Roy M, Kam AJ. A 10-year review of necrotizing fasciitis in the pediatric population: delays to diagnosis and management. Clin Pediatr (Phila). 2017;56:627–33.
29. Moss RL, Musemeche CA, Kosloske AM. Necrotizing fasciitis in children: prompt recognition and aggressive therapy improve survival. J Pediatr Surg. 1996;31:1142–6.
30. Fustes-Morales A, Gutierrez-Castrellon P, Duran-Mckinster C, Orozco-Covarrubias L, Tamayo-Sanchez L, Ruiz-Maldonado R. Necrotizing fasciitis: report of 39 pediatric cases. Arch Dermatol. 2002;138:893–9.
31. Jauregui JJ, Bor N, Thakral R, Standard SC, Paley D, Herzenberg JE. Life- and limb-threatening infections following the use of an external fixator. Bone Joint J. 2015;97-B:1296–300.
32. Tancevski A, Bono K, Willis L, Klingele K. Necrotizing fasciitis in a pediatric orthopedic population. Orthopedics. 2013;36:e741–5.
33. Groupe Francophone de Réanimation et Urgences Pédiatriques (GFRUP), Réseau Mères-Enfants de la Francophonie (RMEF), Dauger S, Blondé R, Brissaud O, Marcoux M-O, Angoulvant F, Levy M. Necrotizing soft-tissue infections in pediatric intensive care: a prospective multicenter case-series study. Crit Care. 2021;25:139.
34. Endorf FW, Garrison MM, Klein MB, Richardson A, Rivara FP. Characteristics, therapies, and outcome of children with necrotizing soft tissue infections. Pediatr Infect Dis J. 2012;31:221–3.
35. INFECT study group, Madsen MB, Skrede S, et al. Patient's characteristics and outcomes in necrotising soft-tissue infections: results from a Scandinavian, multicentre, prospective cohort study. Intensive Care Med. 2019;45:1241–51.
36. Horn CB, Wesp BM, Fiore NB, Rasane RK, Torres M, Turnbull IR, Ilahi ON, Punch LJ, Bochicchio GV. Fungal infections increase the mortality rate three-fold in necrotizing soft-tissue infections. Surg Infect. 2017;18:793–8.
37. Khoury MK, Heid CA, Cripps MW, Pickett ML, Nagaraj MB, Johns M, Lee F, Hennessy SA. Antifungal therapy in fungal necrotizing soft tissue infections. J Surg Res. 2020;256:187–92.
38. Giuliano A, Lewis F, Hadley K, Blaisdell FW. Bacteriology of necrotizing fasciitis. Am J Surg. 1977;134:52–7.
39. Morgan MS. Diagnosis and management of necrotising fasciitis: a multiparametric approach. J Hosp Infect. 2010;75:249–57.
40. Tessier JM, Sanders J, Sartelli M, Ulrych J, De Simone B, Grabowski J, Buckman S, Duane TM. Necrotizing soft tissue infections: a focused review of pathophysiology, diagnosis, operative management, antimicrobial therapy, and pediatrics. Surg Infect. 2020;21:81–93.
41. Hysong AA, Posey SL, Blum DM, et al. Necrotizing fasciitis: pillaging the acute phase response. J Bone Joint Surg. 2020;102:526–37.
42. Frère J, Bidet P, Tapiéro B, Rallu F, Minodier P, Bonacorsi S, Bingen E, Ovetchkine P. Clinical and microbiological characteristics of invasive group A streptococcal infections before and after implementation of a universal varicella vaccine program. Clin Infect Dis. 2016;62:75–7.
43. Hsieh T, Samson LM, Jabbour M, Osmond MH. Necrotizing fasciitis in children in eastern Ontario: a case-control study. CMAJ. 2000;163:393–6.
44. Minodier P, Bidet P, Rallu F, Tapiero B, Bingen É, Ovetchkine P. Clinical and microbiologic characteristics of group A streptococcal necrotizing fasciitis in children. Pediatr Infect Dis J. 2009;28:541–3.
45. Nazir Z. Necrotizing fasciitis in neonates. Pediatr Surg Int. 2005;21:641–4.
46. An TJ, Benvenuti MA, Mignemi ME, Thomsen IP, Schoenecker JG. Pediatric musculoskeletal infection: hijacking the acute-phase response. JBJS Rev. 2016. https://doi.org/10.2106/JBJS.RVW.15.00099.
47. Olsen RJ, Musser JM. Molecular pathogenesis of necrotizing fasciitis. Annu Rev Pathol. 2010;5:1–31.
48. Hietbrink F, Bode LG, Riddez L, Leenen LPH, van Dijk MR. Triple diagnostics for early detection of ambivalent necrotizing fasciitis. World J Emerg Surg. 2016;11:51.
49. Young MH, Aronoff DM, Engleberg NC. Necrotizing fasciitis: pathogenesis and treatment. Expert Rev Anti-Infect Ther. 2005;3:279–94.
50. Fais P, Viero A, Viel G, Giordano R, Raniero D, Kusstatscher S, Giraudo C, Cecchetto G, Montisci M. Necrotizing fasciitis: case series and review of the literature on clinical and medico-legal diagnostic challenges. Int J Legal Med. 2018;132:1357–66.
51. Bakleh M, Wold LE, Mandrekar JN, Harmsen WS, Dimashkieh HH, Baddour LM. Correlation of histopathologic findings with clinical outcome in necrotizing fasciitis. Clin Infect Dis. 2005;40:410–4.
52. Zerr DM, Alexander ER, Duchin JS, Koutsky LA, Rubens CE. A case-control study of necrotizing fasciitis during primary varicella. Pediatrics. 1999;103:783–90.
53. Wang Y-S, Wong C-H, Tay Y-K. Staging of necrotizing fasciitis based on the evolving cutaneous features. Int J Dermatol. 2007;46:1036–41.
54. Goh T, Goh LG, Ang CH, Wong CH. Early diagnosis of necrotizing fasciitis: early diagnosis of necrotizing fasciitis. Br J Surg. 2014;101:e119–25.
55. Kiat H, En Natalie Y, Fatimah L. Necrotizing fasciitis: how reliable are the cutaneous signs? J Emerg Trauma Shock. 2017;10:205.

56. Borschitz T, Schlicht S, Siegel E, Hanke E, von Stebut E. Improvement of a clinical score for necrotizing fasciitis: 'pain out of proportion' and high CRP levels aid the diagnosis. PLoS One. 2015;10:e0132775.
57. Hsiao C-T, Chang C-P, Huang T-Y, Chen Y-C, Fann W-C. Prospective validation of the laboratory risk indicator for necrotizing fasciitis (LRINEC) score for necrotizing fasciitis of the extremities. PLoS One. 2020;15:e0227748.
58. Putnam LR, Richards MK, Sandvall BK, Hopper RA, Waldhausen JHT, Harting MT. Laboratory evaluation for pediatric patients with suspected necrotizing soft tissue infections: a case–control study. J Pediatr Surg. 2016;51:1022–5.
59. Karnuta J, Featherall J, Lawrenz J, et al. What demographic and clinical factors are associated with in-hospital mortality in patients with necrotizing fasciitis? Clin Orthop Relat Res. 2020;478:1770–9.
60. Wong C-H, Khin L-W, Heng K-S, Tan K-C, Low C-O. The LRINEC (Laboratory Risk Indicator for Necrotizing Fasciitis) score: a tool for distinguishing necrotizing fasciitis from other soft tissue infections. Crit Care Med. 2004;32:1535–41.
61. Fernando SM, Tran A, Cheng W, Rochwerg B, Kyeremanteng K, Seely AJE, Inaba K, Perry JJ. Necrotizing soft tissue infection: diagnostic accuracy of physical examination, imaging, and LRINEC score. Ann Surg. 2019;269:58–65.
62. Aboul-Fettouh N, Nguyen KD, Dominguez AR. Retiform purpura as a sign of necrotizing cellulitis in an immunocompetent boy. Pediatr Emerg Care. 2020;36:e646–8.
63. Novoa-Parra CD, Wadhwani J, Puig-Conca MA, Lizaur-Utrilla A, Montaner-Alonso D, Rodrigo-Pérez JL, Morales-Suárez-Varela M. Usefulness of a risk scale based on procalcitonin for early discrimination between necrotizing fasciitis and cellulitis of the extremities. Med Clin (Barc). 2019;153:347–50.
64. Friederichs J, Hutter M, Hierholzer C, Novotny A, Friess H, Bühren V, Hungerer S. Procalcitonin ratio as a predictor of successful surgical treatment of severe necrotizing soft tissue infections. Am J Surg. 2013;206:368–73.
65. Malghem J, Lecouvet FE, Omoumi P, Maldague BE, Vande Berg BC. Necrotizing fasciitis: contribution and limitations of diagnostic imaging. Joint Bone Spine. 2013;80:146–54.
66. Paz Maya S, Dualde Beltrán D, Lemercier P, Leiva-Salinas C. Necrotizing fasciitis: an urgent diagnosis. Skelet Radiol. 2014;43:577–89.
67. Sartelli M, Guirao X, Hardcastle TC, et al. 2018 WSES/SIS-E consensus conference: recommendations for the management of skin and soft-tissue infections. World J Emerg Surg. 2018;13:58.
68. Tso DK, Singh AK. Necrotizing fasciitis of the lower extremity: imaging pearls and pitfalls. Br J Radiol. 2018;91:20180093.
69. Lau JK, Kwok K, Hung Y, Fan C. Validation of finger test for necrotising soft tissue infection. J Orthop Trauma Rehabil. 2020:221049172096154.
70. Ellis Simonsen SM, Van Orman ER, Hatch BE, Jones SS, Gren LH, Hegmann KT, Lyon JL. Cellulitis incidence in a defined population. Epidemiol Infect. 2006;134:293–9.
71. Miller LG, Eisenberg DF, Liu H, Chang C-L, Wang Y, Luthra R, Wallace A, Fang C, Singer J, Suaya JA. Incidence of skin and soft tissue infections in ambulatory and inpatient settings, 2005–2010. BMC Infect Dis. 2015;15:362.
72. Alayed KA, Tan C, Daneman N. Red flags for necrotizing fasciitis: a case control study. Int J Infect Dis. 2015;36:15–20.
73. Shallcross LJ, Hayward AC, Johnson AM, Petersen I. Evidence for increasing severity of community-onset boils and abscesses in UK General Practice. Epidemiol Infect. 2015;143:2426–9.
74. Galli L, Venturini E, Bassi A, et al. Common community-acquired bacterial skin and soft-tissue infections in children: an intersociety consensus on impetigo, abscess, and cellulitis treatment. Clin Ther. 2019;41:532–551.e17.
75. Barbic D, Chenkin J, Cho DD, Jelic T, Scheuermeyer FX. In patients presenting to the emergency department with skin and soft tissue infections what is the diagnostic accuracy of point-of-care ultrasonography for the diagnosis of abscess compared to the current standard of care? A systematic review and meta-analysis. BMJ Open. 2017;7:e013688.
76. Wakhlu A, Chaudhary A, Tandon RK, Wakhlu AK. Conservative management of necrotizing fascitis in children. J Pediatr Surg. 2006;41:1144–8.
77. Gangopadhyay AN, Pandey A, Upadhyay VD, Sharma SP, Gupta DK, Kumar V. Neonatal necrotising fasciitis - Varanasi experience. Int Wound J. 2007;5:108–12.
78. Gangopadhyay A, Sharma S, Kumar V, Gopal S, Gupta D, Pandey A. Surgical considerations in pediatric necrotizing fasciitis. J Indian Assoc Pediatr Surg. 2009;14:19.
79. Pandey V, Gangopadhyay AN, Gupta DK, Sharma SP, Kumar V, Tiwari P. Neonatal necrotising fasciitis managed conservatively: an experience from a tertiary centre. J Wound Care. 2014;23:270–3.
80. Nawijn F, Smeeing DPJ, Houwert RM, Leenen LPH, Hietbrink F. Time is of the essence when treating necrotizing soft tissue infections: a systematic review and meta-analysis. World J Emerg Surg. 2020;15:4.
81. Holena DN, Mills AM, Carr BG, Wirtalla C, Sarani B, Kim PK, Braslow BM, Kelz RR. Transfer status: a risk factor for mortality in patients with necrotizing fasciitis. Surgery. 2011;150:363–70.
82. Khoury MK, Pickett ML, Cripps MW, Park S-Y, Nagaraj MB, Hranjec T, Hennessy SA. Transfer is associated with a higher mortality rate in necrotizing soft tissue infections. Surg Infect. 2020;21:136–42.
83. Stewart SK, Vu J, McCulloch GAJ. Necrotising fasciitis deaths in Australia: patient characteristics and potential areas for improvement in clinical management. ANZ J Surg. 2020;90:2329–33.

84. Farrell LD, Karl SR, Davis PK, Bellinger MF, Ballantine TV. Postoperative necrotizing fasciitis in children. Pediatrics. 1988;82:874–9.
85. Tom LK, Wright TJ, Horn DL, Bulger EM, Pham TN, Keys KA. A skin-sparing approach to the treatment of necrotizing soft-tissue infections: thinking reconstruction at initial debridement. J Am Coll Surg. 2016;222:e47–60.
86. Rüfenacht MS, Montaruli E, Chappuis E, Posfay-Barbe KM, La Scala GC. Skin-sparing Débridement for necrotizing fasciitis in children. Plast Reconstr Surg. 2016;138:489e–97e.
87. Sarani B, Strong M, Pascual J, Schwab CW. Necrotizing fasciitis: current concepts and review of the literature. J Am Coll Surg. 2009;208:279–88.
88. Solomon IH, Borscheid R, Laga AC, Askari R, Granter SR. Frozen sections are unreliable for the diagnosis of necrotizing soft tissue infections. Mod Pathol. 2018;31:546–52.
89. Wong C-H, Yam AK-T, Tan AB-H, Song C. Approach to debridement in necrotizing fasciitis. Am J Surg. 2008;196:e19–24.
90. Siemens N, Chakrakodi B, Shambat SM, et al. Biofilm in group A streptococcal necrotizing soft tissue infections. JCI Insight. 2016. https://doi.org/10.1172/jci.insight.87882.
91. Huang W-S, Hsieh S-C, Hsieh C-S, Schoung J-Y, Huang T. Use of vacuum-assisted wound closure to manage limb wounds in patients suffering from acute necrotizing fasciitis. Asian J Surg. 2006;29:135–9.
92. Iacovelli V, Cipriani C, Sandri M, et al. The role of vacuum-assisted closure (VAC) therapy in the management of FOURNIER'S gangrene: a retrospective multi-institutional cohort study. World J Urol. 2021;39:121–8.
93. Chen M-C, Chao H-C, Yeh P-J, Lai M-W, Chen C-C. Therapeutic efficacy of nasoenteric tube feeding in children needing enteral nutrition. Front Pediatr. 2021;9:646395.
94. Waisman D, Shupak A, Weisz G, Melamed Y. Hyperbaric oxygen therapy in the pediatric patient: the experience of the Israel naval medical institute. Pediatrics. 1998;102:e53.
95. Levett DZ, Bennett MH, Millar I. Adjunctive hyperbaric oxygen for necrotizing fasciitis. Cochrane Database Syst Rev. 2015. https://doi.org/10.1002/14651858.CD007937.pub2.
96. Faunø Thrane J, Ovesen T. Scarce evidence of efficacy of hyperbaric oxygen therapy in necrotizing soft tissue infection: a systematic review. Infect Dis. 2019;51:485–92.
97. Janisch T, Stollenwerk A, Siekmann UP, Kopp R. Treatment of children with Hyperbaric Oxygenation (HBOT): an Europe-wide survey. Minerva Pediatr. 2020. https://doi.org/10.23736/S0026-4946.20.05741-2.
98. Hua C, Bosc R, Sbidian E, De Prost N, Hughes C, Jabre P, Chosidow O, Le Cleach L. Interventions for necrotizing soft tissue infections in adults. Cochrane Database Syst Rev. 2018. https://doi.org/10.1002/14651858.CD011680.pub2.
99. Ward JA, Gibson JAG, Nguyen DQ. Management of necrotising fasciitis within a burns centre: do outcomes differ? Scars Burn Heal. 2020;6:205951312092474.
100. Firth G, Oetzmann von Sochaczewski C, Ramguthy Y, Khalfallah A. Necrotising fasciitis following a supracondylar fracture and an open radius fracture in a child. SA Orthop J. 2018;17:49–53.

Gas Gangrene

37

Parmanand Gupta and Hitesh Shah

Introduction

Gas gangrene derives its name from a condition of toxin-induced tissue necrosis associated with the formation of gas in the myofascial planes. The condition is associated with morbidity and a high incidence of mortality if unrecognized or untreated [1]. Historically, it was described in association with injuries sustained during the war in the pre-antibiotic era. During World War I and II, it was reported to complicate around 5% of all wounds sustained on the battlefield, but with improvement in wound care, antisepsis and the use of antibiotics, the incidence had fallen to 0.1% of war-related wound infections by the Vietnam War [2]. In the current era, the incidence of gas gangrene remains higher in patients with firearm injuries, farmyard injuries, and earthquake-induced injuries, especially those presenting later than 24 hours. Cases have been reported following tight splintage [1, 3–5].

Epidemiology

In the United States, the incidence of myonecrosis is only about 1000 cases per year [6–10]. In less developed countries with decreased access to healthcare and antibiotics, the incidence is probably higher, but the exact number is unknown. The overall incidence of gas gangrene has tremendously reduced due to a good understanding of the pathophysiology and better management of the disease [8, 9]. With the best of care, including early recognition, surgical care, antibiotic treatment, and hyperbaric oxygen therapy, the overall mortality rate is 20–30% [11]; however, if not treated the disease has a 100% fatality. If the infection involves the abdominal soft tissue or chest wall, the mortality rate can be as high as 60% compared to extremity infections with more favorable mortality of 5–30% [6–9]. The reported incidence of gas gangrene in children is much less as compared to adults [12–14].

Etiology

The primary reason for gas gangrene is the entry of pathogenic organisms into injured soft tissues and their proliferation under anaerobic conditions. A reduction in local tissue oxygenation and perfusion facilitates the proliferation of gas-forming bacteria. Reduction of vascular supply to tissues may result from angiopathy, tight casts,

P. Gupta (✉)
Government Medical College and Hospital, Chandigarh, India

H. Shah
Kasturba Medical College, Manipal Academy of Higher Education, Manipal, Karnataka, India

© Springer Nature Switzerland AG 2022
M. V. Belthur et al. (eds.), *Pediatric Musculoskeletal Infections*,
https://doi.org/10.1007/978-3-030-95794-0_37

tight bandages, and compartment syndrome. Tissue oxygenation can also be reduced by tissue necrosis due to infection by other pyogenic bacteria that consume oxygen and by the use of vasoconstrictor drugs like adrenaline. The proliferation of the gas gangrene forming organisms can especially occur in wounds following high energy motor vehicular or agricultural accidents, especially when the closure has been done over undebrided necrosed tissue [15]. Foreign material like mud, gravel, and clothing in a wound increases the chances of developing gas gangrene as these materials can harbor Clostridia [16]. The condition has also been reported in children undergoing treatment by bonesetters using a tight splint with bamboo sticks [15].

Apart from traumatic conditions, gas gangrene can be associated with non-traumatic conditions as well. Spontaneous gas gangrene has been reported in patients undergoing chemotherapy, immuno-compromised children, children with cyclic neutropenia, and in association with pediatric oncological conditions [17, 18].

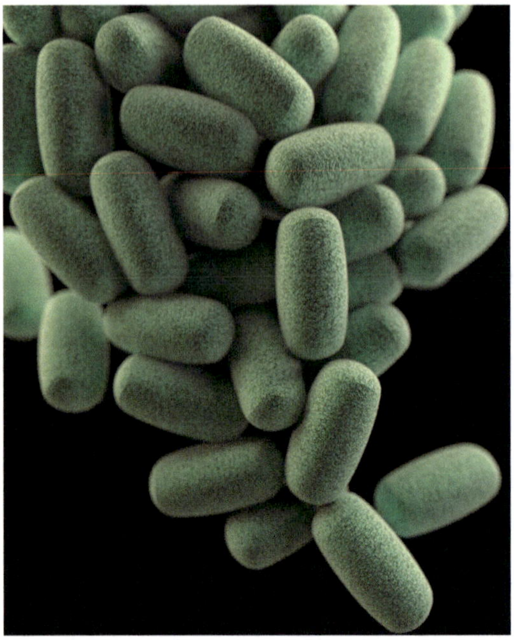

Fig. 37.1 This illustration depicts a three-dimensional (3D), computer-generated image of a cluster of barrel-shaped, *Clostridium perfringens* bacteria. The artistic recreation was based upon scanning electron microscopic (SEM) imagery. (This image is taken from CDC Public Health Image Library, ID # 21913. Courtesy: CDC/ James Archer & Illustrator: Jennifer Oosthuizen)

Causative Organisms

***Clostridium* Species** The most common causative agent is *Clostridium perfringens* (80–95% cases), which is a saprophyte present in the form of spores under normal conditions but proliferates under anaerobic conditions. Other clostridial species that have also been associated with the condition include *Clostridium septicum*, *Clostridium novyi*, *Clostridium bifermentans*, *Clostridium histolyticum*, and *Clostridium fallax* [12, 19]. Clostridium perfringens is a thick gram-positive anaerobic rod that is non-motile. It is also popularly known as *Clostridium welchii* [11] (Fig. 37.1).

Non-Clostridial Organisms Infection by pyogenic organisms like *Klebsiella pneumoniae*, group A *Streptococcus*, *Escherichia coli*, and *Proteus* have also been known to be associated with the production of gas in the tissues, but they rarely cause true gas gangrene with myonecrosis [20].

Pathophysiology

Clostridium is a ubiquitous organism found in the soil and clothing. It is also commonly found on the skin and is present as normal flora of the biliary, gastrointestinal, and female genital tract [16]. The first step is the establishment of the organism in the injured or vascular compromised soft tissue. This can happen through traumatic or non-traumatic means.

Traumatic

1. *High-Velocity Vehicular Accidents*: Trauma, particularly associated with vehicular accidents, remains the leading cause of gas gangrene. Extensive soft tissue damage, with a high probability of organic contamination, results in the seeding of organisms. An open

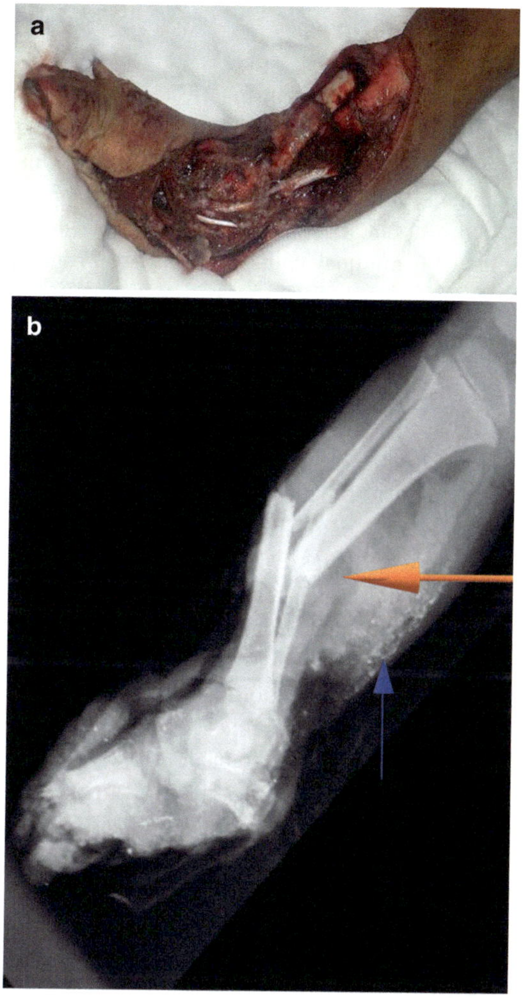

Fig. 37.2 (**a**) Clinical photographs of a five-year-old child with crush injury of right lower limb who presented 12 hours after injury showing open fracture tibia with extensive involvement of soft tissue of leg and foot. (**b**) The radiographs showed a middle third lower third fracture of the right tibia and fibula with foreign bodies (thin arrow) and gas (thick arrow). The child developed gas gangrene and was treated with a right knee disarticulation

fracture, including those with puncture wounds, is also prone to developing gas gangrene (Fig. 37.2a, b). Puncture wounds may present as "grade 1" open fractures. However, failure to recognize extensive underlying soft tissue devitalization with such open fracture may predispose the chances of gas gangrene [11, 16, 21].

2. *Agricultural Accidents*: Farm accidents have a high propensity for developing gas gangrene. This is due to wound contamination with *C. perfringens* from soil [15].
3. *Firearm Injuries*: Gas gangrene is often seen in wounds of gunshot injuries due to extensive soft tissue damage [5].
4. *Surgery*: Muscles with compromised vascularity as a result of surgery makes the limb prone to gas gangrene [19].
5. *Tight Splint*: Tight bandaging and splinting with bamboo sticks by quacks and bonesetters result in compromised vascularity and tissue oxygenation of a compartment making it prone to gas gangrene [4].

After the establishment of bacteria in the soft tissues, in an anaerobic environment caused by stripping of vascularity of tissues by trauma, the bacilli start proliferating (Fig. 37.3a, b). The proliferation of these anaerobic bacteria leads to the formation of gases (carbon dioxide and hydrogen), which move into fascio-muscular planes. The gas can cause separation of myofascial planes leading to stripping and further compromise the vascularity of the tissues, aggravating the anaerobic environment, forming a vicious cycle [16, 19, 22, 23].

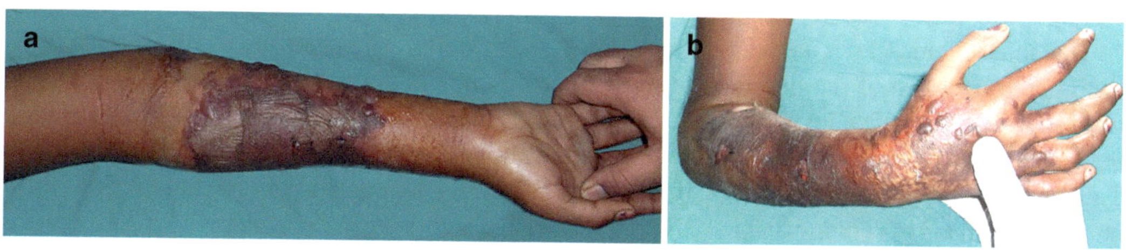

Fig. 37.3 (**a, b**) Clinical photographs of a nine-year-old child with crush injury right forearm. The presence of hemorrhagic bullae and serosanguinous discharge in association with bronze colored discoloration should arouse strong clinical suspicion of gas gangrene

Non-traumatic

Non-traumatic spontaneous cases of gas gangrene have been seen in children with acquired, cyclical, and congenital neutropenia and in children receiving immunotherapy [23]. The commonest organism responsible for non-traumatic etiology is *Clostridium septicum.* The direct seeding can occur from the gut to compromised intestinal tissue leading to spontaneous gas gangrene of the gut. Bacteria can spread from the gut into the bloodstream and lead to seeding at peripheral sites as well. The incubation period ranges from 6 to 96 hours [16]. Non-traumatic gas gangrene has an insidious onset [12, 17, 23]. In contrast, gas gangrene of traumatic origin spreads rapidly and can manifest within 6–8 hours [11, 16].

Formation of Toxins The proliferating clostridia lead to the formation of potent toxins. Many exotoxins are produced; the most notable among them include α-phospholipase C (α-toxin). α-Toxin is a lecithinase and causes disruption of cell membranes leading to hemolysis. It is also cytotoxic to platelets and leukocytes and increases capillary permeability as well. This leads to extensive hemolysis, disseminated intravascular coagulation, and myonecrosis. Systemic effects of α -toxin include reduced myocardial contractility, leading to cardiogenic shock. Another potent toxin is perfringolysin O or the μ-toxin, which is a hyaluronidase causing edema by its action on connective tissue [16, 19, 22, 24].

Pathology Histologically, there is significant tissue necrosis with an absent or minimal inflammatory response. This contrasts with pyogenic infections, where the inflammatory response is profound with little tissue necrosis [24].

The infected muscle is edematous initially. With the progression of the disease, the muscle turns brownish red with a loss of contractility. In the late stages, the muscle turns greenish black. The consistency of the affected muscle is initially mucoid, which later becomes friable [25].

Clinical Features

The symptoms may start manifesting as early as 6 hours after inoculation. The usual time frame is about 1–4 days following an open injury. The initial presenting complaints are usually nonspecific and include a feeling of heaviness in the limb with minimal pain. With disease progression, pain may become out of proportion to the severity of the injury. Locally, the skin appears pale, is cold and clammy. This may progress to a bronze or magenta discoloration. Hemorrhagic bullae appear associated with brownish serosanguinous discharge. The discharge has a characteristic "mousy" odor [25]. Tenderness, tense swelling, and hemorrhagic exudates are the cardinal signs [2] (Figs. 37.4a, b and 37.5). Gas in the myofascial planes results in the characteristic crepitus, appreciable clinically in the late stages of the disease [25].

The child may have normal vital parameters in the early stages. As toxemia sets in, hypotension and alteration of mental status follow. Later there is high-grade fever with rigors. If untreated, shock, renal failure, metabolic acidosis, sepsis, coma, multi-organ failure, and eventually death result [26].

Diagnosis

The most reliable diagnosis of gas gangrene is by the demonstration of the organisms in the tissues by Gram's stain (Fig. 37.6). However, the demonstration of *Clostridium perfringens* does not always mean a diagnosis of gas gangrene. The presence of the offending organism in tissues can present in three ways—contamination of wound without invasion into tissues, clostridial cellulitis, and myonecrosis. Clostridial cellulitis is a common, milder form of the disease wherein the crepitus is more marked, but the gas formation and infection are limited to the fascial plane. Clostridial myonecrosis is the more serious form of the infection wherein there is an invasion of

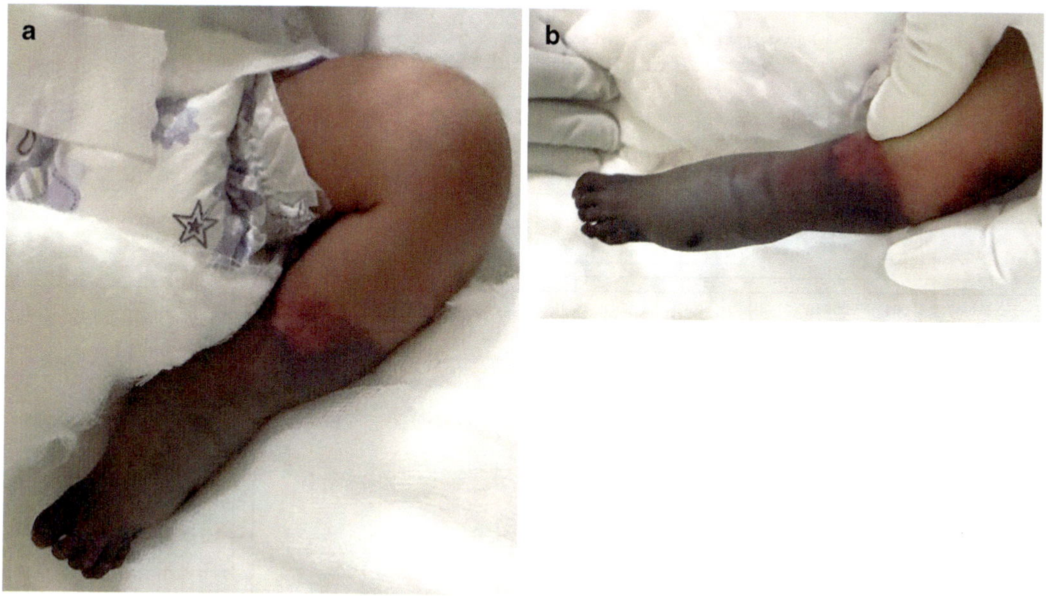

Fig. 37.4 (**a**, **b**) An infant with gas gangrene of the left leg from the front (**a**) and side (**b**). This child was treated with a left below-knee amputation

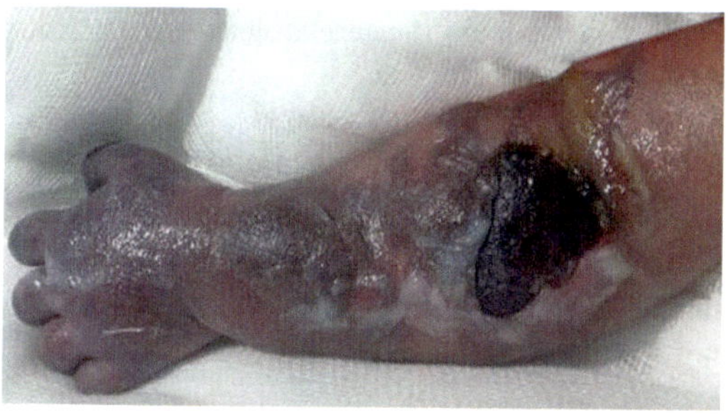

Fig. 37.5 Clinical photograph of a two-year-old child showing established gas gangrene of the left hand. The child was treated with a left through elbow amputation

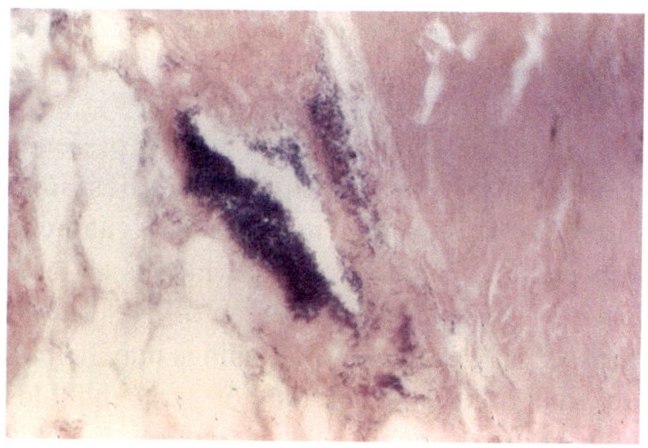

Fig. 37.6 Under a magnification of 80×, this hematoxylin-eosin (H&E)-stained photomicrograph of a necrotic muscle tissue specimen reveals numerous. *Clostridium perfringens*, formerly *C. welchii*, or *Bacillus welchii* bacteria, as well as presence of some gas. (This image is taken from CDC Public Health Image Library, ID# 16291. Courtesy: CDC/ Dr. Robert Fass, Ohio State Dept. of Medicine)

the healthy tissue. The diagnosis of gas gangrene is based on a combination of clinical and radiological features, with confirmation by microbiological testing [2] (Fig. 37.7).

Differential Diagnosis

There are similar infections mimicking gas gangrene (Table 37.1).

Imaging

The presence of gas can be seen on plain radiographs; these changes are not appreciable in the early stages of infection. Gas in the tissues is not

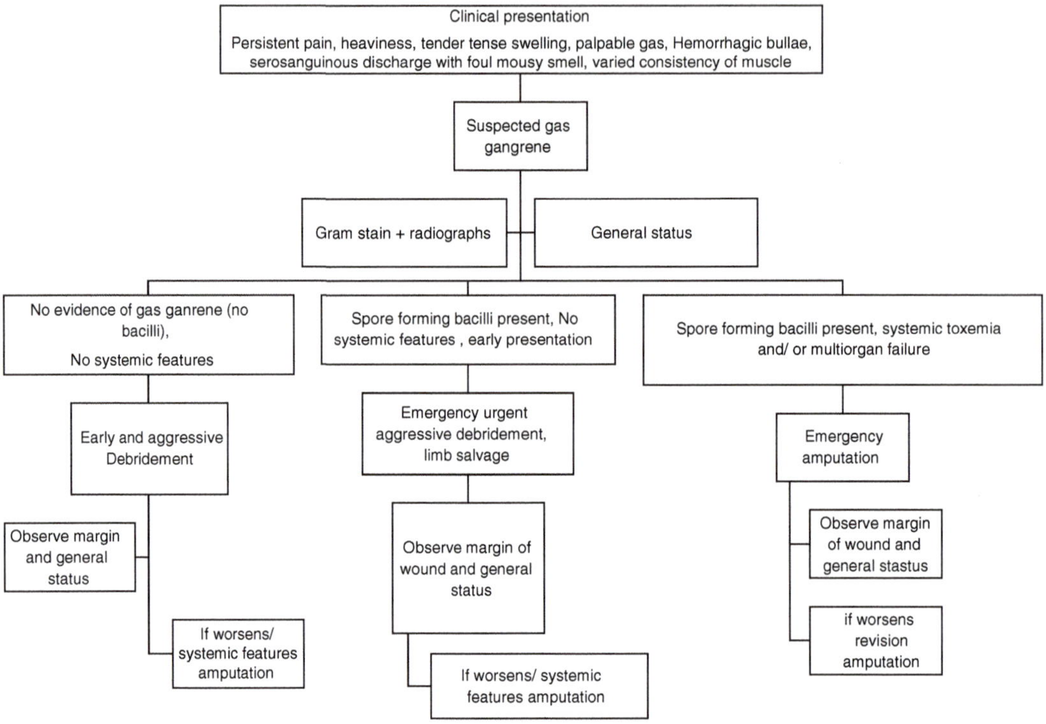

Fig. 37.7 Flowchart showing the clinical presentation of a suspected case of gas gangrene, diagnosis, and decision making of surgical intervention

specific to the diagnosis; however, its presence should raise a strong suspicion of Clostridial infection. Gas in patients with gas gangrene appears in a feathery pattern, which is an indicator of gas entering the region of muscle fascicles. These radiographic findings may help in differentiating it from that of large bubbles seen in open wounds and necrotizing fasciitis [30]. Other causes of gas in tissues include *Peptostreptococcus*, *E. coli*, *Bacteroides*, *Staphylococcus epidermidis*, *Streptococcus*, and diphtheroids [31]. Some air may appear on radiographs in children with open fractures especially in patients with crush injuries (Fig. 37.8a, b). Air may also be carried in the tissues by penetrating injuries and by air hose injuries and wound irrigated with hydrogen peroxide; gas shadows in these radiographs do not spread beyond the zone of injury. A breach in soft tissues may also give the appearance of radiolucent areas, which can be confused with gas shadows. Gas shadows may also be appreciated in subcutaneous emphysema in children with penetrating injuries to the lungs [32]. Advanced imaging techniques, including ultrasound, CT scan, and MRI, do not have additional value in the diagnosis of gas gangrene, do not add to the cost, and do not delay treatment [33].

Microbiological Diagnosis

A wound swab is one of the most important and reliable indicators of gas gangrene by Clostridia. It is more valuable for early diagnosis than any culture. The smears from the wound show presence of thick gram-positive bacilli with scanty inflammatory cells [3, 34] (Fig. 37.9).

Treatment

The best form of management is to prevent the condition of *Clostridial myonecrosis*. This is by having a high index of suspicion in traumatic

Table 37.1 Differential diagnosis of gas gangrene with similar infections [19, 27–29]

Clinical features	Gas gangrene	Anaerobic cellulitis	Necrotizing fasciitis	Progressive bacterial synergistic gangrene	Necrotizing cellulitis	Gangrenous cellulitis
Systemic septic shock	Very high	Absent	Present	Minimal	Present	Present
Fever	High	Mild	High	Not present	Moderate	High
Pain	Severe	Minimal	Mild	Severe	Severe	Minimal
Crepitus	Present in late stage	Absent	Absent	Absent	Occasionally	Absent
Loss of sensation at the lesion	Absent	Absent	Occasionally present	Absent	Absent	Occasionally present
Involved area	Skin, subcutaneous tissue, fascia, muscle	Skin, subcutaneous tissue	Skin, subcutaneous tissue, fascia	Skin, subcutaneous tissue	Skin, subcutaneous tissue	Skin, subcutaneous tissue
Clinical appearance	Yellow-brown skin, bullae, green-black patch, foul mousy smell,	Swelling of skin (edematous)	Necrotic skin and fascia	Necrotic ulcer, dusky margin, and red periphery	Necrotic skin, thick discharge, crepitus, foul smell	Black discharge, erythema
Immunocompromised status	Occasionally	Absent	Absent	Absent	Absent	Present
Microorganism	*Clostridium perfringens, Clostridium septicum*	*Clostridium perfringens, Clostridium septicum*	*Streptococcus pyogenes,* synergistic infection due to facultative and anaerobic bacteria	Anaerobic or microaerophilic streptococci	A mixture of anaerobic bacteria and gram-negative bacilli	*Pseudomonas aeruginosa*

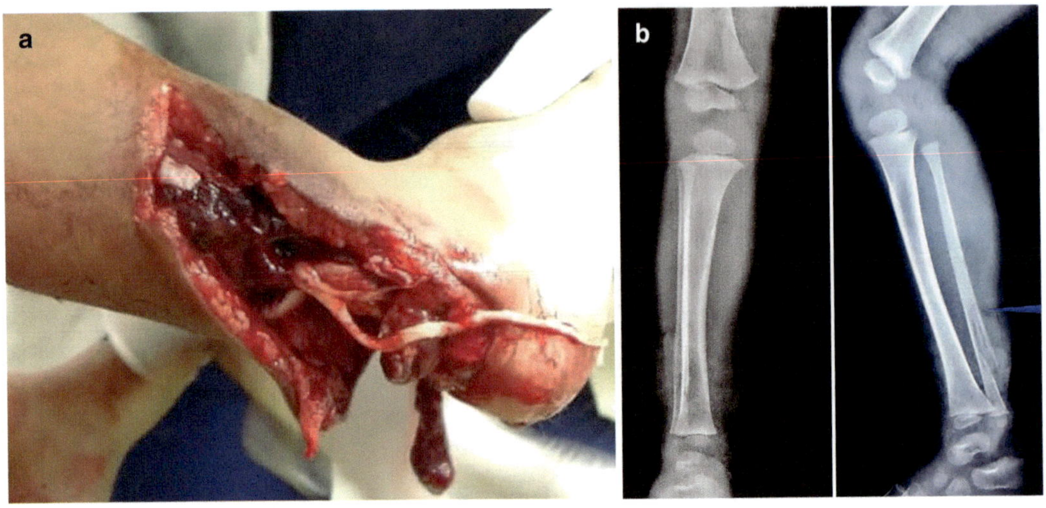

Fig. 37.8 (**a**, **b**) A five-year-old child with crush injury of the distal third of the right leg (**a**). Gas shadows can be appreciated in the tissue planes (**b**). These gas shadows are due to breach in soft tissues (arrow) and should not be confused with the gas shadows seen in gas gangrene

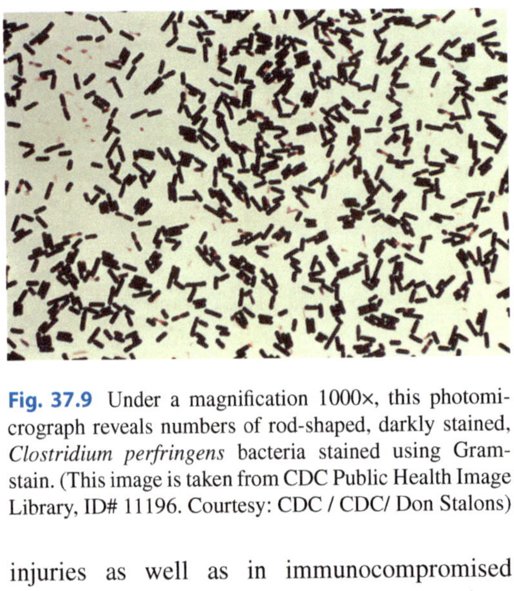

Fig. 37.9 Under a magnification 1000×, this photomicrograph reveals numbers of rod-shaped, darkly stained, *Clostridium perfringens* bacteria stained using Gram-stain. (This image is taken from CDC Public Health Image Library, ID# 11196. Courtesy: CDC / CDC/ Don Stalons)

injuries as well as in immunocompromised patients. Once diagnosed, the management of gas gangrene includes a combination of treatment of septic shock, parenteral antibiotics, hyperbaric oxygen, and early and aggressive surgical debridement [13, 26].

General Management

When the patient presents to the emergency room after securing the airway, the patient must be given high flow oxygen if the patient is in toxemia. If the presentation of the patient is in shock, management must focus on first stabilizing the general condition of the patient. Isotonic crystalloids are the fluids of choice. All the sutures must be removed, and the anaerobic environment must be mitigated. Blood and blood products have a limited role in this due to preexisting hemolysis and toxins circulating in the blood. Local and systemic use of vasoconstrictors must be avoided as they further decrease perfusion and hence oxygen tension. This can ultimately lead to increased proliferation of the microorganisms [25].

Medical Management

Antibiotics

The antibiotic of choice is intravenously administered penicillin G in high doses of 250,000–400,000 U/kg/day in six divided doses. For patients with hypersensitivity to penicillin or where infection with multiple organisms is expected, Metronidazole, Imipenem, Meropenem, and Chloramphenicol or Clindamycin are the commonly used alternatives [11]. Vascular compromise due to gangrenous changes leads to suboptimal delivery of the antibiotic to the desired area. Hence, antibiotics cannot be used as an exclusive modality of treatment [35].

Antitoxin

Antitoxin treatment or anti-gas gangrene serum was introduced in 1918 and was extensively used during wartime. Subsequent studies have shown no benefit of the antitoxin in preventing gas gangrene, and currently, the use of antitoxin or anti-gas gangrene serum is no longer recommended [25].

Hyperbaric Oxygen

Hyperbaric oxygen therapy is based on the concept of raising the oxygen tension of the affected area as clostridia are anaerobic and cannot multiply in aerobic conditions. Due to increased solubility of oxygen under pressure greater than atmospheric pressure, there is increased delivery of oxygen to the tissues. It stops the production of toxins, suppresses peroxidase in the necrotic tissue, promotes capillary angiogenesis, and reduces local edema, leading to faster healing [34].

Hyperbaric oxygen is not a stand-alone therapy. It is always recommended to be used along with medical and surgical treatment. Some researchers have suggested that improved results with hyperbaric oxygen can be attributed to its availability in tertiary care centers, where better medical and surgical facilities are available [15]. A major drawback is the potential toxicity of hyperbaric oxygen and its extremely limited availability in most centers [19, 34]. The current role of hyperbaric oxygen remains controversial [25].

Recombinant Human Granulocyte Colony-Stimulating Factor

Early and empirical use of recombinant human granulocyte colony-stimulating factor plays a role in gas gangrene children with congenital neutropenia [14]. Early administration in the case with congenital neutropenia is associated with a satisfactory outcome [19].

Surgical Treatment

Surgical debridement of the involved area is the mainstay of treatment. Early and aggressive surgical treatment has shown excellent results. Surgical treatment can be divided into limb salvage and limb ablative surgeries [30].

Early, aggressive debridement is limb salvage surgery and is preferred for upper limb gas gangrene. A fasciotomy must be done to reduce the compartment pressure and to mitigate the anaerobic environment of the wound. The debridement should include cleaning of all pockets of the wound, removal of all necrotic parts, including compromised muscles, dirt, and all foreign bodies. Further, the drainage of hematoma and complete hemostasis should be achieved. Thorough debridement of the affected tissue helps to remove the infected tissue, which is the nidus of infection and drains the toxic fluids out of the wound, thus reducing the systemic toxicity. The surgical debridement is the cornerstone of the gas gangrene treatment [30].

Amputation of the extremity may be needed in severe cases with widespread myonecrosis and severe toxemia, in late presenting cases, in cases of progressive gangrene despite early debridement, and with toxemia leading to septic shock [5]. Amputation is usually left open initially, and a delayed primary or secondary closure may be carried out depending on the local tissue condition [34]. The decision of primary closure of amputation can be taken in children with good general status with the amputation level well away from the focus of infection. Revision amputation at a higher level may be considered depending on the response of the child [34].

In cases where gas gangrene occurs as a result of natural calamity like earthquakes, the patients are isolated, and the amputations are not closed till wound smears on three consecutive days do does not show any clostridium bacilli [34].

Complications

The mortality rate may vary from 5% to 25% [30, 34]. Multidisciplinary care may reduce the mortality rate. The morbidity remains high in children requiring extensive debridement and lifesaving amputation. An early and coordinated team approach must be required to prevent irreversible multi-organ failure.

Outcomes

Despite high incidence of these infections and associated sepsis, current day mortality is lower than previously reported. It is due to better understanding of the pathogenesis and advancement in the treatment [36]. Inter-hospital transfer has not proven to be a risk factor for the poor outcome of this type of necrotizing infection [37].

Key learning points, tips and tricks for a successful outcome, and pitfalls to avoid are mentioned in Tables 37.2, 37.3, and 37.4, respectively.

Table 37.2 Key learning points

Gas gangrene is associated with a high incidence of morbidity and mortality
It may present in high-velocity injuries with extensive soft tissue damage. It is not uncommon with atraumatic etiology
The common organisms are *Clostridium perfringens* and *Clostridium septicum*
Pain out of proportion, swelling, crepitus, and systemic toxicity (septic shock) are indicators of gas gangrene
The most typical signs are mousy odor and crepitus
It is a clinical diagnosis. No investigation apart from Gram's stain and plain radiographs are needed
It must be treated as a surgical emergency

Table 37.3 Tips and tricks for a successful outcome

Early and correct diagnosis of gas gangrene is the key to an effective outcome, as it progresses very rapidly
The doubtful gas gangrene must also be treated as a surgical emergency
A high dose of parenteral antibiotics with surgical debridement is the mainstay of treatment
Early and aggressive surgical debridement reduces morbidity and mortality

Table 37.4 Pitfalls to avoid

Gas gangrene must be differentiated from other types of anaerobic infections and gangrene
The typical radiological features are gas in the myofascial plane. However, it is absent in the early stage of the disease
The presence of gas in the radiograph is suggestive but not pathognomonic of gas gangrene

Conclusion

Gas gangrene is a lethal bacterial myonecrosis caused by the Clostridium species. It is associated with high morbidity and mortality, but fortunately, is rare in children. Gas gangrene is commonly associated with high-velocity injuries with severe soft tissue involvement. Symptoms may be non-specific. It should be suspected if there is sudden onset of severe persistent pain, tender tense swelling of muscle with hemorrhagic exudate, and systemic signs of septic shock. Early decisive and aggressive surgical debridement coupled with IV antibiotics is the optimum treatment. Hyperbaric oxygen therapy is of limited use and can be used based on availability.

References

1. Yang Z, Hu J, Qu Y, Sun F, Leng X, Li H, Zhan S. Interventions for treating gas gangrene. Cochrane Database Syst Rev. 2015;(12):CD010577. https://doi.org/10.1002/14651858.CD010577.
2. Buboltz JB, Murphy-Lavoie HM. Gas gangrene. In: StatPearls [Internet]. Treasure Island (FL): StatPearls Publishing; 2020. PMID: 30725715.
3. Wang Y, Hao P, Lu B, Yu H, Huang W, Hou H, Dai K. Causes of infection after earthquake, China, 2008. Emerg Infect Dis. 2010;16(6):974–5. https://doi.org/10.3201/eid1606.091523.
4. Brume J, Ijagha EO. Traditional bone setters and gas gangrene. Lancet. 1985;1(8432):813. https://doi.org/10.1016/s0140-6736(85)91465-5.
5. Nwankwo OE. Causes of gas gangrene seen at the University of Nigeria Teaching Hospital, Enugu, Nigeria. Trop Dr. 2008;38(2):76–8. https://doi.org/10.1258/td.2007.005194.
6. Shindo Y, Dobashi Y, Sakai T, Monma C, Miyatani H, Yoshida Y. Epidemiological and pathobiological profiles of Clostridium perfringens infections: review of consecutive series of 33 cases over a 13-year period. Int J Clin Exp Pathol. 2015;8(1):569–77.
7. Lehnhardt M, Homann HH, Daigeler A, Hauser J, Palka P, Steinau HU. Major and lethal complications of liposuction: a review of 72 cases in Germany between 1998 and 2002. Plast Reconstr Surg. 2008;121(6):396e–403e.
8. Stevens DL, Bryant AE. Necrotizing soft-tissue infections. N Engl J Med. 2017;377(23):2253–65.

9. Garcia NM, Cai J. Aggressive soft tissue infections. Surg Clin North Am. 2018;98(5):1097–108.
10. Finsterer J, Hess B. Neuromuscular and central nervous system manifestations of Clostridium perfringens infections. Infection. 2007;35(6):396–405.
11. Oncel S, Arsoy ES. Rapidly developing gas gangrene due to a simple puncture wound. Pediatr Emerg Care. 2010;26(6):434–5. https://doi.org/10.1097/PEC.0b013e3181e15e4f.
12. Kiser CJ, Urish KL, Boateng HA. Development of Clostridium septicum gas gangrene as an adverse effect of clindamycin-induced Clostridium difficile infection in a pediatric patient. J Pediatr Orthop. 2014;34(6):e19–21. https://doi.org/10.1097/BPO.0000000000000144.
13. Smith-Slatas CL, Bourque M, Salazar JC. Clostridium septicum infections in children: a case report and review of the literature. Pediatrics. 2006;117(4):e796–805. https://doi.org/10.1542/peds.2005-1074.
14. Barnes C, Gerstle JT, Freedman MH, Carcao MD. Clostridium septicum myonecrosis in congenital neutropenia. Pediatrics. 2004;114(6):e757–60. https://doi.org/10.1542/peds.2004-0124.
15. Brummelkamp WH. Treatment of anerobic infections with hyperbaric oxygen. In: Brown IW, Cox BG, editors. Proceedings of the third international conference on hyperbaric medicine. Durham: Duke University Press; 1966. p. 492–500.
16. Cline KA, Turnbull TL. Clostridial myonecrosis. Ann Emerg Med. 1985;14(5):459–66. https://doi.org/10.1016/s0196-0644(85)80292-4.
17. Delbridge MS, Turton EP, Kester RC. Spontaneous fulminant gas gangrene. Emerg Med J. 2005;22(7):520–1. https://doi.org/10.1136/emj.2003.013144.
18. Lu J, Wu XT, Kong XF, Tang WH, Cheng JM, Wang HL. Gas gangrene without wound: both lower extremities affected simultaneously. Am J Emerg Med. 2008;26(8):970.e3–970.e970004. https://doi.org/10.1016/j.ajem.2008.01.051.
19. Brook I. Microbiology and management of infectious gangrene in children. J Pediatr Orthop. 2004;24(5):587–92. https://doi.org/10.1097/00004694-200409000-00023.
20. Bessman AN, Wagner W. Nonclostridial gas gangrene. Report of 48 cases and review of the literature. JAMA. 1975;233(9):958–63. https://doi.org/10.1001/jama.233.9.958.
21. Riddell LA. Gas gangrene in a child. Br Med J. 1936;1(3916):159. https://doi.org/10.1136/bmj.1.3916.159.
22. Stevens DL, Troyer BE, Merrick DT, Mitten JE, Olson RD. Lethal effects and cardiovascular effects of purified alpha- and theta-toxins from Clostridium perfringens. J Infect Dis. 1988;157(2):272–9. https://doi.org/10.1093/infdis/157.2.272.
23. Kukul MG, Ciki K, Karadag-Oncel E, Cengiz AB, Kuskonmaz B, Tavil B, Kesici S. A fatal Clostridium perfringens infection with hemolysis after chemotherapy in an adolescent. Arch Argent Pediatr. 2017;115(2):e92–5. https://doi.org/10.5546/aap.2017.eng.e92.
24. Brook I. Clostridial infections in children: spectrum and management. Curr Infect Dis Rep. 2015;17(11). https://doi.org/10.1007/s11908-015-0503-8.
25. Weinstein L, Barza MA. Gas gangrene. N Engl J Med. 1973;289(21):1129–31. https://doi.org/10.1056/NEJM197311222892107.
26. Darke SG, King AM, Slack WK. Gas gangrene and related infection: classification, clinical features and aetiology, management and mortality. A report of 88 cases. Br J Surg. 1977;64(2):104–12. https://doi.org/10.1002/bjs.1800640207.
27. Wilson CB, Siber GR, O'Brien TF, Morgan AP. Phycomycotic gangrenous cellulitis. A report of two cases and a review of the literature. Arch Surg. 1976;111(5):532–8. https://doi.org/10.1001/archsurg.1976.01360230032005.
28. Husseinzadeh N, Nahhas WA, Manders EK, Whitney CW, Mortel R. Spontaneous occurrence of synergistic bacterial gangrene following external pelvic irradiation. Obstet Gynecol. 1984;63(6):859–62.
29. Strasberg SM, Silver MS. Hemolytic streptococcus gangrene. An uncommon but frequently fatal infection in the antibiotic era. Am J Surg. 1968;115(6):763–8. https://doi.org/10.1016/0002-9610(68)90515-1.
30. Hart GB, Lamb RC, Strauss MB. Gas gangrene. J Trauma. 1983;23(11):991–1000. https://doi.org/10.1097/00005373-198311000-00006.
31. Brucato MP, Patel K, Mgbako O. Diagnosis of gas gangrene: does a discrepancy exist between the published data and practice. J Foot Ankle Surg. 2014;53(2):137–40. https://doi.org/10.1053/j.jfas.2013.10.009.
32. Rhinehart DA. Air and gas in the soft tissues: a radiologic study. Radiology. 1931;17(6):1158–69. https://doi.org/10.1148/17.6.1158.
33. Kan JH, Young RS, Yu C, Hernanz-Schulman M. Clinical impact of gadolinium in the MRI diagnosis of musculoskeletal infection in children. Pediatr Radiol. 2010;40(7):1197–205. https://doi.org/10.1007/s00247-010-1557-2.
34. Wang Y, Lu B, Hao P, Yan MN, Dai KR. Comprehensive treatment for gas gangrene of the limbs in earthquakes. Chin Med J. 2013;126(20):3833–9.
35. Pinzon-Guzman C, Bashir D, McSherry G, Beck MJ, Rocourt DV. Clostridium septicum gas gangrene in a previously healthy 8-year-old female with survival. J Pediatr Surg. 2013;48(4):e5–8. https://doi.org/10.1016/j.jpedsurg.2013.01.033.
36. Mills MK, Faraklas I, Davis C, Stoddard GJ, Saffle J. Outcomes from treatment of necrotizing soft-tissue infections: results from the National Surgical Quality Improvement Program database. Am J Surg. 2010;200(6):790–6.
37. Ingraham AM, Jung HS, Liepert AE, Warner-Hillard C, Greenberg CC, Scarborough JE. Effect of transfer status on outcomes for necrotizing soft tissue infections. J Surg Res. 2017;220:372–8.

Meningococcal Infections

38

Sam Weston-Simons, Mohan V. Belthur, and James A. Fernandes

Introduction

Invasive meningococcal disease (IMD) is a bacterial infection caused by the Gram-negative coccobacteria *Neisseria meningitidis*. It is a condition, too often fatal, that commonly presents as an inflammation of the brain (meningitis) and infection of the blood (septicaemia) with subsequent development of septic shock and purpura fulminans in a subset of patients. IMD continues to be among the leading causes of infant mortality in the developed and developing worlds and has significant short- and long-term impacts on the children it affects [1, 2]. Within Europe, it remains the leading cause of community-acquired sepsis in those admitted to paediatric intensive care units [1].

The advent of antibiotics and supportive measures has led to greater survival of such children, but this has led to significant physical and psychological challenges which the orthopaedic surgeon caring for such children must address [2–4].

This chapter will address the basic science required to understand the impact and consequences of this infection as well as the orthopaedic consequences both in the short and long term.

Epidemiology

There are an estimated 1.2 million cases of meningococcal infections per year with disease patterns varying widely internationally [5]. Meningococcal disease occurs worldwide, with the highest incidence of disease found in the 'meningitis belt' of sub-Saharan Africa. In this region, major epidemics occur every 5–12 years with attack rates reaching 1000 cases per 100,000 population. Other regions of the world experience lower overall rates of disease and occasional outbreaks with annual averages around 0.3–3 per 100,000 population [5].

The incidence of Invasive Meningococcal Disease (IMD) and the predominant disease-causing meningococcal serogroups vary worldwide. The incidence of IMD varies by geographic

S. Weston-Simons (✉)
Evelina London Children's Hospital, Guy's and St Thomas' NHS Foundation Trust, London, UK
e-mail: sam.weston-simons@nhs.net

M. V. Belthur
Department of Child Health & Orthopedics, University of Arizona College of Medicine, Phoenix, AZ, USA

Department of Orthopedics, Phoenix Children's Hospital, Phoenix, AZ, USA
e-mail: mbelthur@phoenixchildrens.com

J. A. Fernandes
Sheffield Children's Hospital NHS Foundation Trust, University of Sheffield, Sheffield, UK
e-mail: james.fernandes@nhs.net

© Springer Nature Switzerland AG 2022
M. V. Belthur et al. (eds.), *Pediatric Musculoskeletal Infections*,
https://doi.org/10.1007/978-3-030-95794-0_38

region and ranges from <0.5 to 0.9 cases per 100,000 population in North America and Europe to 10 to 1000 cases per 100,000 population in the African meningitis belt. Incidence is highest in infants and young children (two-thirds of cases in children <5 years of age), with a second smaller peak in adolescents and young adults [5].

In Europe, since the introduction of a serogroup C conjugate vaccine in 1999, serogroup C IMD has been substantially reduced. Serogroup B predominates in Europe, although cases of serogroup Y IMD have been increasing in recent years. In the United States, with the introduction of quadrivalent (serogroups ACWY) meningococcal conjugate vaccines in 2005, declines in serogroup C and Y disease have been observed; serogroup B persists and is now the most common cause of outbreak associated disease [5]. In the African meningitis belt, a conjugate vaccine for serogroup A has been effective in decreasing meningitis associated with that serogroup. Recent epidemics have been primarily due to serogroups C and W.

Impact

The morbidity and mortality resulting from IMD are substantial, with a case-fatality rate (CFR) approximating 8–15% in developed countries [6, 7]. This may be higher (up to 40%) in resource-poor environments. Up to 10–20% of survivors suffer from serious complications (vision/hearing loss, renal/hepatic/neurologic and developmental complications) and orthopaedic sequelae such as amputation, stump overgrowth, scar contractures, growth plate arrests (resulting in deformity and leg length discrepancy) and soft tissue/bone infections [2, 3].

Etiopathogenesis

Pathogen

Neisseria meningitidis is an aerobic Gram-negative diplococcus that may be encapsulated or unencapsulated with a 'kidney' or 'coffee bean' shape under microscopy (Fig. 38.1). Humans are its only natural host. However, those that cause invasive disease are almost always encapsulated. There are 13 distinct serogroups of which six cause life-threatening disease (A, B, C, W-135, Y and X), which are defined upon their genome, capsular polysaccharides and non-capsular antigens [8]. Three of these serogroups (B, C and Y) cause most of the illness seen in the world. The key virulence factor is the polysaccharide capsule that surrounds the outer membrane, which helps bacteria resist phagocytosis and complement-mediated lysis.

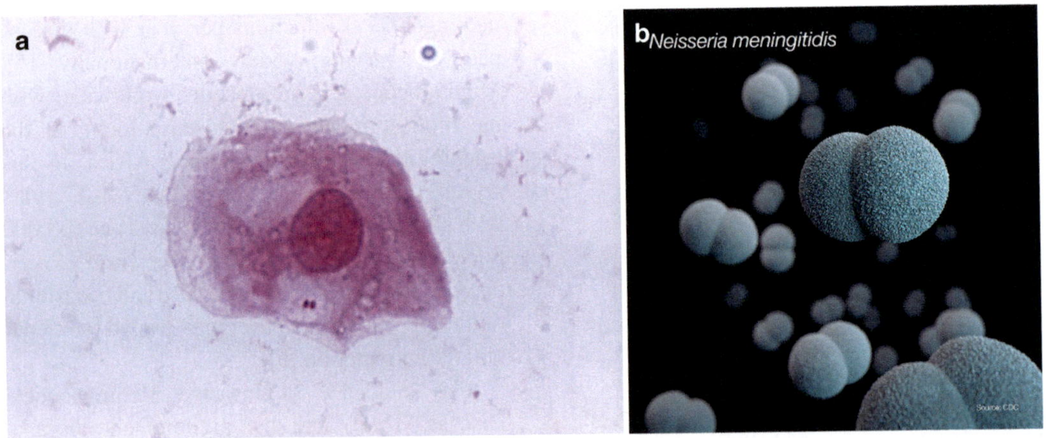

Fig. 38.1 (**a**) Under a magnification of 1125×, this photomicrograph reveals the presence of intracellular, diplococcal, *Neisseria meningitidis* bacteria (Public Health Image Library; CDC/James Volk; 1972). (**b**) A computer-generated 3D image of *Neisseria meningitidis* from an electron microscope image (Public Health Image Library; CDC/Sarah Bailey Cutchin; 2016, Illustrator: Dan Higgins)

Optimal growth of the bacteria occurs at 35–37 °C and it dies within hours on inanimate surfaces. Antibiotic resistance (other than to sulphonamides) is relatively uncommon, although there have been reports of ciprofloxacin-resistant strains and a decrease in penicillin susceptibility [9].

Mode of Infection

IMD is spread through respiratory droplets (e.g. coughing, sneezing) and direct contact with someone who is infected (e.g. kissing). About one in ten people (one out of four in adolescence) have meningococcal bacteria as a commensal. The average incubation period is 3–4 days (usually ranging from 2 to 10 days).

Risk factors associated with developing IMD include age with the highest rates seen in infants, adolescence and young adults. Outbreaks tend to occur in community settings such as college campuses and children summer camps. Immunosuppressed patients such as those with HIV, anatomic and functional asplenia, complement component deficiencies and on complement inhibitors (such as patients with atypical haemolytic uraemic syndrome and generalized Myasthenia Gravis) are at greater risk [5, 10].

Pathogenesis

Neisseria meningitidis releases an endotoxin (a lipooligosaccharide), which also plays a role in adherence of the meningococcus and in activation of the innate immune system. It consists of three distinct parts of which Meningococcal lipid A (a disaccharide of pyranasol N-acetyl glucosamine residues) is the primary driver of biological activity and toxicity.

The endotoxin binds to monocytic and dendritic cells of the innate immune system triggering a variety of cytokines (such as IL-6 and TNF-α) to be released leading to endothelial damage and capillary leakage. There is a direct correlation between endotoxin levels and the severity of disease. Additionally, meningococci are resistant to antimicrobial peptides found in macrophages and neutrophils [11].

Invasive disease usually occurs 1–14 days after bacterial acquisition and, having entered the blood stream, the organism's endotoxin triggers a complex cascade of events including complement activation, the release of interleukin and tumour necrosis factor, diffuse vasculitis, disseminated intravascular coagulation, septic shock and multi-organ failure. The resulting disseminated intravascular coagulopathy (DIC) creates micro-thrombocytosis in small vessels and capillaries and may cause clinically obvious haemorrhagic skin necrosis [11]. Occult damage to bones and growth plates may also occur. An initial vascular occlusive process leads to an inflammatory process that damages the bone and cartilage of the metaphysis, physis and epiphysis [12].

It has also been postulated that growth plate arrests occur under areas of extensive skin necrosis, which can cause a tether effect similar to that of a type-6 physeal injury involving the periphery of the physis and the ring of Ranvier. An indirect mechanism may also be associated with full thickness involvement of the skin and underlying tissue, resulting in an interruption to the angiosomal blood supply [13].

Clinical Presentation

The early symptoms of IMD can be misleading as they are flu-like in nature, making the disease diagnosis difficult. Parents often report a sudden onset deterioration in their child with a possible prodromal illness such as fever and being general unwell. The child may appear lethargic, irritable, have a temperature, be poorly interactive to verbal and physical stimulus and be complaining of a headache, generalized aches and pains and possibly have respiratory symptoms/distress. Classic signs of meningococcal meningitis include fever, headache and stiff neck. Other symptoms include nausea, vomiting, photophobia (being sensitive to light), confusion or on occasion seizures. Meningococcal sepsis is characterized by fever

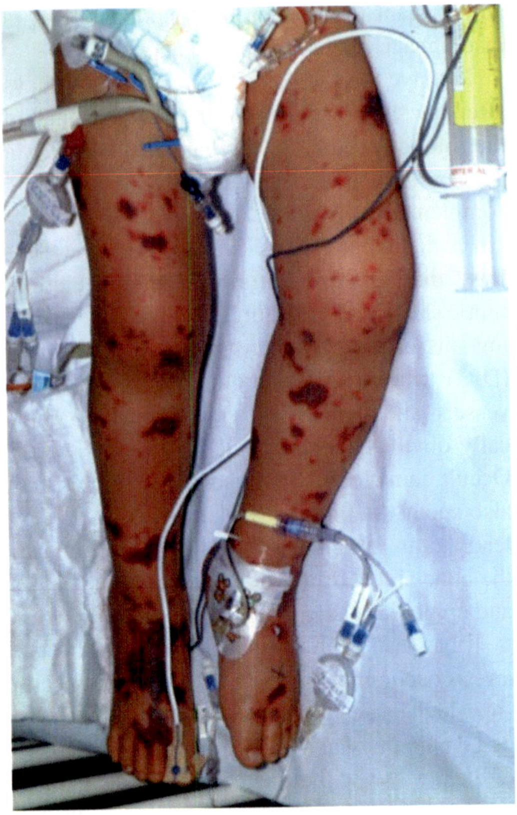

Fig. 38.2 Clinical photograph showing the non-blanching petechial rash

and a petechial or purpuric rash, often accompanied by septic shock, DIC and multiple organ failure.

Orthopaedic surgeons may only be asked to review patients after the child has been stabilized or in conjunction with plastic surgical colleagues. Specifically and clinically, there may the characteristic non-blanching rash (Fig. 38.2), a stiff neck, and evidence of septic shock (hypotension, tachycardia, tachypnoea, reduced capillary refill, cool peripheries and poor urine output). Skin changes (dark purple rash/purpura fulminans) may occur in isolated areas before becoming more fulminant.

Diagnosis

Meningococcal disease can be difficult to diagnose because the signs and symptoms are often similar to those of other illnesses. Initial investigations should be combined with resuscitative measures. The diagnosis of IMD is based on bacteriologic isolation, antigen or DNA detection of *Neisseria meningitidis* in a usually sterile body fluid such as blood, CSF, synovial or pleural fluid. The sensitivity of culture is reduced after the initiation of antimicrobial therapy and polymerase chain reaction-based assays are increasingly used for the diagnosis of meningococcal disease.

Blood should be taken to confirm the diagnosis and assess the severity of the infection including complete blood count, ESR, CRP, basic metabolic profile and a coagulation screen. An arterial blood sample sent for blood gas will help assess the severity of the illness. Blood cultures are taken to confirm the diagnosis and antibiotics given immediately, with samples sent for whole-blood polymerase chain reaction for *N. meningitidis*. A lumbar puncture should be carried out (unless evidence of raised intracranial pressure), and Cerebrospinal fluid should be sent for gram stain, culture and sensitivity with antibiotics not delayed for it [14].

IMD is a notifiable disease in many countries, and clinical, laboratory and epidemiological criteria have been developed by many countries in the world for case definition. Cases are defined as probable (positive clinical criteria), possible (clinical and epidemiologic criteria) and confirmed (clinical, epidemiologic and lab criteria) based on these criteria [15].

Initial imaging focuses on attempting to isolate the source of the infection and a chest X-ray is the mainstay. As the child becomes more stabilized, full body MRI scans may be performed to attempt to identify any collections or surgical targets, particularly in the presence of a child that is not responding to antibiotic treatment.

Subsequent assessment must focus on the musculoskeletal system to identify (after discharge from hospital) areas of growth arrest in the extremities. These should initially focus on the lower limb with long leg alignment views if clinical assessment suggests deformity. Parents should be counselled as to the unpredictable nature of which and how many physes may be affected at the initial review. Once identified, regular (annual), clinical and radiological assessment to assess alignment and limb-length discrepancy is necessary with a low threshold for radiographing other joints if suspicious (Figs. 38.3 and 38.4).

In the presence of instability further evaluation of the joint with computerized tomography (CT) scan may help understand the anatomical geometry (Figs. 38.5, 38.6, and 38.7), bar formation and patient and parent counselling. Magnetic resonance imaging (MRI) scan may also be useful in assessment of the physis for the presence, location and extent of a growth arrest. Clinical photographs and a 3D gait analysis may be helpful to evaluate the child's function before and after surgical reconstruction.

Management

Invasive meningococcal disease is a severe infection and can be deadly in a matter of hours. Prompt recognition of disease, administration of antibiotics, usually beta-lactam and supportive measures are vital to improve the outcome in IMD.

Initial Medical Management

At the initial presentation, if IMD is suspected, intravenous third-generation cephalosporin

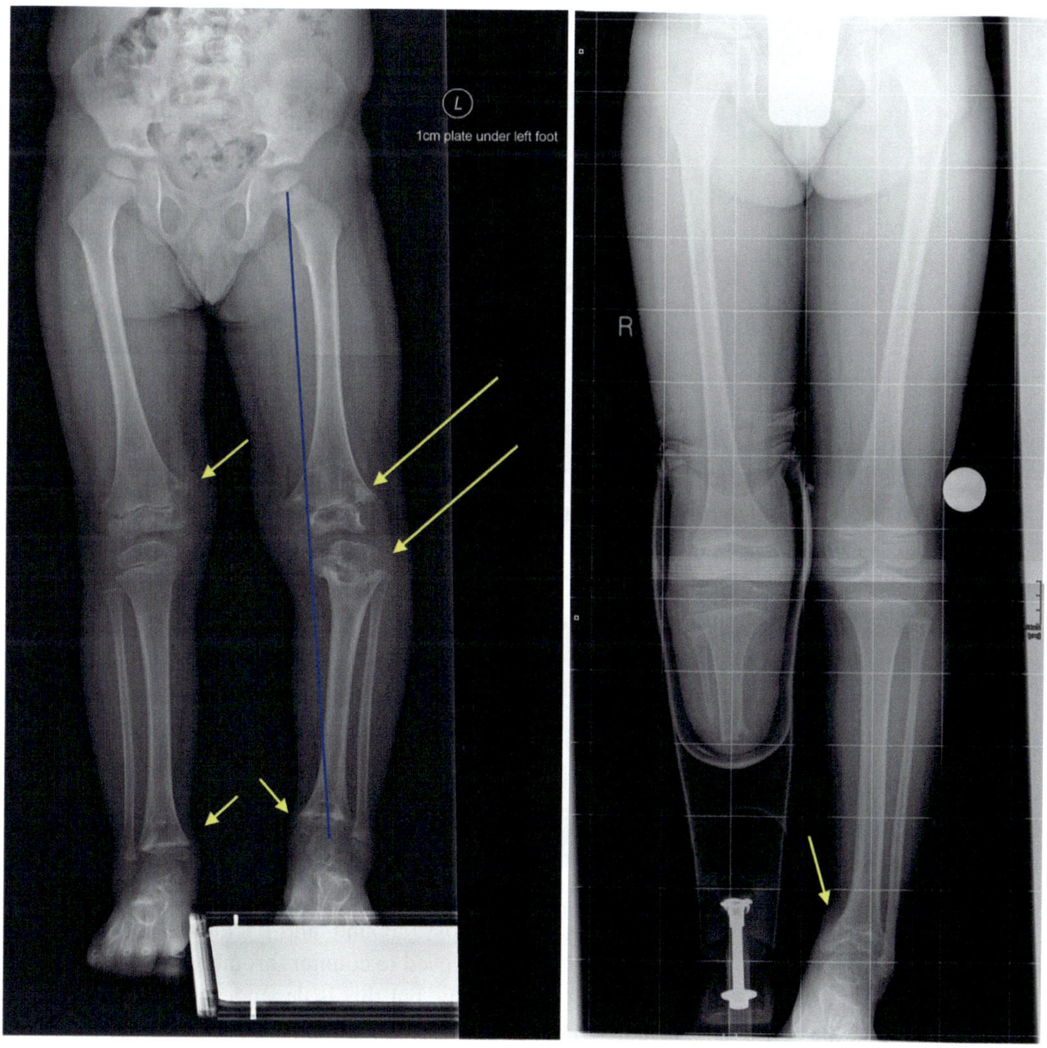

Figs. 38.3 and 38.4 Long leg alignment Radiographs demonstrating multiple growth arrests involving Left distal femur, proximal tibia and distal tibia with varus deformity at all these sites

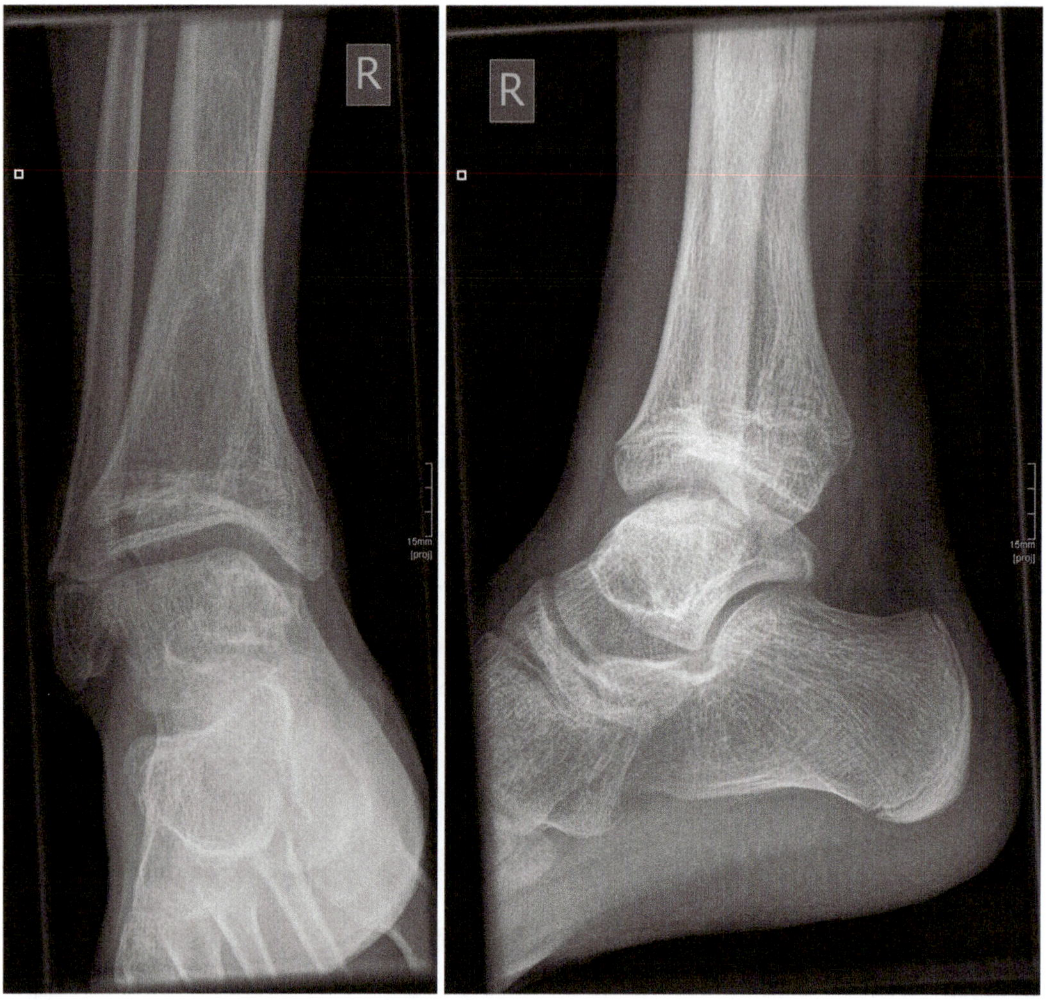

Figs. 38.5 and 38.6 Plain radiographs of the right ankle demonstrating varus, apex posterior deformity (note the relative fibula over growth)

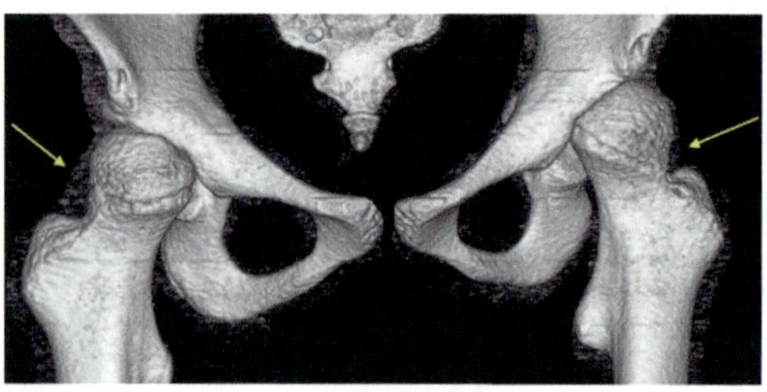

Fig. 38.7 A 3D CT reconstruction demonstrating bilateral lateral proximal femur growth arrests (highlighted by arrows)

should be given at the earliest opportunity. This should not delay transfer to secondary care. Initial supportive measures are directed by the paediatric medical and intensive care teams. Children with severe IMD are transferred to the intensive care unit, often sedated and ventilated to provide multiple organ support, with correction of metabolic disturbances as required. IV crystalloids and inotropes are given to counter septicaemic shock and support the circulatory system. Dexamethasone should be given as soon as possible and anti-haemostatic therapy has been used to counter thrombosis and microangiopathy, but this is dependent on local protocols [14, 16]. Septicaemic shock can result in multiple organ failure including renal failure, peripheral limb ischaemia and gangrene. Despite aggressive medical management, mortality is around 10% [6]. Of the 90% of patients who survive, 20% will have permanent disabilities with a mean length of stay in the ICU being 14 days (SD 7–34 days) [17].

Initial Surgical Management

Initial surgical management is necessary to preserve extremities in the setting of peripheral limb ischaemia and compartment syndrome, debride dead or dying tissue parts and to provide wound management for parts of the body with damaged skin. Consultation with an experienced paediatric orthopaedic surgeon/plastic surgeon in the early stages of the illness is vital for planning surgical approaches for amputation of the resulting necrotic tissue and for minimizing eventual tissue loss.

Necrotic Areas

Tissue injury is primarily ischaemic in nature and related to the three stages of meningococcal disease: poor tissue perfusion, vascular infarction and gangrene. Lower extremity more involved than upper extremity/axial body parts. The first step in treatment is waiting and watching for tissue demarcation, which may take a number of weeks. Aggressive, early debridement has been shown to result in more proximal amputation level and repeated surgeries than those that were watched [18]. Surgical debridement of necrotic tissue is the next step, especially in the presence of a secondary wound infection. Early debridement of large volume dry, necrotic tissue has been advocated to improve renal function if patients are continuing to deteriorate despite medical management [16]. Wound management of extremities with vacuum-assisted dressings and devices to promote healthy new granulation tissue growth and decrease the risk of infection may subsequently be required. Skin grafting or flap (muscle/fasciocutaneous) reconstruction may be necessary in the presence of localized tissue necrosis (in >60% of cases) and are the mainstays of managing cutaneous/soft tissue necrotic lesions [16, 19].

Peripheral Limb Ischaemia and Compartment Syndrome

Multiple authors recommend that compartment pressures are difficult to interpret and advocate clinical judgement following frequent, personal review with subsequent fasciotomy if indicated [20]. There remains some debate over fasciotomy in the presence of compartment syndrome. Fasciotomy for the purpose of decompressing compartment syndrome-like situations is not indicated in the vast majority of these patients because the ischaemic damage, regardless of its aetiology, has already occurred [21]. However, an early fasciotomy in the absence of peripheral ischaemia and raised compartment pressures, especially if the purpuric rash had been present for no more than 24 hours, may be useful [22].

Secondary Infections

Secondary bacterial infections of the soft tissues, bone and joint are common (25%) and are treated by IV antibiotics and debridement of dead tissue [23].

Amputations

It is common for selective and carefully planned digit/limb amputations/disarticulations to be required once the areas of necrosis have fully demarcated. The level of such an amputation is variable from patient to patient, although many authors advocate the need for patience in allowing necrotic demarcation. Younger age has been significantly associated with amputation occurrence. Upper-extremity amputations are less frequent than lower-extremity amputations [19]. Above knee and elbow amputations are seldom required. Amputations may become necessary

Table 38.1 Timing, prevalence and management of sequela following IMD

Treatment phase	Specific sequela	Prevalence	Treatment
Early (50–100%), less than 6 months after IMD	Multiple organ Failure	50–100%	IV antibiotics, ventilation, inotrope support, delayed and selective surgery
	Tissue necrosis	50–90%	Medical management, wait for demarcation, delayed and selective SX
	Peripheral limb ischaemia	50–60%	Wait for demarcation, delayed and carefully planned, selective amputation
	Mortality	10–20%	Multi-Organ Failure, adrenal failure, DIC
	Amputations	8–60%	Follow principles of paediatric amputations
Late (> 60%), more than 6 months after IMD	Partial growth arrest LE > UE, below knee	7–45%	Epiphysiodesis with deformity correction – acute or gradual
	Complete growth arrest LE > UE (femur > tibia)	5–30%	Epiphysiodesis, limb lengthening/ shortening
	Revision amputations	30–60%	Follow principles of paediatric amputations
	Stump overgrowth	23%	Revision amputation, medullary capping
	Scar contractures	15–25%	Soft tissue release, tendon lengthening/ transfer
	Secondary infections		Debridement, antibiotics
	Hip avascular necrosis/ partial growth arrest	10%	Hip reconstruction

within 6 months of survival from IMD and involve multiple limbs [18]. The surgical treatment plan should be guided by paediatric, not adult, limb amputation principles [24] (Table 38.1) (Box 38.1).

Box 38.1 Key Principles of Paediatric Amputations [24]

1. Primary goal is to maximize function with careful consideration of timing of interventions.
2. A multi-disciplinary team involving an orthopaedic surgeon, a rehabilitation medical specialist, prosthetist, physiotherapist and occupational therapist is essential for good outcome.
3. Preserve limb length whenever possible even if soft tissue coverage not initially possible.
4. Physes, particularly around the knee, should attempt to be preserved as without these at skeletal maturity short stumps are challenging for prostheses.
5. If possible, the knee joint should be preserved (even with short tibial stumps) to maximize gait efficiency.
6. Disarticulate rather than through-the-bone amputation whenever possible to avoid complication of overgrowth. Stump length can be controlled by epiphysiodesis.
7. Articular cartilage provides cushioning and associated widening from metaphysis provides better socket suspension.
8. If additional abnormality more proximally further surgical interventions or prosthesis modifications may be needed for improving function.

Late Orthopaedic Management

Patients who survive the initial acute phase of fulminant meningococcemia are at increased risk for serious long-term morbidities, including vision/hearing loss, orthopaedic, dermatological, renal/hepatic, neurological and developmental complications and psychosocial problems [17]. Late orthopaedic sequelae (7–70%) requiring surgical management after 6 months or more following the initial infection include growth disturbances, amputation stump revisions, scar contractures and soft-tissue/bone infections [21, 23]. All patients who survive meningococcal septicaemia should be followed by an orthopaedic surgeon who is experienced in paediatric limb deformities and amputations. Younger age, cutaneous scarring, severity of infection and need for a limb amputation appear to be predictive of orthopaedic sequelae.

Growth Disturbances

Growth plate disturbances (7–70%) occur in the early stage of the disease but may not be recognized for several years and may result in angular deformities or length discrepancies at a later stage. Growth disturbances in the upper extremities are less frequent than in the lower extremities [25–28]. Peripheral growth plate arrests are more common and lead to angular deformities, while central growth plate arrests are less common and lead to limb-length discrepancy. Multiple growth plate arrests are common in children with IMD due to the ischaemic aetiology. In the lower limb, most commonly the physes around the knee and ankle (with sparing of the distal fibula) are affected [20, 23, 27]. Growth arrests may lead to not only extra-articular deformity but also abnormal intra-articular geometry. This may lead to instability of the joint and needs to be fully assessed before embarking on limb reconstruction.

A thorough assessment is crucial with a full clinical examination and complete radiological investigations. Clinical examination, radiographs and CT scans are used to assess the deformity and limb-length discrepancy, and to identify which growth plates are affected and to what extent. It is important to assess the function of the joints affected, particularly the knee and ankle joints, which often present with severe varus deformities. Compensatory deformities at adjacent joints must be included in developing a treatment plan. Prediction of final limb-length discrepancy is also important to anticipate the need for further lengthening. At first presentation, this can be undertaken in a simple manner by using the arithmetic method of Menelaus [29]. Later, with serial measurements, the estimate can be calculated more accurately using the multiplier method of Paley et al. [30].

The surgical approach to correction of deformity depends on the extent and site of damage to the growth plate. If there is central growth arrest, the aim is to achieve limb-length equality by lengthening. If there is a peripheral growth plate arrest, angular correction is also necessary, and we recommend ablation of the growth plate in the lower limb to prevent recurrent angular deformity [27]. In the lower limb angular correction can be either acute, using a dome or transphyseal osteotomy, or gradual using a circular external frame [23]. Follow-up to skeletal maturity is essential to recognize and treat any recurrence. Smaller physeal bars can be excised with fat or cranioplasty insertion and the use of guided growth whenever feasible. The overall goal must be to achieve limb-length equality, normalization of the mechanical axis in the lower limb and restoration of joint alignment with minimal loss of stature (Figs. 38.8, 38.9, and 38.10). The surgeon, the patient and caregivers must be prepared for repeated bone-lengthening surgery (Case Study 1).

The upper limb physes do not appear to be affected as frequently as the lower limb [4, 21]. The principles of management are similar to

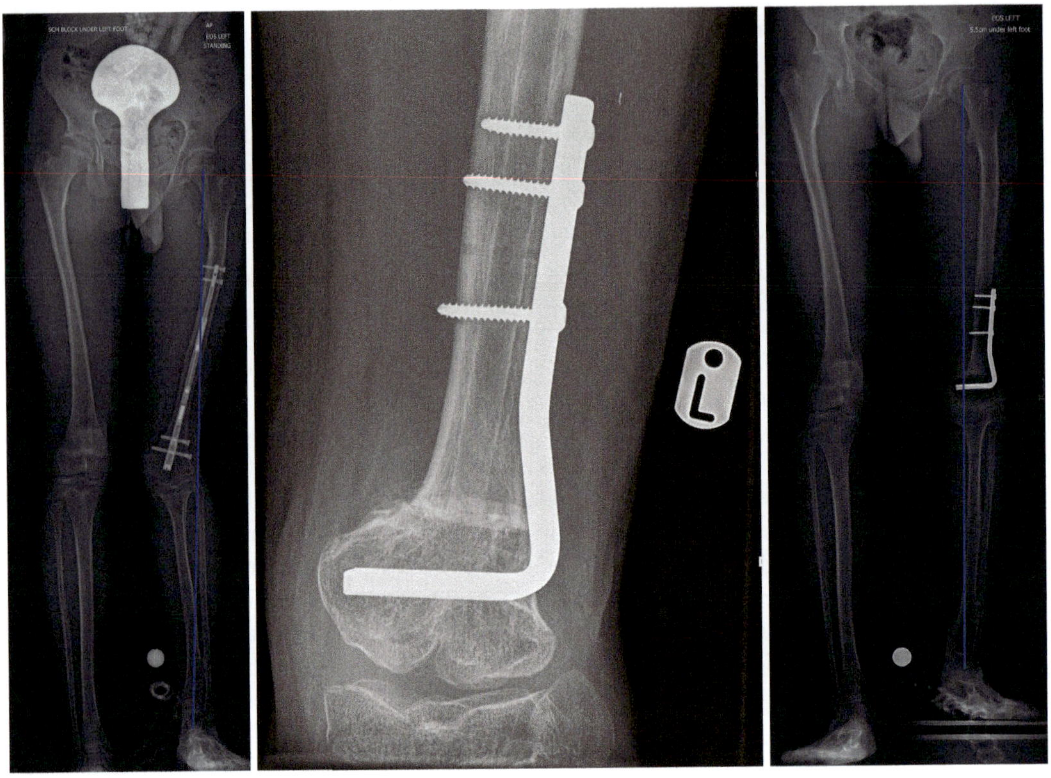

Figs. 38.8, 38.9, and 38.10 Long leg radiographs with intra-medullary device in situ. A left distal femoral osteotomy was carried out post-lengthening to correct the femoral axis with a subsequent plan for tibial lengthening and angular correction with all images demonstrating the mechanical axis deviation

those of the lower limb growth arrests though limb-length discrepancy (up to 4 cm) is better tolerated. Attention though should be paid to the wrist, (specifically the distal radius physis), as patient complaints about wrist function tend to be late when there may be significant distal radial–ulnar joint mismatch (Case Study 2). In such situations the ulna tends to be unaffected and so early recognition of the deformity may lead to pre-emptive ulnar epiphysiodesis, negating the need to reconstruction.

The treatment of deformity in this heterogenous group of patients is different from that of other patients due to the presence of abnormal 'sick physes'. This may explain why the use of guided growth has had limited success, and attempts at physeal resection/physiolysis have also had poorer outcomes (Figs. 38.11 and 38.12). Attention must also be made to both sagittal and coronal elements of the deformity.

Hip Problems

Hip problems are not common but have been reported following IMD. Avascular necrosis of the femoral head and partial growth arrests have been reported and should be monitored for with initial pelvic radiographs to evaluate the hip to see if such a deformity is present. Attempts at guided growth using an inferiorly placed cannulated screw may have limited success as discussed previously. The common form of physeal growth arrest at the proximal femoral physis produces a type 2 Kalmachi and Ogden avascular necrosis sequela and a posterolateral tether. Near maturity hip reconstruction may be required as part the overall limb reconstruction to improve the hip mechanics (Case Study 3). Commonest procedure is relative neck lengthening osteotomy with a modification of the Morscher or Wagner technique for the hip.

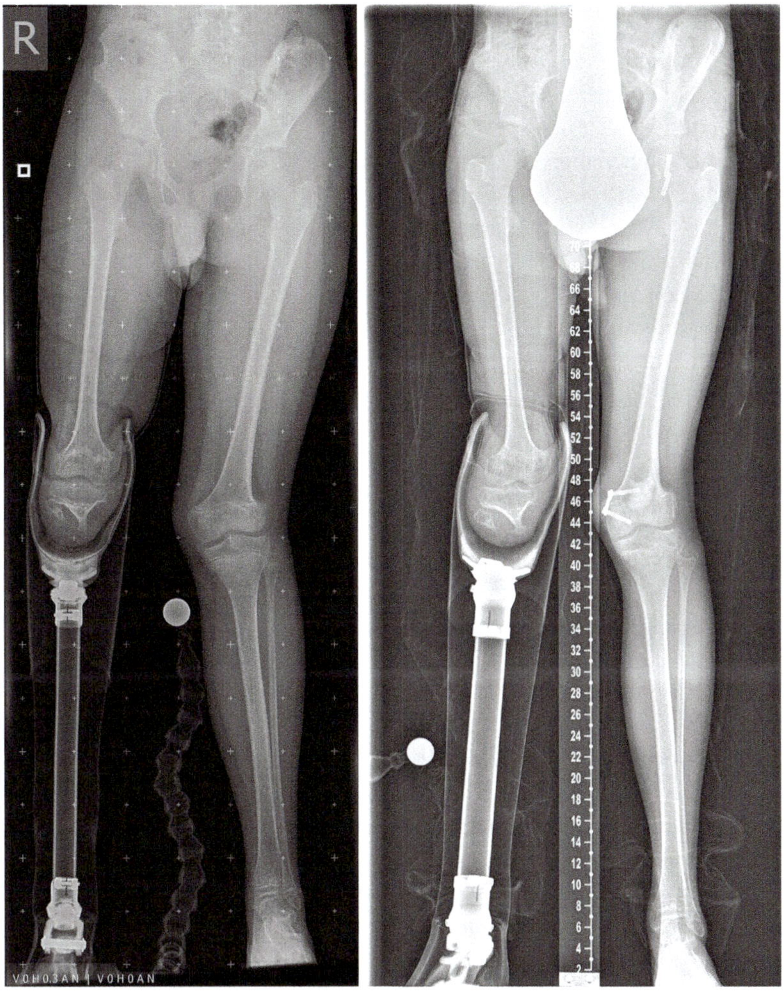

Figs. 38.11 and 38.12 Guided growth attempted on left distal femoral physis that appeared healthy but 2 years later no correction achieved

Prosthetic Fitting Issues

Almost all amputations of the lower limbs and some upper extremity amputations require prosthetic replacement. Compared to patients undergoing standard amputation, these patients present an additional challenge in prosthetic fitting because their residual limbs frequently have poor soft tissue coverage that contains scars and skin grafts. The residual limb may also be short and susceptible to bone overgrowth after trans-osseous amputations [23, 31]. Ischaemic injury to the remaining growth plate adds to the challenge of prosthetic fitting because the growth plate affects normal growth of the remaining extremity. A complete growth arrest results in a short residual extremity and a partial growth arrest can cause angular deformity of the remaining stump [31] (Box 38.2).

Box 38.2 Key Paediatric Prosthetic Management Principles after IMD [31]

1. Input from the multi-disciplinary team is critical for successful management of the patient and prosthesis.
2. Although often an initial concern, prosthesis use only becomes a priority once other issues (such as initial soft tissue management with grafts/flaps) have been resolved.

3. Protection soft tissue and bone with accommodation of deformity must be considered at first prosthetic fitting.
4. Accommodation of deformity/pressure areas with viscoelastic polymer pads and atypical contact points is crucial to maximize pressure distribution.
5. Patient and family education about skin monitoring is key, as repeated tissue breakdown because of fragile tissue and bony overgrowth is not uncommon.
6. Evaluate extremity alignment often as joint malalignment secondary to growth plate disturbances often necessitate atypical prosthetic alignment.
7. Prostheses may often require patient specific customization with physeal disturbance to maintain overall alignment.

Amputation Stump Revisions

Stump revisions are a predictable complication (60%) reported in nearly all studies reviewing such patients [23, 28, 32]. This may be related to bone overgrowth of the stump or soft tissue complications such as the scarring or unstable skin. Stump overgrowth occurs predominantly in patients with lower extremity amputations (23%). Partial growth arrest in the physis proximal to the amputation may result in further deformity or a soft tissue contracture. In young children, below-knee amputation often leads to secondary proximal tibial varus due to differential fibular growth, regardless of the amputation indication. Ablation of the proximal fibular growth plate in children with below-knee amputation is strongly advocated to prevent prosthetic misadaptation [23].

Scar Contractures

The prevalence of scar contractures in the upper extremities was similar to that in the lower extremities. Skin and other soft tissue (muscle/nerve) necrosis frequently leads to scar contractures that affect the range of motion of joints adjacent to the injury. Contracture releases, scar resections, tendon transfers and various plastic surgery procedures may be required to keep the joint reasonably mobile and functional. Volkmann ischaemic contractures following compartment syndrome are addressed with soft tissue release/reconstruction [25].

Soft Tissue and Bone Infections

These patients are susceptible to late infections in their extremities associated both with late surgical or nonsurgical treatment usually at the distal portion of the amputation stump [23].

Complications

(a) *Recurrence of the angular deformity:* Belthur et al. [25] observed that patients with growth arrests around the knee who underwent realignment procedures (either with an osteotomy or by hemicallotasis) without an additional epiphysiodesis had a high rate of recurrence of deformity. Park et al. [33] and Nectoux et al. [28] reported that all patients who had an angular correction and lengthening combined with a percutaneous epiphysiodesis had no recurrence of angular deformity.
(b) Complication's related to the surgery are in keeping with the use of external fixator frames and intramedullary devices. During lengthening with either device, close monitoring of the joints above and below should occur to identify early joint subluxation.
(c) *Revision of amputation* is a predictable complication in this cohort of patients and long-term follow-up to skeletal maturity is essential.
(d) *Late infection of the soft tissues and bone* has been reported. These were primarily associated with the distal portion of the amputation site with *Staphylococcus aureus* being the predominant species.

Outcomes

IMD is associated with neurological sequelae, with a reported incidence of 35% in those discharged from paediatric intensive care. General outcomes reviewing survivors have identified hearing loss in 2–4%, although it has been reported as being as high as 38% [3, 17]. Wheeler et al. [18] found that in their cohort of 21 children, who had a total of 117 procedures, age-appropriate milestones were reached. All those over 5 years of age and who were interviewed attended regular school classes and were active within the context of their physical disabilities. However, an evaluation of 115 child survivors 10 years after hospital admission found although there were no gross neurological deficits and attendance at mainstream schools, when compared with controls there were significantly lower scores in psychometric and behaviour rating scales [34]. However, no statistical difference in overall cognitive function in adults has been reported [35]. Specific data examining the impact of meningococcal disease in survivors has a number of limitations. However, studies have clearly demonstrated that loss of functional ability (from for example digit loss) has a clear impact on quality of life (QoL) [36]. The orthopaedic literature reports outcomes of deformity correction and limb lengthening. Validated HRQOL measures and Patient Reported Functional Outcomes are not available as most are not validated for paediatric/adolescent reconstruction. Most studies report that once growth was balanced with epiphysiodesis or bar resection, angular correction and limb lengthening had good clinical and radiologic outcomes at short- and mid-term follow-up (Box 38.3).

Box 38.3 Key Paediatric Rehabilitation Principles after IMD [31]

(a) Full multi-disciplinary team involvement with emphasis on the need to build a relationship with the child and their family and team involvement throughout child development.
(b) Identify any external challenges to patient care such as socioeconomic concerns, belief systems and family dynamics.
(c) Manage parental expectations at the first appointment with thorough MDT evaluation and goal setting. The need for early patient independence is key. Keep the prosthesis height short initially. Add joints and height, at a later time.
(d) Throughout growth reassess the patient's functional and mobility needs such as the need for a wheelchair in those with higher-level amputations.
(e) With the upper extremity involvement keep patient height low and consider arm span when fitting prostheses for function and safety.
(f) Educate the patient and parents that ongoing rehabilitation and therapy are crucial to optimize function as the child grows and matures.
(g) Consider growth and the delayed effects of the disease.

Conclusion

IMD is an uncommon but devastating disease caused by *N. meningitidis*. One in ten people who develop the disease will die from it and up to 20% of survivors suffer from serious complications and orthopaedic sequelae such as amputations, scars, deafness or brain damage resulting in physical and psychosocial disability. IMD results in significant while underestimated lifetime costs for the society. Early consultation with a paediatric orthopaedist is vital to help patients successfully deal with the orthopaedic sequelae associated with the disease. Careful attention to bone growth and recognition of growth arrests allows for early detection and timely surgical intervention. Evaluation and management by a multi-disciplinary rehabilitation team help these children maximize their functional potential and quality of life (Box 38.4).

Box 38.4 Tips and Tricks to Stay Out of Trouble

1. Early prompt diagnosis of IMD is essential.
2. Transfer to PICU with focus on resuscitative and supportive medical management.
3. Early consultation with ortho/plastics to assess soft tissues with patience and monitoring before surgical intervention.
4. Multi-disciplinary team management throughout childhood till maturity.
5. Physeal disturbances may present throughout growth and so regular clinical and radiological assessment of patients is essential.
6. Epiphysiodesis with angular deformity correction for partial arrests.
7. Epiphysiodesis of opposite limb with lengthening of affected limb for complete arrests.
8. Follow principles of paediatric amputations and subsequent rehabilitation.

Case Studies

Case Study 1

This case study demonstrates the typical journey of a patient affected by meningococcal septicaemia and the need for continual assessment of limb deformity and reassessment of physes throughout growth (Fig. 38.13):

- The patient was initially reviewed after referral at the age of 3 with multiple physeal involvement identified (bilateral proximal femora, bilateral distal tibiae, left proximal tibia). This has led to multiple subsequent limb reconstructive procedures
- Aged 5/6: Staged bilateral bifocal tibial and fibular osteotomies with subsequent distal tibio/fibular epiphysiodeses
- Aged 8: Bilateral proximal medial hip epiphysiodesis and greater trochanteric apophysiodesis
- Aged 10/11: Staged bilateral hip reconstruction (modified Morscher type)
- Aged 12: 4-cm intramedullary lengthening of femur
- Aged 13: Left proximal tibial epiphysiodesis
- Aged 15: Bifocal right tibio/fibular osteotomy hybrid TSF/Ilizarov, with left distal tibial varus requiring planned intervention

Case Study 2

This young man had multiple upper and lower limb amputations related to his initial disease. He was highly functional but had left wrist pain related to relative ulnar overgrowth and abnormal radial sagittal alignment. This was managed with a distal ulnar epiphysiodesis and hexapod correction of the length and deformity (Fig. 38.14).

Case Study 3

This young man had multiple upper and lower limb physes affected including his bilateral proximal femora with lateral growth arrests. Hemiepiphysiodesis was not successful and after monitoring the hips close to maturity definitive interventions were carried out (Fig. 38.15).

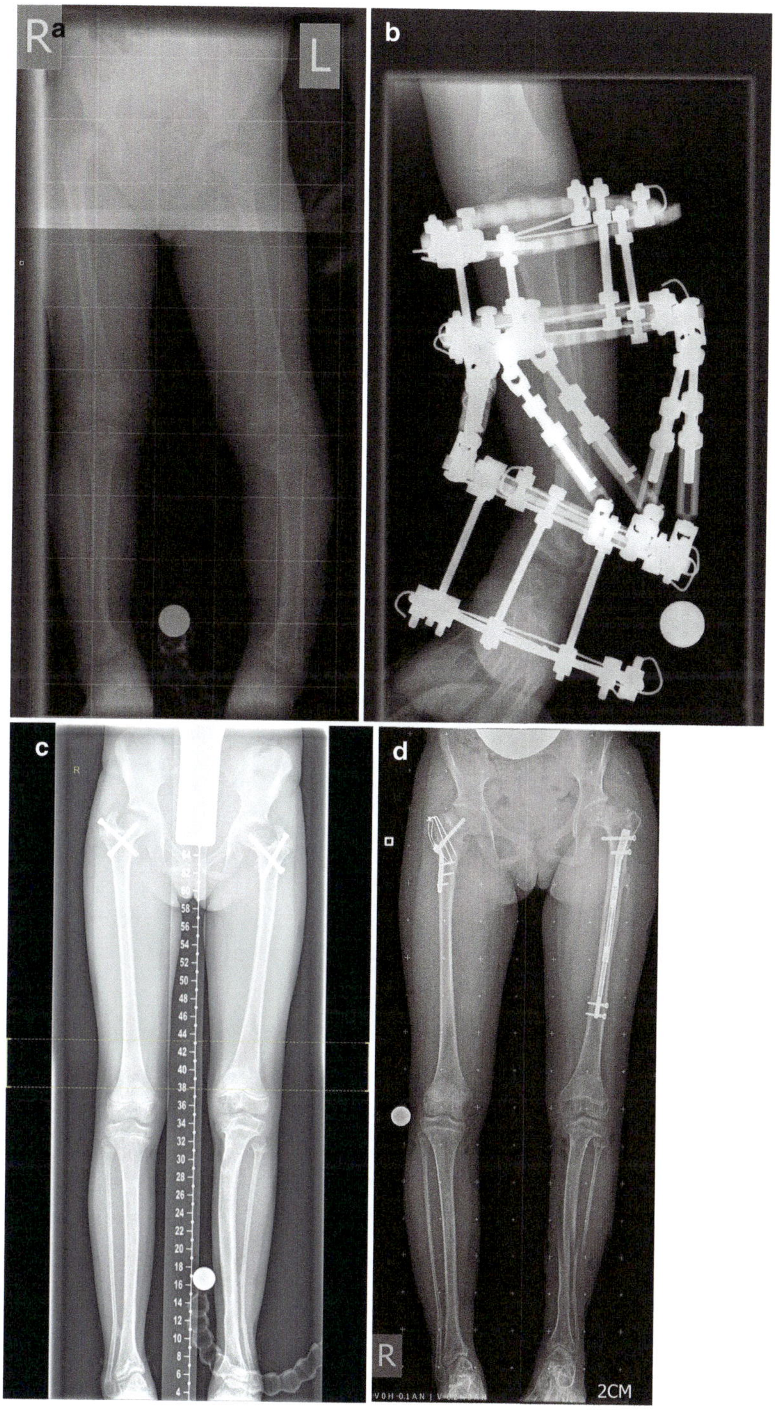

Fig. 38.13 (**a**) Initial presenting long leg radiograph demonstrating the bilateral apparent growth arrests and mechanical axis deviation on the left. (**b**) Left tibia and fibula deformity correction with hexapod frame carried out at the age of 5. (**c**) Long leg radiograph aged 9 after bilateral lower limb frame hexapod deformity corrections and bilateral hip interventions (hemiepiphysiodesis and trochanteric apophysiodesis). Note the now evident left distal femur and proximal tibia physeal arrests which were not clearly apparent at initial presentation). (**d**) Long leg radiograph aged 13 after bilateral hip reconstructions and left femur intramedullary lengthening with recurrent bilateral distal tibia deformities. (**e**) Long leg radiograph aged 15 with current ongoing right tibia hexapod deformity correction and lengthening

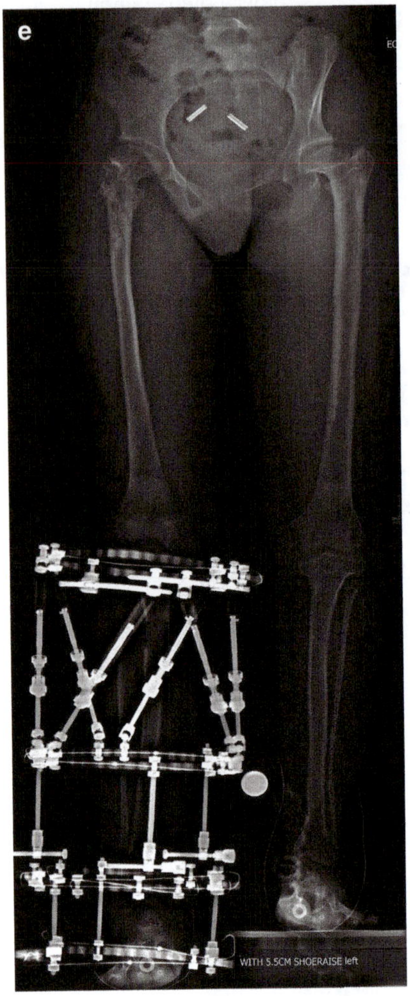

Fig. 38.13 (continued)

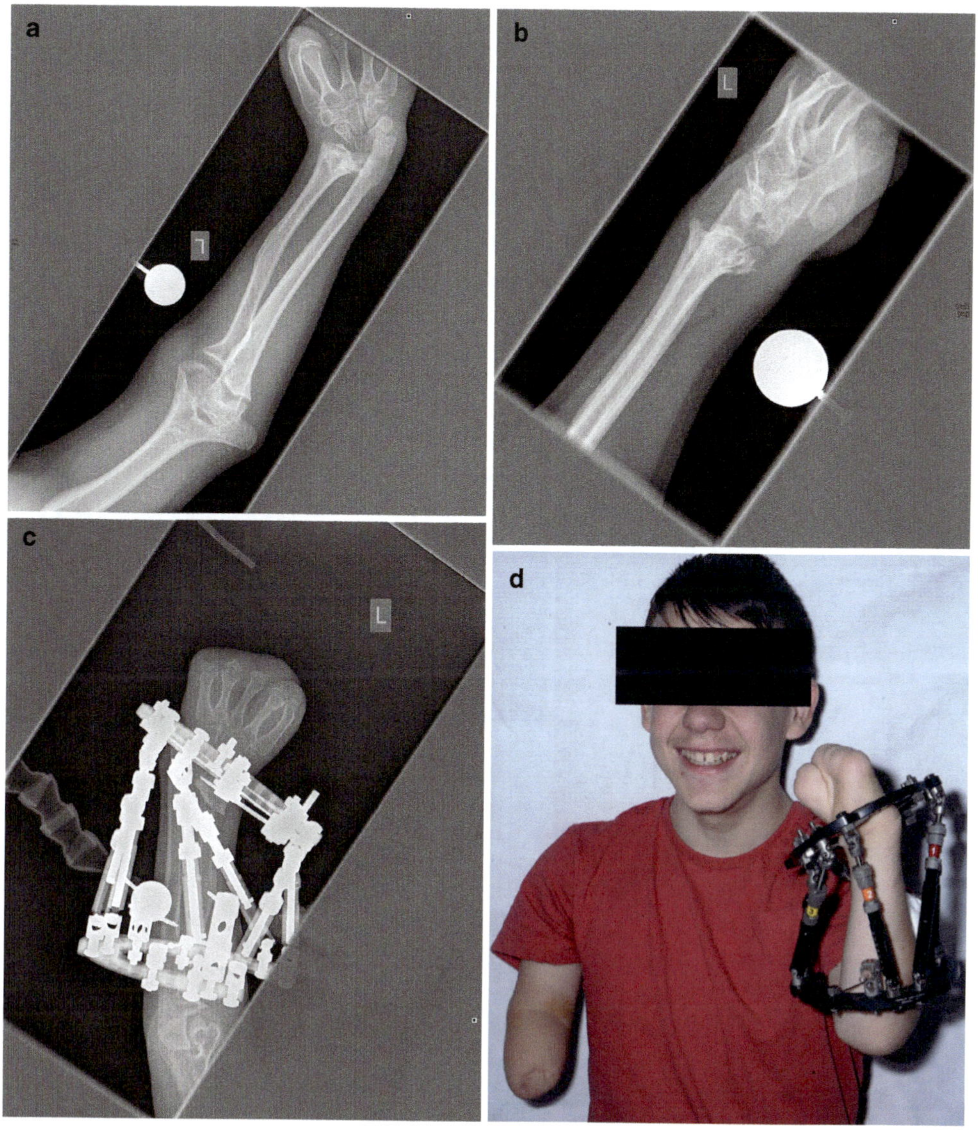

Fig. 38.14 (**a**, **b**) Initial radiographs demonstrating left distal radius growth arrest with relative ulna overgrowth and abnormal carpus. (**c**) Immediate radiographs post application of hexapod fixator and distal radial osteotomy. (**d**) Patient with hexapod frame in situ. During acute admission patient had had right below elbow amputation and multiple digit amputations on the left. (**e**, **f**) Radiographs after removal of the frame and correction

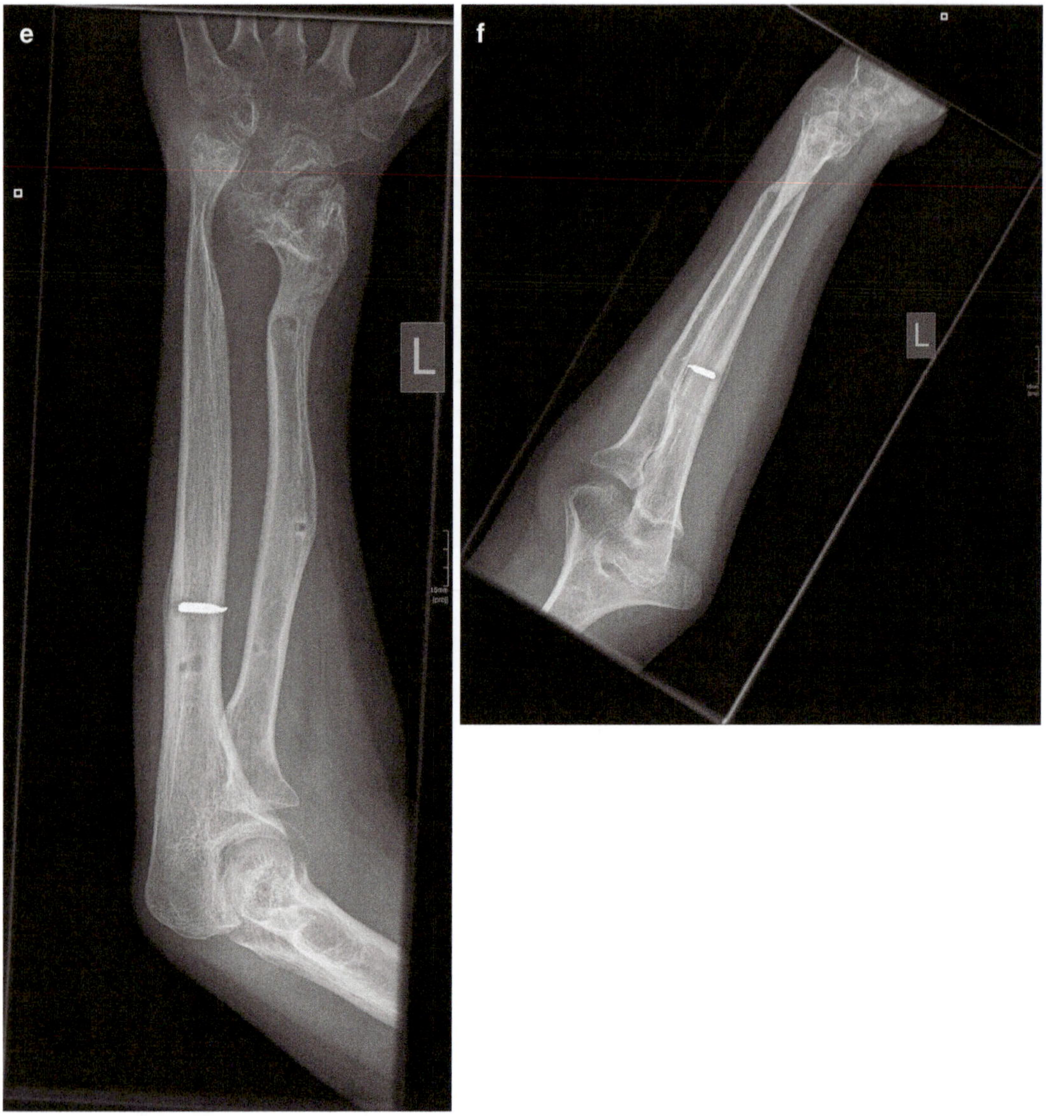

Fig. 38.14 (continued)

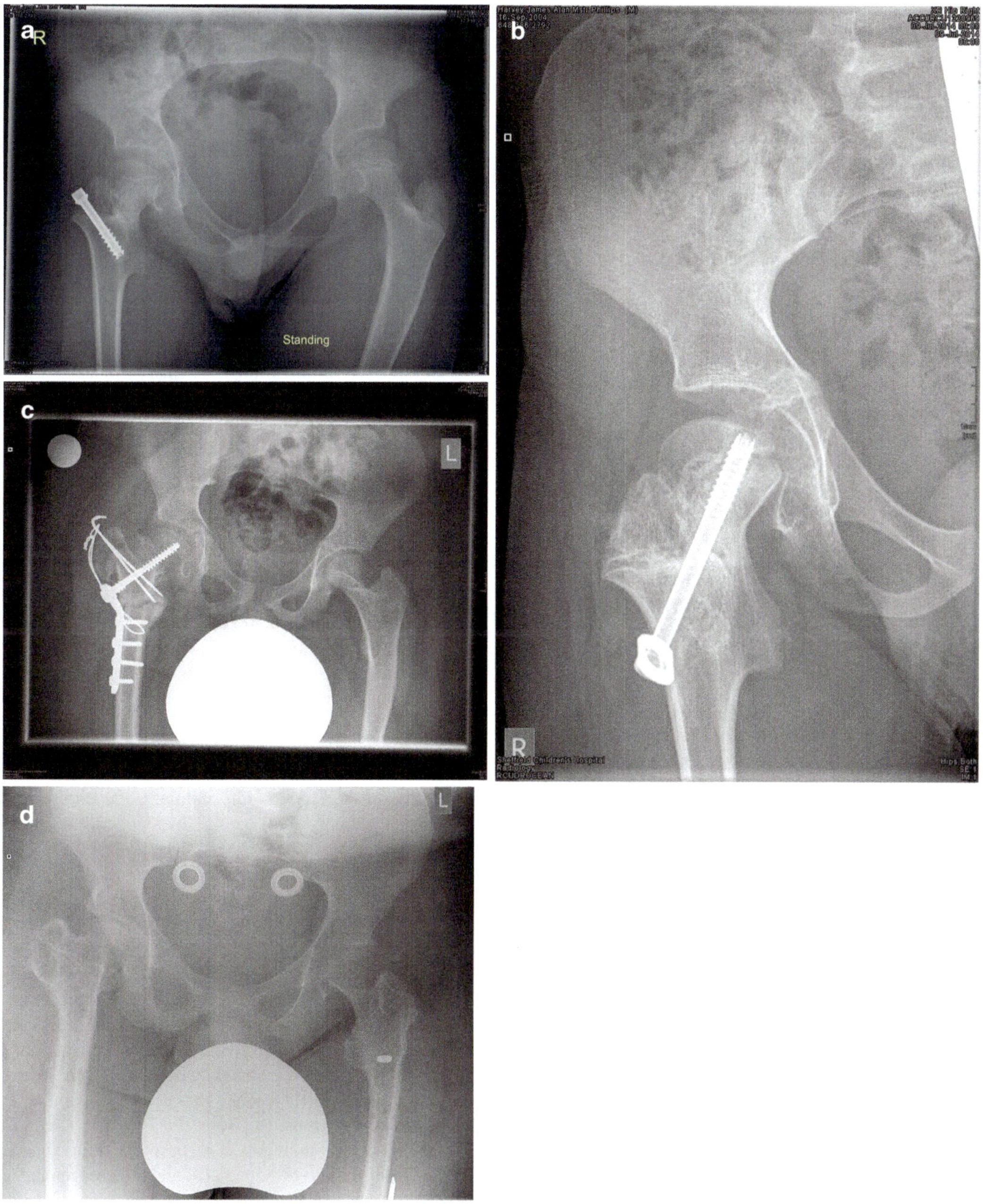

Fig. 38.15 (**a**) Initial attempt made to prevent right relative trochanteric overgrowth with trochanteric epiphysiodesis after identifying right proximal femur lateral growth arrests. (**b**) A further attempt was made to carry out guided growth with hemiepiphysiodesis. (**c**) Bilateral hip deformities with the right hip treated with reconstruction by subtrochanteric varus osteotomy and trochanteric advancement. (**d**) AP pelvis of patient from figure C post-removal of bilateral metalwork

References

1. Martinón-Torres F, Salas A, Rivero-Calle I, Cebey-López M, Pardo-Seco J, Herberg JA, et al. EUCLIDS Consortium. Life-threatening infections in children in Europe (the EUCLIDS project): a prospective cohort study. Lancet Child Adolesc Health. 2018;2(6):404–14.
2. Vyse A, Anonychuk A, Jäkel A, Wieffer H, Nadel S. The burden and impact of severe and long-term sequelae of meningococcal disease. Expert Rev Anti-Infect Ther. 2013;11(6):597–604.
3. Strifler L, Morris SK, Dang V, Tu HA, Minhas RS, Jamieson FB, et al. The health burden of invasive meningococcal disease: a systematic review. J Pediatric Infect Dis Soc. 2016;5(4):417–30.
4. Edwards TA, Bowen L, Bintcliffe F, Aird J, Monsell F. The orthopaedic consequences of childhood meningococcal septicaemia. J Meningitis. 2016;1:109. https://doi.org/10.4172/2572-2050.1000109.
5. Rouphael NG, Stephens DS. Neisseria meningitidis: biology, microbiology, and epidemiology. Methods Mol Biol. 2012;799:1–20.
6. Goldacre MJ, Maisonneuve JJ. Mortality from meningococcal disease by day of the week: English national linked database study. J Public Health (Oxf). 2013;35(3):413–21.
7. Sharip A, Sorvillo F, Redelings MD, et al. Population-based analysis of meningococcal disease mortality in the United States: 1990–2002. Pediatr Infect Dis J. 2006;25:191–4.
8. Branham S. Serological relationships among meningococci. Bact Rev. 1953;17:175–88.
9. Wu HM, Harcourt BH, Hatcher CP, et al. Emergence of ciprofloxacin-resistant *Neisseria meningitidis* in North America. N Engl J Med. 2009;360:886–192.
10. Centers for Disease Control and Prevention Factsheet on Meningococcal Disease. https://www.cdc.gov/meningococcal/about/risk-medical.html. Accessed 16 Dec 2020.
11. de Kleijn E, Hazelzet J, Kornelisse R, et al. Pathophysiology of meningococcal sepsis in children. Eur J Pediatr. 1998;157:869–80.
12. Grogan DP, Love SM, Ogden JA, Millar EA, Johnson LO. Chondro-osseous growth abnormalities after meningococcemia. A clinical and histopathological study. J Bone Joint Surg Am. 1989;71(6):920–8.
13. Watson CH, Ashworth MA. Growth disturbance and meningococcal septicemia. Report of two cases. J Bone Joint Surg Am. 1983;65:1181–3.
14. National Institute for Healthcare and Excellence Meningitis (bacterial) and meningococcal septicaemia in under 16s: recognition, diagnosis and management. 2010. https://www.nice.org.uk/guidance/cg102. Accessed 16 Dec 2020.
15. European Centre for Disease Prevention and Control. Factsheet about meningococcal disease. 2019. https://www.ecdc.europa.eu/en/meningococcal-disease/factsheet. Accessed 16 Dec 2020.
16. Dinh TA, Friedman J, Higuera S. Plastic surgery management in pediatric meningococcal-induced purpura fulminans. Clin Plast Surg. 2005;32(1):117–21.
17. Olbrich KJ, Müller D, Schumacher S, Beck E, Meszaros K, Koerber F. Systematic review of invasive meningococcal disease: sequelae and quality of life impact on patients and their caregivers. Infect Dis Ther. 2018;7(4):421–38.
18. Wheeler JS, Anderson BJ, De Chalain TM. Surgical interventions in children with meningococcal purpura fulminans--a review of 117 procedures in 21 children. J Pediatr Surg. 2003;38(4):597–603.
19. Nectoux E, Mezel A, Raux S, Fron D, Maillet M, Herbaux B. Meningococcal purpura fulminans in children: I. Initial orthopedic management. J Child Orthop. 2010;4(5):401–7.
20. Monsell F. The skeletal consequences of meningococcal septicaemia. Arch Dis Child. 2012;97(6):539–44.
21. Bache CE, Torode IP. Orthopaedic sequelae of meningococcal septicemia. J Pediatr Orthop. 2006;26(1):135–9.
22. Davies MS, Nadel S, Habibi P, Levin M, Hunt DM. The orthopaedic management of peripheral ischaemia in meningococcal septicaemia in children. J Bone Joint Surg Br. 2000;82(3):383–6.
23. Canavese F, Krajbich JI, LaFleur BJ. Orthopaedic sequelae of childhood meningococcemia: management considerations and outcome. J Bone Joint Surg Am. 2010;92(12):2196–203.
24. Krajbich JI. Lower-limb deficiencies and amputations in children. J Am Acad Orthop Surg. 1998;6(6):358–6.
25. Belthur MV, Bradish CF, Gibbons PJ. Late orthopaedic sequelae following meningococcal septicaemia. A multicentre study. J Bone Joint Surg Br. 2005;87(2):236–40.
26. Monsell FP, Barnes JR, Kirubanandan R, McBride AM. Distal tibial physeal arrest after meningococcal septicaemia: management and outcome in seven ankles. J Bone Joint Surg Br. 2011;93(6):839–43.
27. Monsell FP, McBride AR, Barnes JR, Kirubanandan R. Angular deformity of the ankle with sparing of the distal fibula following meningococcal septicaemia: a case series involving 14 ankles in ten children. J Bone Joint Surg Br. 2011;93(8):1131–3.
28. Nectoux E, Mezel A, Raux S, Fron D, Klein C, Herbaux B. Meningococcal purpura fulminans in children. II: late orthopedic sequelae management. J Child Orthop. 2010;4(5):409–16.
29. Menelaus MB. Correction of leg length discrepancy by epiphysial arrest. J Bone Joint Surg Br. 1966;48(2):336–9.
30. Paley D, Bhave A, Herzenberg JE, Bowen JR. Multiplier method for predicting limb-length discrepancy. J Bone Joint Surg Am. 2000;82(10):1432–46.
31. Wick JM, Krajbich I, Kelly S, Dewees T. Meningococcemia: the pediatric orthopedic sequelae. AORN J. 2013;97(5):559–78.
32. Genoff MC, Hoffer MM, Achauer B, Formosa P. Extremity amputations in meningococcemia-

induced purpura fulminans. Plast Reconstr Surg. 1992;89(5):878–81.
33. Park DH, Bradish CF. The management of the orthopaedic sequelae of meningococcal septicaemia. J Bone Joint Surg Br. 2011;93:984–9.
34. Fellick JM, Thomson AP, Sills J, Hart CA. Neurological soft signs in mainstream pupils. Arch Dis Child. 2001;85:371–4.
35. Borg J, Christie D, Coen PG, Booy R, Viner RM. Outcomes of meningococcal disease in adolescence: prospective, matched-cohort study. Pediatrics. 2009;123:e502–9.
36. Erickson LJ, De Wals P, McMahon J, Heim S. Complications of meningococcal disease in college students. Clin Infect Dis. 2001;33:737–9.

Brucellosis, Hydatid Disease, and Viral Osteomyelitis

39

Nirmal Raj Gopinathan, Jagdish Menon, and James A. Fernandes

Brucellosis

Introduction and Epidemiology

Brucellosis is a zoonosis of domesticated livestock and human infection is known by various names, viz. undulant fever, Malta fever, and Mediterranean fever. Although initially thought to be restricted to the Middle East, Mediterranean European countries, south and central Asia, north and east Africa, and central and South America, it is prevalent in many countries across the world and is the most common emerging global zoonosis [1, 2].

The annual occurrence has been estimated to be about more than 500,000 cases per year globally [3]. The epidemiology has evolved over the past two decades because of increased connectivity and travel across the globe, improvement in recognition and reporting, and changing socio-economic parameters. Unfortunately, many countries do not have data on prevalence to confirm the endemicity which creates a situation where the infection is often overlooked. The incidence quoted is much less because of underreporting, mainly attributed to nonspecific clinical presentation and laboratory parameters [4]. The CDC reports the annual incidence of brucellosis to be about 100–200 cases annually.

Complaints pertaining to the skeletal system are the main reason which brings the child to the hospital, and the attending orthopedic surgeon must be vigilant enough to suspect it facilitating early diagnosis.

Microbiology

The *Brucella* species are aerobic, Gram-negative, non-motile, non-spore-forming coccobacilli. *Brucella melitensis* is the most commonly encountered and the most virulent species found in goats, sheep and camels. *Brucella abortus* is found in cows, other bovidae animals, and camels. Dogs and pigs are the reservoirs for *Brucella canis* and *Brucella suis* respectively. Also, very rarely marine species (*B. pinnipedialis* and *B. cataceae*) are found to cause human disease (neuro-brucellosis) [5]. The severity of manifestations of human disease varies according to the infecting species. For example, *B. abortus* is associated with mild disease, whereas *B. melitensis* contributes to severe symptoms [1] (Fig. 39.1).

N. R. Gopinathan (✉)
Division of Paediatric Orthopaedics, Department of Orthopaedic Surgery, Post Graduate Institute of Medical Education and Research, Chandigarh, India

J. Menon
Department of Orthopaedic Surgery, Jawaharlal Institute of Postgraduate Medical Education and Research, Pondicherry, India

J. A. Fernandes
Sheffield Children's Hospital NHS Foundation Trust, University of Sheffield, Sheffield, UK
e-mail: james.fernandes@nhs.net

© Springer Nature Switzerland AG 2022
M. V. Belthur et al. (eds.), *Pediatric Musculoskeletal Infections*,
https://doi.org/10.1007/978-3-030-95794-0_39

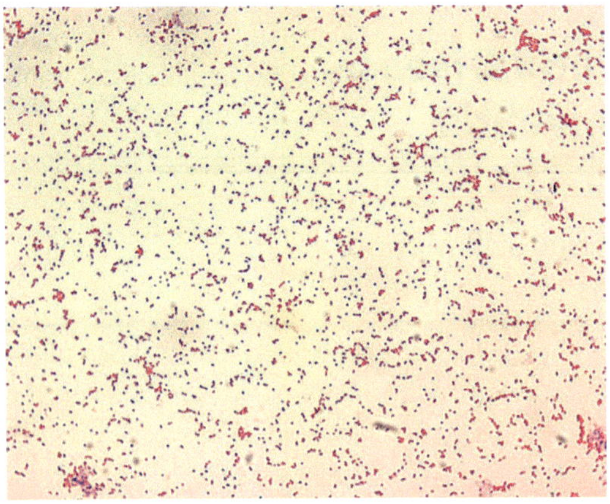

Fig. 39.1 This is an illustration of a photomicrograph of a culture sample, revealing the presence of numerous *Brucella melitensis* coccobacilli. (ID # 1901/Centers for Disease Control USA 2002/CDC/Courtesy of Larry Stauffer, Oregon State Public Health Laboratory; with permission CDC Public Health Image Library [6])

Table 39.1 Modes of human transmission [7]

Route of entry	Source material
Per oral[a]	Consumption of unpasteurized raw milk and other dairy products like butter, soft cheese, cream, and undercooked meat
Direct contact	Open wounds or mucous membrane exposed to secretions of infected animals and products like placenta, aborted tissue, soil contaminated with animal feces and dust contaminated with the microbe
Air borne	Inhalation of aerosolized materials contaminated with *Brucella*-like dust or in laboratories dealing with microorganisms
Vertical transmission	Intrauterine transmission, sexual transmission and through breast milk

[a]Sour milk, yogurt and hard cheese do not transmit disease due to fermentation by-products

Disease Transmission

The endemicity of brucellosis is because of many factors like prevalence of infection in animals, social and cultural preferences—food and milk habits, animal husbandry practices (regular domestic livestock screening and vaccination), etc. Animal handling is the commonest mode of human transmission [1, 2]. Certain occupations are at risk—slaughterhouse workers, employees of meat packing industries, veterinarians, and laboratory workers. The various modes of *Brucella* transmission are enumerated in Table 39.1.

Table 39.2 Presentation pertaining to the involved organ system

Organ system	Involvement, symptoms, and signs
General	Anorexia, myalgia, weight loss, abdominal pain, dyspepsia, headache
Central nervous system	Meningitis, meningo-encephalitis, neck stiffness, drowsiness, ataxia
Eye	Uveitis
Thyroid	Thyroiditis, abscess
Lung	Pneumonia
Abdomen	Hepatomegaly, splenomegaly
Genitourinary	Epididymo-orchitis, nephritis
Hematological involvement	Immune thrombocytopenic purpura, hemophagocytic syndrome

Clinical Presentation and Examination

Human beings are the accidental hosts portray variety of symptoms and signs when contracted with the infection. Childhood brucellosis is not uncommon and in endemic region about 11–56% of individuals affected by brucellosis are lesser than 14 years of age [5, 7].

Brucellosis in childhood has heterogeneous presentation and most often seen in acute and sub-acute forms with approximately 2–4 weeks of symptomatology. Fever is the most common presenting complaint, and the other most common accompaniments are malaise, arthralgia, and myalgia. Arthralgia is the commonest musculoskeletal manifestation followed by myalgia and arthritis [5, 8]. The heterogeneity of presentation results from the possibility of involvement of any organ system. The presentations pertaining to the involved organ systems are summarized in Table 39.2.

Based on endemicity and history, brucellosis must be kept as a differential in any child presenting with fever along with other constitutional symptoms like myalgia, arthralgia and joint swelling [9]. There are more chances that the child may present initially or be referred to an orthopedic surgeon as skeletal system involvement is the most common source of complaint and the frequency of skeletal involvement varies between 6.4% and 73.5% in the affected children [9]. An algorithm for suspecting brucellosis in a child is given below:

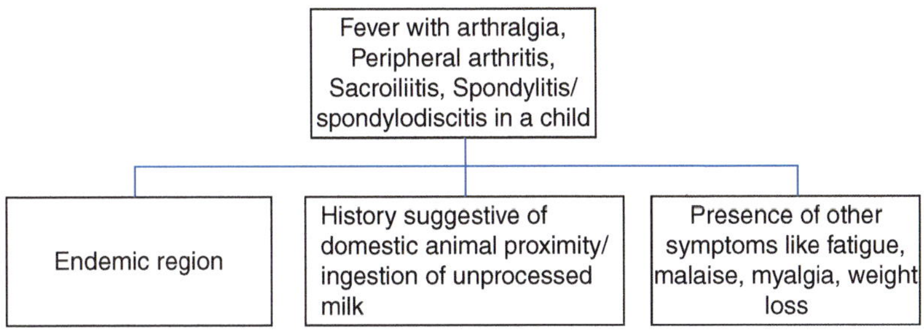

Appendicular Skeletal Involvement

Fever along with joint pain (mono-arthritis > polyarthritis) is the most common presenting complaint. The treating orthopedic surgeon must be aware that brucellosis can involve any of the organ system and must be vigilant for other signs and symptoms. Many a time the presentation is mistaken for septic arthritis and the condition is overlooked.

Ciftdogan DY et al. evaluated clinical and laboratory characteristics of childhood brucellosis with osteo-articular involvement (53/202) in the age group 1–18 years. The descending order of presentation is peripheral arthritis (monoarthritis > polyarthritis) followed by sacroiliitis, spondylitis, and rarely osteomyelitis (only in 1–2% of children) [4]. Peripheral joint involvement in children ranges from 13.6% to 50% and the most common joints involved are knee, hip, ankle, shoulder, wrist, elbow, sternoclavicular joint, and occasionally small joints of hand like proximal interphalangeal joint [9]. Brucella arthritis presents frequently as arthralgia (intermittent or migratory) with no movement restriction. Other uncommon manifestations are bursitis, teno-synovitis, etc. [10].

Axial Skeletal Involvement

In contrary to adults where sacroiliitis is the dominant form of skeletal involvement, it is not as common as peripheral arthritis in the pediatric population. Apart from one study by Geyik et al. [10] which showed frequency of sacroiliitis in children to be 48.7%, rest of the studies found it to be rare, between 4.8% and 8%. Similar to sacroiliitis, spondylitis and spondylodiscitis are also rare in children and are in the range of approximately 17%, and the lumbar region is the most common site of involvement followed by thoracic and cervical region. Back pain is the most common complaint in patients presenting with spinal brucellosis.

Apart from these manifestations rarely epidural abscesses are also seen and should be looked for in these children. Spinal brucellosis should be considered a differential for cases presenting with sciatica and back pain in the endemic region. Spondylodiscitis is the most severe form of skeletal involvement neurological sequelae may persist despite therapy. Also, contiguous and noncontiguous multifocal spinal involvement should be kept in mind and MRI is helpful in the evaluation and localization of the pathology [11].

Investigations/Workup

Vigilance and strong clinical suspicion are the main factors that help in diagnosing brucellosis. Apart from clinical findings, the diagnostic workup for brucellosis comprises the following investigations.

General Workup

Many a time the differential count is within normal limits, but few cases may show leucopenia, anemia, and thrombocytopenia alone or in combination. The erythrocyte sedimentation rate (ESR) might show modest raise and the liver function test may depict deranged transaminases and rarely hyperbilirubinemia.

Investigations Specific for the Diagnosis of Brucellosis

Culture Peripheral joint involvement can be septic with the microbe in the joint or reactive with absence of microbe in the joint. The gold standard investigation for diagnosing brucellosis is positive culture (blood, tissue, pus, bone marrow or body fluids like synovial fluid, pleural fluid, cerebrospinal fluid, etc.). But the yield is sub-optimal, and it reduces after the initial 2 weeks of illness. The current automated, non-radiometric BACTEC or BACT/ALERT culture techniques have shown faster and better yield with positive cultures occurring by 5–7 days of incubation instead of 4 weeks of incubation that was required by conventional methods.

Serological tests Due to the low yield of culture, the next dependable diagnostic investigations are the serological tests. They are the Rose Bengal slide agglutination test, standard agglutination test (SAT) and the antiglobulin or Coomb's test and are based on antibody reactivity against the smooth bacterial lipopolysaccharide.

Standard agglutination test (SAT) It is the commonly used serological diagnostic technique and a positive Brucella serology of 1: ≥160 with symptoms suggestive of brucellosis is diagnostic. In the absence of symptoms of active brucellosis, a titer of 1:320 or more is suggestive of presence of the infection.

The other serological investigations are 2-mercapto-ethanol (ME) test, ELISA, PCR, etc. ELISA is more sensitive in diagnosing brucellosis when compared to the traditional agglutination tests. PCR can be used for species isolation, bio-typing, and also in assessment of treatment efficiency. Remember that despite major joint involvement, serology may be negative and high index of suspicion is required to evaluate further in cases of strong suspicion.

Imaging

Radiography Changes appreciable on radiography develop late in the course of brucellosis and are extremely rare in peripheral arthritis. The changes described in sacroiliitis and spondylitis are commonly found in adults. In sacroiliitis, by 2–3 weeks, the subchondral osseous line gets blurred and becomes indistinct and the interosseous line and space can get narrowed or widened [10].

CT The role of CT again is limited. A CT-guided needle biopsy may be required to confirm the etiology microbiologically and by histopathological assessment.

MRI MRI is the best diagnostic modality to diagnose and localize spondylodiscitis and epidural abscess, cord, or nerve root compression. One of the pathognomonic findings of spondylodiscitis in MRI is destructive lesion at the antero-superior corner of vertebrae along with prominent osteosclerosis called the Pedro Pons' sign.

Radionuclide bone scan again helps in localizing and in differentiating brucellosis from tuberculosis. Increased uptake is seen in Brucellar spondylodiscitis and differentiates it from tubercular spondylodiscitis. Despite all these investigations, strong clinical suspicion is the primary tool that facilitates early diagnosis in these patients.

Differential Diagnoses

Brucellosis in childhood presents commonly as unilateral mono-arthritis and the differentials include septic arthritis, tubercular arthritis, monoarticular inflammatory arthropathy, etc. The commonest differential for spinal brucellosis is tubercular spondylitis and the pyogenic spondylodiscitis becomes another differential in case of associated disk involvement.

Management

Existing literature supports medical management with antibiotics administered in combination and the duration of treatment depends on the system involved [5]. The recommended duration of therapy with respect to skeletal brucellosis is 6 weeks or longer to avoid relapse and the regimen according to the age of child is given in Table 39.3. The preferred regimen is dual or triple drug regimen with an aminoglycoside (streptomycin or gentamycin) given for the first 1 or 2 weeks.

Usually, the child shows improvement within a week and if not, sensitivity to drugs should be checked. Prolonged therapy or surgery is rarely indicated in conditions like deep-seated chronic infections like osteomyelitis refractory to medical management or in case of spondylitis or spondylodiscitis with epidural abscess causing neural compromise. But fortunately, the incidence of these complications is extremely rare in children.

Table 39.3 Medical management of skeletal brucellosis

Age	Management
Children less than 8 years old	Rifampicin[a] and (sulfamethoxazole + trimethoprim)[b] or Rifampicin alone for a period of 45 days along with gentamycin[c] for a period of 7 days
Children more than or equal to 8 years old	Doxycycline[d] and rifampicin or Doxycycline for 45 days along with streptomycin[e] for 14 days/ Doxycycline for 45 days and gentamicin for 7 days

Key: (a) 20 mg/kg/day in two divided doses (max—600 mg), (b) 10 mg of trimethoprim/kg/day (max—480 mg), (c) 5–7.5 mg/kg/day as IM or IV in single dose, (d) 5 mg/kg/day in two divided doses (max—200 mg, only in children 8 years and above), (e) 15 mg/kg IM or IV once a day (max—1 g/day, only in children 8 years and above). (Monitoring for the complications associated with the above antibiotics is advised.)

Complications

Brucellosis in children produces mild-to-moderate disease and rarely persists to chronic forms. Longstanding spinal brucellosis may result in unresolving neurological deficit. Chronic brucellosis results from persistent deep foci and one of the examples is suppurative lesions of the bone [8].

Box 39.1: Brucellosis

- Brucellosis is not restricted to endemic regions and is an emerging global zoonosis.
- Varied clinical presentation leads to overlooking of the infection.
- Incidence quoted is less due to underreporting.

- Childhood brucellosis comprises 50% of affected individuals.
- Musculo-skeletal system complaints are the main reason which brings the child to the hospital.
- Mono-arthritis is the commonest presentation.

- Vigilance and strong clinical suspicion lead to diagnosis.
- Medical management is primary treatment.
- Surgery reserved for epidural abscesses, refractory osteomyelitis.

Hydatid Disease

Introduction and Epidemiology

Hydatid disease is a zoonosis resulting from the tapeworm (*Echinococcus* species) and is endemic in regions where sheep and cattle livestock are raised in proximity with dogs. Like brucellosis hydatid disease is also an emerging global public health concern with significant morbidity and mortality and is not restricted to endemic areas only. The countries labeled as endemic for hydatidosis are Australia, Africa, Latin America and Middle East. It is a parasitic infestation and human beings are the accidental intermediate hosts. The most commonly encountered species is *Echinococcus granulosus* while others are rare (*E. multilocularis* and *E. vogeli*) [12]. Skeletal hydatidosis is exceedingly rare and consists of 0.5–4% of the total cases reported [13].

Microbiology The larval stage of *E. granulosus* and *E. multilocularis* causes cystic hydatid disease and alveolar hydatid disease respectively [14]. Primary extrahepatic localization of metacestodes of *E. multilocularis* is extremely rare and is not dealt with in this chapter as childhood skeletal involvement is exceedingly rare [15] (Fig. 39.2).

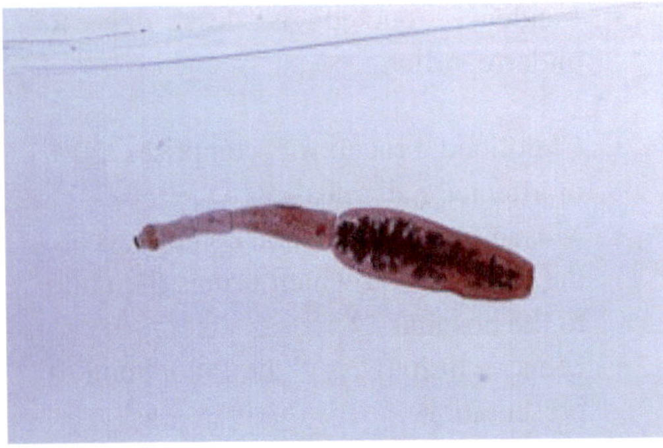

Fig. 39.2 This photomicrograph reveals some of the ultrastructural morphology exhibited by an adult dog tapeworm, *Echinococcus granulosus*, which had been found in a canine. *Echinococcus granulosus* causes what is known as cystic echinococcosis in dogs and other canids. Note the worm's head is on the left, exhibiting its scolex, with its hook-rimmed rostellum. (ID # 11020/ Center for Disease Control USA 1975/Courtesy CDC -Dr. Peter M. Schantz; with permission CDC Public Health Image Library)

Pathogenesis

The definitive hosts for the parasite are dogs, foxes, and other carnivores. The adult tapeworm harbors in the small intestine of these animals and releases eggs. They are excreted by the definitive hosts which are ingested by intermediate hosts commonly sheep (natural intermediate host) while grazing contaminated ground or ingesting contaminated water. Human beings play the role of an accidental intermediate host and get infestation either by close contact with definitive hosts (dogs) or consumption of contaminated food and water. Primary skeletal hydatidosis occurs when the blood borne scolex passes through the hepatic and pulmonary filters and settles in bone [13] (Fig. 39.3).

Childhood Hydatidosis

The lesions are silent without symptoms for decades and are rarely diagnosed in childhood. The disease is usually contracted in childhood and adolescence but presents in adults [12]. Bloomfield reported 55 patients with hydatidosis under the age of 20 years (2 osseous disease) and the disease was more common in boys. According to him, children are at higher risk contracting the disease due to their proximity to floor and lack of knowledge on simple hygiene [16]. Also, the involvement of both male and female is equal in adults, whereas childhood hydatidosis predominantly involves boys. The predominance in boys is said to be because of the differences in behavior and more outdoor activities in boys. Children of all age group are susceptible and there are reports involving infants as young as 6 months of age [12].

Childhood hydatidosis differs from adults by predominant lung involvement, whereas liver is the most common site where the larval forms localize in adults. The reason for predominant pulmonary involvement is the less dense nature of the hepatic tissue in children.

Skeletal Hydatidosis

Liver and lung functions as the primary and secondary capillary filters and other system involve-

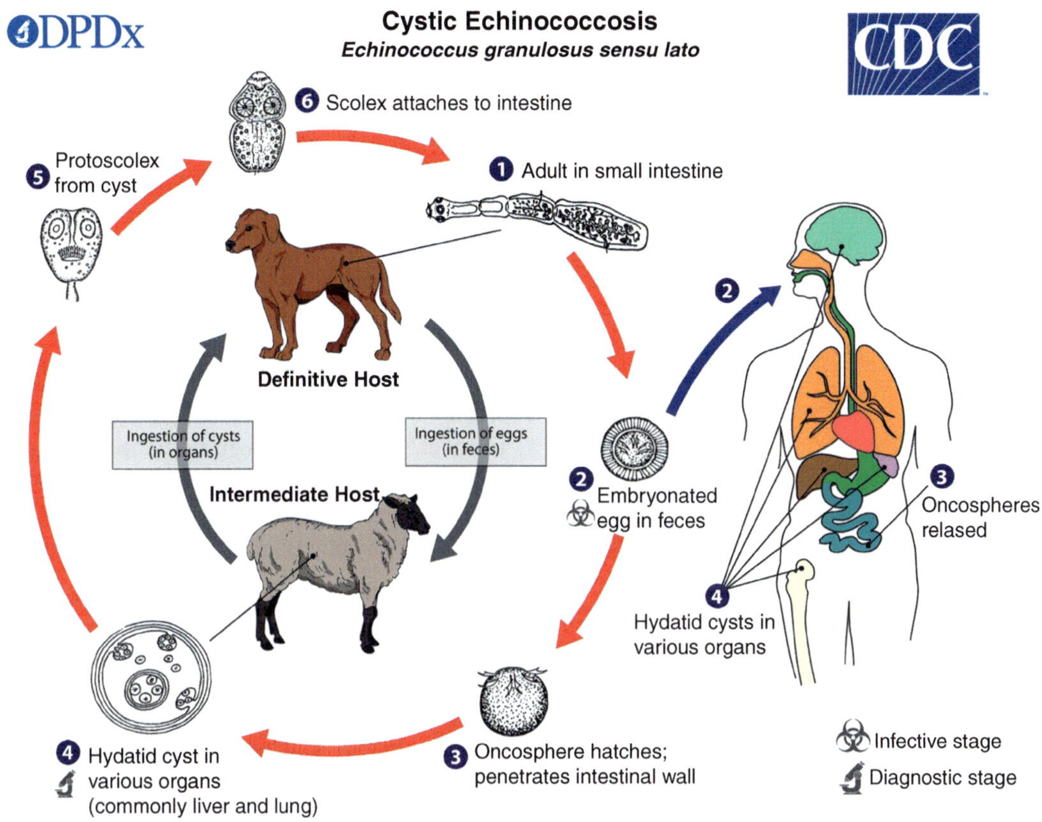

Fig. 39.3 Life cycle of *Echinococcus granulosus*. (Courtesy https://www.cdc.gov/dpdx/echinococcosis/index.html, accessed 22nd August 2021)

ment are exceedingly rare, to the extent of 15% and musculoskeletal system is affected in only 1–4% of cases [17]. The lesions found in the musculoskeletal tissue are usually because of hematogenous spread and not continuum from visceral infections. Skeletal hydatidosis is rare and is chronic in nature commonly presenting as cystic lesions of the bone. It must be kept as a differential diagnosis in endemic regions and even in region, which is not endemic; a high index of suspicion is warranted [16].

Merkle EM reported eight cases of musculoskeletal cystic echinococcosis and one of them is a 10-year-old girl with right frontal bone involvement. In general, skeletal hydatidosis commonly involves spine (thoracic) followed by pelvis, femur, tibia, ribs, skull, scapula, humerus, and fibula. According to von Sinner, spine, pelvis, and hip joint comprise 60% of osseous hydatid cysts, 28% occurring in long bones and rest involving ribs, scapula, and skull [14, 18].

Pathology

Cysts that develop in muscles are solitary with well-defined adventitia, whereas those that develop in bones are multiple without detectable adventitia. The reason proposed is that cyst in muscle expands in soft tissue planes peripherally displacing the adjacent muscle fibers resulting in development of adventitia of the cyst. Bone being a rigid structure does not facilitate expansion like muscle tissue. So, expansion results in rupture of the laminated membrane resulting in formation of new cysts. This results in multiplicity of cysts in skeletal disease [17]. Due to absence of pericyst formation in bone, the cyst proliferates aggressively along the line of least resistance (bone canals) in an irregular branching fashion and spreads to surrounding tissues as the cortex gets destroyed.

Also, the growth in rigid skeletal tissue is slow and rarely exceeds 2 cm in diameter. Bone lesions and deformations are due to the following reasons: (1) expansion and compression of surrounding tissues mechanically, (2) obstruction of nutrient vessels resulting in ischemia, and (3) proliferation of resorptive osteoclasts around the compressed skeletal tissue [19]. Untreated cyst may undergo calcification and spontaneous death in few cases. But majority of them progressively enlarges in size and becomes symptomatic. Multiorgan system involvement is rare in children in comparison to adults [12].

Clinical Features

The lesions are asymptomatic and go unnoticed for a longer period making their diagnosis in childhood extremely rare. This is because of absence of reactive inflammation from bone. As is said for brucellosis, any organ system can be involved by hydatidosis, and the symptoms vary according to the organ system involved. The symptoms are not specific and clinical attention is sought for complications that occur. The possible presenting complaints are pain, deformity, pathological fracture, and swelling/lump in case of muscular involvement or extraosseous expansion. These lumps can be mistaken as tumor or abscess with inadvertent drainage and risk of dissemination.

The lesions in long bones and vertebra can result in pathological fractures. Expanding cysts may infect the surrounding tissue or can lead to pressure effects on the adjacent structures. Spinal involvement results in back pain and neurological deficit depending upon the extent of involvement.

Initially pain associated with the lesion is intermittent and becomes continuous and severe at the later stage of the disease. Tumefaction might be seen in long-standing lesions. Pelvic lesions might expand within or outside the pelvis and causes compressive symptoms on the adjacent structures. Papanikolaou describes it as cold migratory abscess without a fistula which turns hot if infected [14].

Investigations

Many a times, diagnosis is made intraoperatively based on morphology of the specimen unless otherwise a high index of suspicion is maintained [14] (Fig. 39.4).

Radiography

The radiographic appearance is of a single or multiple expansile irregular cystic destructive lesions and as earlier described is frequently multilocular. The lesions might be trabeculated and periosteal reaction denotes pathological fracture. Extraosseous expansion after a cortical breach is visualized as soft tissue mass with calcification [13]. It is repeatedly emphasized that radiographic picture is not characteristic, and diagnosis is delayed unless strong clinical suspicion exists. The long bone lesion, although can occur anywhere between epiphysis and diaphysis, usually starts in the metaphysis and gradually spreads creating an inflated appearance but commonly spares the overall morphology and articular surface integrity [13].

Spinal picture is not specific and usually is irregular destruction of the vertebral body with disk space narrowing. The index lesion starts in

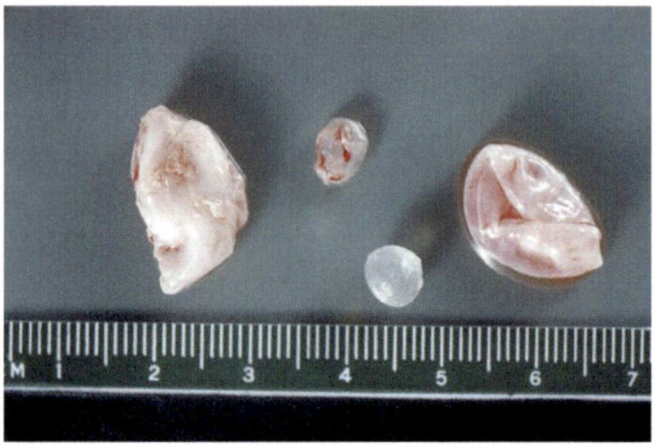

Fig. 39.4 This gross pathology specimen consists of the hyaline membrane or ectocyst of a halved *Echinococcus* sp. hydatid cyst and two hydatid daughter cysts contained inside. This specimen was harvested from a human lung. (ID # 349/Center for Disease Control USA 1961/Courtesy CDC/ Dr. I. Kagan; with permission CDC Public Health Image Library)

the vertebral body or very rarely in the posterior arch and gradually spreads to all vertebral structures, vertebral canal, ribs, adjacent vertebra, etc. The lesion in body gives a "bunch of grapes" appearance.

Suspicion of skeletal lesion calls for an abdominal ultrasonography and chest radiography to identify liver and lung lesions if any. Up to 45% of patients with osseous disease might have a liver or lung lesion which should be looked for [13].

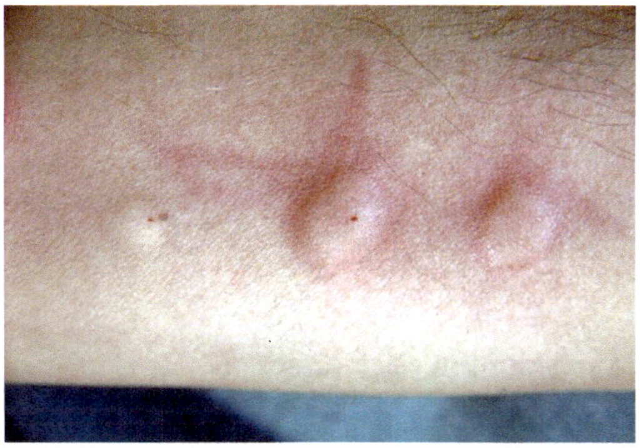

Fig. 39.5 This photograph shows you the clinical appearance of a male patient's arm, which reveals a positive Casoni skin test for hydatid disease, also referred to as cystic echinococcosis (CE). The test is carried out by injecting a tiny amount of sterilized fluid, created from *Echinococcus granulosus* hydatid cysts, into the recipient's forearm, using a subcutaneous technique. (ID # 347 / Center for Disease Control USA 1961/Courtesy CDC/ Dr. I. Kagan; with permission CDC Public Health Image Library)

Computerized Tomography (CT Scans)

They are again not specific and the characteristic finding is the round/oval space-occupying lesion. They help in better visualization of spinal elements and the extent of the lesion which are difficult to appreciate in a radiograph and can guide when aspiration is attempted [13].

Magnetic Resonance Imaging (MRI)

MRI is a better diagnostic modality and shows the following characteristics. The lesions are typically multilocular and both parent and daughter cysts are of high signal intensity in T2-weighted sequence. The appearance resembles a rose or a wheel because of spaces or septi of the daughter cyst. MRI also provides added information on the soft tissue structures including vertebral axis of the spinal canal on the vicinity and the characteristic extent of the lesion. MRH (magnetic resonance hydrography) is another investigation that gives information on the number of daughter cysts and the extent of the disease. MRI is also of particular help in evaluating recurrences [13].

Serological Investigations

The diagnostic tests based on serology can be classified into three categories, viz. detection of circulating antigen (in the cystic fluid and its components), immune complexes, and circulating antibodies in serum. Individually none of them are satisfactory alone in clinching the diagnosis. As a result, multiple tests are to be used together for definitive yield. The antibody detection tests are Casoni test, indirect hemagglutination (IHA), counter-immuno-electrophoresis (CIE), ELISA, and gold labeled antibody test. ELISA being highly sensitive and relatively specific is the commonly used confirmatory test when used alone (Fig. 39.5).

Serological tests are commonly used for screening, follow up after surgery and to assess response to medical therapy and its discontinuation. One more peculiar feature of skeletal lesion is absence of pericyst which leads to more host parasite interaction resulting in higher levels of circulating antigen. Few authors are of the opinion that diagnostic aspiration should be contraindicated for the fear of spillage, anaphylaxis, and dissemination [13, 14].

Differential Diagnoses

Spinal disease might be mistaken for tuberculous spondylitis or a primary neoplasm although the latter is extremely rare in children. Extremity lesion might resemble aneurysmal bone cyst, solitary cyst, fibrocystic disease, osteoclastoma, neurofibromatosis, chondromyxoid fibroma, tuberculosis, osteomyelitis, and at times malignancies like lymphoma, plasmacytoma, and chondrosarcoma [13].

Management

The disease is usually diagnosed at an advanced stage due to the absence of symptoms and hence treatment is difficult and complete eradication might be difficult resulting in more chances of recurrences [13].

The management evolved from injection of scolicidal agents (formalin, hypertonic saline, and 0.5% silver nitrate) with the aim of chemical sterilization. But injections alone were not successful as most of the scolicidal agents are not effective in eliminating microscopic daughter cysts and thereby recurrences. The percutaneous PAIR (puncture, aspiration, injection, and re-aspiration) technique is not frequently used as the skeletal disease is usually multilocular and not effective in disease eradication. Irrigation with scolicidal agents is not without complications. Hypertonic saline might lead to massive tissue necrosis.

Conservative surgical techniques like curettage alone carry the risk of anaphylaxis and contamination of surrounding tissues and nearly 80% recurrence. The absence of adventitia/pericyst formation makes it difficult to demarcate normal tissues from the lesion thereby making excision difficult, which increases chances of recurrences if radical surgery is not performed [14]. Few authors have claimed success with partial cystectomy and drainage in muscular disease, although complete removal is aimed for to prevent recurrences. The aim of managing a skeletal hydatid disease is wide resection (removal of cyst and 1–2 cm of healthy appearing surrounding bone), [20] filling bone defect with bone grafts/bone cement/or replacement with prosthesis under anti-helminthic cover. The wide resection aims in prevention of recurrences.

Pelvic and extremity lesions are managed by wide resection which may at times be even amputation. Complete eradication is difficult in areas where accessibility is an issue like pelvis and the surgical morbidity and chances of recurrence are more [13]. The complications following resection of long-standing extensive lesions are infection, creation of large bone defect, and recurrences which increase long-standing morbidity and are to be managed accordingly [13].

Spinal disease is managed by a combined anterior and posterior approach. The combination of anterior corpectomy and fusion with bone graft removes the diseased anterior segment followed by removal of involved posterior elements and fusion with instrumentation. However, the mean delay in diagnosing spinal disease is 6 months more than other regions and many of them present with neurological deficit. So, the results are poor with more than 50% developing early or late complications which include persistence of neurological deficit. These patients also require repeated procedures which may be as high as four per patient [14].

Musculoskeletal lesions occur in isolation and rarely with concomitant lesions in lungs and liver or other areas. The adjacent soft tissues show cystic changes and morphologically resemble an abscess. Out of the eight cases reported by Merkle, two had concomitant musculoskeletal and hepatic lesions [21]. Concomitant lesions of liver and lungs have therapeutic importance as isolated musculoskeletal lesions can be subjected to curative surgical excision. Surgical excision is the primary management modality for isolated lesions of the musculoskeletal system. If there are multiple foci, the twofold procedure to eradicate all infestation foci must be attempted [22–24].

Chemotherapy

In confirmed cases preoperative adjuvant chemotherapy can be given. Chemotherapy plays a role in local control, prevention of systemic spread, and recurrence when administered in the postoperative period [13]. Benzimidazole derivatives namely mebendazole and albendazole are used for management of human hydatid disease. Albendazole has the advantage of better absorption and achieves higher concentration of active metabolite in blood and the cyst fluid. The bioavailability of albendazole significantly improves when it is combined with drugs like praziquantel (25 mg/kg), cimetidine.

Albendazole (15 mg/kg) daily for 4 weeks followed by a 2-week interval constitutes one course of drug therapy. One course is given preoperatively in confirmed cases followed by six or more courses postoperatively, while few recommend continuous therapy without interruption for osseous hydatidosis. The duration is decided by serological tests and radiological assessment. A treatment period of 2 years may be needed and in certain inoperable cases the treatment might go on lifelong to limit the cystic growth. Medical therapy alone is not preferred for skeletal lesions as the results are not encouraging when given alone [14].

Box 39.2: Skeletal Hydatid Disease

- Diagnosed rarely in childhood.
- Lesions asymptomatic for longer duration.
- Spine followed by hip region is commonly affected.
- Skeletal lesions are multiple/multilocular.
- Skeletal lesions do not have peri cyst/adventitia.
- Muscular lesions have pericyst formation.
- Wide resection with 2 cm margin of normal tissue advocated.
- Anthelminthic cover can be started preoperatively and continued postoperatively.
- Recurrences common due to microscopic daughter cysts.

Viral Musculoskeletal Infection in Children

Musculoskeletal manifestations are typically not the primary presenting feature of viral infections [25]. Common musculoskeletal features of viral infection include arthralgia, arthritis, myalgia, myositis, and tenosynovitis. The commonest viral musculoskeletal infection of significance in children includes viral arthritis and viral myositis [26].

Viral infections are highly transmissible and even have the propensity to become epidemics [27]. The emergence of new human viruses is continuous biological process [28]. The exact prevalence and incidence rates of viral arthritis are not available owing to seasonal and geographic disparity, variations in the causative virus, and the self-limiting nature of the disease. The incidence of certain viral arthritides like those associated with mumps, measles, and rubella has reduced owing to routine immunization [29]. On the other hand, epidemics of virus-related arthritis, especially vector transmitted like chikungunya, dengue, are increasingly being recognized [30].

Microbiology

Many viruses have the ability to cause arthritis; however, the arthritogenic potential of different viruses varies greatly [31]. Viral pathogens commonly implicated in children include rubella, parvovirus B19, arboviruses, and hepatitis B. Other viral pathogens less commonly associated with arthritis are coxsackie, Epstein-Barr, herpes simplex, varicella-zoster, and mumps virus [32]. Current evidence suggests that in children, the SARS Cov2 virus is not arthritogenic [33].

Pathogenesis

The mechanisms by which viruses cause arthritis are diverse and still not precisely defined. Viral arthritis results from one of the following pathomechanisms: [34]

- Direct viral infection of the synovial cells
- Immune response to the viral antigen—both humoral and cellular
- Autoimmune processes—by immune complex formation.

Clinical Manifestations

Most viral arthritis present as an acute self-limiting, transient arthropathy, usually lasting a few weeks. Fever, rash, or malaise may precede or accompany the joint symptoms. Transient arthritis has been reported following viral vaccinations [35]. Viral arthritis may occasionally become prolonged or chronic [30]. Both Rubella and Parvovirus B19 infection affect adolescents but are rare in young children. No particular pattern of joint affliction has been identified. An asymmetric pattern involving both small and large joints is seen in rubella. In young children, a transient, symmetric, arthritis involving the small joints is seen with hepatitis B [36]. Chikungunya virus infection has biphasic presentation, an initial period lasting 1–6 days with fever, nausea, vomiting, and intense pain in one or more joints. The second phase of illness follows an afebrile interval and is characterized by pharyngitis, rash, lymphadenopathy, and persistent arthritis [30].

Investigations

Many arthritides are presumed to be viral in origin by virtue of their clinical presentation, epidemiology, or by exclusion. Confirmatory diagnosis of viral arthritis is not always done due to their self-limiting nature. Serology shows an initial IgM response followed by an increasing IgG response, 2–3 weeks later. Synovial fluid analysis of the afflicted joint is nonspecific. Methods for directly isolating viral organisms are limited and demonstrating the causal relationship of joint symptoms to other clinical features is often difficult to establish.

Differentials

Inflammatory arthritis and other postinfectious (reactive) arthritis may mimic the presentation of viral arthritis. Low-titer autoantibodies, such as rheumatoid factor and antinuclear antibody, can occur in acute viral arthritis.

Treatment

Viral arthritides are generally, but not always self-limiting and antiviral treatment is rarely required. As viral arthritides are self-limiting the treatment is usually no more than a few days of NSAID treatment, combined with rest and other symptomatic measures.

Viral Myositis

This disorder has also been termed as benign acute childhood myositis, *influenza-associated myositis, or acute myositis* [26]. Children usually between 5 and 10 years of age complain of severe calf pain following a prodromal viral illness. An elevated creatine phosphokinase (CPK) level is common finding. The disease is mild and usually resolves within 2–4 days [37].

References

1. WHO Corbel, M. J, Food and Agriculture Organization of the United Nations, World Health Organization & World Organization for Animal Health. 2006. Brucellosis in humans and animals. World Health Organization. https://apps.who.int/iris/handle/10665/43597.
2. Mantur BG, Akki AS, Mangalgi SS, Patil SV, Gobbur RH, Peerapur BV. Childhood brucellosis--a microbiological, epidemiological and clinical study. J Trop Pediatr. 2004;50:153–7. https://doi.org/10.1093/tropej/50.3.153.
3. Pappas G, Papadimitriou P, Akritidis N, Christou L, Tsianos EV. The new global map of human brucel-

losis. Lancet Infect Dis. 2006;6:91–9. https://doi.org/10.1016/S1473-3099(06)70382-6.
4. Çiftdoğan DY, Aslan S. Osteoarticular involvement of brucellosis in pediatric patients: clinical and laboratory characteristics. Turk J Pediatr. 2020;62:199–207. https://doi.org/10.24953/turkjped.2020.02.005.
5. Bukhari EE. Pediatric brucellosis. An update review for the new millennium. Saudi Med J. 2018;39:336–41. https://doi.org/10.15537/smj.2018.4.21896.
6. https://www.cdc.gov/brucellosis/index.html. Accessed 8th Aug 2021.
7. Al Shaalan M, Memish ZA, Al Mahmoud S, Alomari A, Khan MY, Almuneef M, et al. Brucellosis in children: clinical observations in 115 cases. Int J Infec Dis. 2002;6:182–6.
8. Zaks N, Sukenik S, Alkan M, Flusser D, Neumann L, Buskila D. Musculoskeletal manifestations of brucellosis: a study of 90 cases in Israel. Semin Arthritis Rheum. 1995;25:97–102. https://doi.org/10.1016/s0049-0172(95)80022-0.
9. Dashti AS, Karimi A. Skeletal involvement of Brucella melitensis in children: a systematic review. Iran J Med Sci. 2013;38:286–92.
10. Geyik MF, Gür A, Nas K, Cevik R, Sarac J, Dikici B, et al. Musculoskeletal involvement of brucellosis in different age groups: a study of 195 cases. Swiss Med Wkly. 2002;132:98–105.
11. Esmaeilnejad-Ganji SM, Esmaeilnejad-Ganji SMR. Osteoarticular manifestations of human brucellosis: A review. World J Orthop. 2019;10(2):54–62. Published 2019 Feb 18. https://doi.org/10.5312/wjo.v10.i2.54.
12. Jairajpuri ZS, Jetley S, Hassan MJ, Hussain M. Hydatid disease in childhood: revisited report of an interesting case. J Parasit Dis. 2012;36:265–8.
13. Song XH, Ding LW, Wen H. Bone hydatid disease. Postgrad Med J. 2007;83(982):536–42. https://doi.org/10.1136/pgmj.2007.057166.
14. Papanikolaou A. Osseous hydatid disease. Trans R Soc Trop Med Hyg. 2008;102(3):233–8. https://doi.org/10.1016/j.trstmh.2007.09.012. Epub 2007 Nov 9
15. Guidelines for treatment of cystic and alveolar echinococcosis in humans. WHO Informal Working Group on Echinococcosis. Bull World Health Organ. 1996;74(3):231–42. PMID: 8789923; PMCID: PMC2486920.
16. Bloomfield JA. Hydatid disease in children and adolescents. Aust Radiol. 1980;24:277–83.
17. Ammari FF, Khasawneh Z, Salem MK, Mesmar M, Omari H, Masa'deh R. Hydatid disease of the musculoskeletal system. Surgery. 1998;124(5):934–7.
18. von Sinner WN. New diagnostic signs in hydatid disease; radiography, ultrasound, CT and MRI correlated to pathology. Eur J Radiol. 1991;12:150–9.
19. Zlitni M, Ezzaouia K, Lebib H, Karray M, Kooli M, Mestiri M. Hydatid cyst of bone: diagnosis and treatment. World J Surg. 2001;25:75–82.
20. Herrera A, Martinez AA, Rodriguez J. Spinal hydatidosis. Spine. 2005;30:2439–44.
21. Merkle EM, Schulte M, Vogel J, Tomczak R, Rieber A, Kern P, Goerich J, Brambs HJ, Sokiranski R. Musculoskeletal involvement in cystic echinococcosis: report of eight cases and review of the literature. AJR Am J Roentgenol. 1997;168:1531–4. https://doi.org/10.2214/ajr.168.6.9168719.
22. Inayat F, Azam S, Baig AS, Nawaz G, Ullah W. Presentation patterns, diagnostic modalities, management strategies, and clinical outcomes in patients with hydatid disease of the pelvic bone: a comparative review of 31 cases. Cureus. 2019;11(3):e4178.
23. Sioutis S, Reppas L, Bekos A, Soulioti E, Saranteas T, Koulalis D, Sapkas G, Mavrogenis AF. Echinococcosis of the spine. EFORT Open Rev. 2021;6(4):288–96.
24. Cattaneo L, Manciulli T, Cretu CM, Giordani MT, Angheben A, Bartoloni A, Zammarchi L, Bartalesi F, Richter J, Chiodini P, Godbole G, Junghanss T, Stojkovic M, Sammarchi L, Dore R, Vercelli A, Benazzo F, Cuzzocrea F, Tamarozzi F, Brunetti E. Cystic echinococcosis of the bone: a European multicenter study. Am J Trop Med Hyg. 2019;100(3):617–21.
25. Franssila R, Hedman K. Infection and musculoskeletal conditions: viral causes of arthritis. Best Pract Res Clin Rheumatol. 2006;20:1139–57. https://doi.org/10.1016/j.berh.2006.08.007.
26. Magee H, Goldman RD. Viral myositis in children. Can Fam Physician. 2017;63:365–8. PMID: 28500193; PMCID: PMC5429052.
27. Wolfe ND, Dunavan CP, Diamond J. Origins of major human infectious diseases. Nature. 2007;447:279–83. https://doi.org/10.1038/nature05775.
28. Woolhouse M, Scott F, Hudson Z, Howey R, Chase-Topping M. Human viruses: discovery and emergence. Philos Trans R Soc Lond Ser B Biol Sci. 2012;367:2864–71. https://doi.org/10.1098/rstb.2011.0354.
29. Tingle AJ, Allen M, Petty RE, Kettyls GD, Chantler JK. Rubella-associated arthritis. I. Comparative study of joint manifestations associated with natural rubella infection and RA 27/3 rubella immunisation. Ann Rheum Dis. 1986;45:110–4.
30. Nicole R, Markus H, Patrick G. Chikungunya in children. Pediatr Infect Dis J. 2015;34:789–91. https://doi.org/10.1097/INF.0000000000000716.
31. Lund KD, Chantler JK. Mapping of genetic determinants of rubella virus associated with growth in joint tissue. J Virol. 2000;74:796e804.
32. John J, Chandran L. Arthritis in children and adolescents. Pediatr Rev. 2011;32:470–80. https://doi.org/10.1542/pir.32-11-470.
33. Pousa PA, Mendonça TSC, Oliveira EA, Simões-E-Silva AC. Extrapulmonary manifestations of COVID-19 in children: a comprehensive review and pathophysiological considerations. J Pediatr

(Rio J). 2021;97:116–39. https://doi.org/10.1016/j.jped.2020.08.007. PMCID: PMC7508521.
34. Günther F, Fleck M, Bach B. Virusassoziierte Arthritiden [Virus-associated arthritis]. Z Rheumatol. 2017;76:693–704. German. https://doi.org/10.1007/s00393-017-0376-3.
35. Toussirot É, Bereau M. Vaccination and induction of autoimmune diseases. Inflamm Allergy Drug Targets. 2015;14:94–8. https://doi.org/10.2174/1871528114666160105113046.
36. Kappus MR, Sterling RK. Extrahepatic manifestations of acute hepatitis B virus infection. Gastroenterol Hepatol (N Y). 2013;9:123–6.
37. Tippett E, Clark R. Benign acute childhood myositis following human parainfluenza virus type-1 infection. Emerg Med Australas. 2013;25:248–51. https://doi.org/10.1111/1742-6723.12064. Epub 2013 Apr 8

Index

A
Acquired immune deficiency syndrome (AIDS), 302
Acute bone infections, 142
Acute flaccid myelitis, 687, 688
Acute hematogenous osteomyelitis (AHO), 134, 144, 152–154, 159, 201, 392
combined medical and surgical management, 25–26
complications, 199
differential diagnoses, 196–197
duration of therapy, 23–24
empiric therapy, 21–23
epidemiology, 191–192
imaging, 194
initial laboratory evaluation, 194
microbiology, 192–194
pathogen-specific agents, 22
pathology, 192–194
pattern recognition, 195
transition to oral therapy, 24–25
treatment options, 197–199
Acute MSK infection, 172
Acute osteomyelitis, 167
Acute-phase response (APR), 38, 95, 96, 413
Acute respiratory distress syndrome (ARDS), 39
Aminoglycosides, 137
Amputation, 753, 755
Antibiotic-loaded bone cement (ALBC), 137, 142
Antibiotics, 176
Antibiotic therapy, 160–161
Antifungal-impregnated polymethyl methacrylate (PMMA), 719
Antimicrobial agents, 23
Antimicrobial therapy, 18, 24–26, 28, 30, 120, 128, 133, 136, 197, 310, 326, 392, 487, 707, 754, 776
Antimicrobial treatment, 133, 197
Antistaphylococcal therapy, 24
Anti-tuberculous treatment (ATT)
first line drugs, 649
second line drugs, 649, 650
Arthrocentesis, 211–212
Aspergillosis, 724–726
Aspergillus spp., 136
Athlete's foot, 603, 604
Autogenous bone graft, 181
Autoinflammatory disorders, 372
Avascular necrosis (AVN), 41, 412, 486

B
Bacillus Calmette-Guérin (BCG) vaccine, 663, 668–671
BACTEC Mycobacteria Growth Indicator Tube (MGIT) cultures, 646
Bacterial hijacking, 40
Bacterial myositis, 29
Bioabsorbable ceramics, 137–140
Biofilms, 133–136
Bisphosphonates, 379
Blastomyces, 12, 30
Blastomycosis, 687, 732
Bone defects, 520
Bone gap, 512, 514, 515, 543
clinical presentation, 544
Ilizarov transport, 553
investigations, 545
ongoing sepsis, 545
osteomyelitis, 543
vascularised contralateral fibula transfer, 555
vascularised ipsilateral fibula transfer, 553
work-up, 545
Bone marrow biopsy, 78
Bone repermeabilization, 568
Bone scan, 64
Bone transport, 334
Borrelia burgdorferi, 206
Boston Children's septic arthritis, 157
Brodie's abscess, 19, 52, 141

© Springer Nature Switzerland AG 2022
M. V. Belthur et al. (eds.), *Pediatric Musculoskeletal Infections*,
https://doi.org/10.1007/978-3-030-95794-0

Brucellosis
  appendicular skeletal involvement, 797
  axial skeletal involvement, 797
  clinical presentation and examination, 796
  complications, 799
  differential diagnosis, 799
  disease transmission, 796
  epidemiology, 795
  imaging, 798, 799
  investigations, 798
  management, 799
  microbiology, 795, 796
  workup, 798
Bypass grafting, 334

C
Calcium phosphates, 137
Calcium sulfates (CS), 137
Candida osteomyelitis (OM), 718–722
Candida spp., 30, 136
Capital femoral epiphysis (CFE), 462
Carpal tunnel syndrome, 662
Cellulitis, 597
Center for Disease Control (CDC), 281
Cephalexin, 25
Cervical spinal tuberculosis, 636, 651
Cervicodorsal tuberculosis, 651
Charcot neuropathic arthropathy, 89
Chemotherapy agents, 81
Children, 543, 547
Chondroblastoma, 580
Chondromyxoid fibroma, 580
Chronic granulomatous disease (CGD), 717
Chronic hematogenous osteomyelitis (CHOM), 322, 324, 328
  adjunctive therapies, 335
  classification, 323, 324
  clinical presentations, 323
  complications, 335
  epidemiology, 322
  etiology, 322
  focal bone loss, 331
  imaging studies, 325
  laboratory investigations, 325
  pathogenesis, 322, 323
  segmental bone defects, 331, 333
  soft tissue defects, 335
  tissue sampling, 326
  treatment, 326–329
Chronic left anterolateral hip pain, 86
Chronic noninfectious/nonbacterial osteitis (CNO), 69, 73, 76, 77
  autoinflammatory bone disorder, 371
  bone biopsy, 378
  choice of imaging, 375, 377
  clinical presentation, 373
  complications, 380
  differential diagnoses, 373, 374
  investigations, 374
  microbiology, 372
  monitoring response, 379
  treatment, 378, 379
Chronic/neglected MSK infections, 172, 173
Chronic osteomyelitis (CO), 19–20, 56–58, 63, 134, 142, 199, 385, 512, 514, 521, 543, 544, 546
Chronic pediatric diseases, 276
Chronic posttraumatic osteomyelitis, 339, 351
  classification, 341
  clinical presentation, 341
  complications, 357
  epidemiology, 340
  etiology, 340
  imaging studies, 342, 345, 346, 350
  laboratory investigations, 342
  pathogenesis, 340, 341
  prevention, 357
  tissue sampling, 351
  treatment, 351, 353, 355–357
Chronic recurrent multifocal osteomyelitis (CRMO), 73
Clindamycin, 25
Clostridium difficile colitis, 297
Coccidioides, 12, 30
Coccidioidomycosis, 726–728, 731
Community-acquired methicillin-resistant *Staphylococcus aureus* (CA-MRSA), 18, 97, 384
Complete blood cell count (CBC), 158, 240
Complete physiodesis, 557
Complicated osteomyelitis, 174
Continuous ECG monitoring, 117
Continuous renal replacement therapy (CRRT), 124
Conventional bone grafting, 331
Cortical sclerosis, 56
Corticosteroids, 379
Cost-effective analysis (CEA), 6
C-reactive protein (CRP), 43, 74, 117, 142, 158, 194, 209, 255, 288, 325, 662
Crohn's disease, 227–229
Cryptococcosis, 723, 724
Cryptococcus, 12
Crystalloid fluids, 122

D
Debridement, 751, 752
Debridement and implant retention (DAIR), 28
Deep venous thrombosis (DVT), 195, 414
Deficiency of interleukin-1 receptor antagonist (DIRA), 372
Delayed- and late-onset deep infections, 268
Dicloxacillin, 25
Direct inoculation osteomyelitis, 27
Disability adjusted life years (DALYs), 4
Discitis and vertebral osteomyelitis, 19
Disease-modifying antirheumatic agents, 379
Disseminated intravascular coagulopathy (DIC), 775
Distal femur osteomyelitis, 110
Distal tibia, 140
DNA-neutrophil extracellular traps (DNA-NETS), 38

E

Empirical antibiotics, 28
Enterobacter, 7
Enterobacteriaceae, 29
Enteroviruses, 687
Eosinophilic granulomas, 88, 580
Epidural abscess, 288
Epiphyseal disappearance, 442
Epiphyseal osteomyelitis
  clinical manifestations, 578, 579
  complications, 583
  computed tomography, 580
  differential diagnosis, 580
  epidemiology, 578
  laboratory findings, 579
  magnetic resonance imaging, 580
  medical treatment, 581
  pathogenesis, 578
  plain radiographs, 580
  radioisotope scans, 580
  Staphylococcus aureus, 578
  supportive treatment, 581
  surgical interventions, 581
  treatment, 581
  ultrasonography, 580
Erythrocyte sedimentation rate (ESR), 74, 117, 158, 171, 194, 209, 240, 325, 662
Evidence-based management
  antibiotic treatment, 152
  case-by-case approach, 152
  complications, 161–162
  differential diagnoses, 159–160
  essential workflows, 156
  initial assessment, 156
  interdisciplinary communication, 156
  laboratory studies, 158
  pathology and microbiology, 152–155
  radiographic studies, 158–159
  severity of illness, 159
  skin and skin structure infections, 155
  surgical intervention, 152
  treatment options, 160–161
Ewing sarcoma (ES), 74, 79–81, 580
Ewing's tumour, 61
External fixation
  conversion scenarios, 303
  extraperiosteal devices, 303
  intramedullary devices, 303, 304
  lethal scenarios, 303
  location of the pin site, 305
  material properties of the pins and wires, 304–305
  method of pin insertion, 305
  osteomyelitis, 303
  pin site care regimes, 306, 307
  pin site infections, 302
  trauma, 302
  treating pin site infections, 310
Extracellular polymeric substances (EPSs), 135
Extracellular polysaccharides (EPSs), 133, 136
Extracorporeal membrane oxygenation (ECMO), 124
Exuberant survival APR, 40

F

Fasciotomy, 752
FAST-sequence MRI, 37, 38
Femoro-acetabular impingement (FAI), 496
Fibular osteomyelitis, 59
Flexor tenosynovitis, 591, 592
Fluid-refractory shock, 122
Foot infections, 11
Foul smelling wounds, 169
Fungal infections, 12–13
Fungal musculoskeletal infections, 30
Fungal osteomyelitis, 20
Fungi
  aspergillosis, 724–726
  blastomycosis, 732
  candidiasis, 718–722
  classification, 714–716
  coccidioidomycosis, 726–728, 731
  cryptococcosis, 723, 724
  diagnosis, 717
  differential diagnosis, 717
  epidemiology, 714, 715
  etiopathogenesis, 716, 717
  histoplasmosis, 733
  management, 717–719
  mycetoma, 735, 736, 739, 740
  sporotrichosis, 734

G

Ganselen's approach, 609
Gap grafting, 548
Gas gangrene, 770
  causative organisms, 762
  clinical features, 764, 765
  complications, 769
  diagnosis, 764–766
  differential diagnosis, 765, 767
  epidemiology, 761
  etiology, 761, 762
  imaging, 765, 766, 768
  outcomes, 770
  pathophysiology, 762–764
  treatment
    medical management, 768, 769
    surgical treatment, 769
    vasoconstrictors, 768
Global Burden of Disease (GBD), 4
Gonococcal arthritis, 26
Gower's sign, 634
Gram-negative sepsis, 12
Greater trochanteric arthroplasty (GTA), 504
Growth arrest, 412

H

Haemophagocytic lymphohistiocytosis (HLH), 707
Haemophilus influenzae, 7, 237
Hand, foot and mouth disease (HFMD)
  clinical presentation and examination, 602
  differential diagnosis, 602
  investigations/work-up, 602
  outbreaks of, 602
  pathology and microbiology, 602
  treatment options, 602, 603
Hand infections, 11
  anatomy, 588
  animal bites, 595, 596
  cellulitis, 597
  clinical presentation, 588
  complications, 599
  consultation, 588
  deep space infections, 592–594
  epidemiology, 588
  factors, 588
  felon, 590
  flexor tenosynovitis, 591, 592
  herpetic whitlow, 590, 591
  history, 588
  human bites, 596
  mycobacterial infections, 598, 599
  necrotizing fasciitis, 598
  osteomyelitis, 596, 597
  paronychia, 589
  routine utilization, 588
  septic arthritis, 594, 595
Health care systems, 183
Hematogenous osteomyelitis, 536
Hematogenous seeding, 227
Hematogenous septic arthritis
  duration of therapy, 26
  empiric therapy, 26
  oral antibiotics, 26–27
  treating culture negative, 27
Hemophilic hemarthrosis, 90
Histiocytosis, 61
Histoplasma, 12
Histoplasmosis, 733
Hoffman fixator, 178
Hospital-acquired MRSA (HA-MRSA), 97
Humeral bone defects, 539
Humerus, 527
Hydatid disease
  chemotherapy, 804, 805
  in childhood, 800
  clinical features, 802
  computerized tomography (CT scans), 803
  differential diagnoses, 804
  epidemiology, 800
  investigations, 802
  magnetic resonance imaging (MRI), 803
  management, 804
  pathogenesis, 800, 801
  pathology, 801, 802
  radiography, 802, 803
  serological tests, 803
  skeletal hydatidosis, 800, 801
Hydroxyapatite (HA) coating, 304
Hyperbaric oxygen therapy (HBOT), 335
Hyperglycemia, 124
Hypoechoic fluid, 57

I

Iatrogenic fractures, 183
Idiopathic scoliosis, 281, 282, 292
Ilizarov hip reconstruction (IHR), 506
Ilizarov transport, 553
Imaging modalities
  computed tomography, 62, 63
  MRI
    acute infection, 61
    fatty marrow, 60
    general anaesthesia, 62
    osteoid osteoma, 61
    pulse sequences, 60
    transient synovitis, 62
    unossified cartilage, 59
    unossified epiphyses, 60
  radiography
    Brodie's abscess, 55
    chondrolysis, 54
    chronic osteomyelitis, 56
    cortical sclerosis, 56
    joint sepsis, 52
    leucocytic infiltration, 52
    metaphyseal lucency, 53
    permeative lucency, 54
    Perthes' disease, 52
    serpentine sign, 54
    slipped capital femoral epiphysis, 52
  scintigraphy, 63–66
  ultrasonography, 55–59
Immediate bone transport, 549
Immunocompromised child
  acute infection treatment, 706–708
  antibiotics, 709, 710
  caregivers, 696
  causes, 694, 695
  clinical history, 694
  clinical presentation, 693, 694
  examination, 694–696
  hallmark presentation, 694
  PID, 697
  potential treatments, 710
  routine investigations, 701, 702, 706, 707
  secondary/acquired immunodeficiency
    AIDS-related causes, 698, 700
    chemotherapy and cancer, 700
    drug-induced immune incompetence, 700
    malnutrition, 698, 700
    mechanisms of action, 698, 699
    SBD, 700, 701
    SCD, 701, 702
  surgical intervention

child and family education, 709
infection control, 708
nutritional support, 708
perioperative care, 708
physical, emotional or spiritual well- being, 709
risk factors, 709
Induced membrane, 561, 563
Infection mimics
clinical features, 69–74
comprehensive history and exam, 74
diagnosis for pyomyositis, 90
diagnosis for septic arthritis, 90
differential diagnoses for osteomyelitis
Charcot neuropathic arthropathy, 89
chronic noninfectious osteomyelitis, 76, 77
ewing sarcoma, 79–81
langerhans cell histiocytosis, 87–89
leukemia, 82
lymphoma, 85
osteoid osteomas, 86
osteosarcoma, 81–82
scurvy, 89
sickle cell crisis, 78–79
stress injuries, 75, 76
imaging, 74
laboratory studies, 74
osteomyelitis, 70
plain radiographs, 74
radiographic findings, 75
T2-weighted sequences, 75
Infectious Diseases Society of America (IDSA), 28
Ingrown toenails
clinical presentation and examination, 605
differential diagnosis, 605
investigations/work-up, 605
pathology and microbiology, 605
treatment options, 605
Interferon-gamma release assays (IGRA), 663
Interleukin 1 antagonists, 379
Intravenous immunoglobulins (IVIG), 124
Invasive meningococcal disease (IMD), 786
amputations, 780
clinical presentation, 775, 776
complications, 784
diagnosis, 776–778
epidemiology, 773, 774
initial medical management, 777, 779
initial surgical management
amputations, 779, 780
necrotic areas, 779
peripheral limb ischemia and compartment syndrome, 779
secondary bacterial infections, 779
late orthopedic management, 781
growth plate disturbances, 781–783
hip problems, 782
prosthetic fitting issues, 783
scar contractures, 784
soft tissue and bone infections, 784
stump revisions, 784
management principles, 783, 784
mode of infection, 775
outcomes, 785
pathogen, 774, 775
pathogenesis, 775
patient history, 786, 787, 789, 791
rehabilitation principles, 785

J

Japanese encephalitis virus (JEV), 687
Joint communication, 581
Joint sepsis, 52
Juvenile idiopathic arthritis (JIA), 90, 159
Juvenile rheumatoid arthritis, 90

K

Kanavel's signs, 591
Kawasaki's disease, 158
Kingella kingae, 7, 18, 192
Kirschner wire, 12, 142, 143
Kocher criteria, 157, 213

L

Langerhans cell histiocytosis (LCH), 74, 87–89
Legg-Calve-Perthes disease, 212
Leg-length discrepancy (LLD), 496
Leucocytic infiltration, 52
Leukaemia/leukemia, 82, 580
Leukocytosis, 171
Limb length discrepancy (LLD), 412, 415, 485
Limb reconstruction, 302
Linezolid, 25
Local antibiotic drug delivery systems
delivery vehicles
bioabsorbable ceramics, 137–140
PMMA, 137
extended antimicrobial therapy, 133
local antimicrobials
infected non-union, 143–144
osteomyelitis, 142
pathology, 134–137
surgical debridement, 133
Low- and middle-income countries (LMIC's), 124, 166, 412
LukAB assay, 100
Lyme arthritis, 90, 212
arthrocentesis, 211–212
clinical presentation and examination, 207–209
complications, 216–217
differential diagnosis, 212–213
epidemiology, 204
imaging, 210–211
laboratory studies, 209–210
microbiology, 204–207
treatment, 213–216
Lyme disease, 204, 208, 209
Lymphoma, 85

M
Madura foot, 623–625
Malnutrition, 698, 700
Masquelet technique, 561
  bone stabilization, 563
  complications, 570, 571
  physiology, 561
  post-operative care, 566
  preparation of the graft, 569, 570
  second surgical session, 567, 568
  spacer, 563, 564
  surgical site preparation, 563
  wound closure, 565
Mendelian susceptibility to mycobacterial disease (MSMD), 697
Metaphyseal equivalent, 73
Methicillin susceptible/sensitive Staphylococcus aureus (MSSA), 97, 236, 254, 327
Methicillin-resistant *Staphylococcus aureus* (MRSA), 111, 191, 194, 206, 327, 588
Microbiology
  acute osteoarticular infections, 18–19
  Brodie's abscess, 19
  chronic osteomyelitis (CO), 19–20
  discitis and vertebral osteomyelitis, 19
  fungal osteomyelitis, 20
  orthopaedic implants, 20–21
  Pseudomonas aeruginosa, 19
Mimic osteomyelitis, 69
Minimum biofilm eradication concentration (MBEC), 137
Monoarticular arthritis, 90
Monolateral construct, 178
Morselized autograft, 567
Multi-acquisition with variable-resonance image combination (MAVRIC), 346
Multidrug resistance, 133
Multidrug-resistant (MDR) tuberculosis, 10
Multi-organ dysfunction (MOD), 39, 111
Musculoskeletal impairment (MSI), 5
Musculoskeletal infections (MSKI), 4, 412
  avascular necrosis, 486
  bone issues, 459
  classification, 415
  deformity, 465, 473, 480, 483, 484
  epidemiology, 412
  evaluation, 415
  fungi (*see* Immunocompromised child)
  impact, 413
  joint contractures, 459, 460, 463
  limb length discrepancy, 485, 486
  management, 416, 442, 450, 458
  pathogenesis, 413
  presentation, 415
  risk factors, 414
  spectrum of disease, 414
Mycetoma, 623–625, 735, 736, 739, 740
Mycobacteria spp., 29
Mycobacterium tuberculosis, 255, 581
  see also Tuberculosis (TB)

N
Natural resistance-associated macrophage protein gene 1 (NRAMP1), 661
Near-infrared spectroscopy (NIRS), 118
Necrotising fasciitis (NF), 303, 598
  clinical presentation, 747–749
  differential diagnosis, 749, 751
  epidemiology, 743, 744
  etiology, 745, 746
  finger test, 750
  flesh-eating bacteria, 743
  imaging studies, 750
  laboratory tests, 749, 750
  microbiology, 744, 745
  outcomes and complications, 755, 756
  pathology, 747
  pathophysiology, 746, 747
  risk factor, 745, 746
  treatment of
    broad-spectrum intravenous antimicrobial chemotherapy, 754
    conservative treatment, 751, 752
    erythematous skin, 752, 753
    hyperbaric oxygen therapy, 754, 755
    intensive care support, 754
    nutritional support, 754
    principles, 752
    reconstructive procedures, 755
Needle aspiration, 259
Neisseria gonorrhoeae, 7, 26
Neonatal musculoskeletal infections
  antibiotic therapy, 245
  bone and joint infections, 241
  bone scintigraphy, 239
  complications, 245
  CT scan, 240
  elbow and ankle, 243
  knee, 243
  management, 240–242
  microbiology, 236
  MRI, 239
  pathophysiology, 237
  plain radiographs, 238, 239
  Psoas, 244
  risk factors, 237
  shoulder, 243
  signs and symptoms, 238
  site of involvement, 238
  spectrum, 240
  surgical decompression, 242
Neonatal skeletal infections (NSK), 235
Nerve palsy, 183
Neuromuscular scoliosis, 286
Nihilistic, 306
Nocturnal pain, 69
Non-hematogenous osteomyelitis, 19
  contiguous focus, 27, 28
  direct inoculation osteomyelitis, 27
Nontuberculous mycobacteria (NTM), 29, 663
Nontyphoidal *Salmonella* species (NTS), 19

Non-vascularized fibular graft (NVFG), 514, 551
Nuclear medicine imaging, 325
Nutrition, 176

O

Onychocryptosis, *see* Ingrown toenails
Oral antibiotics, 25
Orthopedic hardware infections, 28–29
Osteoarticular infection, 205
Osteoid osteomas, 86
Osteomyelitis, 5, 7, 8, 27, 59, 60, 167, 178–180, 303, 310, 322, 384, 596, 597
  type 1, 173
  type 2, 174
  type 3, 174
Osteomyelitis of hindfoot
  clinical presentation and examination, 608
  complications, 609–616
  diagnosis, 608
  differential diagnosis, 608, 609
  incidence, 607
  pathology and microbiology, 607, 608
  treatment, 609, 610
Osteosarcoma, 81–82
Outpatient parenteral antimicrobial therapy (OPAT), 25

P

Paediatric musculoskeletal infection (MSKI) in LMIC, 166
  build effective review mechanisms, 185
  building capacity, 185
  burden of disease, 166–167
  challenges to optimal treatment, 167–168
  clinical examination, 169–171
  clinical presentation, 169–171
  complications, 181–183
  decision-making and classification, 172–176
  developing referral mechanisms, 185
  differential diagnosis, 172
  education and building awareness, 184
  epidemiology, 166–167
  imaging studies, 172
  impact, 168
  laboratory investigations, 171
  medical treatment, 176
  pathology and microbiology, 168–169
  surgery and MSK infections, 176–178
  surgery in resource-challenged environment, 183–184
  surgical procedures, 178–181
  tissue sampling, 172
  treatment options, 178–181
Paediatric osteomyelitis, 52
Panton-Valentine leukocidin (PVL), 99, 169, 384
Pathogen-associated molecular patterns (PAMPs), 114
Pathological fractures, 384
  clinical presentation, 386
  epidemiology, 385
  investigations, 389
  management, 392, 394–396, 402
Pediatric acute hematogenous osteomyelitis, 133
Pediatric musculoskeletal infection (MSKI)
  "tortuous" vascularity, 35
  assessing the severity
    antibiotic administration, 46
    cellular markers, 44–46
    classification system, 42–43
    identification of pathogen, 41
    laboratory measure, 43–44
    surgical debridement, 46
  cellulitis, 35
  clinical presentation, 36–37
  continuous injury, 38–41
  epidemiology of
    foot infections, 11
    fungal infections, 12–13
    hand infections, 11
    osteomyelitis, 7, 8
    pyomyositis, 8, 9
    septic arthritis, 8
    spine infections, 9–10
    surgical site infections, 12
    tuberculosis, 10
  global burden, 4–7
  hematogenous origin, 4
  imaging, 37–38
  MRSA AND MSSA
    comparative severity of, 102–104
    epidemiology of, 102
  osteomyelitis, 35
  pyomyositis, 35
  septic arthritis, 35, 36
Pediatric outcomes data collection instrument, 484
Pediatric sepsis, 112
Pediatric spinal infections
  acute flaccid myelitis, 687, 688
  blastomycosis, 687
  risk factors, 675
  schistosomiasis, 688, 689
  spinal abscesses (*see* Spinal abscesses (SA))
  spondylodiscitis (*see* Spondylodiscitis)
Pediatric tuberculosis, 630
Pelkan spurs, 89
Pelvic pyomyositis, 225
Pelvic support osteotomy (PSO), 506
Penetrating injuries
  clinical presentation and examination, 606
  complications, 607
  differential diagnosis, 606
  epidemiology, 606
  investigations/work-up, 606
  pathology and microbiology, 606
  treatment options, 606, 607
Percutaneous drainage (PCD), 228
Periacetabular osteotomy (PAO), 500
Perthes' disease, 52
Pigmented villonodular synovitis, 90
Planktonic microorganisms, 136
Plasma exchange (PLEX), 124

Polycaprolactone (PCL), 140
Poly (lactic-co-glycolic acid) (PLGA), 140
Polymerase chain reaction (PCR) analysis, 205
Polymethylmethacrylate (PMMA), 134, 135, 137, 327, 353, 396, 533, 561
Polymorphonuclear leucocytes (PMN), 725
Positron emission tomography (PET-CT), 66
Post-septic hip sequelae, 495
  choi Type IV deformity, 503, 504
  classification, 496
  clinical problems, 496
  greater trochanteric arthroplasty, 505, 506
  radiographic classifications, 496
  salvage, 498
  treatment, 497–499
  type 1 deformity, 499
  type II and III deformity, 499, 500, 503
Post-streptococcal reactive arthritis (PSRA), 159
Pott's disease, 29, 170, 634, 635
Primary epiphyseal osteomyelitis (PEO), 577, 583
Primary immunodeficiency disease (PID), 697
Primary infectious myositis, 154–155
Primary septic arthritis, 154, 159
Propionibacterium, 264
Prosthetic joint infection (PJI), 28
Protruding sequestra, 169
Proximal tibial chronic osteomyelitis, 66
Pseudomonas aeruginosa, 19
Pseudomonas spp., 20
Pseudoparalysis, 170
Psoas, 244
Pulmonary edema, 414
Pulse oximetry, 118
Pyoderma gangrenosum, and acne syndrome (PAPA), 372
Pyogenic arthritis, 372
Pyomyositis, 8, 9, 29, 73, 90, 161
  nonspecific symptoms, 221
  primary pyomyositis
    clinical presentation, 222, 223
    complications, 227
    differential diagnoses, 225
    epidemiology, 221–222
    evaluation, 223–225
    pathology and microbiology, 222
    treatment, 225–227
  secondary pyomyositis
    clinical features, 228
    conventional radiography, 228
    etiology, 227
    osteoarticular infections, 229, 231
    penetrating trauma, 227
    primary osseous pathology, 227
    retroperitoneal space and aspiration, 228
    surgical intervention, 229
    transient bacteremia, 227
    treatment, 228–231

R

Reactive arthritis, 90
Renal replacement therapy, 124
Right hip effusion, 57
Rose gardener's disease, 734

S

Schistosomiasis, 688, 689
Scintigraphy, 63–66
Sclerosing bone dysplasia's (SBD), 700, 701
Scoliosis Research Society (SRS), 281
Scorbutic lattice, 89
Scurvy, 89
Sepsis and septic shock, 110
  age specific pediatric vital sign criteria, 112
  definitions, 111–113
  distal femoral epiphysis and metaphysis, 110
  hyperglycemia, 124
  ICU monitoring
    continuous ECG monitoring, 117
    NIRS, 118
    organ dysfunction, 118
    pulse oximetry, 118
  LMICs, 124–126
  management of
    antimicrobial therapy, 120
    ECMO, 124
    hemodynamic resuscitation, 120–122
    immunoglobulins, 124
    initial management, 119–120
    PLEX, 124
    renal replacement therapy, 124
    source control, 120
  nutrition, 124
  outcomes, 126, 127
  pathophysiology
    arterial oxygen content, 114, 115
    clinical presentation, 115–117
    DO_2-VO_2 graph, 115
    innate and adaptive immunity, 114
    multi-organ dysfunction, 114
    oxygen delivery, 116
  risk factors, 113
Septic arthritis, 6, 8, 36, 52, 71–72, 90, 180, 241, 414, 594, 595
  arthrocentesis, 211–212
  clinical presentation and examination, 207–209
  complications, 216–217
  differential diagnosis, 212–213
  epidemiology, 204
  imaging, 210–211
  laboratory studies, 209–210
  microbiology, 204–206
  pathology, 204–207
  treatment, 213–216
Severe combined immunodeficiencies (SCID), 710
Sickle cell disease (SCD), 8, 701, 702
Silver, 304
Skeletal stabilization, 353
Skin necrosis, 183
Slice encoding for metal artifact correction (SEMAC), 346
Slipped capital femoral epiphysis, 52
Soft tissue deficiency, 557

Soft tissue infections, 754
Spinal abscesses (SA)
  diagnostic tests, 685
  history, 684, 685
  imaging, 685, 686
  outcomes and complications, 687
  pathogenesis, 684
  physical exam, 685
  treatment, 685, 687
Spinal tuberculosis (TB)
  clinical features, 634, 635
  complications, 643, 653, 654
  differential diagnosis, 642, 646, 649
  epidemiology, 630, 631
  investigations/work-up, 636, 639, 641–643, 645, 647, 648
  medical management, 639, 641–643, 649, 650
  pathology, 631–633
  surgical treatment
    cervical spinal tuberculosis, 636, 651
    cervicodorsal tuberculosis, 651
    decision making, 651
    goals of, 651
    indications for, 650
    neurological deficit, 650
    thoracic and thoracolumbar tuberculosis, 652, 653
Spine surgery, site infections, 9–10
  clinical presentation, 287
  complications, 297
  CT scans, 288, 289
  delayed surgical site infection treatment, 296, 297
  epidemiology, 281, 282
  high-performance teams, 294–296
  identification of risk factors, 292
  implementation of best practice guidelines, 293, 294
  investigations, 288
  microbiology, 282, 284, 285
  MRI, 289, 292
  nonidiopathic etiologies, 287
  plain radiographs, 288
Spondylodiscitis (SD)
  antibiotic therapy, 683, 684
  causative pathogens, 676
  computed tomography (CT), 683
  diagnostic tests, 677
  history, 677
  magnetic resonance imaging (MRI), 677–679
  nuclear bone scan, 679
  outcomes and complications, 684
  pathogenesis, 676
  physical exam, 677
  surgical treatment, 684
  X-ray, 679, 681
Sporotrichosis, 734
Stabilization, 396
Staged grafting, 549
Standard agglutination test (SAT), 798
Staphylococcus aureus, 7, 11, 12, 18, 73, 95–98, 134, 154, 236, 307, 384, 512, 543, 544
  antibiotic resistance, 97–99
  toxin-mediated virulence, 99–102
Staphylococcus epidermidis, 136
Streptococcus agalactiae, 18
Streptococcus pneumoniae, 327
Streptococcus pyogenes, 154, 327
Stress injuries, 75, 76
Subacute osteomyelitis
  absence of constitutional symptoms, 254
  clinical presentation and examination, 255
  complications, 261
  differential diagnosis, 255–257, 259
  investigations, 255
  pathology and microbiology, 254–255
  treatment options, 259–261
Surgical debridement, 546
Surgical site infections (SSIs), 6, 12, 281, 282, 288, 292, 294, 296–298
  anatomic space, 263
  bacterial etiologies, 265
  classification, 266
  clinical presentation, 265
  complications, 277
  dental disease, 276
  diagnostic evaluation, 266
  diagnostic imaging, 266
  differential diagnoses, 267
  immediate-onset deep infections, 268
  immediate-onset superficial infections, 267
  implant decision-making, 268
  nutritional status, 275
  optimizing nutritional status, 275, 276
  pediatric orthopedic surgery, 264
  prevention strategies, 275
  resolution, 274
  Staphylococcus species, 264
  surgical factors, 277
  surgical incision, 263
  urinary incontinence, 277
  wound exploration, 268
  wound management, 274
Synovial chondromatosis, 90
Synovitis, acne, pustulosis, hyperostosis, and osteitis (SAPHO) syndrome, 73
Systemic inflammatory response syndrome (SIRS), 111, 112
Systemic lupus erythematosus (SLE), 159

T
Telemetry, 117
Tendon rupture, 662
Thoracic tuberculosis, 652, 653
Thoracolumbar tuberculosis, 652, 653
Tibia, 543, 548
Tinea pedis, 603, 604
Tissue ischaemia, 746, 747
Titanium, 304
Transient synovitis, 90
Traumatic hemarthrosis, 90
Triple diagnostics, 747
Triple innominate osteotomy (TIO), 500
Tubercular arthritis, 90

Tuberculin skin test (TST), 663
Tuberculosis (TB), 6, 10, 169, 170, 181
  evidence, 659
  extrapulmonary, 659
  incidence of, 659
  osteomyelitis (*see* Tuberculous osteomyelitis)
  spinal (*see* Spinal tuberculosis)
  types, 659, 660
Tuberculosis arthritis, 662
Tuberculosis of foot and ankle
  clinical presentation and examination, 617
  complications, 621–623
  differential diagnosis, 619
  epidemiology, 616
  investigations/work-up, 617–620, 622
  pathology and microbiology, 616, 617
  treatment options, 619–621
Tuberculous osteomyelitis
  BCG vaccine, 668–671
  clinical presentation and examination, 661, 662
  complications, 666, 668, 669
  diagnosis, 662
  differential diagnoses, 666
  investigations/workup, 662–667
  pathology and microbiology, 660, 661, 663
  radiographic findings, 665
  treatment options, 667, 668
  treatment outcomes, 668
Tuberculous tenosynovitis, 662

U
Uncomplicated osteomyelitis, 173–174
Unguis incarnates, *see* Ingrown toenails
Upper extremity, 512
  clinical presentation, 512
  complications, 535
  epidemiology, 512
  evaluation, 512, 513
  external fixator, 520, 526, 527
  induced membrane technique, 533, 535
  non-vascularized bone grafts, 514, 518
  single-bone forearm, 535
  Staphylococcus aureus, 512
  treatment options, 514
  vascularized fibular bone graft, 520

V
Vancomycin, 22
Vanderbilt medial approach, 225
Vascularized bone grafting, 331
Venous thromboembolism (VTE), 194
Verruca vulgaris, *see* Viral warts
Vertebral osteomyelitis, 19
Viral arthritis, 805, 806
Viral infection
  clinical manifestations, 806
  clinical presentation, 806
  features, 805
  incidence rates, 805
  investigations, 806
  microbiology, 805
  pathogenesis, 805
  prevalence, 805
  treatment, 806
Viral myositis, 806
Viral warts
  clinical presentation and examination, 603
  differential diagnosis, 603
  pathology and microbiology, 603
  prevalence, 603
  treatment options, 603
von Willebrand factor binding protein (vWBP), 95

W
Water-based hydrogels, 142
Western blot analysis, 212
White blood cell count (WBC), 74, 288
Whole body (WB), 375
Wound dehiscence, 289
Wound management, 274

X
Xpert MTB/RIF assay, 663

Z
Ziehl–Neelsen staining, 663

GPSR Compliance

The European Union's (EU) General Product Safety Regulation (GPSR) is a set of rules that requires consumer products to be safe and our obligations to ensure this.

If you have any concerns about our products, you can contact us on ProductSafety@springernature.com

In case Publisher is established outside the EU, the EU authorized representative is:

Springer Nature Customer Service Center GmbH
Europaplatz 3
69115 Heidelberg, Germany

Batch number: 09036638

Printed by Printforce, the Netherlands